SAGE was founded in 1965 by Sara Miller McCune to support the dissemination of usable knowledge by publishing innovative and high-quality research and teaching content. Today, we publish over 900 journals, including those of more than 400 learned societies, more than 800 new books per year, and a growing range of library products including archives, data, case studies, reports, and video. SAGE remains majority-owned by our founder, and after Sara's lifetime will become owned by a charitable trust that secures our continued independence.

Los Angeles | London | New Delhi | Singapore | Washington DC | Melbourne

Abnormal Psychology

Abnormal Psychology

Neuroscience Perspectives on Human Behavior and Experience

William J. Ray
Pennsylvania State University

Adapted by

Anuradha Sovani
SNDT Women's University, Mumbai, India

SAGE | TEXTS

Los Angeles | London | New Delhi
Singapore | Washington DC | Melbourne

Originally published in 2015 by

SAGE www.sagepublishing.com
Los Angeles | London | New Delhi | Singapore | Washington DC | Melbourne

The South Asia adaptation published in 2018 by

SAGE | TEXTS

SAGE Publications India Pvt Ltd
B1/I-1 Mohan Cooperative Industrial Area
Mathura Road
New Delhi 110 044, India

Published by Vivek Mehra for SAGE Publications India Pvt Ltd, typeset in 9.5/11.5 pt Bookman Old Style by AG Infographics, Delhi and printed at Sai Print-o-Pack, New Delhi.

Library of Congress Cataloging-in-Publication Data

Names: Ray, William J., author. | Sovani, Anuradha, author. | Adaptation of (work): Ray, William J., author. | Abnormal psychology.
Title: Abnormal psychology : neuroscience perspectives on human behavior and experience / William J. Ray; adapted by Anuradha Sovani.
Other titles: SAGE TEXTS.
Description: Los Angeles: SAGE Publications India Pvt Ltd, 2018. | Series: SAGE TEXTS | Adaptation of abnormal psychology / William J. Ray. 2015. | Includes bibliographical references and index.
Identifiers: LCCN 2018009643| ISBN 9789352806829 (pbk.) | ISBN 9781412988124
Subjects: MESH: Mental Disorders | Psychopathology | Culture | Neurosciences | India
Classification: LCC RC454 | NLM WM 140 | DDC 616.89—dc23 LC record available at https://lccn.loc.gov/2018009643

ISBN: 978-93-528-0682-9 (PB)

To Judy, Vicki, & Jim for their insight and dedication to quality
William J. Ray

To all my students at SNDT Women's University and University of Mumbai, and wherever else you came from, to learn
Anuradha Sovani

CONTENTS

Preface xxi
Preface to the Indian Adaptation xxv
Acknowledgments by William J. Ray xxvii
Acknowledgments by Anuradha Sovani xxix
About the Author xxxi
About the Adaptor xxxiii

CHAPTER 1
An Overview of Psychopathology 1

CHAPTER 2
Changing Conceptualizations of Mental Illness 26

CHAPTER 3
Neuroscience Approaches to Understanding Psychopathology 65

CHAPTER 4
Research Methods 115

CHAPTER 5
Assessment and Classification 158

CHAPTER 6
Disorders of Childhood 184

CHAPTER 7
Schizophrenia 231

CHAPTER 8
Mood Disorders 269

CHAPTER 9
Stress, Trauma, and Psychopathology 310

CHAPTER 10
Anxiety Disorders and Obsessive-Compulsive Disorder 346

CHAPTER 11
Dissociative Disorders and Somatic Symptom Disorders **382**

CHAPTER 12
Eating Disorders **407**

CHAPTER 13
Sexuality Disorders and Gender Dysphoria **435**

CHAPTER 14
Substance-Related and Addictive Disorders **475**

CHAPTER 15
Personality Disorders **534**

CHAPTER 16
Neurocognitive Disorders **578**

CHAPTER 17
The Law and Mental Health **612**

Glossary G–1
References R–1
Index I–1

DETAILED CONTENTS

Preface xxi
Preface to the Indian Adaptation xxv
Acknowledgments by William J. Ray xxvii
Acknowledgments by Anuradha Sovani xxix
About the Author xxxi
About the Adaptor xxxiii

CHAPTER 1
An Overview of Psychopathology 1
Mental Health Disorders 6
Stigma and Mental Disorders 8
Stigma of Mental Illness 8
Different Conceptions of Mental Illness 12
The Three Major Themes of This Book 13
Levels of Analysis 14
Biopsychosocial Approach 15
The Relation of Evolution and Culture to Psychopathology 15
Humans and Their Environment 20
Is Psychopathology Universal? 21
Experiential Perspective 22
Plan of the Book 23
Summary 23
Study Resources 24
Review Questions 24
For Further Reading 25
Key Terms and Concepts 25

CHAPTER 2
Changing Conceptualizations of Mental Illness 26
Historical Considerations in Understanding Psychopathology 29
Ancient Greek and Roman Influences—Mental Illness Involves the Brain 29
Thoughts from Ancient India 31
Psychopathology in the Middle Ages 31
From the Renaissance to the 1700s—The Beginning of Modern Science 32
Discovering the Function of the Brain in Behavior and Psychopathology 35
The 1700s to the 1900s 36
The 1800s and Evolution 41
A Search for Organization 42

Care for Those With Mental Disorders 43
From the Past to the Present 48
The Psychological Treatment Perspectives in the 20th Century 48
Psychodynamic Perspectives on Treatment 49
Existential-Humanistic Perspectives 52
Behavioral and Cognitive Behavioral Perspectives 56
Summary 62
Study Resources 62
Review Questions 62
For Further Reading 63
Key Terms and Concepts 64

CHAPTER 3
Neuroscience Approaches to Understanding Psychopathology 65
Diagnostic Considerations of Psychopathology 67
Neuroscience Perspectives 76
What Are Endophenotypes? 78
Genes 78
Neural Networks 79
Neuroscience Techniques and Levels of Analysis 80
The Brain 81
How Does the Neuron Pass Information? 83
Encoding Information 84
Unique Aspects of the Human Brain 85
How Do We Observe the Brain at Work? 85
Electroencephalography 86
Magnetoencephalography 88
Functional Magnetic Resonance Imaging 90
Spatial and Temporal Resolution 92
Networks of the Brain 93
Neurons Connect in a Network 94
What Is the Brain's Default (Intrinsic) Network? 95
Different Networks Are Involved in Different Tasks 96
Major Neurotransmitters in the Brain 98
The Study of Genetics 99
What Do Genes Do? 100
DNA 102
How Do Genes Influence Behavior? 103
Epigenetic Processes 103
Mitochondria and Mitochondrial Inheritance 105
The Themes of Evolution 106
Psychopathology From an Evolutionary Perspective 107
Neuroethics 110
Summary 112
Study Resources 113
Review Questions 113
For Further Reading 114
Key Terms and Concepts 114

CHAPTER 4
Research Methods **115**
What Is Science? 119
The Methods of Science 119
Case Study 120
Naturalistic Observation: Just Looking 122
Correlational Approach: What Goes With What 123
Experimental Method: Making It Happen 126
Logic and Inference: The Detective Work of Science 129
What Do I Expect to Happen? 131
Designing an Experimental Study 132
Single Subject Designs 141
Longitudinal Research 142
Epidemiological Research 144
Research Involving Genetics 145
Clinical and Statistical Significance 148
Replication and Meta-Analysis 149
Ethics and the Scientific Experiment 149
The Experiment as an Ethical Problem 151
Ingredients of the Initial Scientist–Participant Dialogue 151
The Rights of the Research Participant and the Responsibilities of the Experimenter 152
What Is Harmful to a Research Participant? 153
Institutional Review Board 153
The Ethical Relationship 154
Summary 154
Study Resources 155
Review Questions 155
For Further Reading 156
Key Terms and Concepts 156

CHAPTER 5
Assessment and Classification **158**
The Mental Status Exam 160
Cultural Variations Relevant to India 160
Structured Interviews 161
Structured Clinical Interview for *DSM* Disorders 161
Assessing Cultural Dimensions 163
Reliability and Validity in Relation to Psychopathology 164
Reliability 165
Validity 166
Models of Assessment 167
Symptom Questionnaires 167
Personality Tests 167
Use of Empirical Tests in India 170
Projective Tests 170
Use of Projective Tests in India 174
Neuropsychological Testing 174
Using Neuroscience Techniques to Identify Mental Illness 175

Classification 176
Classification Systems for Mental Disorders 177
International Statistical Classification of Diseases and Related Health Problems 177
Diagnostic and Statistical Manual of Mental Disorders 177
Summary 181
Study Resources 182
Review Questions 182
For Further Reading 183
Key Terms and Concepts 183

CHAPTER 6
Disorders of Childhood **184**
Experience 184
Introduction to Childhood Development 185
Brain Development 188
Effects of Early Life Stress 189
Theories of Attachment 190
Imitation Learning 193
Theory of Mind 194
Adolescence 196
Brain Systems Involved in Social Relations 198
Attachment Disorders 202
Autism Spectrum Disorders 203
Special Talents 210
Treatment for Autism Spectrum Disorders 211
Attention Deficit/Hyperactivity Disorder 213
Treatment for Attention Deficit/Hyperactivity Disorder 217
Conduct Disorder 218
Oppositional Defiant Disorder 219
Treatment for Conduct Disorder and Oppositional Defiant Disorder 220
Learning Disabilities 220
Intellectual Developmental Disorder 222
Intellectual Developmental Disorder Related to Chromosomes 223
Intellectual Developmental Disorder Related to Metabolism 224
Intellectual Developmental Disorder Related to Gestation 224
Treatment of Intellectual Developmental Disorder 225
Summary 226
Study Resources 229
Review Questions 229
For Further Reading 229
Key Terms and Concepts 230

CHAPTER 7
Schizophrenia **231**
Experience 232
Schizophrenia 234
Positive and Negative Symptoms 234

Positive Symptoms 235
Negative Symptoms 236
Course of Schizophrenia 237
Historical Perspective 238
Subtypes of Schizophrenia? 239
Schizophrenia From an Evolutionary Perspective 242
Factors in the Development of Schizophrenia 244
Genetic Factors in Schizophrenia 245
Endophenotypes Associated With Schizophrenia 247
Ventricle Changes in Schizophrenia 249
Schizophrenia and Brain Function 249
What Brain Changes Are Seen in Schizophrenia? 252
Schizophrenia and Brain Networks 255
Neurotransmitters Involved in Schizophrenia 257
How Are Cognitive Processes Changed in Schizophrenia? 258
Schizophrenia and the Experience of Emotions 259
Facts of Schizophrenia 259
Treating Individuals With Schizophrenia 260
Antipsychotic Medications 262
Psychosocial Interventions for Schizophrenia 263
Summary 266
Study Resources 268
Review Questions 268
For Further Reading 268
Key Terms and Concepts 268

CHAPTER 8
Mood Disorders **269**
Depressive Disorders 270
Mood Disorders Around the World 271
Developmental Aspects of Depression 273
Cognitive Model of Depression 275
Are Depression and Inflammation Related? 277
Does Depression Run in Families? 277
The Evolutionary Perspective Concerning Depression 278
Prevention and Treatment of Depression 280
Psychological Treatments for Depression 286
Bipolar Disorder 289
Bipolar Disorders 290
Diagnosis of Bipolar Disorder 291
Genetics of Bipolar Disorder 296
Bipolar Disorder and Creativity 297
Brain Imaging of Bipolar Disorder 297
Neurotransmitter Dysregulation 298
Environmental Factors 299
Treatment of Bipolar Disorder 300
Suicide 302
Cultural Differences in Suicide 303
Gender Differences in Suicide and the Type of Attempts 303

Endophenotypes and Suicide 304
Short-Term and Long-Term Factors Related to Suicide 304
Preventing Suicide 305
Summary 305
Study Resources 308
Review Questions 308
For Further Reading 309
Key Terms and Concepts 309

CHAPTER 9
Stress, Trauma, and Psychopathology **310**
Psychological Stress and Psychopathology 315
Does Trauma Produce Mental Illness? 316
Is Social Pain Like Physical Pain? 317
The Physiological Mechanisms Related to Stress and Trauma 318
Trauma Changes Our Genes Through Tagging (Epigenetics) 318
Physical Illness and Concomitant Psychological Stress 320
Psychological Stress and the Immune System 321
What Makes You Run From Bears? Stress and the Hypothalamic-Pituitary-Adrenal Axis 323
The Autonomic Nervous System 325
The Study of Stress 327
Does Fight or Flight Apply Equally to Males and Females? 329
Does Social Stress Produce a Similar Reaction to Physical Stress? 330
Trauma- and Stressor-Related Disorders in *DSM–5* 331
Post-Traumatic Growth 334
Adjustment Disorders 334
Acute Stress Disorder 335
Post-Traumatic Stress Disorder 335
Spirituality and Resilience, Volunteering, and Wellbeing 343
Summary 343
Study Resources 345
Review Questions 345
For Further Reading 345
Key Terms and Concepts 345

CHAPTER 10
Anxiety Disorders and Obsessive-Compulsive Disorder **346**
Anxiety Disorders 346
Overview of Anxiety Disorders 348
Cognitive Processes in Anxiety 351
Neurobiology of Anxiety Disorders 352
Developmental Aspects of Anxiety 353
Anxiety Disorders Around the World 355
Major Types of Anxiety Disorders 359
Separation Anxiety Disorder 359
Generalized Anxiety Disorder 360
Social Anxiety Disorder 364

Agoraphobia 366
Specific Phobia 367
Panic Disorder 370
Obsessive-Compulsive Disorder 373
Brain Processes Associated With Obsessive-Compulsive Disorder 376
Indian Studies on Obsessive-Compulsive Disorder 378
Treatment of Obsessive-Compulsive Disorder 378
Summary 379
Study Resources 381
Review Questions 381
For Further Reading 381
Key Terms and Concepts 381

CHAPTER 11
Dissociative Disorders and Somatic Symptom Disorders **382**
Dissociative Disorders 383
Depersonalization–Derealization Disorder 385
Dissociative Amnesia 387
Dissociative Identity Disorder 389
Relative Paucity of Work in India, Yet Plethora of Cultural Factors 391
Treatment of Dissociative Disorders 392
Somatic Symptom and Related Disorders 393
Somatic Symptom Disorder 394
Indian Studies on Somatic Symptom Disorder 394
Illness Anxiety Disorder 395
Conversion Disorder 396
Factitious Disorder 402
Treatment of Somatic Symptom Disorders 403
Summary 404
Study Resources 404
Review Questions 405
For Further Reading 406
Key Terms and Concepts 406

CHAPTER 12
Eating Disorders **407**
Overview: Feeding Disorders, Obesity, and Eating Disorders 408
Feeding Disorders 409
Pica 409
Rumination Disorder 410
Avoidant/Restrictive Food Intake Disorder 410
The Problem of Obesity 410
Differences in the View of Ideal Weights Between Males and Females 417
The Major Eating Disorders 418
Anorexia Nervosa 420
Treating Anorexia Nervosa 426
Bulimia Nervosa 428
Treating Bulimia Nervosa 430

Summary 432
Study Resources 433
Review Questions 433
For Further Reading 434
Key Terms and Concepts 434

CHAPTER 13
Sexuality Disorders and Gender Dysphoria **435**
Historical Perspectives 436
India—The Land of the Kamasutra 436
Sexual Activities of Americans 438
Indian Epidemiological Data 439
Sexual Arousal and Sexual Drive 439
Your Brain and Sexual Activity 442
Sexual Arousal 444
Normal Sexual Functioning 445
Sexual Dysfunction Disorders 450
Erectile Disorder 452
Female Orgasmic Disorder 453
Delayed Ejaculation 453
Early Ejaculation 453
Female Sexual Interest/Arousal Disorder 454
Male Hypoactive Sexual Desire Disorder 454
Genito-pelvic Pain/Penetration Disorder 454
Treatment Approaches for Sexual Dysfunction Disorders 454
Paraphilic Disorders 457
Exhibitionistic Disorder 458
Frotteuristic Disorder 459
Fetishistic Disorder 459
Pedophilic Disorder 459
Sexual Masochism Disorder 461
Sexual Sadism Disorder 462
Transvestic Disorder 462
Voyeuristic Disorder 463
Other Paraphilic Disorders 463
Treatment Approaches for Paraphilic Disorders 464
Gender Dysphoria 465
Other Indian Work on Gender Dysphoria, Gender Identity Issues and Their Management 469
Interesting Work on Infertility Treatment in India and the Psychosocial Consequences 470
Summary 470
Study Resources 473
Review Questions 473
For Further Reading 474
Key Terms and Concepts 474

CHAPTER 14
Substance-Related and Addictive Disorders **475**
Indian Case: Internet Addiction 476
Indian Statistics on Drug Use 478
Drug Use in the United States 479
Substance Abuse, Dependence, and Addiction 482
Substance Disorders in *DSM–5* and *ICD-10* 482
Explanatory Models for Alcohol Use 483
Who Becomes Addicted? 483
Qualitative Study from India on Onset and Progression of Alcohol Use 485
Pattern of Addiction 486
Can Drugs Change Your Brain? 487
Alcohol 491
An Older Indian Study on Neuropsychological Rehabilitation for Alcohol 492
DSM–5 Alcohol-Related Disorders 492
Effects of Alcohol on the Human Body 496
Moderate, Heavy, and Binge Drinking 498
Rates of Drinking 498
Do People Who Drink More Like It More? 501
Publications from India, Based on the Premium Study 502
Cannabis 503
Cannabis and Psychosis 505
Hallucinogens 506
Opioids 510
Do You Have Opium Receptors in Your Brain? 511
Cocaine 511
Amphetamines 514
Amphetamines as a Medicine 514
Caffeine and Tobacco 516
An Indian Study on Cognitive Dysfunction in Chronic Smokers 517
Gambling 519
Treatment of Substance-Related Disorders 522
Principles of Effective Treatment 523
Psychosocial Therapies and Addiction 525
The 12-Step Program 526
Controlled Drinking Approaches 527
Medications Used to Treat Addiction 528
Summary 529
Study Resources 532
Review Questions 532
For Further Reading 532
Key Terms and Concepts 533

CHAPTER 15
Personality Disorders **534**
Introducing Personality Disorders 536
What Is a Personality Disorder? 536
Comorbidity of Personality Disorders 537

Personality Disorders and Normal Personality Traits 539
The Characteristics of a Healthy Self 540
Normal Personality Traits 541
Evolution and Different Personality Characteristics 543
Personality and Personality Disorders 543
Categories and Dimensions 546
Environmental and Genetic Studies of Personality Disorders 546
Sociocultural Dimensions of Deliberate Self-harm: A Study from Mumbai 547
Odd-Eccentric Personality Disorders 547
Paranoid Personality Disorder 547
Schizoid Personality Disorder 548
Schizotypal Personality Disorder 548
Dramatic Emotional Personality Disorders 551
Antisocial Personality Disorder and Psychopathy 551
Borderline Personality Disorder 556
Histrionic Personality Disorder 566
Narcissistic Personality Disorder 567
Anxious Fearful Personality Disorders 568
Avoidant Personality Disorder 568
Dependent Personality Disorder 569
Obsessive-Compulsive Personality Disorder 569
Treatment of Personality Disorders 570
Treatments for the Other Personality Disorders 573
DSM Future Considerations of Personality Disorders 574
Summary 574
Study Resources 574
Review Questions 576
For Further Reading 577
Key Terms and Concepts 577

CHAPTER 16
Neurocognitive Disorders **578**
Announcement of Alzheimer's Disease by President Ronald Reagan 578
Changes Related to Aging Across the World 580
Prevention of Neurocognitive Disorders 583
Do Cognitive Abilities Change With Age? 583
Brain Changes With Age 584
Can an Individual's Activities Be Protective in Brain Changes? 587
Studies from India on Aging Changes in the Brain 589
Delirium 590
Mild and Major Neurocognitive Disorders 592
Indian Work on Mild Cognitive Impairment 594
Neurocognitive Disorder Due to Alzheimer's Disease 594
Vascular Neurocognitive Disorder 599
Frontotemporal Neurocognitive Disorder 600
Neurocognitive Disorder Due to Traumatic Brain Injury 603
Neurocognitive Disorder Due to Lewy Body Dementia 605
Neurocognitive Disorder Due to Parkinson's Disease 606

Neurocognitive Disorder Due to HIV Infection 607
Substance-Induced Neurocognitive Disorder 608
Neurocognitive Disorder Due to Huntington's Disease 608
Neurocognitive Disorder Due to Prion Disease 608
Summary 609
Study Resources 610
Review Questions 610
For Further Reading 611
Key Terms and Concepts 611

CHAPTER 17
The Law and Mental Health **612**
The Legal System and the Insanity Defense 615
Ethical and Legal Issues in Treatment 618
The Ethical and Legal Aspects of the Initial Contract for Treatment 619
Emergency Commitment 620
New Developments on the Indian Legal Scenario 622
The Protection of Children from Sexual Offences Act, 2012 (POCSO) 623
The Sexual Harassment of Women at Workplace (Prevention, Prohibition And Redressal) Act, 2013 (POSH) 623
The Juvenile Justice (Care and Protection of Children) Act, 2015 (JJ Act) 623
Narcotic Drugs and Psychotropic Substances (NDPS) Act, 1985 623
Neuroscience and Evolutionary Perspectives on the Legal Aspects of Psychopathology 628
Summary 630
Study Resources 631
Review Questions 631
For Further Reading 631
Key Terms and Concepts 631

Glossary G–1
References R–1
Index I–1

PREFACE

Abnormal psychology books from the middle of the last century largely contained descriptions of particular disorders. However, there would not be much written about the experiences of having a mental disorder. Since that time, society has a new conceptualization of what it means to have a mental disorder. There is also a greater awareness of how many people with a mental illness are able to live full lives and have productive occupations. In this text, I want to introduce some of these individuals and describe their experiences.

Also, in a textbook from the last century, there would not be much written about research studies. The research that would be contained would also be focused exclusively on studies related directly to abnormal psychology. It would not be connected with the larger human condition and how mental illness is part of our evolutionary history and related to human cognition, emotion, and motor processes. In many ways the field of abnormal psychology at that time remained disconnected from other areas of psychology as well as the life sciences.

Jumping ahead to the beginning of the 2000s, abnormal psychology textbooks would have contained more research. However, the amount of research related to the neurosciences would have been limited. There would be little in the way of brain imaging and the manner in which different disorders are related to one another on an underlying level. However, there would be a realization that mental illness is a complex process and cannot be explained on a single level such as the possibility of mental illness being produced by a single gene.

Using this broader perspective, the dichotomous positions of nature versus nurture or innate versus learned fuse into the larger question of how aspects of each lead to an understanding of behavior and experience and their relationship to mental illness. Understanding that human behavior and experience take place on a number of different levels of analysis replaces the strict dichotomous approach pitting one level against another. On a molecular level, for example, we know that genes must be turned on and turned off. What this means is that many significant human processes are directed by the environment. On a higher level, the genetics versus culture debate may be of limited value without understanding the manner in which humans both live within a culture and are influenced by historical environments. This brings us to the value of an evolutionary perspective.

DEVELOPMENT OF AN EVOLUTIONARY PERSPECTIVE

An evolutionary perspective examines the close interaction of organisms with their environment. In this close connection, the organism seeks ways to solve the fundamental problems or challenges of its existence. This is true whether one has a mental illness or not. The environment for humans includes not only nature but also culture. Humans throughout their evolutionary history have always lived in groups with other people. The manner in which cultures understand and solve problems related to mental illness is one crucial question I will explore in this book. An evolutionary perspective also can give us insight into why some disorders such as schizophrenia are seen in similar proportions around the world whereas other disorders vary by geographical location.

DEVELOPMENT OF BRAIN IMAGING

As we entered the 21st century, questions of importance to psychology were being embraced by the neurosciences. This allowed for both richness and an integration of scientific information concerning important psychological questions. In the past 20 years, we have seen a shift in focus that has included the "decade of the brain" as well as a real emergence of the cognitive and affective neurosciences. A number of scientists have also begun to ask how neuroscience approaches can influence psychopathology and inform the diagnosis of different types of mental disorders.

In addition to genetic and evolutionary perspectives, recent developments in brain imaging have provided important perspectives on psychopathological processes. These techniques include functional magnetic resonance imaging (fMRI), electroencephalography (EEG), and magnetoencephalography (MEG), and their basics should be understood by students seeking an overview of psychopathology. These techniques are beginning to emphasize the manner in which underlying cortical networks may reflect particular changes in psychopathological conditions and give us a better understanding of the manner in which normal social and emotional processes may become dysfunctional. For example, we know that there are a variety of basic networks in the brain, some of which are involved in internal processes such as mind wandering when there is no external stimulation and others that become activated when interaction with the external world is required. A number of researchers have sought to articulate how these so-called default networks as well as other networks are associated with psychopathology. Other researchers have focused on emotional circuits that are either under- or overactivated in particular psychopathologies.

IMPLICATIONS FOR TREATMENT

Further, an integration of research from the neurosciences as well as traditional psychological research helps to clarify the efficacy and mechanisms of psychological treatments. For example, recent brain imaging research concerning treatment suggests different modes of function mediated by the nature of the therapy. On the one hand, research concerning treatment of depression shows that psychotropic medications work from a bottom-up perspective by influencing the limbic areas that, in turn, influence higher cortical networks. On the other hand, cognitive therapies work in a top-down manner by influencing the prefrontal cortex (PFC), which, in turn, has an inhibitory effect on the lower brain processes. Even within traditional psychotherapy outcome research, there is a new sense of integration of traditionally dichotomous positions. This includes a search for specifying empirically supported procedures such as the successful relationship between client and therapist, which determines treatment outcome. In terms of prevention, there has been a recent increase in neuroscience research that shows the manner in which enriched environments as well as exercise can influence brain development and play an important role in the prevention of both pathophysiology and psychopathology.

NEW PERSPECTIVES IN ABNORMAL PSYCHOLOGY

In the same way that psychology offers important insights into the systems level in terms of human behavior and experience, it is imperative that abnormal psychology texts begin to offer such an integrative perspective. For example, recent perspectives in social neuroscience suggest that it is not productive to teach brain anatomy or emotionality in one chapter and social relationships, influence, and perception in another. Within the community of abnormal psychology researchers, there is an increasing understanding of the manner in which various disorders reflect impairments in social processes and the brain functions associated with them. With such an integrated approach, students can come to understand the nature of impaired relationships on a variety of levels including cognitive, affective, and motor processes.

THIS TEXT

The purpose of this text is to bring together current perspectives in understanding mental disorders. In addition to the traditional psychological literature, additional information from the cognitive and affective neurosciences, ethology, evolution, and genetics will be discussed. The focus is on a unification and integration of these understandings within a broader consideration.

[illegible]

NEW PERSPECTIVES IN ABNORMAL PSYCHOLOGY

[illegible]

[illegible]

PREFACE TO THE INDIAN ADAPTATION*

A human being cannot be understood only as a bunch of diagnostic terms and observable behaviors, based on how he or she interacts with others socially or reacts to situations emotionally. Nor is he or she an unchanging map of social, emotional, and behavioral manifestations. People are changeable beings, and any textbook on abnormal psychology, psychopathology, or the neuroscientific basis of human behavior needs to reflect all these facets of a person.

This is the perspective I have used for over three decades of teaching. I often begin talking about a condition with a case example—a first-person narrative—and I love to watch the class slowly beginning to look at the individual not as a "case" but as a "person." They grow to understand how hard it must be to reside in that person's skin; to see and feel and think how he or she sees, feels and thinks; and to understand how it must feel to see others react to their "different"ness.

"Functional" psychological conditions then pose the next puzzle as you show the class how these conditions are based in the brain and yet are not neurological conditions! The realization that any of us, the teacher or the students, could so easily be in the patient's shoes is rather disturbing to the new learner and yet helps us all to move toward a more empathic understanding of the patient's circumstances and to grasp preventive perspectives more easily. Moving toward a deeper understanding of etiology, symptoms, psychometric test profiles, and therapy processes is but few steps away.

I have enjoyed this shared process of discovery and continue to enjoy it every academic year with every new batch of postgraduates. Who knows, I might find ways to continue doing this even after I retire! I also feel lucky to be in touch with senior researchers and academicians, practitioners in the field all over India who are adding value to the field with their contributions. I take pride in bringing their insights to my classroom and my students, so that they too can be proud of the amazing work happening in India and at the same time be attuned to the global scenario. This is important because the world is growing smaller, and any of them could be in any part of the world a few years hence. What makes me even more proud is to bring work to the classroom that was carried out by my own former students who were in these classroom benches not that many years ago.

When SAGE offered me this opportunity to work on the Indian adaptation of a book that covers all these bases, and to add Indian research as and where appropriate, I felt it was a gift I could not refuse! I hope the readers enjoy the book as much as I enjoyed writing for it.

Anuradha Sovani

*Color images and figures used in this printed edition are available at http://studysites.sagepub.in/ray_AP.zip.

ACKNOWLEDGMENTS

I appreciate the many individuals who have contributed to this book. Ken Levy, Sandy Testa, Mike Wolff, and Cliff Evans discussed their clinical work with me and contributed case studies seen throughout this book. I also appreciate the students in my senior seminar on abnormal psychology from a neuroscience perspective who over the years gave me insight into how to present the information seen throughout this book as well as finding new information and perspectives. Faculty from across the country were extremely helpful in their reviews of this book and suggestions. They include the following individuals:

Cameo F. Borntrager, *University of Montana*

Amy Badura Brack, *Creighton University*

Elysia V. Clemens, *University of Northern Colorado*

Amanda di Bartolomeo, *University of California, Los Angeles*

Fred Ernst, *University of Texas–Pan American*

David M. Feldman, *Barry University*

Brian Fisak, *University of North Florida*

Sarah Fischer, *The University of Georgia*

David E. Gard, *San Francisco State University*

Brian K. Gehl, *Coe College*

Henry J. Grubb, *University of Dubuque*

Rob Hoff, *Mercyhurst University*

Lisa R. Jackson, *Schoolcraft College*

Bruno M. Kappes, *University of Alaska Anchorage*

Lynne M. Kemen, *Hunter College, CUNY*

William Kimberlin, *Lorain County Community College*

Lee Kooler, *Modesto Junior College*

Jason M. Lavender, *University at Albany, SUNY*

Martha Low, *Winston-Salem State University*

Richard Martielli, *Washington University in St. Louis*

Ryan A. McKelley, *University of Wisconsin–La Crosse*

Jan Mendoza, *Golden West College*

Courtney K. Mozo, *Old Dominion University*

Kimberly Renk, *University of Central Florida*

Ashley M. Rolnik, *Loyola University Chicago*

H. Russell Searight, *Lake Superior State University*

Fran Sessa, *Penn State Abington*

Kim Stark, *University of Central Missouri*

Wayne S. Stein, *Brevard Community College*

Philip Yanos, *John Jay College*

I also appreciate the staff at SAGE. Vicki Knight is an excellent editor who knows how to find the appropriate reviewers and bring quality ideas to the project. Jim Strandberg is a creative developmental editor with superb insight. Jessica Miller does an amazing job of keeping track of all of the illustrations and figures for the book and came up with original ideas for graphics. Brittany Bauhaus is excellent as a production editor who carefully brought everything together as a quality book.

William J. Ray

ACKNOWLEDGMENTS

I wish to express my appreciation for the help, support, and partnership offered to me by many of my colleagues in both India and abroad, not only for the Indian adaptation of this book but for my work in general.

Let me begin with "my seniors":

Several persons have contributed richly to the insights I developed and perhaps was able to impart to the field of psychology, both in academic circles and in the community.

Dr. Shubha Thatte, former Clinical Psychologist, KEM Hospital, Mumbai; Senior Trustee, Institute for Psychological Health, Thane, Maharashtra.

Dr. Mitchell Weiss, Professor Emeritus and former Chair, Department of Epidemiology and Public Health, Swiss Tropical and Public Health Institute (Swiss TPH) and University of Basel.

Dr. R. Srinivasa Murthy, Professor of Psychiatry (retd) NIMHANS, Bangalore; former Medical Officer, Mental Health, World Health Organization, Eastern Mediterranean Region, Cairo, Egypt; World Health Organization, Eastern Mediterranean Region, Cairo, Egypt; and Editor-in-Chief, World Health Report (Mental Health) 2001.

Dr. C. R. Mukundan, former Professor and Head of Clinical Psychology and Department of Neuropsychology, NIMHANS, Bangalore; former Professor Emeritus, Institute of Behavioural Science, Gujarat Forensic Sciences University, Gandhinagar; Chairman, Axxonet Brain Research Laboratory, Axxonet System Technologies, Bangalore.

Dr. S. K. Chaturvedi, Dean, Behavioural Sciences; Head, Department of Mental Health Education; Senior Professor, Department of Psychiatry, NIMHANS, Bangalore.

Dr. Roy Abraham Kallivayalil, President, Indian Psychiatric Society; former Professor and Head, Department of Psychiatry, Government Medical College, Kottayam and Trichur; Secretary General, World Psychiatric Association; Co-Chairman, Preventive Psychiatry Section, World Psychiatric Association, Geneva.

Dr. Mohan Agashe, Padma Shri; Consulting Psychiatrist; Stage and Film Artist; Founding Director, Maharashtra Institute of Mental Health (MIMH), Pune; former Director, Film and Television Institute of India (FTII), Pune.

Next, "my contemporaries" in the field of mental health, who have raised the bar so high and ensured that we all continue to deliver quality service and research:

Dr. Vikram Patel, Professor of International Mental Health and Wellcome Trust Principal Research Fellow in clinical science, Centre for Global Mental Health, London School of Hygiene and Tropical Medicine, UK; Sangath, Goa, India; Centre for Chronic Conditions and Injuries, Public Health Foundation of India, India; currently Pershing Square Professor of Global Health at Harvard Medical School. His Sangath team.

Dr. Anand Nadkarni, Founder Director and Managing Trustee, Institute for Psychological Health, Thane, Maharashtra. The IPH team, many of whom are former students and teaching assistants.

Dr. Samir Dalwai, Founder Director, New Horizons Child Development Centre & Research Foundation; Consultant, Nanavati Super Speciality Hospital, NeuroDevelopmental Clinic, Lokmanya Tilak Municipal General Hospital and Medical College. The New Horizons team, many of whom are former students and teaching assistants.

Dr. Seema Mehrotra, Professor, Department of Clinical Psychology, NIMHANS, Bangalore.

Dr. Urvashi Shah, Consultant Neuropsychologist, KEM Hospital and GSMC, Global Hospital, Mumbai, and many young neuropsychologists who work with her.

Dr. Shubhangi Parkar, Dr. Ravindra Kamath, Dr. Nilesh Shah, Professors and Heads of the Department of Psychiatry at the three major BMC Hospitals in Mumbai and their entire departmental team.

Last but not least, my "many former students, masters as well as doctoral," at both University of Mumbai and SNDT Women's University and currently my colleagues in India and abroad whose work is cited in this book, my research assistants, Jagruti Wandrekar and Advaita Nigudkar, and, of course, "my current students," who have always demanded the best in teaching, guidance, and mentoring, which I hope I delivered most of the time.

I would also like to acknowledge the support given by the SAGE India team, who gave me a lot of freedom and space to contribute my best to this book adaptation and yet made sure that timelines were adhered to. I apologize in advance if I have missed any names, since there have been so many people who have given so much as we all worked together over the years. Thank you all.

Anuradha Sovani

ABOUT THE AUTHOR

William J. Ray is a Professor of Psychology at Penn State University. He received his PhD from Vanderbilt University and was a Fellow in Medical Psychology at the University of California Medical Center in San Francisco. He received his undergraduate degree from Eckerd College, where he learned about the value of primary sources and the need to integrate information from a number of perspectives. As part of his clinical training, he has worked in a number of mental hospitals and clinics across the country, where he developed an appreciation of the experiences of those with mental disorders. In his career, he has served as a visiting professor and researcher at the University of Hawaii, Münster University, University of Rome, Tübingen University, and Konstanz University. At Penn State, he is currently the Director of the SCAN (Specialization in Cognitive and Affective Neuroscience) program and was previously the Director of the Clinical Psychology Program. His research has focused on approaching clinical questions from a neuroscience perspective. He has used psychophysiological and brain imaging techniques such as EEG, MEG, DTI, and fMRI to study emotionality, psychopathology, and individual differences. These studies can be found in numerous articles, book chapters, and books. His work has been published in such journals as *Science, Proceedings of the National Academy of Sciences, Journal of Neuroscience, Psychophysiology, Physiological Reviews, Journal of Personality and Social Psychology, Developmental Psychology, Journal of Abnormal Psychology, Cognitive Brain Research, Biological Psychology, NeuroImage,* and *Clinical Neurophysiology*. This work has been funded by both national and international agencies including NIH, NIMH, NASA, NATO, and the DAAD. In addition to research, teaching has been an important part of his career. His textbooks include *Methods Toward a Psychology of Behavior and Experience, Psychophysiological Methods* (with Robert Stern & Karen Quigley), and *Evolutionary Psychology: Neuroscience Perspectives Concerning Human Behavior and Experience.*

ABOUT THE ADAPTOR

Anuradha Sovani is a full Professor of psychology and heads the Department of Psychology at SNDT Women's University, Mumbai. Prior to this appointment, she has headed the Department of Applied Psychology at the University of Mumbai.

She has been a UGC Research Fellow during her MPhil as well as doctoral work at the University of Mumbai, an NCERT scholar through college life, and a Chancellor's Gold Medalist. Teaching is her passion, as is writing; she has written several books, chapters, newspaper columns, and articles in both English and Marathi (the local language of Maharashtra), for both professional and lay readers, and has been sought after as a speaker at national and international meetings.

Having worked as a psychologist in general hospital settings, served on committees for the care of long-stay chronic psychiatric patients, women in distress, and children who come from disadvantaged backgrounds, she has learned to respect hidden sources of resilience and to trust the spirit of human endeavor. Much of this belief as well as her training in cognitive behavioral and rational emotive psychotherapy approaches translates into her teaching, mentoring, and therapeutic work.

Dr Sovani is a trustee and consultant at the Institute for Psychological Health (IPH), and over the 27 years of her work with the institute, many of her research publications draw upon the community mental health and prevention focus espoused by IPH. Her research collaborations, both funded and others, extend beyond India; she has worked with colleagues in the fields of mental health and education from countries including the United States of America, Canada, and the United Kingdom. Twelve doctoral students have completed their work under her guidance in diverse areas ranging from psychosocial aspects of schizophrenia, epilepsy, and mild cognitive impairment on the one hand to speech difficulties, infertility, and parenting issues on the other. Both her own research and that of some of her doctoral and postdoctoral scholars have been funded by the UGC and ICMR.

Integration of the understanding of human behavior from a variety of different perspectives has been a central theme in her approach to psychology and psychopathology, leading to her working closely with psychiatrists, social workers, pediatricians, neuropsychologists, forensic psychologists, and human resource professionals in the corporate world; experts in the field of occupational therapy and speech and language pathology, general medicine, and surgery to deal with anxiety and pain management; and educationists and special educators. Working in the areas of awareness building and de-stigmatization has given her an opportunity to work with all strata of society and different age groups, using live, social, and print media and film-based discussions to ensure that apparently complex concepts are made simple and easy to comprehend.

CHAPTER

1

An Overview of Psychopathology

CHAPTER OUTLINE

- MENTAL HEALTH DISORDERS 6
- STIGMA AND MENTAL DISORDERS 8
- DIFFERENT CONCEPTIONS OF MENTAL ILLNESS 12
- THE THREE MAJOR THEMES OF THIS BOOK 13
- LEVELS OF ANALYSIS 14
- THE RELATION OF EVOLUTION AND CULTURE TO PSYCHOPATHOLOGY 15
- HUMANS AND THEIR ENVIRONMENT 20
- IS PSYCHOPATHOLOGY. UNIVERSAL? 21
- EXPERIENTIAL PERSPECTIVE 22
- PLAN OF THE BOOK 23
- SUMMARY 23
- STUDY RESOURCES 24

The book *A Beautiful Mind* describes the life and experiences of John Nash (Nasar, 1998). The book tells a powerful story and soon was made into a major Hollywood film that won the Academy Award for Best Picture of 2001. John Nash was, indeed, a remarkable figure, who received a PhD in mathematics from Princeton University and taught at both MIT and Princeton. In 1994, Nash won the Nobel Prize in economics for his work on game theory. From what I just told you, you probably assume that John Nash had a very productive career, and in many ways he did. However, there was another aspect to John Nash's life that caused considerable distress to him and puzzlement to others. One day he walked into a room full of others in his department, held up a copy of the *New York Times*, and said to no one in particular that the story in the upper-left

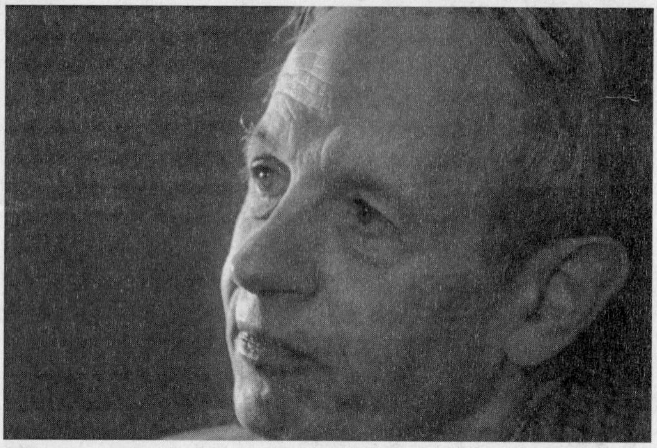

John Nash receiving his nobel prize in 1994
© Najlah Feanny/Corbis SABA

corner contained an encrypted message. Not only was it a message in code but it had been put there by inhabitants of another galaxy and he knew how to decode it (Nasar, 1998, p. 16). He was 30 years old at the time.

From that time on, there were times he was productive, but there were also times where he had disordered thoughts, mumbled to himself without thought of those around him, and experienced delusions of situations that did not exist. He felt there were individuals around him who put him in danger. He even wrote letters to officials in the U.S. government to suggest that these individuals were setting up alternative governments. John Nash suffers from schizophrenia.

Devrai is a film in Marathi, the state language of Maharashtra, India. The film was released in 2004 and later emerged as the first of an interesting trilogy focusing on awareness about mental disorders. *Devrai* is directed by a well-known director duo, Sumitra Bhave and Sunil Sukhtankar, who later went on to direct the entire trilogy. *Devrai* has been produced by K. S. Wani Memorial Trust, a charitable trust working in the area of schizophrenia, and Schizophrenia Awareness Association.

The term "Devrai" represents a forest territory that is a sacred grove, and the story revolves around a brilliant young man who develops schizophrenia and the grove assumes a personalized importance in his delusional world.

The next film in this sensitive trilogy is *Astu* (which means "so be it" in Sanskrit, a classic Indian language). The film is produced by Sheelaa Rao and Dr. Mohan Agashe, an actor and a psychiatrist who also plays the role of a person developing dementia. Finally, the third film *Kaasav*, meaning tortoise in Marathi, uses the creature as a symbol for the person in depression when they retract into their shell.

All three films have won awards and have been used widely for building awareness about mental illnesses. Films are an excellent medium to introduce students to the world of psychopathology, although it is important that the information therein is authentic and that the film screening is followed by a detailed discussion.

Mental disorders are part of our human condition. We have many names for these conditions. We speak of people with *mental illness*. For over a century, psychologists have studied these conditions in terms of **abnormal psychology.** Others have used the term ***psychopathology.*** This is in contrast with *pathophysiology,* or pathology of our physiology. Slang words such as *being crazy* or *nuts* have been around for hundreds of years. One of the oldest words is *insanity,* or *insane,* which comes from the Latin meaning "not healthy." Mental disorders have been with us throughout our human history. Since the time that written language became a part of our experience, humans have included descriptions of mental disorders. We find such descriptions in Egyptian, Greek, Chinese, Indian, and other texts throughout our world history. Today, our films, novels, plays, and television programs often portray problems experienced by those with mental disorders.

The experiences of the individuals just described give us insights into the nature of mental illness. In India, several prominent figures such as actors and sportspersons have shared that they did undergo severe mental health problems, and their stories motivate others to be resilient and cope with their own difficulties. These may lie in the realm of mood disorders such as depression or a learning disability. Laymen and fans identify with these well-known individuals who require vast courage to reveal their condition to a stigmatizing society. When well-known personalities declare that they too suffered from these conditions, the stigma associated with mental health conditions gets diluted with the glamour associated with the famous personalities.

Once again, films made on various disorders such as psychosis and learning disabilities have opened people's minds to accepting people who are "different."

An interesting experiment with what is known as Recovery Awards has also done a great deal to dispel the stigma of mental illness. Internationally, a person called Gayatri Ramprasad has conducted a number of public awareness sessions to make people aware about depression and has also published a book *Shadows in the Sun* (http://www.hazelden.org/web/public/shadows-in-the-sun.page), which has also been translated into multiple languages.

The Marathi translation was released in a function held at the Institute for Psychological Health (IPH), Maharashtra. This institute has also launched its own brand of Recovery Awards, for one of which Ms. Gayatri was present as a guest of honor. This series of awards is called Dwij Puraskar, where *dwij* means "life reborn" and *puraskar* means "award." Thus, one important characteristic of mental illness is the lack of control over one's experience. This can also be described as a loss of freedom or an inability to consider alternative ways of thinking, feeling, or doing.

Another common theme seen in psychopathology is the loss of honest personal contact. Individuals with depression or schizophrenia often find it difficult to experience social interactions as experienced by other people. Just having a simple conversation or talking to clerks in stores may seem impossible. Mental illness not only affects individuals' interpersonal relationships with others but also their relationship with themselves, their intrapersonal relationship. When individuals with schizophrenia or depression talk to themselves, they often think negative thoughts about who they are and what will happen in the future.

Additionally, in most cases, the experience of a mental disorder results in personal distress. Not being able to get out of depression, or feeling that a voice in your head is telling you that you are psychotic, or worrying that even a rice cake or an apple will make you fat all represent different degrees of distress. Thus, we can consider four important body image issues in psychopathology. These are first, a loss of freedom or ability to consider alternatives; second, a loss of honest personal contact; third, a loss of one's connection with one's self and ability to live in a productive manner; and fourth, personal distress. As you will see with the disorders presented in this book, personal distress for a period of time is one of the criteria required for a diagnosis to be made.

The National Sample Survey Organization report estimates the prevalence of mental illness to be between 17.1 and 12.7 per thousand, averaging out at 14.9 per thousand in the overall population of India (https://www.ncbi.nlm.nih.gov/pmc/articles/PMC4244788/). Other research articles also cite that epidemiological findings in India suggest that the incidence of various forms of psychopathology is much like that in the rest of the world.

Given that India has 17.5% of the world's population, this spells a very large figure.

The Government of India has released data based on work done in 2009, estimating Disability Adjusted Life Years (DALYs) and attribution of the same to various causes (https://data.gov.in/catalog/disability-adjusted-life-years-india-estimated-percentage-daly-cause).

Disease	*Total DALY (in '000)*	*Percentage Share of Total*
Communicable, Maternal, Perinatal and Nutritional	134,077.636	43.94374394
Infectious and parasitic diseases	58,836.002	19.28341134
Tuberculosis	7,286.141	2.388021776
STDs excluding HIV	3,000.700375	0.983475044
Syphilis	695.595625	0.227980422
Chlamydia	1,096.115492	0.359250207
Gonorrhea	1,121.886063	0.367696473
HIV/AIDS	3,851.9035	1.26245559
Diarrheal diseases	17,445.007	5.717574858
Childhood-cluster diseases	10,569.8165	3.464241492
Pertussis	4,157.068	1.362472797
Poliomyelitis	2.428426025	0.000795913
Diphtheria	61.17761328	0.020050871
Measles	4,994.00925	1.636779035
Tetanus	1,355.133031	0.444142817
Meningitis	2,361.860625	0.774096274
Hepatitis B (g)	486.9101094	0.159584057
Hepatitis C (g)	192.3068906	0.063028295
Malaria	603.3595625	0.197750191
Tropical-cluster diseases	3,815.4045	1.250493098
Trypanosomiasis	0	0
Chagas disease	0	0
Schistosomiasis	0	0
Leishmaniasis	1,192.448781	0.390823298
Lymphatic filariasis	2,622.956063	0.859669912
Onchocerciasis	0	0
Leprosy	90.86030078	0.029779327
Dengue	192.7909063	0.06318693
Japanese encephalitis	358.5637031	0.117518715
Trachoma	62.57239258	0.020508008
Intestinal nematode infections	610.4946563	0.200088707
Ascariasis	253.7123281	0.083153835

Disease	Total DALY (in '000)	Percentage Share of Total
Trichuriasis	238.0890938	0.078033343
Hookworm disease	109.079543	0.035750656
Perinatal conditions (h)	35,467.658	11.62447167
Respiratory infections	21,702.626	7.113003094
Lower respiratory infections	21,154.9	6.93348672
Upper respiratory infections	247.0063906	0.080955974
Otitis media	300.720125	0.09856057
Nutritional deficiencies	9,854.0035	3.229634855
Maternal conditions	8,217.3465	2.69322298
Prematurity and low birth weight	14,563.595	4.7731964
Birth asphyxia and birth trauma	10,216.822	3.348548074
Neonatal infections and other conditions	10,687.241	3.502727195
Protein-energy malnutrition	4,113.5795	1.348219506
Iodine deficiency	329.7566094	0.108077234
Vitamin A deficiency	73.71108789	0.024158698
Iron-deficiency anemia	5,029.11025	1.648283335
Non-Communicable Diseases	131,255.616	43.01883112
Non-communicable	131,255.608	43.01882849
Neuropsychiatric conditions	35,980.982	11.79271284
Cardiovascular diseases	28,959.663	9.491486077
Sense organ diseases	19,208.785	6.29565045
Respiratory diseases	11,197.8745	3.670086558
Digestive diseases	8,704.877	2.85301037
Malignant neoplasms	8,486.609	2.781473361
Congenital anomalies	5,741.4945	1.881766204
Musculoskeletal diseases	4,557.21775	1.493621277
Genitourinary diseases	2,885.05725	0.945573183
Diabetes mellitus	2,700.758375	0.885169503
Mouth and oropharynx cancers	1,187.14625	0.389085401
Esophagus cancer	724.6046563	0.237488088
Stomach cancer	467.3378906	0.153169292
Colon and rectum cancers	384.1903281	0.125917803
Liver cancer	166.6788359	0.054628738
Pancreas cancer	139.4481328	0.045703916
Trachea, bronchus, lung cancers	675.9392578	0.221538077
Melanoma and other skin cancers	25.90817188	0.008491364

(Continued)

(Continued)

Disease	*Total DALY (in '000)*	*Percentage Share of Total*
Breast cancer	665.926625	0.218256452
Cervix uteri cancer	987.373625	0.323610223
Corpus uteri cancer	33.06529297	0.0108371
Ovary cancer	241.5744688	0.07917567
Prostate cancer	118.3906328	0.038802352
Bladder cancer	121.920041	0.03995911
Lymphomas, multiple myeloma	585.4071406	0.191866312
Leukemia	829.5945	0.271898352
Oral conditions	1,656.238938	0.542829826
Skin diseases	625.8085625	0.205107817
Endocrine disorders	304.2430313	0.099715197
Other neoplasms	245.9990859	0.080625831
Injuries	39,778.63725	13.03738865
Unintentional injuries	32,047.013	10.50336041
Road traffic accidents	6,747.405	2.21145186
Poisonings	1,473.4535	0.482922173
Falls	4,362.4465	1.429785292
Fires	5,147.021	1.686928407
Drownings	1,913.468438	0.627136408
Other unintentional injuries	12,403.2175	4.065135917
Intentional injuries	7,731.62425	2.534028242
Total	305,112	100

Source: Open Government Data Platform, India (data.gov.in), Released under National Data Sharing and Accessibility Policy (NDSAP) (https://data.gov.in/catalog/disability-adjusted-life-years-india-estimated-percentage-daly-cause)

Further, data released by the Ministry of Health and Family Welfare, Government of India, points to large amounts of money spent on mental health (http://www.who.int/macrohealth/action/Report%20of%20the%20National%20Commission.pdf).

In an article in *The Lancet*, Dr. Vikram Patel et al. (2011) have reported DALY findings on chronic diseases and injuries in India and have permitted the reproduction of the tables and material from the paper.

MENTAL HEALTH DISORDERS

Building on an earlier WHO-CHOICE analysis, we analyzed interventions for alcohol misuse as a risk factor for disease, including psychosocial treatment in primary care ($490 per DALY averted) and pricing policies aimed at increasing excise taxation or reducing untaxed consumption (<$22 per DALY averted). On the basis of an estimate of unrecorded consumption of 1.7 liters of pure alcohol per person per year, we calculate that 3 billion liters of illicit alcohol is produced and consumed per year in India, which is why taxation enforcement strategies for illegally produced alcohol are expected to be as effective as increased taxation of legal alcohol.

Clinical interventions for mental health disorders include antipsychotic drugs for schizophrenia (with or without psychosocial support and care) and antidepressant drugs or psychosocial treatment for depression (on an episodic or long-term basis). Methods and assumptions underlying these analyses are reported elsewhere. Because of the high prevalence of depression, treatment for a meaningful population coverage (50%) is expensive but is nevertheless a cost-effective strategy (<$440 per DALY averted). Compared with depression, community-based care and treatment of people with schizophrenia is more expensive (per patient) and not as cost effective—combination treatment with a cheap, generically produced antipsychotic drug (risperidone) and 6–8 individualized psychosocial sessions costs roughly $2200 per DALY averted.

Having a mental disorder results in lost productivity, lost personal enjoyment, and potentially even premature death. The World Health Organization (WHO) estimated that in the United States and Canada mental disorders cause a greater loss in what they refer to as disability-adjusted life years (DALY) than cardiovascular disease or cancer (see *Figure 1-1*). DALYs represent the total number of years lost to illness, disability, or premature death.

With mental illness being so common, you might think that we as humans would have a complete understanding of the factors involved. However, this is not the case. We are not even sure how to refer to individuals with mental disorders. Are they abnormal? Depending on the reference group one uses, one can be normal or abnormal. Many

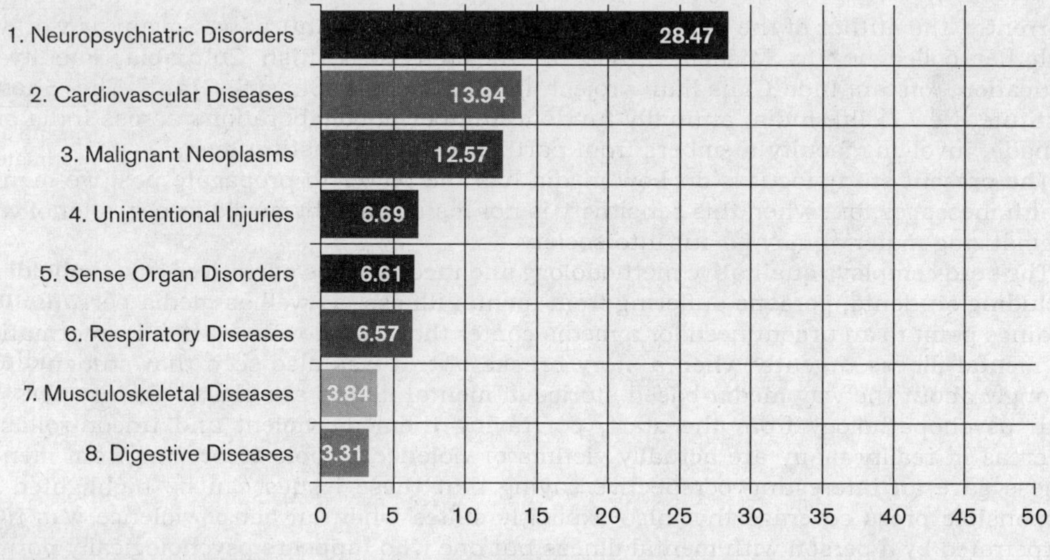

FIGURE 1-1 Leading Contributing Disease Categories to DALYs

Source: WHO; From http://www.nimh.nih.gov/statistics/2LEAD_CAT.shtml

famous artists such as the Impressionists had their work initially rejected because it did not fit into the standards of what was considered good art at the time. However, today we appreciate that these artists showed us another way of viewing the world. Likewise, many movies and music videos today would be rejected as not representing mainstream values at a previous time. Further, what would be acceptable in one culture might be seen as completely "crazy" in another.

STIGMA AND MENTAL DISORDERS

Each of the individuals described in the initial vignettes of this chapter not only has a mental disorder but also has had personal and professional success. As you will see throughout this book, experiencing a mental illness does not mean that one has to live a limited life. These individuals not only have productive careers such as being a writer, lawyer, college professor, or executive but also have successful personal relationships. However, many children, adolescents, and young adults with a mental illness report being told they could never perform in a high-level profession or have the types of relationships that others have.

There is often a **stigma** experienced by those with a mental disorder. Historically, stigma has been defined as a mark of disgrace associated with a particular person. In psychological terms, stigma involves negative attitudes and beliefs that cause the general public to avoid others including those with a mental illness.

Stigma of Mental Illness

Currently, the author of the Indian edition of this book, Dr. Anuradha Sovani, is working with her colleague Dr. Michelle Stack of University of British Columbia, Faculty of Education, on an Indo-Canadian project funded by the Shastri Grant. The Shastri Institute, New Delhi, India, annually funds a number of collaborations across India and Canada, involving faculty members from partner academic institutions.

The present study focuses on how media has the power to propagate positive mental health messages, but when this sensitivity is not maintained by media forces, a lot of very stigmatizing material may go out into society.

The study employs qualitative methodology and incorporates narratives of stakeholders, including students, persons suffering from mental illness, as well as media persons. The findings point to an urgent need for a media center that will provide authentic information on mental illness urgently when a story breaks out. It was also seen that students feel strongly about the way media-based stories of mental illness are biased against persons with psychopathology from the start, portraying them as violent and uncontrollable, whereas in reality many are actually victims of violence. People recovering from mental illness gave an interesting perspective saying that these issues can be highlighted by responsible press coverage that also explicitly states when an act of violence was NOT perpetrated by a person with mental illness but one who "appears psychologically normal or typical." The action research has involved counseling psychology students as well as educational trainers and set off a ripple effect where they, in turn, can spread the message of mental health in the schools and colleges where they work. In many cultures, they are seen as different. When they are thus stigmatized, these individuals are no longer treated as an individual person but only as part of a group who is different. It becomes an "us versus them" way of thinking.

Part of the stigma comes from inaccurate information concerning those with mental illness. For example, many people think that anyone with a mental illness is violent. Dr. Vikram Patel et al. (2012) have published their work in *The Lancet*, focusing on suicide mortality in India.

There has been a spate of farmer suicides in Maharashtra due to high dependency on the monsoon, and many efforts are made by mental health professionals to work through local leaders and train them to work with farmer families. A popular film and film-songs-based program called *Prakashdoot* (messenger of light) has been developed in this context and cited in the *Lancet* article, which is used in the public awareness campaigns. *Prakashdoot* was developed by the IPH (Thane, Maharashtra), funded by Sangath and the Tata Trust, and supported by Public Health Foundation of India.

Dr. Srinivasa Murthy (2012), senior psychiatrist and former professor and head of department of psychiatry at NIMHANS, Bangalore, spoke on the issue of farmer suicides in his N. N. De Oration Award (2011) speech. The oration is published in the *Indian Journal of Social Psychiatry*.

Dr. Murthy (2012) talks about the prevalent narrow view of looking at farmer suicides as a crisis in agriculture (the agricultural dimension) and an issue of farmer loans (the economic dimension). He says, "To date, the third dimension of mental health and psychosocial aspects and the need for a caring community to address the issue of farmers' distress has not been given any attention" and goes on to emphasize the third, psychosocial dimension underlying the crisis. He quotes the National Commission on Farmers (NCF) to emphasize the following:

> There is need for public awareness campaigns to make people identify early signs of suicidal behavior, make them aware of different socially acceptable measures for solving problems and information on helpline centres; develop a group of volunteers from the community to provide counsel, encourage increased communication within families, media education on internationally accepted guidelines for reporting suicides and creation of taluk level mental health services. (NCF, 2006)

He goes on to list 10 potential mental health interventions.

The MacArthur Foundation followed hospitalized individuals with mental illness after their release from the hospital and found that only 2% to 3% of these individuals were involved with violence with a gun. As a general rule, individuals with mental illness do not show more violence than that seen in the general population. There are, however, particular disorders such as psychopathy associated with serial killers in which individuals are violent. Also, substance abuse can increase violence in some individuals. With these exceptions, having a mental illness does not increase violence toward others.

Stigma can be seen on a number of levels. If a society believes that mental illness is the fault of the person—and that the person can change himself by willpower—then it is less likely to spend the money necessary to set up clinics and train professionals. Society may also be less likely to set up school-based programs to help adolescents with bullying or suicide. As well, companies may not be willing to include mental health treatment in their insurance coverage, or they may place limits on benefits for treatment of these disorders. In the United States, attitudes are moving toward less stigma. In 1996, for example, 54% of the U.S. population viewed depression as related to neurobiological causes. During the next 10 years, this increased to 67%. With a better understanding of the disorders presented throughout this book, it is possible to have a more compassionate as well as intellectual understanding of those with mental disorders.

1-1 LENS
Mental Illness Stigma

In a paper published in the *Indian Journal of Psychiatry,* Dr. Sushrut Jadhav et al. (2007) used a case vignette to explore the mental illness stigma.

Readers of this book may try to respond to the questionnaire provided later.

Here is a short account of a person who became ill. Please answer the questions about him:

This young man is 20 years old. He is unmarried and lives with his parents. He is friendly and hard-working. He works in a local factory. One day, he falls ill and starts imagining things that are not true. He cannot do his job properly and eventually loses it. He spends a lot of time by himself. He hears people talking to him when there is no one there. His parents now become anxious, but he does not get better. He starts shouting at the voices that he hears and tells his family that they themselves are trying to hurt him. On one occasion, he hits his father.

The family members are very distressed and frightened and do not know what is happening. They ask their neighbors; nobody thinks this is any sort of religious experience. The family members take him to the local doctor who tells them the young man is ill and gives him some tablets. The tablets do not help him. He does not eat properly. He seems puzzled by what is happening. He does not dress himself properly and is often dirty. He wanders about and says embarrassing things to people whom he meets in the streets.

His parents do not know what he is talking about. His doctor sends him to hospital, where he stays for two months. He gets better on some new tablets but still needs to take them when he leaves hospital. He does not hear the voices anymore nor does he have the strange ideas, but he is very quiet and stays alone for much of the time. He occasionally talks to himself but is usually polite to his family. He goes often to see his doctor to get his tablets and wishes to go back to work.

Here are some questions about this person. Each one must be answered by whether you agree with the question. Tick the appropriate box for each question. Remember this is not a test of knowledge but about how you really feel.

	Yes, very much	Yes, a little	No, not much	No, not at all
1. Would you be frightened if this man came to live next door to you?	☐	☐	☐	☐
2. Would you be content if he was to work together with you in your workplace? (If you do not have a job, answer as if you did.)	☐	☐	☐	☐

	Yes, very much	Yes, a little	No, not much	No, not at all
3. Do you think he will get ill again even if he takes the medicines?	☐	☐	☐	☐
4. Should he take part in meetings of his family that are to make important decisions?	☐	☐	☐	☐
5. Would you be happy if he married your sister?	☐	☐	☐	☐
6. Could he suddenly become physically violent?	☐	☐	☐	☐
7. If he was your brother, would it be important not to let other people know that he had been ill, to avoid shame for your family?	☐	☐	☐	☐
8. If your local hospital opens a clinic for people like him in your neighborhood, would you hope the local council would object?	☐	☐	☐	☐
9. Is the cause of this sort of illness something passing down in the family?	☐	☐	☐	☐
10. Should the doctors tell him not to have any children in case he passes the illness onto them?	☐	☐	☐	☐
11. Should the doctors have let him out of hospital?	☐	☐	☐	☐
12. Is his illness something he might have brought on himself?	☐	☐	☐	☐
13. Should the doctors only let him leave hospital on the condition that he comes to see them regularly?	☐	☐	☐	☐
14. Do you think a sympathetic family and friends can stop him becoming ill again?	☐	☐	☐	☐
15. Will a sympathetic family be more help to him than regularly taking medicine?	☐	☐	☐	☐
16. Would it be wise for this man to inherit his parents' property?	☐	☐	☐	☐
17. If he becomes ill again, do you think it would be better to call the police first than the doctor?	☐	☐	☐	☐
18. Would you be happy if this person became the teacher of your children?	☐	☐	☐	☐
19. Will he be able to return to a completely normal life?	☐	☐	☐	☐
20. Should he stay in hospital for his whole life?	☐	☐	☐	☐
21. Would you eat food cooked by him?	☐	☐	☐	☐

(Continued)

(Continued)

		Yes, very much	Yes, a little	No, not much	No, not at all
22.	Would you avoid talking to him if possible?	☐	☐	☐	☐
23.	Might he have any special powers (to heal, to predict future events, to cause illness)?	☐	☐	☐	☐
24.	Could this illness be caused by some spirits or an enemy harming him?	☐	☐	☐	☐
25.	Could you give a name to this illness?	☐	☐	☐	☐
26.	Has any person you know personally ever had a similar illness? Yes/No	☐	☐	☐	☐

Findings of the paper showed a better prognosis in rural societies and lower income countries.

DIFFERENT CONCEPTIONS OF MENTAL ILLNESS

At one time in our history, professionals made a sharp distinction between physical disorders and mental disorders—physical disorders involved the body and mental disorders involved the mind. Today we have come to see the close connection of the brain with what was previously considered mental processes. Mental disorders are brain disorders. Further, those physiological processes involved in physical disorders such as the immune system, the turning on and off of genes, and the chemical processes of the body are also equally involved in mental disorders.

In this book, I will use the terms *psychopathology*, *mental disorders*, or *mental illness* to refer to those disorders traditionally described in scientific and professional research and practice. *Psychopathology* is the word commonly used in the neurosciences and the one you would want to use when performing literature searches in research and clinical journals. *Abnormal psychology* as a research area has a long tradition in psychology, and I will refer to this tradition by that term.

Concept Check

- What is the status of mental health research in India?
- What is the role of community mental health initiatives?

Within psychology, *The Journal of Abnormal Psychology* was once *The Journal of Abnormal and Social Psychology.* This reflected both practical issues and the overlap of interests. For example, topics such as personality were of interest to both social psychologists and clinical psychologists. Also, understanding normal social functioning helped to clarify the manner in which various psychopathologies interfere with human interactions. Many disorders I will describe in this book are characterized by problems in social relationships and their components.

If we think about our social relationships, we realize that there are a variety of levels that help us to understand our experiences. Part of our reactions may relate to people we have known personally in the past. Part of our reactions may be related to what we have learned to value from our culture. If we realize that humans throughout our history have always lived in groups, then we might see an even larger perspective that would be related to the evolutionary development of humans. Part of this perspective is that we not only pay attention to our own experiences but also try to understand the experiences of others. These are part of the everyday interactions that we all go through.

What do you do when you meet someone for the first time? Most people make a quick assessment about that person. Are we attracted to that person, or do we find ourselves moving away from him? Sometimes we don't even realize we make the judgments that we do. Social psychology research has shown us that we are quick to see others who are like us as attractive and those not like us as unattractive. If the person makes us laugh and feel good, we continue to interact with them. If the person scares us, we move away quickly. If the person treats us in a way we don't like, we may even get angry.

In meeting individuals with mental disorders, we may be unsure of how to react, and stigma can become a problem. If stigma leads to problems with finding jobs or places to live, then individuals with mental disorders have an even more difficult time being part of a community. As you will see in the next chapter, those with mental disorders have been treated differently throughout history.

THE THREE MAJOR THEMES OF THIS BOOK

In this book, there are three major themes I will explore.

The first theme takes a **behavioral and experiential perspective** and relates to the behavior and experience observed in psychopathology. In this theme, I will examine current ways of classifying and describing abnormal behavior. I also want you to consider the experience of having a psychological disorder and will present first person reports from individuals with particular disorders. We will also discuss symptoms and signs. Traditionally, symptoms, such as feeling sad, are seen as subjective, which the individual reports to a professional, whereas signs, such as having a fever, are an objective process that can be measured and would be apparent to a professional. An important aspect of this perspective is the manner in which the signs and symptoms of a particular disorder are seen in a similar manner throughout the world. The universality of mental disorders has been an important consideration for scientists. It is also important to note the role culture plays in the manifestations of behaviors and experiences related to psychopathology.

The second theme examines what we know about particular psychopathological experience from the standpoint of a **neuroscience perspective.** In particular, I will emphasize the structure and function of the brain as it relates to psychopathology. With the advent of neuroscience techniques such as brain imaging, it is becoming clear that mental disorders are also brain disorders. In fact, with every disorder we will consider in this book, it is possible to examine the manner in which the structure and function of the brain is changed. The neuroscience perspective will also help us to consider how certain disorders share a similarity in underlying brain processes. For example, knowing that the same brain networks involved in physical pain are also involved in social rejection help us understand the experience of each and how they are like one another.

The third theme asks a much broader scientific question and examines psychological disorders from an **evolutionary perspective.** In adopting this perspective, we can think about how certain ways of seeing or being in the world might be adaptive. Being afraid of heights, for example, keeps us from taking unnecessary risks. We can ask if there is any advantage to behaving and feeling in certain ways that others consider abnormal. We can also ask if the disordered behavior is secondary to another process that is beneficial. This could include an attempt by our body to protect itself.

Let's look at the ways a disorder may be protective. One classic example is the blood disorder sickle-cell anemia. Although the genetic disorder sickle-cell anemia can cause a variety of physiological problems, its presence also confers a resistance to malaria. Thus, having one disorder may be protective of another. Sickle-cell anemia is most often seen in individuals whose ancestors lived in parts of West Africa, lowland regions of Sicily, Cyprus, Greece, the Middle East, and India. Since this is where malaria exists, it is assumed that its presence evolved as a result of natural selection.

In the same way that we know that having a fever is protective and beneficial to recovering from sickness, we can look for similarities in psychological disorders. We can also ask questions concerning why particular disorders continue to exist. Individuals with schizophrenia, for example, generally have fewer children than those without the disorder. Thus, you might expect that schizophrenia would have gradually disappeared over our evolutionary history through the production of fewer children with the genetics related to the disorder. However, this is not the case, and in fact, schizophrenia occurs in approximately the same percentage (1% of the population) throughout the world in both developed and developing countries. As I will discuss in more detail later in this book, this suggests that schizophrenia is an old disorder that has existed since humans migrated out of Africa some 80 to 100 thousand years ago. It also suggests that the multiple genes associated with schizophrenia may be associated with more positive human traits such as creativity.

In summary, the three themes—behavior and experience, neuroscience, and the evolutionary perspective—give us important perspectives for thinking about psychopathology.

LEVELS OF ANALYSIS

Concept Check

- How has the relationship between physical disorders and mental disorders changed historically?
- Identify the three major themes this book takes in regard to psychopathology.

As we explore together the themes of behavior and experience, neuroscience contributions, and evolutionary perspectives as related to psychopathology, you will see that we will move across a variety of **levels of analysis** ranging from culture to genetics. Higher-level understandings include culture and society as well as our social relationships. From there, we can look at what makes up the social level as well as the individual level, which includes our actions and our experiences. We can then ask what makes up the individual in terms of sensory, motor, emotional, and cognitive systems. We can examine each of these levels as they influence our behavior and experience. From there, we can ask how each of these systems works and look at the physiological processes that make up our central and peripheral nervous systems. This will take us to the cortical network level, and we will see how neurons and their connections form the basis of information transfer and processing. The most basic level we will be introduced to in this book is the genetic level, which in turn will require us to understand how environmental conditions influence genetic processes. We will also learn about a related process, epigenetics, in which genes can be turned on or off by the environment and these mechanisms can be passed on to future generations without actually changing the basic genetic structure. These levels are depicted in the photos and illustrations beginning on this page.

In order to help focus their work, scientists often focus primarily on one of these levels of analysis. However, in this book I want to consider a more integrative approach that draws on a number of these levels. Further, you should not take any one of these levels of analysis as more important or truer than another. A similar plea was made by George Engel in 1977 when he helped to develop the biopsychosocial approach to understanding mental illness (Engel, 1977).

Biopsychosocial Approach

In a paper in the scientific journal *Science*, George Engel introduced the term *biopsychosocial*. He suggested that those with mental illness or even a medical disorder should not be understood from only a biological perspective. Diabetes is a disorder, but it is also related to how the person eats and exercises. Likewise, depression and anxiety can be influenced by social and emotional factors. Thus, it is necessary to see the signs and symptoms of the disorder in a larger context. Otherwise, one has a limited perspective that ignores the social, psychological, and behavioral dimensions of any disorder. Thus, as a mental health professional, you would want to know more about an individual than just the symptoms that the person describes. This could be his or her family life, work conditions, and cultural practices as well as eating habits and how the person exercises. As you will see in this book, since the 1970s researchers have come a long way in understanding how various levels ranging from genetics to culture interact with each other in a complex manner. Let us now begin with a consideration of culture over our longer evolutionary time that will take us to an understanding of behavior and experience on a number of levels. In later chapters, I will introduce you to additional levels of analysis.

THE RELATION OF EVOLUTION AND CULTURE TO PSYCHOPATHOLOGY

Considering psychopathology from evolutionary and cultural perspectives goes beyond the traditional psychological and physiological considerations (Ray, 2013). These perspectives make us realize that for at least the last 100,000 years humans have been social beings who have lived within the context of a group in which there were interactions related to gathering and preparing food, having sexual relations, and being part of a community. Cultures developed from this.

From the **cultural perspective,** current views of culture emphasize the social world in which a person lives (López & Guarnaccia, 2000). In this sense, culture can be viewed as "information capable of affecting individuals' behavior that they acquire from other members of their species through teaching, imitation, and other forms of social transmission" (Richerson & Boyd, 2005). From this perspective, culture can be seen as a system of inheritance. Humans learn a variety of things from others in their culture including skills, values, beliefs, and attitudes. Historically, parents and others taught children how to perform particular jobs such as farming, toolmaking, hunting, and performing other skills. Human culture has also formalized learning in the form of schools and apprenticeships. Cultures also differ in their level of economic development and the amount of resources they devote to mental health. In the LENS 1-2 on page 18, the availability of mental health professionals across the world is described.

For a more complete understanding of psychopathology, it is important to understand the particular rules a culture has for expressing both internal experiences and external behaviors (see Marsella & Yamada, 2007, for an overview). What may be a common experience in one culture may lead to stress and anxiety in another. Even what individuals tell themselves about having a mental disorder can vary from culture to culture. Likewise, artistic and spiritual experiences considered normal in one group may be considered "crazy" in another.

Historically, a simplistic view of culture has emphasized how each culture is locally determined, without reference to universal psychological processes. When universal ways of behaving, feeling, or thinking are suggested, this view assumes that this information is acquired by social learning. Although this is an important aspect of culture, this emphasis will quickly lead you into the outdated nature–nurture debate, which lacks the insights of modern evolutionary and neuroscience perspectives. For example, consider the question of why foods with milk are found in European diets and not in Asian diets. One answer could be cultural preferences. However, a more complete answer includes the fact that Northern Europeans have a gene that allows them to continue digesting milk products after the traditional time of weaning.

A person with such a gene would have had an advantage in Northern Europe since dairy products are a high quality food source, and over time—probably less than 10,000 years—that advantage would have allowed these genes to be passed on to almost all of the European population. Today, 98% of all individuals in Sweden have this gene. In the United States, with its large European migration, 88% of white Americans are lactose tolerant. Native Americans on the other hand are not lactose tolerant. Overall, this suggests a close connection between cultural and evolutionary perspectives.

The picture becomes even more complicated in terms of psychological processes. There is a particular form of a gene (5-HTT) related to the neurotransmitter serotonin, which is associated with being prone to develop higher levels of anxiety and depression. When its occurrence is examined cross-culturally, studies have shown that 70% to 80% of Japanese individuals carry this gene whereas only 40% to 45% of Europeans carry it (see Ambady & Bharucha, 2009, for an overview). Likewise, brain imaging studies have shown that cultural values can influence which areas of the brain are active during self-evaluation (see Chiao, 2011, for an overview).

The larger question raised by these studies is whether this genetic variation influences the manner in which cultural structures formalize social interactions and how this might be related to what is considered mental illness. That is, a society that has more individuals who are prone to anxiety may develop different forms of social interaction than one that does not. Not only can the environment influence genetics but genetics can influence culture. This work is just beginning to be applied to viewing psychopathology from a cultural standpoint (Figure 1.2).

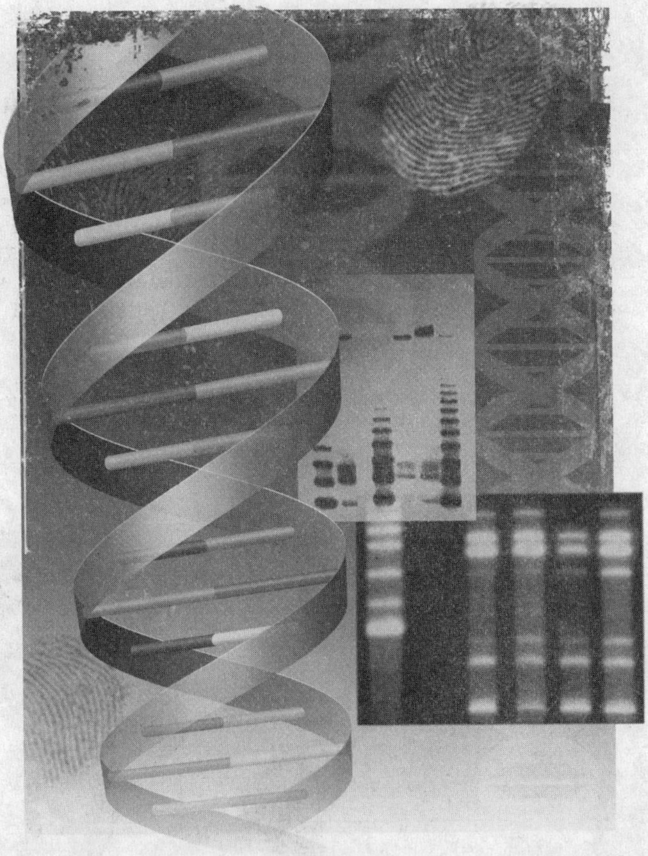

FIGURE 1-2 Genetics—What Are the Possibilities of Our Structure and Experience?

Source: Thinkstock/photos.com

Considering how a condition such as lactose tolerance is found in some groups of individuals around the world and not in others gives us additional insights into when this condition may have developed. Since lactose tolerance is not found throughout the world but is limited to one group, one would assume that it was not part of the human condition when humans migrated out of Africa some 100,000 years ago. We can ask similar questions in terms of psychopathology. One question might be how long, in terms of our human history, a particular psychopathology has existed.

Let's take schizophrenia as an example. A WHO study examined the presence of schizophrenia in a number of countries with very different racial and cultural backgrounds (Sartorius et al., 1986). If schizophrenia had an important environmental component, then you would expect to see different manifestations of the disorder in different cultures. Developed countries would show different rates than nondeveloped countries. Areas with different climates might also show differences, as is the case with multiple sclerosis. What these authors found was that, despite the different cultural and racial backgrounds surveyed, the experience of schizophrenia was remarkably similar across countries. Likewise, the risk of developing schizophrenia was similar in terms of total population presence—about 1%. Further, the disorder had a similar time course in its occurrence with its characteristics first being seen in young adults.

The evolutionary and cultural perspectives help us ask questions such as what function a disorder might serve, as well as how it came about. For example, humans fear animals they have little contact with but do not fear more likely causes of danger such as automobile accidents. Likewise, rejecting a food for years that once made us sick does not seem logical. This is particularly true in a time of food safety conditions available in most

1-2 LENS
Global Mental Health: Available Treatment

Mental health services are available worldwide. However, they differ by country in how available they are as well as the nature of the services offered. In countries in which individuals have a higher income, such as the United States, Canada, England, Germany, France, Japan, and Australia, there are many more mental care workers such as psychologists and psychiatrists than in low-income countries such as India, China, and much of Africa. *Figure 1-3* shows the number of mental health professionals throughout the world. This map shows the number of psychiatrists, psychologists, nurses, and social workers per 100,000 people in the country.

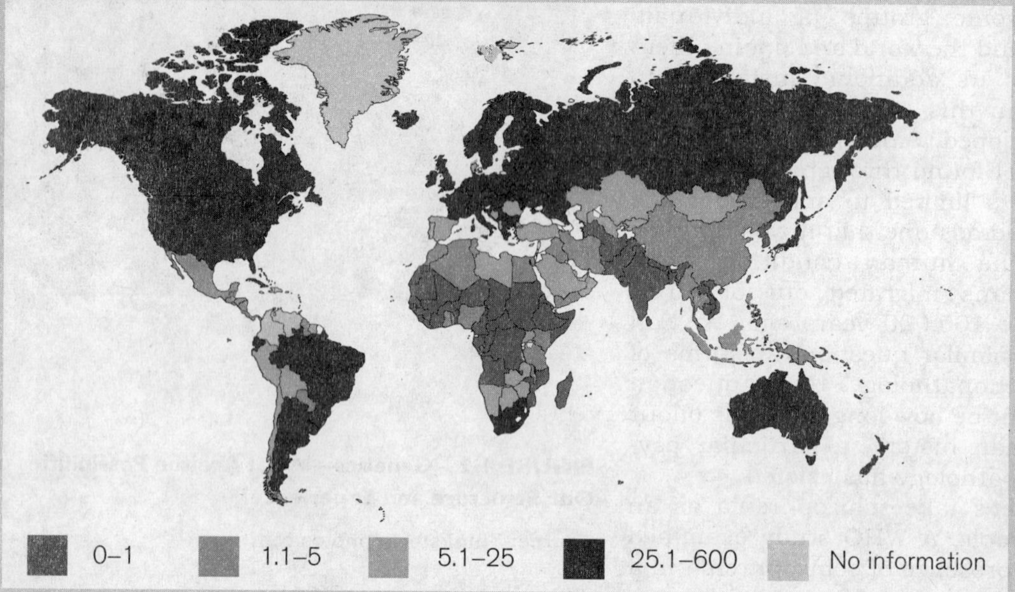

FIGURE 1-3 Human Resources for Mental Health (Psychiatrists, Psychologists, Nurses, and Social Workers) per 100,000 Population

Disclaimer: This figure is not to scale. It does not represent any authentic national or international boundaries and is used for illustrative purposes only.

Reprinted from *The Lancet*, Vol. 370, Shekhar Saxena, Graham Thornicroft, Martin Knapp, and Harvey Whiteford, Global Mental Health 2 Resources for Mental Health: Scarcity, Inequity, and Inefficiency, p. 880. Copyright © 2007, with permission from Elsevier.

High-income countries have the greatest number of mental health professionals and low-income countries the least. *Figure 1-4* shows the number of psychiatrists, psychologists, nurses, and social workers by income level. The governments of about one third of all countries do not have a specific budget for mental health. In many countries, informal networks of families, friends, and other social networks are utilized to care for those with mental illness.

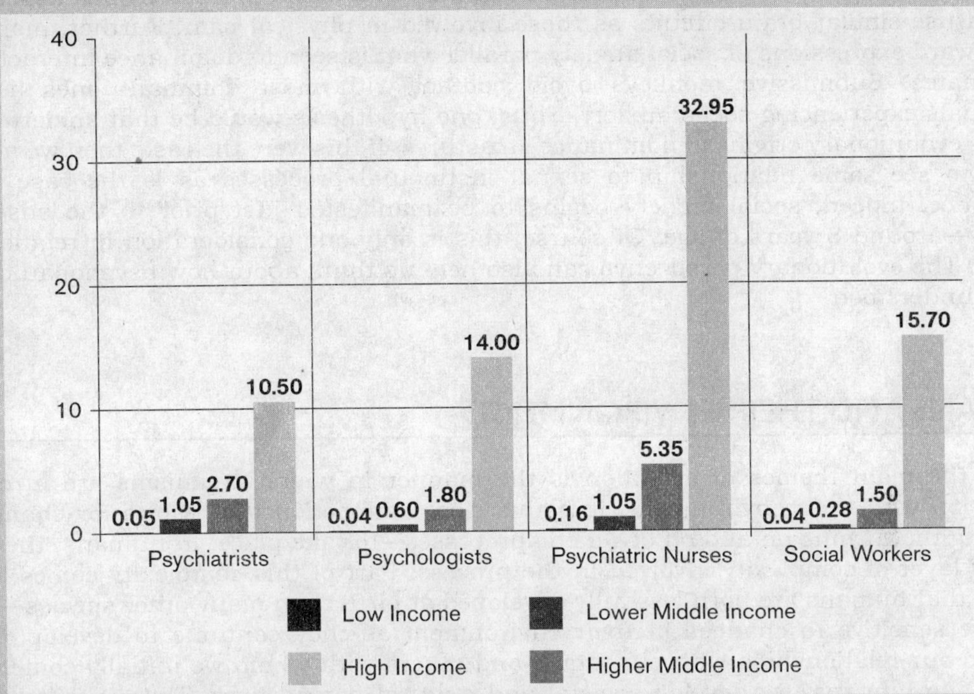

FIGURE 1-4 Human Resources in Terms of Mental Health Professionals in Each Income Group of Countries per 100,000 Population

Reprinted from *The Lancet*, Vol. 370, Shekhar Saxena, Graham Thornicroft, Martin Knapp, and Harvey Whiteford, Global Mental Health 2 Resources for Mental Health: Scarcity, Inequity, and Inefficiency, p. 880. Copyright © 2007, with permission from Elsevier.

developed countries, but it is a common experience. Of course, both experiences make sense if we consider our long evolutionary history.

Considering how many human processes evolved, it is clear that few of the environments in which we live today conform to the environment in which humans developed. Unlike other species, humans live in environments that are different in many respects from those that shaped our early evolutionary history. We have developed large cities and the technological abilities to communicate instantly around the planet. We have also developed ways to mitigate conditions such as the weather that would have played a greater role in our lives thousands of years ago. Compared with other species, humans live less in nature and more in culture. However, it is important in considering psychopathology to remember the environment in which humans as a species developed. John Bowlby (1969) referred to the environment found in our early evolutionary history as the environment of evolutionary adaptedness.

In thinking about our evolutionary history, we can consider how one basic human process developed in relation to an earlier one. For example, in the same way that pain can be seen as a warning system to the body to protect it from tissue damage, anxiety may have evolved to protect the individual from other types of potential threats. In fact, an evolutionary perspective has helped to determine that social processes such as feeling rejected use similar brain circuits as those involved in physical pain. Further, many of the outward expressions of social anxiety parallel what is seen in dominance interactions in primates. Submissive monkeys avoid contact with most dominant ones as do individuals experiencing social anxiety. Thus, one hypothesis would be that anxiety may have its evolutionary origins in dominance structures. If this were the case, then we might expect to see some relationship to sexual instinctual processes as is the case with dominance. Indeed, social anxiety begins to be manifested just prior to the onset of puberty—around 8 years of age. Of course, this is only one consideration in relation to anxiety. The evolutionary perspective can also help us think about how psychopathology can be understood.

HUMANS AND THEIR ENVIRONMENT

One of the main themes of evolution is the manner in which organisms are in close connection with their environment. It is this close connection that allows for change—including the turning on and off of genetic processes—to take place. In humans, there is another layer of complexity involved in the process. Part of this complexity comes from the fact that humans are born less fully developed at birth than many other species—and thus are sensitive to changes in their environment as they continue to develop. This includes our relationships with our family and others with whom we initially come into contact. As humans, we develop societal and cultural perspectives. These perspectives become the backdrop of our environment. Unlike animals that live within nature, we as humans largely live within the backdrop of our culture. Another part of the complexity with humans is our ability to reflect on ourselves and our world. In this way, a layer of thought can be injected between the person and the environment. This allows for expectation and even imagination to play a role in human behavior and experience.

We live in a way that keeps us in close contact with others and with our environment. You wear a coat when it is cold or call a friend when you are lonely. What I want to do in this book is to consider what happens when our interactions with others and with our environment lose this close connection. On an experiential level, we may feel isolated and lonely. In more severe situations, we can experience the exaggerated feelings and distorted thoughts that do not fit the situation in which we live. There are a variety of ways that our close connections can be lost. In some cases, genetic and environmental processes lead to this close connection not developing in the first place. In other cases, the connection develops but becomes broken through a variety of factors including trauma. These experiences and behaviors mark the content area of psychopathology.

Humans not only consider themselves; they also consider others. A positive side of this, as noted previously, is the ability to understand the internal experiences of another. This allows us to experience empathy. We can also consider how we appear to others and other questions of self-image. One aspect of this is related to the sexual instinct. That is, we can say or do things that make us more attractive to a potential mate. In terms of self-preservation, humans also have a personal history that allows each person to learn from the past and develop strategies for living life. These strategies tend to protect us, and even may have saved our lives in exceptional cases.

However, it is also possible for the strategies that work in one environmental situation not to work in another. When a person loses contact with the current environment and applies strategies that worked perhaps in an earlier time, then unsuccessful adaptation is the result. This lack of connectedness to our environment may take place on both external and internal levels. On an external level, the person finds himself or herself different from the group or even seeks to be separate from others. As humans, this is not our historical experience—humans have never lived as isolated individuals. As a species we have always lived in close contact with other humans, leading to the development of societies and cultures. In fact, many of the specific abilities of humans are geared to social interactions on a variety of levels. When we no longer have the connection with the group, we experience a sense of loss. This loss often carries with it the experience of negative affect and depression and a need to withdraw. On an internal level, humans often have the need to explain to themselves the events that have just occurred, which may include anger, distorted perceptions, or a genuine plan for recovery. Extreme cases are referred to as psychopathological.

What is psychopathology? Although there is no one single definition of what represents abnormal processes, five ideas have been critical.

1. The processes involved in psychopathology are maladaptive and not in the individual's best interest.
2. The processes cause personal distress.
3. The processes represent a deviance from both cultural and statistical norms.
4. The person has difficulty connecting with his or her environment and also with himself or herself.
5. There is an inability of an individual with a mental disorder to fully consider alternative ways of thinking, feeling, or doing. That is to say, such individuals often do not see, feel, or think there are alternatives. This results in their psychological processes being rigid and patterned. Having fewer alternatives also suggests that they have less freedom in any given situation.

IS PSYCHOPATHOLOGY UNIVERSAL?

If psychopathology is part of our human makeup, then we expect to see similar manifestations of it worldwide. One classic study in this regard was performed by Jane Murphy (1976) of Harvard University. It dates from the 1970s when mental illness was considered to be related to learning and the social construction of norms. In fact, some suggested that mental illness was just a myth developed by Western societies. In this perspective, neither the individual nor his or her acts are abnormal in an objective sense. One important implication of this view was that what would be seen as mental illness in a Western industrial culture might be very different from what was seen as mental

> **Concept Check**
>
> - Identify seven of the levels of analysis presented for studying psychopathology. Which is the most important?
> - Is the nature–nurture debate outdated? What evidence would you cite to characterize the relationships among genetics, culture, and the environment in human development?

illness in a less developed rural culture. That is to say, mental illness in this perspective was viewed as a social construction of the society. The alternative to this perspective is more similar to other human processes such as emotionality, in which humans throughout the world recognize similar expressions of the basic emotions. If mental illness is part of our human history, as evolutionary psychologists would suggest, then we would expect to find similar manifestations across a variety of cultures.

Dr. Murphy first studied two geographically separate and distinct non-Western groups: the Eskimos of northwest Alaska and the Yorubas of rural tropical Nigeria. Although many researchers of that time would have expected to find the conceptions of normality and abnormality to be very different in the two cultures, this is not what she found. She found that these cultures were well acquainted with processes in which a person was said to be out of their mind. This included doing strange things as well as hearing voices. Jane Murphy concluded that processes of disturbed thought and behavior similar to schizophrenia are found in most cultures and that most cultures have a distinct name in their language for these processes. Additionally, she reported that these cultures had a variety of words for what traditionally is referred to as neurosis although today we would refer to these as affective disorders. Affective disorders include feeling anxious, tense, and fearful of being with others as well as being troubled and not able to sleep. One Eskimo term was translated as worrying too much until it makes the person sick. Thus, it appears that most cultures have a word for what has been called psychosis, what has been called neurosis, and what has been called normalcy. What is also interesting is that many cultures also have words for describing people who are out of their mind but not "crazy." These would be witch doctors, shamans, and artists.

To add evidence to her argument that psychopathology is indeed part of our human nature, Murphy also reviewed a large variety of studies conducted by others that looked at how common mental illness was in different cultures. The suggestion here is that if its prevalence is similar in cultures across the world then it is more likely to be part of the human condition rather than culturally derived. What these studies suggest is that many forms of mental illness such as schizophrenia are found at similar rates the world around. Overall, this research established that mental illness was not a created concept by a given culture but rather part of the human condition in both its recognition and its prevalence. However, culture will play a role in how it is manifested in the larger community.

EXPERIENTIAL PERSPECTIVE

Concept Check

- Is psychopathology universal? What kinds of evidence show that it is? What evidence is there for cultural differences in psychopathology?
- How does reading about the experiences of individuals with mental illness inform our understanding of the nature of psychopathology?

One important aspect for a complete understanding of psychopathology is the experiential perspective—how the individual with the disorder experiences it and sees the world. At the beginning of many of the chapters of this book, you will read first person accounts from individuals with particular disorders. As you will see, sometimes the experience of the person may result from the personal distress related to the disorder or the inability to relate to others. Sometimes the experience may be the result of reduced capacity as in the inability to consider alternative ways of acting or thinking or feeling. Other times, the experience may be of non-normal reality as when hearing voices in one's head or seeing things not seen by others. Recently, there has been an attempt to better document the experience of mental illness. For example, the scientific journal *Schizophrenia Bulletin* has begun to publish first person accounts of individuals with schizophrenia. Likewise, a number of highly successful individuals with particular disorders have published detailed accounts of their experiences. I will draw upon these sources throughout this book.

PLAN OF THE BOOK

In the next chapter, I will introduce you to the historical manner in which psychopathology has been viewed and treated. Following that, I will introduce you to some of the ways scientists research psychopathology and the types of neuroscience measures and research methods they use. I will then introduce you to ways in which psychopathology is assessed and classified. In the United States, the criteria for the diagnosis of mental illness are denoted in the *Diagnostic and Statistical Manual of Mental Disorders (DSM)* published by the American Psychiatric Association (APA). The current version is *DSM–5* (APA, 2013). I will introduce you to these criteria throughout this book in the order similar to how they are presented in *DSM–5*.

SUMMARY

Three major themes—behavior and experience, neuroscience, and the evolutionary perspective—give us important perspectives for thinking about psychopathology. In addition, an integrative perspective ranging across a number of different levels provides a greater understanding of psychopathological processes. These levels range from the highest levels of environment, culture, and society to social relationships to individual behavior and experience to our sensory, motor, emotional, and cognitive systems to the physiological processes that make up our central and peripheral nervous systems to the cortical network level to the most basic level of genetics and epigenetics. The genetic level in turn takes us back up to the highest level to understand how environmental conditions influence genetic processes.

Considering psychopathology from evolutionary and cultural perspectives goes beyond the traditional psychological and physiological considerations. Culture can be seen as a system of inheritance—humans learn a variety of things from others in their culture including skills, values, beliefs, and attitudes. For a more complete understanding of psychopathology, it is important to understand the particular rules a culture has for expressing both internal experiences and external behaviors. Overall, research suggests a close connection between cultural and evolutionary perspectives. Not only can the environment influence genetics; genetics can in turn influence culture. The evolutionary and cultural perspectives help us ask questions such as these: (1) Can genetic variation influence the manner in which cultural structures formalize social interactions and how this might be related to what is considered mental illness? (2) How long, in terms of our human history, has a particular psychopathology existed? (3) What function might a disorder serve and how did it come about? (4) How can a basic human process (e.g., the pain of social rejection) develop in relation to an earlier one (e.g., the brain circuits involved in physical pain)?

One of the main themes of evolution is the manner in which organisms are in close connection with their environment. It is this close connection that allows for change—including the turning on and off of genetic processes—to take place. Humans are born less fully developed at birth than many other species and thus are sensitive to changes in their environment as they continue to develop. Unlike animals that live within nature, humans largely live within the backdrop of our culture. Another part of the complexity with humans is our ability to reflect on ourselves and our world. In this way, a layer of thought, including expectation and imagination, is injected between the person and the environment.

Five ideas are critical to the concept of psychopathology. First, the processes involved are maladaptive and not in the individual's best interest. Second, these processes cause personal distress. Third, the processes are considered to be deviant from cultural and statistical norms. Forth, the individual has difficulty connecting with his or her environment and also with himself or herself. Finally, the individual is not able to consider alternative ways of thinking, feeling, or doing.

STUDY RESOURCES

Review Questions

1. Why do stigmas arise in regard to mental illness? What impacts do stigmas have on individuals with psychopathology as well as their families, communities, and society as a whole?
2. Three major themes—behavior and experience, neuroscience, and the evolutionary perspective—are presented as giving us important perspectives for thinking about psychopathology. What are some of the ideas each of these perspectives offers?
3. What levels of analysis are important to consider in understanding psychopathology? What are the advantages of considering multiple levels and taking an integrated approach?
4. This chapter states that "considering psychopathology from evolutionary and cultural perspectives goes beyond the traditional psychological and physiological considerations." What arguments does the author put forth to explain the importance of these two perspectives in asking critical questions that need to be answered? Do you agree?
5. What are the five critical characteristics to be included in answering the following question: What is psychopathology?

For Further Reading

Open Government Data Platform, India. Released under National Data Sharing and Accessibility Policy (NDSAP).
Mental Health Research in India Indian Council of Medical Research (ICMR). 2005.
Reviews of Marathi film trilogy "Devrai", "Astu" and "Kaasav."

Key Terms and Concepts

abnormal psychology
behavioral and experiential perspective
cultural perspective
evolutionary perspective
levels of analysis
neuroscience perspective
psychopathology
stigma

CHAPTER

2

Changing Conceptualizations of Mental Illness

CHAPTER OUTLINE

- HISTORICAL CONSIDERATIONS IN UNDERSTANDING PSYCHOPATHOLOGY 29
- DISCOVERING THE FUNCTION OF THE BRAIN IN BEHAVIOR AND PSYCHOPATHOLOGY 35
- CARE FOR THOSE WITH MENTAL DISORDERS 43
- FROM THE PAST TO THE PRESENT 48
- THE PSYCHOLOGICAL TREATMENT PERSPECTIVES IN THE 20TH CENTURY 48
- SUMMARY 62
- STUDY RESOURCES 62

My students filled the room. They were interested and eager, unusually so, given that they were second- and third-year law students for whom the fear and trembling that came with the first year had long since faded. The course was "Advanced Mental Health Law." The day's topic: Billie Boggs. A street person who lived over a hot air vent in midtown Manhattan, she threw food at people who wanted to help her and chased them across the street. Her rantings and ravings seemed crazy to most of the students, and we were discussing whether she should be sent to a psychiatric hospital.

I heard myself speak, surprising myself by the steady sound of my voice as I tried to restore my attention to the group before me: "What if Billie Boggs were your sister—would you put her in a psychiatric hospital then?" Up shot the hands.

Concentrate. These are your students. You have an obligation to them. Canceling class would be admitting defeat. But there are explosions in my head. They're testing nuclear devices on my brain. They're very little and they can get inside. They are powerful.

I pulled myself together, enough to point to a young woman who spoke often in class. "I couldn't let my sister live like that," she said from across the classroom, which held the students in curved rows, like a giant palm before me. "I know my sister. That wouldn't be her. There's one and only one of her—and that's the one before she got sick."

Is she trying to kill me? No, she's a student. But what about the others? The voices inside my head, the explosions. What do they want? Are they trying to interdict me, to hit me with the Kramer device? I went to the store and they said "interdiction." Interdiction, introduction, exposition, explosion. Voicemail is the issue.

I knew not to say those thoughts out loud. Not because they were crazy thoughts—they were every bit as real as the students sitting right in front of me—but I kept silent because others would think them crazy. People would think me as deranged as Billie Boggs.

But I'm not crazy. I simply have greater access to the truth.

"Good," I replied. "But why isn't it the case that your sister has two selves, the sick one you see now and the healthy one you've known all your life? Why should you get to pick which is real? Shouldn't your sister make that choice?" Up shot more hands.

My brain is on fire! My head is going to explode right here, right in front of my class!

"But isn't health always preferred to illness?" a bright-eyed young man countered. "We should prefer the healthy self."

Mercifully, the class ended. A law-school dean spotted me as I walked back to my office. He said I looked as if I were in pain. "Just a lot on my mind," I heard myself reply as I continued quickly down the hall. Keys out, door open, door shut. I crumpled into my chair and buried my face in my hands.

That was in September of 1991, and it was one of my worst such incidents. Ten years before, in my mid-20s, during my third psychiatric hospitalization, I had been given the diagnosis "chronic paranoid schizophrenia with acute exacerbation." My prognosis? "Grave." I was, in other words, expected to be unable to live independently, let alone work. At best I would be in a board-and-care, holding a minimum-wage job—perhaps flipping burgers—when my symptoms had become less severe.

That has not turned out to be my life. I am the Orrin B. Evans professor of law, psychology, and psychiatry and the behavioral sciences at the University of Southern California's law school; adjunct professor of psychiatry at the University of California at San Diego's medical school; and an assistant faculty member at the New Center for Psychoanalysis, where I am also a research clinical associate.

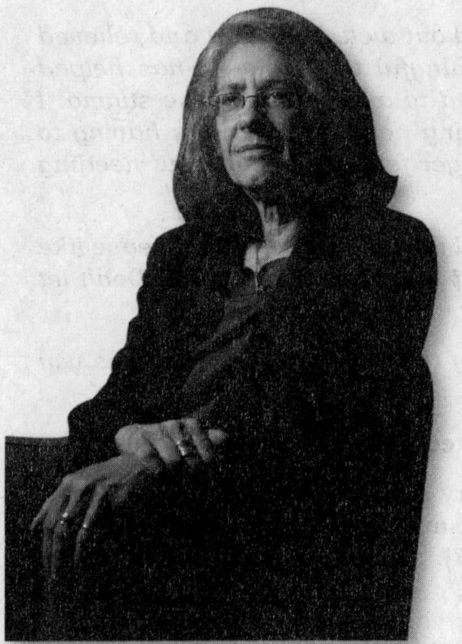

Elyn Saks
© ASSOCIATED PRESS/Damian Dovarganes

My schizophrenia has not gone away. I still become psychotic, as happened in class that day in 1991. Today my symptoms, while not as severe, still recur and I struggle to stay in the world, so to speak, doing my work. I have written about my illness in a memoir and much of the narrative takes place after I had accepted a tenure-track appointment at USC.

Barring a medical breakthrough of Nobel-Prize-winning proportions, I will never fully recover from schizophrenia. I will remain on antipsychotic medication and in talk therapy for the rest of my life. Yet I have learned to manage my illness.

Some are steps that everyone with mental illness should take. First, learn about the illness you have—the typical signs, symptoms, and course. Many excellent sources are available. You may want to start with the Diagnostic and Statistical Manual of Mental Disorders, DSM-IV-TR. Psychiatric textbooks, e.g., Kaplan and Sadock's, can be helpful. I have also discovered excellent lay accounts of mental illness.

Second, understand how your illness affects you. What are your triggers? What are your early warning signs? What can you do to minimize your symptoms when they worsen—e.g., call your therapist, increase your medication, listen to music, exercise? Try to devise some techniques for your own situation. Some colleagues and I are studying how a group of high-functioning people with schizophrenia manage their symptoms. You are in the best position to determine what works for you.

Put a good treatment team in place. You need a therapist you can trust and can turn to in times of difficulty. Does he or she respond if you call in crisis? The same is true of a psychopharmacologist. Make friends and family members part of your team.

Sometimes your team can see early warning signs before you can. For instance, my closest friend, Steve, and my husband, Will, often identify when I am slipping. Will says I become quieter in a particular way that signals all is not well. It's a blessing to have such people in your life. Seek them out.

We also need to put a face on mental illness. Being open about one's own illness will probably do more good than all the laws we can pass.

My own "outing" of myself was a bit of a risk, but has turned out well. I am glad and relieved I no longer have to hide. And my story seems to be meaningful to people—it has helped people understand mental illness more and perhaps has led to a decrease in the stigma. I was lucky in that my law school accommodated my teaching needs without my having to invoke the ADA. My colleagues are supportive, and I no longer feel ashamed about needing their help.

Perhaps most important: Seek help when you need it. Mental illness is a no-fault disease like any other, such as cancer or diabetes. Help is available, but you need to ask for it. Don't let the threat of stigma deter you. You shouldn't have to suffer.

And you shouldn't allow mental illness to stand in the way of the wonderful contributions you are poised to make to your students and to your field.

From *Chronicle of Higher Education*, November 25, 2009 (edited part of a larger article).

Elyn R. Saks is a professor of law, psychology, and psychiatry and the behavioral sciences at the University of Southern California's law school. She is the author of a memoir, The Center Cannot Hold: My Journey Through Madness (Hyperion, 2007).

The previous description of one person's experience with mental illness gives you a quick history of how mental illness has been conceptualized in the past and what the future may offer. When Elyn Saks initially went to the hospital, she was told that her prognosis was "grave." She was also told that she would never live independently, hold a job, find a loving partner, or get married. Her future was described as one in which she would live in a board-and-care facility, spending her days watching TV in a dayroom with other people debilitated by mental illness. For work, she would work at menial jobs when her symptoms were quiet. Following her last psychiatric hospitalization at the age of 28, she was encouraged by a doctor to work as a cashier making change. Not unlike people with cancer who were told in the last century to not expect a long life, individuals with mental illness were not given the possibility of real change.

In this chapter, I will examine our conceptualizations of mental illness over time. I will also show you how as we developed new scientific techniques for understanding human processes, the conceptualizations of mental illness also changed. We have gone from a worldview in which magic, including the idea that you could be possessed by spirits or demons, produced mental illness to a time in which our scientific understanding describes a complex set of processes on many levels that contribute to mental illness. During the current historical period, we have also come to see those with mental illness as whole people with both abilities and deficits. In terms of the future, Elyn Saks described a movement to allow people with mental disorders to have a say in their treatment. A person's high functioning and the ability to make decisions is not totally taken away by having a mental disorder. The person is still able to describe her experiences and, in the best of conditions, to ask others for help. However, I am getting ahead of myself.

HISTORICAL CONSIDERATIONS IN UNDERSTANDING PSYCHOPATHOLOGY

Psychology seeks to describe and understand human behavior and experience. In fact, as humans, we have a long history of trying to understand ourselves. In this section, I will discuss with you some of the historical conceptions that have influenced psychology (see Finger, 2000, or the classic Boring, 1950, for more information). One of these conceptions is the role of the body and its involvement in our mental processes. Some of the ideas we will examine date back thousands of years yet still influence our views today. Some others we may have rejected but we still show their influence in language. For example, no one today would think of the heart being involved in memory as did Aristotle in the fourth century BC. Yet, today we still say that we learn things by heart.

Ancient Greek and Roman Influences—Mental Illness Involves the Brain

Beginning with Pythagoras in the 6th century BCE, whom we know for his theorem concerning the sides of a right triangle, there was an emphasis on identifying the underlying scientific principles that may account for all forms of behavior. Pythagoras not only coined the term *philosophy,* which can be translated as love of meaning or wisdom, but also began to set the stage for understanding human behavior and experience as related to internal processes and natural causes. This is in contrast to a view that human behavior and related disorders reflect the actions of the gods such as the belief that mental illness was a divine punishment. Pythagoras was one of the first to see the brain as the structure involved in human intellect as well as in mental disorders.

In the next century, Hippocrates moved this to the next level with his emphasis on careful observation and a continued articulation of the idea that all disorders, both mental and physical, should be sought within the patient. Hippocrates is often seen as the father of Western medicine. His view of the brain is clearly stated in the following quote:

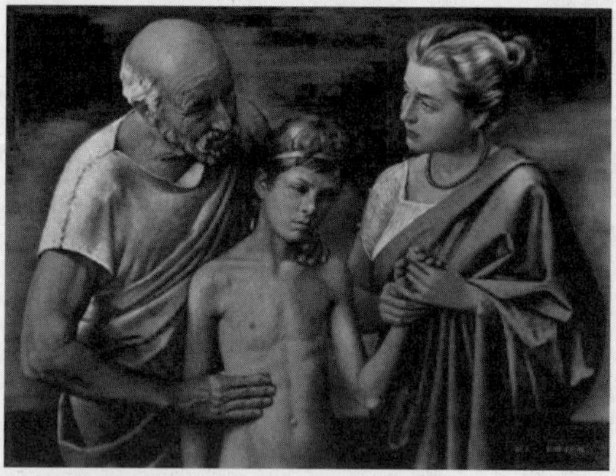

Hippocrates

© Buyenlarge/Archive Photos/Getty Images

> Men ought to know that from nothing else but the brain come joys, delights, laughter and sports, and sorrows, griefs, despondency, and lamentations. And by this, in an especial manner, we acquire wisdom and knowledge, and see and hear, and know what are foul and what are fair, what are bad and what are good, what are sweet, and what unsavory; some we discriminate by habit, and some we perceive by their utility. By this we distinguish objects of relish and disrelish, according to the seasons; and the same things do not always please us. And by the same organ we become mad and delirious, and fears and terrors assail us, some by night, and some by day, and dreams and untimely wanderings, and cares that are not suitable, and ignorance of present circumstances, desuetude, and unskilfulness. All these things we endure from the brain. (Hippocrates, *On The Scared Disease,* 400 BC)

Let's pause for a moment and get a sense of how the Greeks saw the world. They believed, as most scientists do today, that complex processes can be understood by breaking them down into their parts. The Greeks suggested that all things in the world can be understood in terms of just four *elements*—earth, air, fire, and water. In the body, they thought that these four elements took the form of what were called *humors,* which were yellow bile (fire), blood (air), phlegm (water), and black bile (earth). Blood was associated with the heart, black bile with the spleen, yellow bile with the liver, and phlegm with the brain. When the humors were in balance, health resulted. When they were out of balance, disease resulted. The cure for any disease was to restore balance. If the disease was seen to be "wet" or watery as in the case of tuberculosis, then the person might be sent to a dry climate. If the person's blood was seen to be out of balance, then bloodletting was the treatment.

In some ways, the Greeks were using the observations in front of them, as in the case of bloodshot eyes or the yellowing seen in jaundice, to determine the treatment. Some of our current ways of describing temperament and related psychopathology in terms of positive and negative emotions can be traced back to the ideas from the Greeks' understanding of the four humors.

Galen (130–200 CE) was a physician who influenced Western and Islamic thought until the Renaissance. Some see him as a representation of the beginning of experimentation in medicine in that he used dissection to better describe the structure and function of physiological structures. His work as a physician to the gladiators would have also given him firsthand knowledge of the consequences of trauma and its treatment. In the introduction to one of his medical texts, he described how to arrive at an understanding of structure and function of the nervous system.

> How the phenomena revealed in the brain and cord can best be observed in the dead and the living respectively will be made clear in this book. The anatomy of the dead teaches the position,

number, proper substance, size, and construction of the parts. That of the living may reveal the function at a glance or provide premises for deducing them. (Galen, reprinted in Finger, 2000, p. 39)

During his lifetime, Galen wrote a large number of treatises on science, medicine, and philosophy, which some estimate to number between 500 and 600. He was largely a champion of *empiricism,* which stresses the use of direct observation as a means of gaining information. Writing in his treatise *On Medical Experience,* Galen stated, "I am a man who attends only to what can be perceived by the senses . . ."

From chance encounters with human accidents and trauma and his anatomical work using a variety of animals, Galen carefully described the brain; the cranial nerves that are involved in sight, smell, movement, and other functions; and the nerves of the sympathetic nervous system involved in fight or flight reactions, among others. From his experiments with animals, Galen knew that blood was transported throughout the body. He had an early theory of how blood was changed by the organs based on the idea of *spirits.* Galen believed that blood was made in the liver, which gave it *natural spirits.* It then went to the heart where it developed *vital spirits* and then, with the introduction of air to the blood on the way to the brain, it was transformed into *animal spirits.* These animal spirits could be stored in the ventricles of the brain until they were needed. Today, we think in terms of hormones rather than spirits. Galen's works became the encyclopedia of medicine for the next 1,500 years.

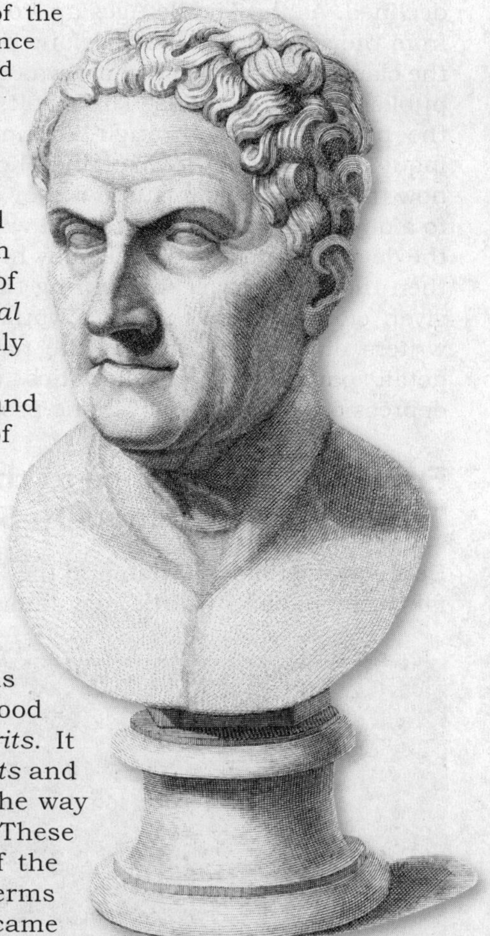

Galen
© Istockphoto/wynnter

Thoughts from Ancient India

Bhugra (1992), Nizamie and Goyal (2010), and Weiss (1986) discuss the role of Ancient Indian thinking and texts that discussed psychopathology and its etiology. All the scholars emphasize the social construction of distress and illness and warn against ethnocentric assumptions made out of context. Mentions of "*unmaada*" or excitement are found in the Vedas and those of "*duhkha*" or distress in Buddhist texts. *Dharmasaastra* and *Nitisaastra,* both ancient Indian texts, examine the various social and legal issues related to insanity.

Psychopathology in the Middle Ages

Although the Greek and Roman periods included individuals who attempted to understand psychopathology in a more humane way, this perspective disappeared as their civilizations declined. As the Middle Ages approached, disease and especially mental illness was seen from the standpoint of a religious perspective with the devil being a major player. One of the classic books in this genre was the *Malleus Maleficarum* (The Hammer of the Witches), published in the 1480s. This book was written by two German priests and approved by the pope. It went through a number of editions and became the handbook of the inquisition. As such, it explained how witches existed and flew through the air as well as how they should be tortured if they did not confess. In a "catch-22," the witches were tied to a device and lowered into cold water. If they floated, they were seen to be possessed by the devil and most likely killed by hanging or fire. If they went to the bottom and drowned, then they were innocent. During the interrogations, witches were not to be left alone or given clothes since the devil would visit them or hide in their clothing. Although the writers did not understand the nature of psychopathology, they did describe in some detail particular characteristics of different disorders including bipolar disorder, depression, and such psychotic processes as hallucinations and delusions.

From the Renaissance to the 1700s—The Beginning of Modern Science

Between the time of Galen and the Renaissance, Western science and medicine remained fairly stagnant with little new knowledge being added. One problem during this period was that authority, which was often the structure of the church, determined what was true or not. Since authority was able to use its own standard of truth, it was difficult to argue another position. For example, the church was able to say that the earth was the center of the universe and that was that.

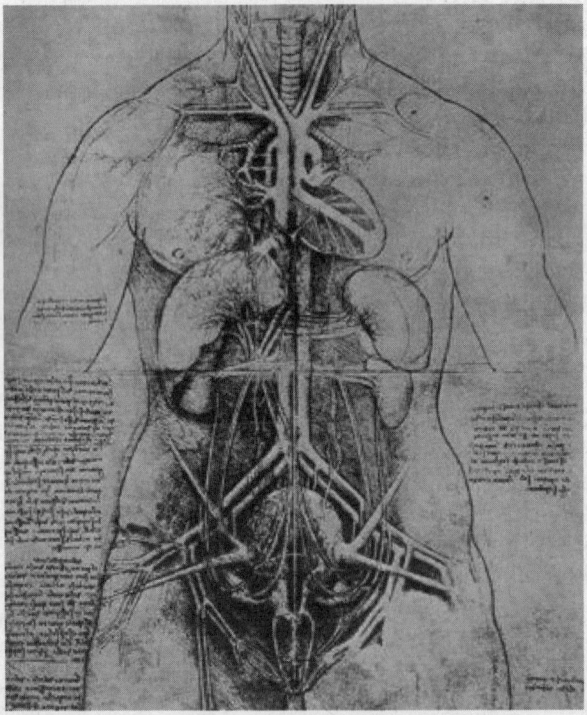

FIGURE 2-1 Leonardo da Vinci Drawing of the Structure of Human Organs

Beginning in the 14th century, however, a new spirit began to emerge in Europe. It influenced art, literature, politics, and science. In art, there was a desire for a sense of realism, which led artists such as Leonardo da Vinci to carefully study the human body. He performed dissections on animals and human cadavers to carefully reveal the structure of organs. *Figure 2-1* shows one of Leonardo da Vinci's drawings.

Leonardo drew on his knowledge of art to perform creative experimental studies. In the early 1500s, he wanted to know the structure of the ventricles in the brain. To determine their structure, Leonardo adapted the process of pouring molten metal into a mold in order to produce a statue. Using a similar procedure, he poured hot wax through a tube into the ventricles of an ox that had just been killed. Another tube allowed the cerebrospinal fluid to flow from the ox's brain. The wax was then allowed to harden and the cortical structure removed from around the wax. His drawings appear similar to what we know of the ventricles today. As can be seen in *Figure 2-2*, the ventricles are hollow structures that contain a clear fluid referred to as cerebrospinal fluid. Today, we note how ventricles may differ in size between healthy individuals and those with schizophrenia and other disorders.

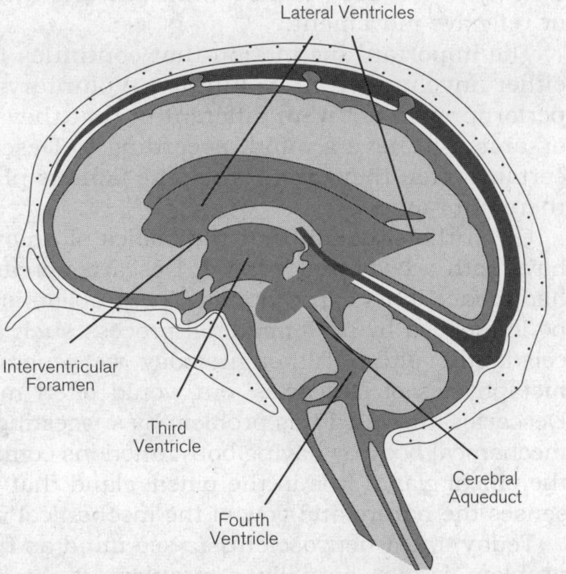

FIGURE 2-2 Structure of the Ventricles in the Brain

Source: Garrett (2010, Figure 3.15).

With the detailed drawings of human anatomy created by the artists of the time, there was now the possibility for the scientists of the 1600s to consider function. One important focus was the manner in which the nervous system allows us to perform both involuntary and voluntary functions. How physiological processes are involved in remembering, moving, feeling, and thinking became topics of consideration. Mechanical models became important as illustrated by William Harvey's 1628 publication describing how blood circulates throughout the body. Another individual who utilized mechanical models along with physics and mathematics was the French philosopher René Descartes (1596–1650).

Descartes was intrigued by mechanical machines such as the large clocks in Europe with moving figures or water displays in large fountains. By analogy, he assumed that reflexes or involuntary actions of organisms were based on similar principles. Thus, moving your hand from a hot stove or even digesting food was seen as a mechanical operation. For Descartes, all animal behavior could be explained by mechanical principles as could human involuntary actions. In *Figure 2-3* from Descartes'

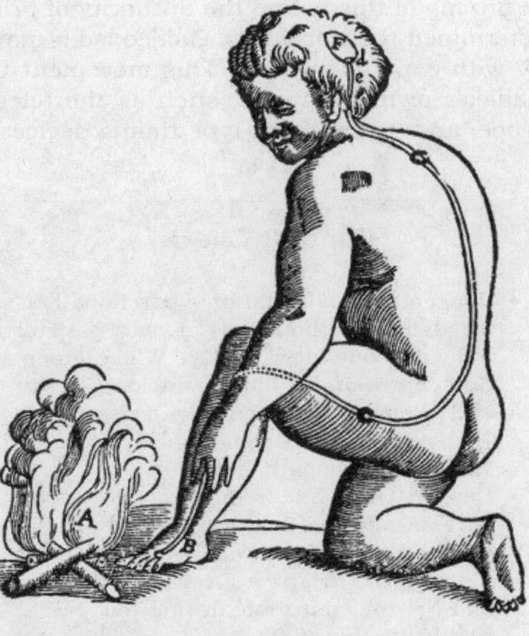

FIGURE 2-3 Descartes' Mechanical Principles of Human Involuntary Actions

work, you can see the mechanical means by which a hot fire would cause an involuntary or reflexive movement.

The important distinction that continues today is that behavior can be categorized as either involuntary or voluntary. Voluntary actions such as thinking or consciously performing an act were different in that they required a mind and humans were the only organism to have a mind, according to Descartes. By thinking, humans can know with certainty that they exist. Thus, the famous philosophical statement of Descartes: "I think, therefore I am."

Given the situation that the bodies of animals are totally mechanical and that humans have both a body and a mind, Descartes created a mind–body distinction that science has had to face in its explanations. The problem is how can a material body including the brain be influenced by an immaterial process such as the mind? How can a thought influence a cell in the brain? Although today we generally talk about the mind–body problem, the metaphysics of Descartes' era would often make the distinction between body and soul. Descartes answered this problem by suggesting that the rational soul was able to control the mechanical body by having both functions come together in one particular organ of the brain, the pineal gland. It is in the pineal gland that the mind not only controls the body but also senses the nature and flow of the mechanical nervous system.

Today, most neuroscientists see mind as resulting from brain and that the mind–body problem is not actually a problem to be solved. However, the question of whether particular behaviors seen in individuals with mental illness represent involuntary processes performed without the benefit of a conscious mind has plagued our legal understanding of mental illness.

In the 1600s, science as a way of knowing about the world began to emerge. At the beginning of this period the authority of prior authorities such as Aristotle or the church determined the worldview. Galileo led a movement that would eventually replace authority with experimentation. This movement toward experimentation was greatly aided by Galileo's own inventions, such as the telescope, the thermometer, an improved microscope, and a pendulum-type timing device. Each of these instruments allowed people to experiment and answer for themselves the questions of nature. After establishing that balls rolling down an inclined plane act similarly to falling objects, Galileo successfully challenged the authority of Aristotle concerning two falling weights. With Galileo's work, a new science based on observation and experimentation was beginning. Galileo was part of a revolution that was to challenge authority. In the 1680s, Newton's classic work *Principia* was published (Newton, 1729/1969). Designated by science historian Gerald Holton (1952) as "probably the greatest single book in the history of science," this work describes Newton's theories of time, space, and motion as well as his rules of reasoning for science.

Concept Check

- Concepts in understanding psychopathology date back thousands of years yet still influence our views today. What important contributions did the ancient Greeks and Romans—particularly Pythagoras, Hippocrates, and Galen—make to current views of psychopathology?
- Describe the shift from authority to science as a way of knowing that happened during the Renaissance. Specifically, what did da Vinci, Harvey, Descartes, Galileo, and Newton contribute during this period that led to this shift?

DISCOVERING THE FUNCTION OF THE BRAIN IN BEHAVIOR AND PSYCHOPATHOLOGY

The developing spirit of science during the 1600s began to set the stage for a new breed of scientists to emerge. One of these scientists was an English doctor, Thomas Willis (1621–1675). He was interested in neurology and in fact coined the term along with a number of anatomical terms such as lobe, hemisphere, pyramid, peduncle, and corpus striatum. He may also have been the first person to use the word *psychology* in English although *psychologia*—meaning study of the psyche or soul—had been used in the late 1500s.

Willis sought to combine the study of structure and function. He suggested that lower brain structures were responsible for more basic functions of life and that these structures could be found across a variety of vertebrates. On the other hand, those structures located higher in the brain must be involved in more advanced processes seen in higher organisms such as humans. Implicit in this idea is a break with Descartes' suggestion that animals are only machines. For Willis, animals could perceive, think, and remember although there were limitations in these abilities in comparison to humans. Willis further suggested that all organisms, including humans, have a corporeal or material soul that can be explored by scientists. Humans also have an immortal soul that can be discussed by theologians but is not in the realm of scientists. Further, he suggested that behavioral problems and mental illness were related to the material soul and not the work of the devil or possession. Thus, mental illness should be studied by scientists and medical professionals.

In his own writings, Willis noted how mania and melancholia (depression) could change into one another and thus gives us a 1600s description of bipolar disorder (previously called manic depression). At a time when witch hunting was epidemic, he presented a clarifying picture of mental illness as having natural causes. He also noted that men were as likely to show hysteria as women. Willis contributed greatly to the beginnings of neurology including his discovery of what is now called the *circle of Willis*, a structure of blood vessels that supplies blood to the brain. He was also the first person to number the cranial nerves. The famous British physiologist Sir Charles Sherrington, who won the Nobel Prize in 1932, suggested that Willis clarified the anatomy and physiology of the brain and nerves and put them on their modern footing.

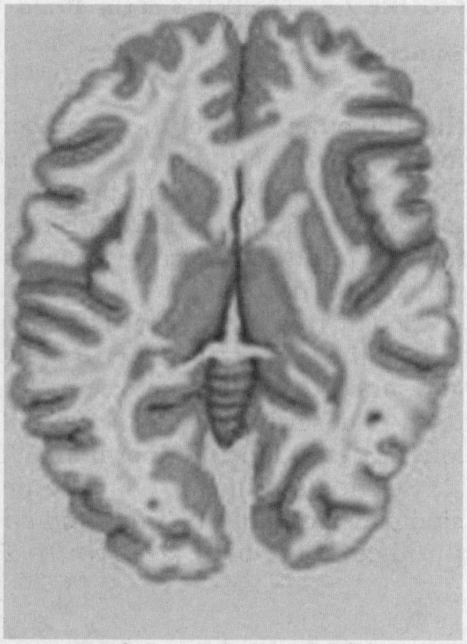

FIGURE 2-4 Gray Matter and White Matter in the Brain

Source: Garrett (2010, Figure 3.9).

By the end of the 1700s, the nervous system had been completely dissected and the major parts described in detail. The brain was seen to be composed of gray matter and white matter (see *Figure 2-4*). White matter was involved in moving information to and from the gray matter. Today, we have a fuller understanding of brain structure with

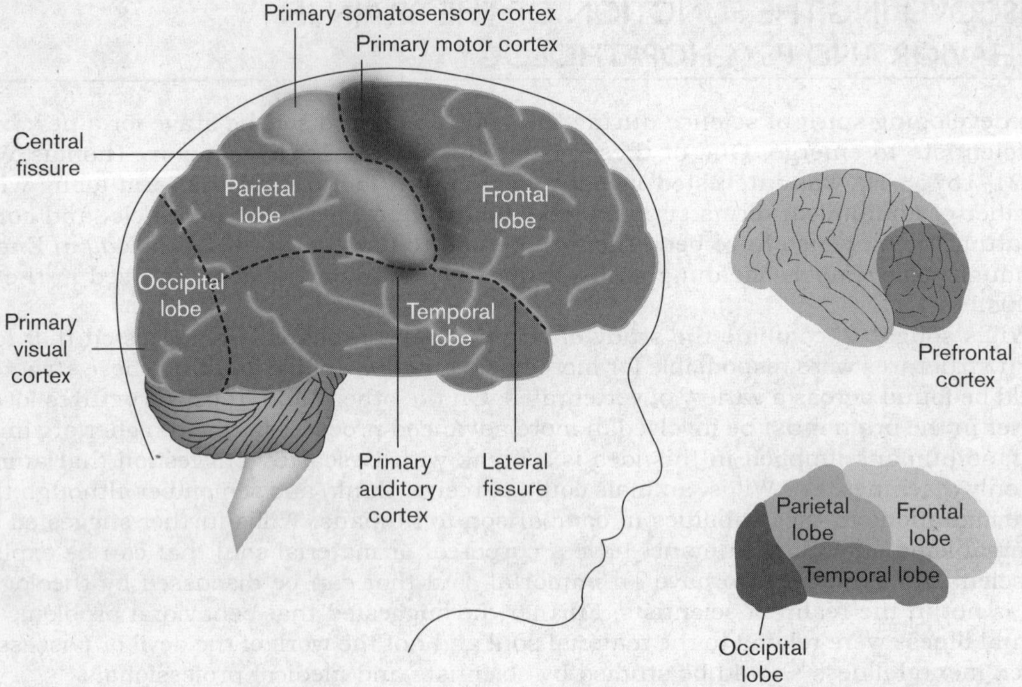

FIGURE 2-5 The Lobes of the Brain

Source: Garrett (2010, Figure 3.8).

the thin outer shell of the brain consisting of cells, which appear a darker color, thus gray matter. Underlying this are the axons, which transfer information throughout the brain. Their myelin sheaths are lighter in color and thus these areas are referred to as white matter. Myelin is made up of fats and proteins and wraps around axons like insulation does around electrical cables and results in an increased speed in information transmissions.

Also by this time, scientists knew that there was a general pattern in all human brains in how the brain was structured in terms of surface structures or bumps, which are called gyri, and the grooves between them referred to sulci and fissures. The present-day terms used to describe parts of the brain come from Latin, so the lobes of the brain are frontal lobe, parietal lobe, temporal lobe, and occipital lobe. This can be seen in *Figure 2-5*.

Scientists of the 1700s also determined that the nervous system had a central division consisting of the brain and spinal cord and a peripheral division consisting of nerves throughout the body (see *Figure 2-6*).

The 1700s to the 1900s

With the basic structure of the nervous system known, the 1700s began a quest to understand how the system developed and how it worked. One of the contributions of this quest was the realization that the body created and used electrical activity in its basic processes. By the middle of the 1700s, individuals such as Benjamin Franklin, experimenting with lightning rods and kites, published works on the nature of electrical activity in general.

Later in the century, such scientists as Luigi Galvani and Emil du Bois-Reymond were able to show that electrical stimulation would cause a frog's leg to twitch. With this demonstration, nerves began to be thought of as wires through which electricity would pass. Further, it was determined that the brain could itself produce electrical activity. The greater impact was that electricity was also something that could be measured, thus setting the stage for following centuries in which experimentation in the electrical activity of the brain and body would play a significant role in physiology and psychology.

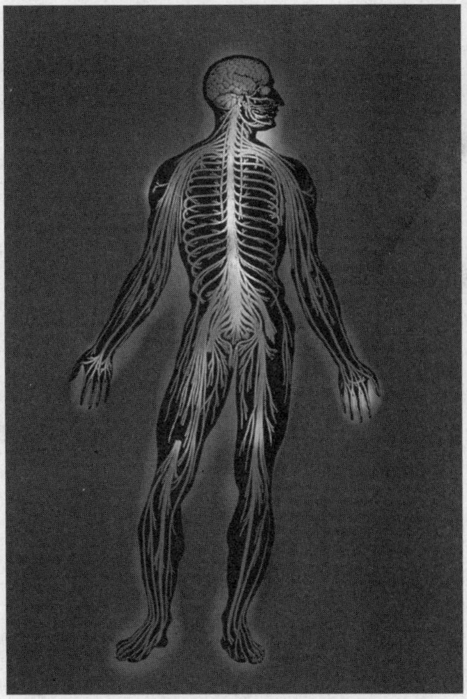

FIGURE 2-6 Distribution of the Nervous System

Source: © M. Kulyk/Science Source.

One of the discoveries during the early part of the 1800s was that there was a system for sending information to the muscle, which resulted in muscle movement, and another system for bringing sensory information back to the brain. When you hold a glass, for example, the sensory or affector system relays information on what the object you are touching feels like whereas the muscular or effector system tells the muscles how to hold and pick up the glass. Thus, in many nerves there are connections for both receiving and sending information. These pathways are referred to as fiber tracts.

At the level of the spinal cord, these **fiber tracts** split, with the sensory information being conveyed by the dorsal root and the action or motor information involving the ventral root. By the 1850s, Hermann von Helmholtz had measured the speed of the nerve impulse and found it to be around 90 feet a second, which is a little more than a mile a minute. Of course, this is much slower than the speed of electricity in a copper wire, which approximates the speed of light (186,000 miles per second). However, the advantage of the nerve impulse—as shown in later research—is that it is not diminished over the length of its travels.

One important realization of the 1700s was that particular functions could be localized to different parts of the brain. One person often cited today is Joseph Gall. Although Gall was correct in suggesting that the frontal part of the brain involved higher cognitive processes and social determinations, he was wrong in assuming that somehow brain function would be reflected in the shape of the skull. If an individual were good at a particular ability, Gall assumed that his or her skull would look different from another person's skull who was not as talented. To support this idea, he examined the skulls of people at the extremes, such as great writers, statesmen, and mathematicians as well as criminals, the mentally ill, and individuals with particular pathologies. Overall, he defined 19 processes that he thought humans and animals both performed and another 8 that were unique to humans (see *Figure 2-7*).

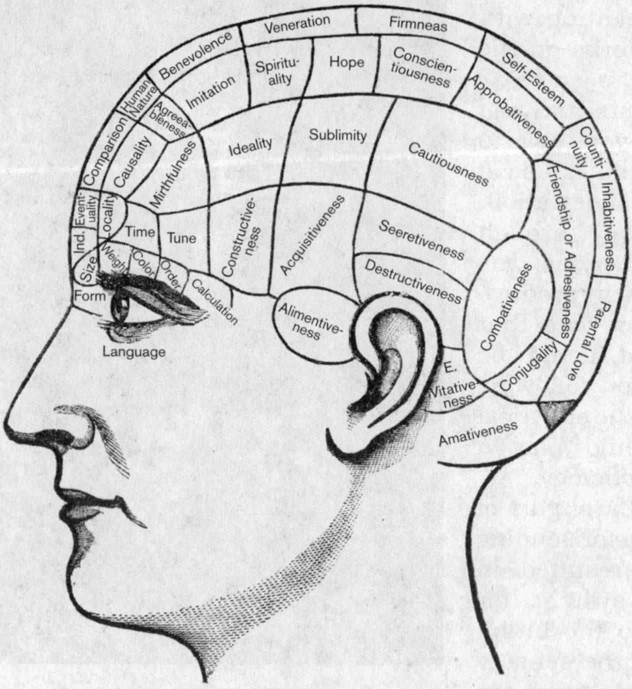

FIGURE 2-7 Gall's Structure of the Head

Source: © iStockphoto.com/Chris Price

Although Gall and his followers never scientifically tested their ideas, research by others did not support their ideas about the structure of the head. What Gall did that was supported was to suggest that an important idea was to view the brain as capable of performing a variety of functions and these functions could be localized in different parts of the brain.

Abilities related to understanding and producing language greatly aided specific discoveries related to cerebral localization of function. Individuals like Jean-Baptiste Bouillaud in France collected considerable information on patients who had a variety of difficulties with language. Some patients could understand language but could not produce speech. Others had trouble remembering words. Still others could not understand language. Overall, he suggested that word memory and the executive aspects of speech are located more frontally in the brain. An area located below this area was seen to be involved in the muscle movements necessary for speech. Partly because of the problems associated with Gall and his study of bumps on the head, the idea of localization of function in the brain was also hotly debated.

The debate changed when Paul Broca examined a patient who could understand language but could not speak. In 1861, this patient was sent to Broca with a much more serious medical condition and died shortly thereafter. This allowed Broca the opportunity to perform an autopsy and report an abnormality in an area on the left side of the frontal lobe. Based on a variety of cases, Broca was able to show that language is a left hemispheric process and that damage to the frontal areas of the left

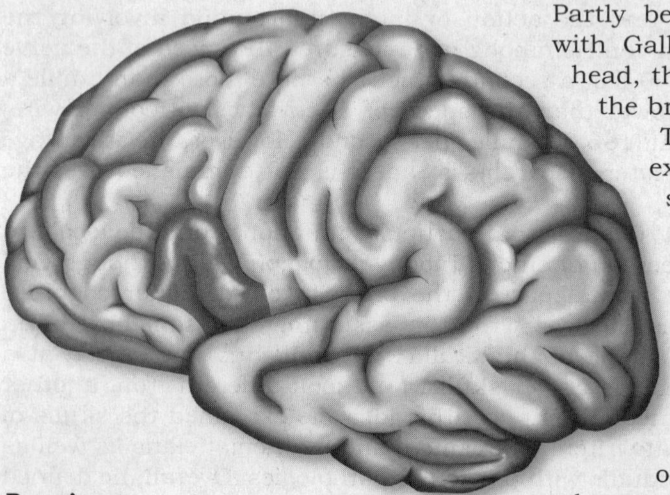

Broca's area
© BSIP/Science Source

hemisphere also results in problems in higher executive functions such as judgment, the ability to reflect on a situation, and the ability to understand things in an abstract manner. Today, the area related to language production in the left hemisphere is called *Broca's area* and is shown above.

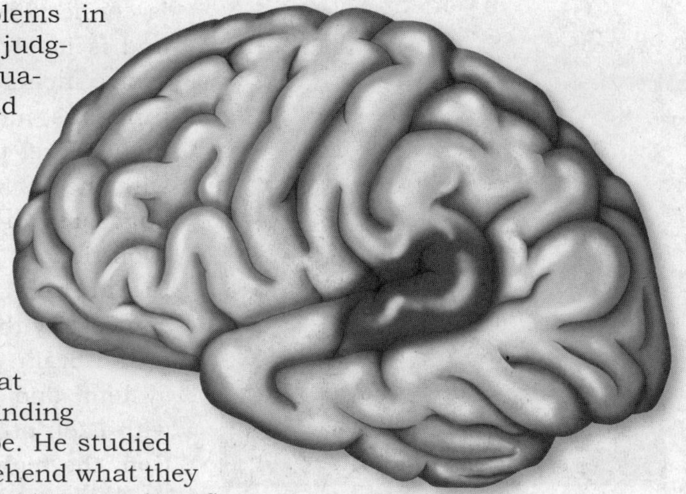

Wernicke's area
© BSIP/Science Source

In 1874, some 15 years after Broca made his discovery related to language production, Carl Wernicke published a paper that suggested that language understanding was related to the left temporal lobe. He studied patients who were unable to comprehend what they heard. At the same time, they were able to produce fluent speech although it was incomprehensible and included nonexistent words. The specific area identified by Wernicke is now called *Wernicke's area* and is located in the left temporal lobe as seen in the figure on this page. The discoveries of Broca and Wernicke helped the scientific community understand that language was made up of different processes, including the ability to understand language and the ability to produce language. Modern case studies show even more complicated processes. Texting appears to use different parts of the brain than other language processes. A 40-year-old man had no trouble reading, writing, or understanding language. However, he did have problems sending coherent text messages on his cell phone. Brain imaging showed that he had had a stroke. A healthy 25-year-old woman also showed garbled texting following a stroke (Ravi, Rao, & Klein, 2009).

In 1868, Broca went to the United Kingdom for a scientific meeting where he met John Hughlings Jackson, a well-known British neurologist. Having learned of Broca's work in Paris some 4 years earlier, Jackson examined some cases of individuals who showed problems with speech. In almost all of these cases, Jackson found that the person had a paralysis on the right side of his or her body, which would suggest that the damage to the brain was in the left hemisphere, thus supporting Broca's idea of which cortical areas were involved in language production. Jackson also noted that patients with left hemisphere damage did not show problems in performing perceptual tasks whereas those with right hemisphere damage did. He reported on particular patients with right hemisphere damage, one of whom could not recognize people, including his wife, and another who had difficulty with finding his way through a town he knew. In doing this, Jackson became the first scientist to realize that language is processed by the left hemisphere and spatial abilities by the right.

Throughout his career, Hughlings Jackson examined the brain from a developmental and evolutionary perspective (see Williamson & Allman, 2011, for an overview. Jackson saw the brain as composed of three levels. The earliest part of the brain to evolve was the spinal cord and brain stem, which controlled the vegetative functions such as breathing, sleep, and temperature control. The next level to evolve included the basal ganglia, which

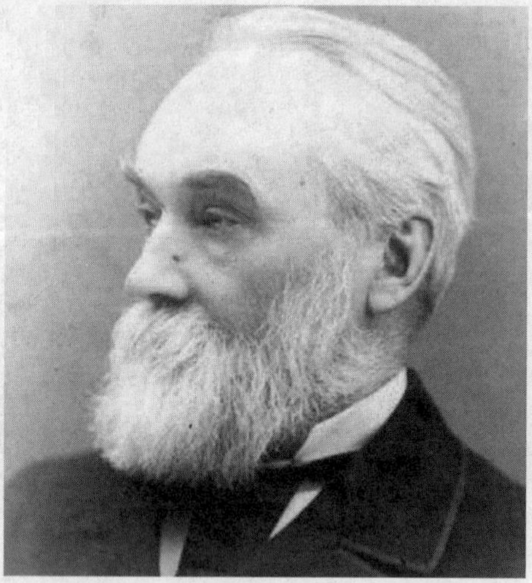

Hughlings Jackson

Source: Swash, M., & Evans, J. (2006). Hughlings Jackson's clinical research: Evidence from contemporary documents. Neurology, 67, 666–672.

is connected to various other parts of the brain and is involved in movement. The third level to evolve included areas involved in higher cortical functions, including thought. It is the task of the higher level to keep the person in close contact with the environment. Within this framework, he suggested two principles based partly on evolutionary analysis. The first principle is **hierarchical integration** through inhibitory control. By this, he means that the various levels of the brain, such as the brain stem, the limbic system, and the neocortex, are able to interact with each other. Further, the type of interaction from the higher levels is restricting or inhibiting the lower levels.

In terms of mental illness, Jackson (1894) suggested that symptoms such as illusions, hallucinations, and delusions are not in themselves the result of disease. Rather, it is when higher-level processes no longer inhibit the earlier evolved processes of the brain that these symptoms appear. Jackson referred to this process as dissolutions. Dissolutions are the reversal of the normal process of evolution. Thus, the primitive experiences seen in psychosis, for example, represent the primitive parts of the brain working normally. What is missing is the relationship of these primitive areas with higher mental processes. The disease process produces negative symptoms such as lack of affect or disordered thought in the areas of the brain that evolved later. Without inhibition, the earlier evolved layer of the brain functions on its own. The result is the symptoms of illusions, hallucinations, and delusions. Jackson referred to these symptoms as positive symptoms in that they represent the emergence of a lower-level process as opposed to negative symptoms, which reflect loss of higher-level control. Jackson further suggested that problems with different parts of the higher centers result in different types of mental disorders. Jackson thus connected mental illness with problems found in the most recently evolved parts of the human brain. He stated, "In every insanity . . . the highest cerebral centres is out of function" (Jackson, 1894, p. 615).

Current research has supported Jackson by showing that there are many more inhibitory pathways going from the higher levels of the brain to the lower brain structures than vice versa. This suggests that we use higher-level processes to inhibit more simple ones. Some suggest that when this inhibition is reduced, as during sleep, then less patterned types of processes, such as those seen in dreams, become possible. Another simple example of this is that when a human infant is first born she displays a number of simple reflexes. One of these is the *Babinski reflex.* If you take your finger

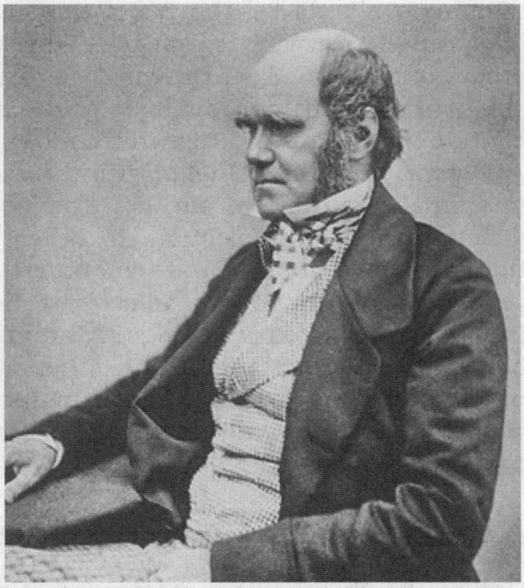

Charles Darwin

and run it along an infant's foot, the toes will curl up. As the infant matures, the reflex disappears. If there is cortical damage at a later point in life, then this reflex can reappear. Jackson assumed that the higher-level structures, which evolved later than the reflexive ones, serve the purpose of inhibiting and modulating these basic reflexes.

Jackson's second principle is **encephalization.** This is the principle by which systems in the brain that perform one task, for example, over evolutionary time are taken over by a general purpose control system that is involved in a number of different tasks. That is, more recently evolved higher-level centers control the older lower-level centers. It also suggests that the higher levels of the brain are able to include more information than lower-level ones. Over evolutionary time, sensory processes are gradually transferred from the lower centers to higher centers in the brain, and human brains have developed a more general purpose processing system without replacing the earlier special purpose processing mechanisms seen in the lower levels.

The 1800s and Evolution

Another big idea that emerged in the 1800s was the idea that all of nature is in constant flow and that things, including organisms, change. This idea focused on the evolution of species and is most often associated with the work of Charles Darwin (1809–1882). **Variation** was to become one of the major components of Darwin's thinking concerning evolution. In fact, he began his thinking with the assumption that heritable variations can and do occur in nature. Darwin then presented the important realization that not all plants or animals that come into existence survive. Many organisms such as sea stars, for example, produce millions of eggs of which only a limited number survive. Depending on climate conditions, food supply, predator population, and a host of other factors including disease, only a limited number of births survive to maturity. Consequently, Darwin suggested, "There is a frequently recurring struggle for existence." Who is to survive in this struggle? Darwin suggested that if an individual has even a slight variation that helps it to compete successfully for survival, then over time the species will be made up more and more of members with these characteristics and less and less of individuals lacking these features. This process is referred to as **natural selection.** Darwin described this process in his book *On the origin of species by means of natural selection* (Darwin, 1859).

Darwin later extended the theory of natural selection to include **sexual selection,** or the manner in which males and females choose a mate. This work is described in his book *The Descent of Man.* Darwin noted that males and females differ not only in terms of organs of sexual reproduction but also in secondary sexual characteristics such as mammary glands for the nourishment of infants in females or physical size in males. According to Darwin, sexual selection depends on the success of certain individuals over others of the same sex. Darwin also saw that besides same-sex competition, there is also competition to attract members of the opposite sex. As you can imagine, there has been continuous debate and research concerning what attraction means for males and females.

Darwin began the *Origins* with the question of natural selection especially as it related to animals. In the *Descent*, he expanded these ideas to humans and also examined the question of sexual selection. In other works, such as his notebooks, he extended his thinking to cognitive and emotional processes. The broad question is how might psychological functions have evolved. One answer he gives is that living in social groups produces an increase in cognitive ability. Darwin also presents notes on memory and habit, imagination, language, aesthetic feelings, emotion, motivation, animal intelligence, psychopathology, and dreaming (Gruber, 1974). One important question is the manner in which self-preservation, sexual selection, and social processes are reflected in psychopathology.

A Search for Organization

One of the themes of the sciences of the 1800s was the search for organization. One example of this in chemistry was the publication of the periodic table of elements in 1869 by the Russian scientist Dmitri Mendeleev. In the periodic table, elements were organized by their atomic weight. The basic idea was to find families of elements that displayed similar properties. A similar search was going on in medicine in terms of disease as well as in clinical neurology, which today we refer to as abnormal psychology, psychopathology, or mental illness.

One of the men associated with this search was the Paris physician Jean-Martin Charcot (1825–1893). Charcot came into the world at a time in which neurological disorders were often classified on the basis of a single feature such as a tremor or not being able to move a limb. What we see today as different disorders might have been classified together by this single feature.

In the second half of the 1800s, Charcot sought to bring organization to an understanding of neurological disorders through a variety of methods. One important technique was careful observation. This observation was of both what the patient said, which we refer to today as **symptoms,** as well as what the clinician observed, or what we refer to as **signs.** The overall search was for determining which signs and symptoms go together to form a **syndrome.** An additional technique—autopsy—further allowed for the connection of syndromes with underlying anatomy. Autopsies allowed for the determination of which tissue showed signs of pathology. Using this method, Charcot was able to show the correctness of Jackson's thoughts on neurological organization. Overall, Charcot showed that the human motor cortex is organized similarly to that of other animals with the left hemisphere controlling the right side of the body and vice versa.

Charcot is best known for initially describing brain disorder relationships for a number of motor-related disorders including Parkinson's disease, amyotrophic lateral sclerosis (ALS or Lou Gehrig's disease), and multiple sclerosis. Charcot also established Tourette's disorder as a separate disease when he asked his assistant Gilles de la Tourette to help him. Gilles de la Tourette wrote of these cases that included a teenage boy who would show involuntary movements and scream swear words.

Charcot was also able to show that conversion reactions in which the person shows outward signs of trouble hearing or seeing or not be able to experience pain in the hand were without any underlying pathology. During Charcot's time, conversion reactions were referred to as hysteria. Sigmund Freud heard Charcot's lectures on hysteria including the observation that psychological trauma could trigger these reactions. This became the initial basis of Freud's psychoanalytic work.

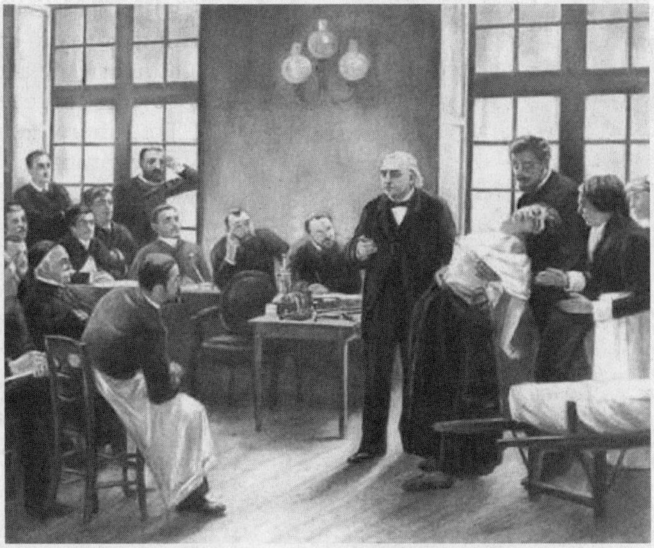

Charcot demonstrates a case of hysteria (Painting by André Brouillet)

In this manner, Charcot helped to integrate symptoms of a disorder with both psychological processes and brain processes. He also emphasized that, as in the case of hysteria, much of what had been seen as possession by demons could be seen as resulting from natural causes. Thus, there was no need for faith healers or church rituals to remove evil spirits. This also let society view these people as someone with a disorder rather than as an evil person. Much of Charcot's work took place at the Salpêtrière, a hospital for the poor in Paris.

CARE FOR THOSE WITH MENTAL DISORDERS

In 1330, a convent of the order of St. Mary of Bethlehem became the first institution for the mentally ill in England. Two hundred years later, King Henry VIII gave the institution a royal charter although there is some suggestion other royal commissions came earlier. Over the years, the word *Bethlehem* became *Bedlam,* and the institution was referred to as "Old Bedlam." The English word *bedlam* comes from this institution. Various reports suggested that the inmates were often chained and treated cruelly without proper food or clothing. As depicted in novels of the day, people of the 1700s would go to Bedlam to see the inmates as an outing in much the same way today we would go to a zoo. Such an outing is depicted in a 1796 illustration.

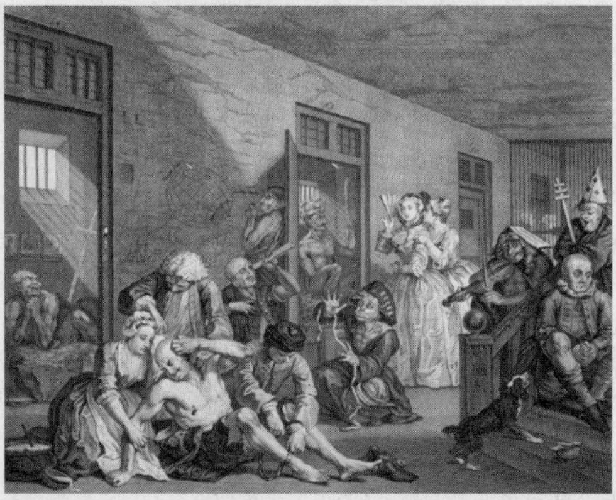

Illustration of Bedlam
© Burstein Collection/Corbis

In 1814, some 96,000 people visited the asylum. Another common illustration of the day depicts the seaman James Norris, who was shackled for 14 years.

In the 1800s, there was a campaign in England to change the conditions of the patients,

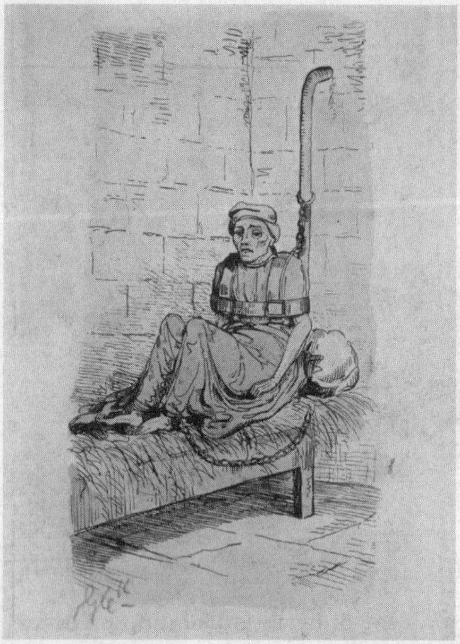

Illustration of James Norris shackled

© Eileen Tweedy/The Art Archive at Art Resource, NY

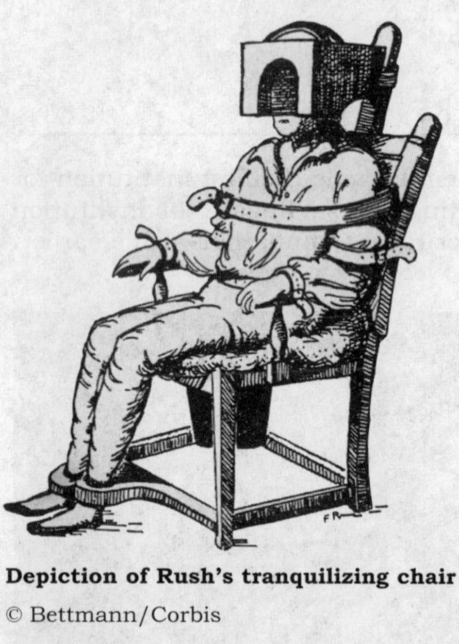

Depiction of Rush's tranquilizing chair

© Bettmann/Corbis

which led to the establishment of the Committee on Madhouses in 1815. This issued in a period of concern for the patients rather than seeing them as objects of curiosity as in the previous century. Treatment for patients during the 1800s brought new practices including the therapeutic value of work.

During this period, there was a spirit throughout the world to adopt a "moral treatment of the insane." Three important individuals were Benjamin Rush (1745–1813) in the United States, Phillipe Pinel (1745–1826) in France, and Vincenzo Chiarugi (1759–1820) in Italy (see Gerard, 1997). In the United States, Rush, who had signed the Declaration of Independence, later established a wing at the Pennsylvania Hospital in Philadelphia for the treatment of mental illness. He is often considered to be the father of American psychiatry and saw mental illness as a problem of the mind. However, he continued to practice bloodletting as the best treatment for mental illness. As shown on this page, he developed a tranquilizing chair that he believed would change the flow of blood. Professionals tend to view this invention as neither helpful nor hurtful to the patient. He also wrote the first psychiatric textbook published in America.

In France, Pinel sought to change the way the insane were treated. Pinel engaged the idea that mental illness could be studied by the methods of the natural sciences. In 1793, Pinel became the director of the Bicêtre Asylum in Paris. As director, he reviewed the commitment papers of the inmates, toured the building, and met with each patient individually. The building was in bad shape, and the patients were chained to walls. As Pinel himself described the institution, "everything presented to me the appearance of chaos and confusion." As Pinel petitioned the government and received permission to remove the chains as portrayed in the painting on the left. He also abandoned the practice of bloodletting.

He began to carefully observe patients and also interact with them. In these discussions, he attempted to create a detailed case history and to better understand the development of the disorder. This led to a classification system that he published in his *Nosographie philosophique ou méthode de l'analyse appliquée à la médecine* in 1789, which sorted mental diseases into five categories: melancholia, mania without delirium, mania with delirium, dementia, and idiocy. In 1795, Pinel became the chief physician at the Hospice de la Salpêtrière, where he remained for the rest of his life. For many, Pinel is seen as the father of scientific psychiatry.

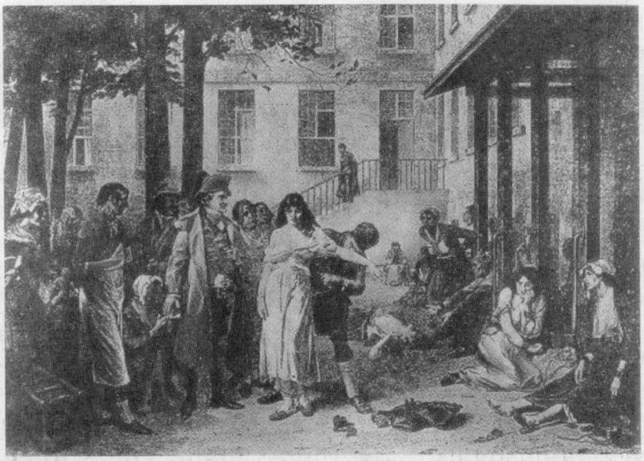

Illustration of pinel removing the chains

Vincenzo Chiarugi had been less well known outside of Italy until a paper in the middle of the last century, which brought his name to the attention of Americans (Mora, 1959). Some 8 years earlier than Pinel, Chiarugi began removing chains from his patients. Early in his career, Chiarugi became the director of a large hospital in Florence, which included special facilities for the mentally ill. This resulted from the passage of a law in 1774 in Italy that allowed individuals seen as mentally ill to be hospitalized. As director of the hospital, Chiarugi created guidelines concerning how patients were to be treated. One of his rules suggested that patients were to be treated with respect. He also suggested that if restraints were required, they should be applied in a manner to protect the patient from sores and be made of leather rather than chains. He also used psychopharmacological agents such as opium for treatment.

In addition to mental health professionals, the humane care of individuals with mental illness was moved forward by a number of other individuals. William Tuke (1732–1822) was a successful merchant of tea, coffee, and cocoa in England. He was a Quaker philanthropist, and friends had told him of being turned away from an asylum in York when they had tried to visit a fellow Quaker who had been confined there. Within a few days, the patient was reported dead. Tuke visited the asylum and found the conditions deplorable. Having retired, he decided to devote his life to creating alternative places where "the unhappy might find refuge."

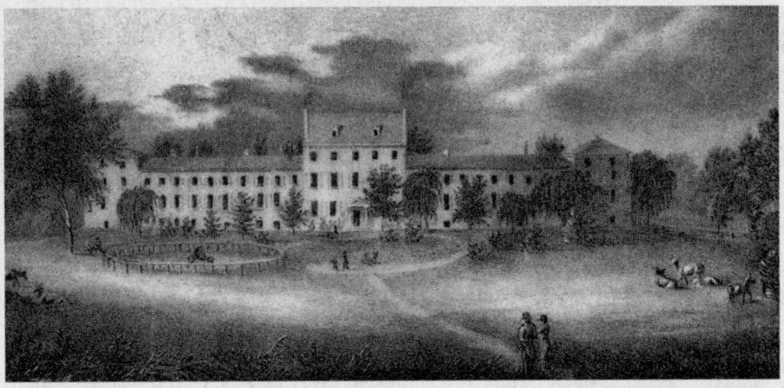

Friends hospital Philadelphia

Source: *Friends' Asylum for the Insane* near Frankford, printed by Lehman & Duval, 1836 (litho), Lehman, George (d.1870)/Library Company of Philadelphia, PA, USA/The Bridgeman Art Library.

In 1796, near York, England, he created a *Retreat for Persons Afflicted With Disorders of the Mind.* This Quaker retreat, as it was called, carried with it the idea that the individuals who were there should be given respect as well as good food and exercise. There were to be no chains or manacles. The model for the retreat was a farm and the patients performed farm duties as part of their treatment. Others visited to learn of its operation. In 1813, the Quakers of Philadelphia founded the Friends Asylum for the Use of Persons Deprived of the Use of Their Reason, which was the first private psychiatric hospital in the United States. Both the retreat in York and the Friend's Hospital of Philadelphia continue to function as places for mental health treatment.

Another individual who contributed to the American mental health movement was Dorothea Dix (1802–1887). Dix became a schoolteacher but contracted tuberculosis and needed to find a less than full-time position. She found a job teaching women at the East Cambridge House of Correction in Massachusetts. This position opened her eyes to the terrible conditions these women faced. Dix also realized that a number of these women had some type of mental illness. From this experience, she devoted her life to crusading for the improved treatment of the mentally ill. As part of this crusade, she visited every state east of the Mississippi River and testified before local and national legislatures. She encouraged the U.S. Congress to give federal land to the states to establish mental hospitals in the same way they created land grant colleges in the 1860s. Both houses of Congress passed the bill only to have it vetoed by President Franklin Pierce. Although this bill was not passed, it is estimated that her work led to the establishment of some 40 mental hospitals in the United States and Europe.

By the 1950s, there were a number of hospital facilities in the United States for those with mental illness. These were administered by both state governments and private organizations. This changed in the 1950s as described in LENS 2-1.

2-1 LENS

Long Stay Institutions for Persons with Mental Illness: Status in America and India

During the first half of the 20th century, state mental hospitals were the main source of treatment and care for those with serious mental disorders in the United States (see Fisher, Geller, & Pandiani, 2009; Torrey, 1997, for overviews). By the 1950s, there were more than a half million individuals in these hospitals. However, during the 1950s and 1960s a number of events occurred that changed the way individuals with mental disorders were treated in the United States.

One significant event was the introduction of antipsychotic medication. Prior to this, individuals with serious mental disorders such as schizophrenia needed a high level of care and protection. With the introduction of medications that would help treat the disorder, it was possible for some of these individuals to live outside the hospital.

The Community Mental Health Act of 1963, signed into law by President John F. Kennedy, reflected the growing understanding that all but a small portion of those in mental hospitals could be treated in the community. The basic idea was that community mental health centers would offer a variety of programs to those with mental illness.

Although the population of the United States increased by 100 million between 1955 and 1994, the number of individuals in mental hospitals decreased from 550,239 to 71,619. The process of moving individuals from mental hospitals to the community was known as *deinstitutionalization. Figure 2-8* shows this drastic change.

For some of the individuals today who would have been placed in a hospital in the 1950s, their quality of life in the community is much better than it would have been. However, for many individuals, the ideals of the community mental health movement were never fulfilled. The community facilities for those with mental illness were never fully funded or were not even built. This left many individuals not receiving the type of treatment they needed. Some of these individuals have found themselves homeless and on the streets. Others, who were disruptive or concerned the community, found themselves in

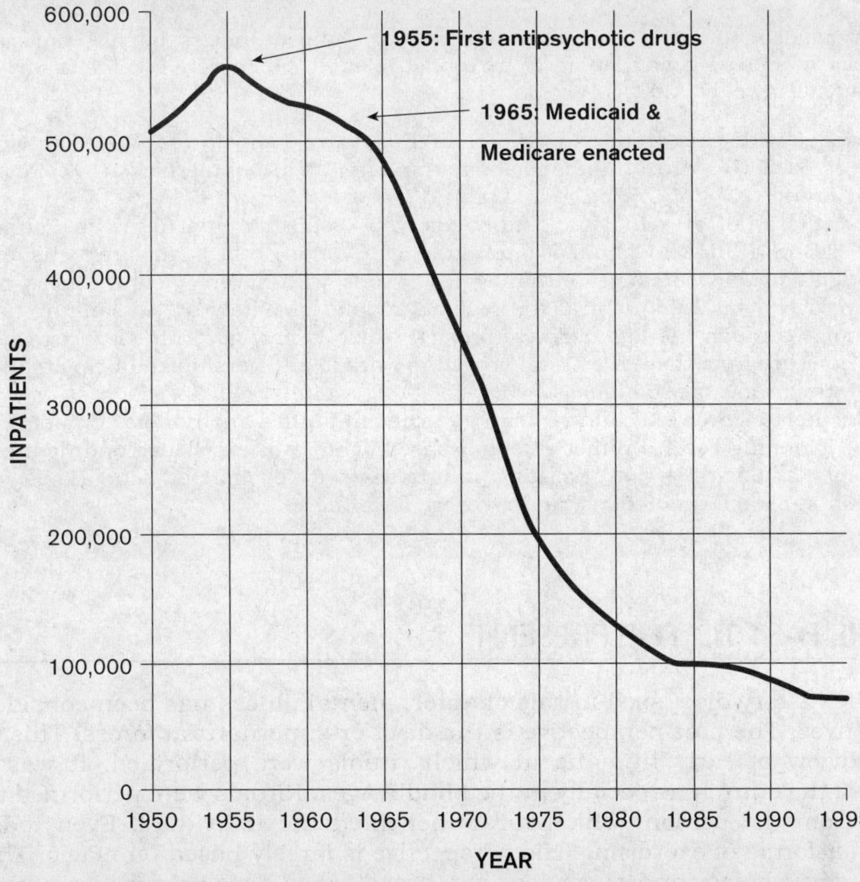

FIGURE 2-8 Number of Individuals in a Mental Hospital by Year

Source: E. Fuller Torrey. *Out of the Shadows: Confronting America's Mental Illness.* New York: John Wiley & Sons, 1997.

jails and prisons with little mental health treatment and care. Similar deinstitutionalization occurred in the United Kingdom and other developed countries.

The Indian Scenario

There is also a great shift in India from Inpatient care to Rehabilitation and Recovery and the LENS section could focus on this. An article in the *Indian Journal of Psychiatry* (2000) focuses on the changes in mental hospitals in India over the decades (Krishnamurthy, Venugopal, & Alimchandani, 2000).

> The changing role of mental hospitals also needs to be reconsidered. This is because earlier, hospitals were primarily used to sequester 'dangerous' lunatics form the society. With the advancement of our knowledge regarding mental illnesses, mental hospitals need to take a

(Continued)

(Continued)

more expanded role in the community—not only as treatment centres, but also as facilitators of social awareness and training of personnel to meet community mental health needs. (Krishnamurthy et al., 2000)

In keeping with this trend, NIMHANS in Bangalore has started Recovery Oriented Services or ROSeS. (http://nimhans.ac.in/nimhans/sites/default/files/u197/Roses%20Brochure_Front%20%26%20Back_Final.pdf)

Other centers, all over India, including Banyan, Schizophrenia Research Foundation (SCARF), IHBAS, PGIMER Chandigarh, Muktaangan, among others, too are focusing more on rehabilitation and cognitive retraining of persons with severe mental illness moving towards recovery. In Maharashtra, the regional mental hospitals are attempting to bring about change through the *Saptasopaan* project, which is now government recognized and borrows expertise from the IPH's Tridal project to work in partnership and help mainstream persons with chronic mental illness.

Many centers all over the country, both government funded and non-governmental organizations, including several public hospital-based centers of excellence and de-addiction departments, among others, are working hard to deal with drug de-addiction, tobacco cessation, non-substance addictions, and recovery from these.

FROM THE PAST TO THE PRESENT

In light of the history discussed in this chapter, mental illness has been considered from two perspectives. The first perspective is the devil or supernatural forces. This was seen in the worldview of early humans in which rituals were performed. It was also the perspective of the church, especially in the Middle Ages. Rituals were performed to remove the demon from the person, which rarely benefited the individual. Even today, some churches offer forms of exorcism. This perspective is largely based on magic. The second perspective is psychology and physiology in a broad sense. This perspective uses research and the sciences to understand what mechanisms lead to mental disorders. Treatment involves the manipulation of these mechanisms through psychotropic medications and psychotherapy. In the next section, I will examine psychological factors involved in developing, maintaining, and treating mental disorders. What a person learns in interacting with other people as well as his or her environment is crucial. Additionally, what individuals tell themselves or how they experience significant others in their lives is an important aspect of this perspective.

THE PSYCHOLOGICAL TREATMENT PERSPECTIVES IN THE 20TH CENTURY

As you read in Elyn Saks's description of her schizophrenia, there are two sides to every person with a mental disorder. One side is how the person herself has tried to respond to her own symptoms. How can I treat myself? she often asks. The other side comprises the treatments that mental health professionals have developed to treat the disorder. There is now evidence that both aspects are important and that a crucial aspect of treatment is the willingness of the person to be actively involved in her own treatment.

In this section, I want to discuss three approaches for the psychological treatment of mental disorders. These are the psychodynamic approach, the existential-humanistic approach, and the cognitive behavioral approach. These approaches were developed somewhat independently and often in opposition to one another. For that reason, I will initially discuss each independently. I will introduce you to a historical understanding of the approach including its broad principles and then present one specific treatment that has been tested in a scientific manner.

> **Concept Check**
>
> - The research of John Hughlings Jackson has contributed much to our understanding of the brain. How would you describe his concepts of localization of function, three levels of the brain, hierarchical integration through inhibitory control, and encephalization?
> - Describe the primary aspects of Charles Darwin's theory of evolution. How might those processes be reflected in psychopathology?
> - Do you agree or disagree: Large institutions for treating the mentally ill should be closed and all treatment given in the community. Choose one side of the debate, and present evidence for your position.

Before the middle of the 20th century, very little formal research was performed to see how effective psychological interventions were. This was also true of traditional medical procedures. Beginning in the 1950s and 1960s, there were the beginnings of a movement to determine the effectiveness of both medical and psychological treatments in a scientific manner. In medicine, this came to be known as *evidence-based medicine.* In psychology, the terms *empirically based treatments* or *empirically based principles* refer to treatments and their aspects for which there is scientific evidence that the treatment is effective.

Three websites have been developed that list treatments for specific mental disorders. The first is maintained by the Clinical Psychology section of the American Psychological Association (APA) (http://www.div12.org/PsychologicalTreatments/index.html). The second is maintained by the U.S. Substance Abuse and Mental Health Services Administration (SAMHSA), which is part of the U.S. Department of Health and Human Services. This website contains a searchable online registry of mental health and substance abuse interventions that have been evaluated (http://www.nrepp.samhsa.gov/Index.aspx). The third website is devoted to effective treatments for children and adolescents (http://effectivechildtherapy.com/). This site is maintained by the Society of Clinical Child and Adolescent Psychology section of the APA.

As researchers and clinicians began to focus more on approaches and principles for which there was scientific evidence that they were effective, there began a movement to develop effective treatments for particular disorders. There has been more willingness to integrate techniques from the three different approaches as well as from other perspectives. For example, in the chapter on personality disorders, you will see that one of the most researched treatments—dialectical behavior therapy (DBT)—is based on techniques from each of the three approaches described in this chapter. This effective treatment uses aspects of cognitive behavioral techniques, dynamic techniques, and humanistic existential techniques.

Psychodynamic Perspectives on Treatment

The **psychodynamic perspective** is based on the idea that psychological problems are manifestations of inner mental conflicts and that conscious awareness of those conflicts is a key to recovery. Historically, Sigmund Freud laid the foundation for this perspective.

By the beginning of the 20th century, there was an understanding that psychological processes were an important source of information concerning mental illness. Sigmund Freud had worked with Charcot in Paris and observed individuals with hysteria. In this disorder, the experience, such as not feeling pain in a limb or difficulty hearing, did not match the underlying physiology. For example, with glove amnesia the person would not feel pain in the area of the fingers covered by a glove even when pricked with a pin. However, the nerves related to this pain followed a different pattern, which meant that the pain experience could not have a totally physiological cause. These types of experiences led Freud to seek psychological explanations for the cause and treatment of mental disorders.

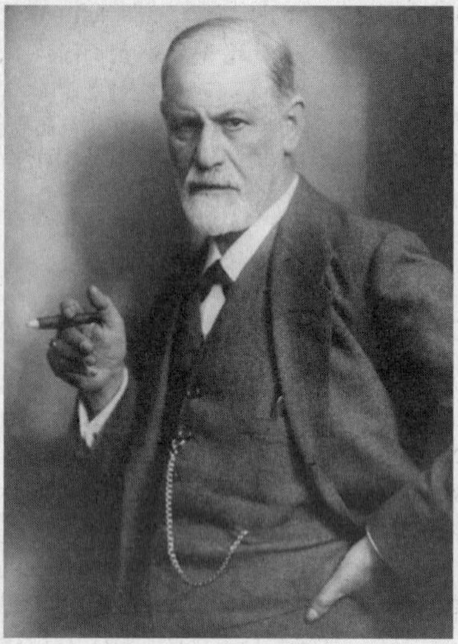

Sigmund Freud

Sigmund Freud was initially trained as a zoologist before he completed medical school. The nature of the neuron was just being discovered, and Freud based his early theories on the neuroscience of his day. Freud was an enthusiastic reader of Darwin and credited his interest in science to an early reading of Darwin. A number of Freud's ideas can be seen as coming from Darwin (Ellenberger, 1970; Sulloway, 1979). Although Freud incorporated Darwin's emphasis on instinct into his work, he emphasized sexual selection over natural selection. For Freud, the sexual instinct becomes the major driving force for human life and interaction. Freud was also influenced by the suggestion of the neurologist John Hughlings Jackson that in our brains we find more primitive brain areas underlying more advanced ones. Thus, it is quite possible for the psyche to be in conflict with itself or at least to have different layers representing different processes.

To understand the nature of these more primitive processes, Freud looked to the description of dreams and wish fulfillment. One of his works, *The Project for a Scientific Psychology*, utilized these ideas and sought to place psychology on a firm scientific basis. The *Project* was based on three separate ideas. The first was reflex processes. For example, organisms withdraw when confronted with unpleasant stimuli. Freud extended this idea to cognitive and emotional processes to suggest that, mentally, humans avoid ideas or feelings that are unpleasant to them. The second principle Freud used was associationism. That is to say, ideas that are presented together in time will be mentally called forth together. Freud suggested that if as a child you experience a fearful situation such as falling out of a carriage, then riding in a carriage could make you feel fearful or anxious. The third idea is that the nervous system is capable of retaining and discharging energy. This energy was initially called "Q" but Freud later identified it as libido or sexual energy.

This psychic manipulation of energy allowed for the possibility that higher cortical processes could inhibit the experience of lower ones, a process that would come to be called *repression.* Anxiety is the result of society and culture having inconsistent rules for the expression of sexuality and aggression. This anxiety and our inability to acknowledge these instinctual experiences lead to defense mechanisms and neurosis. The *Project* sees the brain as basically a blank slate upon which experiences become connected with one another driven by instinctual processes of sexuality and self-preservation. Some see

Freud's ideas in the *Project* as anticipating Donald Hebb's concept that use modifies neuronal connection in the brain (Schott, 2011). The human for Freud becomes the real-life laboratory in which nature and nurture struggle. The *Project* was finished in 1895. After this period, Freud mainly spoke of mental illness in terms of psychological processes and did not return to brain-based ideas.

Treatment for Freud was based on the search for ideas and emotions that are in conflict and the manner in which the person has relationships with other people. His specific treatment came to be called **psychoanalysis.** One basic procedure was free association in which an individual lay on a couch with the therapist behind him and said whatever came to mind. It was the therapist's job to help the client connect ideas and feelings that he was not aware of. One thing Freud was searching for was connections within the person's psyche when external stimulation was reduced. Dreams were also analyzed in this way since they are produced outside of daily life.

Other aspects of psychoanalysis were to examine resistance or what the client is unwilling to say or experience and transference or the manner in which a person imagined how another person thought about him or sought a certain kind of relationship with that person. Since the job of the therapist was to only ask a few questions or make interpretations during a session, the client knew little of how the therapist felt. Thus, the client's view of the therapist, such as "he is critical of me" or "does not like my ideas," were seen to come from the client's psyche. Freud has greatly influenced therapies based on insight. Insight therapy, which has been used to treat disorders such as anxiety and depression, is based on the principle of bringing patterns of behavior, feelings, and thoughts into awareness. In order to do this, it is necessary to discuss past patterns and past relationships to determine how they are being replayed or influencing the present.

Although many people think of Freud as being outdated, there is currently a resurgence of interest in the interface between dynamic approaches and neuroscience. Eric Kandel, who won the Nobel Prize for his work on learning and memory, described his interest in Freud and the manner in which dynamic principles can be viewed in terms of brain functioning (Kandel, 2005, 2012a, 2012b). Carhart-Harris and Friston (2010) have also updated Frued's ideas in terms of the brain networks discovered in current brain imaging techniques. One important concept in both Freud's *Project* and current neuroscience research is the manner in which the brain conserves and uses energy to perform psychological functions including the development of mental illness.

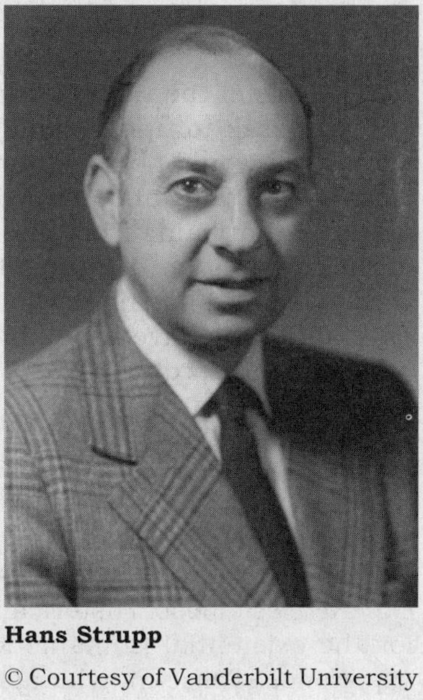

Hans Strupp

A number of dynamically orientated therapies have been shown to be effective (Barber, Muran, McCarthy, & Keefe, 2013). One empirically supported therapy based on dynamic principles was developed by Hans Strupp and his colleagues. Strupp was a researcher who throughout his career sought to understand what were the important components of successful therapy and how to perform therapy outcome research (Strupp, 1971). He was particularly interested in the psychoanalytic or psychodynamic perspective as it is sometimes called. Strupp embodied the dynamic principles in a therapy of a few months' duration (Strupp & Binder, 1984). The focus of this therapy is the relationship between the client and other individuals in her life. It is assumed that the client's problems are based on disturbed relationships.

The therapeutic relationship between the client and the therapist offers an opportunity to see disturbed relationships in a safe environment. Transference is an important mechanism in which the client tends to see the therapist in terms of significant others in her life. As the client talks with the therapist, she will replay prior conflicts and enact maladaptive patterns. For example, if one of your parents was very critical of your ideas, than you may initially find it difficult to tell the therapist feelings or thoughts that are very important to you or related to how you see yourself. You could have another situation in which a parent never allowed you to engage in tasks in which you could fail or would save you whenever you encountered problems. These past situations would leave you with unrealistic expectations as to what to expect from the world and others. In these situations the person has never really learned what the world has to offer and may act as a child expecting someone to protect her and thus miss out on new experiences and learning.

Strupp and Binder illustrated how they might initially discuss interpersonal transactions with a client.

Therapist: How do you feel about yourself at those times?
Client: I feel like I don't have anything to offer.
T: That you have nothing to offer. What do you imagine people are thinking about you then? What's their attitude toward you when you're with them and you feel like you have nothing to say?
C: Really, that I'm present and that's about all.
T: Really, that I'm present. They're not attracted to you or they have negative feelings toward you. They just don't feel about you one way or the other?
C: Right.
T: Like you're invisible.
C: Just like I'm not there. It doesn't really matter whether I'm there or not. (from Strupp & Binder, 1984, p. 115)

The role of the therapist from this approach is mainly to listen. As you listen to a client, you seek to understand what she is saying and how she feels as she describes her world. You would note to yourself when she finds talking to you difficult or experience distress as she talks about her life. On a larger level, the therapist is looking for themes and patterns that came from one's past. In a relaxed, nonjudgmental manner, it is the task of the therapist to help the client understand the patterns and to see how they interfere with living and having rewarding relationships with others. Different versions of dynamic psychotherapy have been shown to be effective for a number of disorders, especially the personality disorders.

Existential-Humanistic Perspectives

The **existential-humanistic perspective** begins by asking, What is the nature of human existence? This includes both the positive experiences of intimacy and the negative experiences of loss. Historically, two clinicians influenced by Freud helped to set the stage for the existential-humanistic movement in that they emphasized the value of internal experience. These individuals were Carl Jung and Karen Horney.

Whereas Freud emphasized the drives of the sexual and self-preservation instincts within the context of experience, Jung, a Swiss psychiatrist and a colleague of Freud, viewed human behavior and experience in much broader terms. Jung asked this question: In the same way that there is an evolutionary history of the body, is there also one of consciousness? He spent a great amount of time examining old myths, stories, and artifacts in an attempt to reconstruct a history of the psyche. Jung was particularly interested in the close connection between instinctual processes and the environmental factors that influence them. Like Darwin, Jung examined human universals. He spent time in Africa, the American Southwest, and other non-European areas to determine if the psychic structure of all humans was similar. For example, one question that Jung asked was the following: Do individuals throughout the world have similar dream patterns? He answered this question in the affirmative and suggested that humans throughout the world showed similar cognitive, emotional, and reflexive patterns. One important aspect of therapy for Jung was to bring together discrepant aspects of one's personality to create a unified self, which would give meaning to one's life. Jung also introduced the terms *introversion* and *extraversion* to reflect a person's tendency to value internal or external information. By noting that introversion in itself is not a sign of mental illness, Jung helped to set up the valuing of internal experience that existential-humanistic therapy focuses on.

Karen Horney, a German-born psychoanalyst, felt that Freud's approach did not fully present a psychology that applied to women as well as men. Overall, for both men and women she differentiated between healthy growth in which a person developed to her full potential and neurotic growth in which a person limited her development by unrealistic ideas and feelings. These ideas would include the idea that "everyone should love me," "I should never make mistakes," or "the world should always give me what I want." Horney's (1950) final book, *Neurosis and Human Growth*, described how these types of unrealistic ideas along with an idealized self-image leave the person feeling out of touch with herself and others. In contrast to an idealized self-image in which one is always perfect and loved by everyone, Karen Horney created the concepts of **self-realization** and a **real self.** A real self includes who one is and what one appreciates. It is the alienation from the real self that is seen to constitute a key process of neurotic development. It also requires energy to present a false self, which leaves few resources for developing healthy human growth. Her ideas were echoed later in the century by Abraham Maslow.

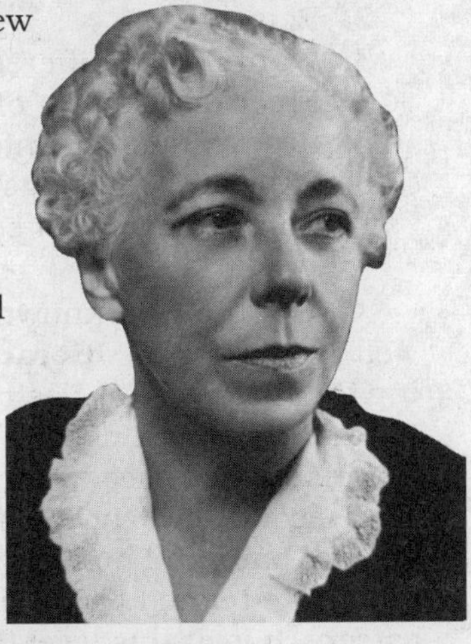

Karen Horney

As the existential-humanistic movement grew, a number of themes became critical. The first is an emphasis on human growth and the need for a positive psychology, which moves beyond the discussion of stress and neurosis seen in the psychodynamic approaches. A second emphasis is that psychological health is more than just the absence of pathology. Not having a problem is not the same as finding meaning in one's life. The third theme stresses the importance of not only considering the external world and a person's relationship to it but also the internal world. In the humanistic existential perspective, the internal world of a person and his or her experiences are valued. With the emphasis on experience, you will also see the therapies that developed from this approach referred to as humanistic-experiential therapies.

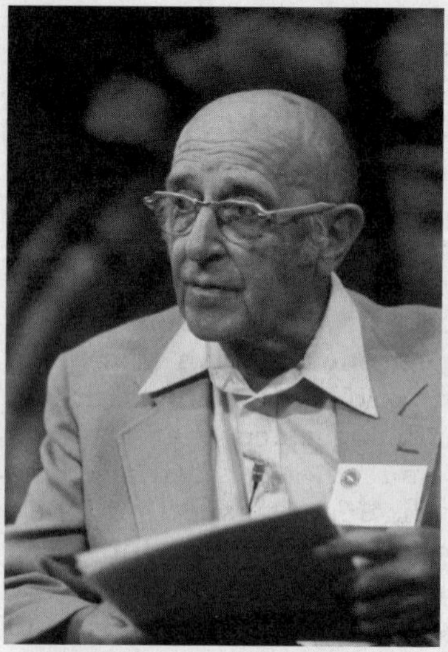

Carl Rogers

© Roger Ressmeyer/Corbis

Carl Rogers brought the humanistic movement to the forefront by creating **client-centered therapy,** also referred to as **person-centered therapy.** He was also one of the first psychologists to record therapy sessions so that they could be used for research. Rogers continued on the theme of potential by saying that psychotherapy is a releasing of an already existing capacity in a potentially competent individual. In fact, it was the interaction with the therapist that allowed for the person to experience himself and come to understand his potential. In this way, Rogers emphasized the relationship between the therapist and client as a critical key to effective therapy.

There are three key characteristics of the client-centered approach. The first is empathic understanding. As the therapist reflects back what the client says, the client begins to experience his innermost thoughts and feelings. The second is what Rogers referred to as unconditional positive regard. That is, the therapist accepts what the client says without trying to change the client. For some individuals who had experienced significant others in their lives as critical of them, to be accepted by the therapist is a new experience. The third characteristic is for the therapist to show genuineness and congruence. In this way, the therapist models what interactions between two real people could be like.

As a person continues in therapy, Rogers suggested that the client goes through seven stages. These stages begin with an unwillingness to share one's internal world. This is followed by blaming things on others and accepting one's own experiences. The next set of stages begins with a freer description of feeling and ends with the client's being comfortable with himself. The stages are as follows:

1. Unwillingness to reveal self, feeling not recognized
2. Externalizes
3. Wants to be different (not accepting past feelings)
4. Freer description of feelings
5. Recognition of conflict between feelings and thoughts
6. Experience feelings without denial, more willing to risk in relationships
7. Comfortable with self and with having new feelings

One of the best known of the humanistic psychologists is Abraham Maslow. Maslow is well known for his **hierarchy of needs.** Although there are few empirical studies examining the hierarchy, it has remained an important theoretical concept for understanding the nature of human needs. The first level is physiological needs such as hunger and thirst. Before one can seek higher-level psychological needs, physiological needs must be met. The second level needs are safety, which includes the desire for safety and the avoidance of pain and anxiety. The third level of needs includes belongingness and love. These needs are related to intimacy, affection, and being part of a peer group. The fourth level is esteem. It is at this level that one seeks self-respect, adequacy, and mastery of one's skills. The fifth and highest level is a search for **self-actualization.**

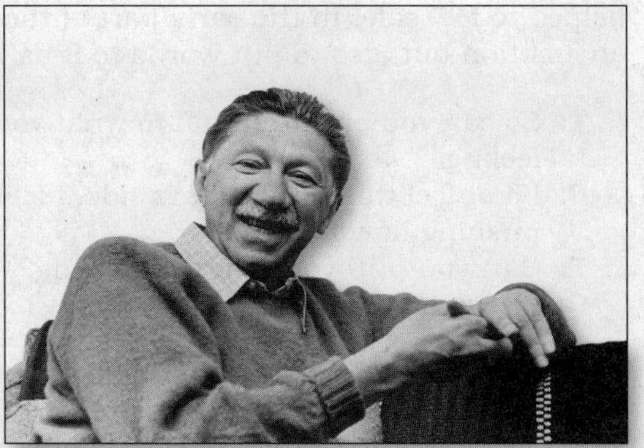

Abraham Maslow

© Bettmann/Corbis

Self-actualization, according to Maslow, is the situation in which one lives one's life to the fullest. At times, one may experience peak experiences or flow states in which everything appears to go perfectly with little effort, but this is not a constant state. In general, self-actualized individuals are reality- and problem-centered. It is not their desire to blame others but rather to solve the problem at hand. They also accept others as well as themselves. In their actions, they tend to be spontaneous and live a fairly simple life.

A number of humanistic-experiential orientated therapies have been shown to be effective (Elliott, Greenberg, Watson, Timulak, & Freire, 2013). One of these empirically supported therapies based on humanistic principles was developed by Leslie Greenberg and his colleagues. This approach is known as **emotion-focused therapy** or **process experiential therapy** (Greenberg, 2002). In this therapy, emotion is viewed as centrally important in the experience of self. Emotion can be either adaptive or maladaptive. However, in either case, emotion is the crucial element that brings about change in therapy. In therapy, clients are helped to identify and explore their emotions. The aim is to both manage and transform emotional experiences.

Greenberg described five principles that relate emotion-focused therapy to a humanist approach concerning human nature (Pos & Greenberg, 2007). These principles are as follows:

1. Experiencing is the basis of thought, feeling, and action.
2. Human beings are fundamentally free to choose how to construct their worlds.
3. People function holistically while at the same time are made up of many parts, or self-organizations, each of which may be associated with quite distinctive thoughts, feelings and self-experiences.
4. People function best and are best helped by a therapist who is psychologically present and who establishes an interpersonal environment that is empathic, unconditionally accepting, and authentic.
5. People grow and develop to the best of their abilities in supportive environments.

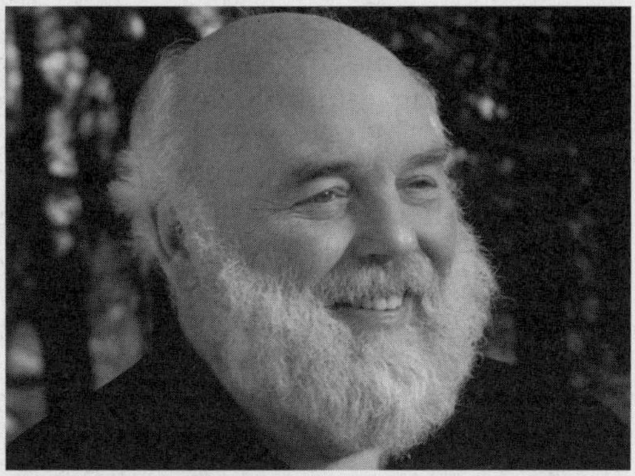

Leslie Greenberg

Photo courtesy of Leslie Greenberg

Emotion-focused therapy can be thought of in three phases (Greenberg & Watson, 2006). The first phase is one of bonding and awareness in which it is the job of the therapist to create a safe environment in which emotional experience can take place. Empathy and positive regard are part of the way the client is helped to feel safe. In the early part of therapy, the client is helped not only to experience an emotion but also to put words to it as illustrated below.

T: So can you pay attention to what you feel inside in that place where you feel your feelings?
C: I just feel this heaviness inside. I feel the weight of all the things I have to do just pushing down on me.
T: Can you put words to that feeling?
C: I have no choice.

The second phase is evocation and exploration. At this point, emotions are evoked and even intensified. The therapist also helps the client to understand how she might be interfering with her own experience of emotion. Such examples of interference would include changing the subject and beginning to talk about the emotion in a cognitive manner as a way to distance one's self from the experience. The third phase is transformation and generation of alternatives. It is at this point that the therapist helps the client construct alternative ways of thinking, feeling, and doing, which are more consistent with her real self. Empirical studies have shown that emotion-focused therapy is effective with depression and emotional trauma (Greenberg & Watson, 2006).

Another therapeutic technique that has gained popularity and been empirically shown to be effective is **mindfulness.** Mindfulness techniques were originally meditation techniques developed in Theravada Buddhism. These techniques involve an increased focused purposeful awareness of the present moment. The idea is to relate to one's thoughts and experiences in an open, nonjudgmental, and accepting manner (Kabat-Zinn, 1990). The basic technique is to observe thoughts without reacting to them in the present. This increases sensitivity to important features of the environment and one's internal reactions. This leads to better self-management and awareness as an alternative to ruminating about the past or worrying about the future. This reduces self-criticism.

Nonjudgmental observing allows for a reduction in stress, reduction in reactivity, and more time for interaction with others and the world. Also, feelings of compassion for another person become possible. This broadens attention and alternatives. Meta-analysis performed by Hofmann and his colleagues examined 39 studies of mindfulness (Hofmann, Sawyer, Witt, & Oh, 2010). He found significant reductions in anxiety and depression following mindfulness techniques. Grossman and his colleagues examined 20 studies and found overall positive changes following mindfulness approaches (Grossman, Niemann, Schmidt, &, Walach, 2010; see also Hofmann, Grossman, & Hinton, 2011). Empirical evidence using mindfulness techniques has shown positive change with a number of disorders including anxiety, depression, chronic pain, and stress. Mindfulness is also a component of DBT that is an effective treatment of borderline personality disorder.

Overall, the existential-humanistic perspective emphasizes the emotional level. There is also an emphasis on the value of internal processes and the manner in which the exploration and experiencing of these internal processes can lead to changes in behavior and experience.

Behavioral and Cognitive Behavioral Perspectives

The **behavioral perspective,** as the name implies, has focused on the level of actions and behaviors. Most histories of behaviorism begin with a discussion of Ivan Pavlov, the Russian physiologist who won the Nobel Prize in 1904 for his work on the physiology of digestion. Pavlov noted in his Nobel Prize speech that the sight of tasty food makes the mouth of a hungry man water. However, what became of interest to behavioral psychologists was not the salivary reflex itself but the fact that other objects associated with the presentation of food could also produce salivation. For example, in his work with dogs, the sound of the door of the lab being opened preceding the dogs being presented with food would also produce the reflex. In a variety of studies, it was shown that any sensory process such as sound that was paired with the food would produce salivation. After a number of pairings, the sound alone without the food could produce this reflex. This came to be known as **classical conditioning.**

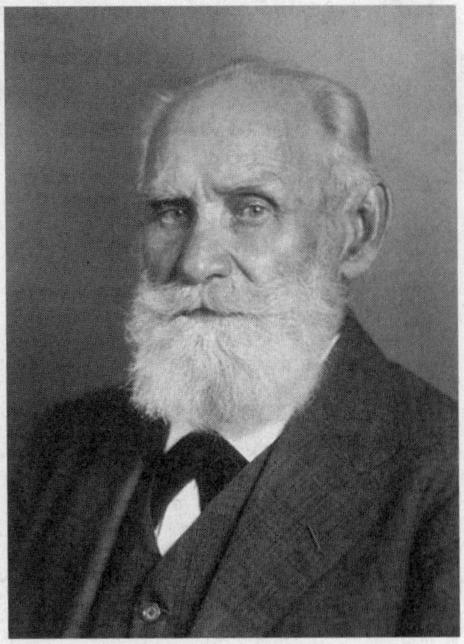

Ivan Pavlov

Classical conditioning is the situation in which an unconditioned stimulus such as food will result in an unconditioned response such as salivation. If this unconditioned stimulus is paired with a neutral stimulus a number of times, then the neutral stimulus will produce the response. Technically, this is referred to as a conditioned stimulus producing a conditioned response. After a period of time, the conditioned stimulus such as sound when presented alone will no longer produce the response. This process is referred to as **extinction.** Behaviorists saw classical conditioning as one mechanism underlying the development of mental illness. It should be noted, however, that Pavlov saw mental illness as resulting from stress, which he studied in dogs. Also, Pavlov saw disorders such as schizophrenia resulting from weakness in neuronal activity in the brain. The disorder itself actually protected the weakened brain according to Pavlov.

John Watson is often described as America's first behaviorist. His work set psychology on the course of emphasizing environmental explanations for behavior and rejecting the theoretical value of internal concepts. This called into question the value of studying such topics as consciousness and other internal processes. John Watson set the course of only studying observable behavior with his 1913 paper *Psychology as the Behaviorist Views It.* Watson suggested that the proper study of psychology was behavior and not the mind. Further, Watson saw the goal of psychology as identifying environmental conditions that direct behavior. Under no circumstances should the theory make reference to consciousness, mind, or other internal unobservable events. Partly as a reaction against those who sought to infer conscious processes from behaviors in animals and partly from the failure of introspection in humans as a technique for describing mental processes, Watson created a psychology based on observable behaviors alone. This position allowed for and supported the development of a strong stimulus-response psychology. Watson's statement emphasizing the role of the environment in development is well known.

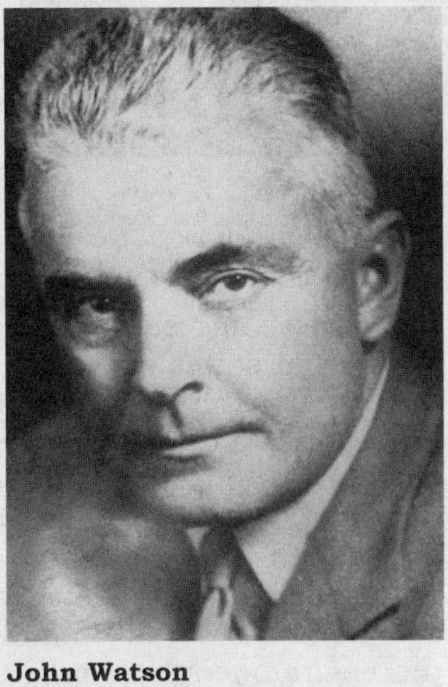

John Watson

> Give me a dozen healthy infants, well-formed, and my own specified world to bring them up in and I'll guarantee to take any one at random and train him to become any type of specialist I might select—doctor, lawyer, artist, merchant-chief, and yes, even beggar-man and thief, regardless of his talents, penchants, tendencies, abilities, vocations, and race of his ancestors. (Watson, 1924)

As the quote implies, Watson assumed that there existed "talents, penchants, tendencies, abilities" that were part of an individual but that these could be overridden by environmental factors. In fact, Watson demonstrated that an 11-month-old infant named Little Albert could be conditioned to fear an animal such as a lab rat that the infant had previously enjoyed playing with (Watson & Rayner, 1920). The procedure (which would be considered unacceptable and unethical today) was to create a loud noise when the infant was observing the animal. A loud noise will produce a startle response. In a classical conditioning manner, the pairing of the aversive noise and the animal led to conditioned fear. Behaviorists used classical conditioning as a mechanism for understanding phobias and other processes seen in mental illness.

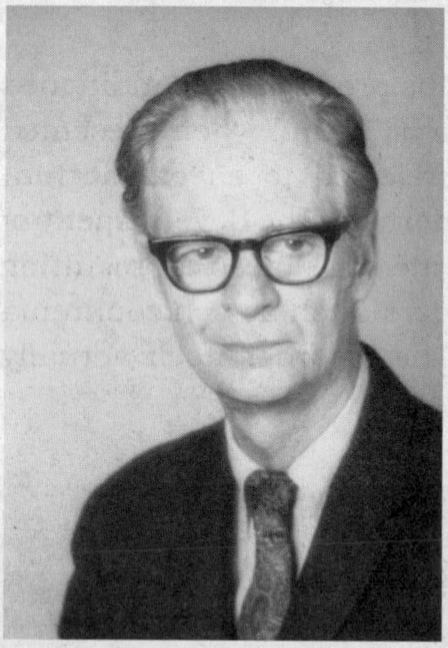

B. F. Skinner

© Bettmann/Corbis

B. F. Skinner became the 20th century's most vocal proponent of behaviorism. Beginning with his 1938 book, *The Behavior of Organisms,* Skinner played a significant role in experimental psychology until his death in 1990. His exemplar experimental procedure was to demonstrate that an animal, generally a laboratory rat or pigeon, could be taught to make specific responses if, after the occurrence of the desired response, the animal was given a reward, generally food. This procedure came to be known as **operant conditioning.** The basic idea was that behavior could be elicited or shaped if **reinforcement** followed its occurrence. Consequently, if these behaviors ceased to be rewarded, the occurrence would decrease. Thus, the emphasis was on behaviors and the rewards that follow them as opposed to the environmental stimuli evoking them. These techniques were applied to the management of individuals with mental disorders in institutional settings. In these procedures, called token economies, individuals with schizophrenia were rewarded with products they sought for behaviors such as cleaning their room or taking a bath.

Skinner suggested that freedom, will, dignity, and other concepts referring to the mind or internal states have no explanatory value. Psychologists should only be interested in the relationship between behavior and consequences, according to Skinner. Even processes such as language learning were seen as the result of words being reinforced and learned one at a time. In this manner any type of complex behavior was seen as the result of learning simple behaviors, which were then chained together. The larger implication was that humans came into the world ready to be influenced by the reinforcement contingencies of the environment to determine their development and actions in the world. Both Skinner and Watson left us with a psychology that emphasized the environment and ignored any discussion of internal processes or mechanisms for understanding life. Their real contribution for understanding mental illness was not their mechanisms per se since it is difficult for learning theory to adequately describe psychopathology across the life span but their emphasis on experimental research and the necessity to evaluate treatment procedures in a scientific manner.

In the middle of the last century, a number of psychologists began to see the limitation of strict behaviorism in that it ignored internal processes. Simple demonstrations such as offering a 6-year-old a candy bar if he would do a particular task showed that the idea of a reward was enough to motivate behavior. Also, behaviorally oriented psychologists such as Albert Bandura showed that humans would imitate the behaviors of others even without reinforcement. This type of learning was called **observational learning** or **modeling.** One classic set of studies involved children hitting a Bobo doll after seeing cartoon characters being aggressive. In another study, children watched an adult interact with the Bobo doll in an aggressive or nonaggressive manner. Those children who watched the aggressive adult later showed more aggression than those who watched a nonaggressive adult.

Nonclinical areas of research in psychology such as the study of cognitive processes and social processes were demonstrating that humans often make quick decisions based on information that is outside of normal awareness. Humans make these decisions without actually realizing there are alternative ways of thinking. Further, evolutionary thinking was showing how humans come into the world with an evolutionary history such that they develop fears and phobias to some objects such as snakes or spiders more readily than to a toy truck or a flower. Arne Öhman at the Karolinska Institute sought to determine the basis of fear learning and how it relates to psychopathology (e.g., Öhman, 1986). Others emphasized the fact that humans talk to themselves and pay attention to their own thoughts, which can influence behavior. Individuals such as David Barlow at Boston University and Tom Borkovec at Penn State University used cognitive and behavioral research to develop empirically supported treatments for anxiety (Barlow, 1988; Borkovec, 2006).

The **cognitive behavioral perspective** suggests that dysfunctional thinking is common to all psychological disturbances. By learning in therapy how to understand one's thinking, it is possible to change the way one thinks as well as one's emotional state and behaviors. One basic feature of our thinking is that it is automatic. Ideas just pop into our mind such as "I can't solve this" or "it is all my fault." A number of therapies based on be cognitive principles along with behavioral interventions have been shown to be effective (Hollon & Beck, 2013).

Aaron Beck developed a cognitive therapy for depression in the early 1960s (Beck, 1967; see also Beck, 2011, for an overview and update). The model is described in terms of a cognitive triad related to depression (see *Figure 2-9*).

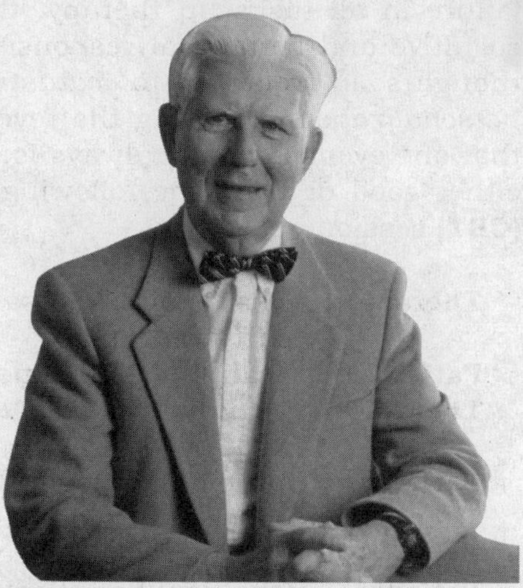

Aaron Beck

Courtesy of the Beck institute for cognitive behavior Therapy: www.beckinstitute.org

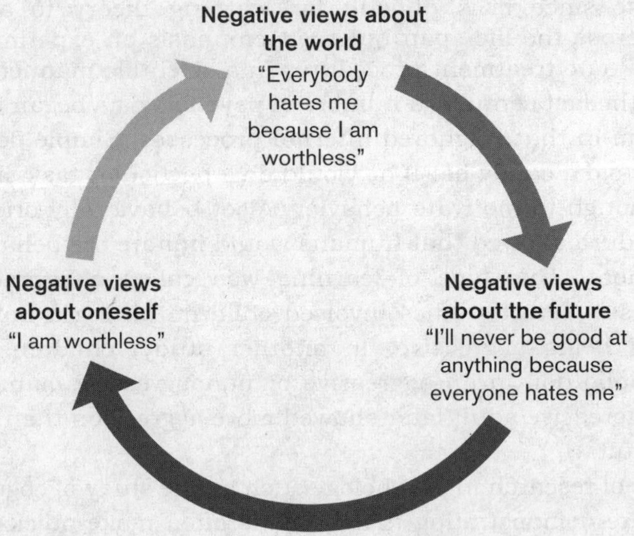

FIGURE 2-9 Beck's Cognitive Triad

The first component of the triad is the individual's negative view of self. This is when the individual attributes unpleasant experiences to his own mental, physical, and moral defects. When something negative happens, the person says it is his or her fault. In therapy, the client can become aware of the content of his thinking. The second component is the individual's tendency to interpret experiences in a negative manner. That is, the person tailors the facts to fit negative conclusions. The basic idea is that thinking influences emotion and behavior. The third component is that the person regards the future in a negative way. He envisions a life of only hardships and anticipates failure in all tasks. In therapy, the basic idea is that the individual can modify his cognitive and behavioral responses. Overall, the therapy is directed at the automatic thoughts in relation to *catastrophizing*—believing that nothing will work out; *personalization*—believing that everything relates to you; *overgeneralization*—believing that one event is how it always is; and *dichotomous thinking*—believing that things are either good or bad. The following is an example of a **cognitive behavioral therapy (CBT)** session:

Therapist: Okay, Sally, you said you wanted to talk about a problem with finding a part-time job?
Patient: Yeah. I need the money . . . but I don't know.
Therapist: [*noticing that Sally looks more dysphoric*] What's going through your mind right now?
Patient: [automatic thought] I won't be able to handle a job.
Therapist: [labeling her idea as a thought and linking it to her mood] And how does that thought make you feel?
Patient: [emotion] Sad. Really low.
Therapist: [beginning to evaluate the thought] What's the evidence that you won't be able to work?
Patient: Well, I'm having trouble just getting through my classes.
Therapist: Okay. What else?

Patient: I don't know . . . I'm still so tired. It's hard to make myself even go and *look* for a job, much less go to work every day.

Therapist: In a minute we'll look at that. [suggesting an alternative view] Maybe it's actually harder for you at this point to go out and *investigate* jobs than it would be for you to go to a job that you already had. In any case, is there any other evidence that you couldn't handle a job, assuming that you can get one?

Patient: . . . No, not that I can think of.

Therapist: Any evidence on the other side? That you *might* be able to handle a job?

Patient: I did work last year. And that was on top of school and other activities. But this year . . . I just don't know.

Therapist: Any other evidence that you could handle a job?

Patient: I don't know. . . . It's possible I could do something that doesn't take much time. And that isn't too hard.

Therapist: What might that be?

Patient: A sales job, maybe. I did that last year.

Therapist: Any ideas of where you could work?

Patient: Actually, maybe the [university] bookstore. I saw a notice that they're looking for new clerks.

Therapist: Okay. And what would be the *worst* that could happen if you did get a job at the bookstore?

Patient: I guess if I couldn't do it.

Therapist: And if that happened, how would you cope?

Patient: I guess I'd just quit.

Therapist: And what would be the *best* that could happen?

Patient: Uh . . . that I'd be able to do it easily.

Therapist: And what's the most realistic outcome?

Patient: It probably won't be easy, especially at first. But I might be able to do it.

Therapist: Sally, what's the effect of believing your thought, "I won't be able to handle a job"?

Patient: Makes me feel sad. . . . Makes me not even try.

Therapist: And what's the effect of changing your thinking, of realizing that possibly you could work in the bookstore?

Patient: I'd feel better. I'd be more likely to apply for the job.

Therapist: So what do you want to do about this?

Patient: Go to the bookstore. I could go this afternoon.

Therapist: How likely are you to go?

Patient: Oh, I guess I will. I will go.

Therapist: And how do you feel now?

Patient: A little better. A little more nervous, maybe. But a little more hopeful, I guess. (Beck, 2011, pp. 23–25)

Concept Check

- What does *empirically based treatments* mean? Why is it important, and what impacts has the concept had on treatment for psychopathology?
- Describe the basic principles underlying each of these perspectives on psychological treatment, and give an example of an empirically based treatment from each: psychodynamic perspective, existential-humanistic perspective, and cognitive behavioral perspective.

The cognitive behavioral movement sought to understand how cognitions were disordered or disrupted in mental disorders. Whereas humanistic therapies emphasized emotional processing, cognitive behavioral approaches emphasized thoughts and the manner in which a person thought about her life and experiences. The basic idea is that psychological disturbances often involve errors in thinking. One real value of many cognitive behavioral approaches is that they have been tested empirically and presented in books and manuals that describe the steps involved in therapy. CBT has been developed for a variety of disorders, which will be described in the appropriate chapters of this book.

SUMMARY

Mental disorders have been with us throughout our human history. Since the time that written language became a part of our experience, humans have included descriptions of mental disorders. Examples of historical conceptions of psychopathology are included from Pythagoras and Hippocrates in ancient Greece; Galen from the period of the Roman Empire; advances in anatomy by da Vinci in art and Harvey and Descartes in science from the Renaissance; advances in understanding the brain and nervous system in the 1700 to 1900 period; and Darwin's description of the theory of evolution and Charcot's classification of psychological and brain disorders in the 1800s. Historically, the care and treatment of individuals with mental illness also advanced as did our understanding of the experience of these disorders. Although the Greeks saw mental illness as a disorder involving the brain, it is only within the past 100 years that scientific support began to clarify this position.

There are two sides to every person with a mental disorder—the person responding to her own symptoms and mental health professionals treating the disorder. There is now evidence that both aspects are important and that a crucial aspect of treatment is the willingness of the person to be actively involved in her own treatment. There are currently three broad perspectives for the psychological treatment of mental disorders: the psychodynamic perspective, the existential-humanistic perspective, and the cognitive behavioral perspective. They were developed somewhat independently and often in opposition to one another. Beginning in the 1950s and 1960s, however, there was a movement to determine the effectiveness of both medical and psychological treatments in a scientific manner. Researchers and clinicians began to focus more on approaches and principles for which there was scientific evidence on effectiveness. This led to developing effective treatments for particular disorders as well as greater integration of techniques from the three different approaches as well as from other perspectives.

STUDY RESOURCES

Review Questions

1. How does reading about the experiences of individuals with mental illness inform our understanding of the nature of psychopathology?

2. Describe how mental illness was understood in each of the following historical periods and how that understanding was advanced: Ancient Greece, Roman Empire, Renaissance, and 1700s to 1900s. Give examples of the individuals and ideas critical to each period.
3. How were individuals with mental illness treated during those same historical periods: Ancient Greece, Roman Empire, Renaissance, and 1700s to 1900s? Who were some of the people who played a critical role in advancing treatment?
4. Descartes created a mind–body distinction that science since that time has had to address: How can a material body including the brain be influenced by an immaterial process such as the mind? How can a thought influence a cell in the brain? How would you handle the mind–body problem?
5. What we now know about the structure and function of the human brain and nervous system has developed across many times and places. Bring together in a model the pieces you consider important to your current understanding of the human brain and nervous system.
6. Describe the contributions of the following individuals from different perspectives to the field of psychological treatment as a whole: Sigmund Freud, Hans Strupp, Carl Jung, Karen Horney, Carl Rogers, Abraham Maslow, Leslie Greenberg, B. F. Skinner, Albert Bandura, and Aaron Beck.

For Further Reading

Andreasen, N. (2001). *Brave new brain.* New York: Oxford University Press.

Freud, S. (1966). Project for a scientific psychology. *Standard Edition, 1,* 281–397. (Original work published 1895)

Greenberg, L. (2011). *Emotion-focused therapy.* Washington, DC: American Psychological Association.

Horney, K. (1945). *Our inner conflicts.* New York: W. W. Norton & Co.

Jung, C. (1968). *Analytical psychology: Its theory and practice.* New York: Random House.

Kandel, E. (2005). *Psychiatry, psychoanalysis, and the new biology of mind.* Washington, DC: American Psychiatric Publications.

Kandel, E. (2012). *The age of insight: The quest to understand the unconscious in art, mind, and brain, from Vienna 1900 to the present.* New York: Random House.

Maslow, A. (1971). *The farther reaches of human nature.* New York: Viking Press.

Pribram, K., & Gill, M. (1976). *Freud's "project" Re-assessed.* New York: Basic Books.

Rogers, C. (1951). *Client-centered therapy, its current practice, implications, and theory.* London: Constable & Robinson.

Skinner, B. F. (1974). *About behaviorism.* New York: Random House.

Strupp, H., & Binder, J. (1984). *Psychotherapy in a new key.* New York: Basic Books.

Key Terms and Concepts

behavioral perspective
classical conditioning
client-centered therapy
cognitive behavioral perspective
cognitive behavioral therapy (CBT)
emotion-focused therapy
encephalization
existential-humanistic perspective
extinction
hierarchical integration
hierarchy of needs
mindfulness
modeling
natural selection
observational learning
operant conditioning
person-centered therapy
process experiential therapy
psychoanalysis
psychodynamic perspective
real self
reinforcement
self-actualization
self-realization
sexual selection
signs
symptoms
syndrome
variation

CHAPTER 3

Neuroscience Approaches to Understanding Psychopathology

CHAPTER OUTLINE

- DIAGNOSTIC CONSIDERATIONS OF PSYCHOPATHOLOGY 67
- NEUROSCIENCE PERSPECTIVES 76
- NEUROSCIENCE TECHNIQUES AND LEVELS OF ANALYSIS 80
- THE BRAIN 81
- HOW DOES THE NEURON PASS INFORMATION? 83
- ENCODING INFORMATION 84
- HOW DO WE OBSERVE THE BRAIN AT WORK? 85
- NETWORKS OF THE BRAIN 93
- THE STUDY OF GENETICS 99
- HOW DO GENES INFLUENCE BEHAVIOR? 103
- THE THEMES OF EVOLUTION 106
- PSYCHOPATHOLOGY FROM AN EVOLUTIONARY PERSPECTIVE 107
- NEUROETHICS 110
- SUMMARY 112
- STUDY RESOURCES 113

The neuroscientist V. S. Ramachandran told about an individual who came to see him at the medical center (Ramachandran, 1998). This individual who was named David appeared completely normal. He had no problems with ***memory,*** *engaged easily in conversation, expressed emotions, and otherwise appeared as anyone you might meet every day. However, he did one very puzzling thing. When he saw his mother, he said, "That woman looks exactly like my mother, but she is not my mother!"*

As a clinician, how might you understand this? You might ask if this was some type of psychosis in which he had the delusion that his mother was not his mother. However, David showed no other signs of disorganization or problems with functioning. You might also ask if David had any type of emotional conflict with his mother. The answer was no. After more information gathering, it was discovered that David, at times, also thought his father was not his real father. Additional information revealed that David did indeed experience his parents as his parents when talking to them on the phone.

The formal name for this condition is the Capgras syndrome, named after the physician who first described the symptoms in the 1920s. However, the mechanisms involved were not known. Since David had previously had a motorcycle accident, it was possible that normal brain processes were not functioning correctly. In order to understand David, Ramachandran asked himself what was missing in David's experience of his mother. His answer was that there was no emotional response.

The normal emotional response to seeing someone like our parents is as follows. Our visual system gives us the experience of seeing the person. In humans, one particular part of the temporal lobe is sensitive to seeing faces, the fusiform face area (FFA). In turn, this information goes to a variety of areas including the limbic system, which is involved in emotional processing. One particular structure, the amygdala, is involved in perceptions that are emotionally important to us. The amygdala has rich connections with other cortical areas, which together give us the experience of emotion.

If David had no emotional response to seeing a face, how might this be tested? Emotion is processed not only in the brain but also in the autonomic nervous system (ANS), which prepares the body for dangerous situations. If we see a bear and run, it is the sympathetic part of the ANS that makes us feel excited and moves blood to our muscles for a quick getaway. One easy way to measure the sympathetic nervous system is to pass a small electrical current along the skin, usually between the palm and the finger. This procedure is referred to as electrodermal activity (EDA). If we are excited, then our skin sweats slightly. This, in turn, makes it easier for the electrical current to pass between the two electrodes. Whenever we have an emotional response to what we see, we get changes in the EDA. David did not show any EDA differences when viewing pictures of those close to him. This suggested to Ramachandran that there was a disconnection between his visual face perception areas and the emotional centers of the brain. Since the auditory system is wired differently, that would also explain why David did not have the same experience when talking with his parents on the phone. The point of the story of David, as strange as it may seem, is to suggest that one important way to understand our mental processes is through their underlying mechanisms.

We can discuss David on different levels. We can consider his actual behavior of saying his mother was not his mother. We can also ask David to tell us what he experiences when he sees his parents. In this case, David said that he sees them as nice people but that he does not expect from them what he expects from his parents. We can discuss how this affects other people, such as his parents, to be told they are not his parents. We can also look at the interaction between him and his parents. From another standpoint, we can consider cognitive and emotional mechanisms involved such as the memory of his mother and his emotional feeling for her. In other chapters of this book, I will include discussions of mental illness from the levels just described. In this present chapter, I will focus on current neuroscience approaches to understanding mental illness with an emphasis on brain imaging, genetics, and evolutionary perspectives.

DIAGNOSTIC CONSIDERATIONS OF PSYCHOPATHOLOGY

The historical considerations of psychopathology emphasized careful observation and interaction with the afflicted individuals as important methods for understanding the nature of the disorder. Based on these observations of symptoms and signs, individuals were diagnosed and classified as falling into discrete categories of disorders. This is an important level of analysis and one I will emphasize throughout this book. However, there are other levels of analysis for understanding psychopathology.

With progress in the neurosciences in general and brain imaging and genetics in particular, other levels of analysis have become possible. The new levels of analysis offer different perspectives for the field of mental illness. What seemed like discrete categories of psychopathology previously are now seen to cluster in new and different ways when considered from the standpoint of genetics. Still, additional groups have emerged as scientists have considered the neural networks involved in particular manifestations of psychopathology. This has led to the realization that mental disorders can be described in both a **categorical** and a **dimensional** manner.

As shown in the physical sciences, there are times in which a phenomenon can be described in both a categorical and a dimensional manner. For example, when water is heated the rise in temperature can be described in a dimensional manner in terms of a certain number of degrees. However, at a critical point, the water turns to steam, which is a categorically different state from water. Likewise, a reduction in temperature changes water into a different categorical state—ice. The question for the study of psychopathological disorders is to determine the underlying dimensional changes that are associated with categorical-like transformations leading to a disordered state. Further, different underlying processes may actually allow for the presence of more than one disordered state at the same time.

Technically, when an individual is seen to have more than one disorder at the same time, the disorders are referred to as **comorbid.** In the National Comorbidity Survey, a large number of individuals with one disorder were found to have one or more additional diagnoses (Kessler et al., 1994). For example, individuals with generalized anxiety disorder will often also show symptoms of depression. Further, these two disorders have overlapping genetic and environmental risk factors (Kendler, Neale, Kessler, Heath, & Eaves, 1992). The number of diagnoses found in the National Comorbidity Survey was associated with the severity of the symptoms. This has suggested to researchers that there exists a general underlying vulnerability to psychopathology that may be independent of the particular symptoms expressed (Pittenger & Etkin, 2008). This is similar to the idea of Griesinger in the 19th century that there is a general psychiatric disorder whose expression in different individuals is modulated by continuous variable traits.

A related approach is to consider which disorders co-occur with one another. In general, two clusters have been found. The first is referred to as **internalizing disorders.** These disorders include anxiety and depression. The second cluster is referred to as **externalizing disorders.** These disorders include conduct disorder, oppositional defiant disorder, antisocial personality disorder, substance use disorder, and in some studies attention deficit/hyperactivity disorder (ADHD). These types of studies have led scientists to search for common factors such as genetics, brain processes, and environmental risk profiles that might be associated with each cluster.

A lot of work has been done in India the lines of understanding the biological basis of psychiatric disorders. A summary of this appears in the *Indian Journal of Psychiatry* (Shrivastava, 2010).

The article speaks of some prominent Indian academic institutions and describes the work that began there. For example, the author writes about the establishment of psychophysiological and clinical psychopharmacology department at the King Edward Memorial Hospital, Mumbai. The same hospital has a WHO collaborative center of excellence for de-addiction. It is a large multi-specialty teaching hospital in Mumbai. Four such centers of excellence were set up in India for the research on and treatment of addictions, two of them being Muktangan in Pune, Maharashtra and the Department of Addiction Psychiatry at the All India Institute of Medical Sciences (AIIMS), New Delhi.

Also, very important is the establishment of the National Institute of Mental Health and Neurosciences (NIMHANS), Bangalore, which made cutting-edge contributions to the clinical and experimental studies in neurochemistry, genetics, and neuroimaging. Equally significant is the establishment of WHO collaborative center at the King George's Medical College at Lucknow.

The prestigious Madras Medical College set up a biological psychiatry unit in early days, and a neurochemistry unit came up at the equally well-known CMC, Vellore. Central Institute, Ranchi, set up their Department of Electroencephalographic studies.

The Indian Council of Medical research also contributed significantly to the growth of biological psychiatry by supporting the ICMR Center of Research in Geriatric Psychiatry, Madurai. There were many ICMR, Ministry of Health, Government of India, research initiatives as well as Department of Science and Technology (DST) initiatives in advanced neurosciences.

Interestingly, the same article (i.e., Shrivastava, 2010) from the *Indian Journal of Psychiatry*, rather painstakingly, lists some of the early works in biological underpinnings of mental illness details, which may be considered trivia by some but nevertheless list some of the important classic works from India. The table is reproduced below.

Topic	Sub-topic	First author	Year of publication
ECT	Ectonus	Murti D. L. N. Rao	1958
	Electric and chemical convulsive	David J. Impastato	1960
	Analysis of 5021 ECT	A. V. Shah	1962
	Four techniques	V. N. Bagadia	1962
	Memory and intelligence	H. Narayan Murthy	1966
	Unilateral and bilateral	L. G. Kiloh	1971
	ECG changes	R. K. Jain	1976
	The efficacy of spaced v/s daily	D. K. Deshmukh	1980
	Propanidid	M. R. Kulkarni	1980
	ECT Phenothiazine combination	A. K. Agarwal	1985
	A review	G. D. Shukla	1989
	Althesin and thiopentone	R. K. Mahendru	1989
	Psychobiological frontiers	Chittaranjan Andrade	1990
	E.C.T. a need of reappraisal	A. K. Agarwal	1990
	Seizure duration estimates	D. K. Subbakrishna	1992

Topic	Sub-topic	First author	Year of publication
	Seizure duration	Chittaranjan Andrade	1993
	ECT induced EEG seizure	B. N. Gangadhar	1993
	Physical morbidity	Prathap Tharyan	1993
	Merits of EEG monitoring during ECT	K. Girish	2002
	Molecular mechanisms underlying		
	electroconvulsive therapy-induced		
	amnestic deficits: A decade of research	Chittaranjan Andrade	2008
	Psychosomatics blood glucose	T. H. Seth	1958
Neuropsychiatry EEG			1958
	The Neurology and bio-chemistry of behavior	Satya D. Nand	1960
	Cerebral arteriosclerosis	A. K. Chatterjee	1965
	Temporal lobe epilepsy	G. D. Shukla	1981
	Cerebral laterality in schizophrenia	R. K. Gaur	1985
	Epileptic psychosis	Antony Fernandez	1988
	Neurological "Soft signs"	Alice Cherian	1989
	Eye movements	Ram Sharan	1990
	Neuroanatomical correlates	S. Sabhesan	1990
	Temporal lobe focus	Jambur Ananth	1990
	Neurological abnormalities	K. S. Shaji	1990
	Visual information processing deficits	C. V. Ananthanarayanan	1993
	Cerebral blood flow and metabolism	Roy J. Mathew	1994
	Neuropsychiatric model of psychosis	Shrivastava Amresh	1996
	Progressive multifocal leukoencephalopathy in AIDS	Pradeep Kumar	2006
	The limbic system	V. Raj Mohan	2007
	Fronto-temporal dysfunction in schizophrenia: A selective review	John P. John	2009
Neurochemistry	Body fluids	R. B. Davis	1960
	Guaiacol Glyceryl Ether (GGE)	C. H. Mehta	1960
	Phosphate and creatinine excretion	P. Subrahmanyan	1962
	Acetyl methyl carbinol metabolism	Mc C. W. Anderson	1962
	Functional hypoglycemia	Sankara A. Rao	1963
	Extra-cellular fluid volume Liver function tests, serum oxidation	Harish Verma	1966
	Tests, serum ascorbic acid and copper levels	B. S. Sridhara Rama Rao	1970
	Blood histamine, histaminase levels and tissue sensitivity to histamine	R. K. Sanyal	1970

(Continued)

(Continued)

Topic	Sub-topic	First author	Year of publication
	Metabolic defect	Sridhara B.	1974
	N-Acetylneuraminic acid levels in the cerebrospinal fluid	B. S. Sridhara	1975
	Excretion of 3, 4-Dimethoxy Phenyl–Ethylamine	B. S. Sridhar Rama Rao	1976
	ABO blood groups	Gurmeet Singh	1979
	Plasma and erythrocyte sodium, potassium	N. Pradhan	1983
	Renal and extra-renal functions	V. N. Puri	1984
	Serum lipids	T. K. Mishra	1984
	Platelet MAO activity	A. K. Gupta	1985
	Serum immunoglobulins	I. V. L. Narasimha Rao	1985
	Electrolyte profile	M. S. Bhatia	1987
	Renal function tests	Kuruvilla Mathew	1988
	Renal function	M. K. Dhar	1988
	Phenylketonuria	H. S. Narayanan	1988
	Blood groups	P. Lakshmi Reddy	1988
	Rheumatoid factor		1988
	Platelet MAO activity	J. K. Trivedi	1989
	Immunoglobulins and viral antibodies	S. C. Tiwari	1990
	Platelet MAO activity	I. Sharma	1990
	Pharmacokinetics	A. D. Bhatt	1991
	Platelet MAO	Indira Sharma	1991
	Effect of negative ion	Chitra Andrade	1992
	Immunomodulator in the treatment of schizophrenia	S. Agarwal	1992
	Serum acetylcholinesterase level	Nilesh Shah	1992
	Australia antigen (HBsAG)	S. Chaudhury	1993
	Psychoimmunology and functional psychoses	S. C. Tiwari	1994
	Serum lipid profile	Sandeep Verma	1999
	CSF amines and their metabolites in first episode drug NaÃve schizophrenic	Anand L.	2002
	Evaluation of antioxidant deficit in schizophrenia	Gora Dadheech	2008
	Oxidative stress and interrelationship of important antioxidants	Om Prakash Singh	2008
Neurotransmitter	5 HT	K. S. Sachdev	1960
	Central dopamine and serotonin turnover	R. S. Pandey	1987
	Dopamine postsynaptic receptor	Chittaranjan Andrade	1990

Topic	Sub-topic	First author	Year of publication
	Single electroconvulsive shock and dopamine autoreceptors	B. N. Gangadhar	1990
	Serotonin and its metabolites	J. K. Trivedi	1992
	Alpha-2 noradrenergic and dopamine postsynaptic receptor functioning	Chittaranjan Andrade	1993
	Glucocorticoid receptor dysfunction	Aju Abraham	2003
	Platelet serotonin level	Devasis Ghosh	2008
	Cognitive neurosciences Cognitive effects of chronic bhang	A. K. Agrawal	1975
	Cannabis (Ganja) and cognition	A. Venkoba Rao	1975
	Memory in depression	S. Chandra	1982
	Cognitive dysfunction in depression	I. Sharma	1984
	Complex motor programming	Sumant Khanna	1987
	Cognitive disorder and depression	A. Venkoba Rao	1989
	Cognitive dysfunction in depression	Sajiv John	1992
	Luria-Nebraska neuropsychological battery	Alaka Nizamie	1992
	Cognitive functions in epileptic patients	M. R. Nainian	1993
	Neurocognitive impairment in HIV infection	Tony Edwin	1999
	Schizophrenic Luria-Nebraska neuro-psychological battery	B. P. Mishra	2002
	Neuro-psychological profile of epilepsy	B. P. Mishra	2002
	Executive functions in depression	Rajul Tandon	2002
	Neurocognitive dysfunction in mood disorders	Brian P. Moore	2003
	Executive functions in schizophrenia	S. Sabhesan	2005
	Neuropsychological impairment in bipolar affective disorder	Mubeen Taj	2005
	Neurocognitive function in women affected by the Bhopal gas disaster	R. N. Sahu	2005
	Cognitive dysfunction and associated factors in patients with chronic schizophrenia	Latha Srinivasan	2005
	Cognitive deficits in psychiatric disorders: Current status	J. K. Trivedi	2006
	Cognitive and emotional effects of renal transplantation	A. A. Pawar	2006
	Neuropsychological disposition and its impact on the executive functions and cognitive style in patients with obsessive-compulsive disorder	Sreemoyee Tarafder	2006
	Wisconsin card sorting test: Normative data and experience	Adarsh Kohli	2006

(Continued)

(Continued)

Topic	Sub-topic	First author	Year of publication
	The trail making test in India	Triptish Bhatia	2007
	Cognitive deficits in children of alcoholics	Melvin Chagas Silva	2007
	Neuropsychology of prefrontal cortex	Shazia Veqar Siddiqui	2008
Genetics	Schizophrenia—A genetic study	R. Ponnudurai	1989
	Fragile Xq-27	S. K. Murthy	1989
	Genomic imprinting	Ratanendra Kumar	2000
	Genetics of schizophrenia—An overview	R. Ponnudurai	2003
	The future of psychiatric genetics	Vishwajit L. Nimgaonkar	2003
	Serotonin transporter gene polymorphism	Mushtaq A. Margoob	2008
Clinical Research in biological psychiatry	Sedation threshold test	N. S. Vahia	1965
	Thyroid disorder	A. K. Chatterjee	1965
	Electroplexy	Dinshaw R. Doongaji	1966
	Electrically induced sleep	Kirpal Singh	1966
	Patterns in dreams	S. S. Nathawat	1973
	Family study of atypical lymphocytes		1973
	Teratogenic study	N. Sethi	1974
	Buccal and dermatoglyphic studies	S. S. Agarwal	1975
	Habitual use of cannabis indica	V. N. Bagadia	1976
	Palm prints	G. Eswaraiah	1978
	Tetratogenic effects	N. Sethi	1980
	Negative symptoms	Santosh Chaturvedi	1985
	Work performance of schizophrenic	P. S. Gopinath	1985
	Season of birth	Rakesh Kumar Jangid	1989
	Dermatoglyphics	H. P. Jhingan	1989
	Dermatoglyphics	H. P. Jhingan	1990
	Finger pulse volume	P. Bharathi	1992
	Finger pulse volume during Co_2 induced panic states	P. Bharathi	1992
	Alcohol dependence: biological and clinical correlates	Pratima Murthy	2003
	Neurobiological basis of Ganser syndrome	Daniel Ouyang	2003
	Sleep disorders in children with attention-deficit hyperactivity disorder	Subhash C. Bhargava	2005
	Impact of vocational rehabilitation on social functioning, cognitive functioning, and psychopathology in patients with chronic schizophrenia	P. N. Suresh Kumar	2008
	Neurobiology of Alzheimer's disease	E. Mohandas	2009

Topic	Sub-topic	First author	Year of publication
Neurophysiology, psychophysiology and electrophysiology	Emotional stress		1960
	Autonomic response	Abraham Verghese	1970
	Eosinophil rhythm	Parvathi S. Devi	1971
	Concepts of patanjali	N. S. Vahia	1973
	Skin conductance responses	P. K. Biswas	1981
	EMG bio-feedback	M. T. Gada	1984
	Psychobiology of depression	M. T. Gada	1987
	Psychobiology of suicide	A. Venkoba Rao	1987
	Electrocardiographic changes	S. Haque	1988
	E.E.G. abnormality	Alice Cherian	1990
	EMG biofeedback	D. Sargunaraj	1990
	EMG biofeedback	D. Sargunaraj	1991
	Efficacy of meditation	Vihang N. Vahia	1993
	Electromyography feedback	A. Abraham	1994
	Biology of addictions	N. G. Desai	1995
	P300 event related potential	R. Shukla	2000
	P300 event related potential	R. Singh	2000
	EEG alpha coherence and psychopathological dimensions	John P. John	2002
	Spirometry and airway reactivity	R. B. Galgali	2002
	EEG fractal dimension and spectral	Jagadisha	2003
	REM sleep latency and neurocognitive dysfunction in schizophrenia	Mrinmay Das	2005
	Psychoneuroendocrine Dexamenthasone	S. Kumar	1970
	Plasma cortisol	Abraham Verghese	1973
	Pineal gland responses	S. Parvathi Devi	1976
	Pineal gland RNA	N. Hariharasubrmanian	1976
	Thyroid function	G. C. Boral	1980
	Pineal gland in clinical cases of psychological stress	P. M. Singh	1980
	Pineal response to lithium	S. Parvathi Devi	1982
	Dexamethasone suppression test	R. Ghulam	1985
	Psychoendocrinology and behavior	G. C. Boral	1986
	Dexamethasone suppression test	M. Saikumar Reddy	1986
	Serum prolactin levels	K. Kuruvilla	1986
	Dexamethasone suppression test	G. Prasad Rao	1987
	Dexamethasone suppression test	S. L. Varma	1987
	Dopamine related hormone levels in acute schizophrenia	S. B. Chatterjee	1988

(Continued)

(Continued)

Topic	*Sub-topic*	*First author*	*Year of publication*
	Adrenocortical dysfunction in depression	K. C. Gurnani	1988
	Serum prolactin	P. Tharyan	1988
	Dexamethasone suppression test	S. Chaudhury	1989
	DST	A. Agarwal	1989
	Post dexamethasone plasma cortisol	R. Ghulam	1990
	ACTH and the dexamethasone suppression test	Ashok Kumar Jainer	1992
	Multiple endocrine responses to clonidine	Sumant Khanna	1992
	Concentrations of homovanillic acid and gonadal hormones	S. L. Gong	1993
	Serum prolactin level	Amresh Shrivastava	2000
	Thyroid hormones	Jalaj Saxena	2000
	Is estrogen a biological neuroleptic?	Subhagata Chattopadyay	2003
Neuroimaging	Structural changes in the brain in schizophrenia: a computed tomographic study	S. K. Jayaswal	1987
	ECT and T2 relaxometry: A static Walter proton magnetic resonance imaging study	K. Girish	2001
	Reduced caudate volume in never-treated schizophrenia	Ganesan V.	2003
	Enlargement of the third ventricle in affective disorders	Rano Bhadoria	2003
	Regional brain metabolism in schizophrenia: An FDG-PET study	R. Seethalakshmi	2006
	Study of childhood onset schizophrenia (COS) using SPECT and neuropsychological assessment	Savita Malhotra	2006
	MRI T 2 relaxometry of brain regions and cognitive dysfunction following electroconvulsive therapy	Girish Kunigiri	2007
Therapeutics	Lithium and adrenal cortex	S. Parvathi Devi	1973
	Lithium and kidney	Venkoba Rao	1981
	Lithium and renal functions	N. Sethi	1987
	24-hour serum lithium level	K. Kuruvilla	1989
	Lithium psychiatry	S. K. Khandelwal	1991
	Bioavailability of lithium carbonate	S. K. Tripathi	1993
	Long term effects of lithium	Baljinder Singh	2000
	Lithium toxicity	Ratanendra Kumar	2001
Conceptual, Thematic, Educational and Research	Research training in psychiatry	B. B. Sethi	1968

Topic	Sub-topic	First author	Year of publication
	WHO Collaborating Centre for Psychopharmacology		1974
	Teaching of psychopharmacology	J. V. Ananth	1976
	Handbook of biological psychiatry		1980
	Research in psychiatric genetics in India	R. Srinivasa Murthy	1983
	Psychiatric research	S. M. Channabasavanna	1987
	International collaborations in psychiatric research	S. M. Channabasavanna	1988
	Postpartum psychiatric syndromes: Are they biologically determined?	Shiv Gautam	1989
	National workshop on “ECT: Priorities in research and practice”		1989
	The practice of ECT in India: Issues relating to the administration of ECT	A. K. Agarwal	1992
	The practice of ECT in India: II. The practical administration of ECT	Chittaranjan Andrade	1993
	Do Indian researchers read Indian research?	Chittaranjan Andrade	1994
	Evidence based medicine in psychiatry	J. K. Trivedi	2000
	Clinical methods in psychiatry	Mukul Sharma	2000
	Evidence-based psychiatry: A distant dream?	N. G. Desai	2000
	Your research project	J. S. Srivastava	2001
	Research in biological psychiatry in India	V. Palaniappun	2002
	Research endeavors in child and adolescent psychiatry in India	Shoba Srinath	2002
	Practice of ECT in India		2002
	Mind in Indian philosophy	A. Venkoba Rao	2002
	Glimpses of neurobiological underpinnings of bipolar disorder		2003
	Publication of mental health research from poor income countries: Resolving the information divide!		
	Why “publish or perish?” Why not “publish and prosper?”		
	Perspectives from developing countries	Nimesh G. Desai	2005
	Social origins, biological treatments	Vikram Patel	2005
	Mild cognitive impairment: The dilemma	Charles Pinto	2009

Given these new perspectives, it is not surprising that with new scientific discoveries the field of mental illness is in flux. In this section, I want to describe the nature of some of the current considerations of how we should approach the field of psychopathology from these larger perspectives. In later chapters of this book, I will describe specific approaches in greater detail.

NEUROSCIENCE PERSPECTIVES

Over the past 100 years, there have been a variety of debates on how to diagnose and classify mental disorders. In the past 50 years, the emphasis has been on reliability of diagnosis such that mental health professionals in one location would diagnose the same individual in the same manner as professionals in another location. As part of this emphasis, there has been a push for observable characteristics that would define a specific disorder. Such characteristics as depressed mood over the day, diminished interest in activities, weight loss, insomnia, fatigue, feelings of worthlessness, difficulty thinking, and thoughts of suicide would be considered in the diagnosis of depression. These types of criteria make up the structure of the ***Diagnostic and Statistical Manual of Mental Disorders (DSM),*** published by the American Psychiatric Association (APA), and the ***International Classification of Diseases (ICD),*** published by the World Health Organization (WHO). The *DSM* is used in North America whereas the *ICD* is used in Europe. In general, the criteria used in *DSM* and *ICD* are signs and symptoms that are delineated through observation of, and conversation with, the individual.

More recently, there has been a push to find more objective markers that can be used in the diagnosis and treatment of mental disorders. One approach has been to utilize neuroscience research. With the advent of the various levels of analysis available to neuroscientists including brain imaging, genetics, biochemical and electrophysiological processes, brain networks, behavior, and experience, a variety of researchers have sought to describe cognitive, emotional, and motor processes in both health and illness. This has resulted in a better articulation of what underlies these processes.

One such process is memory. It is possible to describe its underlying process including specific brain areas such as the hippocampus, the brain networks involving memory, and the biochemical and structural changes among neurons as new information is retained. With this knowledge, it is also possible to explore psychopathological conditions such as amnesia or delusions that involve the memory system.

Another example is the **reward system.** Humans seek rewards from a variety of sources, including food, sex, power, acclaim, and affiliation, as well as drugs. A number of studies show that particular brain structures, especially the nucleus accumbens part of the ventral striatum, are influenced by an increase in dopamine during reward (see *Figure 3-1*). In fact, all addictive drugs result in dopamine release in the nucleus accumbens (Pittenger & Etkin, 2008). Individuals with alcoholism show greater activation to alcohol-related cues in the nucleus accumbens and the anterior thalamus. The activation of the nucleus accumbens also correlates with the degree of craving. One approach involving the reward system is to note its involvement in active reward processes such as those seen in addiction or mania as well as those disorders in which reward is reduced such as depression or schizophrenia (Russo & Nestler, 2013).

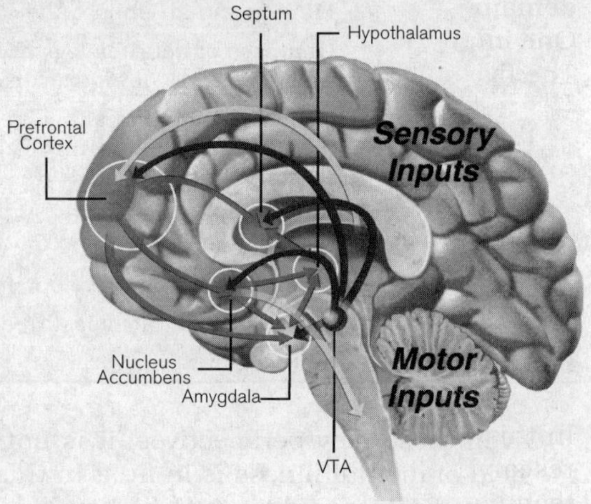

FIGURE 3-1 Reward System of the Brain

Since the beginning of the 21st century, a number of researchers and clinicians have asked whether it would be possible to use neuroscience approaches to classify mental illness and inform its treatment (see Cuthbert & Insel, 2010; Halligan & David, 2001; Hyman, 2007, 2010; Insel, 2009; Miller, 2010; Sanislow et al., 2010, for overviews). Part of this desire stems from the fact that not all individuals with depression, for example, report the same symptoms. This suggests to some researchers that there might be different underlying brain processes involved in what appears as a single disorder. By knowing the underlying processes involved in a particular disorder, it would be possible to create a treatment that was specific to a given individual.

Neuroscience perspectives can also help validate theoretical constructs used in a variety of theoretical orientations. For example, Carhart-Harris and Friston (2010) examined the relationship between brain network processes and Freudian constructs. Likewise, DeRubeis, Siegle, and Hollon (2008) examined the different pathways of treatment found for cognitive therapy versus medication in the treatment of depression. These researchers suggested that cognitive therapy works from a top-down approach by increasing higher cortical functioning associated with the frontal lobes whereas medication works in a more bottom-up approach by decreasing excessive emotional responsiveness associated with the amygdala.

In India, as listed here, several large institutions help to take forward the work of establishing biopsychosocial underpinnings of abnormal behavior. NIMHANS is one of these.

As can be seen, the objectives are designed to identify the manner in which brain processes are involved in a specific disorder, to better describe the course of a mental disorder including when the first signs appear—even if abnormal processes are not yet seen—to use this knowledge to create a treatment related to a given individual, and to make these treatments available to all members of society. Thus, traditional neuroscience perspectives that reflect action on the level of genetics, the neuron, and neural networks are integrated with research perspectives related to more system-level cognitive, emotional, and behavioral processes.

More specific research domains referred to as **Research Domain Criteria (RDoC)** have been articulated by a variety of conferences supported by NIMH. At this point, five domains have been established to better clarify our understanding of psychopathology. One important aspect is to consider how these systems are disrupted in psychopathology. The five domains are as follows:

1. Negative affect—includes fear, distress, and aggressions
2. Positive affect—includes reward seeking, learning, and the creation of habits
3. Cognition—includes how individuals conceptualize and think about themselves and their environment
4. Social processes—includes how individuals experience and view others
5. Regulatory systems—includes the variety of individuals' regulatory systems ranging from sleep–wake cycles to the manner in which they regulate their emotions

In this book, I will follow the current *DSM* classification system as well as include critical research from the neurosciences. This chapter will describe specific neuroscience techniques and broad theoretical considerations. But first, let us briefly consider some important perspectives that will be expanded upon throughout this book.

What Are Endophenotypes?

In a move to go beyond using only the signs and symptoms of psychopathology, there has been a search for stable internal physiological or psychological markers for a disorder (see Gottesman & Hanson, 2005; Gottesman & Shields, 1972; Insel & Cuthbert, 2009; Miller & Rockstroh, 2013). Such markers have been called **endophenotypes.** Unlike symptoms that can be observed, endophenotypes cannot be seen except with special equipment and computational analysis such as seen in brain imaging procedures or patterns of performance on neuropsychological tests. For example, individuals with a particular disorder may show particular types of electroencephalogram (EEG) responses to certain stimuli or a particular pattern of brain activity that is different from that seen in healthy individuals. Endophenotypes are patterns of processes that lie between the gene (the genotype) and the manifestations of the gene in the external environment (the phenotype).

Like genes, the presence of the endophenotype itself does not mean that the disorder itself will be present. For example, a specific endophenotype may be seen in both first degree relatives and a person with schizophrenia although the relatives themselves do not have schizophrenia. As such, an endophenotype can help to identify the systems involved in a particular disorder as well as note which genes are influenced by environmental and other internal factors related to a disorder. The potential of endophenotypes is their ability to better articulate the relationship between genetic and environmental factors in the development of psychopathology and to clarify which processes are influenced. Some interesting work on endophenotypes in schizophrenia has been reported from India (Solanki, Kumar, Satija, Gupta, & Singh, 2016).

Genes

Genes form the blueprint that determines what an organism is to become. HOX genes, for example, lay out the basic structures in all organisms. In fact, HOX genes are found in the order that the body parts are structured, that is, going from head to tail. It is the same genes that produce the long neck of a giraffe as the short neck of a turtle. The difference lies in the manner in which they are turned on and turned off. Other genes are less involved in the structure of an organism and more involved in function. For example, the learning of songs in some birds is influenced by the turning on and off of specific genes. In some species, this is a onetime event in which the song remains the same throughout the bird's life. In others, the songs can change.

Specific genes have been associated with a variety of disorders as will be described throughout this book. However, the original hope of finding a few genes that were involved in particular mental disorders has not panned out. What has become apparent is that there is a complex interaction of genetic and environmental factors involved in mental illness. Just having a gene does not mean that it is active—it turns on or off under a complex set of circumstances.

As the factors involved have become more complicated, there has been a search for particular processes related to psychopathology. For example, there exists a gene (SERT) that is involved in the removal of the neurotransmitter serotonin from the synapse. A variant of the SERT gene has been associated with depression, alcoholism, eating disorders, ADHD, and autism (see Serretti, Calati, Mandelli, & De Ronchi, 2006, for an overview). Likewise, a variant of the gene (DßH), which is associated with the synthesis of norepinephrine from dopamine, is associated with schizophrenia, cocaine-induced paranoia, depression, ADHD, and alcoholism (Cubells & Zabetian, 2004). It is suggested that the lower level of the **proteins** produced by the DßH gene is associated with a vulnerability to psychotic symptoms.

As researchers discover genes related to specific forms of mental illness, there may be a need to reorganize the manner in which we view mental illness. One study analyzed the genes from 33,332 individuals with a mental disorder in comparison with 27,888 without a disorder (*Cross-Disorder Group of the Psychiatric Genomics Consortium* et al., 2013). This research suggests that similar genetic risk factors involved in calcium channel signaling exist for what we have considered to be separate disorders. These five disorders are autism spectrum disorder, schizophrenia, bipolar disorder, major depressive disorder, and ADHD. This study suggests that a particular genetic makeup may put some individuals at higher risk for developing a variety of disorders. There is also research that suggests that having certain mental disorders such as schizophrenia may actually protect these individuals from having certain types of cancer (Tabarés-Seisdedos & Rubenstein, 2013).

How Does the Environment Play a Role in Genetics?

As researchers studied how genes turn on and off and what factors influence this, the story became even more complicated—the processes that determine which genes turn on and off could themselves be passed on to the next generation. Of course, which factors turn the genes on and off are largely influenced by the environment of the organism. Thus, although the genes themselves could not be influenced by the environment, it was possible for the environment to influence future generations through its changes to those processes that turn genes on and off. This is referred to as **epigenetics** and will be described later in this chapter.

Overall, current genetic research suggests a complicated relationship between genetic conditions and environmental factors. For example, the MAOA gene, which is located on the X chromosome, makes the **neurotransmitters** serotonin, norepinephrine, and dopamine inactive and is associated with aggression in mice and humans. Caspi and his colleagues (2002) performed a longitudinal study and found that mistreatment as a child influenced some boys differently from others later in adulthood. Those boys who were mistreated in childhood and had a particular form of the MAOA gene were more likely to be violent and engage in a variety of antisocial behaviors as adults including problems with law enforcement officials. Those without this particular form of the gene did not display antisocial behaviors even if they had been mistreated as children. Thus, environmental influences in terms of maltreatment modulate the expression of specific genetic structures but not the expression of others.

Neural Networks

Given that the human brain has some 100 billon neurons with 50 to 200 trillion connections, it is clear that a higher-level analysis is necessary. A variety of brain imaging techniques have allowed for a network analysis that describes which areas of the brain are involved in specific tasks. The first step has been to describe the normal processing of networks such as those involved in reward or fear. The next step is to understand how these networks become involved in addiction and anxiety. In delineating networks involved in psychopathology, the task is to understand how the basic network becomes involved in psychopathological processes. Is it a lack of connections between brain areas, or is there a reorganization of normal processes that underlie specific psychopathologies? This is one question scientists are asking.

Networks have been studied in terms of a variety of cognitive and emotional tasks (Bressler & Menon, 2010). Three specific networks have been examined in terms of psychopathology (Menon, 2011). These are the baseline or default network (also called the intrinsic network), the **central executive network,** and the **salience network.** The default network is active when an individual is not performing a particular task such as when one's mind wanders or is processing internal information. The central executive network is involved in higher order cognitive and attentional tasks. The salience network is important for monitoring critical external events as well as internal states. As will be described in detail later, psychopathological disorders such as schizophrenia, depression, anxiety, dementia, and autism have been shown to have problems in turning networks on or off as well as problems in the connections within the network itself.

The historical considerations of psychopathology emphasized careful observation and interaction with the afflicted individuals as important methods for understanding the nature of the disorder. However, with progress in the neurosciences, brain imaging, and genetics, other levels of analysis have become possible. The new levels offer different perspectives for the field of mental illness, but because many of these discoveries are so new, it is not surprising that our understanding of the field of mental illness is currently in flux. Neuroscience research has been used to find more objective markers in the diagnosis and treatment of mental disorders. It has also helped describe cognitive, emotional, and motor processes in both health and illness. This has resulted in a better articulation of what underlies these processes such as problems in setting goals, having relationships with others, thinking, and feeling, as well as deficits in the memory system and the reward system. Let us now move from a higher-level consideration of the systems involved in psychopathology to some of the specific techniques that are used to understand psychopathological processes.

NEUROSCIENCE TECHNIQUES AND LEVELS OF ANALYSIS

As described in terms of the story of David who did not recognize his mother as his mother, there are a number of levels to describe human behavior. In this book, I take an integrative perspective that draws on a number of levels. I do not consider any one of these levels of analysis as more important or more true than another. We can both ask a person what he is experiencing as well as observe what he is doing. By considering a number of levels at the same time, it is possible to obtain a more complete picture. For example, it is possible to image brain activity while an individual is solving a cognitive problem or recognizing facial

Concept Check

- What does it mean that mental disorders can be described in both a categorical and a dimensional manner? Discuss some of the advantages of including underlying processes in the study of psychopathology.
- Why is the reliability of diagnosis an important aspect of psychological treatment? What has been the contribution of the *DSM* and the *ICD* in improving reliability?
- Identify three specific ways in which neuroscience approaches have been utilized to classify mental illness and inform its treatment.
- Which three specific networks have been examined in terms of psychopathology? How do these networks become involved in psychopathology?

emotions. In doing this, it is possible to see how individuals with a particular mental disorder perform cognitive and emotional tasks differently from those without the disorder. One word of warning—currently, we have no neuroscience technique that can definitively diagnose a given individual in terms of mental disorders. What we can say is that a group of individuals with a particular disorder appear differently on certain measures than a group of individuals without the disorder.

To understand mental illness as a brain disease, we need methods for showing how the brain is involved in psychopathology (see Andreasen, 2001). Within the past two decades, a variety of research techniques have been developed that allow us to better specify the nature of mental disorders from the standpoint of the brain. Most of these techniques are described as neuroscience approaches. In general, these approaches have allowed researchers to study individuals with mental disorders on a number of levels simultaneously.

Historically, what we now consider neuroscience approaches to psychopathology were limited. Broca for example in the 1800s needed to wait until his patients died before he could study the nature of their brains. In the early part of the 20th century, work with animals was the major way of understanding how the various structures of the brain influenced behavior. Some scholars such as Carl Jung added EDA to reaction time research. Jung used the word association test developed by Wilhelm Wundt to better understand psychopathology and how individuals with different disorders process cognitive and emotional information. The second part of the 20th century expanded a tradition that used psychophysiological measures such as **electroencephalography (EEG)** and EDA to study psychopathology. Within the current century, a variety of noninvasive techniques allow researchers and clinicians to obtain a better view of how the brain and other physiological systems function in psychopathology. These will be reviewed in this current chapter.

THE BRAIN

The brain works in terms of one basic element, the neuron. Over millions and even billions of years of evolution, the neuron has served as the basic building block of organisms. Although neurons come in a variety of sizes and shapes, there are some basic characteristics as shown in *Figure 3-2*:

1. The cell body contains a nucleus, which includes **deoxyribonucleic acid (DNA)** and other processes including mitochondria which are involved in supplying energy.
2. The axon comes from the cell body and is involved in conveying information. Axons can be fairly short as found in the human brain or four or five feet in length such as those that go from the spinal cord to the arms and legs.
3. The dendrites receive information from other cells.

The dendrites receive information from other neurons, which terminate at different locations on the dendrites. Although illustrations in textbooks usually show only a few connections between neurons, there are generally thousands of these connections. The terminal branches from these other neurons do not actually touch but make a biochemical

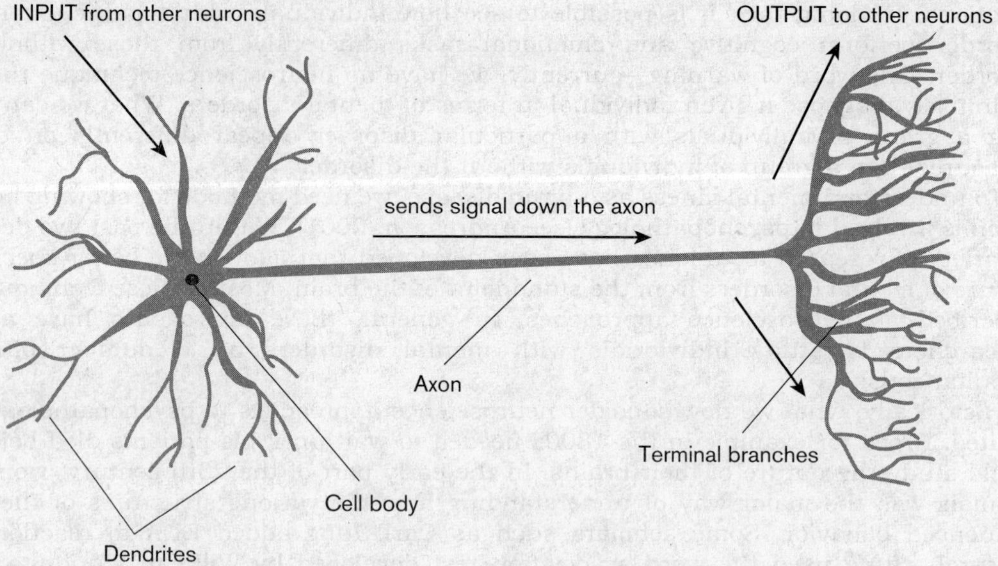

FIGURE 3-2 Basic Characteristics of Neurons

Source: Sobel and Li (2013).

connection through a small gap filled with fluid, which is referred to as a synapse. These biochemical connections can release molecules (ions) with an electrical charge.

As more of these electrical charges add together, it increases the size of the electrical potential. At a critical point, an action potential is produced at a location near the cell body, which travels quickly down the axon in one direction. An action potential is referred to as an "all or none" signal since above the critical value an action potential is produced whereas below the critical value, no electrical activity is sent down the axon.

The speed at which the action potential travels down the axon depends on two factors:

1. The width of the axon. Action potentials travel faster in larger diameter axons.
2. Whether the axon is covered with an insulating material called the myelin sheath. Action potentials travel faster in axons surrounded by myelin.

Thus, an axon with a larger diameter and wrapped in myelin would have the fastest conduction times. Disorders such as multiple sclerosis and autism show deficits in axonal connections.

It should be noted that there are two major types of synapses:

1. One type, referred to as a chemical synapse, involves secretion from the previous neuron of various types of neurotransmitters. These neurotransmitters create a current flow. This changes the physiological state of the next (postsynaptic) neuron such that it is more likely (excitatory) or less likely (inhibitory) to create an action potential (see *Figure 3-3*).
2. The second type of synapse is electrical in nature. Current flows through special channels that connect the gap between the two neurons.

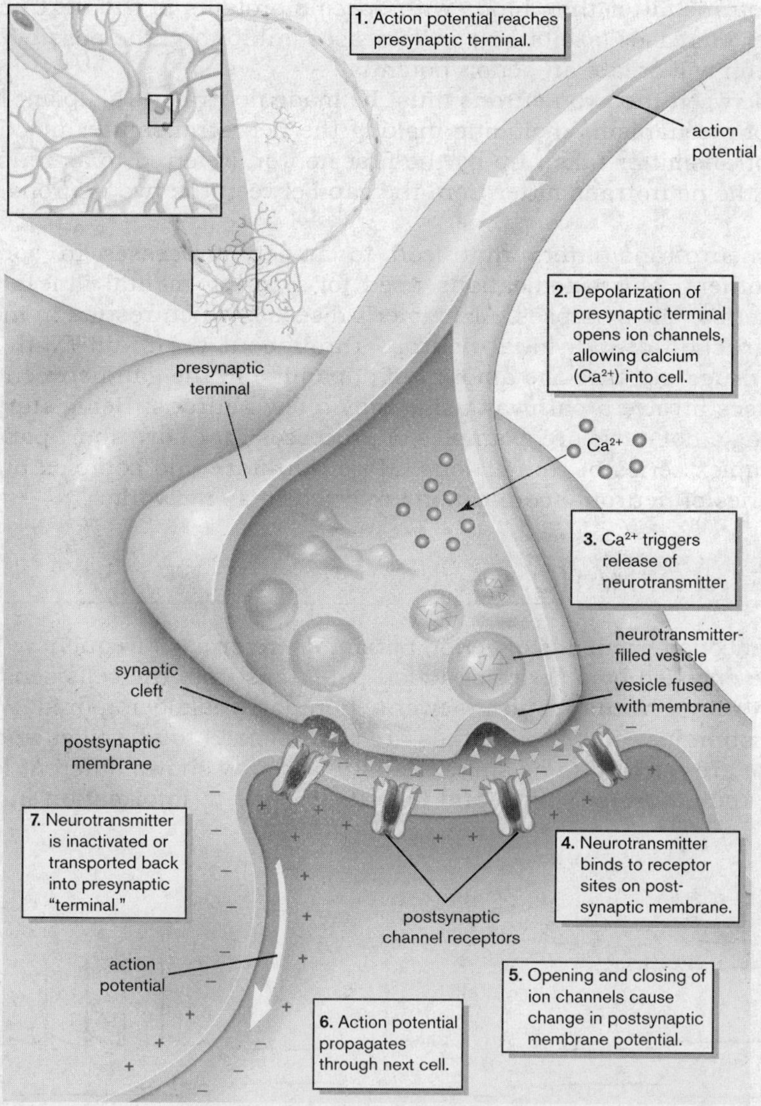

FIGURE 3-3 Depiction of the Structures and Processes of Synapses

Source:

HOW DOES THE NEURON PASS INFORMATION?

Passing information from one neuron to another involves a number of steps:

1. Neurotransmitters need to be created and stored.
2. An action potential travels down the axon to the terminal.
3. Through a variety of processes a neurotransmitter is released into the gap between the two neurons.

4. The neurotransmitter then binds with specific proteins in the next neuron.
5. This either increases (excitatory) or decreases (inhibitory) the possibility that the next neuron will create an action potential.
6. The gap between the two neurons must be made neutral at this point by any of a number of mechanisms including making the neurotransmitter inactive, having the neurotransmitter taken up by the first neuron (referred to as reuptake), and removing the neurotransmitter from the gap between the two neurons.

It is these neurotransmitters that lead to anxiety processes in some cases but depression in others. Most medications used for treating mental illness influence the neurotransmitters at the synapses. Alzheimer's disease, which results in memory loss, is caused by destruction of individual neurons throughout the brain (Nath et al., 2012). Most addictive drugs increase the amount of dopamine in the gap between the neurons.

Some processes involve a pathway using only a few neurons. Being startled by a loud noise or touching a hot stove are examples of processes that have short pathways. Others use a more complex series of connections. More voluntary and complex processes use a much larger series of neuronal connections referred to as networks.

ENCODING INFORMATION

Information is encoded by means of action potentials in terms of frequency. That is, a loud sound would be encoded by a series of action potentials from the cells sensitive to sound intensity. A soft sound would result in fewer action potentials being fired. When observed in relation to a stimulus, action potentials are also referred to as spikes and a number of spikes over time are referred to as spike trains. *Figure 3-4* shows different levels of firing. Understanding the nature of spikes and how they relate to information in the brain has

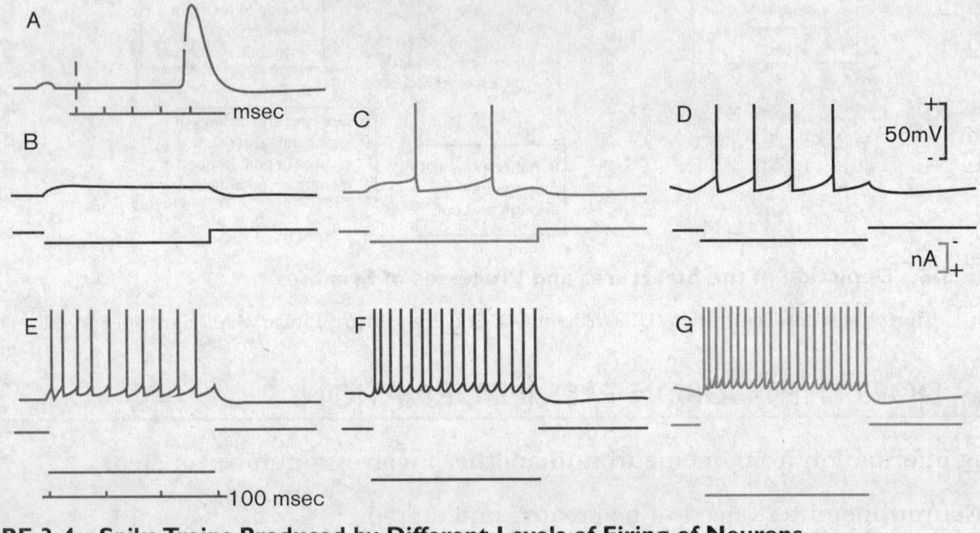

FIGURE 3-4 Spike Trains Produced by Different Levels of Firing of Neurons

Source: Spencer, W. (2011). The Physiology of Supraspinal Neurons in Mammals. *Supplement 1: Handbook of Physiology, The Nervous System, Cellular Biology of Neurons*, pp. 969–1021. First published in print 1977.

been an important question since the beginning of the 20th century when they were first recorded (see Rieke, Warland, van Steveninck, & Bialek, 1999, for an overview).

The early work on spike trains was performed at Cambridge University in the United Kingdom by Lord Adrian (see Adrian, 1928, for an overview). From this work, three important observations were obtained:

1. Although there are a variety of sensory systems (e.g., vision, audition), the neurons connected to these all produce similar action potentials to external stimuli. This universality is seen across a variety of species.
2. The rate of spiking increases as the stimulus becomes larger.
3. If a given stimulus is continued for a long period of time, the spiking will decrease (referred to as habituation).

Unique Aspects of the Human Brain

One common conviction of neuroscientists is that there is something unusual about the human brain that leads to our abilities to perform a variety of tasks (Northcutt & Kaas, 1995; Preuss & Kaas, 1999). The human brain has been estimated to contain 100 billion neurons and more than 100,000 kilometers of interconnections (Hofman, 2001). Estimates in mammals suggest that a given neuron would directly connect to at least 500 and probably more other neurons. This, in turn, would suggest there are 50 trillion different connections in the human brain!

Regardless of how exact this estimate may be, the conclusion is that the human brain has an extremely complex set of networks. Neurons created before birth follow chemical or other pathways in the brain to create the necessary connections to allow for vision, hearing, and other processes. There is also the suggestion that neurons are created in humans after birth. A 1-year-old infant has more neurons than she will have throughout her life.

In infancy, use is important. In the first year of life, an individual can recognize any sound used in any language in the world. However, the ability to hear those sounds that are not part of the languages one hears is lost after infancy. Likewise, if a child is born unable to hear, the normal initial babbling behaviors will be produced during the first year of life but then lost. These types of disuse and loss take place on a neuronal level. Unused neurons die.

Concept Check

- We think of neuroscience techniques as being new and "high tech," but throughout history researchers have used various neuroscience approaches to study the brain and psychopathology. Identify four of these approaches, and describe how they advanced our understanding of psychopathology.
- "The brain works in terms of one basic element, the neuron." What are the different parts that form the structure of the neuron, and what roles do they play?
- How does the neuron pass information on to other neurons, and how is that information encoded?

HOW DO WE OBSERVE THE BRAIN AT WORK?

With 100 billion neurons and 50 to 200 trillion connections between neurons in the human brain, understanding these connections on a neuronal level would be an impossible task. However, scientists have been able to use the manner in which neurons work as a window into their function. A variety of techniques for observing activity in the brain have been developed.

Currently, the major types of brain imaging techniques are EEG, **magnetoencephalography (MEG), positron emission tomography (PET),** and **functional magnetic resonance imaging (fMRI).** EEG is a technique for recording electrical activity from the scalp related to cortical activity. MEG measures the small magnetic field gradients exiting and entering the surface of the head that are produced when neurons are active. PET is a measure related to blood flow in the brain, which reflects cognitive processing. fMRI is based on the fact that blood flow increases in active areas of the cortex. It is also possible to use the magnetic resonance imaging (MRI) magnet to measure cortical connections in the brain, which is referred to as **diffusion tensor imaging (DTI).**

Electroencephalography

EEG is a technique for recording electrical activity from the scalp related to cortical activity. It reflects the electrical activity of the brain at the level of the synapse (Nunez & Srinivasan, 2006). It is the product of the changing excitatory and inhibitory currents. Action potentials contribute very little to the EEG. However, since changes at the synapse do influence the production of action potentials, there is an association of EEG with spike trains (Whittingstall & Logothetis, 2009).

The EEG was first demonstrated in humans by Hans Berger in 1924 and published 5 years later (Berger, 1929/1969). Since the neurons of the brain and their connections are constantly active, EEG can be measured during both wake and sleep. In fact, EEG serves as an objective measure of depth of sleep (see *Figure 3-5*).

EEG can be measured with only two electrodes or as a high density array of more than 200 electrodes. EEG activity has been used to infer brain processing. The actual measure of EEG is the difference between the signals at any two electrodes. Traditionally, the second or reference electrode was placed at a location not considered to produce electrical signals, for example, the ear lobe.

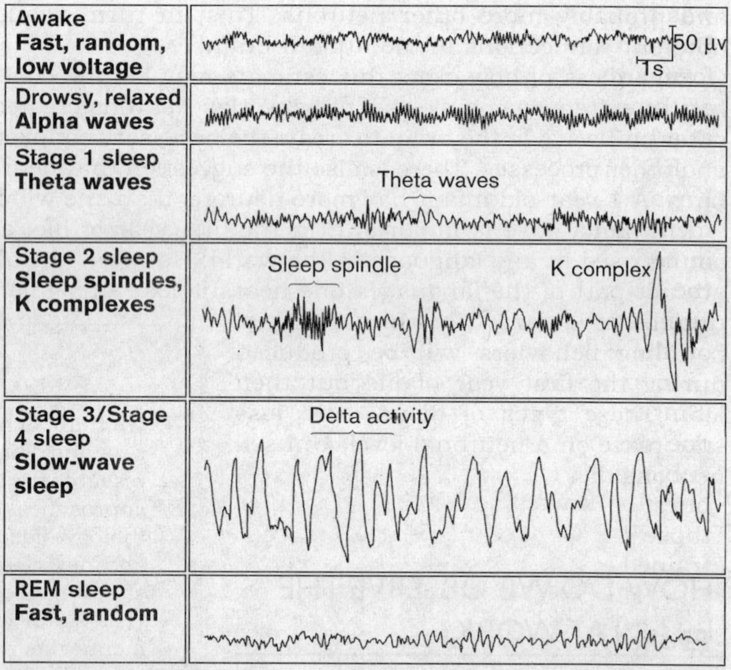

FIGURE 3-5 Electroencephalogram as an Objective Measure of Sleep

Source: *Current Concepts: The Sleep Disorders*. P. Hauri, 1982, Kalamazoo, MI: Upjohn.

Today, a common practice is to average the signals in all of the electrodes available and compare that with each specific electrode.

Some aspects of the EEG signal may appear almost random while other fluctuations appear periodic. Using signal processing techniques, it is possible to determine the major frequency and amplitude seen in the signal. Amplitude refers to how large the signal is, and frequency refers to how fast the signal cycles measured in cycles per second, or Hertz (Hz). Over the years, researchers have noticed that specific patterns of EEG activity were associated with a variety of psychological states (see *Figure 3-6*). When an individual is relaxed with his or her eyes closed, high amplitude regular activity is seen in the EEG at a frequency of 8 to 12 Hz. Alpha activity in the 8 to 12 Hz range was the first pattern of EEG activity Hans Berger noted. If the person begins to perform some mental activity such as mental arithmetic, lower amplitude EEG is seen at a higher frequency above 20 Hz.

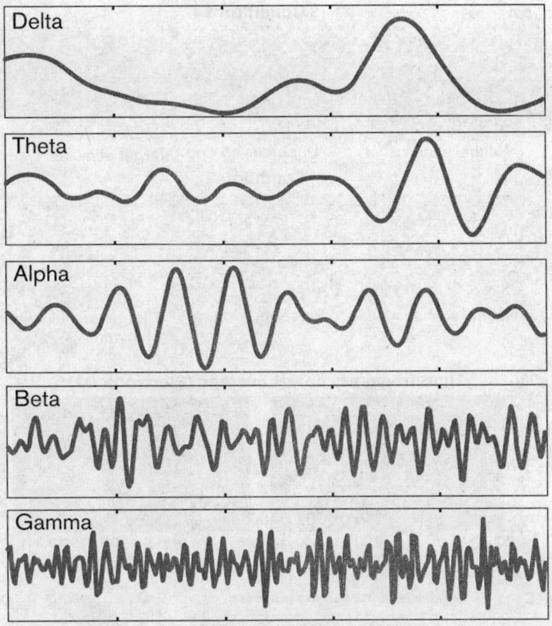

FIGURE 3-6 Depiction of Specific Patterns of Electroencephalography Activity

Source: Hugo Gambo (2005), Wikipedia.

EEG oscillations are one way in which information is transferred in the brain (see Knyazev, 2007, for an overview). For example, theta oscillations are associated with memory performance (Liebe, Hoerzer, Logothetis, & Rainer, 2012). Theta is also involved in coordinating emotional information between the limbic areas and the frontal areas of the brain. Delta oscillations are seen in motivational processes such as drug use. Drugs such as cocaine produce changes in a number of EEG frequency bands. Alpha oscillations, on the other hand, are involved in inhibiting the activity of various brain areas.

In recent years, researchers have become interested in the processing of a percept (Singer, 2009; Singer & Gray, 1995; Tallon-Baudry & Bertrand, 1999). For example, when one sees the Dalmatian dog against the black-and-white background, there is usually a subjective experience of having the image "pop out." Associated with this perception is a burst of EEG gamma activity. This figure compares the amount of EEG gamma activity in those individuals trained to see the Dalmatian as compared with those who were not trained (see *Figure 3-7*).

Evoked Potentials

Event-related potentials (ERPs), also known as **evoked potentials (EP),** show EEG activity in relation to a particular event. Imagine taking a continuous EEG signal during which a picture or tone is presented to an individual a number of times. If we were to take the EEG in the half second following the stimulus presentation and average these together,

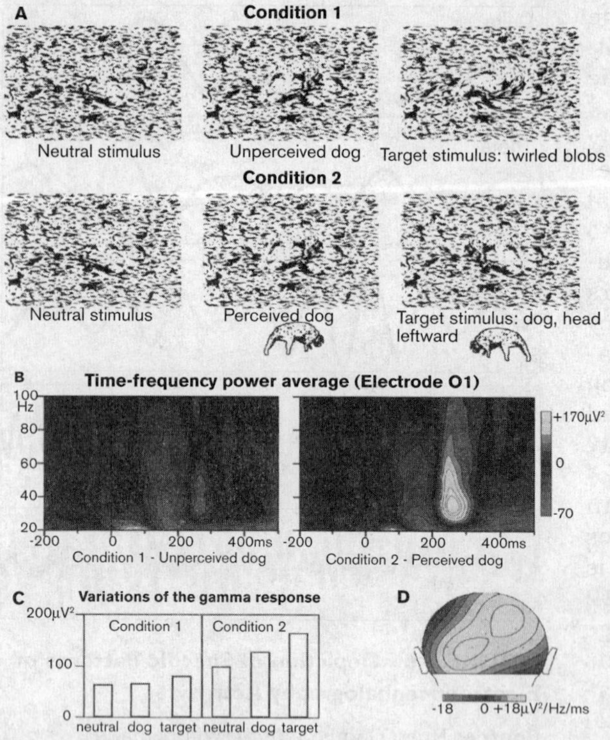

FIGURE 3-7 Wavelet Analysis Associated With Seeing the Dalmatian Dog

Reprinted from *Trends in Cognitive Sciences*, Vol. 3, Catherine Tallon-Baudry and Olivier Bertrand, Oscillatory gamma activity in humans and its role in object representation, pp. 151–162, Copyright © 1999, with permission from Elsevier.

we would have the brain response to the stimulus (see *Figure 3-8*).

The waveform of the ERP is described in terms of positive and negative peaks and the time elapsed from the stimulus presentation. Thus, a P300 waveform is a peak in the ERP in the positive direction occurring 300 milliseconds after the stimulus presentation. Based on early recording equipment characteristics, positive peaks are often shown pointing downward and negative peaks upward. For simplicity, P300 is sometimes referred to as P3 since it represents the third positive peak following a stimulus presentation. Thus, one sees both N1 or P3 as well as N100 or P300 in the literature.

Magnetoencephalography

MEG measures the small magnetic field gradients exiting and entering the surface of the head that are produced when neurons are active. It uses a SQUID (superconducting quantum interference device) to detect small magnetic activity that results from the activity of neurons. As shown above, the person simply puts her head in a device that contains magnetic sensors.

MEG signals are similar to EEG signals but have one important advantage. This advantage stems from the fact that magnetic fields are not distorted when they pass through the cortex and the skull. This makes it possible to be more accurate in terms of spatial location of the signal with MEG. For example, youth with bipolar disorder show greater activation in the frontal gyrus and less in the insula following negative feedback than do control participants (Rich et al., 2011).

Positron Emission Tomography

PET is a measure related to blood flow in the brain that reflects cognitive processing. PET systems measure variations in cerebral blood flow that are correlated with brain activity. It is through blood flow that the brain obtains the oxygen and glucose from which it gets its energy. By measuring changes in blood flow in different brain areas, it is possible to infer which areas of the brain are more or less active during particular tasks. Blood flow using PET is measured after participants inhale, or are injected with, a tracer (a radioactive isotope) that travels in the bloodstream and is recorded by the PET scanner (a gamma ray detector). *Figure 3-9* shows a PET scan in which individuals with

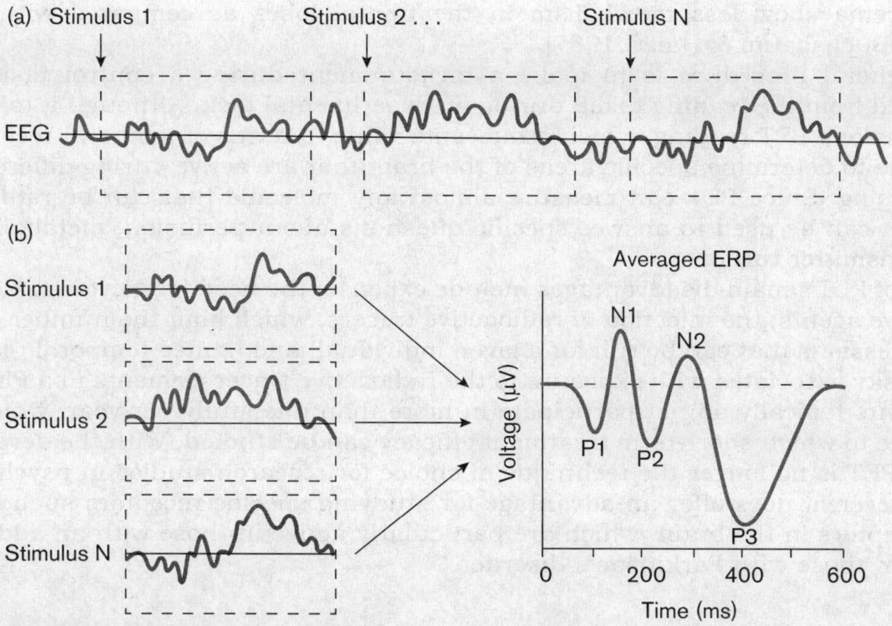

FIGURE 3-8 Extraction of the Event-Related Potential Waveform From the Ongoing Electroencephalography

Reprinted from *Trends in Cognitive Sciences,* Vol. 4, Steven J. Luck, Geoffrey F. Woodman, and Edward K. Vogel, Event-related potential studies of attention, pp. 432–440, Copyright © 2000, with permission from Elsevier.

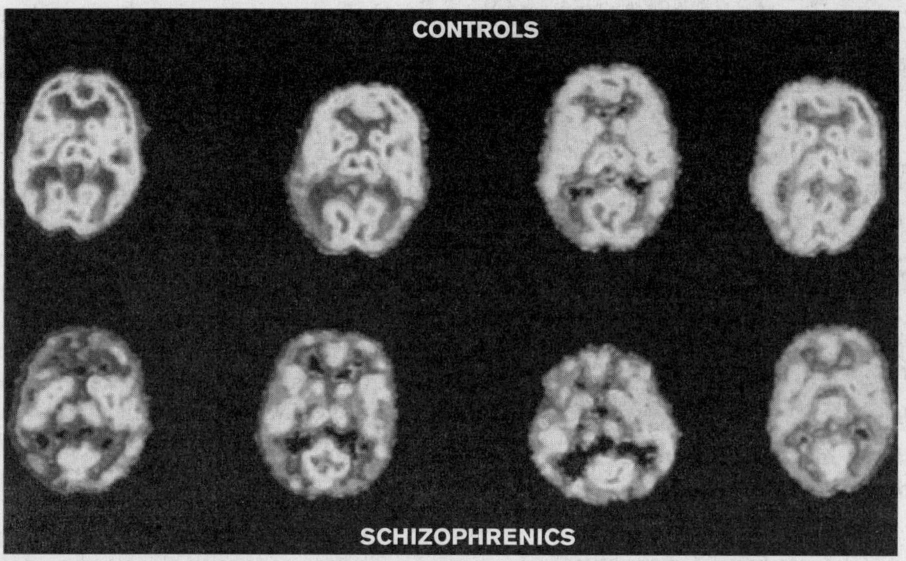

FIGURE 3-9 Comparing Positron Emission Tomography Scans Between Schizophrenics and Controls

Source: Buchsbaum, M. S., & Haier, R. J. (1987). Functional and Anatomical Brain Imaging: Impact on Schizophrenia Research. *Schizophrenia Bulletin, 13*(1), 115–132.

schizophrenia show less metabolism in the frontal lobes as compared with healthy controls (Buchsbaum & Haier, 1987).

The general procedure is to make a measurement during a control task that is subtracted from the reading taken during an experimental task. Although it takes some time to make a PET reading, which reduces its value in terms of temporal resolution, it is possible to determine specific areas of the brain that are active during different types of processing. Since PET can measure almost any molecule that can be radioactively labeled, it can be used to answer specific questions about perfusion, metabolism, and neurotransmitter turnover.

Some of PET's main disadvantages include expense; the need for a cyclotron to create radioactive agents; the injection of radioactive tracers, which limit the number of experimental sessions that can be run for a given individual; and limited temporal resolution. Due to risks associated with exposure to the radioactive tracer elements in a PET study, participants typically do not participate in more than one study per year, which limits the degree to which short-term treatment efficacy can be studied. With the development of fMRI, PET is no longer the technique of choice for research studies in psychopathology. However, it does offer an advantage for studying specific receptors such as dopamine receptors in the brain, which are particularly active in those with an addiction or inactive in those with Parkinson's disorder.

Functional Magnetic Resonance Imaging

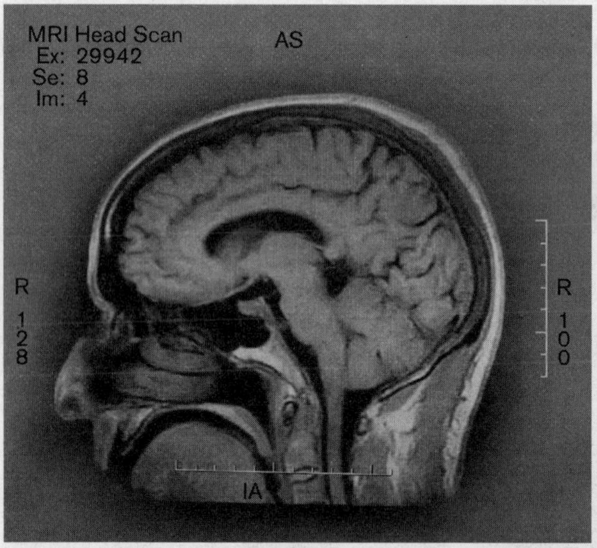

FIGURE 3-10 Magnetic Resonance Imaging Shows the Anatomy of the Brain but Does Not Reflect Activity

Source: ©iStockphoto.com/CGinspiration

fMRI is based on the fact that blood flow increases in active areas of the cortex. Specifically, hemoglobin, which carries oxygen in the bloodstream, has different magnetic properties before and after oxygen is absorbed. Thus, by measuring the ratio of hemoglobin with and without oxygen, the fMRI is able to map changes in cortical blood and infer neuronal activity.

Measurements using fMRI are made by having a person lie on his back inside a large magnet and radio frequency device, which measures changes in blood oxygen levels. Initially a structural image of the brain is created (see *Figure 3-10*). A structure image (MRI), like an X-ray, shows the anatomy of the brain but does not reflect activity. However, a reduction in brain volume is seen in a variety of disorders including schizophrenia. These measures can be determined from the MRI.

Brain activity can be determined with the fMRI, or functional MRI. A common procedure for showing brain activity is to take a baseline in which the person just relaxes. Following this baseline period, specific tasks are performed. The fMRI response recorded during the task is subtracted from that during baseline. This shows which specific areas of the brain are involved in performing a task. This information is then placed on the structural MRI image of the brain as shown in *Figure 3-11*. The color used reflects the amount of activity seen in a particular brain area. As you will see throughout this book, fMRI has been used with almost every disorder discussed. You can also compare one group of individuals with another. For example, *Figure 3-12* shows that women with post-traumatic stress disorder (PTSD) activate different areas of the brain (the amygdala and insula) when processing emotional information compared with women without PTSD (Bruce et al., 2013).

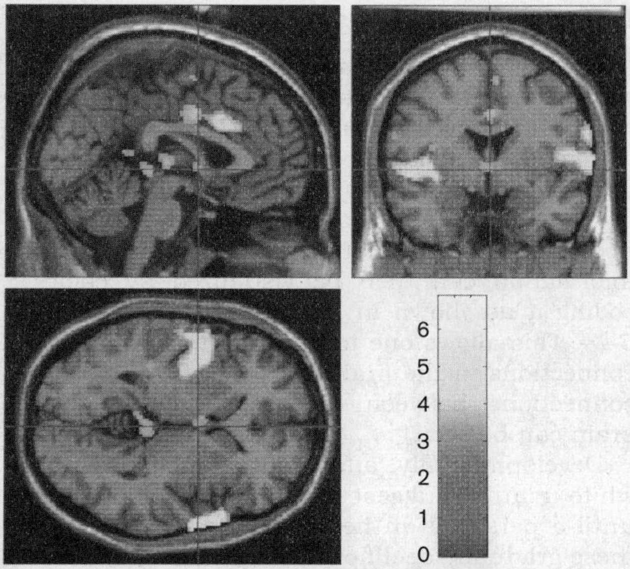

FIGURE 3-11 Functional Magnetic Resonance Imaging—Color Reflects the Amount of Activity Seen in a Particular Brain Area

Source: © Zephry/Science Source.

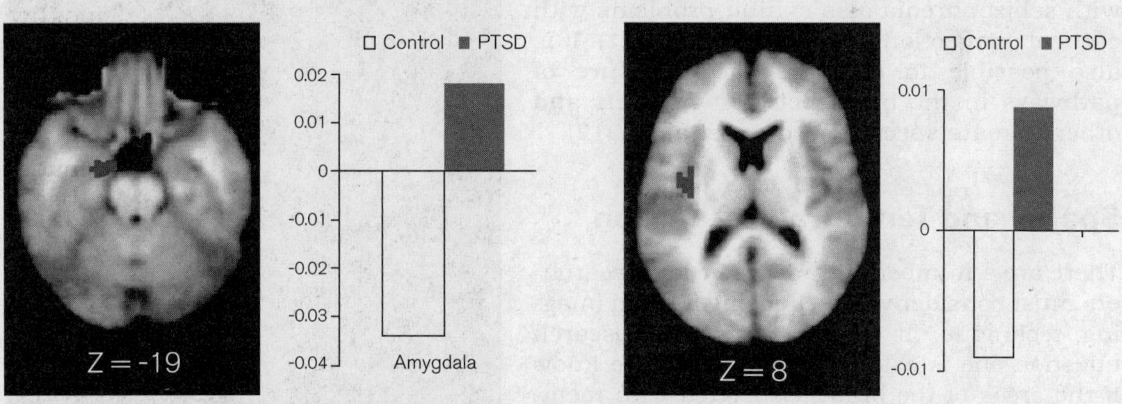

FIGURE 3-12 Brain Activation Differences in the Amygdala and Insula for Those With Post-Traumatic Stress Disorder Compared With Healthy Controls

Reprinted from *NeuroImage:* *Clinical,* Vol. 2, Steven E. Bruce, Katherine R. Buchholz, Wilson J. Brown, Laura Yan, Anthony Durbin, and Yvette I. Sheline, Altered emotional interference processing in the amygdala and insula in women with post-traumatic stress disorder, pp. 43–49, Copyright © 2013, with permission from Elsevier.

Diffusion Tensor Imaging

It is also possible to use the MRI magnet to measure cortical connections in the brain, which is referred to as DTI. DTI is available with most MRI imaging systems (see Thomason & Thompson, 2011, for an overview of DTI and psychopathology). It is a procedure for showing fiber tracts (white matter) in the brain. This information can then be visualized by color coding it as shown in *Figure 3-13* and *Figure 3-14*. This allows one to map the white matter connections in the brain. In these figures, the connections between different parts of the brain can be seen.

Developmentally, after infancy measures of white matter suggest a linear development until a person is in her 30s. After a plateau, these gradually decline with age. Using DTI, it is possible to map the mild cognitive impairment seen in dementia and the more severe impairment seen in Alzheimer's disorder. Disconnections are seen between the major areas involved in memory such as the hippocampus and the temporal lobes (Stebbins & Murphy, 2009). As would be expected, this loss of connectivity is greater in Alzheimer's than in mild cognitive impairment. Individuals with schizophrenia also exhibit problems with cortical connections (Phillips et al., 2011). It is also possible to compare the structure of pathways in the brain between humans and other primate species (Wedeen et al., 2012).

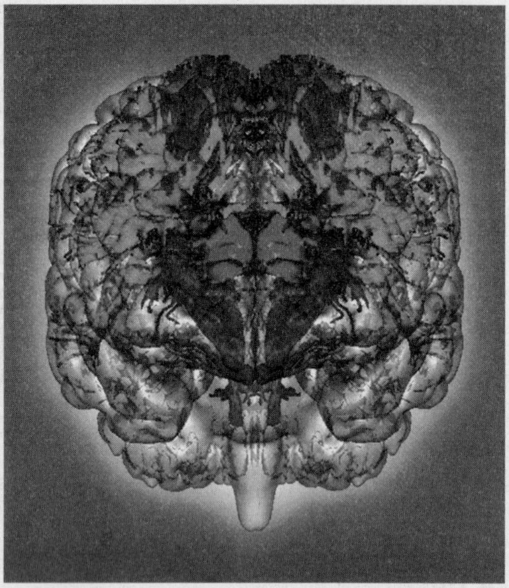

FIGURE 3-13 Mapping White Matter Connections in the Brain With Diffusion Tensor Imaging

Source: © Zephyr/Science Source

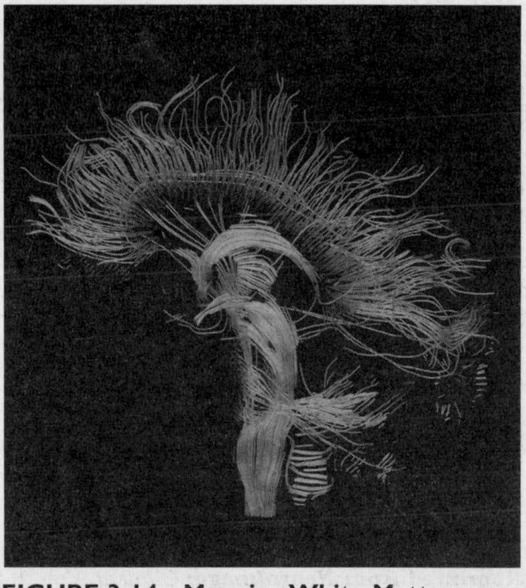

FIGURE 3-14 Mapping White Matter Connections in the Brain Using Color Coding

Source: Thomas Schultz (2006), Wikipedia.

Spatial and Temporal Resolution

There are a number of trade-offs that researchers must consider when choosing a brain imaging technique. It begins with the research question one is asking. If you wanted to know if the areas of the brain associated with memory such as the hippocampus are larger or small in those with PTSD, then you would want a measure of structure. If you wanted to know if those with autism quickly viewed different emotional faces in a different way, then you would want a measure that reflects changes in brain processes.

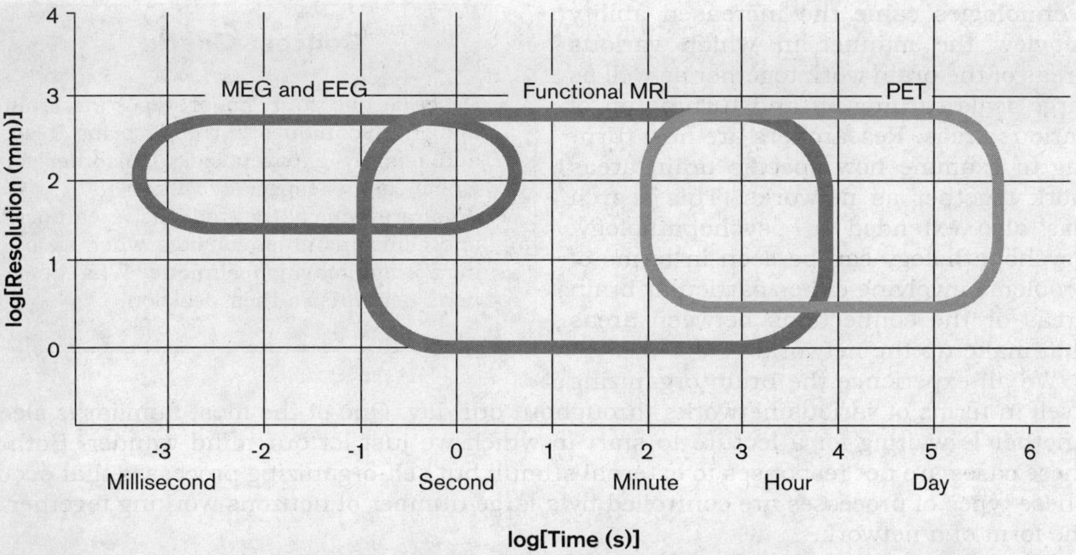

FIGURE 3-15 Spatial and Temporal Resolution of Imaging Techniques

Source: Meyer-Linderberg (2010, p. 194).

One important question is how fast a particular technique can measure change. This is referred to as temporal resolution. EEG and MEG, for example, can measure quick changes in the brain on the millisecond level. PET, on the other hand, can only record changes that take place in a period of a few minutes or more. Another consideration is spatial resolution—that is, what size of brain area can a technique measure? PET and fMRI are better able to pinpoint the location of activity in the brain whereas with EEG it is less possible to know specifically where in the brain activity came from. The relationship between spatial and temporal resolution is shown in *Figure 3-15.*

There are several centers in India that carry out cutting-edge research in imaging. Jaslok Hospital and Research Center, Mumbai, started this journey early with a large the Department of Nuclear Medicine. NIMHANS has excellent imaging facilities and research being conducted in brain imaging.

Some important epidemiological work on epilepsy is reported from NIMHANS (Amudhan, Gururaj, & Satishchandra, 2015; Santhosh, Sinha, & Satishchandra, 2014). Some linkages between epilepsy and genetics are reported as well (Fong et al., 1998). Pediatric epilepsy too is an important area of research in India (see *Journal of Pediatric Neurosciences*, 3, Jan–Jun, 2008). Research is also being done in India on cognitive and behavioral changes in epilepsy (Raha, Shah, & Udani, 2012).

NETWORKS OF THE BRAIN

With the discovery of brain areas involved in particular functions such as Broca's area in the 1800s, researchers searched for specific areas involved in particular cognitive, emotional, and motor processes. With the increased sophistication of brain imaging technologies came the increased ability to view the manner in which various areas of the brain work together as well as large-scale turning off and turning on of various areas. Researchers are now turning to examine how specific brain areas work together as networks. This search has also extended to psychopathology. Psychopathology can be seen in terms of problems involving either particular brain areas or the connections between areas that make up the network.

Concept Check

- Describe the four major types of brain imaging techniques currently being used, and identify a psychological disorder for which each is especially valuable.
- What are some of the tradeoffs researchers and clinicians must consider when choosing a brain imaging technique? What questions help inform their decision?

We all experience the brain organizing itself in terms of various networks throughout our day. One of the most familiar is sleep. Another is waiting for a lecture to start in which we just let our mind wander. Both of these cases are not responses to external stimuli but self-organizing processes that occur. These types of processes are controlled by a large number of neurons working together in the form of a network.

Networks allow our brains to process information efficiently (Laughlin & Sejnowski, 2003; Sporns, 2011). Overall, cortical networks are influenced by experience and designed to be efficient in terms of connections between neurons in the network. This efficiency allows for less use of energy. One way energy is conserved is through not having every neuron connect with every other neuron.

Neurons Connect in a Network

How are neurons connected in a network? The answer may seem strange. Neurons are neither totally random in their connections with other neurons nor totally patterned. It appears that neurons are connected to one another in the same way that all humans on this planet are socially connected.

In the 1960s, the social psychologist Stanley Milgram (Travers & Milgram, 1969) asked the question, "What is the probability that any two people randomly selected from a large population of individuals such as the United States would know each other?" He answered this question by giving an individual a letter addressed to another person somewhere in the United States. This individual was to send the letter to someone he knew who might know the other person. In turn, this person was to send the letter to someone she knew who might know the person. Surprisingly, it only required five or six different people for the letter to go from the first individual to the final individual. This phenomenon has been referred to as the small world problem; more recently, the phrase *six degrees of separation* has been used.

Various studies have shown that the neurons in the brain can also be considered within a **small world framework** (Sporns, 2011). Neurons have numerous short distance local connections, which taken together can be considered as a hub or module. From these hubs are more long-distance connections to other hubs.

Local hubs can be made up of neurons that connect with each other over very short distances. Such connections are seen in gray matter. Underlying this are the axons, which transfer information throughout the brain. Their myelin sheaths are lighter in color, and thus, these areas are referred to as white matter. Myelin is made up of fats and proteins and wraps around axons like insulation does around electrical cables and results in an increased speed in information transmissions. About 44% of the human brain is white matter. White matter generally represents longer connections between neurons. This allows for cortical networks over larger areas of the brain. Knowing this, it is possible to examine the network connections in individuals with a particular disorder and their matched controls. A lot of work has also been done in this realm in India. The nationally recognized association, SCARF, holds a niche biennial international conference known as the International Conference on Schizophrenia (IConS). These conferences have been held regularly for the last one and a half decades, and draw academicians and researchers in schizophrenia from all over the world.

Schizophrenia research involves studying some interesting aspects such as facial emotion recognition, interpersonal interaction in groups, and caregiver burnout too, since this has tremendous implications in the course of rehabilitation (*Indian Journal of Psychiatry*, 57(3), Jul–Sep, 2015; Sovani & Apte, 2012; Sovani & Thatte, 1994).

As noted previously, three specific networks have been examined in terms of psychopathology (Menon, 2011). These are the baseline or default network, the central executive network, and the salience network. The default network is active when an individual is not performing a particular task such as when one's mind wanders. The central executive network is involved in higher order cognitive and attentional tasks. If you are thinking about how to write a paper or build a building, you will use your executive network. The salience network is important for monitoring critical external events as well as internal states. Other researchers (e.g., Raichle, 2011) have also noted the presence of networks for basic sensory and attentional processes. Some of these that have been identified include a visual network, a sensorimotor network, an auditory network, and a dorsal attentional network.

What Is the Brain's Default (Intrinsic) Network?

What does your brain do when you are just sitting and waiting or daydreaming or talking to yourself? This is a question that is just now beginning to be explored. In psychology, most of the research you read about involves a person doing something. Reacting to emotional pictures or solving cognitive problems are common examples. In these cases, one's attention is focused on a task in the external world.

In the same way that the brain is organized to process spatial and verbal material differently and involve different cortical networks, it also appears that different circuits are involved with internal versus external information. A variety of studies have examined brain imaging procedures in which individuals performed internal tasks versus external tasks (e.g., Ray & Coles, 1985).

However, we all know that even without an external task to do, our mind is constantly working. It jumps from one thought to another. William James called this process the stream of consciousness. Recent researchers refer to this process as mind wandering.

Those neural networks that are active during internal processing have come to be referred to as the brain's **default or intrinsic network** (see Buckner, Andrews-Hanna, & Schacter, 2008; Raichle, 2011; Raichle & Snyder, 2007, for an overview). However, it has been suggested that intrinsic is a better term than default since a variety of internal tasks use this network (Kelly, Biswal, Craddock, Castellanos, & Milham, 2012). The default network is separate from, but one that can be understood as similar to, other networks such as those involved in visual perception or motor activities. It is made up of a set of interacting brain regions. Those areas involved are pictured in *Figure 3-16* and represent periods of brain imaging when individuals are not engaged in any active task.

Overall, the default network is involved during internal or private considerations that do not require processing external sensory information. In fact, it appears as if there is a negative correlation between activities in the default network versus networks associated with processing information from the environment. That is, when someone begins some cognitive activity then new networks associated with that task become active and the default network becomes less active. Overall, this suggests that separate brain mechanisms evolved for dealing with information involving the external environment as opposed to considerations internal to the person. A variety of psychopathology disorders show problems with the default network in terms of being able to turn it off and engage in a more active external task. People with schizophrenia are one group that has difficulty turning off the default network and moving to an active task that uses a different network.

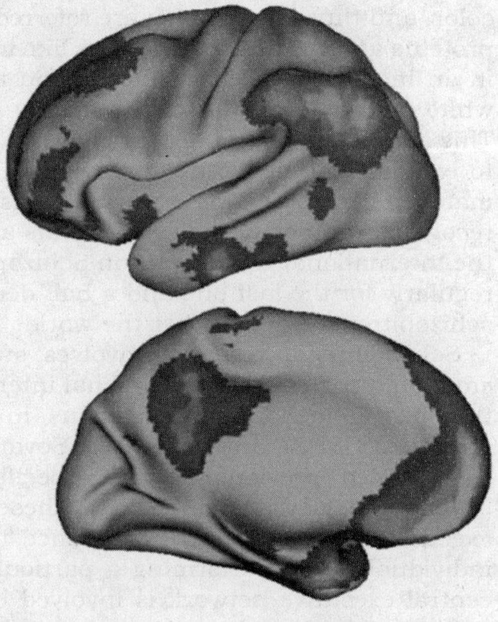

FIGURE 3-16 Brain's Default Network as Constructed From a Meta-Analysis of Positron Emission Tomography Studies

Source: Buckner et al. (2008, p. 4).

Different Networks Are Involved in Different Tasks

In addition to the default network, the executive and salience networks are dysfunctional in different psychopathologies (Menon, 2011). The central executive network is involved in performing such tasks as planning, goal setting, directing attention, performing, inhibiting the management of actions, and the coding of representations in working memory (see Eisenberg & Berman, 2010, for an overview). These are sometimes referred to as frontal lobe tasks since damage to the frontal areas of the brain compromise performance in these tasks. These tasks are also referred to as **executive functions** since they are involved in planning, understanding new situations, and having cognitive flexibility. The salience network as the name implies is involved in monitoring and noting important changes in biological and cognitive systems.

The three networks—default, executive, and salience—show deficits in individuals with specific psychopathologies. Menon (2011) has reviewed the research literature and suggests that these networks play a prominent role in schizophrenia, depression, anxiety, dementia, and autism. As you will see throughout this book, the role of these networks may be dysfunctional in the network itself or in the ability to activate or deactivate specific networks in changing situations.

Figure 3-17 shows those areas of the brain that Menon found to be associated with each of these networks. The figure shows a structural image of the brain shown in

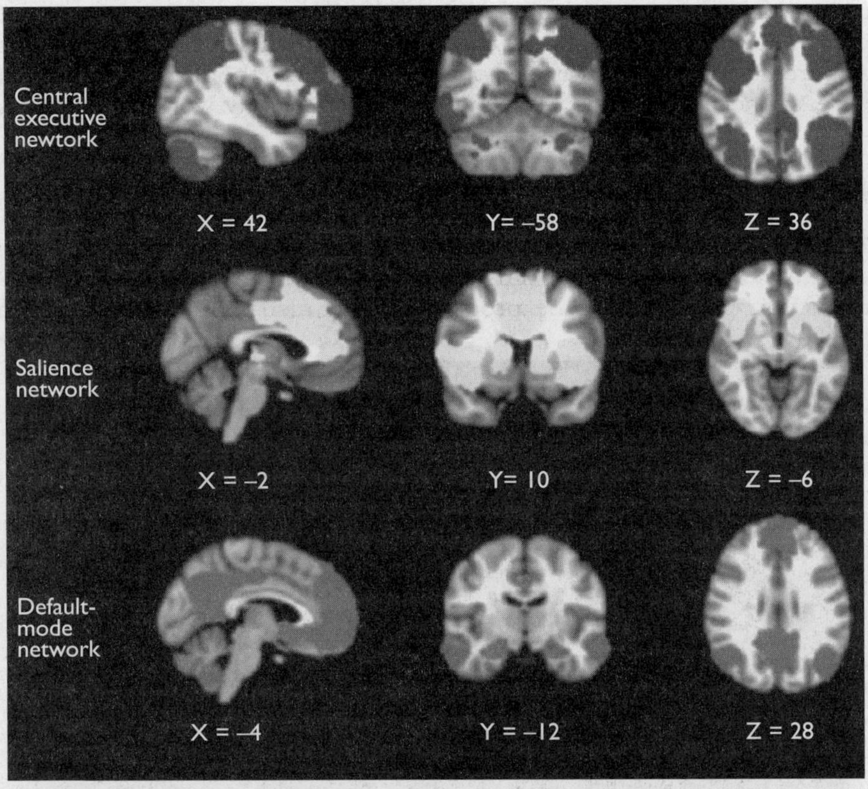

FIGURE 3-17 Structural Image of the Brain With Networks Shown in Color

Source: Reprinted from *Trends in Cognitive Sciences,* Vol. 15, Vinod Menon, Large-scale brain networks and psychopathology: A unifying triple-network model, pp. 483–506, Copyright © 2011, with permission from Elsevier.

black-and-white. The areas shown to be activated during the task are displayed in color. The brain is shown in terms of a three-dimensional image along an x-, y-, and z-axis. The x-axis shows the brain from the side. The y-axis shows the brain from the back. The z-axis shows the brain from above. The numbers below the image represent the location along each axis the image is from. Using these three numbers, brain imaging programs can identify the areas in terms of traditional anatomical structures.

In *Figure 3-17*, the central executive network, which is involved in higher order cognitive and attentional demands including planning for the future and remembering concepts, is shown in blue. The salience network, which is important for monitoring critical external events and internal states, is shown in yellow. The default network, which is active during mind wandering and when the person is not engaged in active problem solving, is shown in red.

Let's take a moment and understand how researchers describe brain function in terms of networks. One important concept is **modularity.** This describes how specific areas of the brain are dedicated to certain types of process. For example, we know that a particular part of the temporal lobe, the FFA, is involved in processing the human face. fMRI measures for example would show greater brain activation in this area when observing the human face as opposed to nonhuman faces.

Another important concept is **connectivity.** This asks how different areas of the brain work together in specific conditions. To determine connectivity, researchers examine fMRI or EEG measures from a large number of locations throughout the brain. It is assumed that those areas whose activity is correlated are in some way working together.

Major Neurotransmitters in the Brain

In the chemical synapse, neurotransmitters play a critical role (see *Figure 3-18*). Neurotransmitters are chemicals that are involved in increasing or decreasing the potential for action potentials to be produced. They also maintain the communication

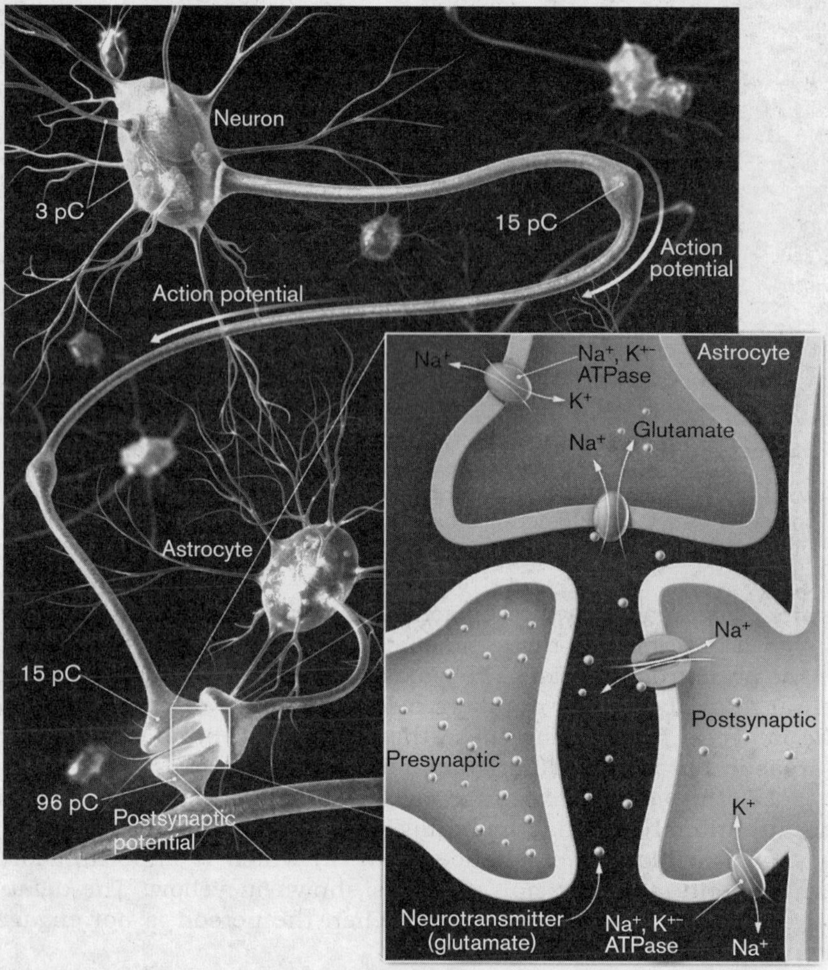

FIGURE 3-18 The Role of Neurotransmitters in Synaptic Processes

Source: Magistretti, P. J. (2009). Low-cost travel in neurons. *Neuroscience Science, 325*(5946), 1349–1351. doi:10.1126/science.118102. Retrieved from http://www.sciencemag.org/content/325/5946/1349.short. Reprinted with permission from American Association for the Advancement of Science (AAAS).

across the synapse. Neurotransmitters largely influence a variety of processes including those associated with psychopathology. For example, cocaine blocks the ability of a neuron to remove the neurotransmitter dopamine from the synapse, which increases the experience of addiction. It is also the case that psychotropic medications largely have their influence at the site of the synapse.

At this point, more than 100 different neurotransmitters have been identified. Neurotransmitters have been classified in terms of both structure and function. Most neurons utilize more than one type of neurotransmitter for their functioning.

1. In terms of structure, neurotransmitters can be classified in terms of size (Purves et al., 2013). This results in two broad categories:
   a. Small molecule neurotransmitters such as glutamate, which is excitatory, and GABA, which is inhibitory, are often composed of single amino acids. These small molecule neurotransmitters tend to be involved in rapid synaptic functions. Glutamate is considered to be the most important neurotransmitter in normal brain function. In abnormal conditions, the firing of rapid glutamate neurons can lead to seizures in a number of areas of the brain. GABA is inhibitory, and drugs that increase the amount of GABA available are used to treat such disorders as anxiety.
   b. Larger protein molecules referred to as neuropeptides can be made up of 3 to 36 amino acids. Neuropeptides tend to be involved in slower ongoing synaptic functions.
2. In terms of function, neurotransmitters can be categorized into three broad groups:
   a. The first category includes those neurotransmitters such as glutamate and GABA that mediate communication between neurons.
   b. The second category includes those neurotransmitters, such as opioid peptides in the pain system, which influence the communication of information.
   c. The third category includes those neurotransmitters such as dopamine, adrenaline, noradrenaline, and serotonin that influence the activity of large populations of neurons.

Concept Check

- How is the brain's default or intrinsic network different from the central executive and salience networks?
- Researchers are concerned with modularity and connectivity in terms of neural networks. What are modularity and connectivity, and how are they important in thinking about psychopathology?
- Why is the role of neurotransmitters important in the development of psychotropic medications to treat mental disorders?

THE STUDY OF GENETICS

The study of genetics begins with the work of Gregor Mendel (1823–1884). Being curious as to how plants obtain atypical characteristics, Mendel performed a series of experiments with the garden pea plant. Peas are a self-fertilizing plant, which means that the male and female aspects needed for reproduction develop in different parts of the same flower. Therefore, successive generations of peas are similar to their parents in terms of particular traits such as their height or the color of their flowers.

Mendel found that when combining peas with white flowers with those with purple flowers, the next generation had all purple flowers. Allowing this generation to self-fertilize brought forth plants that had purple flowers but also some that had white flowers. Mendel explained these findings by suggesting that a plant inherits information from each parent, the male and female aspect. Mendel was hypothesizing that information must be conveyed. He further suggested that one unit of information could be dominant in comparison to the other, which we now call recessive. In this case, the unit of information that coded for purple would be dominant.

Mendel did not know about genes but hypothesized the existence of a specific structure he called elements. From his experiments, he determined the basic principle that there are two elements of heredity for each trait (e.g., color in the previous example). Mendel also assumed that one of these elements can dominate the other and if it is present then the trait will also be present. Mendel also suggested that these elements can be nondominant, or recessive. For the trait to appear, both of these nondominant elements must be present. These ideas are referred to as **Mendel's first law or the law of segregation.**

Put in today's language, Mendel suggested that variants of a specific gene exist, which account for variations in inherited characteristics, and that an organism receives one of these from each parent. Further, one of these can be dominant or recessive, which determines which characteristics are expressed. Mendel also realized that the inheritance of the gene of one trait is not affected by the inheritance of the gene for another trait. In the previous example illustrating the inheritance of color and height, those factors influencing color do not affect height, and vice versa. That is, the probability for each occurs separately. This fact is known as **Mendel's second law or the law of independent assortment.**

Since Mendel's time, we have learned a great deal concerning the process of inheritance. What he referred to as elements or units of information, we now call genes (see *Figure 3-19*). We also know that genes can have alternative forms, which we call alleles. Independent researchers, Walter Sutton and Theodore Boveri, in 1903 suggested the now-accepted fact that genes are carried on **chromosomes.** We now know that each of the approximately 20,000 human genes occurs at a specific site, called a locus, on one of our 23 different pairs of chromosomes. As genetics progressed in the 20th century, it became clear that it was necessary to go beyond the two laws suggested by Mendel to a more complex understanding of how traits are passed from generation to generation. For example, if two genes are located close to one another on the same chromosome, then the result is different from that predicted by Mendel's second law.

What Do Genes Do?

Genes form the blueprint to describe what an organism is to become. Over our evolutionary history, a majority of human genes reflect little variation. This is why all humans have two eyes and one nose and one mouth. However, perhaps one fourth of all genes allow for variation. What makes things interesting is that the two genes of these pairs are usually slightly different. The technical name for the unique molecular form of the same gene is an **allele.** It has been estimated that of our approximately 20,000 genes, some 6,000 exist in different versions or alleles (Zimmer, 2001).

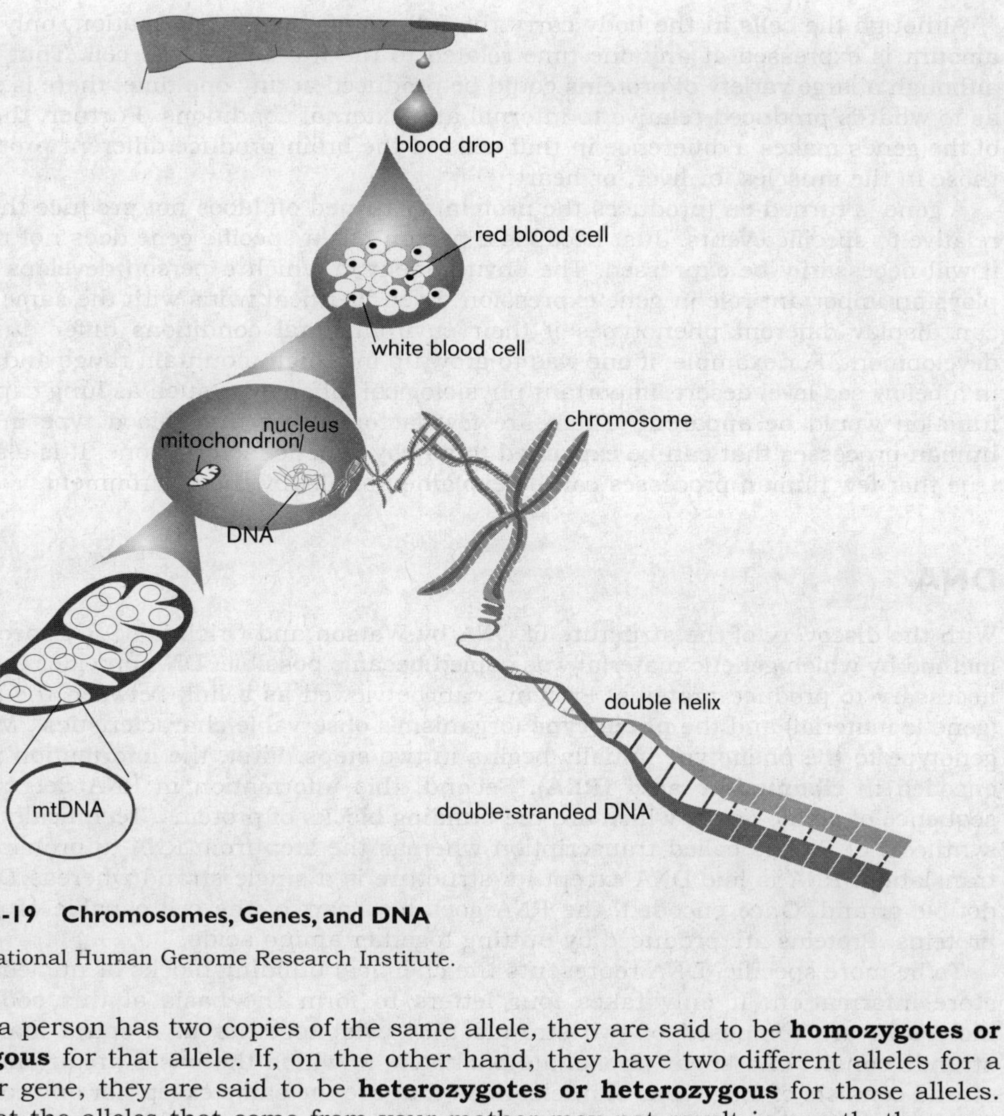

FIGURE 3-19 Chromosomes, Genes, and DNA

Source: National Human Genome Research Institute.

When a person has two copies of the same allele, they are said to be **homozygotes or homozygous** for that allele. If, on the other hand, they have two different alleles for a particular gene, they are said to be **heterozygotes or heterozygous** for those alleles. Given that the alleles that come from your mother may not result in exactly the same characteristics as those from your father, variation is possible. It is these variations that allow for the process of natural selection to have its effect.

The job of a gene is to lay out the process by which a particular protein is made. That is, each gene is able to **encode** a protein, influencing their production. Proteins, which do the work of the body, are involved in a variety of processes. Functionally, proteins in the form of enzymes are able to make metabolic events speed up whereas structural proteins are involved in building body parts. Similar proteins in insects are involved in creating such structures as spider webs and butterfly wings. Proteins are diverse and complex and found in the foods we eat as well as made by our cells from some 20 amino acids. Proteins serve as signals for changes in cell activity as illustrated by hormones. Proteins are also involved in health and disease as well as in development and aging.

Although the cells in the body carry the full set of genetic information, only a limited amount is expressed at any one time related to the function of the cell. That is to say, although a large variety of proteins could be produced at any one time, there is selectivity as to what is produced relative to internal and external conditions. Further, the location of the genes makes a difference in that cells in the brain produce different proteins from those in the muscles, or liver, or heart.

A gene is turned on (produces the protein) or turned off (does not produce the protein) relative to specific events. Just because a person has a specific gene does not mean that it will necessarily be expressed. The environment in which a person develops and lives plays an important role in gene expression. Even identical twins with the same genotype can display different phenotypes if their environmental conditions differ during their development. For example, if one was to grow up in a high mountain range and the other in a below sea level desert, important physiological differences such as lung capacity and function would be apparent. There are few factors other than blood type in terms of human processes that can be explained totally by genetic factors alone. It is also equally true that few human processes can be explained totally by the environment.

DNA

With the discovery of the structure of DNA by Watson and Crick in 1953, specifying the method by which genetic material was copied became possible. DNA provides information necessary to produce proteins. Proteins can be viewed as a link between the **genotype** (genetic material) and the **phenotype** (organism's observable characteristics). Moving the genotype to the phenotype initially begins in two steps. First, the information in DNA is encoded in **ribonucleic acid (RNA).** Second, this information in RNA determines the sequence of amino acids, which are the building blocks of proteins. Technically, the DNA synthesis of RNA is called transcription whereas the step from RNA to protein is called translation. RNA is like DNA except its structure is a single strand whereas DNA has a double strand. Once encoded, the RNA goes to a part of the cell capable of producing proteins. Proteins are produced by putting together amino acids.

To be more specific, DNA represents the chemical building blocks or nucleotides that store information. It only takes four letters to form the basis of this coding. DNA molecules are composed of two strands that twist together in a spiral manner. The strands consist of a sugar phosphate backbone to which the bases are attached. Each strand consists of four types of nucleotides that are the same except for one component, a nitrogen-containing base. The four bases are adenine, guanine, thymine, and cytosine. These are generally referred to as A, G, T, and C. To give you some sense of size, each full twist of the DNA double helix is 3.4 nanometers (i.e., one billionth of a meter). Said in other terms, if we took the DNA in the 46 chromosomes of a single human cell and stretched it out, it would be around 6 feet long. This measurement gives you some idea of the thinness of DNA.

DNA, which is the information storage molecule, transfers information to RNA, which is the information transfer molecule, to produce a particular protein. Further, change in the rate at which RNA is transcribed controls the rate at which genes produce proteins. The expression rate of different genes in the same genome may vary from 0 to approximately 100,000 proteins per second. Thus, not only do genes produce proteins, but they do so at different rates. The crucial question becomes what causes a gene to turn on or off.

HOW DO GENES INFLUENCE BEHAVIOR?

In terms of behavior and experience, the production of proteins can be transitory. For example, touching a cat's whiskers causes changes in gene expression in the cells of the sensory cortex of the brain (Mack & Mack, 1992). This is just a momentary change. Changes can also be long-term. Turning on one set of genes may have lasting influence on the ability of other genes to produce specific proteins. For example, when a songbird first hears the specific song of its species, a particular set of genes comes into play which when once set, determines the song produced by that bird for its entire life. This process has been mapped by a number of researchers (cf. Mello, Vicario, & Clayton, 1992; Ribeiro & Mello, 2000). Likewise, raising mice in an enriched environment—that is, one with lots of toys and stimulation—will cause increased gene expression in genes that are associated with learning and memory (Rampon et al., 2000).

How do we know which genes are involved? In this study, the genes of mice in enriched environments were compared with those of control mice who did not have this experience. Another way to know which genes are involved in a process is to actually change the genes in a particular organism. So-called "knockout" mice are genetically engineered mice in which particular genes have been turned off by breeding them in specific ways. Research shows that simple genetic changes made experimentally in animals can result in protein changes, which influence social behavior. Some examples of such behaviors are increased fear and anxiety, increased grooming, hyperactivity, and even increased alcohol consumption when stressed.

With the beginning of genetic research during the 20th century in relation to psychopathology, it was assumed that one day genes would be able to explain the development of psychopathology. However, after decades of research, it is clear that simple genetic explanations will not be forthcoming. Mental disorders disrupt a variety of cognitive, emotional, and motor processes that are developed during a person's lifetime and that are guided by thousands of genes (see State & Levitt, 2011, for an overview).

Epigenetic Processes

One basic idea from Mendelian genetics was that genes are not changed by experience. What is passed on, except in the case of damage to the gene, is exactly the same gene that was received by the organism from its parents. This came to be called the central dogma of molecular biology as described by Francis Crick. He basically stated that information flow was one-directional. That is, it went from the gene to the protein. What came to be called reverse translation was seen as impossible. Thus, the gene could not be influenced or changed by changes in proteins. This was the basic view from the 1950s until even today.

As researchers became interested in how genes turn on and off and what factors influence this, it became apparent that the story was more complicated. What was discovered was that the processes that determine which genes turn on and off could themselves be passed on to the next generation. Of course, which factors turn the genes on and off are largely influenced by the environment of the organism. Thus, although DNA itself could not be influenced by the environment, it was possible for the environment to influence future generations through its changes to those processes that turn genes on and off.

This possibility of another form of inheritance came to be called **epigenetic inheritance** (see Hallgrímsson & Hall, 2011; Nestler, 2011, for overviews). Instead of actually changing the gene itself, epigenetic modifications mark a gene. This alters how it is turned on and off. Briefly, DNA is wrapped around clusters of proteins called histones. These are further bundled into structures called chromosomes. Being tightly packed keeps genes in an inactive state by preventing access to processes that turn genes on. When action is needed, a section of DNA unfurls and the gene turns on. Whether a segment is relaxed and able to be activated or condensed resulting in no action is influenced by **epigenetic marks or tags** (see *Figure 3-20*). As a tag, histone acetylation tends to promote gene activity and is called a writer. Histone methylation and DNA methylation tend to inhibit it and are called erasers.

The environment can influence these writer and eraser tags. Tags help an organism respond to a changing environment. Some tags last a short time whereas others can last a lifetime. In a now classic study, researchers observed that some rat mothers displayed high levels of nurturing behavior, licking and grooming their pups, whereas others were less diligent (Weaver et al., 2004). Behaviorally, the offspring of the more active mothers were less anxious and produced less stress hormone when disturbed than pups cared for by more passive mothers. Further, the females raised by nurturing mothers became nurturing mothers themselves.

The intriguing part of this study was that the offspring of the rat mothers who showed more licking and grooming differed in epigenetic factors. Pups raised by passive mothers showed more DNA methylation than aggressively groomed pups in the regulatory sequences of

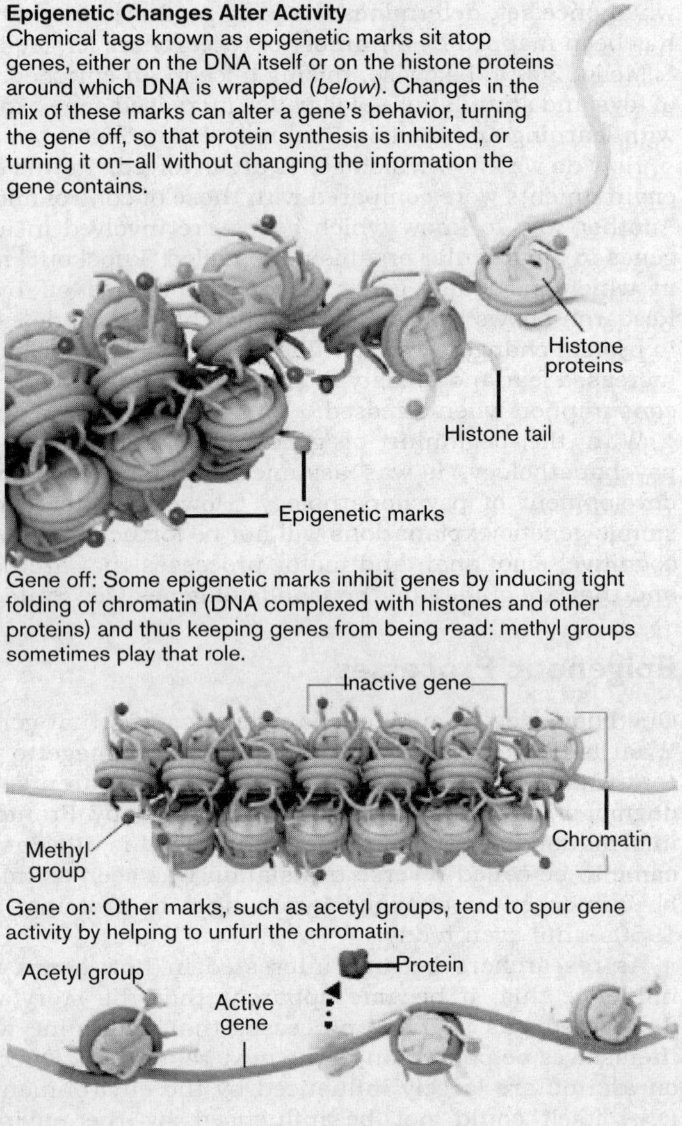

FIGURE 3-20 Epigenetic Changes Alter Gene Activity

Source: Nestler (2011).

a gene encoding the glucocorticoid receptor, which is a protein present in most cells in the body, which mediates an animal's response to the stress hormone cortisol. This excessive methylation was detected in the hippocampus, a brain region involved in learning and memory, which causes nerve cells to make less of the receptor. Activation of the glucocorticoid receptor in the hippocampus actually signals the body to slow production of cortisol. The epigenetic reduction in receptor number exacerbated the stress response in the animals. This made the animals more anxious and fearful. Further, these traits persisted throughout their lifetime. Overall, attentive mothers cause the methyl marks to be removed. Inattentive mothers, on the other hand, caused methyl marks to be added. Thus, rats inherit certain behaviors based on experience. The genes had not been changed but the tags were.

At this point, a variety of studies have shown other examples of epigenetic mechanisms at work. For example, the diet of a mouse mother before conception can influence the hair color of her infants and even her infants' infants (e.g., Cropley, Suter, Beckman, & Martin, 2006). One interesting aspect of this research is the suggestion that a mother's diet can influence future generations, independent of later changes in diet.

Fathers can also influence their offspring. It has been shown that a mouse will develop a diabetes-like disease if her father's diet before her conception was high in fat (Skinner, 2010). Also, if a mouse father is overweight, then gene activity in the pancreas of his offspring is abnormal (Ng et al., 2010). Since the pancreas makes insulin, which regulates blood sugar, this may set up the possibility of future diabetes. The opposite is also the case. If the father's diet results in an underweight condition, then genes in the liver associated with fat and cholesterol synthesis were shown to be more active in their offspring (Carone et al., 2010). Another study suggests that whether a human father smoked early in life was associated with his sons being heaver in weight at age 9 (Pembrey et al. 2006).

Overall, this type of research suggests that behavior and environmental experiences at critical periods could later influence characteristics for future generations. Current health research related to such disorders as diabetes and cancer, as well as types of psychopathology, is suggestive of such a relationship (see Katsnelson, 2010; van Os, 2010, for overviews). Both addiction and depression have been shown to have an epigenetic component (see Nestler, 2011, for an overview). Thus, epigenetic inheritance, which involves tags or marks that determine when genes are turned off or on, offers a parallel track to traditional Mendelian inheritance for influencing phenotypes. Further, a new area of research uses identical twins to study specific epigenetic mechanisms with the goal of determining how genetic and environmental factors influence epigenetics (e.g., Bell & Spector, 2011). This approach may offer better insight into the expression of complex traits as seen in normal and psychopathological processes.

Mitochondria and Mitochondrial Inheritance

Mitochondria are structures within a cell that are involved in the production of energy. It is assumed that mitochondria descended from bacteria that began to live inside single-celled organisms more than a billion years ago. As such, mitochondria have their own DNA (see next paragraph), which contains 13 coding genes with about 16,000 base pairs. Thus, a given cell in your body contains both the nuclear DNA and mitochondria and their DNA.

What is interesting is that generally **mitochondrial DNA (mtDNA)** is inherited only from the mother, clearly a violation of Mendelian inheritance. Because mtDNA does not recombine sections of DNA from the mother and father, it is very stable and mutates very slowly. This gives mtDNA a special application in the study of evolution. This has helped researchers to discover the genetic link of certain disorders that show maternal or **mitochondrial inheritance** patterns, such as Leber's hereditary optic neuropathy, a disorder that results in rapid loss of vision beginning in adolescence.

Evidence is also accumulating that mitochondrial dysfunction is involved in specific mental disorders (see Regenold et al., 2009; Rossignol & Frye, 2012, for overviews). This is referred to as the mitochondrial dysfunction hypothesis. Mitochondrial dysfunction has been identified using a number of different techniques. One technique is to identify structural changes in mitochondria. A second is to examine the manner in which the mitochondrially related genes produce proteins. And a third is the use of metabolic studies. Since mitochondria are involved with energy production, it is possible to measure glucose concentration in cerebrospinal fluid. These studies have shown differences in mitochondrial functioning in individuals with bipolar disorder, schizophrenia, and autism spectrum disorders from healthy controls.

THE THEMES OF EVOLUTION

One of the main themes of evolution is the manner in which organisms are in close connection with their environment. It is this close connection that allows for change to take place, including the turning on and off of genetic processes. In humans, there is another layer of complexity involved in the process. Part of this complexity comes from the fact that humans are born less fully developed at birth than many other species and thus are sensitive to changes in their environment as they continue to develop. This includes our relationships with our family and others that we initially come in contact with. As humans, we also develop societal and cultural perspectives. These perspectives become the backdrop of our environment. Unlike animals that live within nature, we as humans largely live within the backdrop of our culture. Thus, we are influenced by our culture and pay close attention to it.

Another part of our complexity as humans is our ability to reflect on ourselves and our world. In this way, a layer of thought can be injected between the person and the environment. This allows for expectation and imagination to play a role in human behavior and

Concept Check

- What are the two important principles of Mendelian genetics? What evidence led Mendel to their discovery?
- What do genes do and how and where do they do it? What are the roles of DNA and RNA in that process?
- How do we know that genes change behavior? What kinds of research have been done with animals to identify the specific genes involved?

experience. Some have even suggested that humans may be the only species to imagine the world and themselves differently from how it appears. In this sense, our inner world of thoughts and feelings becomes another environment in which we live. For example, you can tell yourself you are wonderful or you are stupid, and there is no one there to dispute this. One positive aspect of this is that your inner world allows you to plan future actions and reflect on past ones, but it can also be experienced as distress when your internal thoughts reflect such states as anxiety or hopelessness. Our internal thoughts at times may lead to interpretations of the environment or ourselves that may not be productive. What should lead to successful survival, sexuality, and social relations leads instead to interactions that reduce the close connection between the individual and his or her internal and external environment. As we will see, this lack of connectedness lies at the heart of psychopathology.

As noted in Chapter 1, humans not only consider themselves but also consider others. A positive side of this is the ability to understand the internal experiences of another. This allows us to experience empathy. We can also consider how we appear to others and other questions of self-image. One aspect of this is related to sexual processes. That is, we can say or do things that make us more attractive to a potential mate. In terms of self-preservation, humans also have a personal history that allows each individual to learn from the past and develop strategies for living. These strategies tend to protect us and may even have saved our lives in exceptional cases. However, it is also possible for the strategies that work in one environmental situation not to work in another. When a person loses contact with the current environment and applies strategies that worked perhaps in an earlier time, then unsuccessful adaptation is the result.

This lack of connectedness to our environment may take place on both an external and an internal level. On an external level, the person finds herself different from the group or even seeks to be separate from others. This is not our historical experience since individual humans have never lived in isolation. As a species, we have always lived in close contact with other humans, which has led to the development of societies and cultures. In fact, many of the specific abilities of humans are geared to social interactions on a variety of levels. When they no longer have the connection with the group, many individuals experience a sense of loss. This loss often carries with it the experience of negative affect and depression and often a need to withdraw. On an internal level, humans often have the need to explain to themselves the events that have just occurred, which may include anger, distorted perceptions, or a genuine plan for recovery. The extreme cases we refer to as psychopathology.

PSYCHOPATHOLOGY FROM AN EVOLUTIONARY PERSPECTIVE

Psychopathology from an evolutionary perspective goes beyond the traditional psychological and physiological considerations. Considering the evolutionary perspective, we ask additional types of questions. One question might be how long in terms of our human history has a particular psychopathological disorder existed. As noted in Chapter 1, a WHO study examined the presence of schizophrenia in a number of countries with very different racial and cultural backgrounds (Sartorius et al., 1986). What these authors found was that despite the different cultural and racial backgrounds surveyed, the experience of schizophrenia was remarkably similar across countries. Likewise, the risk of developing schizophrenia was similar in terms of total population presence (about 1%).

Further, the disorder had a similar time course in its occurrence with its characteristics first being seen in young adults.

If you put these facts together, it suggests that schizophrenia is a disorder that has always been part of the human experience. Because it is found throughout the world in strikingly similar ways, this suggests that it existed before humans migrated out of Africa. The genes related to schizophrenia were carried by early humans who migrated from Africa, and thus, its presence is equally likely throughout the world. Given these estimates as to the history of the disorder, one might ask why schizophrenia continues to exist. We know, for example, that individuals with schizophrenia tend to have fewer children than individuals without the disorder. Thus, we might assume that schizophrenia would have disappeared over evolutionary time in that it reduces reproductive success and has a genetic component. However, this is not the case.

This creates a mystery for evolutionary psychologists to solve. In order to answer this question, we can draw on many considerations. Perhaps, in the same way that sickle-cell anemia is associated with a protection against malaria, schizophrenia protects the person from another disorder. Or, perhaps like the reaction of rats to stress, which results in depression-like symptoms, the symptoms seen in schizophrenia are the result of a long chain of stressful events in which the organism breaks down in its ability to function. Psychopathology could even go in a more positive direction and be associated with creative and nontraditional views of the world. For example, there are a number of accounts that have noted greater creativity in families of individuals with schizophrenia.

The evolutionary perspective helps us ask such questions as what function a disorder might serve as well as how it came about. In the same way that pain can be seen as a warning system to the body to protect it from tissue damage, anxiety may have evolved to protect the person from other types of potential threats. For example, many of the outward expressions of social anxiety parallel what is seen in dominance interactions in primates. Submissive monkeys avoid contact with most dominant ones as do human individuals experiencing social anxiety avoid dominant members of their group. This suggests the possibility that anxiety may have its evolutionary origins in dominance structures. If this were the case then we might expect to see some relationship to sexual instinctual processes—as is the case with dominance. The evolutionary perspective also helps us think about what might be solutions as to how psychopathology should be treated. These are some of the questions I will discuss in this book.

One perspective of the evolutionary approach has been to redirect psychology back to the basic processes of human existence such as survival, sexual processes, and social behavior. We can then ask what types of disorders are found within each broad category. We can also consider the developmental and social processes and ask how these processes may be involved in psychopathology. Thinking in these terms, we may come to discover that disorders that have very similar end states may have developed from distinct beginning conditions. A prominent neuropsychologist from India, Professor C. R. Mukundan, has proposed an interesting hypothesis about the biobehavioral basis of emotion. He has included these theories in his 2017 book. He explains that an action is automatically initiated when emotional arousal or drive reaches a Critical Level of Potentiation. One has the choice and freedom to learn to control emotional arousal well before it reaches the critical level, and thereby control the actions (Mukundan, 2016; Mukundan, 2017).

Another psychopathology that has been approached from an evolutionary perspective is the category of personality disorders. Personality disorders reflect a rigid approach to dealing with social relationships. Two commonly discussed personality disorders are psychopathic personality and hysteria. Psychopaths are described as manipulative, callous, dishonest, and self-centered. They are antisocial in the sense they display no need to follow the traditional rules of a society and display little remorse or guilt for their actions. For example, they would contract and collect money for a job they would never do. They would clearly qualify for who evolutionary psychologists refer to as cheaters. On the other hand, individuals with a histrionic personality disorder overly seek the attention of others and are very emotional in their reactions. They can be manipulative in their interpersonal relationships.

Harpending and Sobus (1987) suggested that the psychopathic and the histrionic personality styles represent different adaptive strategies in relation to sexuality. Both of these personality types were viewed by Harpending and Sobus as cheaters. Given that it is more common to see male psychopaths and female hysterics, these researchers suggest that this results from different reproductive strategies. A male cheater in a sexual relationship should be able to persuade a female to copulate with him while deceiving her about his commitment to her and his willingness to offer resources for the offspring. A female cheater, on the other hand, would exaggerate her need for the male and make herself appear helpless and in need so that he would give her additional attention and resources. She would also be willing to put her own needs ahead of those of her offspring even to the extent of abandoning them. The work of Harpending and Sobus shows how evolutionary thinking can help to explain the motivational factors of a particular disorder as well as the demonstrated gender differences.

Let's look at another well-studied process—sleep—as a model for thinking about psychopathology. Since sleep disturbance is often associated with a variety of psychopathological disorders, this will let us consider how normal processes may be influenced to appear pathological. Most people would like to go to sleep when they want to and not be awakened during the night. However, evolution is not always about what makes us feel good. The critical question from an evolutionary perspective is what function sleep plays. In considering this question, we can look at sleep as a model for how we might approach other basic psychological processes.

One initial question to ask is this: Has sleep been shaped by natural selection? Some researchers answer yes to this question (Nesse & Williams, 1995). They offer at least five reasons for why this is so. First, sleep is found in a variety of organisms and is perhaps universal among vertebrates. However, not all animals sleep in the same way. Elephants and cows spend most of their sleep time standing up. Dolphins sleep with one half of their brain while the other half remains awake. Second, all vertebrates share similar mechanisms that control sleep and dreaming. These mechanisms are found in the more primitive areas of the brain. Third, the pattern of sleep seen in mammals with periods of rapid eye movement and faster EEG activity within the sleep period is also seen in birds. Since the evolution of birds went down a different pathway before the time of dinosaurs, this suggests that sleep is a very primitive and basic mechanism. Fourth, in examining the sleep patterns across species, there appears to be support for the idea that these patterns adapted to match the ecological niche of that particular animal. And fifth, all animals show deficits in response to a lack of sleep. Currently a variety of researchers are seeking to determine the function of sleep. The best evidence suggests that it allows for restoration of certain physiological processes. There is also evidence that sleep consolidates information learned during waking hours. One conceptual idea is that, given the light–dark cycle produced by the earth's rotation around the sun, sleep developed as a protective mechanism during the night.

In summary, we can ask critical questions concerning psychopathology that relate to other evolutionary processes:

1. First, we ask if the experience of mental illness is universal. If it were not universal, then it would be difficult to argue that we should study psychopathology from an evolutionary perspective. If it is a universal process such as emotionality or language then we can begin to ask about the nature of mental illness and how its existence fits into our history as humans.
2. Second, we ask if there is an adaptive value to the behaviors and experiences displayed in psychopathology. It is easy to see that there is a value in not trusting what someone tells you some of the time, but is there any adaptive value in not trusting what anyone tells you all of the time or to think that everyone is always out to get you?
3. Third, we look for evidence of psychopathology across human history. This includes the question of whether we see signs of psychopathology in nonhuman species.
4. Fourth, we seek to understand the nature of psychopathology. That is to say, should we consider psychopathology to be qualitatively different from normal functioning, or is it the situation in which normal processes have been taken to the extreme. We know, for example, that allergic reactions are situations in which our immune system is overreactive. We also know that fever is the process in which body temperature is raised to fight infection. However, the fever uses energy and can damage the body.
5. Fifth, we ask if it is protective in some manner. Like sickle-cell anemia, does having schizophrenia or depression for example make you less likely to experience another disorder?
6. Sixth, we ask if psychopathology is a recent process. That is, should we consider psychopathology as the result of a mental system designed in the Stone Age interacting with a high paced modern environment? For example, aggression in teenage gangs may reflect behaviors that were adaptive in previous times but are no longer adaptive for society today.

These questions are not mutually exclusive. As you will see, they also represent some of the ways scientists and others have sought to understand psychopathology. From an evolutionary perspective, the study of psychopathology begins with the three instincts of survival, sexuality, and socialness. From this perspective, psychopathology becomes a disturbance of these instinctual processes.

NEUROETHICS

When we read in the newspapers about new discoveries in the neurosciences, they are often presented in an optimistic manner. We are told they will help us treat medical disorders or learn more about how we think and feel. This is true. However, traditionally, societies have based codes of conduct and the law on observable behaviors. An important question that is currently being asked is who should have access to your internal processes. The following LENS examines the field of inquiry that is asking these questions. It is referred to as **neuroethics.**

3-1 LENS
Neuroethics—Ethical Considerations When Using Neuroscience Techniques

Through genetics, brain imaging, and other neuroscience procedures, it is now possible to know not only about one's behaviors but also about one's internal processes. For example, predictions can be made from genetics about certain types of medical and psychological disorders that are more likely to develop in one's future. This raises ethical questions concerning who should have access to this information and how it may be used by a society.

In the first half of the 20th century, certain Western societies attempted to make changes in future populations. This was referred to as *eugenics*. The basic idea was that it was possible to improve the human race by discouraging reproduction among those considered to be inferior and encouraging reproduction among those who were considered to be healthy. Individuals with mental disorders and mental retardation were among those sterilized. This took place in America, Britain, and Germany and reached its extreme in Nazi Germany during World War II.

Although today eugenics is thought of as a disreputable crusade of the past, ethical issues in terms of one's own genetic information raise important questions. Should a man and a woman who want to have children be told about the possible characteristics, including potential disorders such as autism, of their future child? Should an insurance company know whether you might have the potential to experience schizophrenia or depression in your lifetime? Should companies be able to patent human genes that could prevent disease? Should people be told early in their life which disorders they might develop 40 or 50 years in the future? These are just a few of the complex questions to be considered.

There are also a number of questions related to brain imaging techniques. For example, with millions of MRI scans being performed for research, scientists may discover what are referred to as *incidental findings*. Should an individual be told that he or she has a non-normal brain if a neurologist does not consider the findings related to the person's physical health?

At this point in time, brain imaging techniques cannot absolutely determine if one individual has a mental disorder or not. What neuroscientists can say is that a group of individuals with a particular disorder will show different patterns of brain activity than another group of individuals who do not have the disorder.

Neuroethics takes us beyond the questions of traditional research ethics and focuses on the ethical, legal, and social policy implications of neuroscience (Illes & Bird, 2006). Because of this, a number of scientific neuroscience groups and governmental agencies have sought to understand the ethical problems that neuroscience will bring our society.

SUMMARY

Historically, individuals were diagnosed and classified as falling into discrete categories of disorders based on careful observation of symptoms and signs. With progress in the neurosciences in general and brain imaging and genetics in particular, other levels of analysis have become possible. This has led to the realization that mental disorders can be described in both a categorical and a dimensional manner. The question for the study of psychopathological disorders is to determine the underlying dimensional changes that are associated with categorical-like transformations leading to a disordered state. Developments in the neurosciences also offer the potential of finding more objective markers that can be used in the diagnosis and treatment of mental disorders.

The basic element of the brain is the neuron that is connected to other neurons. Since the human brain has been estimated to contain 100 billion neurons and more than 100,000 kilometers of interconnections, scientists have analyzed them in terms of networks. Three specific networks have been examined in terms of psychopathology—the default network (also called the intrinsic network), the central executive network, and the salience network. Psychopathological disorders have been shown to have problems in turning networks on or off as well as problems in the connections within the network itself.

Scientists have been able to use the manner in which neurons work as a window into their function. A variety of techniques for observing activity in the brain have been developed. Currently, the major types of brain imaging techniques are EEG, MEG, PET, and fMRI. There are a number of tradeoffs that researchers and clinicians must consider when choosing a brain imaging technique. It begins with the research or clinical question one is asking whether the appropriate measure is one of structure (spatial resolution) or how fast a process can be measured (temporal resolution). With the opening of this window into individuals' internal processes, the new field of neuroethics has started asking questions concerning who should have access to that information.

Genes form the blueprint that determines what an organism is to become. They are found on chromosomes in every cell of the body. Within each gene, DNA—the information storage molecule—transfers information to RNA—the information transfer molecule—to produce a particular protein. The location of the genes in the body makes a difference in that cells in the brain produce different proteins from those in the muscles, or liver, or heart. A gene is turned on (produces the protein) or turned off (does not produce the protein) relative to specific events.

The basis of evolution is genetic variations that occur in response to the environment and that can be inherited and passed on to future generations. The study of genetics begins with the work of

Concept Check

- One of the main themes of evolution is the manner in which organisms are in close connection with their environment. Animals live in nature, but for humans there is another layer of complexity. Describe three uniquely human characteristics that impact our connectedness to our environment. What role do they play in psychopathology?
- What are five critical questions an evolutionary perspective asks concerning psychopathology?
- Neuroethics focuses on the ethical, legal, and social policy implications of neuroscience and asks complex questions. Choose a position on one of the questions presented in the LENS just shown and present evidence to support that position.

Gregor Mendel in the 1800s who established the initial principles of genetic inheritance. Subsequent research has added complexity to that initial conceptualization. Mitochondrial inheritance, for example, involves the mtDNA that generally is inherited only from the mother. Epigenetic inheritance is based on the fact that the processes that determine which genes turn on and off can be passed on to the next generation. Thus, although DNA itself could not be influenced by the environment, it was possible for the environment to influence future generations through its changes to those processes that turn genes on and off. Given this complexity, it is no wonder the original hope of finding a few genes that were involved in particular mental disorders has not panned out. Currently, one promising focus of research has been to identify endophenotypes—patterns of processes lying between the gene (the genotype) and the manifestations of the gene in the external environment (the phenotype)—for particular psychological disorders.

One of the main themes of evolution is the manner in which organisms are in close connection with their environment. It is this close connection that allows for change to take place including the turning on and off of genetic processes. In humans, there is another layer of complexity involved in the process. Part of this complexity comes from the fact that humans are born less fully developed at birth than many other species and thus are sensitive to changes in their environment as they continue to develop. Unlike animals that live within nature, we as humans largely live within the backdrop of our culture. Another part of our complexity as humans is our ability to reflect on ourselves and our world. In this way, a layer of thought can be injected between the person and the environment. This allows for expectation and imagination to play a role in human behavior and experience. This lack of connectedness to our environment may take place on both an external and an internal level.

From an evolutionary perspective, the study of psychopathology begins with the three instincts of survival, sexuality, and socialness. From this perspective, psychopathology becomes a disturbance of these instinctual processes. The evolutionary perspective goes beyond the traditional psychological and physiological considerations and asks some critical questions concerning psychopathology. First, is the experience of mental illness universal? Second, is there an adaptive value to the behaviors and experiences displayed in psychopathology? Third, can we see evidence of psychopathology across human history as well as in nonhuman species? Fourth, what is the nature of psychopathology—is it qualitatively different from normal functioning or have normal processes been taken to the extreme? Fifth, is psychopathology protective in some manner? Sixth, is psychopathology a recent process—a result of a mental system designed in prehistory interacting with a thoroughly modern environment?

STUDY RESOURCES

Review Questions

1. What are genotypes, phenotypes, and endophenotypes? How are these three concepts used in understanding the development of psychopathology?
2. This chapter states that there is a complicated relationship between genetic conditions and environmental factors. How are these two concepts involved in

the development and maintenance of psychopathology? How is it made even more complex by epigenetic processes?

3. How have the discoveries of epigenetic inheritance and mitochondrial inheritance enriched our understanding and added to the complexity of Mendel's initial theory of genetic inheritance?
4. How does the small world framework from social science help us understand how neurons are connected in a network? What implications does this have for the transmission of information within a network and across networks?
5. Historically, those interested in neuroscience research have focused more on the universality of human processing rather than the diversity found in different cultures. What evidence can you present to show that culture creates diversity in human psychological processing?

For Further Reading

Ramachandran, V. S., & Blakeslee, S. (1998). *Phantoms in the brain.* New York: William Morrow.

Key Terms and Concepts

allele
categorical
central executive network
chromosomes
comorbid
connectivity
default or intrinsic network
deoxyribonucleic acid (DNA)
Diagnostic and Statistical Manual of Mental Disorders (DSM)
dimensional
diffusion tensor imaging (DTI)
electroencephalography (EEG)
encode
endophenotypes
epigenetic inheritance
epigenetic marks or tags
epigenetics
event-related potentials (ERPs)
evoked potentials (EP)
executive functions
externalizing disorders
functional magnetic resonance imaging (fMRI)
genes
genotype
heterozygotes or heterozygous
homozygotes or homozygous
internalizing disorders
International Classification of Diseases (ICD)
magnetoencephalography (MEG)
memory
Mendel's first law or the law of segregation
Mendel's second law or the law of independent assortment
mitochondrial DNA (mtDNA)
mitochondrial inheritance
modularity
National Institute of Mental Health (NIMH)
neuroethics
neurotransmitters
phenotype
positron emission tomography (PET)
proteins
Research Domain Criteria (RDoC)
reward system
ribonucleic acid (RNA)
salience network
small world framework

CHAPTER

4

Research Methods

CHAPTER OUTLINE

- WHAT IS SCIENCE? 119
- THE METHODS OF SCIENCE 119
- ETHICS AND THE SCIENTIFIC EXPERIMENT 149
- SUMMARY 154
- STUDY RESOURCES 155

Let us begin with a story that took place in Europe about 150 years ago. At that time, Hungary and Austria were part of a single empire, the Austrian Empire. At the Vienna General Hospital, a physician named Ignaz Semmelweis faced a serious problem when he noticed that previously healthy women who had just given birth to healthy children were dying. The women died of a condition that included fever, chills, and seizures. As you can imagine, numerous theories were offered. Some thought the deaths were related to the diet of the women. Perhaps they drank bad water. Maybe the flowers that were brought to their rooms were the problem.

Observing the overall conditions in the hospital, Semmelweis saw that other women in the same hospital who ate the same food, drank the same water, and smelled the same flowers did not die. Consequently, he reasoned, it was not the food, water, or flowers that caused the deaths. Yet the fact remained that women who had just given birth died of the mysterious condition. Semmelweis became aware of a crucial clue when he learned that an assistant who had accidentally cut his hand during an autopsy later died. Further, this assistant displayed the same symptoms as the mothers. What was the connection between the death of the assistant and the deaths of the mothers? Was there any connection at all?

Where this assistant worked was one of the first questions Semmelweis asked. Perhaps the autopsy laboratory where the assistant had worked might be the cause of the mysterious deaths. To evaluate this notion, he traveled to other hospitals and recorded what physicians did just before delivering babies. From these observations, he learned some physicians gave pathology lectures to the interns in the hospital as part of their daily duties. He also noted that when the physicians who delivered the babies came directly from a pathology lecture in which they handled diseased tissue or performed an autopsy, the death rate was highest.

Semmelweis suggested that it was the physicians who were transferring the diseases from the pathological tissue to the healthy mothers, just as the assistant had accidentally infected himself with the knife cut. The physicians of the day were outraged at the suggestion that they were the cause of the women's deaths. Semmelweis found further evidence by demonstrating that in hospitals where some births were assisted by midwives rather than physicians, the mothers assisted by midwives survived at a much higher rate.

In a rather striking, though not totally controlled, experiment, Semmelweis is said to have placed himself at the door to the delivery ward and forced all physicians who entered to wash their hands first. The number of deaths decreased dramatically. Although not everyone accepted Semmelweis's findings, these data spoke for themselves, and modern medical practice has been shaped by this event (Glasser, 1976).

In many ways, those who study psychopathology are faced with dilemmas similar to those that faced Semmelweis. We can observe and describe the various disorders. However, researchers are still trying to determine which are the more important factors and which factors they can rule out.

In India, in the city of Chandigarh, it was the year 1960 and a psychiatrist, Dr. N. N. Wig (1960), who was trained abroad, was making a mark in the Indian psychiatry with many new approaches to OPD treatment as well as psychotherapy. He began to notice that young males of low or medium socioeconomic status reported with a curious mix of four sets of symptoms that fell neither neatly into somatoform nor into anxiety/depression and were of sexual origin. He and his colleagues soon realized that this was a culture-bound syndrome, related to beliefs held about sexual prowess and functioning in the subculture. In India, it is labelled as Dhat syndrome, which later found parallels in other Asian cultures, such as, Indonesia, Malaysia, China, and Sri Lanka, and even in Europe and the Americas. The syndrome in India appeared to be prevalent in young men who were unmarried or recently married, came from rural backgrounds, and had a fairly conservative attitude towards sex. Malhotra and Wig (1975) explained the clustering as a consequence of differential information and knowledge base of the individuals who seemed to belong to groups where discussions about sexuality were a taboo. Add to the mix the tradition of the Indian medical system of Ayurveda, according to which health of the body is due to the balance between seven *dhatus* or essential components of the body. The science of Ayurveda further held that imbalance in these *dhatus* would be the cause of wide range of physical disorders. These include *rasa*, fluid from digested food; *rakta*, blood; *mamsa*, muscle; *meda*, fat; *asthi*, bone; *majja*, marrow; and *sukra*, semen. Of these, ancient texts held that semen is the perfect substance (*dhatu*) and is a source of all physical and mental power. Indigenous practitioners then created their own interpretations that said something to the effect that "it takes 40 drops of food and 40 days to form one drop of blood; 40 drops of blood to form one drop of marrow and 40 drops of marrow to form one drop of semen."

Patients reported with a puzzling mix of symptoms: Somatic complaints such as body ache and burning sensation, increased frequency and difficulty in micturition, loss of control over body and mind, hollowing of eyes, abdominal distension and belching, etc. Anxiety complaints such as palpitations, tachycardia, dryness of mouth, and fear of losing vital component of the body. Depressive complaints such as weakness, guilt, lethargy, disturbed sleep, and loss of appetite, interest, memory, weight loss, suicidal ideation, and feelings of shame. And finally, sexual complaints such as distortion of shape of penis, genital itching, loss of libido and fear of sexual activity, erectile dysfunction, premature ejaculation, and impotence. It required some cultural understanding and putting together of all the traditions and beliefs to understand the culture-bound syndrome of dhat. In such a cultural milieu of beliefs about sexual excess causing dhat disorder, it was then not surprising that patients reported their dhat syndrome to be due to reading erotic literature or pictures, watching pornographic movies, unfulfilled longings or desires, bad company, premarital or extramarital affairs, homosexuality, increased frequency of heterosexual sex, betrayal in love, black magic by wife, intercourse during menstruation, and bad habits such as alcoholism, among many other "possible causes." Similar patterns were also later unearthed among women patients once again due to the reluctance to talk about problems associated with reproductive tract and sexuality.

In a recent publication, the issue was discussed once more in the light of globalization and rapid industrialization.

> It will be important to explore whether such anxiety has disappeared from industrial nations and the subsequent role globalization is likely to play in eliminating such anxieties or whether, on the other hand, it may further contribute to it. Urbanization is also likely to play a role as increased access to education spreads and higher levels of education and changes in understanding masculinity may well lead to a further reduction of the condition. (Ventriglio, Ayonrinde, & Bhugra, 2016)

Dr. Mitchell Weiss (2017) has written about the new emerging field of cultural epidemiology in his paper "The Promise of Cultural Epidemiology." Rooting his arguments in his previous work on explanatory models (Weiss, 2011), Dr. Weiss outlines various EMIC interview frameworks and ends the paper saying, "The logic and benefits of synergies from linking anthropology and epidemiology as complementary basic sciences for mental health and global health are compelling and ultimately perhaps inexorable" (Weiss, 2017). What are some of the characteristics of the scientific approach?

First, **science** involves detective work. An important aspect of both science and good detective work is careful observation. In his case, Semmelweis observed how doctors in different hospitals went about their day and what experiences preceded other experiences. He also observed others such as midwives who were also involved with births. Thus, careful observation is an important first step.

Second, science involves valid logic. In this case, Semmelweis reasoned that if food, water, or flowers were involved, then they should have affected all of the mothers. However, since there were other mothers who did not get sick and ate the same food and water as the mothers who did, it was possible to conclude this assumption was not supported.

Third, luck often plays a role in science. In this case, the event was the fact that the assistant cut his hand during an autopsy and had similar symptoms as the mothers who died. Although this was unlucky for the assistant, his death gave Semmelweis an important clue as to which variables were involved.

Fourth, science involves **hypothesis** testing. Semmelweis had the hypothesis that the disease was carried on the hands of the physicians. To test this hypothesis, he had the physicians wash their hands and determined how this influenced the wellness of the mothers. If washing the hands of the physicians did not make a difference, then this hypothesis could be determined false. However, washing did make a difference, which allowed for further experimentation as well as establishing techniques for the prevention of the disorder.

You may find it surprising that the physicians at first did not believe Semmelweis. Although we do not know if they did not believe that they had germs on their hands or that a doctor could be responsible for a patient's death, one key ingredient in psychological research is the need to understand how other people understand themselves and their world.

In a situation similar to that of Semmelweis, in the 1990s some babies at a hospital in the United States were found to have a particular type of infection. After some investigation, it was realized that this was an infection that was transmitted from pets. Of course, there were no pets in the hospital. How did it get to the babies? You might first guess the parents of the babies brought these pathogens in. However, since they only handled their own baby, this could not explain how all babies had the infection. What are the other alternatives? Who does go from baby to baby? The health care workers in the ward were one strong possibility.

When the health care workers were asked if they washed their hands, they said yes. They did indeed wash their hands. However, when they were observed it became clear that the workers did not wash their hands after handling each baby but only about one third of the time. This and other similar situations led to the requirement that health care workers today wear gloves, which they change after each patient contact.

Tim Eckmanns and his colleagues studied a modification of medical personnel's hand-cleaning procedures (Eckmanns, Bessert, Behnke, Gastmeier, & Rüden, 2006). This study sought to determine if knowing that you had been chosen to be studied would influence your hand-cleaning procedures in an intensive care unit (ICU). The study was performed in five ICU units in a 2,200-bed hospital. In the first part of the study, medical personnel were observed without their knowledge in terms of how often they engaged in hospital prescribed hand-cleaning procedures. Later, a letter was sent to the head of physicians and head of nursing personnel of the ICU, which stated that someone would be observing the "hygienic performance" of the staff. All of the staff of the ICUs were informed of the observation. The same person who was part of the staff made the observations in both the first and second part of the study. What difference do you think it made for the staff to know that they could be observed as part of the study? As you might imagine, the second observation period in which the staff knew they could be observed resulted in a 55% increase in compliance.

Similarly, while "decoding" the dhat syndrome, it requires a scientific temper to realize why these four types of symptoms are being reported simultaneously, consistently by a patient group that hails from similar cultural and educational backgrounds.

What we learn from these types of situations is that in designing research we need to take human nature into account. One important aspect of the human experience is that we think in a psychological way rather than a logical way. For example, most of us tend to remember good times better than bad times. However, in terms of mental illness, some individuals such as those with depression tend to remember the bad times more often.

We also remember events that put us in a good light rather than in a bad one. Sometimes like the health care workers, we remember things differently than the way they may have happened or perform differently if we know we are being observed. Thus, psychological researchers look for a variety of techniques for obtaining information including self-report, direct observations, and reports of mental health workers, as well as indirect measures such as neuroscience techniques.

The case study approach too can lead to the unearthing of an interesting phenomenon of psychopathology, as was demonstrated in the works from Chandigarh, India, earlier in the chapter. In this manner, as physicians, mental health professionals and other researchers come across a problem in a series of cases and start piecing the whole jigsaw together. This case study approach is discussed at length later in the chapter.

WHAT IS SCIENCE?

In general, there is no single scientific method, yet there is a general process called science. This process consists of experiencing the world and then drawing general conclusions (called **facts**) from observations. Sometimes these conclusions or facts are descriptive and can be represented by numbers. For example, we say that the moon is 238,000 miles from the earth or that the average human heart rate is 72 beats per minute. Other times these facts are more general and can describe a relationship or a process. For example, we say that it is more difficult to learn a second language after puberty than before puberty or that as we age we hear fewer high-frequency sounds. Whatever the topic, the known facts about a particular subject are called **scientific knowledge** (see Ray, 2012, for more information).

There is another aspect to science that many people do not think about. This is the aspect of **doubt.** In science, we use doubt to question our ideas and our research and ask whether factors other than the ones that we originally considered might have influenced our results. By doing this, we come to see that science is a combination of interaction with the world and logic.

The logic of science leads us to the realization that one of the real strengths of science is showing us when we are wrong. If someone says that all swans are white, for example, seeing a white swan does not actually prove this to be the case. However, a black swan would clearly show that the statement was wrong. In this spirit, Einstein is reported to have said, "No amount of experimentation can ever prove me right; a single experiment can prove me wrong." The philosopher of science Sir Karl Popper referred to this approach as **falsification.** Thus, one important aspect of doing science is to ask yourself, how would I know if I was wrong?

THE METHODS OF SCIENCE

The methods of science closely parallel our ways of learning about the world: We can think about these in terms of three stages.

First, scientists begin with an idea or expectation. A formally stated expectation is called a hypothesis**.** The scientist says, "I expect this to happen under these conditions," and thus states the hypothesis.

Second, scientists look to experience to evaluate the accuracy of their ideas or expectations about the world. That is, they try to find or create the situation that will allow them to observe what they are interested in studying. Through observation and experimentation, scientists can begin to evaluate their ideas and expectations about the world. Learning about the world through observation and experimentation is an example of **empiricism,** which means nothing more than the acceptance of sensory information as valid.

Third, on the basis of their observations and experiments, scientists seek to draw conclusions or inferences about their ideas and expectations. They reorganize their ideas and consider the impact of the new information on their theoretical conceptualizations.

Overall, science is a way of determining what we can infer about the world. In its simplest form, the scientific method consists of asking a question about the world and then experiencing the world to determine the answer. When we begin an inquiry, what we already know about our topic leaves us in one of a number of positions. In some cases, we know little about our topic, or our topic may be very complex. Consequently, our ideas and questions are general. For example, how does our memory work? What causes mental illness? What factors make a fruitful marriage? How can we model the brain? Can experience change our brain?

Case Study

The **case study** is one of the most widely used methods for studying individual participants. It is based on the logic of describing, analyzing, interpreting, and evaluating a set of events and relationships within a framework or theory (Bromley, 1986). The typical descriptive case study focuses on either problematic or exceptional behaviors. Indeed, for years the case study approach has been the primary method for studying phenomena in clinical medicine, clinical psychology, and the neurosciences. It has a particularly important history in the study of mental disorders.

The case study method has a rich tradition in studying unique situations that do not lend themselves to traditional experimental procedures. Much of our initial understanding of brain function came from careful study of individuals who had accidents or experienced war injuries. With psychopathology, the case study offers a means of examining in some depth the manner in which a person understands and experiences his or her disorder. Further, the case study offers a means of helping researchers develop new questions to be asked concerning a disorder in terms of how it developed and might be treated.

In psychopathology research, the advantage of the case study is its ability to present the clinical implications of a particular disorder. One classic example that Freud discussed was the case study of Anna O. Another example is described in Morton Prince's book *The Dissociation of a Personality* (1913). Prince described a case of multiple personality (now called dissociative identity disorder) at a time when the existence of that diagnostic category was in question.

An advantage of such extended discussions is the ability to describe processes not easily reduced to a single variable. For example, Luria (1972) described in great detail the attempt of one man to overcome a neuropsychological deficit that left him with "a shattered world." This is a story about a brilliant young Russian scientist, Zasetsky, who became a soldier in World War II and was shot in the head. Zasetsky's wound was such that areas of the brain that help one move in space or understand complex language were damaged whereas areas that allow one to reflect on one's condition were not. Luria's intriguing work describes both his and the patient's own experiences over a 25-year period. Initial case studies from battlefield experiences also helped to clarify the nature of post-traumatic stress disorder (PTSD).

Another famous case study in the history of neuropsychology is Phineas Gage. In 1848, Phineas Gage was a railroad construction supervisor in Vermont. Part of his job was to prepare the charges to blast rocks so that the railroad tracks could be laid. To do this, a hole would be drilled in the rock and then gunpowder would be placed in the hole followed by sand. This would then be tamped down with a long iron rod. On September 13, 1848, Phineas Gage did not realize that the sand had not been added and began to drop the iron rod into the hole. As the rod went into the rock, a spark ignited the gunpowder and the 13-pound iron rod went through Phineas Gage's brain, as shown in *Figure 4-1*, and landed some 30 feet away.

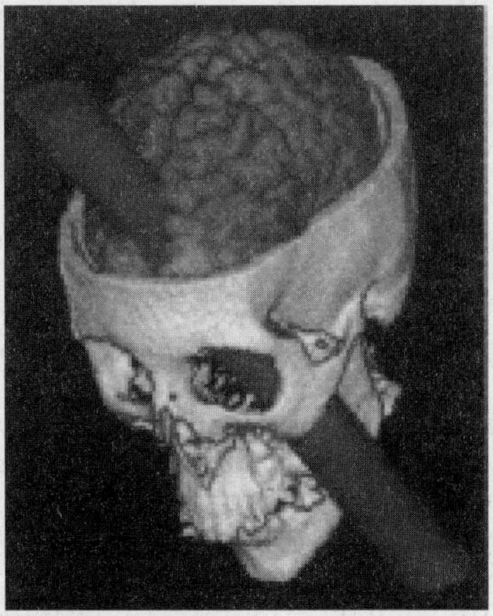

FIGURE 4-1 Depiction of the Rod in Phineas Gage's Brain

Source: Damasio H, Grabowski TJ, Frank RJ, Galaburda AM, Damasio AR, "The Return of Phineas Gage: Clues About the Brain from the Skull of a Famous Patient," Science, Vol 264, 20 May 1994. Reprinted with permission from AAAS.

Amazingly, after being momentarily stunned, Gage regained full consciousness and was able to talk and walk with help. He was taken back to his boardinghouse and seen by a local doctor. What was surprising was that over time Phineas Gage was able to recover from his physical injuries. He continued to be able to speak and do the everyday motor processes required. His intelligence and ability to learn new information remained as before the accident. However, his personality showed such a drastic change that his coworkers said he was "no longer Gage." Whereas he was a mild-mannered person before the accident, afterward he was prone to angry outbursts. Gage also lacked social conventions and frequently used profanity. The accident had influenced his emotional processing. This case study as described by his physician, Dr. Harlow, has helped scientists understand the manner in which brain damage can influence social and emotional processes seen in other types of mental disorder. This helped later scientists to consider which areas of the brain might be involved in mental disorders that show deficits in social and emotional processing. The iron rod and his skull have been retained at the Medical Museum at Harvard University.

Modern researchers have sought to use the case of Phineas Gage to illustrate types of brain damage. Hanna Damasio and her colleagues, using photographs and X-rays of the skull, created a three-dimensional reconstruction including the entry and exit points of the iron rod (Damasio et al., 1994). From this, they described the suggested damage to the left and right prefrontal cortex (PFC), which would include a lack of inhibition as shown by his angry outbursts, a lack of planning, memory problems, and deficits in social cognition. Peter Ratiu and his colleagues performed computerized axial tomography (CAT) scans on the skull of Phineas Gage to determine the manner in which the rod was projected through his skull (Ratiu, Talos, Haker, Lieberman, & Evert, 2004). Using these same CAT scans, John Van Horn and his colleagues sought to model damage to the white and gray matter of the brain (Van Horn et al., 2012). In order to estimate the damage to Gage's brain, these researchers examined the white matter connections of 110 healthy male individuals 25 to 36 years of age using brain imaging techniques. They suggested that Gage suffered from damage to the left frontal cortex and that network connectedness between the left frontal area and other brain areas would have been considerable. This modeling is shown in *Figure 4-2.*

The basis of every case study is the clinical notes of the professionals. Diagnosis and treatment notes are kept for each individual they see. The case study offers an opportunity for an in- depth examination of an individual's manifestation and experience of psychopathology. It is particularly important for the description of rarer conditions in which the important factors are not yet well understood. However, it is difficult from a case study to know whether the relationships described were unique to that individual or could be generalized to others with the disorder. As such, it is useful for directing future research concerning the critical variables involved in the disorder.

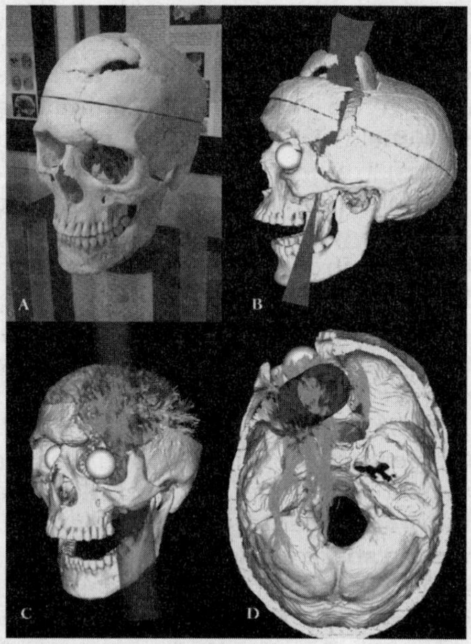

FIGURE 4-2 Full Modeling of the Rod in Phineas Gage's Brain

Source: Van Horn et al. (2012, e37454).
Note: A. The skull of Phineas Gage on display at the Warren Anatomical Museum at Harvard Medical School. B. CT image volumes were reconstructed, spatially aligned, and manual segmentation of the individual pieces of bone dislodged by the tamping iron (rod). C. A rendering of the Gage skull with the best fit rod trajectory and example fiber pathways in the left hemisphere intersected by the rod. D. A view of the interior of the Gage skull showing the extent of fiber pathways intersected by the tamping iron in a sample subject (i.e., one having minimal spatial deformation to the Gage skull). The intersection and density of white matter fibers between all possible pairs of gray matter parcellations were recorded, as was average fiber length and average fractional anisotropy (FA) integrated over each fiber.

Naturalistic Observation: Just Looking

If little is known about a particular phenomenon, it often is useful simply to watch the phenomenon occur naturally and get a general idea of what is involved in the process. Initially, this is accomplished by observing and describing what occurs. This scientific technique is called **naturalistic observation.** A classic example of this approach is Charles Darwin's observation of animals in the Galápagos Islands. He carefully noted their appearance and environment. The observations formed the basis of his theory of evolution. Psychologists have used naturalistic observation techniques to study children and adults, as well as the interactions of those in a mental hospital. New technologies such as video or audio capture have allowed for even greater possibilities.

Using a naturalistic observation study, Rachel Tomko and her colleagues collected data from individuals with borderline personality disorder (BPD) and other individuals with depression (Tomlo et al., 2012). These researchers wanted to better understand the social and emotional interactions of individuals with these disorders. As you will read in later chapters, individuals with BPD may show emotional instability such as an angry outburst. Those with depression do not.

The researchers used a device that periodically recorded 50-second snippets of sound. What these researchers reported was that individuals with depression were more likely to spend time alone if they had previously been angry. Individuals with BPD did not display withdrawal from others after anger and at times showed the opposite.

The naturalistic observation method has four characteristics:

1. Noninterference is of prime importance. Scientists using this method must not disrupt the process or flow of events. In this way, they can see things as they really are, without influencing the ongoing phenomenon.
2. This method emphasizes the invariants or patterns that exist in the world. For example, if you could observe yourself in a noninterfering manner, you might conclude that your moods vary with the time of day, particular weather patterns, or even particular thoughts.
3. This method is most useful when we know little about the subject of our investigation. It is most useful for understanding the "big picture" by observing a series of events rather than isolated happenings.
4. The naturalistic method may not shed light on the factors that directly influence the behavior observed. The method provides a description of a phenomenon; it does not answer the question of why it happened.

Correlational Approach: What Goes With What

The **correlational approach** is designed to help us understand how specific factors are associated with one another. As with much of human behavior, there are complex relationships between psychological variables and factors associated with them. The correlational approaches help us see what factors are related to one another. For example, you can ask if having friends is associated with better physical and psychological health or if negative experiences in one's past are associated with becoming depressed. Thus, we ask if one aspect of a system is associated with another aspect. It should be noted that both the statistical methods used to determine the degree of association and the research designs used to research the relationship between variables use the same term: *correlational.*

How would you go about answering these questions? Let's begin with the relationship between friends and health. You would first need to determine how you know how many friends someone has. One way is to ask them or you could ask how many friends they have on their Facebook page. What about health? One approach is to determine the number of times they went to the health center. If you did this with a number of individuals, you would have two numbers for each person—their number of friends and their health center visits.

What would you do with these data? One helpful technique is to create a scatterplot of the data. A scatterplot is a graph on which the data from each person is plotted. In this way, we would use the y-axis to display the number of friends on Facebook (e.g., 0–150) and the x-axis to display the number of visits to the health center during the past year (e.g., 0–20). We could then look at these measures for each person and plot that point on the graph. This scatterplot is shown in *Figure 4-3.* It is now possible to look at the graph and visually determine if there is a relationship.

Occasionally, cross-cultural comparisons of correlational studies conducted across two diverse cultures can yield a major difference in findings, which can then be attributed to the one factor that differs across both cultures. As a case in point, the widely studied phenomenon of expressed emotion being correlated with relapse in persons with schizophrenia seemed to have been attributable to higher social support in Indian families (Leff et al., 1987).

Although humans are good at determining patterns, a statistical technique would allow for better precision. Such a technique is the **correlation coefficient.** The correlation coefficient gives both the strength of the relationship and its direction.

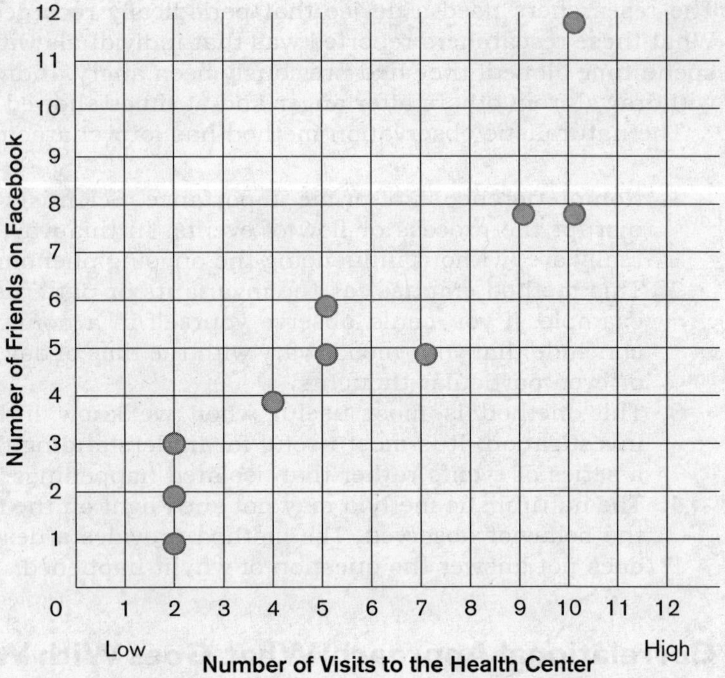

FIGURE 4-3 Scatter Diagram Showing Positive Relationship Between Two Measures

If the number of friends on Facebook was associated with more health center visits then this relationship would be called a **positive correlation.** However, if fewer friends were associated with more visits then this relationship would be called a **negative correlation.**

In the real world, few relationships are perfectly related to one another. Thus, the correlation coefficient is also able to reflect the degree of an association between two variables. Technically, the degree of relationship determined by the correlation coefficient is denoted by the letter *r*. Whether the relationship between the variables is positive or negative is denoted by the + and – signs. The correlation coefficient can range from –1 to +1. A perfect positive relationship would be $r = +1$, and a perfect negative relationship would be $r = -1$. If there was no relationship, it would be $r = 0$. *Figure 4-4* shows a variety of relationships and their *r* values.

What are the basic ideas of correlational studies? In correlational studies, the researcher is interested in asking whether there is an association between two variables, but he or she does not attempt to establish how one variable influences the other, only that a relationship exists. Establishing that such an association exists may be the first step in dealing with a complex problem.

My colleagues and I used a correlational technique to understand whether being tortured influenced the brain differently if one experienced dissociative experiences (Ray et al., 2006). Although not much is known concerning neuroscience measurements of individuals who have been tortured in their native country, there has been some suggestion that torture leads to different types of psychopathological disorders. There is also some evidence to suggest that torture victims adopt psychological mechanisms to

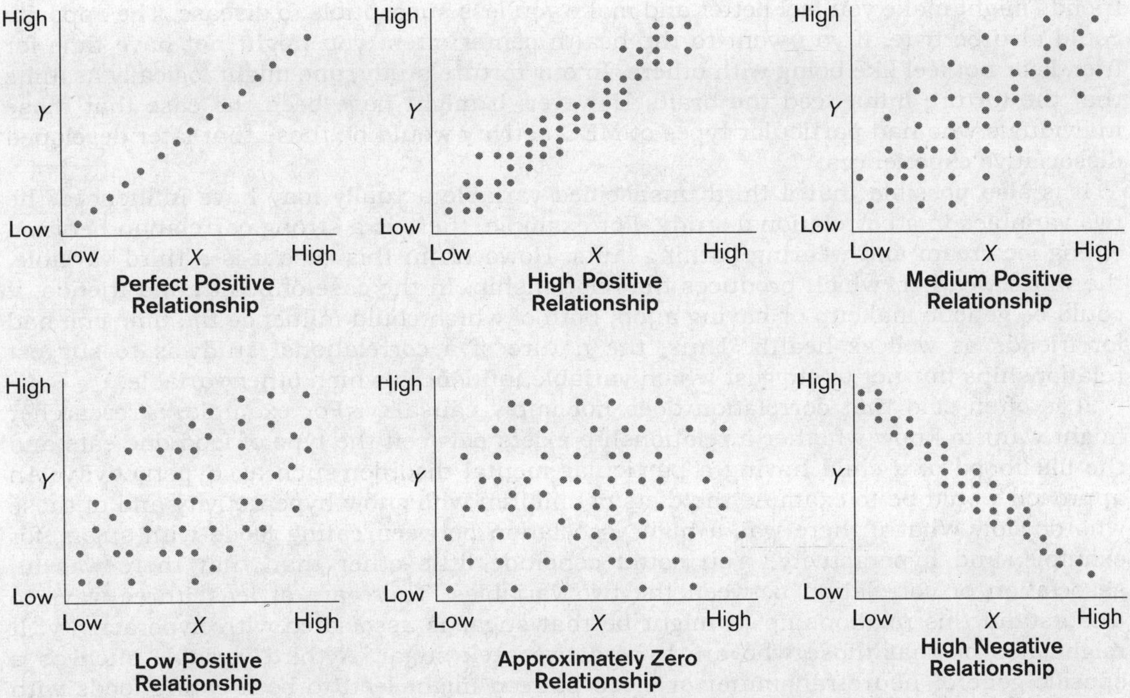

FIGURE 4-4 Scatter Diagrams Showing Various Relationships That Differ in Degree and Direction

escape the experience of the situation. Dissociation is one such mechanism in which individuals are able to distance themselves from such extreme negative experiences as torture or rape. We developed a dissociative scale that asked individuals about dissociative experiences they had experienced. Since some other neuroscience work had shown that non-normal MEG (magnetoencephalography) activity was seen in different areas of the brain in disorders such as schizophrenia, depression, and PTSD (e.g., Rockstroh, Wienbruch, Ray, & Elbert, 2007), we used MEG as the variable to correlate with dissociative experiences. We found a positive correlation of .60 between our measure of MEG activity and the dissociation scale for the left hemisphere as a whole and a negative correlation of –.61 for the right hemisphere as a whole. More precise analysis showed the involvement of the left ventral region of the anterior cortical areas.

What we cannot know from correlational research is whether either variable influences the other directly. There are a variety of ways that one can see a high correlation. It might be that there is a direct relationship. That is, having lots of

Concept Check

- What are four characteristics of the scientific approach? What are two additional key ingredients in psychological research?
- What are the three stages of the scientific process?
- Why has the case study been particularly valuable in psychopathology research?
- What are the four characteristics of the naturalistic observation method?
- If a research study reports that two variables are correlated, what do you know about their relationship? What don't you know about their relationship?

friends might make you feel better and make you less susceptible to disease. The opposite could also be true. If you went to the health center often, you might not have time for friends or not feel like being with others. In our torture study, one might logically assume that the torture influenced the brain. However, it might have been the case that those individuals who had particular types of MEG activity would be those that later developed dissociative experiences.

It is also possible that a third unspecified variable actually may have influenced the two variables in a correlational study. For example, there is a strong correlation between eating ice cream and wearing bathing suits. However, in this case it is a third variable, the warm weather, which produces the relationship. In the case of health and friends, it could be genetic makeup or having a job, both of which could influence the time one had for friends as well as health. Thus, the nature of a correlational study is to suggest relationships but not to suggest which variable influences which other variable.

It is often said that correlation does not imply causality. For example, a researcher might want to know whether a relationship exists between the type of food one eats and the likelihood of a child having a particular mental disorder such as hyperactivity. An approach would be to examine the diets of children who show hyperactivity and of those who do not. What if there was a high association between eating foods with sugar, for example, and hyperactivity? You could conclude little other than that there was an association or correlation between the two variables. There are at least three ways to understand this relationship. It might be that sugar is associated with hyperactivity. It might also be that those who are hyperactive seek sugar. A third variable such as a specific gene or neurotransmitter or sleep pattern might lead to both eating foods with sugar and showing hyperactivity.

The association of two factors does not in itself imply that one influences the other. However, if there is a *low* correlation between the events, you can infer that one event does *not* cause the other. A high degree of association is always necessary for establishing that one variable influences another; a correlational study is often the first step for providing the needed support for later experimental research, especially in complex areas.

Experimental Method: Making It Happen

Just finding that a relationship exists between two events does not allow us to determine exactly what that relationship is, much less to determine that one event actually caused the other event to happen. If we want to state that one event produced another event, we need to develop a much stronger case for our position.

To do this, we could see how some single event over which we have control affects the phenomenon we are studying. In this way, we begin to interact with the phenomenon. We structure our question in this form: If I do this, what will happen? Numerous questions can be asked in this way, such as, Will people with depression learn words better in a foreign language if each word is of the same class (e.g., negative emotional words) than if they are from a variety of different classes (some emotional, some objects, some neutral words)?

As our knowledge grows, we may even get to the point of formulating specific predictions. In this case, our questions are structured in this form: If I do this, I expect this will happen. Sometimes our predictions are more global, and we predict that one factor will be stronger than another. We might predict that more people are likely to help a stranger if they perceive the environment to be safe than if they think it is dangerous. Sometimes, however, we may know enough about an area to make a more precise prediction or point prediction. For example, we might predict that 3 months of exercise will lead to a drop in self-reported depression on a standard scale. These approaches, in which we interact directly with the phenomenon we are studying, are examples of the **experimental method.**

Definitions in the Experimental Method

What if we want to know if exercise affects depression? The hypothesis, or idea being tested, is that exercising would influence depression. To test the hypothesis, we could have one group exercise and another not exercise. The group that performs the exercise is called the **experimental group.** The group that does not is called the **control group.** A control group is a group that is treated exactly like the experimental group except for the factor being studied. In this case, the factor being studied is exercise and its influence on depression.

Depression can be viewed on a number of different levels, so we need to have a definition of what depression means in our study. These representations of psychological events in the physical world are called operational definitions. An **operational definition** defines events in terms of the operations required to measure them and thus gives our idea a concrete meaning. Depression could be defined as the score received on a measure of depression such as the Beck Depression Inventory (BDI).

Cultural context is also important while planning an intervention for depression in an experimental pre-post own control design.

A better understanding of the community's viewpoints about mental illness and health can also help the process of de-stigmatization. For example, to quote R. Thara of SCARF, India, "the community's explanatory model of schizophrenia often shifts from a magico-religious to a medico-social viewpoint" (Patel, Farooq, & Thara, 2007) after the patient has improved with correct pharmacotherapy and psychosocial intervention. Much is currently being done in India to assist this process of de-stigmatization, using a pre-post own control research design. A grassroots community-based study, VISHRAM, for example, cited the use of Prakashdoot videos to raise awareness about Depression: "The Authors would also like to thank Anand Nadkarni, Anuradha Sovani and Shubha Thatte from the IPH, Thane, for developing Prakashdoot videos which played a significant role in improving mental health awareness during VISHRAM implementation" (Shidhaye et al., 2017).

The idea that watching violence on television or playing video games with violent content increases aggression is certainly a reasonable and potentially important notion. The popular press has often tried to link violent video games with those who perform school shootings. Yet before we can test this idea, we must define exactly what is meant by violence on television or in video games. Is a program with an unseen murder more violent than an exciting boxing match? Should violence be rated by how many minutes it appears on the screen, by the particular type of act, by how much blood is shown, or by a combination of all three? Likewise, to perform this research we need to devise some measure of aggression. We would have to adopt operational definitions.

An operational definition takes a general concept, such as depression or aggression or effectiveness, and places it within a given context. That is, it redefines the concept in terms of clearly observable operations that anyone can see and repeat. For example, as with the Bobo doll study (see Chapter 2), we might define *aggression* as the number of times a child hits a toy after watching a violent video.

In an experimental study, we want to know how one variable that we manipulate affects another variable. In the example of coffee affecting memory, whether or not someone drank coffee was the manipulated variable. This is also called the **independent variable (IV).** Memory in this example is the variable influenced by the coffee and is called the **dependent variable (DV).** That is, it depends on or is influenced by the IV.

What other factors could influence a memory test? If we suspect that some unintended factor may also be operating, then the truth or **validity** of the experiment is seriously threatened. Thus, the conclusion that the IV influenced the DV could be questioned. In the memory experiment, if the control group was run in the morning and the experimental group in the afternoon, then time of day could have an effect. Whenever two or more IVs are operating, the unintended IVs (those not chosen by the experimenter) are called **confounding variables.**

Other confounding variables may **covary** with the IV and be more difficult to notice. For example, assume that a researcher compared a new medication against a problem-solving approach for the treatment of anxiety. If she found the problem-solving approach to show a greater reduction in anxiety, could she conclude that problem solving produced the reduction? Although that is one possibility, it also may have been the case that spending time with a professional produced the reduction in anxiety. That is, because giving medications requires less time with a patient than discussing problem-solving techniques, the results found may not have been due to the IV as planned in the study but rather to a confounding variable of time with the patient.

Does Playing Music Change the Brain?

Let's examine a specific study in which both experimental and correlational procedures were used. Thomas Elbert and his colleagues began with the idea that experience could change the manner in which connections in the brain were established (Elbert, Pantev, Weinbruch, Rockstroh, & Taub, 1995). What these researchers needed to do was find a task that would allow them to measure change and make logical inferences. Since they were interested in long-term changes, they sought to find a skill that people learn in childhood. They decided on an experiment that involved playing a musical instrument.

What musical instrument would you choose—piano, saxophone, violin, or another instrument? They chose the violin. Here is where logic and experimental design came in. By choosing the violin, these researchers were able to compare the differences between the violinists' left and right hands and their representation in the brain. Violinists use their left hand to continuously finger the strings. The right hand moves the bow back and forth and does not require the same fine motor skills. If playing a violin for 20 years would affect the brain, then it should affect those areas involved with the left hand in a different manner than those involved with the right. This is exactly what they found.

To measure neuronal activity in the brain, these researchers used a brain imaging device, the MEG. They found that neuronal activity in the brain was different between the areas of the brain related to the left and right fingers of musicians. Further, they found that the brain areas of the musicians' right hands were not different from those of the control group who did not play a musical instrument. Thus, the experimental comparison was between individuals who had played a musical instrument since childhood and the control group, those who had not. There was also a comparison between the brain areas involved with the left and right fingers of the musicians. Further, these researchers examined the correlation between neuronal activity and the length of time an individual had played an instrument. *Figure 4-5* shows this relationship. As you can see, this is a negative correlation in that the earlier (lower number) one began to play an instrument the stronger the neuronal activity was. The experimental and correlational aspects of this research helped the researchers logically conclude that previous experience can influence brain organization. The major point here is that prior experience can influence the brain, which will be an important consideration in fully understanding the development of mental illness and its treatment. For example, therapy for depression changes the flexibility of the brain connections whereas stress restricts flexibility (Castrén & Hen, 2013).

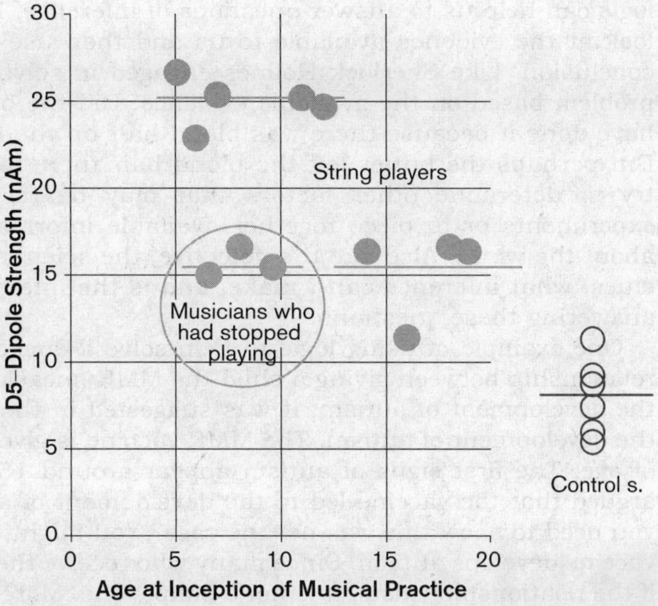

FIGURE 4-5 The Relationship Between Neuronal Activity (Dipole Strength) and the Length of Time an Individual Had Played an Instrument

Source: Elbert, T., Pantev, C., Wienbruch, C., Rockstroh, B., & Taub, E. (1995). Increased Cortical Representation of the Fingers of the Left Hand in String Players, *Science*, 270(5234), 305–307.

Logic and Inference: The Detective Work of Science

Perhaps you have heard the story of our friend from Boston who got up every morning, went outside his house, walked around in a circle 3 times, and yelled at the top of his voice. His neighbor, being somewhat curious after days of this ritual, asked for the purpose behind his strange behavior. The man answered that the purpose was to keep away tigers. "But," the neighbor replied, "there are no tigers within thousands of miles of here." To which our friend replied, "Works quite well, doesn't it?"

How could we demonstrate to our friend that his yelling is not causally related to the absence of tigers? One strategy might be to point out that the absence of tigers might have come about for other reasons, including the fact that there are no tigers roaming in the greater Boston area. Our friend's reasoning was incorrect because it overlooked many other plausible explanations for the obvious absence of tigers. Although our friend sought to infer a relationship between his yelling and the absence of tigers, his **inference** was weak.

Logic is particularly important in science as an aid to answering this question: What question should my experimental study answer to test my ideas about the world? That is, logic can help us to answer questions of inference. Inference is the process by which we look at the evidence available to us and then use our powers of reasoning to reach a conclusion. Like Sherlock Holmes engaged in solving a mystery, we attempt to solve a problem based on the available evidence. Did the butler do it? No, the butler could not have done it because there was blond hair on the knife and the butler had black hair. But perhaps the butler left the blond hair there to fool us. Like a detective, scientists try to determine other factors that may be responsible for the outcome of their experiments or to piece together available information and draw general conclusions about the world. Also like the detective, the scientist is constantly asking, "Given these clues, what inference can I make, and is the inference valid?" Logic is one method for answering these questions.

One example of using logic to help solve a question in psychopathology involved the relationship between giving a child the MMR (measles, mumps, and rubella) vaccine and the development of autism. It was suggested in the media that the MMR vaccine led to the development of autism. The MMR vaccine is given to a child around 12 to 15 months of age. The first signs of autism appear around 15 to 18 months of age. Thus, it was argued that the vaccine led to the development of autism. What type of evidence would you need to show this was not the case? You might first ask if everyone who receives the vaccine develops autism. Since many who receive the vaccine do not develop autism, then if the relationship exists, it is not a simple one. More important from a logical standpoint, you might ask if there exists a child who did not receive the vaccine but did develop autism. This would help to rule out vaccination being the single cause of autism. As you will see in Chapter 6, a critical finding is that there are signs of autism in children before the age of vaccinations. Thus, logically researchers were able to rule out vaccines as the cause of autism.

Validity

Logical procedures are also important for helping us understand the accuracy or validity of our ideas and research. Valid means true and capable of being supported. In studying mental illness, one important way to show that our ideas can be supported is to replicate them with different individuals in different locations. If we hypothesized that a certain type of stress led to depression, for example, then we would need to show that this is the case not only in our research clinic but also in other clinics.

Historically, we have discussed various types of validity in psychology, which arise from differing contexts. These contexts range from developing types of tests to running experiments. The overall question is "Does a certain procedure, whether it is a test of mental illness or an experiment, do what it was intended to do?" There are two general types of validity (Campbell & Stanley, 1963).

The first is **internal validity.** The word *internal* refers to the experiment itself. Internal validity asks the following question: Is there another reason that might explain the outcome of our experimental procedures? Students are particularly sensitive to questions of internal validity, for example, when it is time for final exams; they can make a number of alternative suggestions about what the exam actually measures and why it does not measure their knowledge of a particular subject. Like students, scientists look for reasons (threats to internal validity) that a particular piece of research may not measure what it claims to measure. In the case of our friend from Boston, the absence of tigers near his house could have reflected a long-standing absence of tigers in his part of the world rather than the effectiveness of his yelling.

The second type of validity is **external validity.** The word *external* refers to the world outside the setting in which the experiment was performed. External validity often is called **generalizability.** Remember the story of Semmelweis. His finding that the deaths of the mothers who had just given birth were the result of physicians touching them after handling diseased tissue was true not only for his hospital but also for all other hospitals. Thus, in addressing the question of external validity of Semmelweis's work, we would infer that his answers could be generalized to other hospitals with other women and not just to his own original setting. External validity, however, refers to the possibility of applying the results from an internally valid experiment to other situations and other research participants.

We logically design our research to rule out as many alternative interpretations of our findings as possible and to have any new facts be applicable to as wide a variety of other situations as possible. In many real-life situations in which external validity is high, however, it is impossible to rule out alternative interpretations of our findings. In a similar way, in laboratory settings in which internal validity is high, the setting is often artificial, and in many cases our findings cannot be generalized beyond the laboratory. Consequently, designing and conducting research is always a trade-off between internal and external validity. Which one we emphasize depends on the particular research questions being asked.

Before continuing, let's clear up one misconception. It is the idea of designing "the one perfect study." Although we strive to design good research, there are always alternative explanations and conditions not included in any single study. It is for this reason that Donald Campbell, who introduced scientists to the idea of internal and external validity, also emphasized the importance of replicating studies. If the same study is performed a number of times with similar results, then we can have more assurance that the results were valid. Even better, if the study is performed in a variety of settings around the world, we have even more confidence in our results.

What Do I Expect to Happen?

One characteristic of human beings is that we seek to determine what will happen next. When we are talking with someone we anticipate the next word they will say. The same is true in psychological experiments. Participants imagine what they are expected to do. If their expectation interferes with the influence of the IV then the study could give inaccurate results.

In research terminology, this type of bias is referred to as **demand characteristics.** Demand characteristics occur when a participant's response is influenced more by the research setting than by the IV. For example, a study might examine the effects of a drug as compared with exercise on reducing hyperactivity in adults. Many participants might believe the drug to be most effective, especially if the drug was given by a mental health professional and the exercise by a non–mental health professional. Those who received the drug might look for signs the drug was reducing hyperactivity. They might then pay more attention to the task used as the DV. If demand characteristics play an important role in the experiment, then they pose a significant threat to internal validity and offer an alternative explanation for understanding the influence of the IV.

Concept Check

- What is the difference between the experimental group and the control group? Why is the control group important?
- What is an operational definition? How does it help advance scientific knowledge?
- How are the IV, the DV, and confounding variables related?
- What is a double-blind experiment, and what are we trying to control for by using that design?

A related phenomenon is referred to as the **placebo effect.** The term *placebo* comes from the Latin verb *placere:* "to please." It refers to the phenomenon that some people show psychological and physiological changes just from the suggestion that a change will take place. How could this be accomplished in a treatment study to reduce anxiety?

Experimenters also have expectations. For example, knowing that one set of subjects has been assigned to one condition rather than another could result in those participants being treated differently. Such situations are referred to as **experimenter effects.**

To control for the placebo effect in research as well as experimenter effects, various procedures have been used. One is to use a control group that receives either no treatment or a treatment previously shown to be ineffective for the particular disorder under study. In medical research, it is common to give a "sugar" pill that looks exactly like the medicine with the active ingredient. In psychotherapy research, a control group could be given relaxation training, which has been shown not to be effective on its own.

A more powerful control is to use a **double-blind experiment** in which the experimental group is divided into two groups. One group is given the actual treatment, and the other is given a treatment exactly like the experimental treatment but without the active ingredient. Neither the placebo group nor the experimental group would know which treatment they are receiving, and in this way, these research participants are said to be **blind controls.** The term *double blind* indicates that the experimenters giving the medication also do not know which treatment is experimental and which is placebo.

In order to sort through the results of our experiments, we must be like detectives who constantly ask if there is another way to understand what was found. Our way of doing that is though research, logic, and doubt. We use research to design a study to consider alternative possibilities. We use logic to consider if our conclusions follow from the results. We use doubt to ask if there is a way to know if we are wrong.

Designing an Experimental Study

One goal of experimental research is to determine the relation between the IV and the DV. The less bias in terms of demand characteristics related to both the participant and the experimenter aids in creating a logical relationship between the IV and DV.

There are an additional four factors that are critical to sound inference (*Figure 4-6*). These are as follows:

1. Participant selection
2. Participant assignment
3. Design of experiment
4. Interpretation of relation of IV to DV

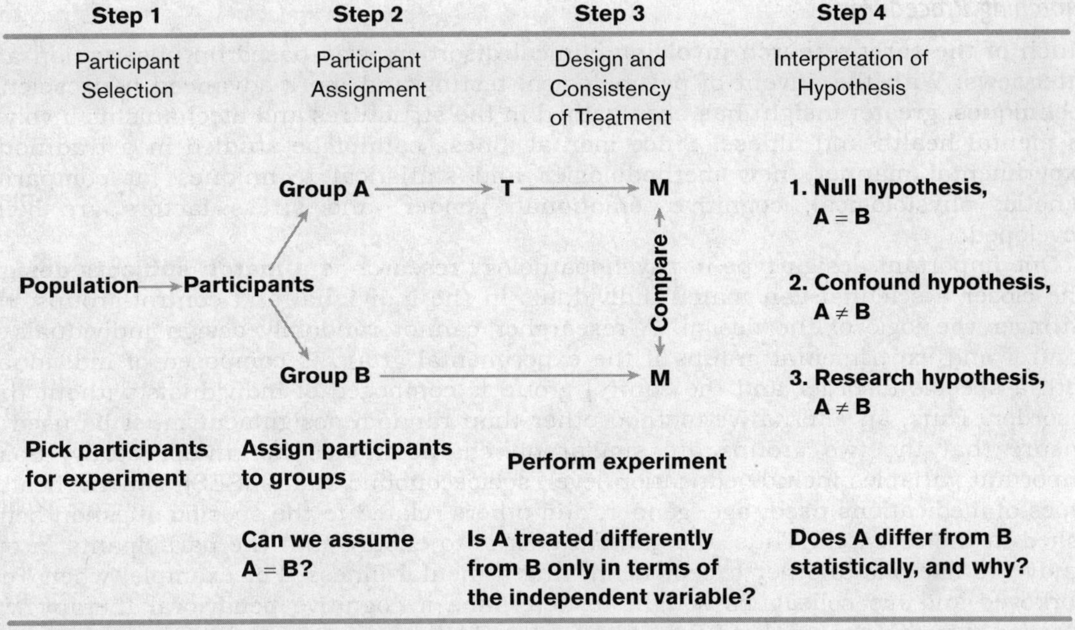

FIGURE 4-6 The Four Conceptual Steps in Experimentation

Participants in the Study

It may seem simple to select subjects for an experiment. However, this is often a greater problem than it appears. The individuals selected for the study should be directly related to the hypothesis being tested. If you want to know if individuals with schizophrenia perform better on a memory test after having drunk coffee, then of course you select individuals with schizophrenia. If you want to be able to apply the results to the **population** of all adults, then it is necessary for adults of all ages, genders, and ethnic backgrounds to be included in the study.

Researchers use a variety of means for selecting participants. The best is some form of random sampling. You might choose every tenth person in the college directory, or every fourth person admitted to the ward for treatment of schizophrenia, for example. When the selection is not random—that is, every person is not equally likely to be chosen—then bias can appear.

Putting Participants in Groups

After the participants have been randomly selected from the larger population under study, they can then be randomly assigned to experimental and control groups. This ensures that the groups are equal before the experiment begins. **Randomization** *controls for both known and unknown potentially confounding variables.* Randomization leaves solely to chance the assignment of our participants to a group. In this way, any differences—even unknown or unsuspected differences—will also be nullified by being randomly distributed between our two groups.

Matching Procedures

Much of the early research involving clinical disorders was based on observation and interviews. With the advent of psychological testing and more advanced neuroscience techniques, greater insight has been gained in the structures and mechanisms involved in mental health and illness. Since mental illness cannot be studied in a traditional experimental manner, new methodologies and statistical techniques for comparing genetic, physiological, cognitive, emotional, gender, and stress factors are being developed.

One important design type in psychopathology research is a **match subjects design.** The closer a scientist can match individuals in the individual and control groups, the stronger the logic of the design. A researcher cannot randomly assign individuals to control and experimental groups if the experimental group is composed of individuals with a specific disorder and the control group is composed of individuals without that disorder. Thus, an alternative method other than random assignment must be used to ensure that the two groups are similar on characteristics not under study. Some important variables include education level, socioeconomic status (SES), general health, types of medications used, age, gender, and others related to the specific question being asked in the research. Thus, the general task is to ensure that the participants in our study are like one another except for having a mental illness. For example, when Tom Borkovec and his colleagues sought to determine if cognitive behavioral therapy was effective in treating generalized anxiety disorder (GAD) as compared with other treatments, it was important that those with anxiety were matched in terms of age, gender, income, education level, and other such variables in terms of the experimental conditions (Borkovec & Ruscio, 2001).

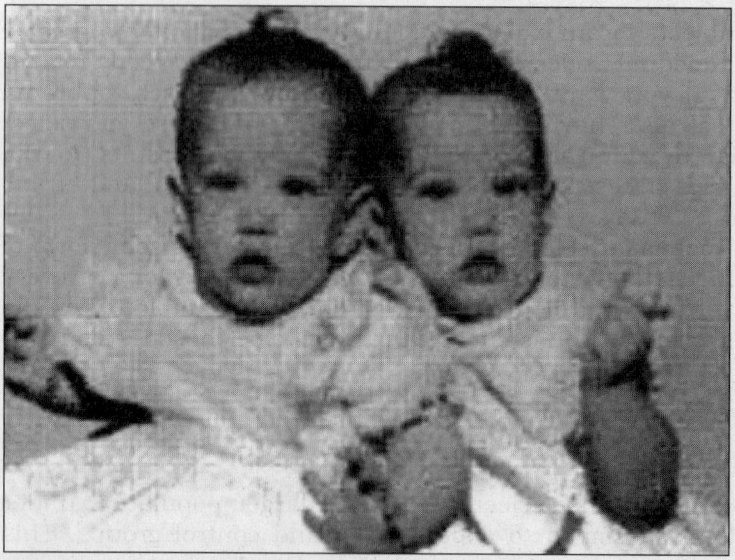

Identical twins as children. Later in life, the one on the right developed bipolar disorder and the one on the left remained well

The strongest version of matching is to use identical twins. The situation in which one has a particular disorder and the other does not helps to focus on the critical variables. One classic study involving these twins was performed by E. Fuller Torrey and his colleagues in the 1990s. They studied individuals who developed schizophrenia or bipolar disorder (manic depression). Twins who lived together would be matched in terms of such factors as genetics, family history, SES, and a number of other factors. However, twins are not always available and thus researchers need to match those with a disorder and those without.

Designing the Study

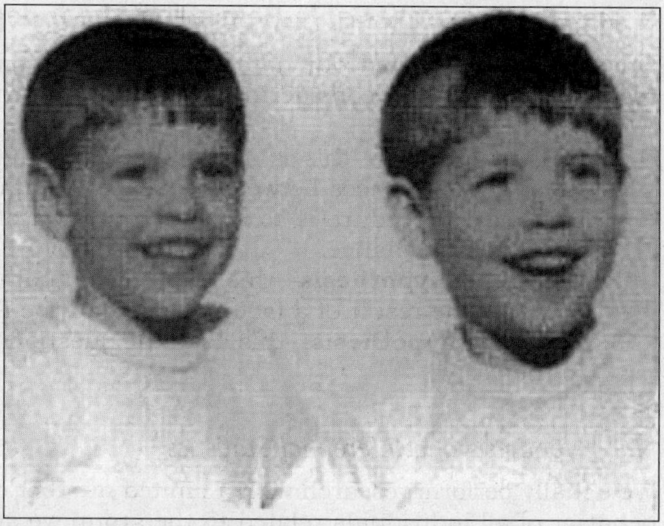

Identical twins as children. Later in life, the one on the right developed schizophrenia and the one on the left remained well.

Science is a way of asking questions about the world. The quality of the answers we receive is influenced by several factors, one of the most important being the experimental design that we use. Somewhat like a blueprint, the experimental design directs the procedures and gives form to the experiment. In essence, an experimental design is a plan for how a study is to be structured.

In an outline form, a design tells us what will be done to whom and when. To be evaluated favorably, a design must perform two related functions. First, it must provide a logical structure that enables us to pinpoint the effects of the IV on the DV and thus answer our research questions. Second, it must help us rule out confounds as an alternative explanation for our findings.

A sound design must allow us to determine logically the effect of the IV on the DV and to rule out alternative explanations.

Imagine a study in which a clinical psychologist was interested in determining if teaching children with autism to look at a person's face would increases their interaction with others. Thus, the question asked would be whether looking at a face (IV) results in the participant interacting more with others (DV). After the subject was taught to look at a face, he or she could be placed in situations in which other individuals were present. The researcher could measure the number of interactions that the child engaged in.

If we were to diagram the design of this study, it would be as follows:

Select the group	Teach facial focus	Measure number of interactions

If we performed the experiment with just Group A, what could we conclude? We could determine if our participants had a certain number of interactions. However, this would not help us determine if this was related to the facial focus procedure. Such a design would not be much help in pinpointing the effect of the IV on the DV, nor would it rule out confounds.

A stronger design would use a control group. This design would appear as follows:

Experimental group	Teach facial focus	Measure number of interactions
Control group	No treatment	Measure number of interactions

Since the control group had not received the treatment, we would have stronger evidence that the treatment was related to differences in number of interactions.

Is the Dependent Variable Related to the Independent Variable?

Once we have collected our data, we want to know how to interpret our experimental results. We do this by considering three separate hypotheses:

1. **Null hypothesis**—this is a statistical hypothesis that is tested to determine if there are differences between our experimental and control groups. Part of this statistical procedure is to ask the question of whether our results could have happened by chance.
2. **Confound hypothesis**—this is a conceptual question that asks if our results could be the result of a factor other than the IV.
3. **Research hypothesis**—this asks the question of whether our results are related to the IV.

Null Hypothesis and Inferential Statistics

We usually perform research with a limited number of individuals so that we can infer the behavior of all individuals related to the group we studied. For example, we might study how a group of individuals with depression responded to mindfulness meditation in terms of measures of distress.

What are the odds that the individuals with depression in our group are like all those with depression everywhere? To determine this **probability,** we use **inferential statistics.** Technically, we refer to all individuals with depression as the population and the particular participants in our study as the **sample.** Inferential statistics concerns the relationship between the statistical characteristics of the population and those of the sample.

One way of viewing the inferential process conceptually is to assume that the same experiment was run an infinite number of times, each time with a different sample of individuals chosen from the entire population. If we were to plot the statistics from each experiment, the population of estimates would then represent all the possible outcomes of the experiment.

In more technical language, inferential statistics is used to infer, from a given sample of scores on some measure, the parameters for the set of all possible scores. All possible scores would be that of the population from which our particular sample was drawn. Implicit in this statement is the assumption that the sample we are discussing is the result of random sampling or some systematic form of sampling. That is, each person in the population of all people is equally likely to be included in the sample, with some known probability.

The important thing to remember is that inferential statistics constitutes a set of tools for inferring from a particular sample to larger populations. One way of viewing this conceptually is to ask how the statistics of our sample (that is, the mean and the standard deviation) match what we expect to be the same measures in the larger population.

Conceptually, we ask if our control and experimental groups could be considered equal before any treatment (IV) was introduced. That is, would we expect them to be drawn equally from the larger population? One way in which we seek to make our experimental and control groups equal is through random assignment to the groups. One critical question that is asked in terms of empirically supported treatments (see Chapter 2) is whether the participants were randomly assigned to the treatment condition. If so, then we take the support for a particular treatment as being more valid.

Given a group of potential subjects, we could expect some of them to be motivated to be part of the experiment, others to be tired, some to be more intelligent, some to have faster reaction times than others, and so forth. By randomly assigning these individuals to groups, we would expect to make the two groups equal.

Another part of the statistical treatment of the null hypothesis is related to probability. If you were to toss a coin a large number of times, you would expect that you would have an equal number of heads and tails. The idea of no differences forms the basis of the null hypothesis, which was developed by Sir Ronald Fisher (1935). He sought to determine whether a set of results differed from what would be expected.

What we need, of course, is a technique for determining if a set of results is different from what would be expected. One of the common statistical techniques used for this is called the *t* test. It was actually developed near the beginning of the last century by William Gosset, who worked for the Guinness Brewery in Dublin. Gosset wanted a way of knowing if all the batches of beer were the same. In this case, he actually wanted the null hypothesis to be true. Fisher developed the *F* test, which is conceptually similar to the *t* test. In fact, mathematically $t^2 = F$.

In our experiment, we can think of the *t* test or *F* test, asking the question of what is the difference in reaction time between the experimental and control groups. The larger the difference, the more certain we can be that the IV had an effect. However, this needs to be mathematically related to the normal variation we find in reaction time in all individuals as well as the number of participants that took part in our experiment. If normal variation in reaction time was high, then it would be more difficult for our IV to show an effect. Likewise, the more participants that are part of our experiment, the less likely factors other than the IV influenced the results.

In the end, we are never fully certain that our results are or are not due to chance. Instead, we use statistics to help us to make a best guess by assigning a probability to the statement that our results are not due to chance alone. That is, we may say that results from our study could have happened by chance less than 1 time out of every 100. Said in other words, if we ran the same study 100 times with a different set of subjects drawn from the total population, what are the odds we would not obtain the same results.

In the published literature, this will be written as $p < .01$. The probability is less than 1 in 100. The actual *t* or *F* ratio in published papers will be written as *t* or *F* equals some number (e.g., $F = 5.8$). In the "Results" section of published papers, the ratio and probability are put together as $F = 21.54$, $p < .001$. In that example, we would expect that the particular differences between the groups would occur by chance less than 1 time in 1,000.

Confound Hypothesis

The second question asked is whether our results are due to a **confound** rather than the IV. What is a confound? Almost anything can be a confound. A confound is something that systematically biases the results of our research.

It may be the fact that women are more likely to go to their mental health provider than men. Thus, a study that looks at rates of a particular disorder based on provider reports may be biased in terms of a gender difference. Since the amount of sunlight can influence the experience of depression, a confound may be introduced into a depression experiment if one group is studied in the winter when there is less light and another group is studied in the summer when there is more sunshine. A confound may also be introduced when one group is made up of more men than women if the disorder under study shows gender differences. In one treatment study, the control group was instructed by young, inexperienced technicians whereas the experimental group was instructed by an older, more experienced professional. This difference may have produced a confound in the results.

Some confounds can be prevented or controlled. However, other factors can never be controlled. You cannot control world events, but you can ask whether there is any reason to believe that a particular event that took place inside or outside of the laboratory could have influenced one group more than another and thus introduced a confound.

Research Hypothesis

After ruling out the null hypothesis and the confound hypothesis, we can assume that the results reflect the action of the IV. Our next step is to consider what this means. We begin to generalize from our set of data and consider both the implications of our results for other groups of people and the theoretical implications of the data. Sometimes we are led to new ideas, which in turn generate new research hypotheses, which can be interpreted with additional experiments.

Figure 4-7 presents a simplified outline of this procedure, which reflects the evolutionary nature of science. The steps include (1) the development of the hypothesis, (2) the translation of this hypothesis into a research design, (3) the running of the experiment, and (4) the interpretation of the results. You will notice that there is also an arrow from Step 4 back to Step 1. Researchers take the results and interpretations of their studies and create new research studies that refine the previous hypotheses.

In psychological research, we have some powerful techniques to help us achieve this goal. Unlike the detective who must

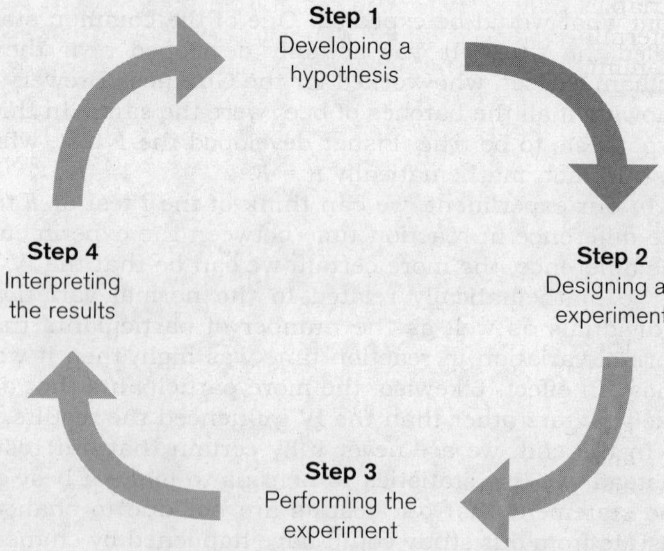

FIGURE 4-7 Schematic Representation of the Four Major Steps in the Experimentation Process

Concept Check

- What are five factors critical to enabling sound inference in determining the relation between the IV and the DV in an experiment?
- Why is randomization important to selecting participants and assigning them to groups in an experimental study?
- What is a match subjects design? When would you use this design instead of a randomized study?
- What roles do the following hypotheses play in interpreting experimental results:
  - Null hypothesis?
  - Confound hypothesis?
  - Research hypothesis?

always reconstruct events after the fact, the researcher has the advantage of being able to create a new situation in which to test ideas. This is comparable to a homicide detective's being able to bring a dead man back to life and place him in the presence of each suspect until the murder is reenacted. Such a reenactment might lack suspense and not make it in prime time, but it would increase the certainty of knowing who committed the murder.

Increased certainty is a large part of the experimental process. Scientists increase certainty by creating an artificial situation—the experiment—in which important factors can be controlled and manipulated. Through control and manipulation, participant variables may be examined in detail, and the influence of one variable on another may be determined with certainty. The follow LENS describes randomized controlled trials (RCTs), examining treatments for mental illness in low- and middle-income countries.

4-1 LENS
Randomized Controlled Trials of Global Mental Health Treatments in Low- and Middle-Income Countries

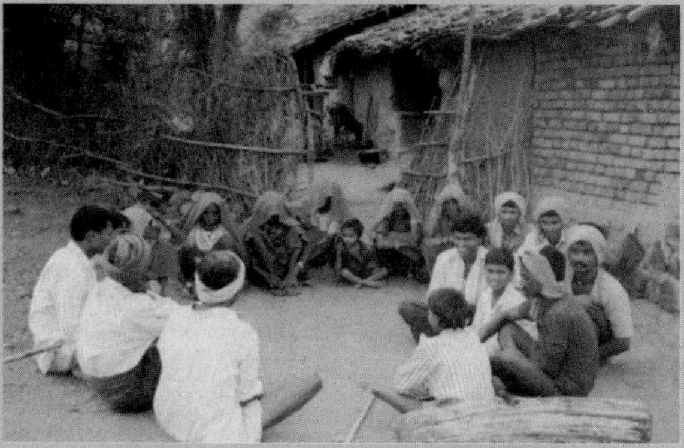

Mental health workers meeting with patients and their families

Source: Reprinted from The Lancet, Vol. 370, Patel, et al, "Treatment and prevention of mental disorders in low-income and middle-income countries," 991–1005, Copyright (2007), with permission from Elsevier.

There is a large difference in mental health treatment in high-income countries like the United States, England, Germany, France, Japan, and Australia as compared with low- and middle-income countries such as India, Pakistan, China, Chile, Mexico, and many countries in Africa. In high-income countries, there are a larger number of professionals who can deliver mental health services. Treatment procedures such as medications and psychological therapies have also been developed and tested in these higher-income countries. There are fewer mental health professionals in low- and middle-income countries. Thus, family members and nonprofessionals are often involved in the treatment of mental disorders. It is critical that low-income countries use treatments that are both effective and available at low costs.

Performing treatment studies in low- and middle-income countries is not only of benefit to the community but also helps research programs to establish the generalizability of the treatment worldwide. To achieve the greatest scientific benefit, it is important that the participants in the program be assigned to groups using an RCT design. That is, the participants in the study must be randomly assigned to the treatment group.

Treatment research does exist, which suggests that local communities can offer effective treatment for depression and schizophrenia. In low- and middle-income countries, these disorders often go untreated. This LENS focuses on depression, although similar positive results have been shown for schizophrenia, particularly in China. Depression is a common disorder throughout the world, so having effective treatments for depression worldwide is critical. Effective treatments are available for depression in terms of both psychotherapy and antidepressant medication. Both of these approaches can be delivered in a relatively inexpensive manner in low-income countries using community individuals with training in that one procedure. These trained individuals also have the advantage of understanding the culture in which the clients live. Not only does the treatment improve the individuals who have the disorder and their community; it also has a positive effect on the economy by a reduction in days lost from work. A number of researchers have begun to evaluate the treatment of depression in low- and middle-income countries (Patel et al., 2007). Some examples of this research are shown in *Table 4-1*.

Thus, if the person's family and community can be involved in the treatment, the results are more positive. Performing treatment studies in low- and middle- income countries is not only of benefit to the community but also helps the researchers to establish the generalizability of the treatment worldwide. Similar research with medical disorders in Africa by the Gates Foundation also suggests that successful interventions developed in low- income countries can also be applied in low- income areas of the United States.

TABLE 4-1 Randomized Controlled Trials for Treatment of Depression in Low-Income and Middle-Income Countries Since 2001

Country	*Setting*	*Study Design*	*Sample*	*Intervention*	*Comparison Group*	*Main Results*
Uganda	Villages	Cluster RCT	248 villagers of both sexes with depression	Group interpersonal psychotherapy	Villages without intervention groups	93.5% recovered with intervention vs. 45.3% in comparison group at the end of treatment, and 88.3% vs. 45.1% at 6 months ($p < 0.001$)
India	General medical outpatients at a district hospital	RCT	450 adults with common mental disorders	Fluoxetine or individual problem-solving treatment	Placebo	70% of antidepressant group recovered at 2 months compared with 54% of placebo group ($p = 0.01$); no difference between psychotherapy and placebo

Country	Setting	Study Design	Sample	Intervention	Comparison Group	Main Results
Chile	Primary care	RCT	240 depressed women living in deprived urban areas	Multi-component stepped-care programme including psychoeducational groups for all and antidepressants for more severe only	Usual care	70% recovered with intervention vs. 30% in usual care at 6 months ($p < 0.001$)
Pakistan Karachi	Urban community	RCT	366 lower middle class women with depression or anxiety	8 individual counselling sessions at home by minimally trained counsellors	No intervention	Reduction in mean symptom scores ($p < 0.001$) at the end of intervention (8 weeks)
Mexico	Community mental-health centres in Mexico City	RCT	135 female patients with depressive symptoms	6 psycho-educational group session	One session of information	Both groups improved but no differences between groups at 4 months and deterioration at 2 years (only 39 women included in final analysis)

RCT= Randomized controlled trial.
Source: Reprinted from The Lancet, Vol. 370, Patel, et al, "Treatment and prevention of mental disorders in low-income and middle-income countries," 991–1005, Copyright (2007), with permission from Elsevier.

Single Subject Designs

Single subject designs, also referred to as small-N designs, use the data from each participant without averaging it as part of a group of participants. It is assumed that the topic under study is accurately reflected in the single individual and can be controlled appropriately. With this approach, statistical tests are typically replaced with graphical changes. For example, if you wanted to know if a child with autism would respond to a particular type of praise, you could determine this by having a condition in which you give praise and a baseline condition in which you do not. A stronger design referred to as ABAB would have a baseline condition (A) followed by the treatment condition (B). Such a design would appear as in *Figure 4-8.*

Hersen and Bellack (1976) used a multiple-baseline design to demonstrate the effects of a treatment program for a schizophrenic patient. The patient made little contact with

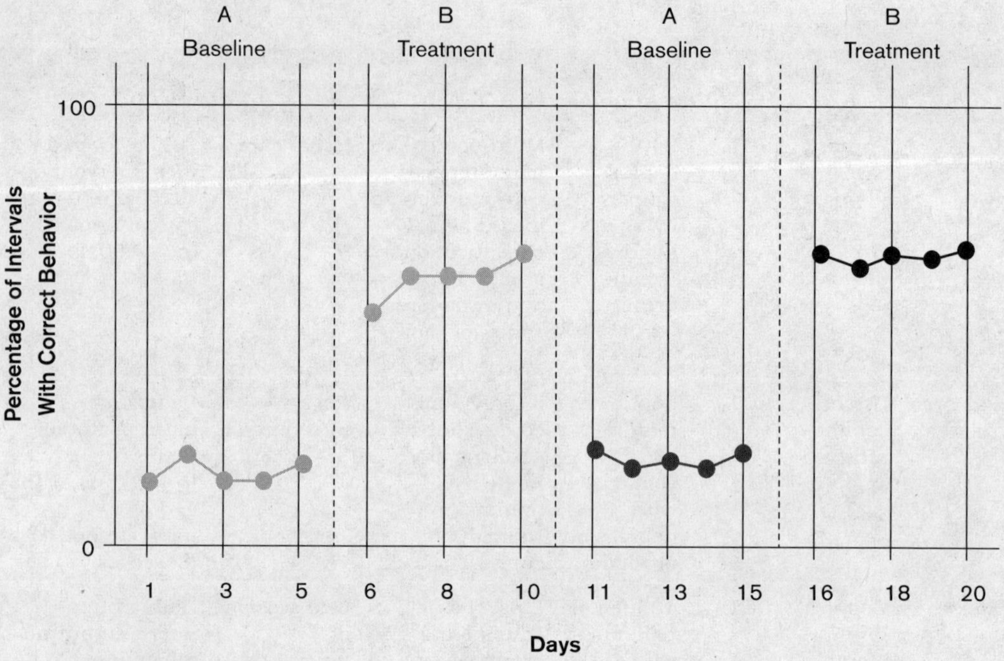

FIGURE 4-8 This Figure Represents an Alternative Method of Diagramming an ABAB Single-Subject Reversal Design

Source: Dyer, Dunlap, and Winterling (1990).

others, rarely engaged in conversation, and was compliant even to unreasonable requests. The treatment consisted of training in the development of assertiveness skills and skills for making contact with others. The measures taken over the baseline and treatment sessions were the amount of eye contact while talking, the amount of speaking without prolonged pauses, the number of requests made of another person, and the number of unreasonable requests not complied with. This design requires that baselines be taken for the four measures and that treatments be introduced at different sessions for each of the behaviors to be changed, while measurements of all behaviors are continued. This type of design helps us to determine whether the treatment was specific to a particular behavior (see *Figure 4-9*). Notice that the treatment was introduced at a different time (dotted vertical line) for each of the four targeted behaviors.

Longitudinal Research

A **longitudinal design** allows the researcher to follow a specific group of individuals across a period of time to document any changes that take place during that time. For example, one study followed children diagnosed with attention deficit/hyperactivity disorder (ADHD) for 9 years and noted changes in specific symptoms (Lahey & Willcutt, 2010). By comparing the children with ADHD to children without the disorder, it was possible to determine normal developmental changes as opposed to changes related to ADHD itself. These researchers were also interested in knowing if ADHD symptoms in year 1 were predictive of symptoms and teacher ratings in later years, which they were.

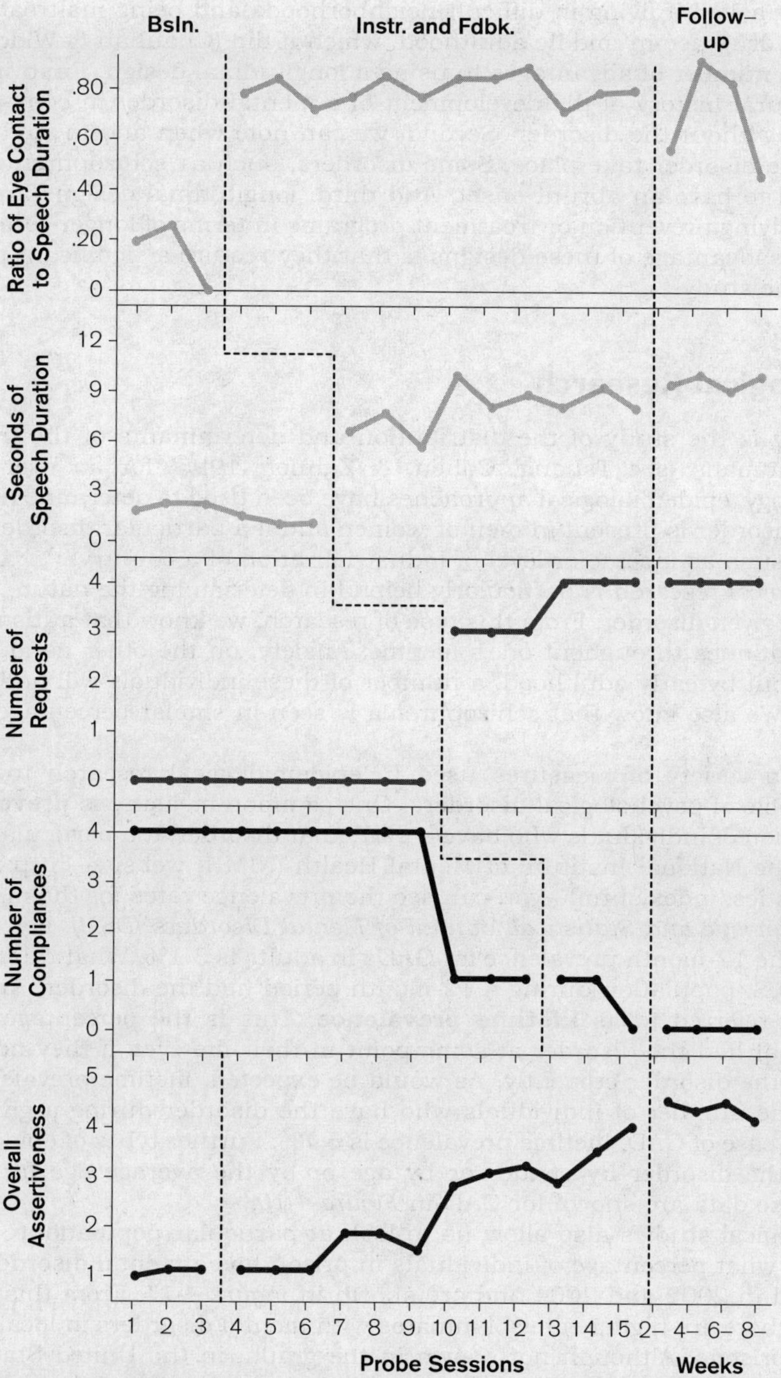

FIGURE 4-9 Probe Sessions During Baseline, Treatment, and Follow-Ups for Subject 1. Data Are Presented in Blocks of Eight Scenes

Source: Hersen and Bellack (1976, p. 243).

Another study asked if living in difficult neighborhoods and being maltreated as a child would predict drug use in middle adulthood, which it did (Chauhan & Widom, 2012).

There are a number of advantages to using a longitudinal design. First, it allows us to study the natural history of the development of a mental disorder in comparison with a similar group without the disorder. Second, we can note when and in what manner the changes in the disorder take place. Some disorders, such as schizophrenia and bipolar disorder, tend to have an abrupt onset. And third, longitudinal designs are particularly useful for studying prevention or treatment programs in terms of longer-term changes. Of course, the disadvantage of these designs is that they require a significant period of time to complete the study.

Epidemiological Research

Epidemiology is the study of the distribution and determinants of the frequency of a disorder in humans (see Tsuang, Cohen, & Zahner, 1995, for an overview). Within psychopathology, epidemiological approaches have been used to determine how frequently a particular disorder is present in men or women and if a particular disorder is related to other factors such as income or level of industrialization of a country.

Epidemiological research is particularly helpful in determining the nature, etiology, and prognosis of a given disorder. From this type of research, we know that autism begins early in life and continues throughout one's lifetime. Anxiety, on the other hand, can begin in adolescence, but by early adulthood, a number of these individuals will no longer display the disorder. We also know that schizophrenia is seen in similar percentages throughout the world.

There are a variety of measures used in epidemiological research to describe the statistical profile of psychological disorders. One common measure is **prevalence,** which is the proportion of individuals who have a particular disorder at a particular time period. If you go to the National Institute of Mental Health (NIMH) website—http://www.nimh.nih.gov/statistics/index.shtml—you can see the prevalence rates for the major disorders from the *Diagnostic and Statistical Manual of Mental Disorders (DSM).* For example, you will see that the 12-month prevalence for GADs in adults is 3.1%. What this means is that 3.1% of the U.S. population during a 12-month period had the disorder. Another type of prevalence is referred to as **lifetime prevalence.** This is the percentage of a specific population that had the disorder at some point in their life even if they no longer show symptoms of the disorder currently. As would be expected, lifetime prevalence is always larger than the number of individuals who have the disorder during a given 12-month period. In the case of GAD, lifetime prevalence is 5.7%. Further types of epidemiology data can include the disorder by gender or by age or by the average age for onset of the disorder. These data are shown for GAD in *Figure 4-10.*

Epidemiological studies also allow us to look at particular populations. For example, we could ask what percentage of individuals in prison has a mental disorder. These data were collected in 2002 and 2004 and are shown in *Figure 4-11.* From this graph, it can be seen that there are higher rates of inmates with mental disorders in local as compared with federal prisons. Although not shown in the graph, in the United States, there are now more than 3 times more seriously mentally ill individuals in jails and prisons than in hospitals (Torrey, Kennard, Eslinger, Lamb, & Pavle, 2010).

Another epidemiological measure is **incidence.** Incidence refers to the number of new cases of a disorder that develop during a certain period of time. Another way of thinking

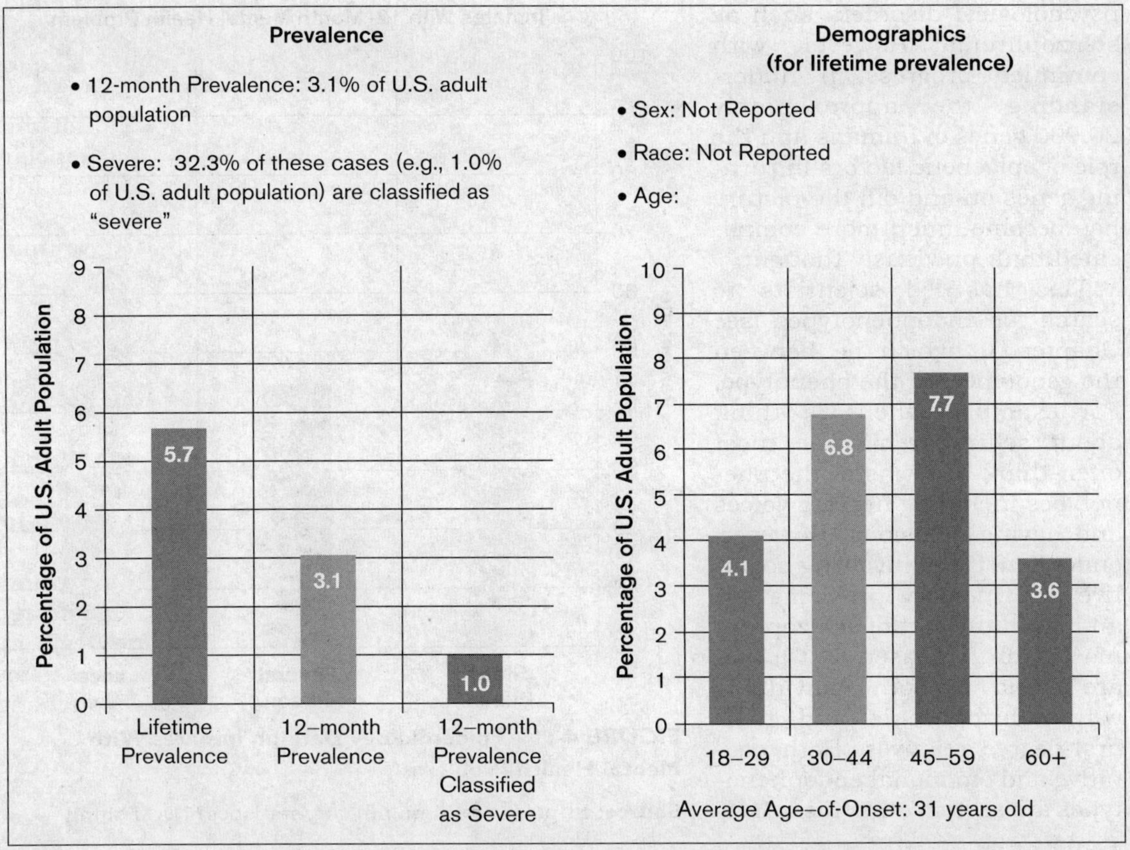

FIGURE 4-10 Describing the Statistical Profile of Psychological Disorders in Epidemiological Research Published in 2005

Source: http://www.nimh.nih.gov/statistics/1GAD_ADULT.shtml

about incidence is to describe it as **risk.** That is, what is the risk of someone in a specific population developing the disorder in a given time period?

Risk is also considered in a statistical manner in terms of correlation or association. For example, you can ask if there is a relationship between environmental variables such as abuse in childhood and development of a particular disorder such as depression. Subject variables such as gender are also used in this way. For example, 1 in 4 females and 1 in 10 males will have depression in their lifetime. Thus, there is a greater risk factor for females as compared with males in terms of developing depression. As with all measures of association, the presence of a relationship does not imply causation.

Research Involving Genetics

Traditional genetics studies have sought to determine which aspects of a person's behavior can be attributed to genetic factors and which can be said to be related to environmental factors. Early research sought to find the single gene or genes involved in psychological disorders such as schizophrenia. However, with continued progress in understanding the approximately 20,000 genes of humans and the role of epigenetic factors in turning genes on and off, the picture has become much more complicated than previously thought.

This has led scientists to search for endophenotypes (see Chapter 3), which lie between the genotype and the phenotype. For example, when we think about schizophrenia, we most often think in terms of the phenotypes including hearing voices and having delusions. However, endophenotypes involving cognitive and memory problems are an important part of schizophrenia (Barch & Ceaser, 2012) and are found in both individuals with schizophrenia and their first-degree relatives. Both cognitive and emotional endophenotypes are seen in other disorders.

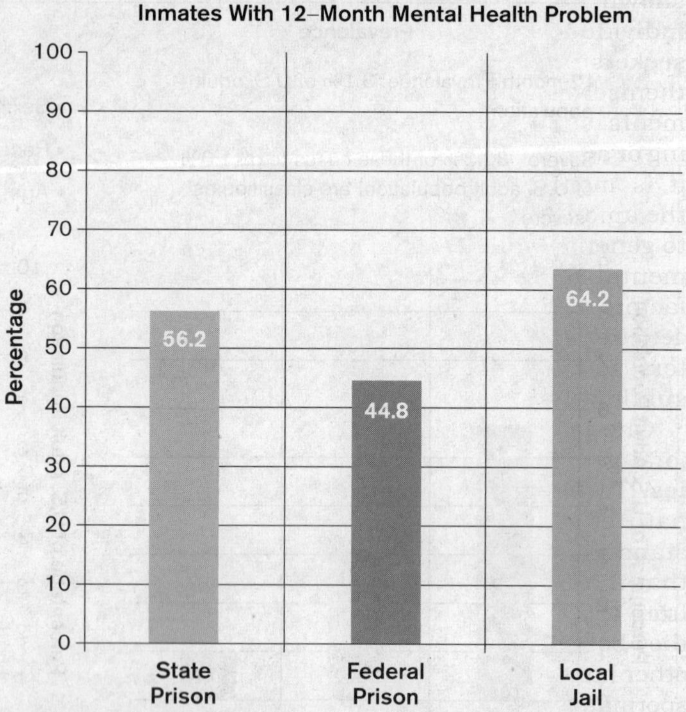

FIGURE 4-11 Epidemiology Data on Inmates With Mental Health Problems

Source: http://www.nimh.nih.gov/statistics/1DOJ.shtml

Behavioral Genetics

One type of genetics research involving psychopathology is **behavioral genetics.** Behavioral genetics is the study of genetic and environmental contributions to organisms' behavior (see Carey, 2003; DiLalla, 2004; Plomin, DeFries, McClearn, & McGuffin, 2008; Kendler, Jaffee, & Romer, 2011, for overviews). One large question is the manner in which genes and the environment work together to shape behavior. Researchers use a variety of behavioral genetic approaches to quantify the amount of variance, which can be attributed to genetic influences and the amount attributed to environmental influences.

One traditional distinction has been between **gene by environment interaction** as opposed to **gene by environment correlations** (see Plomin, DeFries, & Loehlin, 1977). Gene by environment interaction refers to the possibility that individuals with different genotypes may respond to the same environment in different ways. For example, some children respond to stress differently from others based on their genotype. As noted, mistreatment as a child influenced some boys differently from others later in adulthood (Caspi et al., 2002). Those boys who were mistreated in childhood and had a particular form of the MAOA gene were more likely to be violent and engage in a variety of antisocial behaviors as adults.

A gene by environment correlation concerns how certain genotypes and certain environments occur together. For example, sensation seeking as a personality trait has been

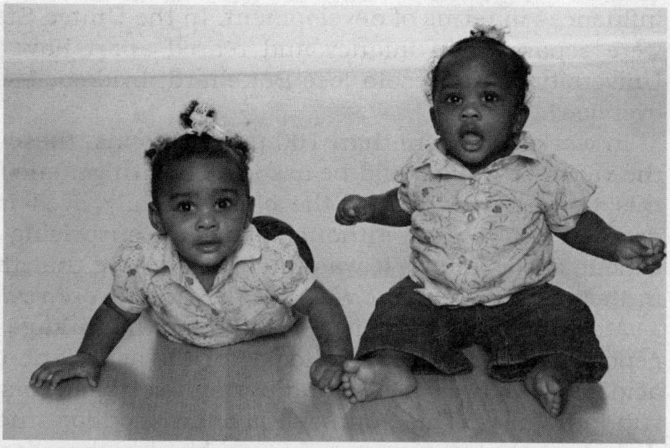
Identical twins
© iStockphoto/video1

shown to be inherited. Those individuals who are sensation seekers are more likely to put themselves in high risk environments such as mountain climbing or auto racing. In this example, it is more difficult to determine the amount of variance attributed to genetic influences and environmental influences as separate factors. Thus, it is possible for genetic and environmental factors to influence each other in subtle ways.

One major paradigm of behavioral genetics involves **twin studies.** Twins offer an occurrence in nature that allows for understanding critical factors related to genetic influences. This is largely based on the fact that there are two types of twins. **Monozygotic (MZ) twins** are identical twins resulting from the zygote (fertilized egg) dividing during the first two weeks of gestation. Because they both come from the same egg, their genes are identical. **Dizygotic (DZ) twins,** on the other hand, arise from the situation in which two different eggs are fertilized by two different spermatozoa. These are called fraternal twins since their shared genes are approximately 50%—the same as that between any two siblings. DZ twins can be either same sex or opposite sex whereas MZ twins must always be same sex. By comparing the psychological traits of MZ and DZ twins it is possible to obtain an estimate of heritability.

A classic research design is to compare the responses of MZ twins with DZ twins on particular behavioral traits such as intelligence or personality characteristics. Since it is assumed that both DZ and MZ twins would have had similar environmental influences in their family, then differences between MZ and DZ twins would be seen to be the result of genetic influences. For example, Gottesman (1991) has studied schizophrenia with this design. In these studies, a particular MZ twin was more likely to have schizophrenia if the other twin also did. In DZ twins, this was not the case.

Statistically, researchers examine the statistical degree to which twins are identical to each other as a function of genetic influences and environmental influences. To answer this question, researchers create correlation coefficients for MZ twins and DZ twins. This correlation reflects how similar each type of twin is on a particular trait. From this, it is possible to determine the percentage of contribution to the trait that comes from environmental influences and the percentage of contribution that comes from genetic influences. For example, personality factors such as extraversion have been shown to have a 50% contribution of genetic factors and a 50% contribution of environmental factors.

Another important type of behavioral genetics research is the **adoption study.** This is the situation where DZ and MZ twins have been raised apart. During World War II, for example, children from England were often sent to Canada to allow them to grow up in a less dangerous situation. By studying those children who were twins and were raised in different environments, it was possible to better determine the environmental and genetic influences in terms of development. In the United States since 1979, a series of twins who were separated in infancy and reared apart have been studied by researchers at the University of Minnesota (see Bouchard, Lykken, McGue, Segal, & Tellegen, 1990, for an overview).

In work with more than 100 pairs of twins, these researchers found that about 70% of the variance in IQ could be associated with genetic factors. Later studies have supported this finding. However, if the child's family lived in poverty, the degree of association dropped drastically. Although it is not surprising to find IQ or temperament to have genetic associations, it was intriguing to see that the leisure time interests of each twin in the pair were similar whether the twins were reared together or reared apart.

A third type of study is referred to as the **linkage analysis.** Linkage analysis examines generations of families and looks for the association between particular deoxyribonucleic acid (DNA) marker alleles and particular traits. This is commonly done for disorders that run in families. This approach is often used for studying psychological and physiological disorders such as depression or bipolar disorder. As part of this type of research, scientists may examine the manner in which traits associated with the disorder are also apparent in first- and second-degree relatives.

Work from India has also underlined the importance of genetic studies of schizophrenia.

Dr. Smita Deshpande, G. Prasad Rao, and Vishwajit L. Nimgaonkar (2016) underline the importance of Indian researchers partnering with international efforts since findings from India are often at variance with worldwide findings. (Department of Psychiatry, Postgraduate Institute of Medical Education and Research, Dr. Ram Manohar Lohia Hospital, New Delhi, India)

Clinical and Statistical Significance

When performing research studies, we use inferential statistics to determine whether the IV influences the DV. By using statistics, we ask if we performed the same experiment 100 times, what is the probability we would obtain the results seen in the present study? If the answer is less than 5 in 100 times ($p < .05$), we say that the results of the study are **statistically significant.** However, when considering medical or psychological disorders, we also want to know if the results of the study are **clinically significant.**

Consider a study in which a researcher wants to determine whether performing exercise would reduce depression. In this study, the experimental group would receive the exercise training for 2 months and the control group would not. Assume that the exercise did indeed reduce the depression score on a particular measure of depression from 21 to 20 whereas the control group's depression did not change. Statistics might show a significant relationship between the two sets of data. However, clinically it would not be worth the effort of having participants exercise for 2 months to have depression change by only 1 unit. Thus, a distinction is often made in clinical work between results that are statistically significant and those that are also clinically significant.

One way to measure the magnitude that a treatment has on the DV is referred to as **effect size.** A common measure of effect is Cohen's *d.* In essence, Cohen's *d* reflects the difference in the mean scores of the control and experimental groups divided by the standard deviation of the measure from the two groups. Effect size measures are important to clinical researchers for two reasons. First, they describe in quantitative terms the influence of the treatment. And second, they aid a researcher in knowing how many participants need to be included in a research study to determine an effect. Effect size is an important measure of the effects of a treatment on a mental disorder. One could compare two different types of psychotherapy for example, or even a psychotherapy with a particular medication.

Replication and Meta-Analysis

Although researchers seek to design studies to rule out alternative hypotheses, they cannot consider every possibility. When a study is performed in different laboratories with different participants, referred to as **replicated,** we can have more certainty that the results found reflect the true nature of what we are studying. Thus, scientists seek to find a number of different studies from different laboratories that answer the same research question. For example, a number of studies from around the world have shown structural brain differences in individuals with schizophrenia including enlarged ventricles in the brain (Faludi & Mirnics, 2011). A number of journals, such as *Clinical Psychology Review* and *Psychological Bulletin,* are designed to publish reviews of research in the field.

Once the literature in a particular area has been reviewed, it is possible to examine statistically the results of all the studies taken together. This technique is referred to as **meta-analysis.** Meta-analysis is a statistical technique for combining a number of studies to improve the reliability of the results. For example, a large number of studies have examined depression and how it can be treated with cognitive behavioral therapy (Butler, Chapman, Forman, & Beck, 2006). With a meta-analysis, it can be asked what if we consider all of these studies to be one study. Then we could calculate the common effect size of all of the available studies. A similar meta-analysis was performed to examine interpersonal psychotherapy for depression (Cuijpers et al., 2011). Another meta-analysis examined results on tests of executive functioning and sustained attention to symptoms seen in individuals with schizophrenia (Nieuwenstein, Aleman, & de Haan, 2001). Overall, the results showed that disorganization seen in schizophrenia was related to executive function but not attention. On the other hand, symptoms of reality distortion in schizophrenia were not related to either executive function or attention.

ETHICS AND THE SCIENTIFIC EXPERIMENT

Ethics is the study of proper action. Ethics examines relationships between human beings and provides principles regarding how we should treat each other. The ultimate decision in ethical questions resides in judgments of value. Ethical considerations of psychological experimentation have at their heart the idea that people participating in research should not be harmed (see Ray, 2012, for

Concept Check

- What kinds of research questions could you explore using each of the following research designs? What are the advantages and disadvantages of each?
  - Single subject design?
  - Longitudinal research?
  - Epidemiological research?
- What is the overall goal of behavioral genetics research? What are the three primary types of research designs used in behavioral genetics research?
- Which is more important: statistical significance or clinical significance? Why?
- If a research study has already been conducted and its results have been communicated, why should it be replicated?

an overview). Specifically, at the end of an experiment, participants should not be affected in a way that would result in a lower level of human functioning. This includes emotional distress.

In most cases, the scientist has a question that he or she wants to ask and that the participant is willing to help answer. In some cases, the participants learn something about themselves from the experience and they are glad to have participated. In brain imaging studies, for example, participants often report that they enjoy seeing their brain activity (e.g., functional magnetic resonance imaging [fMRI], electroencephalography [EEG]) displayed. Thus, they are willing to participate in research in exchange for these types of experiences.

If these experiences were always pleasant and any changes in the participant always positive, participants would participate gladly in experiments, and scientists would face few ethical questions. However, at times the scientist may want to answer a question that requires that the participant experience psychological or physiological discomfort. In terms of psychopathology, we need to be especially certain that the individual with a particular disorder understand her what is being asked of and can freely respond. These situations raise a number of questions:

1. What are the responsibilities of the scientist toward the participant?
2. What are the rights of the participant?
3. Are there guidelines for reconciling conflicts between the rights of the participant to pursue happiness and the rights of the scientist to pursue knowledge?
4. What type of relationship or dialogue would be most productive for helping the scientist and participant to fulfill their needs and desires?

Since the 1950s, the American Psychological Association (APA) has published a set of guidelines. This is available online at www.apa.org/ethics/. In 1974, the National Research Act was signed into law in the United States. This law sought to protect human research participants. In response to the law, the Department of Health, Education, and Welfare held a conference in 1976 and produced a report. This report is referred to as the Belmont Report (http://ohsr.od.nih.gov/guidelines/belmont.html). The Belmont Report identifies three basic ethical principles—respect for persons, beneficence, and justice.

1. Respect for persons includes the idea that people can choose on their own. Further, people with diminished autonomy are entitled to protection. This suggests that all individuals with mental disorders must be protected in research. An important consideration is to determine if individuals can speak for themselves and are able to agree to part of an experiment.
2. Beneficence is to be understood in a strong sense meaning that researchers should do no harm as well as maximize possible benefits and minimize potential negative experiences.
3. The third principle of justice is a statement that research should be available to all people and not just to special classes or groups. This principle is operative in at least two different ways: first, that researchers use more than an easily accessible or compromised sample such as people in a mental hospital and second, that groups of individuals not be excluded. For example, during the

middle of the 20th century, little was known about the manner in which different types of treatments for mental disorders were influenced by cultural factors. Part of the problem was that individuals from some ethnic origins were not recruited into research studies. Another problem was that clinicians tended not to offer African Americans the same choice of treatment alternatives offered to white Americans.

The Experiment as an Ethical Problem

Let's begin with an extreme case of conflictual experimentation: the Nazi medical experiments during World War II. In several concentration camps, such as Ravensbrück, Dachau, and Buchenwald, prisoners were injected with a virus or bacterium and then received drugs to determine the drugs' effectiveness against the injections. Although medical knowledge was gained from these experiments, the world judged the experiments to be unethical and criminal.

During the trials of these scientist–physicians, held at Nuremberg, it was determined that they were guilty of war crimes. Seven of them were later hanged, and eight received long prison sentences. As a result of these trials, a code of ethics for medical experimentation with human participants (called the Nuremberg Code) was adopted as a guideline for future research. What was unethical about the experiments at the Nazi concentration camps was not that human beings were given a virus. Almost all of our current procedures of preventive medicine (the polio vaccine as historical example) require that the procedure eventually be tested on human beings. These physicians were convicted of conducting experiments *without the consent of their participants.*

Ingredients of the Initial Scientist–Participant Dialogue

One of the first principles of research is that the participants must consent to being part of an experiment. Furthermore, they must also be informed of the experiment's purpose and its potential risks. Thus, major ingredients that the witness looks for in the dialogue between the scientist and the research participant are **voluntary participation** and **informed consent.**

Voluntary Participation

In the initial dialogue between the scientist and the prospective participant, the scientist must ask the participant to be a part of the experiment. This is the principle of voluntary participation. In essence, the voluntary participation principle suggests that a person should participate in an experiment only by free choice. In addition, this principle states that a participant should be free to leave an experiment at any time, whether or not the experiment has been completed.

As you think about voluntary participation, you will become entangled in the question of whether anyone can ever make a free decision and, if so, under what circumstances. As you might have realized already, this question becomes even more complicated for someone interested in developmental psychology, which requires research with children, or for someone interested in psychopathology, which requires research with clients or patients who are mentally impaired. In terms of ethical concerns involving research with children, a number of recommendations have been put forward by the National Academies of Science, including how to obtain informed consent and ensure voluntary participation in research (Field & Behrman, 2004).

Informed Consent

Assuming for a moment that someone can agree freely to participate in research, the scientist in the initial dialogue should inform the prospective participant about what will be required of him or her during the study. The scientist must also inform the prospective participant about any potential harm that may come from participation. Thus, the prospective participant must be given complete information on which to base a decision. This is the principle of informed consent. As you can imagine, the principle of informed consent raises the issue of how much information about an experiment is enough.

From the principles of voluntary participation and informed consent, one can see that it is the initial task of the scientist to fully discuss the experimental procedure with prospective participants and to remind them that they are human beings who do not give away their rights just because they are taking part in a psychological experiment.

The Rights of the Research Participant and the Responsibilities of the Experimenter

In our society, research participants have the same rights during an experiment that they have outside the experimental situation. One major one is the **right to privacy.** Most of us at first think of the right to privacy as the right to spend time by oneself or with others of one's choosing, without being disturbed. This is the external manifestation of the right to privacy. But there is also an internal or intrapersonal manifestation of this right (see Raebhausen & Brim, 1967). This is the right to have private thoughts or, as it is sometimes called, a **private personality.** This means that the thoughts and feelings of a participant should not be made public without the participant's consent. It also means that a conversation between a participant and a scientist should be considered a private event, not a public one. This is an important consideration when studying those with mental disorders as private events are often the focus of the research.

How can the scientist ever report her or his findings? There are two considerations that are part of the scientist's responsibility to the participant: **confidentiality** and **anonymity.**

The principle of confidentiality requires that the scientist not release data of a personal nature to other scientists or groups without the participant's consent. Even during the experiment, researchers keep any personal data in a secure location and often destroy personal information once the experiment is completed.

The principle of anonymity requires that the personal identity of a given participant be kept separate from his or her data. The easiest way to accomplish this is to avoid requesting names in the first place; however, there are times when this may be impossible. Another alternative is to use code numbers that protect the identities of the participants and to destroy the list of participants' names once the data analysis has been completed.

What Is Harmful to a Research Participant?

As stated earlier, it is the right of a participant not to be harmed. In most psychological research, physical pain and harm present no problems, either because they are absent completely or because the participant is fully informed of the particular procedure that will be used, such as making a loud noise or placing the participant's hand in cold water to measure physiological responsiveness.

However, the question of psychological harm presents a much larger issue—one that will continue to be debated for years to come. This may be especially true when working with those with a psychopathology. Is it harmful to show participants something true but negative about themselves? Is it harmful to create situations in which participants feel negative emotions such as fear or anger? Is it harmful to make participants feel like failures in order to determine how this affects their performance? These are the types of questions that are being debated currently.

As a scientist, where do you go for help? There are two major sources: the APA's guidelines on ethics and the **institutional review board (IRB),** also known as the human subjects committee or office of research compliance, at the institution in which you study or work. In addition, many specialty organizations have adopted guidelines for specific populations. For example, the Society for Research in Child Development has established ethical standards for research with children.

Institutional Review Board

The U.S. Department of Health and Human Services requires that each scientist whose institution receives federal funds must seek a review of the ethical considerations of research with human participants, whether or not there is a deviation from the APA guidelines. This type of review is required not only of psychological research but of any type of research with human participants. The committee that reviews the research is to be made up of people who work at the same university, hospital, school, or other institution as the scientist and to also include members of the community where the institution is located.

The main task of the IRB is to determine whether the participants are adequately protected in terms of both welfare and rights. One major question that the committee asks is the following: Are there any risks—physical, psychological, or social—associated with participating in a given piece of research? Almost everything we do each day involves varying degrees of risk, so the committee attempts to determine when a risk is unreasonable.

The committee also considers the potential long-term effects of a particular treatment on a person. For example, asking a participant to run a mile, to give a small sample of blood, to have his or her heart rate measured, or to discuss his or her sexual preference or childhood involves some risks in the way the term is used by most internal review committees. However, the committee may decide that, in light of the information that would be gained, these risks are not sufficient to prevent the study from being performed. Thus, a second major question that a review committee asks is the following: Are the risks to the participants outweighed by the potential benefits to them or by the estimated importance to society of the knowledge to be gained? If the committee determines that the answer to this question is yes, a third question is asked: Has the experimenter allowed the prospective participants to determine freely whether they will participate in the experiment? And finally, has the experimenter obtained the participants' informed consent?

The Ethical Relationship

As we conclude our considerations, let's remind ourselves that ethical questions have at their base issues of relationships and traditions. As scientists, we ask what *is* and what *ought to be* our relationship with our participants and our society with regard to research. To answer this question, we stress that part of our ethical responsibility is to consult with others about our research. In this context, we described the manner in which internal review committees evaluate the ethics of research and the guidelines (e.g., those of the APA and the federal government) used to direct our evaluations. With both humans and animals, we are only beginning to develop methods for the study of inner experience that can help to inform our ethical considerations.

Concept Check

- "Ethical considerations of psychological experimentation have at their heart the idea that people participating in research should not be harmed." What four questions does every scientist need to consider in designing a research study?
- Which four sources of ethical and legal guidelines help the scientist in designing and conducting psychopathology research?
- What are "voluntary participation" and "informed consent" in the context of scientific research? What are some of the specific issues they raise in terms of psychopathology research?
- How do "confidentiality" and "anonymity" figure into the experimenter's responsibility to protect the research participant's right to privacy?
- What are the questions an IRB asks in regard to the risks of a psychopathology research study?

SUMMARY

In general, there is no single scientific method, yet there is a general process called science. This process consists of experiencing the world and then drawing general conclusions (called *facts*) from observations. In science, we use doubt to question our ideas and our research and ask whether factors other than the ones that we originally considered might have influenced our results. By doing this we come to see that science is a combination of interaction with the world and logic. There are three stages to the scientific method: (1) develop an idea or expectation (hypothesis), (2) evaluate the ideas and expectations about the world through observation and experimentation, and (3) draw conclusions or inferences about the ideas and expectations and consider the impact of the new information on theoretical conceptualizations. There are many research designs, and which one to select begins with the question the scientist wants to answer. Some of the research designs used to study psychopathology include case study, naturalistic observation, correlational approaches, experimental method, single subject design, longitudinal research, epidemiological research, and behavioral genetics designs. Logic can help us answer questions of inference, which is the process by which we look at the evidence available to us and then use our powers of reasoning to reach a conclusion. Logical procedures are also important for helping us understand the accuracy or validity of our ideas and research.

Increased certainty is a large part of the experimental process. Scientists increase certainty by creating an artificial situation—the experiment—in which important factors can be controlled and manipulated. Through control and manipulation, participant variables may be examined in detail, and the influence of one variable on another may be determined with certainty. There are four steps to the experimental process, which reflect the evolutionary nature of science: (1) the development of the hypothesis, (2) the translation of this hypothesis into a research design, (3) the running of the experiment, and (4) the interpretation of the results. Researchers take the results and interpretations of their studies and create new research studies that refine the previous hypotheses, and the cycle begins anew. One goal of experimental research is to determine the relation between the IV and the DV. It is the task of the experiment to reduce extraneous factors not related to the IV that can influence the DV. Additional factors critical to sound inference are participant selection and assignment, the design of the experiment, and the interpretation of the relationship of the IV to the DV. The experimenter considers three hypotheses in interpreting whether the DV is related to the IV: the null hypothesis, confound hypothesis, and research hypothesis. Both statistical significance and clinical significance are important in interpreting research results. Replication of studies in different locations with different participants increases the certainty that the results found reflect the true nature of what is being studied. Meta-analysis is a statistical technique for combining a number of studies to improve the reliability of the results.

Ethical considerations of psychological experimentation have at their heart the idea that people participating in research should not be harmed. In addition, research participants have a right to privacy including the right to a private personality. To protect those rights, participants must be informed of the experiment's purpose and its potential risks (informed consent) and then voluntarily agree to participate in the experiment (voluntary participation). Confidentiality and anonymity are two additional considerations that are part of the scientist's responsibility to the participant. Guidelines for reconciling conflicts between the rights of the participant to pursue happiness and the rights of the scientist to pursue knowledge are provided by such resources as the APA, U.S. National Research Act, Belmont Report, and IRBs.

STUDY RESOURCES

Review Questions

1. What does the author mean by "science is a combination of interaction with the world and logic"? What key role does doubt play in the process of science?
2. Why can't you design "the one perfect study"? What trade-offs do you need to consider in designing an experimental study in the real world? What can you do to improve the quality of your study?
3. Your research group has been asked by the World Health Organization (WHO) to develop a research program to study anxiety in children around the world using multiple research methodologies. Taking into consideration the

characteristics of each of the following methods, what is a research question you could study using each approach:
- Case study?
- Naturalistic observation?
- Correlational approach?
- Experimental approach?
- Single subject design?
- Longitudinal research?
- Epidemiological research?
- Twin study?

4. How is a scientist conducting psychopathology research like a detective solving a mystery? How are they different?
5. If we think about psychopathology research as an ethical problem, what are the rights of the research participant, and what are the responsibilities of the experimenter in ensuring the protection of those rights? What legal and ethical resources are available to guide this effort?

For Further Reading

Kandel, E. (2006). *In search of memory: The emergence of a new science of mind.* New York: W. W. Norton & Company.

Kuhn, T. (1970). *The structure of scientific revolutions* (2nd ed.). Chicago: University of Chicago Press.

Sacks, O. (1985). *The man who mistook his wife for a hat and other clinical tales.* New York: Summit Books.

Thomas, L. (1979). *The Medusa and the snail: More notes of a biology watcher.* New York: Viking.

Key Terms and Concepts

adoption study
anonymity
behavioral genetics
blind controls
case study
clinically significant
confidentiality
confound
confound hypothesis
confounding variables
control group
correlation coefficient
correlational approach
covary
demand characteristics
dependent variable (DV)
dizygotic (DZ) twins
double-blind experiment
doubt
effect size
empiricism
epidemiology
ethics
experimental group
experimental method
experimenter effects
external validity
facts
falsification
gene by environment correlations
gene by environment interaction
generalizability
hypothesis
incidence
independent variable (IV)
inference
inferential statistics
informed consent
institutional review board (IRB)

internal validity	operational definition	risk
lifetime prevalence	placebo effect	sample
linkage analysis	population	science
logic	positive correlation	scientific knowledge
longitudinal design	prevalence	single subject designs
match subjects design	private personality	statistically significant
meta-analysis	probability	twin studies
monozygotic (MZ) twins	randomization	validity
naturalistic observation	replicated	voluntary participation
negative correlation	research hypothesis	
null hypothesis	right to privacy	

CHAPTER

5

Assessment and Classification

CHAPTER OUTLINE

- THE MENTAL STATUS EXAM 160
- STRUCTURED INTERVIEWS 161
- ASSESSING CULTURAL DIMENSIONS 163
- RELIABILITY AND VALIDITY IN RELATION TO PSYCHOPATHOLOGY 164
- MODELS OF ASSESSMENT 167
- CLASSIFICATION 176
- SUMMARY 181
- STUDY RESOURCES 182

Elyn Saks told of her time as a graduate student at Oxford after graduating from Vanderbilt University. As a student at Oxford, she began to have a hard time concentrating on academic work and lectures. She turned in papers that her tutor did not understand. A friend of hers who was a nurse asked her fiancé, who was a physician who specialized in neurology, to talk with Elyn. Elyn Saks remembers the conversation as follows:

"Jean and I are very concerned about you," he said quietly. "We think you may be quite sick. Would you mind if I asked you some questions?"

"I'm not sick," I responded. "I'm just not smart enough. But questions, yes. Ask me questions."

"Are you feeling down?"

"Yes."

"Loss of pleasure in daily activities?"

"Yes."

"Difficulty sleeping?"

"Yes."

"Loss of appetite?"

"Yes."

"How much weight have you lost in the last month?"

"About fifteen pounds."

"Do you feel like a bad person?"

"Yes."

"Tell me about it."

"Nothing to tell. I'm just a piece of shit."

"Are you thinking of hurting yourself?"

I waited a moment before answering, "Yes."

From The Center Cannot Hold: My Journey Through Madness by Elyn Saks. © 2007 by Elyn Saks. By permissions of Hachette Book Group, Inc. All rights reserved.

After a number of other questions, Elyn Saks was referred to a mental health professional to diagnosis her distress and formulate a treatment plan.

As a clinician, people come to see you in a variety of ways. Some people set up an appointment and tell you about how they are feeling distressed. They may tell you about feeling anxious or sad. If you work in a hospital, people may be brought to you by others who are concerned by the behaviors the person displays or the experiences he or she describes. As a clinician, it is your job to make sense of the information you are given. The first task is that of **assessment.**

Assessment is simply the process of gathering information about a person so that you can make a clinical decision about that person's symptoms. In the process, you may create a variety of hypotheses about the possible causes of the symptoms. Had the person taken drugs that were causing the behavior? Did the person suffer a negative experience such as being robbed or raped? Is the behavior part of an underlying physical or mental disorder? Part of the task of the clinical assessment is to gather data necessary to rule out or support the possible causes of the symptoms.

Most mental health professionals use a clinical interview to initially gather information concerning the status of an individual they are working with. Since the interview is also an interaction between two people, it is a chance for the professional to establish rapport, which will lead to more complete information. This information includes not only the individual's present symptoms but also the social and cultural context in which these symptoms appear. This includes the individual's social support, family connections, and connections within his or her community. It is also important to assess the individual's attitudes, emotions, and experiences of others in his or her world. The clinical interview further offers the opportunity to assess the current ability of the individual to care for him- or herself.

Overall, the major areas of consideration in a clinical interview are (1) the current areas of distress and their history; (2) any past mental health problems; (3) social history including social support; (4) the manner in which cultural factors may influence the current condition; and (5) any way in which previous family, medical, or psychological factors may influence the current situation.

THE MENTAL STATUS EXAM

Throughout the world, the clinical interview has been organized into major categories and referred to as the **mental status exam.** This exam is often given quickly to gain initial information.

The first major category of the exam is the individual's appearance and behavior. In the report, the mental health professional would note such factors as the individual's clothing, grooming, and posture. Motor activity, such as slow movements, may be part of a later diagnosis of depression whereas quick, abrupt movements may be associated with mania.

The second major category of the exam is mood and affect. Affect refers to the emotions that the individual is expressing during the interview. The person might seem happy or sad. The professional might note that the person laughs or cries in describing situations where other individuals would not laugh or cry. Such affect would be described as inappropriate. It should also be noted if the individual shows no affect when describing situations such as receiving a large raise in pay or losing a friend where others would be happy or sad. Such affect is said to be flat. Mood as compared with present affect is more long term. In this sense the professional notes how the individual reports he or she has been feeling recently. Has the individual been feeling blue or sad or angry?

The next category is speech quality. Here, the professional notes the manner in which an individual speaks. Is the person speaking quickly or very slowly? Does the person's manner of speaking feel pressured? Does the person speak very quietly or with great volume? These are the types of speech characteristics the professional can note.

Cultural Variations Relevant to India

Every country and every community in it has its own ways of communication that are considered culturally acceptable. Local languages spoken in India would often contain unique words used to describe various problems, including pain, appetite and digestive problems, sleep difficulties, and sexual difficulties. It is important for a clinician to be completely aware of these and use the correct colloquial expression, or understand it when it is expressed by the patient.

Also, as in many eastern cultures, discussing sexual problems, addictive behaviors, etc. with the opposite gender may be difficult for many patients. This must be taken into account while taking history or an important set of facts may be missed.

It is not unusual for patients, more often women than men, to present with somatic symptoms when the root cause of their distress is in fact emotional in nature (Shidhaye, Mendenhall, Sumathipala, Sumathipala, & Patel, 2013). It is a meta analytic study which included three studies, each were reported from India, Pakistan, and Turkey, two studies were conducted in Sri Lanka, and one each was reported from Brazil, Chile, Ethiopia, and China.

The next major category is thought processes. In describing thought processes, the professional can note if the individual can answer the questions that are asked and adds additional information when appropriate. On the other hand, some individuals will produce responses that are not related to the question asked or tell a narrative in which each sentence is not related to the one that came before it. This is referred to as a **flight of ideas.** The content of the individual's thought is also important. Is there a theme to the thoughts, such as the CIA is out to get the individual? This would be referred to as **delusional thinking.** Does the individual keep repeating a certain theme? For example, some individuals keep being concerned that they will have a heart attack or that their spouse is cheating on them. This is referred to as **obsessional thinking.** The professional should also take particular note if the person is talking about suicide or homicide. This may require an intervention.

Another major category is perceptions and a general awareness of the surroundings. Distortions of perceptions can include hallucinations in which the individual perceives experiences without external stimulation. Individuals with a psychotic disorder may hear a radio program talking to them directly or respond to voices in their head. General awareness of the surroundings includes the question of whether the person knows who and where he or she is and the present date and time.

The final categories describe intellectual functioning and insight. Intellectual functioning is generally noted in terms of current vocabulary used in the interview as well as previous academic achievement. The professional can also note if the person has an abstract understanding of the information he or she is reporting. Insight refers to the individual's awareness of his or her own self and the factors related to his or her current situation and distress.

STRUCTURED INTERVIEWS

A **structured interview** is, as the name implies, an interview that is highly structured in terms of the questions asked. The idea is that by asking clients the same set of questions, it is possible to have better consistency across interviewers. Likewise, because every client receives the same questions, it is assumed that there will be more consistency across clients.

Structured Clinical Interview for *DSM* Disorders

With the development of the current classification manual, the *Diagnostic and Statistical Manual of Mental Disorders (DSM–5*) (American Psychiatric Association [APA], 2013), with specific criteria for each category of disorder, it is possible to ask questions in an interview that directly probe for the existence of these criteria. The **Structured Clinical Interview for *DSM* Disorders (SCID)** sets forth these questions along with a decision tree for directing follow-up questions. For example, if you want to determine if a person displayed an obsessive-compulsive disorder, you would begin with a general question concerning the occurrence of thoughts that kept recurring. If the person said yes, you would then ask what they were. The decision tree would help you to determine if these thoughts were seen by the individual as something produced in his or her own mind or were imposed on the person by an outside agent. Thoughts experienced as not from oneself would be more characteristic of a psychotic disorder whereas those recognized as coming from one's own mind might indicate a possible obsessive-compulsive disorder. Individuals with anxiety may also experience worries as thoughts coming into their mind, and the SCID would help to determine whether the person experiences obsessive- compulsive disorder or anxiety. The next set of questions would help the professional determine whether compulsions were also present. The SCID would instruct the interviewer to ask if there was anything the person had to do over and over again such as hand washing or checking something several times.

5-1 LENS
Cultural Sensitivity in Understanding Behavior and Experience

For thousands of years, humans have traveled and been fascinated at the diversity of human behavior and thinking around the world. Historically, those interested in psychopathology and neuroscience research have focused more on the universality of human processing rather than the diversity found in different cultures. This is beginning to change with an integration of human diversity and neuroscience perceptives on human behavior and experience (see Chiao, 2009, 2011; Kitayama & Cohen, 2007, for overviews).

In terms of assessment and **classification** of mental disorders, it is critical when working with individuals from different cultures to understand the rules of expression as well as the labeling of mental disorders. This is especially true if the rules for expression of distress and emotion differ greatly from the interviewer's culture. It is also important to understand what would be considered a mental disorder in another culture. For example, in some cultures such as the Shona of Zimbabwe there is a disorder referred to as thinking too much (*Kufungisisa*). Thinking too much is seen to cause anxiety and depression as well as headaches and dizziness. A common theme in Latin America is to speak of nerves (*nervios*) as a common idiom of distress. People may say that they cannot function because of nerves. In Japan, there is a broad concept of social concern when interacting with others (*taijin kyofusho*). This can include concern that one is making too much or too little eye contact, has an unpleasant body odor, or is making inappropriate body movements.

In terms of the cultural display of emotional expression, it has been shown that although individuals from different cultures may display their emotions differently, the underlying experience of the emotion may be similar. Some of this early work was performed by Paul Ekman and his colleagues (Ekman & Oster, 1979). In these studies, individuals from North America and Asia were shown emotionally arousing films that brought forth feelings of disgust or happiness. Although in private both cultural groups showed similar facial expression, the situation changed drastically when another person was present. When another person was present, those from Asia showed fewer facial expressions to the films than when they were alone. Western individuals, on the other hand, showed similar reactions to the films both alone and in the presence of another. Thus, different cultures have different display rules for the expression of similar underlying emotions.

Neuroscience research has shown that human reactions are also culturally sensitive. We know that the amygdala shows increased activity in response to emotional activity—especially fear. Native Japanese and Caucasian Americans show greater amygdala responses to fear expressions of those of their own culture. That is, a person shows less response when viewing an emotional expression of someone who is not part of his or her own culture (see *Figure 5-1*).

The previous chapter also threw light on the recent thoughts about how culture-bound symptoms may gradually disappear as industrialization and globalization bring education and health awareness into cultures.

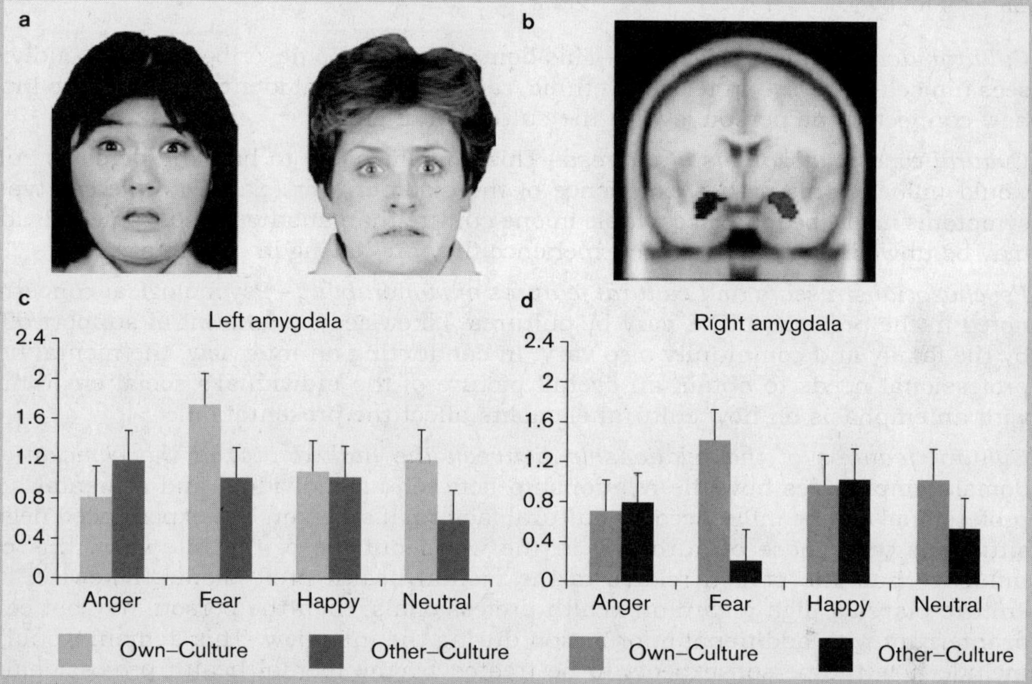

FIGURE 5-1 Cultural Specificity in Bilateral Amygdala Response to Fear Faces

Source: Chiao (2009).

Note: a = examples of Japanese and Caucasian American fear faces; b = illustration of bilateral amygdala; participants show greater left (c) and right (d) amygdala response to fear expressed by members of their own cultural group.

ASSESSING CULTURAL DIMENSIONS

Over the past 40 years, there has been an increasing awareness that mental illness takes place within the context of a particular culture (see Marsella & Yamada, 2007, for an overview). Initially, there was a realization that specific disorders such as depression, schizophrenia, and stress-related disorders are understood differently in different cultures (Draguns, 1973; Draguns & Tanaka-Matsumi, 2003). That is to say, a fuller understanding of mental illness requires an understanding of context. Although every culture has words for severe mental illness such as psychosis, mood disorders such as anxiety, and depression, there is also variation in what is considered normality and deviance. This chapter's LENS notes that culture not only informs one as to how one should view one's distress but also influences how that distress is expressed.

With the fifth edition of *DSM (DSM–5),* a **Cultural Formulation Interview (CFI)** has been developed to help mental health professionals obtain information concerning the person's culture. In general, the CFI focuses on five domains. These are described in *DSM–5* as follows:

Cultural identity of the individual—This domain in *DSM–5* describes how the individual sees himself or herself in terms of ethnic, racial, or cultural identity. It can also include how connected the person is with the culture of origin.

Cultural conceptualizations of distress—This domain refers to how the person's culture would influence his or her experience of the disorder. For example, different types of symptoms might be more acceptable in one culture than another. Also, some individuals may be unwilling to describe the experience they are having in certain areas.

Psychosocial stressors and cultural features of vulnerability—Psychological concerns as noted in the previous LENS vary by cultures. Likewise, the amount of support offered by the family and community also vary. In conducting an interview, the mental health professional needs to obtain an overall picture of the individual's social environment with an emphasis on how cultural elements affect the presentation.

Cultural features of the relationship between the individual and the clinician—This domain emphasizes how the relationship between an individual and a mental health professional can be influenced by cultural factors. If a person has experienced negative situations with those of authority in the world outside of the interview, this could influence how the person relates to the mental health professional. Likewise, if the culture places a high regard on health professionals, then the person may not correct or interrupt with additional information during the interview. This domain would also include how the person expects to be treated by the mental health professional and expectations for future treatment.

Overall cultural assessment—This domain represents an overall assessment and implications of what was identified in the previous domains. Treatment preferences can be described that may be incorporated into the treatment plan.

Understanding the cultural context of a disorder helps increase the validity of the assessment and diagnosis procedure. The CFI asks 16 questions related to culture indirectly. For example, the mental health professional would ask the person how his or her family, friends, or community view what is causing the problems. In this manner, people can describe their understanding of their problems with a direct or indirect reference to their culture.

RELIABILITY AND VALIDITY IN RELATION TO PSYCHOPATHOLOGY

Concerns about the accuracy of assessment and classification of psychopathology require us to consider two very different questions. The first has to do with the person who is being interviewed. We need to know if the person is giving us information that is accurate or not. Sometimes, individuals will "fake bad" if there is some advantage such as receiving a larger disability payout. Other times individuals will "fake good" and deny there are any problems.

The second question is the instrument itself. An assessment instrument can be an interview, an inventory, a mood scale, and so forth. In considering instruments, we think about measurement. Measurement considerations help to define the variety of instruments that we use and the theoretical variables that these reflect.

Traditionally, the two key measurement issues are **reliability** and validity. That is, does an instrument measure the construct consistently (reliability) and accurately (validity)? The measurement of temperature, for example, is based on the kinetic theory of heat, which helped define the type of devices used for the measurement of temperature. With psychopathology, we lack exact formal definitions that tell us exactly how to make measurements. In fact, we are both trying to learn about disorders and creating techniques for making diagnoses of the disorders. This makes reliability and validity considerations both more difficult and more important.

Reliability

Reliability asks the question of whether the instrument is consistent. We would expect, for example, that the odometer in our car would reflect that we drove a mile each time we drove 5,280 feet. We would also expect our bathroom scale to show the same weight if our weight had not changed. Researchers interested in questions of measurement discuss a number of types of reliability.

Internal reliability—Internal reliability asks whether different questions asked on an instrument relate to one another. If we were seeking a general measure of depression, for example, we would seek to find questions that would relate to one another. Questions related to feeling sad, not having energy, and wanting to stay in bed would be expected to show internal reliability.

Test-retest reliability—Test-retest reliability asks whether two measurement opportunities result in similar scores. A key consideration with test-retest reliability is the nature of the underlying construct. Constructs seen as stable, such as intelligence or hypnotizability, would be expected to show similar scores if the same instrument was given on more than one occasion. In psychopathological research, measures of long-term depression or trait anxiety would be expected to show a higher index of test-retest reliability than measures that reflect momentary feelings of mood.

Alternative form reliability—As the name implies, alternative form reliability asks whether different forms of an instrument give similar results. If you were giving an IQ test, for example, you would not want to ask the same question each time since the individual could learn the answers from taking the test. Thus, it would be important to create alternative forms that reflect the same underlying construct.

Inter-rater reliability—Inter-rater reliability asks how similar two or more individuals are when they observe and rate specific behaviors. Psychopathology researchers often rate the emotional responses of children as they engage in various activities. An index of inter-rater reliability would measure how consistent different observers would be in rating the same situation. Historically, one of the motivating factors for developing the *DSM* classification system was the discovery that different clinicians in different locations diagnosed a film of a person with a mental health disorder in different ways.

Validity

Validity asks whether the instrument we are using is accurate. A clock, for example, could be reliable if it was always 5 minutes fast, but it would not be accurate. Unlike time, for which there is a definition in terms of atomic clocks, psychopathological disorders lack exact unchanging definitions. Although measures such as neuropsychological tests, brain images, and molecular and genetic changes suggest possible variables to be considered, there is currently no exact measure by which to diagnose psychopathology. This makes validity an important but complex concept. Partly for this reason, we consider a number of types of validity.

Concept Check

- What are five critical areas mental health professionals cover in an initial clinical interview?
- Why is it important for mental health professionals to understand the cultural context of an individual's mental disorder? What kinds of information does the CFI help mental health professionals obtain?
- In terms of assessment, what are four types of reliability you should be concerned with, and why?
- In terms of assessment, what are five types of validity you should be concerned with, and why?

Content validity—Content validity refers to the degree to which an instrument measures all aspects of the phenomenon. If a final exam only had questions from 1 week of the course, it would not be representative of what the students had learned. A variety of psychopathological disorders, such as depression, for example, have cognitive, emotional, and motor components. A measure that just asks if a person felt negative about the future would be seen as a less good measure of depression than one that also asks about feeling sad and thoughts about suicide and self-worth.

Predictive validity—Predictive validity refers to the degree to which an instrument can predict cognitions, emotions, or actions that a person will experience in the future. If an IQ test in high school predicted college performance, then it would be seen to have predictive validity. Many medical tests such as cholesterol measurements are designed to predict who is at risk for later medical conditions such as cardiovascular problems.

Concurrent validity—Concurrent validity refers to the ability of an instrument to show similar results as other established measures of the construct.

Construct validity—Construct validity refers to the extent that an instrument measures what it was designed to measure (Cronbach & Meehl, 1955). If a test was designed to measure what students learned in a course, then it would be a problem if the test was also sensitive to other factors such as intelligence or the ability to understand test questions asked in terms of double negatives.

Ecological validity—Ecological validity refers to the manner in which data collected has been considered beyond the local context. For example, considering which cultural factors could be influencing the information obtained would improve the ecological validity of the data. This would also hold true in research studies involving mental illness in different cultures. That is, the meaning of a concept in one culture may be different from that in another.

Significant work has been done by Dr. Mitchell Weiss from the University of Basel in the Indian context on the Explanatory Model Interview Catalogue (EMIC) (see Weiss et al., 1992; Weiss, 1997; Weiss, 2001). Work has also been done in the context of physical ailments and illness meanings (see Tandon, Mehrotra, & Vallikad, 2010).

MODELS OF ASSESSMENT

In this section, we will consider different ways of assessing signs and symbols. These range from simply asking a person about his or her symptoms to comparing the person to others who have a similar disorder.

Symptom Questionnaires

At times, it is important to know what a person's symptoms are and how that person may compare with others in terms of reporting these symptoms. A variety of questionnaires have been developed that focus on particular sets of symptoms such as those associated with pain, sleep disorders, anxiety, and depression.

The **Beck Depression Inventory (BDI)** has been used in both clinical and research settings to assess symptoms associated with the experience of depression (Beck & Beck, 1972). The BDI has 21 items, each of which is presented in a four-choice format where the individual is asked to indicate which choice best fits his or her current experience. Here is an example:

I am not particularly discouraged about the future.
I feel discouraged about the future.
I feel I have nothing to look forward to.
I feel the future is hopeless and that things cannot improve.

A questionnaire such as the BDI is useful for determining the level of depressive symptoms that a person is reporting. Given that the measure has been in use for more than 40 years, there is considerable clinical and research data available in terms of level of depressive severity. The measure is also useful for noting changes in depression level during various types of treatment. During psychotherapy, for example, the measure could be given weekly to document changes in depressive experiences. It should be noted that a newer version of the scale (BDI-II) replaced items related to weight loss, changes in body image, and somatic preoccupation in order to better assess depression.

Personality Tests

For at least the past 2,000 years, there has been an understanding that individuals have a particular style for relating to the world and others. At the beginning of the last century, the personality styles of introversion and extraversion were studied. There was also a search to examine the relationship between personality styles and psychopathology. A number of questionnaires have been developed to this end. One of the best known of these is the **Minnesota Multiphasic Personality Inventory (MMPI).**

Minnesota Multiphasic Personality Inventory

The MMPI is composed of more than 500 items of a true–false nature. The person taking the test simply answers yes or no to questions such as "I have trouble falling asleep." The test was developed in an interesting manner. The authors, S. R. Hathaway and J. C. McKinley, began with a large pool of items and then reduced these to 504 items that were determined to be independent of one another. They then gave these items to psychiatric inpatients at the University of Minnesota Hospital. These inpatients were further divided by diagnosis and the responses of each group were compared with nonpatients who had come to the hospital as visitors or relatives. The idea was to develop a scoring scheme that would differentiate those with mental disorders from those without. In this sense, the content of the item was less important than its ability to discriminate between those individuals with a specific disorder and those without as well as between disorders.

In 1989, a new version of the MMPI, the MMPI-2, was released, which improved the generalizability of the test. The new test was normed on a better representation of the general population in terms of race, age, occupational level, income, and geographic location. The new version contains 567 items and uses a true, false, or can't say format. One real advantage of the MMPI and MMPI-2 is that they were developed in a more empirical manner by comparing how the pattern of responding matched populations with specific disorders versus healthy individuals rather than the content of the items. It is also possible using a normal statistical curve to determine how extreme an individual's responses are. Thus, the scales are presented in a dimensional manner and it's easy to determine if a person endorses more or less of a category of experiences than the general population.

The clinical scale in the MMPI uses the following categories:

- *Hypochondriasis*—Individuals who endorse these items show an excessive concern with bodily symptoms.
- *Depression*—Individuals who endorse these items display characteristics of depression such as trouble sleeping, loss of appetite, feeling sad, suicidal thoughts, and loss of interest in positive events.
- *Hysteria*—Individuals who endorse these items tend to view and experience the world in an emotional manner. They may overdramatize their situation. They may also experience emotional difficulties through bodily symptoms such as headaches or upset stomach when in a difficult psychological situation.
- *Psychopathic deviate*—Individuals who endorse these items display antisocial tendencies and experience conflicts with their environment. They may also exploit others without remorse.
- *Masculinity–femininity*—These items reflect the degree to which an individual endorses the traditional gender role of males or females.
- *Paranoia*—Individuals who endorse these items display suspiciousness of others. They also view the world in terms of "who is out to get them."
- *Psychasthenia*—Individuals who endorse these items display excessive anxiety and obsessive behavior.
- *Schizophrenia*—Individuals who endorse these items display bizarre disorganized thoughts along with a lack of normal contact with reality including social aloofness. Various sensory problems such as hallucinations may be present.
- *Hypomania*—Individuals who endorse these items experience high-energy states associated with poor judgment and impulse control.
- *Social introversion*—These items reflect social introversion and extraversion.

Note: The above bulleted list is adapted from MMPI®-2(Minnesota Multiphasic Personality Inventory®-2) Manual for Administration, Scoring, and Interpretation, Revised Edition.

By placing each of the categories on a normal distribution, it is possible to see which categories deviate from responses seen in the general population (see *Figure 5-2*). In addition to the clinical scales, the MMPI also contains validity scales. These scales were designed to determine whether the person is trying to skew the results by either "faking good" or "faking bad." One type of item included in these scales would be one that most healthy individuals would not agree to such as "I have never told a lie." This last item would be found on the lie or L scale. The infrequency or F scale is composed of items that are infrequently endorsed by the general population. Endorsing these items could come about because the person wanted to look as if they had psychological problems. It could also be the case that the individual was confused or could not read or understand the items. The defensiveness, or K scale, seeks to identify individuals who deny having any psychological problems. The number of times the person responds with "can't say" can be noted to help determine the validity of the MMPI. Further, as might be expected after more

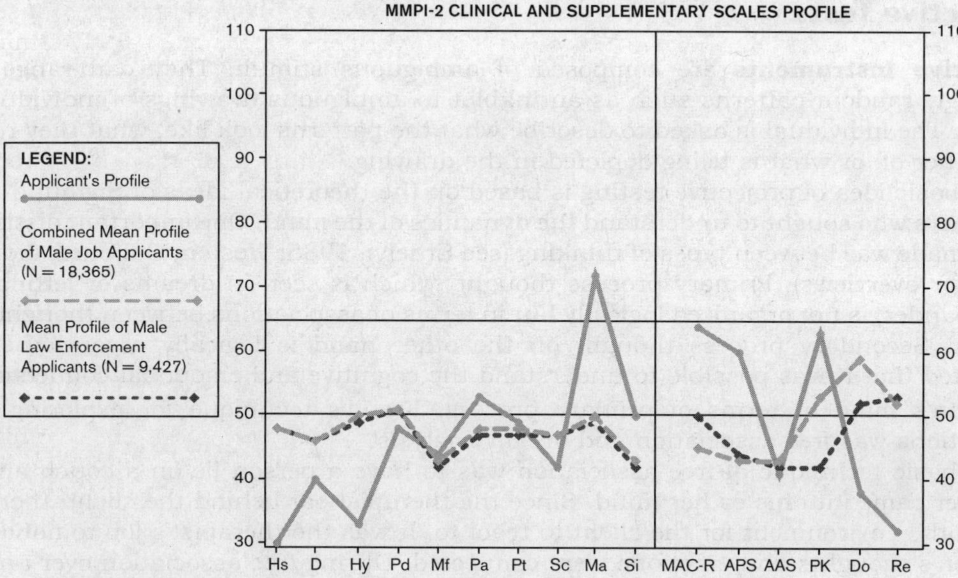

	Hs	D	Hy	Pd	Mf	Pa	Pt	Sc	Ma	Si	MAC-R	APS	AAS	PK	Do	Re
General Applicant Sample Mean Score: ---	48	46	50	51	43	48	48	47	50	43	45	43	43	53	59	52
Law Enforcement Sample Mean Score: ---	48	46	49	51	42	47	47	47	49	42	50	44	42	42	52	53
Applicant's Raw Score:	1	14	11	20	23	11	20	16	27	25	27	27	1	16	13	13
K Correction Score: ----	3			2			6	6	1							
Applicant's T Score: ---	30	40	33	48	44	53	49	42	72	50	64	60	41	63	38	32
Non-Gendered T Score: ----------	30	39	32	48		53	48	42	73	49	67	60	43	62	38	30
Response %: --------	100	100	100	98	100	98	100	100	100	100	98	100	85	100	100	97

Welsh Code: 9'+-6<u>0/74</u>582:31# F:LK#

Profile Elevation: 45.9

FIGURE 5-2 MMPI-2 Profile

than 70 years of use, a variety of additional scales have been developed which have been used for both clinical and research purposes.

Use of Empirical Tests in India

There is limited published work on the use of MMPI 2 and MCMI III in India and Asia due to difficulty in obtaining permissions for language translations, etc. However, a large number of experience is available with these tools in India, accomplished with persons who are familiar with English and have completed the tools. It becomes clear from the work done at multiple public hospitals, university settings, and patient care institutes that the existing versions of these tools are culturally compatible with the current urban, educated populations in India seeking mental health help.

Projective Tests

Projective instruments are composed of ambiguous stimuli. They can range from seemingly random patterns such as an inkblot to ambiguous drawings of individuals or objects. The individual is asked to describe what the patterns look like, what they remind him or her of, or what is being depicted in the drawing.

The basic idea of projective testing is based on the theoretical ideas of Sigmund Freud and others who sought to understand the dynamics of the mind. One important distinction Freud made was between types of thinking (see Erdelyi, 1985; Westen, Gabbard, & Ortigo, 2008, for overviews). Primary process thought, which is seen in dreams or letting your mind wander, is not organized logically but in terms of associations between thoughts and feelings. Secondary process thought on the other hand is logically organized. Freud suggested that it was possible to understand the cognitive and emotional connections of a person's mind in terms of primary process. Freud's technique for exploring these connections was free association and dream analysis.

The basic technique of free association was to have a person lie on a couch and say whatever came into his or her mind. Since the therapist sat behind the client, there was little in the environment for the client to react to. It was the therapist's job to notice how a person's thoughts and emotions were connected. During free association over a period of months, it was assumed that patterns of responding would emerge. It could be, for example, that whenever a client talked about his pet, he would feel sad, or whenever someone began to describe a certain event, he would change the topic.

Projective techniques were formally introduced in the first half of the 1900s as a means of detecting primary process types of thinking and feeling including instinctual and motivational processes. Since there were few techniques for understanding the connections in one's mind at this time, professionals saw projective techniques as having potential for understanding how thoughts and feelings formed a cognitive network. It was assumed that projective techniques would give a window into the thought processes of those with mental disorders and how they differ from the thought processes of healthy individuals.

Historical Examples of Projective Techniques

Two of the most well-known projective techniques are the **Rorschach Inkblot** and the **Thematic Apperception Test (TAT).** Both of these tests have a long history of use although various researchers have been critical of the Rorschach and other projective techniques and suggest clinical situations in which these types of techniques are not useful (Garb, Wood, Lilienfeld, & Nezworski, 2005).

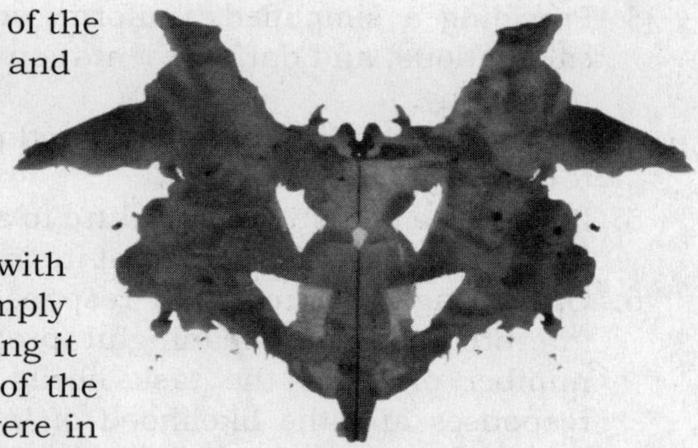

Rohrschach inkblot: Black-and-white

During the early part of the 1900s, Herman Rorschach, a Swiss psychiatrist, experimented with using inkblots. The inkblots were made by simply dripping ink on a piece of paper and then folding it in half to create a symmetrical design. Some of the inkblots were in black-and-white and others were in color. He initially gave his inkblots to a large number of schoolchildren (Ellenberger, 1970). Rorschach was interested in the sensory process of these images, which he connected with Carl Jung's idea of introversion and extraversion.

Rorschach saw introversion as focusing on the inner world of kinesthetic images and creative activity. Extraversion, on the other hand, was a focus on color, emotion, and adjustment to reality. For Rorschach, the content of what was seen in the inkblot was less the focus of the interpretation than the elements used, such as whether the person saw whole images or focused on small details of the blot. Viewing the image as containing movement and the use of the colors was also seen as important. A limited number of 10 plates were selected, and Rorschach published a book in German, *Psychodiagnostics*, in 1921. He died some months later at age 37. His book was translated into English in 1942.

Following his death, various clinicians used the Rorschach in their clinical practice. For a number of years, there was little scientific data concerning the reliability and validity of the measure. Since the late 20th century, there has been a movement to standardize the presentation of the test and the manner in which it is scored. Exner (1986, 2003) offered one such system. Various studies have examined the reliability and validity of the measure with specific diagnostic groups and theoretical constructs (see Hunsley & Mash, 2011; Meyer, 2001; Meyer & Archer, 2001, for overviews). In 2001, a special issue of the journal *Psychological Assessment* was devoted to clarifying the utility of the Rorschach along with its problems from an evidence-based position. In order to address questions of reliability and validity, a series of norms using the Exner system based on more than 5,800 people from 17 countries have been published (Meyer, Erdberg, & Shaffer, 2007). This review showed consistency across samples for adult Rorschach responses but problems with data from children. Overall, the Rorschach and its scoring is a complicated process that continues to be the focus of scientific debate.

In order to respond to the problems of the Exner scoring system, professionals interested in the Rorschach created a simpler scoring system referred to as the Rorschach Performance Assessment System (R-PAS) (http://www.r-pas.org/Docs/Manual_Chapter_1.pdf). The basic idea was to create a scoring system with strong psychometric properties such as reliability and validity. The developers of the R-PAS state their goals as follows:

1. Selecting and highlighting those variables with the strongest empirical, clinical, and response process/behavioral representational support while eliminating those with insufficient support.
2. Comparing test takers' scores to a large international reference sample, using a graphic array of percentiles and standard score equivalents.

3. Providing a simplified, uniform, and logical system of terminology, symbols, calculations, and data presentation in order to reduce redundancy and increase parsimony.
4. Describing the empirical basis and psychological rationale for each score that is to be interpreted.
5. Providing a statistical procedure to adjust for the overall complexity of the record and a graphical illustration of its impact on each variable.
6. Optimizing the number of responses given to the task in order to ensure an interpretable and meaningful protocol, while drastically reducing both the number of times the task needs to be readministered because of too few responses and the likelihood of inordinately long and taxing administrations because of too many responses.
7. Developing new and revised indices by applying contemporary statistical and computational approaches.
8. Offering access to a scoring program on a secure, encrypted web platform from any device that can interface with the Internet (e.g., PC, Notebook, smartphone, iPad).

The R-PAS system was developed around 2006 and continues to be tested worldwide. An initial review and meta-analysis article was published in *Psychological Bulletin,* which described Rorschach variables with research support and those with little or no support (Mihura, Meyer, Dumitrascu, & Bombel, 2013).

Other researchers have begun to use neuroscience techniques such as brain imaging and electrophysiology to understand physiological processes underlying Rorschach responses. For example, Giromini and his colleagues examined movement responses on the Rorschach and how these were reflected in the EEG (Giromini, Porcelli, Viglione, Parolin, & Pineda, 2010).

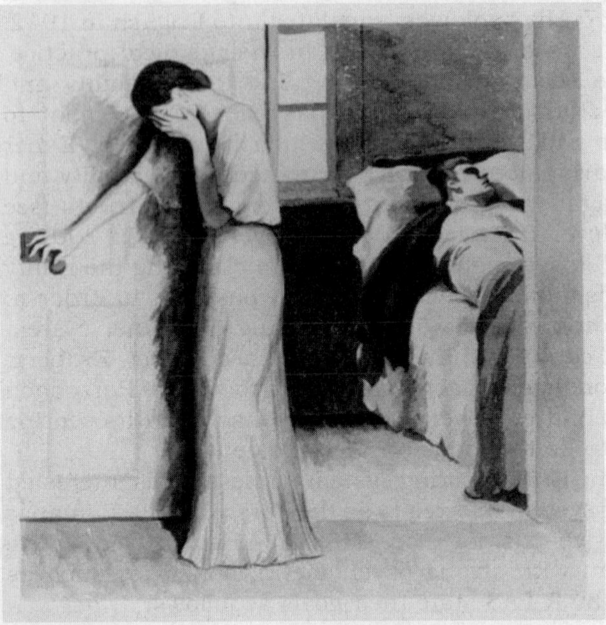

TAT Drawing
Source: Explorations in personality: A clinical and experimental study of fifty men of college age by Murray et al. (1938) "TAT drawing" p. 622. By permission of Oxford University Press, USA.

The TAT is composed of 30 black-and-white drawings of various scenes and people. The instrument was developed by Christiana Morgan and Henry Murray in the 1930s. Typically, an individual is shown 20 of the cards, one at a time, and asked to create a story about what is being depicted on the card. The basic idea is that by noting the content and emotionality of the individual's responses, it is possible to gain insight into his or her thoughts, emotions, and motivations including areas of conflict. For example, if someone described many of the cards in terms of someone leaving another person, the clinician might ask if abandonment was an important issue for the person. Although the TAT technique may be useful to gain additional information concerning a person such as suicidal thoughts, it lacks scientific evidence to make it useful in obtaining a formal diagnosis. Similar problems of reliability and validity exist with the TAT as with the Rorschach.

Overall, projective techniques have been the subject of great debate and controversy. Frick, Barry, and Kamphaus (2010) presented some of the major pros and cons concerning the use of projective techniques (see *Table 5-1*). Some professionals see their value not in terms of giving exact diagnoses but in their ability to allow a professional to see how an individual responds to ambiguous stimuli—especially in terms of suicidal ideation as well as disorganized thought processes. This may lead to further discussions of areas that a professional would not normally discuss. The major disadvantage of projective techniques centers on questions of validity in terms of both the tests' ability to identify specific disorders and the reliance of the test interpretation on a specific population such as children.

TABLE 5-1 Pros and Cons of Projective Tests

The Projective Debate	
Pro	***Con***
Less structured format allows clinician greater flexibility in administration and interpretation and places fewer demand characteristics that would prompt socially desirable responses from an informant.	The reliability of many techniques is questionable. As a result, the interpretations are more related to characteristics of the clinician than to characteristics of the person being tested.
Allows for the assessment of drives, motivations, desires, and conflicts that can affect a person's perceptual experiences but are often unconscious.	Even some techniques that have good reliability have questionable validity, especially in making diagnoses and predicting overt behavior.
Provides a deeper understanding of a person than would be obtained by simply describing behavioral patterns.	Although we can at times predict things we cannot understand, it is rarely the case that understanding does not enhance prediction (Gittelman-Klein, 1986).
Adds to an overall assessment picture.	Adding an unreliable piece of information to an assessment battery simply decreases the overall reliability of the battery.
Helps to generate hypotheses regarding a person's functioning.	Leads one to pursue erroneous avenues in testing or to place undue confidence in finding.
Non-threatening and good for rapport building.	Detracts from the time an assessor could better spend collecting more detailed, objective information.
Many techniques have a long and rich clinical tradition.	Assessment techniques are based on an evolving knowledge base and must continually evolve to reflect this knowledge.

Source: Frick et al. (2010), with kind permission from Springer Science+Business Media B.V.

Use of Projective Tests in India

It is very clear that the Rorschach inkblot method and other projective tools such as the Thematic Apperception Test (TAT) and the Children's Apperception Test (CAT) continue to be widely used in India. An Indian modification of the TAT created by Dr. Uma Choudhury (1960) several decades ago is available, where the pictures are adapted for the urban and rural Indian context. Similarly, Indian adaptations for CAT are also available in regular and colored forms, and also for special populations (Chaudhury et al., 2006).

Neuropsychological Testing

Neuropsychological tests have been developed to help mental health professionals assess a person's general level of cognitive functioning. Intelligence tests, for example, are able to compare a given individual with his or her peers to determine level of functioning. The common intelligence tests, such as the **Wechsler Adult Intelligence Scale (WAIS),** have a number of subscales designed to measure verbal and performance tasks. The verbal tasks include measurements of acquired knowledge, verbal reasoning, and comprehension of verbal information. The performance tasks include nonverbal reasoning, spatial processing skills, attention to detail, and visuomotor integration.

The Wechsler tests for intelligence evaluation are widely used in India. Indian authors such as Fr. Malin (MISIC: Malin's Intelligence Scale for Indian Children) and Dr. Mahendrika Bhatt have developed adaptations of the tools using Indian standardization samples.

Several manuals for use with Indian populations have been developed by NIMH, Secunderabad. The most recent edition of the WAIS India norms in use is WAIS IV, and the most recent India normed WMS is WMS III. WISC IV is also used with India norms.

Other neuropsychological tests have been designed to assess specific types of brain functioning including brain damage. These include memory, attention, reasoning, emotional processing, and motor processes including inhibition of action. One advantage of traditional neuropsychological tests is that they have been given to a large of number of people so that norms could be established. Thus, it is possible to know whether a 70-year-old individual is showing a normal memory decline in certain areas or if there might be the beginning of a neurocognitive disorder or Alzheimer's disease.

Although neuropsychological testing was initially developed to assess brain damage resulting from accidents, strokes, or war, it is now finding a use in delineating deficits in those with mental illness. Today, there is a coming together of neuropsychological tests, measures of cognitive processes in normal individuals, and brain imaging techniques. For example, the **Wisconsin Card Sorting Test (WCST)** requires that an individual sort cards into four piles. Each card has a specific shape on it, such as a circle or square. Each card has a specific number of these shapes, and each card is printed in a specific color. Thus, you could sort the cards by shape, by number, or by color. The person administering the test states that the individual is sorting each card correctly or not. After a number of sorts, the administrator changes the correct sort category. Individuals with frontal lobe damage have difficulty responding to changing demands. Individuals with schizophrenia also have difficulty responding to changing task requirements.

Another test that is commonly used in psychopathology research is the **Continuous Performance Test (CPT).** This is a test that measures attentional characteristics. In one version of the test, participants are shown a series of letters and must respond whenever a particular letter is displayed. The test then requires that the person respond when one particular letter followed by another letter is displayed. Children with attention deficit/hyperactivity disorder (ADHD) have problems with this task. Thus, neuropsychological tests are also being used to understand brain processes in those with mental illness.

Indian Contributions to Neuropsychological Assessment

Much work has been done in India on neuropsychological assessment. The NIMHANS neuropsychological battery has been a major contribution to the field (see Kar, Rao, Chandramouli, & Thennarasu, 2004; Tripathi, Kumar, Bharath, Marimuthu, & Varghese, 2013). Neuropsychological batteries have also been developed by AIIMS, New Delhi, and PGI, Chandigarh (Pershad & Verma, 1990).

Neuropsychological Tests and Mental Illness

Neuropsychological tests can help identify cognitive changes associated with a particular disorder. For example, there is a rare occurrence of four sisters who all developed schizophrenia in their 20s. The Genain sisters were monozygotic quadruplets born in the United States in the early 1930s. These sisters have been studied throughout their life in terms of genetic makeup as well as cognitive functioning. When the sisters were 66 years of age, Allan Mirsky and his colleagues readministered a number of neuropsychological tests including the WAIS, the CPT, and WCST (Mirsky et al., 2000). The scores of each sister at age 66 were compared with their performance at age 27 and 51. By showing that the test scores of the sisters over their lifetime had not changed, these researchers were able to show that cognitive decline is not part of schizophrenia.

Using Neuroscience Techniques to Identify Mental Illness

As more and more researchers and clinicians have come to see mental illness as representing problems with the brain, there has been a variety of projects to utilize neuroscience approaches to describe psychopathology (see Andreasen, 2001, for an overview). These have ranged from identifying the presence of certain genes and the manner in which they turn on and off in psychopathology to structural and functional descriptions of brain processes and psychophysiological changes measured throughout the body. The potential

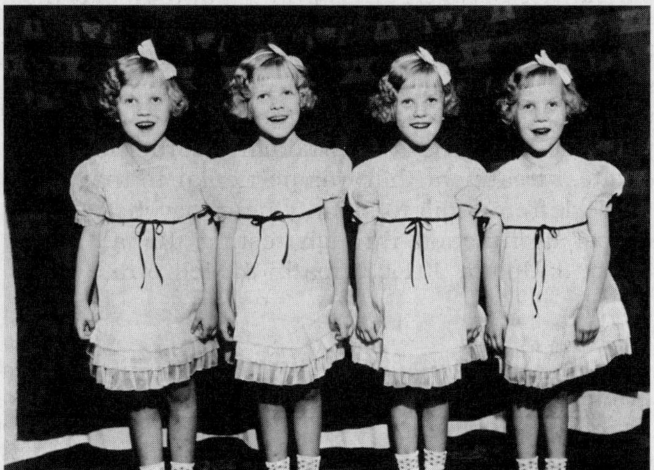

The genain sisters were identical quadruplets who all developed schizophrenia by age 24

for using neuroscience approaches to classify mental illness and inform its treatment is an important one (see Cuthbert & Insel, 2010; Halligan & David, 2001; Hyman, 2007, 2010; Insel, 2009; Miller, 2010, for overviews).

Traditionally, psychopathology has been defined in terms of signs and symptoms. The experiences of the client and what is observed by the professional is one level of analysis. In general, the mental health professional identifies symptoms that group together and the time of their appearance. Neuroscience techniques offer another level of analysis. From a research standpoint, scientists have sought to identify underlying markers associated with specific mental disorders. Using various brain imaging techniques we described in Chapter 3, such as magnetic resonance imaging (MRI), functional magnetic resonance imaging (fMRI), electroencephalography (EEG), and magnetoencephalography (MEG), there has been a search for structural and functional changes associated with psychopathology. For example, researchers have been able to distinguish individuals with autism (Ecker et al., 2010) and with bipolar disorder (Rocha-Rego et al., 2013) from those without the disorder based on fMRI data.

Part of the potential for using neuroscience markers results from the fact that not every individual with schizophrenia, for example, reports the same symptoms. Some individuals describe auditory hallucinations whereas others describe visual hallucinations. This is also the case with depression in that some individuals report different types of depressive symptoms than others. This suggests to some researchers that there might be different underlying brain processes involved in these variations. What now is considered as a single disorder may be better represented as separate disorders based on underlying mechanisms. Further, certain mental disorders also show gender differences. Females develop schizophrenia later than males but both males and females show similar rates of the disorder. However, females do show higher rates of mood and anxiety disorders.

Overall, neuroscience methods may lead to better diagnostic procedures as well as understanding the mechanisms of the disorder. For example, genetic research suggests similarities between schizophrenia and bipolar disorder in terms of the genes involved. It is also possible to use neuroscience techniques to follow the course of a disorder over time. One study (Raj, Kuceyeski, & Weiner, 2012) based on brain imaging methods suggests that neurocognitive disorders follow specific pathways in the brain. Another potential for neuroscience methods is that by knowing the underlying brain and genetic processes involved in a particular disorder for a particular person, it would be possible to create a treatment that was particular to that individual.

Work from India to identify neuropsychological dysfunction through testing (Raha, Shah, & Udani, 2012; Tripathi & Mehrotra, 2015).

CLASSIFICATION

Classification is a way to organize the diversity seen in mental disorders. Blashfield and Draguns (1976; see also Blashfield, Flanagan, & Raley, 2010, for an overview) suggest five different purposes of classification:

Concept Check

- For each of the following types of assessment, what kinds of information can you obtain from it and what is one example of it?
  - Symptom questionnaire
  - Personality test
  - Projective test
  - Neuropsychological test
  - Neuroscience technique

1. As a *nomenclature*—the purpose here is to present a way for mental health professionals to describe and discuss the clients they see.
2. As a *basis of information retrieval*—this allows for individuals who may not be professionals to search for information concerning mental disorders.
3. As a *descriptive system*—this is the case in which the name of the disorder summarizes the behaviors, thoughts, and emotions of individuals with the disorder.
4. As a *predictive system*—in this case, the classification allows one to know the course of the disorder if untreated and particular treatments that may be effective.
5. As a *basis for a theory of psychopathology*—the focus in this case is to use classification to understand the disorder.

Classification Systems for Mental Disorders

Over the past 200 years, numerous systems have been developed concerning the diagnosis and classification of mental disorders (see *Figure 5-3*). In the past 50 years, the emphasis has been on reliability of diagnosis such that mental health professionals in one location would diagnose the same individual in the same manner as professionals in another location. As part of this emphasis, there has been a push for observable characteristics that would define a specific disorder. These types of criteria make up the structure of the *DSM,* published by the APA, and the *International Classification of Diseases (ICD),* published by the World Health Organization (WHO). The *DSM* is used in North America whereas the *ICD* is used in Europe. In general, the criteria used in the *DSM* and *ICD* are signs and symptoms that are delineated through observation of, and conversation with, the individual. Since *ICD* codes are used by many health facilities in the United States, I will note the similarities and differences for *ICD* and *DSM* criteria of mental disorders throughout this book.

International Statistical Classification of Diseases and Related Health Problems

The *ICD* is managed by the WHO and used throughout Europe and other parts of the world. It was created at the beginning of the 20th century as a system for classifying traditional medical disorders. The sixth edition of the *ICD* was published in 1949. This was the first edition to include a section devoted to mental disorders. *ICD-10* is currently in use but is being updated for the 11th edition in 2015. Mental disorders in the *ICD-10* are more of a short narrative describing the condition rather than specific criteria as seen in the *DSM–5.*

Diagnostic and Statistical Manual of Mental Disorders

The *DSM* was created by a group of psychiatrists in the 1940s who had been involved in directing mental hospitals, directing the mental health services for the U.S. Army and Navy during World War II, and others who were part of the APA. The first version of *DSM*

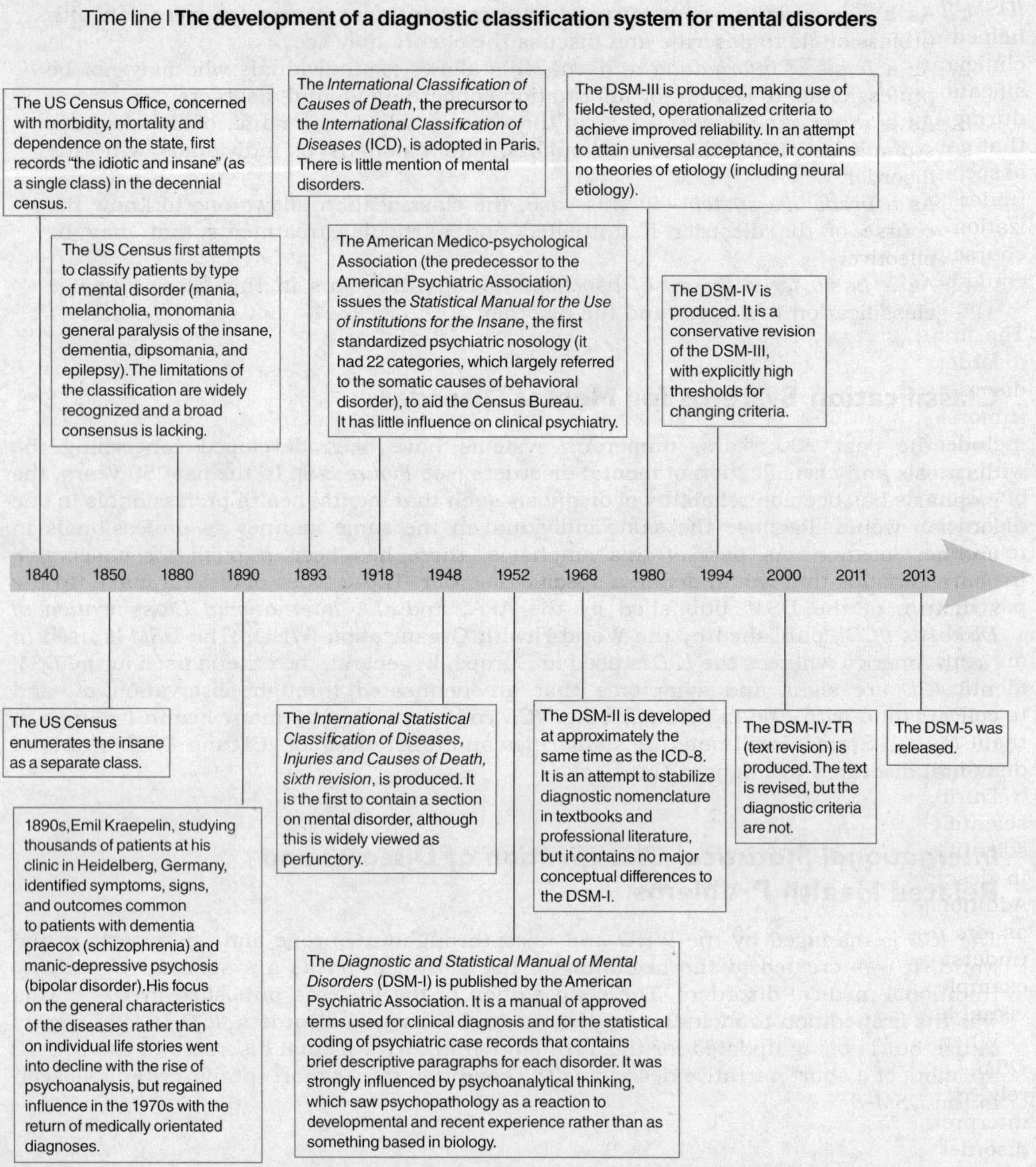

FIGURE 5-3 Time Line Reflecting the Development of a Classification System for Mental Disorders

Source: Hyman (2007).

(DSM–I) was published in 1952 (see Grob, 1991, for an overview). A number of factors helped to create the initial *DSM.* One was the search for consistency in diagnosis across clinicians throughout the country. In this sense, *DSM–I* sought to bring together the classifications used in state and private mental hospitals, those classifications developed during World War II, and those used by professionals in private practice. Another factor that gained emphasis during World War II was the realization that environmental stress associated with combat was related to the expression of mental disorders. A related understanding was that these disorders could be treated without prolonged institutionalization. Additionally, treatment worked best if the treatment was begun early in the course of the disorder. This required that professionals be able to differentiate those who could be treated and sent back to battle and those who needed long-term care.

The classification system used by *DSM–I* divided disorders into two broad categories. The first category was those disorders such as Huntington's chorea or neurocognitive disorders (then called dementias) resulting from brain pathophysiologies. These were disorders that resulted from hereditary origins, infections, long-term drug addictions, tumors of the brain, and other such factors. The second category was those disorders that included an environmental component in which the individual found it difficult to cope with his or her world. This second category was further divided into three different types of disorders. The first was psychosis including schizophrenia and other psychotic disorders. The second was neurosis, such as anxiety disorders. And the third was referred to as character disorders such as psychopathy, which were involved in forensic decisions. In general, it was assumed that the neurotic disorders would be more amenable to psychological treatment.

DSM–II was released in 1968. Although it did not differ greatly from *DSM–I,* it did offer an opportunity for the mental disorder categories of *ICD-8* and *DSM–II* to be almost identical. This allowed for a worldwide classification system, which increased the ability to collect statistics on particular mental disorders. One difference that did exist was that the *ICD* manual just listed the disorders whereas the *DSM* included brief definitions of the disorders.

During the 1970s, there were a variety of changes in issues of importance to both the scientific and larger lay community that influenced the next version of *DSM.* In the scientific study of psychopathology, there was an increased emphasis on greater precision in describing the signs and symptoms associated with a particular psychopathology. Additionally, there was an emphasis on differentiating one disorder from another as well as on using experimental research to inform these definitions. There was also an understanding that some individuals manifest a particular disorder in different ways. For example, some individuals with schizophrenia will hear voices while others will have visual hallucinations.

When *DSM–III* was released in 1980, it included a number of major changes from *DSM–I* and *DSM–II* (see Blashfield et al., 2010). One major change was that it sought to rely on observable evidence to create a scientific system rather than just focus on the interpretations of experts in the field. Another change was that *DSM–III* described disorders in terms of specific criteria rather than the more general descriptions of a disorder seen in *DSM–I* and *DSM–II. DSM–III* also introduced a five-level system or axes to give a more complete picture of the person. Axis I described the individual's psychopathological symptoms. Axis II described the person's personality or mental retardation. Axis III described any medical disorders that the person had. Axis IV described significant environmental factors in the person's life. And Axis V described the person's level of functioning and any significant role impairment. Overall, *DSM–III* sought to be theory neutral and only use observable terms. *DSM–III* was adopted in a number of countries and translated into 16 languages. In 1987, *DSM–III* was revised in terms of diagnostic criteria and referred to as *DSM–III–R.*

In 1994, *DSM–IV* was released. One goal of this release was to coordinate this revision with ICD-10. There was also an attempt to increase the scientific evidence underlying the diagnostic criteria. To achieve this goal, a steering committee composed of 27 members oversaw the work of 13 different work groups. The task of the work groups was a three-step process. The first step was to extensively review the scientific literature related to a particular disorder. The second step was to utilize and reanalyze descriptive data from researchers who studied particular disorders. The third step was to conduct a series of field trials using the diagnostic criteria and to modify the criteria based on these trials. *DSM–IV* was expanded in 2000 with the publication of *DSM–IV–TR. TR* stands for text revision. *DSM–IV–TR* did not make major changes to the diagnostic criteria but did expand the text information describing each disorder.

DSM–5 was released in May of 2013, and the rationale for the changes can be viewed at the website (www.psychiatry.org/dsm5). You may note that *DSM* went from the roman numerals used in previous editions to a numerical one for this edition. According to the *DSM–5* development website (www.dsm5.org), *DSM–5* sought to expand the scientific basis of diagnosis begun in *DSM–III* by working with the National Institute of Mental Health (NIMH). An initial conference was held in 1999. Participants developed a series of reports that sought to examine a variety of broad topics beyond diagnosis itself. These topics included developmental issues, gaps in the current system, disability and impairment, neuroscience, nomenclature, and cross-cultural issues. In later papers, age and gender issues were also considered. Further, international organizations such as WHO offered input into the composition of *DSM–5,* and 13 conferences were held.

One overall change in the *DSM–5* is the use of dimensional assessments and spectrum-related disorders. Dimensional assessment is designed to determine severity of a particular symptom rather than just presence or absence. Additionally, what have been considered to be separate disorders may be better viewed as part of a spectrum. For example, although individuals with autism, childhood disintegrative disorder, pervasive developmental disorder, and Asperger's syndrome may vary in their symptoms and abilities, there are similarities to the disorders. Thus, it would be more accurate to describe autism as falling on a spectrum ranging from mild to severe. In *DMS–5,* the term *Asperger's* is no longer used. Another example is bipolar disorder. Someone diagnosed with bipolar disorder may have a number of severe mood episodes involving mania and depression or just a few. In either case, there is a single category of either having the disorder or not. Dimensional analysis allows for more accurate representation of the disorder by reflecting the severity of the conditions.

The *DSM–5* suggests that every case begins with a careful clinical history as well as the social, psychological, and

Concept Check

- What are some of the reasons for setting up a classification system for mental illness, such as *ICD* or *DSM*?
- How are *ICD* and *DSM* similar? How are they different?
- What are two major changes in the way disorders are classified in the most recent edition of *DSM–5* compared with its predecessor, *DSM–IV*?

biological factors that have contributed to the development of the disorder. It is important to understand the nature of the distress that the person is experiencing as distress is a critical component of a *DSM* disorder. It is also important to understand if the distress and the individual's behavior should be considered as part of a mental disorder or simply deviant from the individual's cultural, religious, or other significant groups. Thus, *DSM–5* is more than just a list of symptoms to be checked off by the mental health professional. It is seen as a manual for organizing types of symptoms, which can suggest treatment approaches. However, *DSM–5* does not specify any particular treatment. Although *DSM–5* suggests that the person be considered within a larger context, it dropped the multiaxial system seen in *DSM–III* and *DSM–IV*. A clinician may continue to note cultural, environmental, and other conditions related to a given disorder, but Axes III, IV, and V are now eliminated. Further, personality disorders are no long described on a separate axis (Axis II).

Another change is in the organization of *DSM–5*. The placement of disorders is based on underlying vulnerabilities as well as symptom characteristics. The chapters are organized by general categories such as neurodevelopmental, emotional, and somatic to reflect how a variety of disorders may have some common underlying similarities. Recent advances in brain imaging, genetics, and the neurosciences have suggested similarities not understood previously. For example, genetic research suggests a closer connection between schizophrenia and bipolar disorder than previously assumed. However, these still remain as separate disorders in *DSM–5*. Throughout this book, I will note changes made from *DSM–IV* to *DSM–5*. A detailed list of changes can be found on the website (www.psychiatry.org/dsm5).

SUMMARY

Assessment is the process of gathering information about a person to be able to make a clinical decision about that person's symptoms. Most mental health professionals use a clinical interview to initially gather information concerning the status of an individual they are working with. Worldwide, the clinical interview, referred to as the mental status exam, has been organized into major assessment categories including the person's appearance and behavior, mood and affect, speech quality, thought processes, perceptions and general awareness of surroundings, and intellectual functioning and insight. With the most recent edition of *DSM (DSM–5)*, the SCID has been developed to set forth specific assessment questions in a structured approach along with a decision tree for directing follow-up questions. Over the past 40 years, there has been an increasing awareness that mental illness takes place within the context of a particular culture, and a fuller understanding of psychopathology requires an understanding of this context. With *DSM–5*, a CFI has been developed to help mental health professionals obtain information concerning the person's culture.

Concerns about the accuracy of assessment and classification of psychopathology require us to consider questions of reliability and validity: (1) whether the person being assessed is giving us accurate information and (2) whether the assessment instrument measures the construct consistently (reliability) and accurately (validity). In terms of assessment, there are a number of types of reliability: internal reliability, test–retest reliability, alternative form reliability, and inter-rater reliability. Although measures such as neuropsychological tests, brain images, and molecular and genetic changes suggest possible variables to be considered, there is currently no exact measure by which to diagnose psychopathology. This makes validity an important but complex concept. In terms of assessment, there are a number of types of validity: content validity, predictive validity, concurrent validity, and construct validity.

There are several models of assessment that represent different ways of assessing signs and symbols. These include symptom questionnaires, personality tests, projective tests, and neuropsychological testing. Neuroscience techniques offer an additional level of analysis to the models of assessment that focus on signs and symbols. Scientists have sought to identify underlying markers associated with specific mental disorders. Using various brain imaging techniques such as MRI, fMRI, EEG, and MEG, there has been a search for structural and functional changes associated with psychopathology. There might be different underlying brain processes involved in what appears as a single disorder. Thus, neuroscience methods may lead to better diagnostic procedures. It is also possible to use these techniques to follow the course of a disorder over time. Another potential for neuroscience methods is that by knowing the underlying brain and genetic processes involved in a particular disorder for a particular person, it would be possible to create a treatment particular to a given individual.

Classification is a way to organize the diversity seen in mental disorders. Over the past 200 years, numerous systems have been developed; however, in the past 50 years, the emphasis has been on reliability of diagnosis. There has been a push for observable characteristics that would define a specific disorder—signs and symptoms delineated through observation of, and conversation with, the individual. In general, these types of criteria make up the structure of the *DSM,* published by the APA and used in North America, and the *ICD,* published by the WHO and used in Europe. One overall change in the most recent edition of *DSM (DSM–5)* is the use of dimensional assessments and spectrum-related disorders. Another change is in the placement of disorders based on underlying vulnerabilities as well as symptom characteristics to reflect how a variety of disorders may have some common underlying similarities. Beginning in Chapter 6, I will focus on particular disorders.

STUDY RESOURCES

Review Questions

1. What are some of the advantages of conducting a structured interview for an initial mental health assessment? In addition, what specific advantages do the mental status exam and the SCID offer?
2. How do reliability and validity relate to the assessment and classification of psychopathology?
3. How can neuropsychological testing help us understand mental illness?
4. What important areas of potential do neuroscience techniques offer in the assessment and classification of mental illness?

5. "Classification is a way to organize the diversity seen in mental disorders." From what you have read about *ICD* and *DSM,* the advantages of classification are clear, but are there any disadvantages or things that are overlooked?

For Further Reading

Meehl, P. E. (1954). *Clinical versus statistical prediction.* Minneapolis: University of Minnesota Press.

Key Terms and Concepts

assessment
Beck Depression Inventory (BDI)
classification
Continuous Performance Test (CPT)
Cultural Formulation Interview (CFI)
delusional thinking
flight of ideas
mental status exam
Minnesota Multiphasic Personality Inventory (MMPI)
obsessional thinking
projective instruments
reliability
Rorschach Inkblot
Structured Clinical Interview for *DSM* Disorders (SCID)
structured interview
Thematic Apperception Test (TAT)
Wechsler Adult Intelligence Scale (WAIS)
Wisconsin Card Sorting Test (WCST)

CHAPTER

6

Disorders of Childhood

CHAPTER OUTLINE

- EXPERIENCE 184
- INTRODUCTION TO CHILDHOOD DEVELOPMENT 185
- ATTACHMENT DISORDERS 202
- AUTISM SPECTRUM DISORDERS 203
- ATTENTION DEFICIT/HYPERACTIVITY DISORDER 213
- CONDUCT DISORDER 218
- OPPOSITIONAL DEFIANT DISORDER 219
- LEARNING DISABILITIES 220
- INTELLECTUAL DEVELOPMENTAL DISORDER 222
- SUMMARY 226
- STUDY RESOURCES 229

EXPERIENCE

"Look me in the eye, young man!"

I cannot tell you how many times I heard that shrill, whining refrain. It started about the time I got to first grade. I heard it from parents, relatives, teachers, principals, and all manner of other people. I heard it so often I began to expect to hear it.

To this day, when I speak, I find visual input to be distracting. When I was younger, if I saw something interesting I might begin to watch it and stop speaking entirely. As a grown-up, I don't usually come to a complete stop, but I may still pause if something catches my eye. That's why I usually look somewhere neutral—at the ground or off into the distance—when I'm talking to someone. Because speaking while watching things has always been difficult for me, learning to drive a car and talk at the same time was a tough one, but I mastered it.

And now I know it is perfectly natural for me not to look at someone when I talk. Those of us with Asperger's are just not comfortable doing it. In fact, I don't really understand why it's considered normal to stare at someone's eyeballs.

Excerpt from LOOK ME IN THE EYE: MY LIFE WITH ASPERGER'S by John Elder Robison, copyright © 2007, 2008 by John Elder Robison. Used by permission of Crown Books, an imprint of the Crown Publishing Group, a division of Random House LLC. All rights reserved.

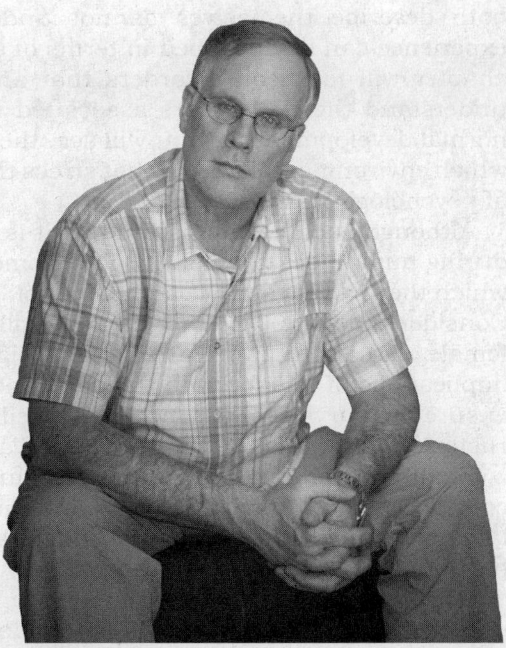

John Robison

© Mark M. Murray/The Republican/Landov

I was my mother's first child, and I was like a little wild animal. I struggled to get away when held, but if I was left alone in the big baby carriage I seldom fussed. Mother first realized that something was dreadfully wrong when I failed to start talking like the little girl next door, and it seemed that I might be deaf. Between nonstop tantrums and a penchant for smearing feces, I was a terrible two-year-old.

I can remember the frustration of not being able to talk at age three. This caused me to throw many a tantrum. I could understand what people said to me, but I could not get my words out. It was like a big stutter, and starting words was difficult. . . . Tantrums also occurred when I became tired or stressed by too much noise, such as horns going off at a birthday party. My behavior was like a tripping circuit breaker. One minute I was fine, and the next minute I was on the floor kicking and screaming like a crazed wildcat.

From Temple Grandin. (2010). *Thinking in Pictures and Other Reports From My Life With Autism* (pp. 43–44). New York: Doubleday.

My mind is similar to an Internet search engine that searches for photographs. I use language to narrate the photo-realistic pictures that pop up in my imagination. When I design equipment for the cattle industry, I can test run it in my imagination similar to a virtual reality computer program. All my thinking is associative and not linear. To form concepts, I sort pictures into categories similar to computer files. To form the concept of orange, I see many different orange objects, such as oranges, pumpkins, orange juice and marmalade.

From Temple Grandin. (2009). How Does Visual Thinking Work in the Mind of a Person With Autism? A Personal Account. *Philosophical Transactions of the Royal Society B, 364,* 1437–1442.

INTRODUCTION TO CHILDHOOD DEVELOPMENT

Everyone's childhood is different. Some have had a stress-free time while others have experienced difficulties, including lack of basic needs or loss of parents. Some of us have found ourselves easily valuing the experiences of our culture while others have felt left out and different. John Robison and Temple Grandin, whose words we just read, both describe themselves as not understanding how others experienced life. Their experience can be described in terms of someone with an autism spectrum disorder. This chapter will focus on disorders that are associated with childhood. In order to better understand these disorders associated with development, I will describe the process of normal development. As you will see, there are particular times in normal development in which environmental factors that stress the individual can lead to increased manifestations of psychological disorders.

Although each human is unique, it is also the case that there are universal situations during human development. Unlike some other species, humans are born into a world in which they cannot survive alone. In fact, human infants are born in an undeveloped state. Consider that a 200-pound female gorilla gives birth to a 4-pound baby while a human female of half to two thirds that weight gives birth to a 6- to 9-pound baby. The implications of this for both the baby and the mother are that mechanisms are needed to ensure the survival of the mother as well as the protection and development of the infant. Historically, it is the group, the family, and the mother who have given this support.

From an evolutionary perspective, human infants display an amazing ability to form connections with their caregivers and maintain a close connection with others. We learn language quickly, know how to understand nonverbal expressions, and later grow to be part of a larger social community. Every infant learns to talk and walk at a different rate and express emotions at a different rate. Mental health professionals have a difficult task in determining what might just be delayed development in certain skills and what represents a developmental disorder. Even with discrete disorders such as autism spectrum disorder, treatment can influence greatly the course of development of the individual. In general, the criteria for diagnosis of a development disorder are in terms of severity, duration, pervasiveness, and degree of impairment.

There are a number of sensitive periods in which disruptions can lead to long-term effects. For example, what happens when events such as war or natural disasters interrupt the normal caregiving patterns? A British psychiatrist, John Bowlby, sought to determine what would happen if a young child had his or her physical needs such as food and housing satisfied but did not experience a close emotional connection. His early work examined children who became orphans during World War II. They were physically cared for but lacked the emotional attention given from a caregiver, such as a mother dealing with her own infant. His and later research has shown that these infants display patterns of interpersonal behaviors that have been associated with psychological problems. He referred to the infant–mother relationship as **attachment.**

Other sensitive developmental periods are directly related to the brain and to the turning on and off of genes. If genetic or other malfunctions happen at these times, psychopathologies or other developmental problems may develop later in the child's life. The brain is also dynamic in the sense that experiences can influence brain development. This can be positive, as seen in the study presented earlier that shows that early experience with music changes the manner in which brain areas develop. As you will see, treatment can significantly improve a number of developmental disorders, which also shows the plasticity of the brain in early life. It can also be negative in which trauma can influence brain structures as well as epigenetic processes in which the environment influences the manner in which genes turn on and off. However, as noted by Caspi and others (Caspi et al., 2002; Caspi, Hairi, Holmes, Uher, & Mofitt, 2010), variations in genetic makeup make some individuals more sensitive to maltreatment and stress than others, which in turn can lead to psychological disorders. Overall, early environmental experiences have been shown to influence brain development, neurotransmitter functioning, and neuroendocrine function, which in turn can influence psychopathological behaviors (Burnette & Cicchetti, 2012).

TABLE 6-1 Categories in *DSM–5* in Which Selective Childhood Disorders Are Described

Trauma- and stressor-related disorders
reactive attachment disorder
disinhibited social engagement disorder
Neurodevelopmental disorders
autism spectrum disorder
ADHD
disorders of learning
motor disorders
Disruptive, impulse control, and conduct disorders
conduct disorder
oppositional defiant disorder

Current research has shown detrimental effects on both physical and mental conditions in relation to physical and sexual abuse, neglect, exposure to domestic violence, and having a parent who is depressed. Bullying or peer verbal abuse, even in children without any history of trauma or abuse, was associated with elevated psychiatric symptoms (Teicher, Samson, Sheu, Polcari, & McGreenery, 2010). Further, the degree of peer verbal abuse was correlated with white matter differences (diffusion tensor imaging, or DTI) in the corpus callosum, which is the large fiber tract connecting the right and left hemispheres of the brain. Middle school years appeared to be a more sensitive period for bullying to have an effect. On the positive side, having friends in elementary school has been shown to be related to having fewer symptoms of depression even when there is genetic risk (Brendgen et al., 2013).

Although brain changes can take place at any point in development, there are two critical periods in which the brain is more sensitive to external and internal factors. The first is the period during gestation and infancy when the cortical connections are initially being organized. The second is adolescence when the brain reorganizes itself. Understanding when brain changes take place in development or whether specific genetic factors prevent normal pathways from being developed is crucial to understanding the nature of developmental psychopathologies. For example, knowing that early brain development patterns are different in children who later develop autism from those who do not helps to rule out environmental factors that occur just prior to symptoms being present. Further, infants who will develop autism are less responsive to social cues than other infants who are developmentally delayed as well as those who show normal developmental patterns (Baranek et al., 2013).

DSM–5 describes disorders of childhood in a number of separate categories (see *Table 6-1*). In this chapter, I will emphasize three of these. The first grouping is **trauma- and stressor-related disorders.** It is in this group that disorders of attachment are included. The second grouping is under the rubric of **neurodevelopmental disorders.** The autism spectrum disorder and **attention deficit/hyperactivity disorder (ADHD)** are included here. This group also includes disorders of learning, intelligence, and communication. Motor disorders such as tics and Tourette's disorder are also included in this group. The third grouping is **disruptive, impulse control, and conduct disorders.**

Before discussing psychopathologies that occur in childhood, I will examine the normal development process and the types of events that can disrupt this process. These can include a number of factors such as family and social relationships, one's culture, and one's genetic makeup. These factors can interact with developmental changes at different ages. Thus, it is important to understand normal development processes and how they can be involved in psychological disorders. Social and emotional processes are particularly important. Using brain imaging and other techniques, our understanding of social relationships and their involvement in psychopathology has increased greatly.

Brain Development

As noted previously, there are two critical periods in terms of brain development. The first is during gestation and the early years of life when the brain is establishing its cortical connections. Within this period, children develop the ability to process sensory information, language, and cognitive skills (see *Figure 6-1*). These skills develop in a particular order, and there is some suggestion that disorders such as autism may be related to a mistiming of this development (see Bardin, 2012, for a summary). Brain connections remain stable until about 12 years of age. During adolescence, there is another critical period when the brain rewires itself in a different manner. At both of these times, external or internal events including genetic processes can happen which may lead to physical or mental disorders (see *Figure 6-2*).

Before a child is born, the brain has begun to form the connections necessary to perform basic sensory and motor functions (see Konrad & Eickhoff, 2010, for an overview of connectivity in the brain). Overall, the first areas to develop in an infant are involved in movement and vision. After that, the brain develops from back to front. The last area to develop is the frontal lobes, which continue to develop into early adulthood.

In India, there is another set of issues with regard to child development that needs to be looked at carefully. Malnutrition is a huge factor that may affect development in a child. Samir Dalwai et al. (2013) have published a Consensus statement on integrated management of severe acute nutrition as an Indian Academy of Pediatrics position statement. Malnutrition at an early stage in life can affect body and brain growth and thus can have an impact on the mental health as well. The authors of the cited paper estimate severe acute malnutrition (SAM) to be a major public health issue in India, afflicting an estimated 8.1 million under-five children in the country.

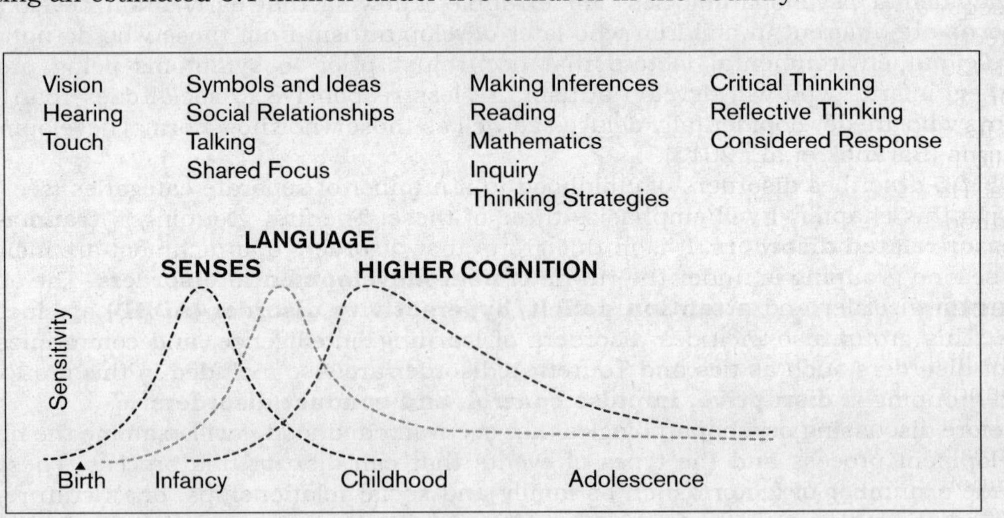

FIGURE 6-1 Timing of Different Types of Learning in Children

Source: Bardin (2012, p. 25).

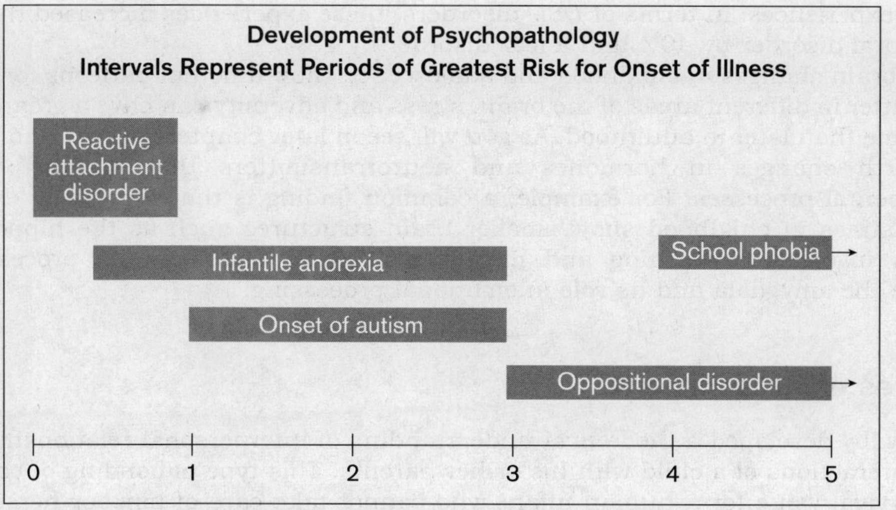

FIGURE 6-2 Onset of Psychopathology During First Five Years of Life

Source: Tasman et al. (2008, p. 107).

> Dietary interventions using WHO F-75 and F-100 formulae (or analogues) in the management of inpatient care of SAM have improved outcomes including reduced mortality, early recovery and higher weight gain. It is possible to implement this intervention in hospitals and healthcare facilities. Community-based programs have shown success in the management of SAM in emergency and non-emergency situations. (Dalwai et al., 2013)

Another serious issue is that of child abuse and neglect. Indian practitioners now mandatorily follow the guidelines subsumed in the Protection of Children from Sexual Offenses (POCSO) Act, 2012, which helps protect a child from sexual abuse. As we are aware, emotional and physical abuse and neglect can have very far-reaching negative consequences for a child. (http://indiacode.nic.in/amendmentacts2012/The%20Protection%20of%20Children%20From%20Sexual%20Offences%20Act.pdf) Aggarwal et al. (2010) have published recommendations for pediatric professionals in this regard.

Dr. Srinivasa Murthy (2014) has written a scholarly paper on child abuse and neglect and its impact on adult mental health. He underlines that child abuse and neglect is a public health priority and rues the poor documentation of child abuse and neglect in India. He goes on to underline the impact of childhood bullying and other abuse faced in childhood, and asserts that it manifests throughout life.

Effects of Early Life Stress

Early life stress reflects the situation in which the child is unable to cope given the demands that he or she experiences (see McLaughlin et al., 2012; Pechtel & Pizzagalli, 2011, for overviews). These situations range from disasters to death of a parent to child mistreatment. In 2009, about 22.5% of all children in the United States came to the attention of child protective services. However, not all of these reports from teachers, the police, and others were substantiated. Child abuse or neglect is estimated to be around 10% in the United States. By the age of adolescence, some 58% of all adolescents reported experiencing some type of adversity during their lifetime with over half of these reporting multiple experiences. In terms of *DSM* disorders, these experiences increased the risk for a behavioral disorder by 40% and a fear disorder by 15%.

Since brain changes in childhood and adolescence show different patterns for gray and white matter in different areas of the brain, stress and adversity can have a greater impact at this time than later in adulthood. As you will see in later chapters, stress and adversity bring forth changes in hormones and neurotransmitters that in turn influence developmental processes. For example, a common finding is that those who experience extreme stress in childhood show smaller brain structures such as the hippocampus, which is involved in learning and memory. Likewise, stress-related processes may influence the amygdala and its role in emotional processing.

Theories of Attachment

John Bowlby developed a theoretical understanding of interpersonal relationships based on the interactions of a child with his or her parents. This type of bonding of course has great survival value for a human infant who cannot take care of him- or herself. Along with a number of other instincts such as the *rooting reflex* in which an infant begins sucking when the cheek or mouth is touched, attachment is seen as the basis of early emotional relationships between a mother and her child. It initially begins in terms of nursing as the mother and her child learn how to respond to one another. Both internal and external processes and their constant interplay lead to mother–infant bonding. Bowlby (1969) named this process *attachment* rather than the traditional term used in psychoanalysis, which was *object relations*. As you will see throughout this book, lack of successful attachment patterns has been associated with anxiety, depression, dissociation, and personality disorders.

Bowlby considered the process of attachment as a social–emotional behavior equally as important as mating behavior and parental behavior. He saw attachment as a multifaceted process involving a variety of developmental mechanisms over the first year of life. Attachment for Bowlby was a process in which the mother was able to reduce fear by direct contact with the infant and provide support, called a secure base. This secure base would allow for later exploratory behaviors. Bowlby suggested that there were five universal attachment behaviors in human infants. These are sucking, clinging, crying, following, and smiling. Bowlby assumed that the relative immaturity of the human infant resulted in attachment being a slower process in humans than in other primates.

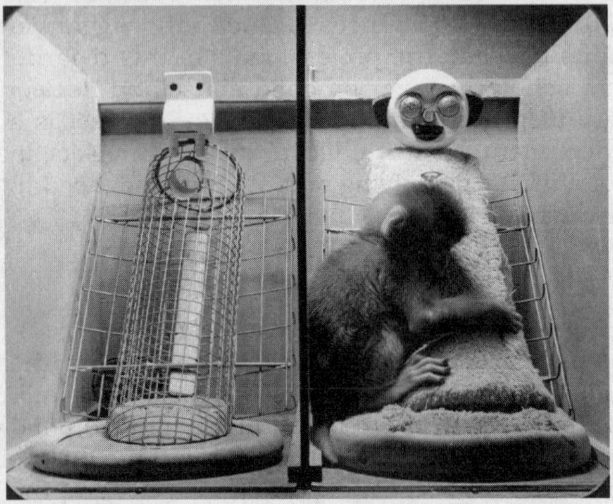

Surrogate mothers
© Photo Researchers, Inc.

In a classic series of experiments, Harry Harlow, in the 1950s, initially examined the mechanisms of attachment with primates. At that time, there was a real debate between whether the infant's response to its mother is learned or whether certain inherent properties of the mother elicit infant attachment (Harlow, McGaugh, & Thompson, 1971). To better understand the nature of attachment in monkey infants, Harlow (1958) separated infant monkeys from their mothers after birth and placed them in isolated cages. In the cage were two surrogate mothers—one made of wire and the other made of terry cloth. The wire surrogates had bare bodies of welded wire whereas the cloth surrogates were covered by soft, resilient terry cloth. Both surrogates had long bodies that could be easily clasped by the infant rhesus monkey.

For half of the infants, a nipple by which they could feed themselves was attached to the wire mother, and for the other half, the nipple was attached to the terry cloth mother. In either surrogate mother, the infants had the nutrition that they needed. If one thought that attachment was totally learned through reinforcement, then the infant monkeys should go to the mother from which they were fed. What do you think happened? What happened was a finding completely contrary to the learning theory interpretation. As the infants who fed on the wire mother grew, they showed decreasing responsiveness to her and increasing responsiveness to the cloth mother even though this mother had no food to offer (see *Figure 6-3*). From this, Harlow concluded that it is the contact comfort and not the feeding per se that binds the infant to the mother.

Although they were in different fields of research, there developed a relationship between Harlow, who worked in the United States, and Bowlby, who worked in the United Kingdom. This can be seen in the letters between the two men and their presence together at international conferences (van der Horst, LeRoy, & van der Veer, 2008). Part of Bowlby's original interest in attachment came from observations of children in orphanages

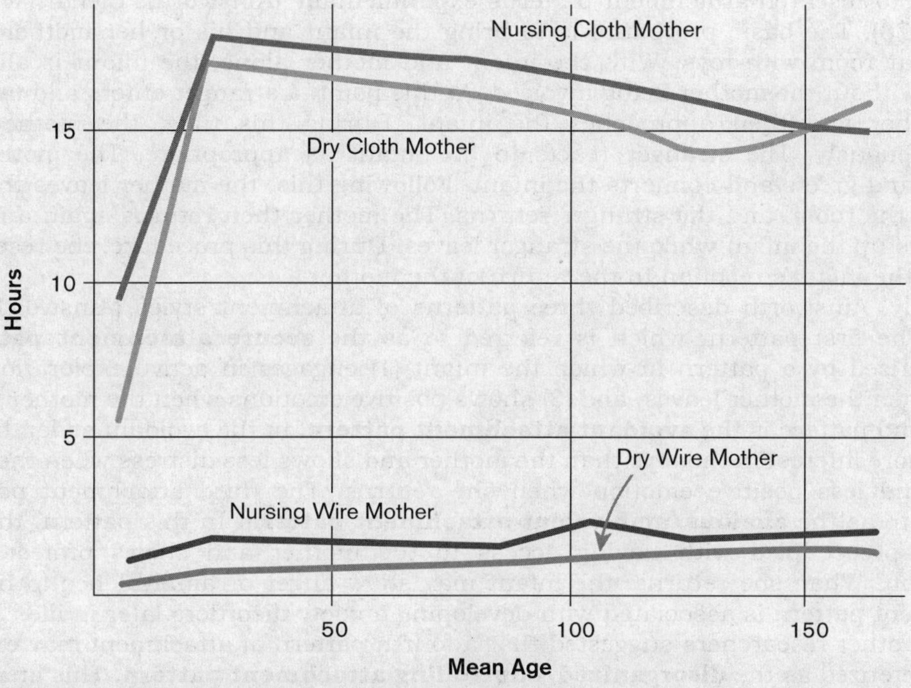

FIGURE 6-3 Time Spent on Cloth and Wire Surrogate

Source: Harlow et al. (1971, p. 59).

following World War II. Like the peer-reared monkeys, these children had all of their physical needs met but lacked a form of emotional and social connectedness. As part of a World Health Organization (WHO) project, Bowlby concluded that children deprived of their mothers were at risk for physical and mental illness. In particular, he concluded that separation from emotional caregivers could lead to severe anxiety and psychopathic personality (Bowlby, 1951).

Bowlby carefully observed children and recorded his observations in a series of books and articles focused on secure attachment as well as loss and separation anxiety (Bowlby, 1961, 1982, 1988). Bowlby had been influenced by *ethology,* which is the study of animal behavior. One classic example as described by Konrad Lorenz is the *imprinting* of newborn ducks on their mother such that they will follow her wherever she goes. Thus, Bowlby interpreted attachment from an evolutionary perspective emphasizing the survival value of attachment, especially as the human infant begins to crawl or walk on his or her own.

In terms of the general characteristics of attachment, Bowlby reported that children who develop a secure bond, or attachment, with a caregiver or parent, who is usually their mother, display patterns of activity that are especially strong from the end of the first year of life until about 3 years of age in relation to that caregiver. First, the infant shows distress when the caregiver leaves. Second, the infant smiles, makes noises, or shows other signs of pleasure when the caregiver returns. Third, the infant shows distress when approached by a stranger, unless the caregiver encourages the interaction. And fourth, the infant shows more exploratory behaviors in an unfamiliar situation when the caregiver is present.

Based on infants' reactions to their caregiver, Mary Ainsworth developed the *strange situation* to research attachment patterns experimentally (Ainsworth, Blehar, Waters, & Wall, 1978). The basic procedure is to bring the infant and his or her mother into an unfamiliar room with toys. With the infant and mother alone, the infant is allowed to explore without the mother being involved. At this point, a stranger enters and talks with the mother and then approaches the infant. During this time, the mother leaves inconspicuously. The stranger reacts to the infant as appropriate. The mother then returns and greets and comforts the infant. Following this, the mother leaves the infant alone in the room, and the stranger returns. The mother then returns again and greets and picks up the infant while the stranger leaves. During this procedure, the researchers observe the infant's reaction to the return of the mother.

Initially, Ainsworth described three patterns of attachment styles (Ainsworth et al., 1978). The first pattern, which is referred to as the **secure attachment pattern,** is characterized by a pattern in which the infant (1) engages in active exploration, (2) is upset when the mother leaves, and (3) shows positive emotions when the mother returns. The second pattern is the **avoidant attachment pattern.** In the avoidant style, the infant shows more interest in the toys than the mother and shows less distress when the mother leaves and less positive emotion when she returns. The third attachment pattern is referred to as the **anxious/ambivalent attachment pattern.** In this pattern, the infant appears preoccupied with having access to the mother and shows protest on her separation. When she returns, the infant may show anger or ambivalence to her. This attachment pattern is associated with developing anxiety disorders later in life.

Later, other researchers suggested that a fourth pattern of attachment may exist that is characterized as the **disorganized/controlling attachment pattern.** This attachment category was added when it was observed that some infants show disruptions in processing during the strange situation (Main & Solomon, 1990). That is, when their parent is present, these infants show disorganized behavior patterns or disorientation. Children with this attachment style tend to have problems dealing with psychological stress and a tendency to develop dissociative disorders later in life.

Of course, infants do not grow up in a vacuum, so it is also important to characterize the mothering style of the caregiver. With infants displaying secure attachment patterns, the style of the mother is consistent and responsive to her infant's signals. On the other hand, mothers of infants showing avoidant patterns tend to be more rejecting and rigid and, in general, insensitive to the infants' signals, including requests for bodily contact. Anxious or ambivalent patterns tend to be associated with inconsistent mothers who may be intrusive. Disorganized or controlling patterns tend to be associated with parents who show unpredictable abusive behavior or other behaviors that are frightening to the child. Mothers of these children are also more likely to experience depression (O'Connor, Bureau, McCartney, & Lyons-Ruth, 2011). Of course, the complexity of the situation is highlighted by the fact that some infants are easier to care for than others. That is to say, some infants appear to be temperamentally more irritable than others and thus could be more difficult for a caregiver to approach positively.

Attachment patterns can be seen as an internal road map or schema through which the person interprets his or her experiences. As such, they are part of a larger overall developmental sequence that can be considered in the development of psychopathology. An attachment pattern gives insight into how a person deals with psychological stress and loss. Is the person able to regulate his or her reaction to a stressful situation? A secure attachment pattern is protective and associated with successful regulation. On the other hand, insecure attachment patterns reflect one aspect of the complex process that leads to psychological disorders. Since attachment patterns tend to be stable, the effects they portray can be cumulative. This can include the type of statements that people make to themselves including negative evaluations of themselves and their abilities, as often seen in depression. It can also include the manner in which a person deals with emotional regulation, whether in an overreaction as seen with personality disorders or not experiencing the emotion as seen in dissociative disorders.

Research has shown children with insecure patterns of attachment to be at risk for several forms of childhood psychopathology (see DeKlyen & Greenberg, 2008, for an overview). Specifically, the avoidant attachment style is associated with aggressiveness in middle childhood, and the anxious or ambivalent attachment style is associated with passive withdrawal. The disorganized or controlling pattern of attachment has been associated with personality disorders and dissociative disorders. The anxious or ambivalent pattern of attachment has also been associated with later mood disorders such as anxiety and depression (see Dozier, Stovall-McClough, & Albus, 2008, for an overview).

Imitation Learning

What happens in your brain when you see someone wave or clap her hands? One intriguing answer to this question comes from research that suggests the neurons in your brain fire as if you had performed the same actions. These neurons are called **mirror neurons.** Mirror neurons were first discovered in monkeys. These neurons were shown to fire not only when the monkey performs a particular action, but also when it just observes another monkey, or even a human, perform that action. These mirror neurons were first discovered in areas of the brain referred to as F5, which is a part of the premotor cortex.

Some researchers suggest that this brain process may lie at the basis of **imitation learning,** as well as other human social phenomena, including language and empathy (Rizzolatti & Craighero, 2004; Sinigaglia & Rizzolatti, 2011). A number of studies have suggested a link between mirror neurons, empathy, and psychopathologies such as autism and psychopathy (Gonzalez-Liencres, Shamay-Tsoory, & Brüne, 2013).

The basic idea for imitation learning is as follows:

- Each time an individual sees an action done by another, the neurons that would be involved in that action are activated.
- This, in turn, creates a motor representation of the observed action.
- That is, we see an action and consider how we might make it ourselves although we don't do this consciously.
- In essence, the observer's brain turns a visual image into a motor plan.

This process can explain one aspect of how imitation learning can take place. That is, by seeing something, I also come to know how I can do it. Since the same neurons fire in my brain as I watch another do a task, my brain is able to create an action pattern when I wish to produce the motor response. Even more important for Sinigaglia and Rizzolatti (2011) is that such a network puts the organism at an advantage. This is because this network helps the organism understand not only "what" others are doing but also "why" they are doing it. By having my brain work similarly to another's brain, I have some understanding of what he or she is experiencing.

It has also been suggested that the mirror neurons lead not only to an understanding of another's actions but also to empathy (see Iacoboni, 2009, for an overview). That is to say, through connections between the mirror neurons system and the limbic system and insula, it would be possible to recognize emotions and thus empathy. In a series of studies, it was shown that the more someone imitates your actions, the more you like that person and report that you care about her (Chartrand & Bargh, 1999). Thus, imitation, liking, and caring go together.

Overall, the mirror neuron system offers a basis of imitation and understanding of another's actions. In the same way that individual neurons in the visual system fire to specific features of a stimulus, and these, in turn, become integrated into a larger perception, the mirror neuron system can be seen as part of a larger cortical network involving the insula and limbic system, which relates to person perception and feelings toward another. This, in turn, could form the basis of interpersonal relationships and more complex social interactions. Over the past decade, research has focused on the manner in which the mirror neuron system is involved in autism spectrum disorder (Dapretto et al., 2006; Williams, Whiten, Suddendorf, & Perrett, 2001).

Theory of Mind

Theory of mind is the study of one's ability to understand one's own or another person's mental state. As you will see later, delays in the development of theory of mind are seen in children with autism spectrum disorder. A number of tasks have been used to study theory of mind. One common one involves a cereal box. If I show you a box of cereal and ask you what is in it, you would probably say cereal. However, if I opened it and pulled out ribbons, you would no longer say it contained cereal. What if I asked you what friends of yours would say? You would, of course, say cereal because they did not see the ribbons being pulled out of the box.

However, young children, as well as individuals with autism, would not give this answer. They would say ribbons because they are unable to understand that what someone else knows could be different from what they know. This ability to take another's perspective is referred to as theory of mind or mind reading. It is an ability that develops over the preschool years, generally between 3 and 5 years of age. Theory of mind has also been seen as a prerequisite for the ability to engage in pretend play and the ability to lie. Some theories of autism suggest that part of the disorder is a deficit in theory of mind (Baron-Cohen, 2009; Baron-Cohen & Belmonte, 2005).

Concept Check

- Why is it important to understand the normal course of human development when learning about the psychological disorders of childhood?
- Every human learns to talk and walk at a different rate and express emotions at a different rate. What implications do these individual differences have for the definition, diagnosis, and treatment of childhood disorders?
- What are the two critical periods of brain development in humans? What changes are taking place in the brain during those periods?
- What neurological evidence can you cite to show that experiencing stress and adversity in childhood and adolescence has a greater impact than experiencing it later as an adult?
- What are the general characteristics of attachment? What three problematic styles of attachment have been described, and what implications do these styles have for future psychopathology?
- What brain processes are involved in imitation learning? How is imitation learning related to the development of empathy?
- Theory of mind develops over time. What are the four stages described by Baron-Cohen, when do they occur, and how are they related to the development of empathy?

The experimental procedure with the cereal box is formally called the *false-belief task* and has been used to assess theory of mind. In this procedure, a cereal box is shown to the child. The child is then asked what is in the box. Of course, the child responds by naming the type of cereal, such as Cheerios. The experimenter then opens the box and shows the child it contains something else, such as ribbons. The child is then asked what another child out in the hall would think is in the box. Three-year-old children tend to respond ribbons whereas 4-year-olds would say Cheerios. Thus, the 4-year-olds understand what others would believe whereas 3-year-olds would not. The final part of the task is where the experimenter asks the child what they initially thought was in the box. Four-year-olds say Cheerios whereas 3-year-olds say ribbons. When theories of mind types of tasks have been given around the world, it is observed that theory of mind develops at about the same time. Few 3-year-olds correctly understand what another knows, and few 5-year-olds are incorrect in their ability to understand what another child would experience.

Researchers have sought to describe theoretically the developmental aspects of inferring mental states in another person. Simon Baron-Cohen's model suggests four components (Baron-Cohen, 2005). The first aspect that the child begins to develop during the first nine months of life is an intentionality detector. What is meant by this is that an infant tends to interpret movement in a two-person relationship as a desire and goal directed. The second aspect that begins to develop during this time is an eye direction detector. What this means for a theory of mind is that the infant infers that another person is looking at him or her versus looking at something else. The third aspect is seen at the end of the first year of life. This aspect is referred to as a shared attentional mechanism. The idea of a shared attentional mechanism is that the infant is able to know that the mother, for example, knows where she is looking. If the infant could put this into adult language, she would say something like "Mother sees that I see the cup." In real life, infants during the second year of life are not surprised when their mother notices that they are looking at a particular object. Built on these aspects, the fourth mechanism, a theory of mind mechanism, is seen after at least 2 years of age. This allows a child to infer what one knows by observing what one sees. For example, if one child sees another child seeing an adult hide a toy under the pillow, then the first child could infer that the second child knows where the toy is.

In order to understand the development of empathy in children, Simon Baron-Cohen has suggested two additional aspects in the theory of mind model. The next aspects are an emotion detector and an empathy system. In theory of mind terms, the emotion detector comes within the first year of life and recognizes emotional signs in another person. The empathy system goes beyond recognition of emotion; it is the ability on some level to know how another person feels. This, of course, signals the beginning of empathy. A lack of the development of empathy would be seen in children with autism and psychopathic individuals. This will be described in more detail later in this chapter.

Adolescence

Adolescence is a time of great change, in both the brain and body, as well as in culture. It is a time of change to one's body and the awakening of new interests and desires associated with brain changes (see Sturman & Moghaddam, 2011, for an overview). An increase in risk taking also leads to various types of accidents, unprotected sex, and use of drugs. This risk taking or impulsivity involves distinct brain networks related to the ability to inhibit that may form an endophenotype related to psychopathology (Whelan et al., 2012). As such, adolescence marks the peak onset of many psychopathologies (Paus, Keshavan, & Giedd, 2008). These psychopathologies include anxiety and mood disorders, eating disorders, personality disorders, substance abuse, and psychosis.

Specifically, data from the National Comorbidity Survey replication study show impulse control disorders, phobias, and separation disorders begin in childhood around the age of 5 whereas panic, generalized anxiety disorder, post-traumatic stress disorder (PTSD), substance abuse, mood disorder, and schizophrenia are most commonly seen to begin around adolescence (see *Figure 6-4*). It is assumed that these later disorders develop as the result of anomalies or exaggerations of typical adolescent maturation processes. These processes include hormonal changes during puberty, adolescent social relationships, and impulsivity, which increase the abuse of certain drugs.

Hormonal changes during puberty are thought to be related to the findings that there are an equal number of males and females experiencing anxiety and depression prior to puberty, which changes to a 2-to-1 female to male ratio after puberty. These differences can also be amplified by the increased emotional reactivity to social situations including peer influence during adolescence. Further, recreational drugs influence the trajectory of brain development during adolescence.

When brain development is examined, it becomes clear that each area has its own time course (Tau & Peterson, 2010). Overall, subcortical areas mature earlier than cortical areas. In considering psychopathology, individuals with ADHD show delays in cortical

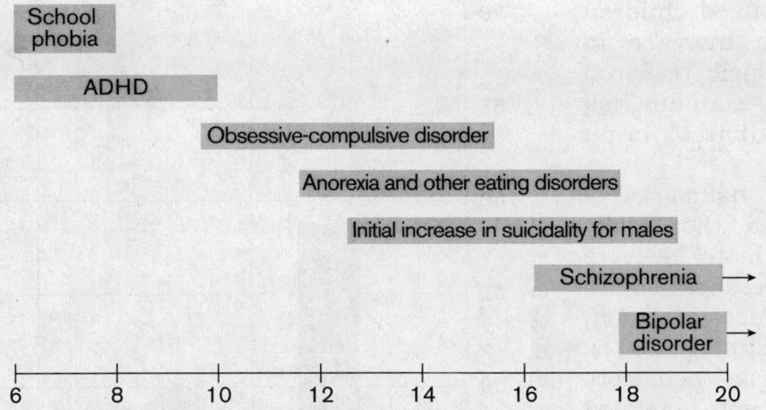

FIGURE 6-4 Onset of Psychopathology From Age 6 Through 20

Source: Tasman et al. (2008, p. 107).

development that are no longer apparent by adulthood. Schizophrenia, on the other hand, is associated with an earlier pruning of neurons as compared with normal children.

In terms of responses to particular tasks, research suggests that from childhood to adulthood, the brain goes from a largely undifferentiated system to one composed of specialized neural networks. It is also the case that there is a reduction of brain energy requirements from childhood to adulthood. In one study (Jolles, van Buchem, Crone, & Rombouts, 2011), functional connectivity in adolescents (11 to 13 years of age) was compared with that of young adults (19 to 25 years of age). These researchers found that similar networks occurred in both groups although the size and strength of the connectivity in the network was greater in adults. Mood and anxiety disorders, which increase dramatically during adolescence, have been associated with the dysfunction of the network involved in social processing (Nelson, Leibenluft, McClure, & Pine, 2005).

Social Brain in Adolescence

Adolescence has been characterized as a time in which an individual moves from a more family oriented frame of reference to one of peer relations. Peer relationships at this period involve meeting and understanding new individuals as well as determining the types of relationships available. Sexuality and romantic interests develop during this period. Concomitant with these social and emotional changes are large changes in the brain. These brain changes also appear to allow for an increase in psychological disorders—especially mood and anxiety disorders. Anxiety disorders, for example, are seen as an abnormal regulation of fear (Hyman & Cohen, 2013). Overall, adolescents show an increased sensitivity to both positive and negative rewards than do either adults or younger children (Galván, 2013).

Risk Taking in Adolescence

Risk taking can play both direct and indirect roles in adolescence in relation to psychopathology. The direct role can lead to substance abuse of illegal drugs and other substances. The indirect role combines taking risks with a psychological disorder, resulting in suicide. Abused children also show an increase in risk taking. Basic research has begun to examine risk taking in relation to brain activation.

One of the hallmarks of adolescence is that risky decisions are more likely to occur in the presence of one's peers (Chein, Albert, O'Brien, Uckert, & Steinberg, 2011). One of the risky behaviors seen in adolescents is related to driving. Using a stoplight driving game and functional magnetic resonance imaging (fMRI), Jason Chein and his colleagues compared the results of adolescents (14–18 years of age), young adults (19–22 years of age), and adults (24–29 years of age). The goal of the stoplight game is to drive through 20 intersections as fast as possible. At each intersection, the driver can either stop for the light and experience a short delay or take a risk and go through the red light without any delay. However, running the red light could result in a crash. All participants were also asked to bring a friend of their same age with them. Compared with young adults and adults, adolescents showed more risky decisions and crashes when they were observed by a friend (see *Figure 6-5*).

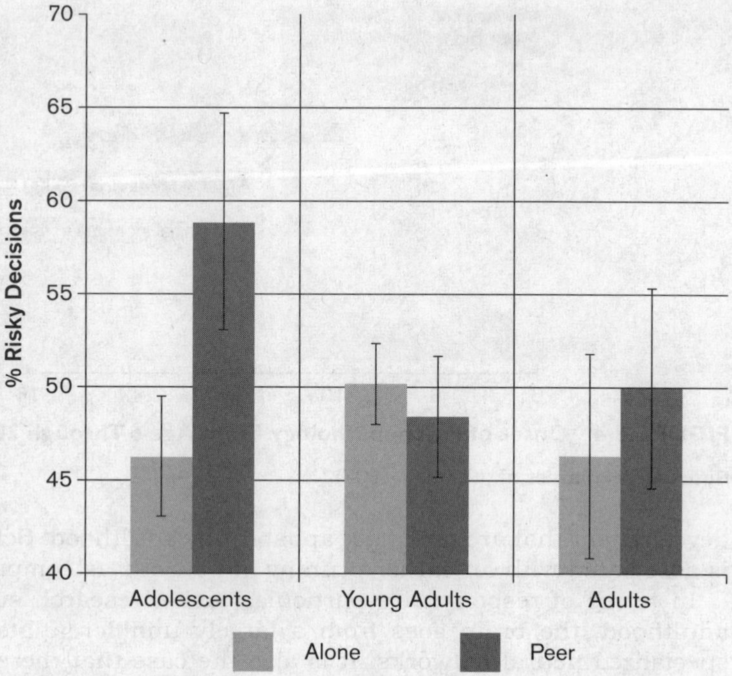

FIGURE 6-5 Risky Decisions on the Stoplight Driving Task When Alone or Being Watched by a Friend by Age-Group

Source: Jason Chein, Dustin Albert, Lia O'Brien, Kaitlyn Uckert, and Laurence Steinberg. "Peers increase adolescent risk taking by enhancing activity in the brain's reward circuitry." *Developmental Science.* 2011 March; 14(2): F1–F10.

The fMRI results showed differences in the left prefrontal cortex (LPFC) by age (see *Figure 6-6*). There were also differences in the right ventral striatum (VS) and the left orbitofrontal cortex (OFC) in terms of age and whether a friend was present. These areas are associated with making a decision in a social context. The greater activation of these areas suggests that adolescents saw risk taking as more rewarding in the presence of a friend. Overall, this research shows that peer presence makes a greater difference in risk taking which is also seen in brain processes in adolescents compared with those beyond adolescence.

Brain Systems Involved in Social Relations

Our present-day emotionality has largely evolved within a social context. In terms of brain structure, many of the structures involved in the processing of emotion are also important for social behavior. Brain structures involved in social interactions can be organized in terms of three processes (Adolphs, 2003; Brothers, 1990; Nelson et al., 2005). The first

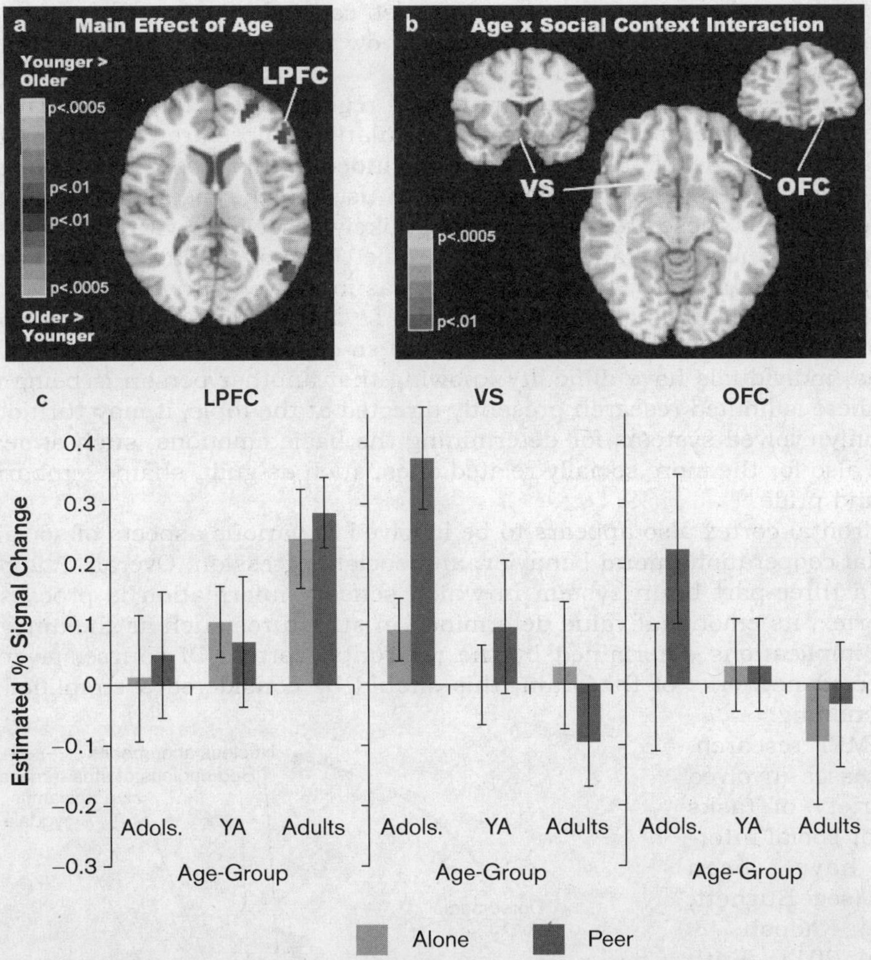

FIGURE 6-6 The Brain Image in A Shows Left Prefrontal Differences in Terms of Age-Group. The Brain Image in B Shows the Areas Affected in Terms of Age and Peer Presence. The Graphs in C Show the Signal Strength Changes by Group and Peer Presence

Source: Chein et al. (2011).

process involves higher-level neocortical regions in the processing of sensory information. This is how we know who we experience through vision, hearing, touch, and other sensory processes. Research suggests when looking at a face, we process broad categorizations related to gender and to the emotion expressed before we complete the detailed construction of the entire face and determine who we are seeing.

Second, our affective system will help us predict what people will do socially. As we see a social interaction, what happens on the level of the brain? What happens first involves the amygdala, striatum, and orbitofrontal cortex. The amygdala is involved in processing the emotional significance of an event. This includes positive emotions such as a person you care about smiling at you as well as negative emotions such as seeing someone angry or fearful. Activation also takes place if a person looks untrustworthy. This determination occurs independent of gender, race, eye gaze, or emotionality expressed. Through its connections to other areas, the amygdala also can influence memory, attention, and decision making. Overall, these areas help us know the emotional context of our perceptions and what we need to do about them.

The third process involves the higher cortical regions of the neocortex. These regions are involved in cognitive understanding and regulation. These are the regions that let us construct an inner model of our social world. Included in this model would be some social understanding of others, their relationship with us, and the meaning of our actions for the social group. It is these areas that are most likely associated with theory of mind, our ability to attribute mental states to other people. Indeed, damage to the orbitofrontal cortex does reduce our ability to detect a faux pas in a given situation.

The prefrontal cortex has also been shown to be activated during humor, social-norm transgressions resulting in embarrassment, and so-called moral emotions. With damage to this area, individuals have difficulty knowing that another person is being deceptive. Although there is limited research presently directed at the topic, it may turn out that we have not only evolved systems for determining the basic emotions, such as fear, joy, or anger, but also for the more socially related ones, such as guilt, shame, embarrassment, jealousy, and pride.

The prefrontal cortex also appears to be involved in various aspects of social relationships, social cooperation, moral behavior, and social aggression. Overall, Adolphs (2003) described a three-part brain system in which sensory information is processed in the sensory cortex, its emotional value determined in structures such as the amygdala, and the social implications determined by the prefrontal cortex. Of course, given the rich interconnected networks of the brain, this should be considered a simplified model of social functioning.

Using fMRI research, brain processes involved in the variety of tasks required for social interactions have been identified (see Burnett, Sebastian, Kadosh, & Blakemore, 2011; Frith & Frith, 2010; Nelson et al., 2005, for overviews). As can be seen in *Figure 6-7*, the social brain can be seen as composed of areas involved in the detection of social processes including face recognition (the fusiform face area [FFA]), emotional recognition (the amygdala, insula, and anterior cingulate cortex [ACC]), and regulating cognitive processes involving the frontal areas of the brain.

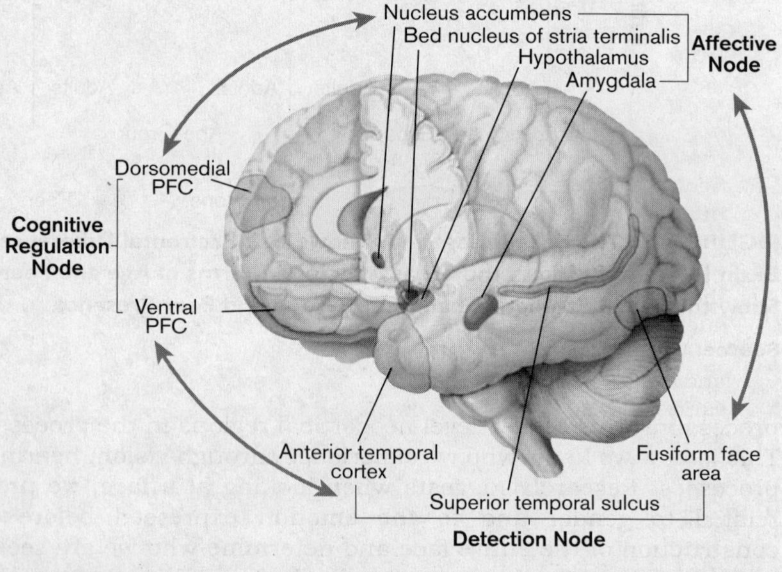

FIGURE 6-7 Regions of the Social Brain Involved in Social Processing

Source: Nelson et al. (2005, pp. 163–174).

Note: Regions of the social brain involved in social processing including a detection node which receives information from brain areas involved in emotional processing. These areas interact with the frontal areas related to cognitive regulation.

Preference for human faces begins shortly after birth in humans. As the child matures, cortical areas such as the FFA in the temporal lobe show greater differentiation. Through its connections comes the ability to recognize and remember faces, which continues into adulthood. As will be noted in this chapter, individuals with autism spectrum disorder do not focus on the faces—especially the eyes—of others. Increased differentiation of emotional facial expression involves the amygdala. Interestingly enough, adolescents show greater reactivity to emotional faces than adults.

One area of the brain that is gaining interest from researchers is the ventromedial prefrontal cortex (vmPFC) (see Roy, Shohamy, & Wager, 2012, for an overview). The vmPFC appears to be important when affective responses are influenced by conceptual information about specific outcomes. In this way, it serves as a hub that links this affective-conceptual information with the brain stem, which is involved in emotional responses of the entire organism through autonomic and endocrine regulation. This includes emotion, emotion regulation, fear conditioning and extinction, episodic and semantic memory, prospection, economic valuation, self-directed cognition, and understanding the feelings and intentions of others. As such, it is an evolutionarily important structure that coordinates information important for survival. The disruption of this system is associated with PTSD, depression, and dysregulation related to chronic stress and pain.

Before examining specific disorders, the following LENS asks the question of how society should deal with one horrific problem seen in adolescence: that of school shootings. Is it a mental health problem, a statement of alienation and revenge, or a combination of both? Of course at this point, society does not know the answer to these questions but can consider if prevention is possible.

6-1 LENS
School Shootings Around the World

School shootings have been recorded in America for at least the past 150 years although the number has increased in the past 20 years. The mass shooting at Sandy Hook Elementary in Newtown, Connecticut, in 2012 by Adam Lanza, which resulted in 26 deaths, and the attack of Seung-Hui Cho at Virginia Tech in 2007, which resulted in 33 deaths, brought to the forefront the need to understand why individuals perform such acts. Quick answers such as the side effects of drugs or violent video games have been part of the discussion.

Others have considered how mental illness plays a role in these cases. Both Adam Lanza and Seung-Hui Cho showed difficulties in previous situations. In a number of press articles, various psychopathologies have been suggested. However, blaming horrific situations such as these school shootings on a mental disorder does not serve society well. Experiencing a mental disorder does not lead directly to violence although society tends to believe that those with mental disorders are more prone to violence. In general, data does not support this generalization.

Overall, these terrible situations offer society an opportunity to consider how to recognize those with difficulties and offer them the necessary help. This requires considerations on a number of levels. Teachers and other professionals need to be trained to recognize individuals with mental health problems. As a society, we need to consider ways to fund mental health services so that individuals without money are not left on their own. We also need to consider laws that recognize when individuals need to be treated. Although stigma appears to be part of the human condition, allowing bullying or making fun of those who are odd does not strengthen the fabric of society.

This map shows where school shootings have occurred since 1996. Although there are examples of shootings worldwide, the majority have happened in America. The occurrence of such violence is a critical topic to understand.

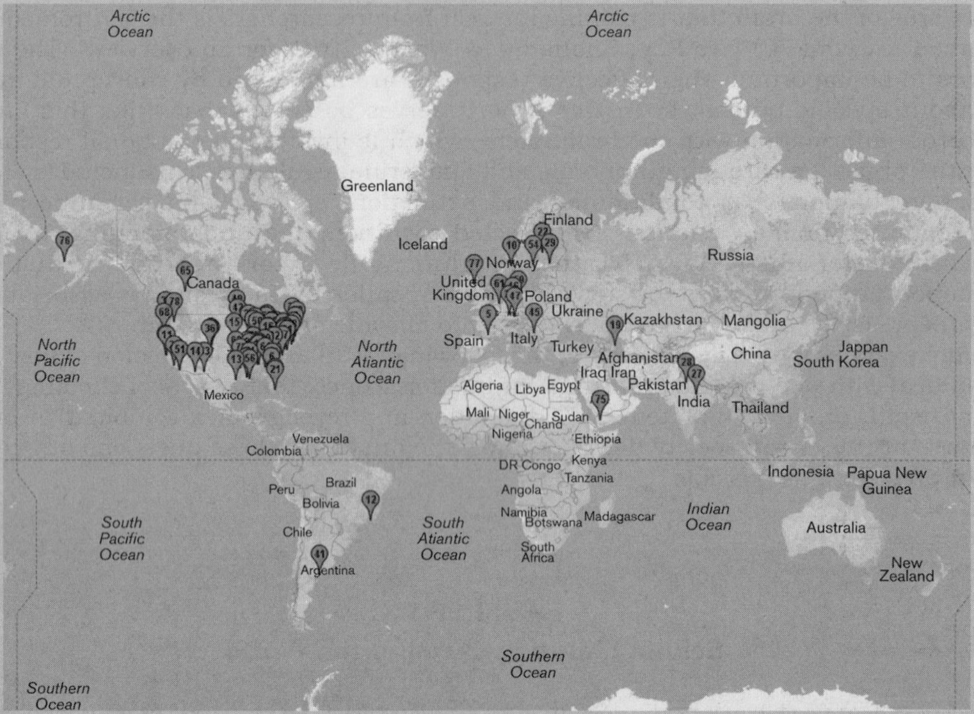

School Shootings Around the World Since 1996

Source: Created by Virender Ajmani, using Google Maps and Source Information Please® Database, © 2012 Pearson Education.
Disclaimer: This figure is not to scale. It does not represent any authentic national or international boundaries and is used for illustrative purposes only.

ATTACHMENT DISORDERS

Beginning in *DSM–III,* an attachment disorder referred to as **reactive attachment disorder (RAD)** was included (see Zeanah & Gleason, 2010, for an overview). The disorder is the result of inadequate caregiving, which may include institutional settings. Although the prevalence is not known, it is generally the result of young children being exposed to neglect before being placed in foster care or an institution. Much of the research with this disorder has focused on children raised in institutions. Two clinical patterns can be present. The first is the emotionally withdrawn or inhibited type, and the second is the indiscriminately social or disinhibited type. The question for a clinician to answer is whether attachment is the primary clinical problem that impairs the child beyond interactions with the attachment figure, which would then qualify as RAD. An alternative is that there is another type of psychopathology present that interferes with a number of developmental processes including attachment. Autism would be such an example.

DSM–5 describes a child with RAD as one who does not seek comfort or support from a traditional attachment figure when distressed. Further, this child will not accept comfort when offered. Overall, there is a lack of emotional responsiveness and positive affect. There may also be negative emotions seen in interactions with adults that are not related to the nature of the interaction. For a diagnosis of RAD, it is also required that the child was not well cared for. If a child is worried about losing a significant attachment figure, this is referred to as separation anxiety disorder in *DSM–5,* which is an anxiety disorder.

The second clinical pattern described in *DSM–IV,* disinhibition, has been classified as a separate disorder in *DSM–5* where it is called **disinhibited social engagement disorder.** This is a disorder in which the child is willing to accept strangers who are not attachment figures. This may include going off with strangers and being overly familiar. As with RAD, it is also required that the child was not well cared for. However, there is no evidence if the neglect begins after age 2 that this disorder will be manifested. There is little data on the prevalence of the disorder although it is assumed to be rare.

RAD and disinhibited social engagement disorder have not been studied empirically in terms of treatment procedures. Typically, treatment procedures have focused on helping the child develop a relationship with a caregiver. The goal is for the child to develop an emotional relationship that represents a more secure attachment relationship. If the child was moved from an institution to a foster family, then the mental health professional would work with the family to develop a new attachment relationship. This treatment would seek to develop more productive internal schema in the child. Additionally, behavioral techniques can be used to modify nonproductive specific behaviors such as those used with aggressive behaviors in children with **conduct disorder (CD).** These will be described later in this chapter. Since maltreatment also results in developmental delays in areas such a language and speech, specific treatments for these deficits are also used.

AUTISM SPECTRUM DISORDERS

Autism spectrum disorders are a group of neurodevelopmental disorders (see Coleman & Gillberg, 2012; Geschwind, 2009; Newschaffer et al., 2007; Sigman, Spence, & Wang, 2006; South, Ozonoff, & Schultz, 2008, for overviews). Autism was initially described by Leo Kanner (1943) as an innate disorder in which children do not show normal development in emotional contact with others. Autism spectrum disorders have achieved a significant place in clinical and research programs and will be discussed in more detail in this chapter.

Individuals with autism spectrum disorders have difficulty in three separate areas. The first is social interactions. Children with autism do not connect with other children or adults in the manner that other children do. They do not look others in the eye or may appear to ignore others while being more interested in other aspects of their environment. The second area is communication. The communication patterns of those with autism spectrum disorder do not usually show the give-and-take of most conversations. The third area is behavioral processes. Individuals with autism spectrum disorder often display stereotypical behaviors and the desire to engage in the same behavior in a repetitive manner (Baron-Cohen & Belmonte, 2005; Kamio, Tobimatsu, & Fukui, 2011). About 30% of children with autism may also show additional complications such as seizure disorders, intellectual disabilities of various kinds, and gastrointestinal problems.

DSM–5 includes what were previously separate disorders—autistic disorder, Asperger's disorder, and a general pervasive developmental disorder—as part of autism spectrum disorders. On the spectrum, Asperger's disorder portrays a milder situation in which developmental language delays may not be present. Also, these individuals show average to above average cognitive skills. General pervasive developmental disorder was characterized in *DSM–IV* as a disorder in which the full criteria for autism were not met. Some researchers suggest that the autism spectrum disorders offer us a way to study brain development that takes a non-normal route (Wicker & Gomot, 2011). *ICD-10* continues to describe **Asperger's syndrome** as a separate disorder. Those with the Asperger's side of autism spectrum disorder report that they do not see the world as others do.

Concept Check

- What characteristics of adolescence contribute to the fact that that period marks the peak onset of many psychopathologies? Does that mean that adolescence "causes" psychopathology? Why, or why not?
- What evidence can you cite to show the importance of the social context to risk taking among adolescents?
- The brain structures involved in social interactions can be organized into three processes. What are these processes, what specifically do they do, and how are they represented in the brain?
- What are the two attachment disorders described in *DSM–5*? How are they differentiated in terms of diagnostic criteria, and what treatments are available for them?

Asperger's syndrome, attributed to Hans Asperger, was added to *DSM* in 1994. The disorder has generated considerable debate as to its relationship with autism. Individuals with Asperger's syndrome tend to be more intelligent and display higher functioning in terms of social processes than those diagnosed with autism. Gillberg (1991) developed a set of diagnostic criteria based on Asperger's original description of specific cases. These include social impairment in the form of egocentricity, a narrowing of interests, compulsive need for introducing routines, speech and language peculiarities, nonverbal communication in the form of limited facial and gesture expression, and motor clumsiness. It should be noted that these are different criteria than those found in *DSM–IV,* which did not specify speech and language problems.

An example of a person who would have been diagnosed with Asperger's syndrome is Temple Grandin. At the beginning of this chapter, Temple Grandin described her experiences of being a person who experienced an autism spectrum disorder (Grandin, 2009, 2010). She described how at age 2 and a half she did not speak and performed actions in a repetitive manner. She was also very sensitive to certain sounds and would respond to these by rocking or staring at sand dribbling through her fingers. Later as a child, she had no understanding of how people relate to each other. She would watch others, trying to understand how she should behave.

Temple Grandin also described herself as thinking totally in pictures (Grandin, 2009). In fact, she described her mind as an Internet search engine set to locate photos. She described this as follows:

> *My mind is associative and does not think in a linear manner. If you say the word "butterfly," the first picture I see is butterflies in my childhood backyard. The next image is metal decorative butterflies that people decorate the outside of their houses with and the third image is some*

butterflies I painted on a piece of plywood when I was in graduate school. Then my mind gets off the subject and I see a butterfly cut of chicken that was served at a fancy restaurant approximately 3 days ago.

From Temple Grandin. (2009). How Does Visual Thinking Work in the Mind of a Person With Autism? A Personal Account. *Philosophical Transactions of the Royal Society B, 364*, 1437–1442.

She has used the ability to think in images to help design humane animal livestock facilities.

I credit my visualization abilities with helping me understand the animals I work with. Early in my career I used a camera to help give me the animals' perspective as they walked through a chute for their veterinary treatment. I would kneel down and take pictures through the chute from the cow's eye level. Using the photos, I was able to figure out which things scared the cattle, such as shadows and bright spots of sunlight. Back then I used black-and-white film, because twenty years ago scientists believed that cattle lacked color vision. Today, research has shown that cattle can see colors, but the photos provided the unique advantage of seeing the world through a cow's viewpoint. They helped me figure out why the animals refused to go in one chute but willingly walked through another.

From Temple Grandin. (2010). *Thinking in Pictures and Other Reports From My Life With Autism* (p. 4). New York: Doubleday.

Temple Grandin is clearly a person who has been very productive in that she received her PhD and is a professor of animal sciences at Colorado State University. She has consulted with many companies concerning how to design environments that treat livestock in a humane manner. She, herself, describes individuals with autism as *specialized thinkers* (Grandin, 2009). For her, they are specialized in one of three types of thinking. The first is *visual thinking,* which allows one to view the world and even words in terms of images. The second is *pattern thinking,* in which the thinking is in terms of patterns such as those seen in music and mathematics. The third is *word and fact thinking,* in which the individual displays an ability to know a large number of facts such as baseball scores or the names of films and who their stars were. More formal research articles have also shown that hypersensitivity to sensory information along with strong logical reasoning ability may be at the basis of talent seen in individuals with autism spectrum disorder (Baron-Cohen, Ashwin, Ashwin, Tavassoli, & Chakrabarti, 2008).

Individuals with autism have often been reported to show a lower IQ than matched control children or adults using traditional IQ tests. Traditional IQ tests have both verbal and spatial components on which normal children tend to show similar scores. Similar scores to traditional IQ tests are also seen on measures of fluid intelligence such as the Raven's Progressive Matrices for those without autism. *Figure 6-8* shows an example of a problem from the Raven's Progressive Matrices.

When adults and children with autism were given the Raven's Progressive Matrices, they showed scores much higher than they obtained with traditional IQ tests. Their scores on the Raven's were more similar to matched controls (Dawson, Soulières, Gernsbacher, & Mottron, 2007). These researchers concluded that intelligence may have been underestimated in those with autism. Others have suggested that many geniuses such as Isaac Newton, Albert Einstein, George Orwell, and H. G. Wells show traits associated with

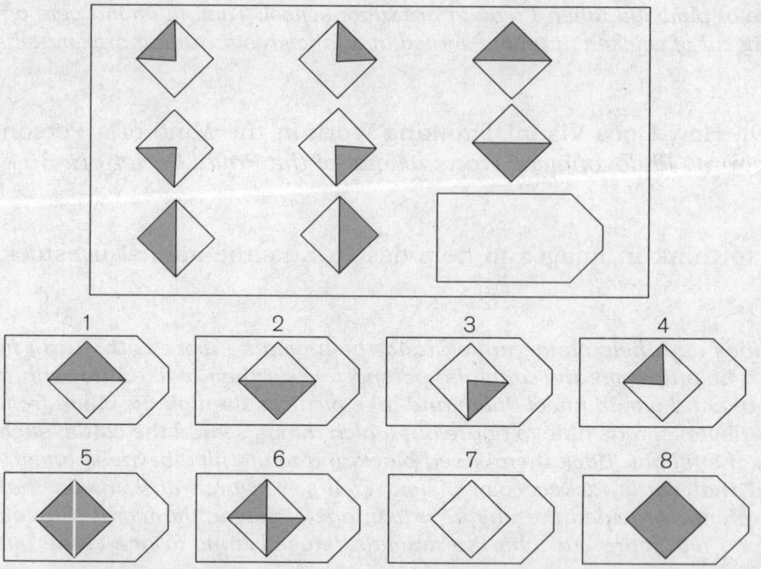

FIGURE 6-8 Example of a Problem From the Raven's Progressive Matrices

Source: From Clancy Blair, David Gamson, Steven Thorne, David Baker. "Rising mean IQ: Cognitive demand of mathematics education for young children, population exposure to formal schooling, and the neurobiology of the prefrontal cortex." *Intelligence*, Volume 33, Issue 1, January–February 2005, Pages 93–106, with permission from Elsevier.
Note: 8 is the correct answer.

Asperger's syndrome, also referred to as high functioning autism (Wicker & Gomot, 2011).

DSM–5 also describes autism spectrum disorder as characterized by problems in the social realm that began in childhood, exemplified in terms of interacting and talking with others. Individuals with an autism spectrum disorder have a difficult time holding typical everyday back-and-forth conversations especially in terms of emotional interchanges. They also lack eye contact and a normal understanding of body language. These problems in social processes tend to leave individuals with autism spectrum disorder with fewer emotionally connected relationships and difficulties in changing social contexts.

The interests and behavior patterns of individuals with autism spectrum disorder are more repetitive and fixed. An individual with autism, for example, may watch the same TV show over and over. These individuals also follow routines and may show sensitivity to normal sensory input such as sound or light. Adults with autism tend to choose occupations that have fewer interpersonal interactions and more focus on manipulating objects. Thus, you would see these individuals designing car engines or programming computers rather than being salespeople. The *DSM–5* criteria for autism spectrum disorder are shown in *Table 6-2*.

Developmentally, symptoms of autism are generally not seen until 8 to 12 months of age (Dawson, Sterling, & Faja, 2009). By the toddler–preschool stage, the traditional symptoms such as social impairment, imitation, responses to emotions, and face processing become apparent. Along with these impairments in social relationships, language delays and repetitive behaviors may also be present. Additionally, infants with autism show a non-normal pattern of growth of the head. At birth, these infants show a small to normal head size. This is followed by an accelerating pattern of growth at about 4 months of age, which results in a larger head size around 1 year of age. Magnetic resonance imaging (MRI) studies suggest 2- to 4-year-old children with autism have larger total cerebral volume compared with healthy controls.

Autism has been shown to have a strong genetic component (see Dawson et al., 2009, for an overview). Concordance rates from numerous studies of twins in terms of autism

TABLE 6-2 ***DSM–5*** **Diagnostic Criteria for Autism Spectrum Disorder**

A.	Persistent deficits in social communication and social interaction across contexts, as manifested by the following, currently or by history. 1. Deficits in social-emotional reciprocity; ranging from abnormal social approach and failure of normal back and forth conversation; to reduced sharing of interests, emotions, or affect; to failure to initiate or respond to social interactions. 2. Deficits in nonverbal communicative behaviors used for social interaction; ranging from poorly integrated verbal and nonverbal communication; to abnormalities in eye contact and body-language, or deficits in understanding and use of gestures; to a total lack of facial expression and nonverbal communication. 3. Deficits in developing, maintaining and understanding relationships, ranging, for example, from difficulties adjusting behavior to suit various social contexts; to difficulties in sharing imaginative play and in making friends to an apparent absence of interest in peers.
B.	Restricted, repetitive patterns of behavior, interests, or activities as manifested by at least two of the following, currently or by history: 1. Stereotyped or repetitive motor movements, use of objects, or speech (e.g., simple motor stereotypies, lining up toys or flipping objects, echolalia, idiosyncratic phrases). 2. Insistence on sameness, inflexible adherence to routines or ritualized patterns of verbal or nonverbal behavior (e.g., extreme distress at small changes, difficulties with transitions, rigid thinking patterns, greeting rituals, need to take same route or eat same food every day). 3. Highly restricted, fixated interests that are abnormal in intensity or focus (e.g., strong attachment to or preoccupation with unusual objects, excessively circumscribed or perseverative interests). 4. Hyper or hypo-reactivity to sensory input or unusual interest in sensory aspects of environment (e.g., apparent indifference to pain/temperature, adverse response to specific sounds or textures, excessive smelling or touching of objects, visual fascination with lights or movement).
C.	Symptoms must be present in early childhood (but may not become fully manifest until social demands exceed limited capacities, or may be masked by learned strategies in later life).
D.	Symptoms cause clinically significant impairment in social, occupational, or other important areas of current functioning.
E.	These disturbances are not better explained by intellectual disability (intellectual developmental disorder) or global developmental delay. Intellectual disability and autism spectrum disorder fequencyly co-occur; to make comorbid diagnosis for autism spectrum and intellectual disability, social communication should be below that expected for general development level.

Reprinted with permission from the *Diagnostic and Statistical Manual of Mental Disorders*, Fifth Edition (Copyright 2013). American Psychiatric Association.

show a range from 69% to 95% for monozygotic (MZ) twins and 0% to 24% for dizygotic (DZ) twins. Also, relatives of those with autism show higher rates of autism-like symptoms. The farther a relative is from the person with autism, the fewer symptoms that are seem. This suggests that autism involves a genetic pathway involving a number of genes in a complex manner.

Autism was initially thought to be largely influenced by environmental factors. Initially, it was suggested that bad parenting was related to developing autism spectrum disorders. This has been shown to be completely false. Another study suggested that measles, mumps, and rubella (MMR) vaccinations produced changes in the infant that led to autism. Not only has this been shown to be false; it was discovered that the original research was fraudulent.

What has been shown is a complex relationship involving environmental factors such as the age of the mother (see Waterhouse, 2012, for an overview). Younger mothers have the lowest risk for having children with autism and older mothers the highest risk. Fathers over 50 years of age have 4 times the risk of having a child with autism. There is also some suggestion that the mother's health during pregnancy is associated with autism although the exact factors remain ambiguous.

In terms of the brain, it is suggested that the autism spectrum disorders reflect dysfunction with areas associated with the social brain (see Minshew & Williams, 2007, for an overview). Briefly, these are the amygdala, specific areas of the frontal lobes, and areas of the temporal lobe. Further, those with autism were shown to have less activity in the mirror neuron system when viewing emotional expressions of faces (Dapretto et al., 2006). In those with autism, there was a negative correlation between cortical activity during this task and the severity of symptoms in the social domain. Another characteristic of autism is the desire to have a stable set of routines, which results in problems shifting attention.

Current neuroscience studies show that by the time of full brain development, a person with autism shows deficits in the areas that make up the social brain. For example, whereas individuals without autism tend to scan the eyes when looking at another person, those with autism focus on the mouth (Pelphrey & Carter, 2008). The photo to the right shows the focus of eye movements on the faces of adults with and without autism. Since various features of the eyes give both emotional and social information, those with autism miss out on this information.

Coupled with the inability to empathize is the superior ability to *systemize* in autism. Systemizing is the ability to analyze objects or events in terms of their structure and future behavior. This involves understanding the rules that govern the object. These rules could be a timetable of trains and planes, how animals are classified, the pattern of tides in the ocean, and how things work such as an automobile engine. These deficits and abilities make up the **empathizing-systemizing theory of autism** (Baron-Cohen, 2009; Baron-Cohen & Belmonte, 2005).

There is some suggestion that those with autism switch their focus of attention to the

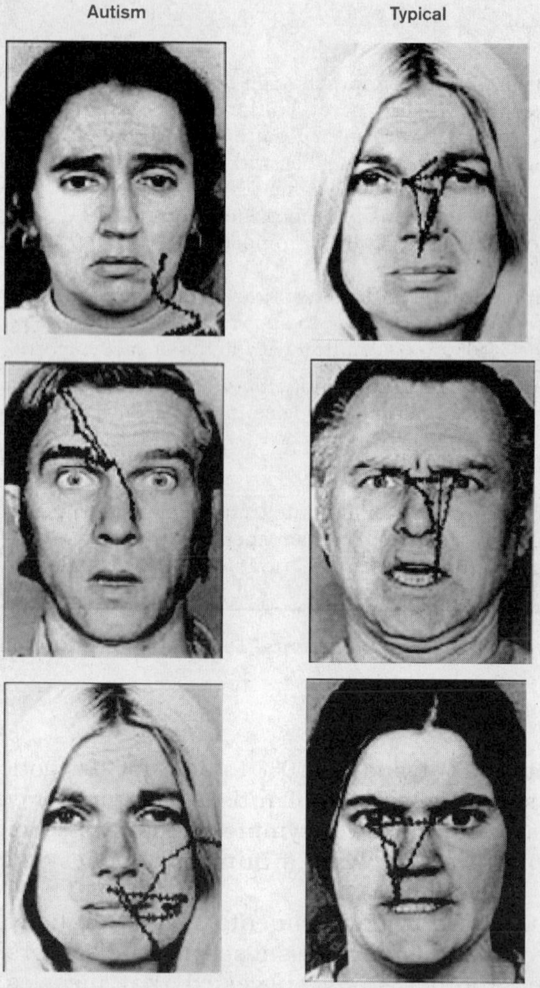

Focus of eye movements on the faces of adults with and without autism

Source: Pelphrey et al. (2002).

mouth between 6 and 12 months of age. This suggests to some researchers that brain changes in terms of facial focus may serve as a marker to predict who will develop autism (Pelphrey & McPartland, 2012; Walsh, Elsabbagh, Bolton, & Singh, 2011). In one study, Mayada Elsabbagh and her colleagues (2012) measured electroencephalogram (EEG) components evoked in response to viewing faces in infants 6 to 10 months of age. These researchers found that these event-related potential (ERP) components were associated with being diagnosed with autism at 36 months of age.

It appears that the higher order frontal lobe functions required to adapt to life fail to fully develop in individuals with autism. Physically, infants who were to develop autism were shown to have an increase in head circumference by the end of the first year of life. MRI studies during the 2nd to 4th year of life showed increases in total brain volume in children with autism. This was seen in both total white and gray matter. It also has been noted that this cortical overgrowth coincided with the onset of the signs and symptoms of autism.

Behaviorally, individuals with autism display problems in three areas (Baron-Cohen & Belmonte, 2005). These areas are social functions, communications, and restrictions in behaviors and interests. Those previously described by the term *Asperger's syndrome* show social impairments and restricted behaviors but fewer problems in terms of language and communication. One current theory of autism centers on problems related to empathy. In particular, it is suggested that individuals with autism fail to develop a theory of mind. As you remember, theory of mind refers to one's ability to infer the mental states of others in relation to their actions or situations. In a variety of studies, individuals with autism were able to describe what was going on in someone else's behavior on the perceptual level but showed difficulties when asked to describe the social–emotional processes that would be expected to accompany the behaviors. This appears to be a general lack of ability since they also have problems reflecting on these aspects of their own behavior. Another characteristic of autism is the desire to have a stable set of routines and problems shifting attention. Overall, individuals with autism show a variety of symptoms including differences in brain size, emotional recognition, ability to understand perspective in others, and knowledge of self (see Lombardo et al., 2011, for an overview).

In the 1960s and 1970s, individuals with autism were considered to have a form of psychosis similar to childhood schizophrenia. Consistent with the historical view at that time, environmental factors such as bad parenting were suggested to be a cause of the disorder although today parenting or social factors are seen to play little role at all. Today, genetic factors are seen to place a larger role in the development of the disorder. However, as you will see in the section on treatment of autism, environmental factors can influence in important ways the progression of the disorder and its remission.

In terms of genetics, twin studies of individuals with these social difficulties show 92% concordance for MZ twins versus 10% for DZ pairs. There is some suggestion that autism spectrum disorder shares common genetic processes with schizophrenia. There is also a connection with ADHD. A large-scale study of more than 10,000 twin pairs in Sweden reported that an MZ twin with autism spectrum disorder had a 44% chance of also being diagnosed with ADHD whereas a DZ twin had only a 15% chance (Lichtenstein, Carlstrom, Råstam, Gillberg, & Anckarsäter, 2010).

Although autism spectrum disorder was initially considered to be rare, current estimates suggest that around 1 in every 100 children have the disorder with it being more common in boys as compared with girls. Depending on the study, the exact gender ratio varies from 2 to 1 to 5 to 1. The ratio of males to females is about 8 to 1 in cases in which there is no intellectual disability (Frith, Happé, Amarakm, & Warren, 2013). More than half of the cases of autism show intellectual disabilities. The exact number of individuals with autism spectrum disorder is related to how broad or narrow the diagnostic criteria were specified in a particular study. One difficulty with diagnosis is that it relies on observations of social interactions of a toddler. Further, different children may show different profiles as well as have varying intellectual abilities. Professional support and special education programs can produce marked improvement. Some children who show the characteristics of autism before the age of 5 show few of the signs some 10 years later (Coleman & Gilberg, 2012). However, social situations still prove difficult for individuals with autism spectrum disorder.

At this point, there are a number of suggestive factors related to the development of autism spectrum disorder. One correlational factor is that males—and in some studies females—who are older are more likely to have children with autism spectrum disorder than younger individuals. Whether this is related to the older males having a different quality of sperm is not known. Another factor is that although infants who later develop autism have similar size heads to other babies at birth, they do show larger heads during the first year of life. Enlargement of the brain by 3% to 10% is one of the most consistently reported observations (South et al., 2008). The overgrowth of cortical tissue takes place more in the frontal and temporal lobes than other areas of the brain. It is these areas that are involved in social and language functions as well as facial processing. Although overgrowth has been shown, there is also a consistent finding of less activity in those cortical areas related to facial processing. This overgrowth and reduced activity may lie at the basis of later social problems.

To summarize, the cortical areas involved in individuals with autism display differential responding on brain imaging tasks. Amaral and his colleagues have described the neuroanatomy of autism (Amaral, Schumann, & Nordahl, 2008). In particular, they depict the cortical structures involved in the three major characteristics of autism. These are problems in social interactions, problems in communication, and the use of repetitive behaviors. *Figure 6-9* shows these areas.

Special Talents

It is estimated that about 10% of individuals with autism spectrum disorder have special abilities in terms of music, art, calculation, or memory (Treffert, 2009). There are more males than females with these abilities. This has been called the *savant syndrome* and was portrayed in the 1988 movie *Rain Man* by the actor Dustin Hoffman. The real-life person on which the movie was based could name all U.S. zip codes, had memorized maps and could tell you how to go from one city to another in the United States as well as move about a city in terms of street names. He had also memorized more than 6,000 books and could repeat facts from a variety of areas. He could also tell you which day of the week a certain date would occur in any year. Another savant artist was Nadia, who drew the horse in *Figure 6-10* at age 5. At this point, there is no single theory that can explain savants. However, it appears that sensory and perceptual areas of the brain are overrepresented in terms of cortical processing. This results in an emphasis on detail and a lack of emotional and social processing.

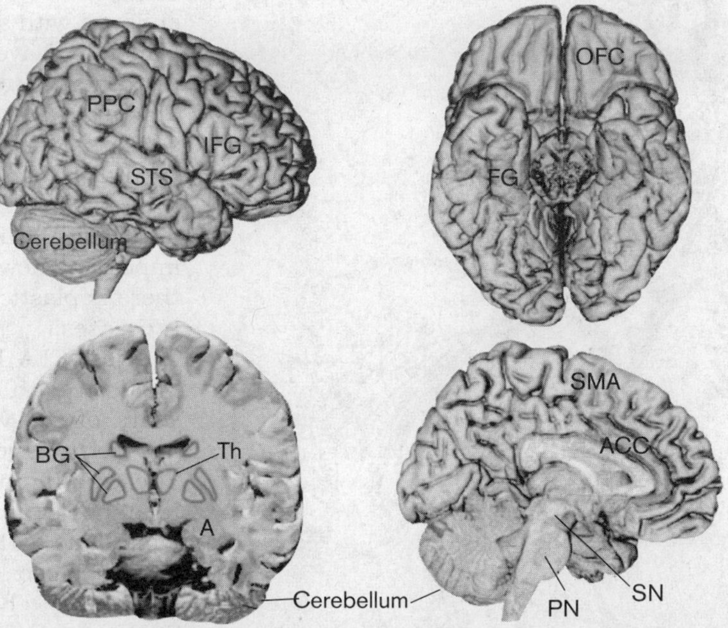

Social impairment	Communication deficits	Repetitive behaviors
OFC: Orbitofrontal cortex ACC: Anterior cingulate cortex FG: Fusiform gyrus STS: Superior temporal sulcus A: Amygdala mirror neuron regions IFG: Interior frontal gyrus PPC: Posterior parietal cortex	IFG: Inferior frontal gyrus (Broca's area) STS: Superior temporal sulcus SMA: Supplementary motor area BG: Basal ganglia SN: Substantia nigra Th: Thalamus PN: Pontine nuclei cerebellum	OFC: Orbitofrontal cortex ACC: Anterior cingulate cortex BG: Basal gangila Th: Thalamus

FIGURE 6-9 The Neuroanatomy of Autism

Source: Amaral et al. (2008).

Treatment for Autism Spectrum Disorders

Since autism spectrum disorders appear early in a child's life, parents turn to a number of different professionals for help. Depending on the initial problems of development noted, these professionals can include kindergarten teachers, special education teachers, speech pathologists, child clinical psychologists and psychiatrists, and pediatricians.

The first empirically supported treatments were developed by Lovaas and his colleagues in the 1960s (Lovaas & Smith, 2003). This approach, which was based on behavioral principles, was referred to as the UCLA Young Autism Project. This project has reported around

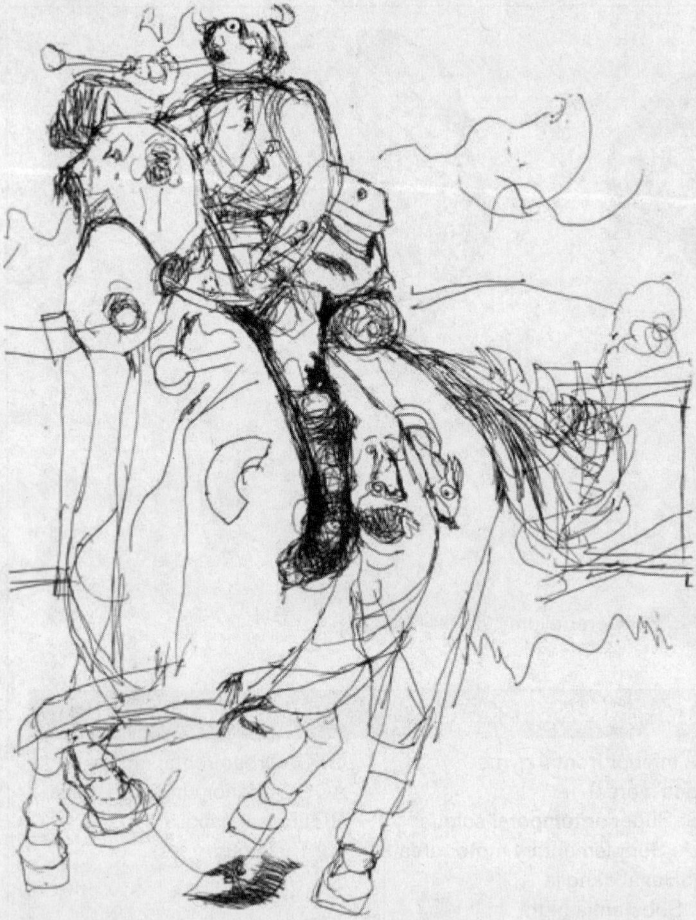

FIGURE 6-10 Drawing by Nadia at Age 5

Source: Selfe (2011, p. 32).

50% "recovery" rates of young children with autism and these principles have been supported in other studies (Rogers & Vismara, 2008). Besides the success with individual children, this approach helped the field to understand that children with autism can learn important new skills and thus there is plasticity to their brain processes.

The UCLA Project accepted children with autism under 4 years of age with the average age being 2 years 10 months. These children also needed not to show major medical problems such as hearing or vision loss. These children then received 40 hours a week of one-to-one interventions. This treatment lasted for about 3 years, depending on the individual child. Based on behavioral principles, the treatment was designed to maximize positive outcomes and reduce failure experiences. This included giving the child short and clear instructions and immediate reinforcement for each correct response. Parents are also an important part of the process.

There are five major stages of treatment in the Lovaas treatment program. The first is establishing a teaching relationship, which lasts from 2 to 4 weeks. Since many of these children have previously avoided situations through tantrums and other means, the therapist works with the child in following simple directions. The second stage, which lasts from 1 to 4 months, involves teaching foundational skills in terms of following directions, imitating behaviors, and identifying objects. The third stage lasts for around 6 months and focuses on beginning communication. This includes initial speech processes and identifying objects and actions. The fourth stage, which lasts for about a year, continues communication processes such as labeling colors and shapes and developing the basic concepts of language. The fifth stage, which also lasts about a year, is designed to continue communication processes and help the child adjust to school situations, including peer interactions. The program ends as the child becomes part of a school situation.

Rogers and Vismara (2008) reviewed the treatment literature for autism spectrum disorder in terms of empirically supported treatments. They found a number of child characteristics were associated with successful treatment outcomes. One characteristic was the age at which treatment was begun. Those children who began treatment before the age of 4 had better outcomes than those who started at age 5 or older. Also, higher IQ was associated with better outcomes. Overall, it appears that early intervention in language skills, communication, and peer relationships along with a reduction in negative behaviors allows many children with autism spectrum disorder to successfully move through a normal school sequence. However, at this point, it is difficult to estimate the percentage of children that are successfully treated.

In addition to psychosocial treatment approaches, medications have been used to address specific disruptive behaviors seen in autism. These behaviors include hyperactivity, inattention, repetitive thoughts and behaviors, and aggressive behaviors against others and self. Medications include antidepressants, stimulants, and antipsychotic medications. These medications are typically given to older rather than younger children with autism spectrum disorder.

There is much work being done in India with young people suffering from Autism Spectrum Disorders (ASD). Kasarpalkar, Kothari, and Dave (2014) found significantly higher ($p < 0.001$) levels of Serum Brain-derived neurotrophic factor (BDNF) in atypical autistic subjects as compared to controls, but not in typical ASD cases. "BDNF levels were significantly lower in females with typical/Rett Syndrome ($p < 0.05$), but not in males with typical autism ($p > 0.1$), as compared to controls. Lower BDNF levels indicate impairment in neuroprotective mechanism, while higher levels may imply a manifested protective response," according to Kasarpalkar et al. (2014).

Mhatre, Bapat, & Vrajesh Udani (2016), in Mumbai, have opined based on their findings that lower disease severity, parent participation, and higher maternal education were associated with better outcomes in ASD. The work focused on a cohort of children treated in a large tertiary care center from 1992 onwards to date, requesting parents either telephonically or via letter for a follow up assessment meeting. Assessment tools such as CARS, GARS, and VSMS were used.

Concept Check

- Individuals with autism spectrum disorder have difficulty in three separate areas. What are those areas and what specific types of difficulty do these individuals encounter in each area?
- Is autism associated with a lower IQ? What evidence can you cite to support your answer?
- What are the primary developmental, genetic, and environmental factors related to autism?
- What is the savant syndrome, and what are its defining characteristics?
- What are the five major stages of treatment for autism spectrum disorders in the Lovaas treatment program?
- What are three characteristics associated with successful treatment outcomes for autism spectrum disorders?

ATTENTION DEFICIT/ HYPERACTIVITY DISORDER

ADHD is a disorder of childhood that tends to develop before the age of 12. Although the conceptualization of ADHD has changed over the years, it currently includes two major dimensions (see Frick & Nigg, 2012, for an overview). The first dimension is *inattention*. Children and adults with inattention problems tend to exhibit these in a cognitive realm such as letting their mind wander or not paying attention. As shown with the inattention diagnostic criteria these individuals may have difficulty paying close attention to details or focusing on activities such as schoolwork or lectures, appear disorganized, be unwilling to engage in activities that require mental effort, and be easily distracted. Individuals with this type of ADHD may also show learning problems.

The second dimension is *hyperactivity and impulsivity*. Children with hyperactivity and impulsivity tend to show these symptoms in a behavioral or motor realm. As shown in the hyperactivity and impulsivity diagnostic criteria (see *Table 6-3*), these individuals may have difficulty waiting their turn, waiting to respond, keeping still, and remaining in their seat. Children with this type of ADHD may also show conduct problems. There is some suggestion that hyperactivity problems may lessen as a child grows older whereas attentional problems may increase resulting in increasing difficulty with schoolwork. It is also possible that individuals with ADHD show characteristics of both inattention and hyperactivity.

TABLE 6-3 *DSM–5* Diagnostic Criteria for Attention Deficit/Hyperactivity Disorder

AD/HD consists of a pattern of behavior that is present in multiple settings where it gives rise to social, educational or work performance difficulties.
A. Either (A1) and/or (A2).
A1. Inattention: Six (or more) of the following symptoms have persisted for at least 6 months to a degree that is inconsistent with developmental level and that impact directly on social and academic/occupational activities. a. Often fails to give close attention to details or makes careless mistakes in schoolwork, at work, or during other activities (e.g., overlooks or misses details, work is inaccurate). b. Often has difficulty sustaining attention in tasks or play activities (e.g., has difficulty remaining focused during lectures, conversations, or reading lengthy writings). c. Often does not seem to listen when spoken to directly (e.g., mind seems elsewhere, even in the absence of any obvious distraction). d. Often does not follow through on instructions and fails to finish schoolwork, chores, or duties in the workplace (e.g., starts tasks but quickly loses focus and is easily sidetracked; fails to finish schoolwork, household chores, or tasks in the workplace). e. Often has difficulty organizing tasks and activities (e.g., difficulty managing sequential tasks; difficulty keeping materials and belongings in order; messy, disorganized, work; poor time management; tends to fail to meet deadlines). f. Often avoids, dislikes, or is reluctant to engage in tasks that require sustained mental effort (e.g., schoolwork or homework; for older adolescents and adults, preparing reports, completing forms, or reviewing lengthy papers). g. Often loses things necessary for tasks or activities (e.g., school materials, pencils, books, tools, wallets, keys, paperwork, eyeglasses, or mobile telephones). h. Is often easily distracted by extraneous stimuli (for older adolescents and adults, may include unrelated thoughts). i. Is often forgetful in daily activities (e.g., chores, running errands; for older adolescents and adults, returning calls, paying bills, keeping appointments).
A2. Hyperactivity and Impulsivity: Six (or more) of the following symptoms have persisted for at least 6 months to a degree that is inconsistent with developmental level and that impact directly on social and academic/occupational activities. a. Often fidgets with or taps hands or feet or squirms in seat. b. Often leaves seat in situations when remaining seated is expected (e.g., leaves his or her place in the classroom, office or other workplace, or in other situations that require remaining seated). c. Often runs about or climbs in situations where it is inappropriate. (In adolescents or adults, may be limited to feeling restless).

d. Often unable to play or engage in leisure activities quietly.
e. Is often "on the go," acting as if "driven by a motor" (e.g., is unable or uncomfortable being still for an extended time, as in restaurants, meetings, etc; may be experienced by others as being restless and difficult to keep up with).
f. Often talks excessively.
g. Often blurts out an answer before a question has been completed (e.g., completes people's sentences and "jumps the gun" in conversations, cannot wait for next turn in conversation).
h. Often has difficulty waiting his or her turn (e.g., while waiting in line).
i. Often interrupts or intrudes on others (e.g., butts into conversations, games, or activities; may start using other people's things without asking or receiving permission, adolescents or adults may intrude into or take over what others are doing).

B. Several inattentive or hyperactive-impulsive symptoms were present prior to age 12.

C. Criteria for the disorder are met in two or more settings (e.g., at home, school or work, with friends or relatives, or in other activities).

D. There must be clear evidence that the symptoms interfere with or reduce the quality of social, academic, or occupational functioning.

E. The symptoms do not occur exclusively during the course of schizophrenia or another psychotic disorder and are not better accounted for by another mental disorder (e.g., mood disorder, anxiety disorder, dissociative disorder, or a personality disorder).

Specify Based on Current Presentation

Combined Presentation: If both Criterion A1 (Inattention) and Criterion A2 (Hyperactivity-Impulsivity) are met for the past 6 months.

Predominantly Inattentive Presentation: If Criterion A1 (Inattention) is met but Criterion A2 (Hyperactivity-Impulsivity) is not met and 3 or more symptoms from Criterion A2 have been present for the past 6 months.

Inattentive Presentation (Restrictive): If Criterion A1 (Inattention) is met but no more than 2 symptoms from Criterion A2 (Hyperactivity-Impulsivity) have been present for the past 6 months.

Predominantly Hyperactive/Impulsive Presentation: If Criterion A2 (Hyperactivity-Impulsivity) is met and Criterion A1 (Inattention) is not met for the past 6 months.

ADHD is reported to be the most common emotional–behavioral disorder treated in youth (see Wilens, Biederman, & Spencer, 2002, for an overview). Epidemiological studies suggest a prevalence rate of 4% to 5% of children in the United States, New Zealand, Australia, Germany, and Brazil. Of those with ADHD, some 20% to 30% have the inattentive subtype, less than 15% have the hyperactive-impulsive subtype, and 50% to 75% have a combination of both. Although long-term studies show different rates, it is assumed that over 50% of the children with ADHD will show continued ADHD into adolescence. A smaller proportion will show ADHD symptoms in adulthood. Adults with ADHD show more symptoms related to inattention as compared with hyperactivity and impulsivity (Kessler et al., 2010). Specifically, almost half (45.7%) of the individuals studied who had childhood ADHD continued to meet full *DSM–IV* criteria for current adult ADHD, with 94.9% of these cases having attention deficit disorder and 34.6% hyperactivity disorder. According to the Centers for Disease Control and Prevention (CDC), boys are more likely (13.2%) than girls (5.6%) to be diagnosed with ADHD (see www.cdc.gov/ncbddd/adhd/data.html).

Epidemiological studies have also shown a comorbidity of ADHD with a variety of other disorders (see Aguiar, Eubing, & Schantz, 2010; Takeda et al., 2012, for overviews). Often, childhood disorders are referred to as either **externalizing disorders** such as CD and **oppositional defiant disorder (ODD)** or **internalizing disorders** such as anxiety and mood disorders. In youth, the comorbidity of ADHD and ODD was greater than 32%. Anxiety disorders were comorbid with ADHD at greater than 22% with a higher proportion of girls compared with boys showing the disorder. CD was comorbid with ADHD at greater than 7%.

Examining neuropsychological functions through a meta-analysis, children and adolescents with ADHD showed problems in a variety of cognitive processes (Aguiar et al., 2010). These include verbal working memory, spatial working memory, response inhibition in which the individual must inhibit a response, cognitive flexibility, and planning. Vigilance was also shown to be a problem. Those with ADHD have difficulty paying attention and inhibiting their responses.

In terms of brain function related to ADHD, it is suggested that dysfunctions exist in networks involving the frontal, striatal, and cerebellar regions (see Hart, Radua, Nakao, Mataix-Cols, & Rubia, 2013; van Ewijk, Heslenfeld, Zwiers, Buitelaar, & Oosterlaan, 2011, for overviews and meta-analysis). These networks are related to executive function, which is seen to be dysfunctional in ADHD.

Various studies have also found differences in gray matter and white matter in those with ADHD. Overall, children with ADHD showed a 7% decrease in total cerebral volume and 8% decrease in total cortical volume in all four major lobes of the brain compared with controls (Wolosin, Richardson, Hennessey, Denckla, & Mostofsky, 2009). DTI studies also showed disturbed white matter connections in children, adolescents, and adults with ADHD.

Neurons in the brain have been shown to be connected in an efficient and economical manner. These connections have been described in terms of small-world properties (Sporns, 2011). Children with ADHD have been shown to have different network properties than children without ADHD (Wang et al., 2009). Although children both with and without ADHD had economical small-world network properties, their networks differed in terms of long-distance and short-distance neural connections. Using brain imaging techniques, children with ADHD showed more efficient short-distance connections as compared with long-distance ones.

Overall, a variety of studies have shown dysfunctional connectivity during both rest and cognitive tasks in the brains of children with ADHD (see Castellanos & Proal, 2012; Konrad & Eickhoff, 2010, for overviews). Cognitive tasks such as having a child inhibit a motor response are associated with less cortical activity in the circuits involving the frontal, striatal, and cerebellar networks in children with ADHD. One common hypothesis directing fMRI research with ADHD is the idea that individuals with ADHD have a more difficult time switching from resting state conditions to those of active task management.

There is evidence to suggest that ADHD is influenced by genetic components (Sharp, McQuillin, & Gurling, 2009). The disorder is more prevalent in identical as compared with fraternal twins. Adoption studies also suggest a genetic component, especially in first-degree relatives. More than 20 research studies suggest a heritability rate of 76%. Further, at least 25% of the adults with a history of hyperactivity have biological children who show hyperactivity. Overall, genetic studies with ADHD show little influence from the family environment. Genes related to dopamine regulation appear to be involved with ADHD.

Treatment for Attention Deficit/Hyperactivity Disorder

The major treatment for ADHD is medications that are stimulants. Although it may seem paradoxical to give a stimulant to a person who is hyperactive, these medications have been shown to be effective (see Bidwell, McClernon, & Killins, 2011; Fredriksen, Halmøy, Faraoned, & Haavik, 2013, for overviews). The most common drugs used in ADHD treatment are methylphenidates, which include the trade name Ritalin, and amphetamines including dextroamphetamine, which are known as Adderall and Dexedrine. These drugs reduce the symptoms of ADHD, such as disruptive and noncompliant behavior. They also increase the ability to focus attention. These medications may also improve physical coordination. It has been estimated that 70% of children with ADHD will show symptom reduction with stimulant medications.

Psychosocial treatments are often used in combination with medication, with the best treatment results seen with a combination of both (see Hoza, Kaiser, & Hurt, 2008). With older adolescents and adults, psychological therapies may be useful in allowing the person to talk about the experience of having ADHD and create cognitive and behavioral strategies for managing his or her environment. For example, reducing distraction allows the person to function more effectively.

For children with ADHD, involving parents in the treatment of their child's ADHD has been shown to be empirically effective (Anastopoulos & Farley, 2003). This cognitive behavioral training approach for parents involves 10 components. These are as follows:

1. Get an overview of the characteristics of ADHD and clarification of the parents' understanding of the disorder.
2. Review behavioral management techniques and the problems associated with escalating negative interactions with the child.
3. Increase positive attention to the child's desired behaviors as well as develop skills to allow the parents to ignore certain behaviors that compromise relationships.
4. Learn how to help the child to comply with simple requests and present requests clearly.
5. Set up a home reward system.
6. Add costs for minor rule violations to the home reward system.
7. Use time-out period for serious rule violations.
8. Learn how to manage behavior in public.
9. Consider potential problems in the future and the removal of the home reward system.
10. Have a booster session to review progress and troubleshoot situations.

The basic idea is to create the situation in which the parents and the child are not arguing with each other, which only leads to escalating negative interactions. Rather, using behavioral principles, the goal is to increase positive interactions and to help the child be less impulsive. This also allows the parents to communicate more effectively with school personnel such that the child receives a consistent message in his or her life. Other similar programs have been developed for classroom management, which have been shown to be empirically supported. It has been shown that involving other children without ADHD in the classroom can be effective.

One of the important ways to deal with ASD, ADHD, and other childhood disorders is the involvement of parents, teachers, and other caregivers. Work with parents of children with multiple disabilities is very necessary. NHCDC is a Mumbai-based multidisciplinary child therapy center that has published a qualitative analysis of counseling inputs for caregivers where they underline the role of contextually relevant advice

> tapping on contextual advantages, for example, domestic chores are often assigned to children in Indian homes as compared to their Western counterparts. In case of children with developmental disorders, these tasks can play important roles to improve a sense of responsibility and self-esteem in children. Counsellors thus encourage parents to assign simple household tasks to their children. The improved motivation thus, translates into greater undertaking of academic responsibilities among children, for example: initiating and completing school home-work. (Dalwai, Kanade-Modak, Siddiqui, Gajria, & Chatterjee, 2016)

They also encourage harnessing the relationships typically seen in Indian families, to get children with communication barriers to write letters or make phone to near and dear relatives.

The same group (Dalwai, Modak, Bondre, & Gajria, 2016) has also published work in the Academic Journal of Pediatrics and Neonatology on the assessment tools for ASD in the Indian context including the Indian Scale for Assessment of Autism (ISAA) and the revised Autism Diagnostic Interview (ADI-R).

CONDUCT DISORDER

Although all children and adolescents seek to assert their independence, children and adolescents with CD display more extreme behaviors that reflect little regard for those around them. They actively violate the rights of others. These violations can include bullying or threatening others. These threats may involve a weapon or object that could do serious physical harm. They may also be cruel and begin physical fights and take things from other people. Children and adolescents with CD also violate the rules of society. Such violations can include destroying property, breaking laws such as stealing, and conning others. Their relationships in school and family situations also show a lack of connectedness such as skipping school or running away from home. As these children get older, violations of a sexual nature can also be seen. The behaviors associated with CDs also lead to problems in other areas of development. These children are often left behind in academic achievement and have difficulties with interpersonal relationships. These children often come from homes with marital discord and high stress levels in terms of neighborhood, financial difficulties, and inconsistent parenting. A consistent relationship has been found between harsh and ineffective parenteral discipline and aggressive problems in children. It is estimated that 5% to 10% of children and adolescents have significant persistent oppositional, disruptive, or aggressive behavior problems in developed countries (Moffitt & Scott, 2008). Some of these children and adolescents will no longer show these behavior problems as they mature into young adulthood while others will continue disruptive behaviors and qualify for an antisocial personality disorder, which will be discussed in Chapter 15.

The *DSM–5* criteria for a CD require that the youth show a persistent and repetitive pattern of behavior. This pattern of behavior includes violating the rights of others and the rules of society during the past 12 months. Some of these violations can include aggression toward people and animals such as bullying or physical fights or cruelty. Other types of violations include destruction of property, including setting fires. Theft and lying are other forms of violation of society's rules. Finally, *DSM–5* includes in the violations such examples as before the age of 13 running away from home or being truant from school. Overall, a youth will demonstrate three of these criteria over the past year and these behaviors will lead to significant impairment in the person's life.

In an early *Psychological Review*, it was suggested that early-onset CD is a neurodevelopmental disorder involving the brain whereas onset in adolescence involves social mimicry (Moffitt, 1993). However, with the advent of brain imaging studies, it has been shown that both early- and late-onset CD showed abnormal activation of the amygdala when viewing emotional human faces (Passamonti et al., 2010). Of course, these brain changes can also be influenced by environmental factors and stress. In a study comparing individuals with early-onset CD, late-onset CD, and matched controls, the researchers found reduced amygdala volume in both early- and late-onset individuals in comparison with controls (Fairchild et al., 2011). For the individuals with CD, a negative correlation was found between number of CD symptoms and insula volume. Since the insula is involved in awareness of one's own self-including affective states, a reduction in volume may be related to deficits in empathy associated with CD.

OPPOSITIONAL DEFIANT DISORDER

Children who mainly show anger and defiance but do not act aggressively toward other people or animals or destroy property are described as having ODD. These children lose their temper easily and often argue with adults. They may do things to annoy others, blame others for their problems, and be vindictive. The prevalence of the disorder is around 3.3% with slightly more males than females showing the disorder (American Psychiatric Association [APA], 2013).

The *DSM–5* criteria for ODD require that the youth engage in four of eight behavioral characteristics. These are grouped in terms of three categories. The first is that of an angry or irritable mood, which includes losing one's temper, being easily annoyed, and being resentful and angry often. The second category of behaviors is that of being argumentative and defiant. These behaviors would include arguing with authority figures or refusing to do what they say as well as deliberately annoying others and blaming others. The third category is that of being vindictive. Overall, these behaviors interfere with the youth's social and educational development.

The criteria for both CD and ODD are based on observed behaviors rather than internal processes. As researchers have sought to understand if there are underlying processes that are common to a number of childhood disorders, particular groupings have been discovered. For example, a number of studies suggest that disorders including ODD, CD, hyperactivity, impulsivity, and substance use tend to cluster together (Lahey et al., 2008; Lahey & Waldman, 2012). Inattention was not part of this grouping. This dimension is referred to as the *externalizing or disinhibition dimension*. This dimension also seems to share substantial genetic influences (Lahey, Van Hulle, Singh, Waldman, & Rathouz, 2011; Markon & Krueger, 2005). Other studies have shown that anxiety and depressive disorders cluster into an internalizing or emotional dimension (Lahey et al., 2008).

Treatment for Conduct Disorder and Oppositional Defiant Disorder

Similar treatments have been developed for the treatment of CD and ODD. Unlike ADHD in which the treatment is centered on the individual's relation with the family, the school, and the clinic, the child or adolescent with oppositional behavior patterns may also be involved with the community and law enforcement facilities. By the very nature of the disorder, there is often an adversarial relationship with those who seek to offer treatment. Additionally, a given individual with these disorders may show a number of other conditions that make a single treatment approach difficult.

Empirically supported interventions and treatment for young children with oppositional behavior patterns are largely family based (see Brinkmeyer & Eyberg, 2003; McMahon & Kotler, 2008, for examples). In essence, the parents are taught to use behavioral techniques to alter the oppositional behaviors. One of these programs, parent–child interaction therapy, has an underlying attachment perspective. Thus, the initial part of the therapy is based on the interaction between the parent and child with the goal of helping the child to develop a secure attachment pattern with the parent. In this approach, this is referred to as PRIDE. PRIDE refers to *praising* the child's behavior, *reflecting* the child's statements, and *imitating* and *describing* the child's play using *enthusiasm*. This is followed by teaching the parent behavioral management techniques based on social learning theory. In particular, this phase is designed to replace critical and commands with positive strategies. Part of this is helping the parent to know to talk to the child in a direct and specific manner in a way that the child can understand.

Treatment approaches with older children and adolescents may also be conducted in the clinic, inpatient, or correctional facilities (see Boxer & Flick, 2008; Kazdin, 2005, for examples). As the child becomes older, there becomes more opportunity for them to engage in property destruction, vandalism, theft, and verbal and physical assault. One empirically supported approach is referred to as multisystemic therapy (MST). As the name implies, this approach seeks to involve the family and other agencies that the youth would be involved with. This could include schools, youth agencies, probation offices, and other such facilities. The overall treatment seeks to have those involved with the youth give a consistent message and a set of skills in terms of family interaction, problem-solving skills, and interpersonal relationships. A single therapist is needed to monitor the youth in terms of these different facilities.

Other empirically supported treatments for older children are focused on a single facility such as a clinic setting. One of these is problem-solving skills training (PSST). This is a cognitive therapy designed to help the youth determine what they are supposed to do in a given situation, examine possibilities, concentrate and evaluate the situation, make a choice, and then evaluate the choice. This basic approach can be applied to a school situation, a family situation, or other life situations.

LEARNING DISABILITIES

Learning disabilities refer to the situation in which a child's achievement is lower than that expected from his or her scores on achievement or intelligence tests (see Naglieri, Salter, & Rojahn, 2008, for an overview). The term *learning disability* was first used in the 1960s and replaced the term *minimal brain dysfunction* in federal regulations in the

CASE OF ROBERT
Conduct Disorder

Prior to the initial diagnostic evaluation, Robert had been suspended from school on four occasions due to behavioral misconduct and had been caught stealing an expensive portable compact disc player from his grandmother. Although this specific incident of theft prompted Ms. Johnson to seek mental health treatment, she had observed over the prior months that Robert had begun to lie to her frequently and to display a negative, callous, and "hard" attitude toward others. Robert acknowledged the validity of his grandmother's concerns and, during the individual interview portion of the evaluation, reported a more elaborated recent history of engagement in aggressive and antisocial behavior, including unprovoked aggression (i.e., "jumping" peers on the street with his currently incarcerated older brother, Jake) and shoplifting (also with his older brother). The persistence and intensity of Robert's conduct problems, and the extent to which he expressed a fondness for and identification with his delinquent older brother, were of serious concern. Along with the primary diagnosis of CD, Robert carried a preexisting diagnosis of ADHD for which he had been receiving pharmacotherapy through his pediatrician. Robert had experienced a fairly extensive social history of family conflict, traumatic loss, and early deprivation. He was removed from his mother's custody at 18 months due to neglectful conditions accruing from his mother's substance abuse and had endured the murders of his father and uncle. At age 5, Robert was exhibiting very high levels of verbal and physical aggression in his kindergarten classroom, in addition to hyperactive behaviors, and consequently during that year was seen for 20 sessions of psychotherapy and psychiatric consultation in our clinic. Unchecked, it was quite likely that Robert's behavior would progress to far more serious manifestations, with significantly more deleterious consequences.

Source: Paul Boxer and Paul Flick. (2008). Treating Conduct Problems, Aggression, and Antisocial Behavior in Children and Adolescents: An Integrated View. In Ric Steele, T. David Elkin, & Michael C. Roberts (Eds.), *Handbook of evidence-based therapies for children and adolescents.* New York: Springer.

United States. The Department of Education in the United States has defined the services required to be provided to students with learning disabilities through the **Individuals with Disabilities Education Act (IDEA).** Various states and local school districts have also set up regulations related to learning disabilities. For each of the years 2005 through 2009, the U.S. Department of Education reported that 5% of all children had a specific learning disability and 3% had a speech or language impairment (nces.ed.gov/fastfacts/display.asp?id=64).

Concept Check

- What are the two primary dimensions of ADHD, and what is their prevalence?
- What are the primary *DSM–5* diagnostic criteria for CD and ODD? What is the difference between them?
- What effective treatments are available for individuals with ADHD, CD, and ODD? What is the role for parents in these treatments?

DSM–5 formally categorizes learning disabilities as **specific learning disorder.** A child who has specific learning disorder would show problems in one of the major school tasks.

These include reading aloud, understanding what is read, spelling, writing, remembering number facts, doing arithmetic calculations, reasoning in a mathematical manner, or the avoidance of these activities. Although there is no precise definition of what constitutes a difficulty, comparisons are made in terms of the child's age, intelligence level, cultural group, gender, and grade.

Work with Pediatric Epilepsy

Since this book does not separate out a chapter on organic disorders, rather seeking the neuropsychological underpinnings of each group of disorders, epilepsy as such has not been handled in details elsewhere. However, much work is done by several research groups on childhood epilepsies and imaging studies (Ursekar, 2008). Work has also been done by the Epilepsy Unit of GS Medical College and KEM Hospital, Mumbai, linking childhood absence epilepsy to Chromosome 8q24 (Fong, 1998).

INTELLECTUAL DEVELOPMENTAL DISORDER

Prior to *DSM–5,* the term ***mental retardation*** was used to refer to intellectual disabilities, and *ICD-10* continues to use the term *mental retardation. Intellectual disabilities* is a term widely used in schools throughout the world. They are estimated to affect between 1% and 2% of the population in Western countries. In *DSM–5,* those with intellectual disabilities are said to have an **intellectual developmental disorder (IDD).** An IDD is defined by three aspects. The first criterion is a deficit in mental abilities such as reasoning, problem solving, planning, abstract thinking, judgment, and ability to learn in both academic and practical settings. The second criterion is referred to as a lack of adaptive functioning in relation to one's age and sociocultural background. Adaptive functioning refers to how an individual copes with the problems of everyday life. These are described in terms of conceptual, social, and practical domains. This would include problems in terms of social communication, being part of a group, school and work functioning, and ability to be independent in an age-appropriate manner. The third criterion is that the onset of the disabilities took place prior to adolescence.

Unlike those with learning disabilities in which a child's achievement is lower than that expected from his or her scores on achievement or intelligence tests, individuals with IDD would be performing consistently with their scores on intellectual and achievement tests. They also tend to show more global deficits rather than difficulties with a specific area of functioning such as mathematical reasoning. Problems are generally seen in cognitive abilities, adaptive processes, social interactions, and reading situational and cultural norms.

Problems with intellectual development are considered to occur on a continuum described in terms of mild, moderate, and severe levels of disability. Unlike previous *DSM* definitions, an actual IQ score is no longer specified. Previously, only those individuals who scored below 70 on an IQ test would be diagnosed as mentally retarded. However, it is assumed that intelligence testing will be part of the overall assessment that would describe the person in terms of cultural, social, economic, and other factors.

The mild level of functioning would show some problems in the conceptual domain. This would include difficulties with academic skills such as math, writing, and reading.

Older students and adults with an IDD may show a more concrete approach to problems and solutions in comparison with peers. In the social domain, these individuals may have more difficulty reading social cues and expressing their emotions. In the practical domain, these individuals may need help in tasks such as grocery shopping, taking buses, and matters involving money such as banking and bill paying. Support would also be needed for making medical and legal decisions and raising a family.

The moderate level of functioning would show an adult who conceptually is functioning more like an elementary school student than a high school student. Younger individuals would lag in comparison with their peers. In the social domain, the person may show less complex relationships while still seeking relationships with family and peers. Social cues would be more difficult to interpret. In the practical domain, the person would need support from others. With this support, various types of jobs that have limited conceptual requirements are possible.

The severe level of functioning would require caregivers for an understanding of concepts involving time and money. Written language may be difficult. Social domains remain on a very concrete level. The relationship is less of a give-and-take nature and more of a simple attachment relationship. Practical tasks generally require a caregiver for most activities of daily living including meals and basic bodily tasks.

Most types of IDD can be traced to biological causes (see Mefford, Batshaw, & Hoffman, 2012, for an overview). However, the variation is huge. Examining genetic, chromosomal, and metabolic abnormalities has led researchers to identify more than 1,000 forms of impairment (Dykens & Hodapp, 2001). It has been suggested that mild disorders are more related to environmental influences and more severe forms are more related to biological factors (see Shapiro & Batshaw, 2011, for an overview). One way to organize these disorders is in terms of those directly related to chromosomes, those related to metabolism, and those related to events that take place in the womb such as malnutrition or the mother taking drugs such as alcohol or crack.

Intellectual Developmental Disorder Related to Chromosomes

The most common form of IDD is **Down syndrome,** which was described by the British physician Langdon Down in 1866. The disorder results in both physical and intellectual problems. The IQ is generally around 50 or below but can vary. There is a characteristic appearance of individuals with Down syndrome that includes a flat face with an upward slant of the eyes and smaller hands and feet. Cardiovascular problems are common in these individuals. There are a number of projects to help individuals with Down syndrome find work. The Special Olympics also offers an opportunity for these individuals to compete in sports.

The disorder occurs during pregnancy with cell division, which results in an extra copy of chromosome 21 (see *Figure 6-11*). The CDC estimates that 1 out of every 691 babies born in the United States has Down syndrome, which results in approximately 6,000 births per year (www.cdc.gov/ncbddd/birthdefects/DownSyndrome.html). This number is lower for young mothers and higher for women over age 35. It is possible to identify a fetus with Down syndrome through a procedure referred to as amniocentesis. Additional tests examine DNA material and are referred to as noninvasive prenatal testing. Brand names of this test include Harmony Prenatal Test and MaterniT21 PLUS. These tests are recommended in the United States and parts of Europe for pregnant women over the age of 35.

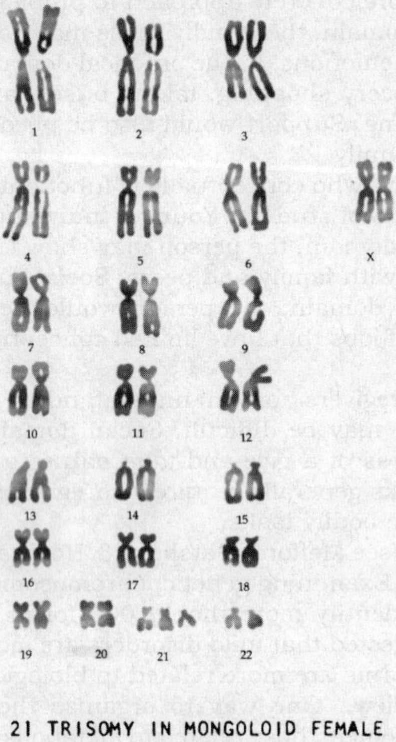

FIGURE 6-11 Karyotype From a Female With Down Syndrome

Source: © Leonard Lessin / Science Source.

Another chromosome disorder that results in IDD is called **fragile X syndrome.** This results from a particular gene, the FMR1, producing too little of a protein needed for brain development. As the name implies, this takes place on a fragile area of the X chromosome. Since males have only one X chromosome, they show more severe problems than females with the disorder. The symptoms include problems in intellectual development, emotional outbursts, and delays in motor development. Current estimates by the CDC are that about 1 in 4,000 males and 1 in 6,000 to 8,000 females have the disorder.

Intellectual Developmental Disorder Related to Metabolism

Phenylketonuria (PKU) is a situation in which a particular liver enzyme does not function correctly. This, in turn, can lead to IDD by preventing myelination of the neurons in the brain. Fortunately, the disorder can be treated through diet by restricting foods such as milk and eggs that contain phenylalanine. In the United States, mandated testing for PKU at birth is required for all infants using a blood test. The disorder appears to be carried by a recessive gene. Thus, both parents must have the gene for the disorder to appear.

Intellectual Developmental Disorder Related to Gestation

The period from conception to birth is a critical one for the fetus. Some researchers see morning sickness as a natural way in which the fetus is protected. That is, this period in which a pregnant woman is sensitive to a variety of foods and feels nauseous and vomits reduces potential danger to the fetus. However, it is possible for the mother to engage in substance abuse, experience malnutrition, or have an infection that can lead to a number of disorders including IDD. Prevention is designed to reduce environmental risk factors in pregnant women.

The extent to which there are intellectual, emotional, or motor deficits is largely related to the degree of exposure the fetus experiences. Greater exposure may lead to a miscarriage or stillbirth. Less exposure may lead to fewer developmental problems. Maternal malnutrition such as iron, zinc, or iodine deficiency will lead to slower developmental processes. Iodine deficiency results in a disorder known as cretinism. Children with this disorder show slower development including cognitive processes. This disorder is less common today with the addition of iodine to table salt. Substance abuse on the part of the mother can also influence the child's developmental processes. Alcohol, for example, will enter the fetus's bloodstream. Heavy use of alcohol will result in fetal alcohol syndrome (FAS), which includes low birth weight, lower intellectual functioning, and problems with cognitive processes such as attention and memory. Likewise, the use of cocaine leads to a phenomenon known as "crack babies" in which the child has problems with language and other cognitive processes. Finally, a variety of infections put the fetus at risk for later developmental problems.

Treatment of Intellectual Developmental Disorder

Treatment for individuals with IDD takes place on a number of levels and varies by age. In the middle of the last century, it was not uncommon for the child to be placed in a state school for the mentally retarded. This was a residential institution in which children would spend most of their lives. Today, most of these state institutions have been closed. In the 1970s, laws were passed that gave people with IDD the right to receive their treatment in the least restrictive setting.

Depending on the level of function of the child, there are a large number of alternatives. With those individuals who have difficulty performing daily tasks, some communities have residential programs that are run by nonprofit agencies designed to help individuals learn how to function and perform these daily tasks. Often behavioral techniques are used to teach the child to learn to use a spoon and fork to eat or how to dress herself. The settings of these residential programs look more like houses with rooms than the large institutional settings of the last century.

Children who are able to function at a higher level typically live at home with their parents or in a foster setting. A number of treatment programs have been set up to help the caregiver learn techniques for educating and managing a child with IDD. For example, some children show angry outbursts with the need to be managed. As the child becomes older, the school system becomes involved in the child's education. Schools in the United States have special education programs designed to help children with developmental disorders. Some school systems place higher functioning individuals into regular classrooms, a process referred to as mainstreaming. As the child becomes older, some school systems teach the child not only traditional educational material but also life skills. Such skills could include how to buy a candy bar or toothpaste in a store or ride a bus. Programs such as the Special Olympics also involve such life skill techniques as practicing for an event, competing, and learning to be with others.

Young adults with IDD are often helped to learn how to be part of a workplace either through a sheltered workshop or jobs in the community. It is estimated that about one third of all adults with IDD are employed. These individuals are covered by the Americans with Disabilities Act (see www.eeoc.gov/facts/intellectual_disabilities.html). Some communities have created apartments with a live-in coach to help these individuals function in practicing life skills and performing successfully at work. This can include helping the person know how to buy food, put their payroll check in the bank, use an ATM, and get to work on time.

Although medications are not generally given to children and adults with IDD, there are exceptions. If the child is aggressive or seeks to hurt himself, then neuroleptic medications may be used. If the child shows patterns of seizure, then epileptic medications are appropriate. There are also new medications being developed to modify the lack of protein production with fragile X syndrome. Other biochemical changes are produced by modifying the diet of those with PKU.

Concept Check

- What are the *DSM–5* diagnostic criteria for a specific learning disorder, also known as a learning disability?
- What three criteria define an IDD?
- What are the three primary causal categories into which IDD is organized, and what is an example of each?

Several Consensus guidelines operative in India have been developed and published by the Indian Academy of Pediatrics for the evaluation and management of ADHD (Dalwai et al., 2017a), ASD (Dalwai et al., 2017b) and LD (Nair et al., 2017). Interestingly, sensory disabilities such as hearing impairment has also been looked at, and similar guidelines are developed for Newborn Hearing screening (Paul et al., 2017).

Several groups, including the apex All India Institute of Speech and Hearing (AIISH), Mysore, the Ali Yavar Jung National Institute of Speech and Hearing Disabilities (Divyangjan) (AYJNISHD) at Bandra, Mumbai, also do a lot of promotional work to build awareness about hearing impairment and its developmental impact, the cognitive, behavioral and emotional comorbidities that may emerge.

SUMMARY

Unlike some other species, humans are born into a world in which they cannot survive alone. In fact, human infants are born in an undeveloped state. Every infant learns to talk and walk at a different rate and express emotions at a different rate. There are a number of sensitive periods in which disruptions can lead to long-term effects—for example, interrupting the normal caregiving patterns. Other sensitive developmental periods are directly related to the brain and to the turning on and off of genes. Current research has shown detrimental effects on both physical and mental conditions in relation to physical and sexual abuse, neglect, and exposure to domestic violence, as well as having a parent who is depressed. Attachment patterns are part of a larger overall developmental sequence that can be considered in the development of psychopathology. Since attachment patterns tend to be stable, the effects they portray can be cumulative. Research has shown children with insecure patterns of attachment to be at risk for several forms of childhood psychopathology. Three problematic attachment patterns have been identified in addition to the normal secure attachment pattern: (1) avoidant, (2) anxious or ambivalent, and (3) disorganized or controlling. In terms of *DSM* disorders, early life stress increases the risk for a behavioral disorder by 40% and a fear disorder by 15%. Stress and adversity can have a greater impact on changes in childhood and adolescence than later in adulthood.

Although brain changes can take place at any point in development, there are two critical periods in which the brain is more sensitive to external and internal factors: (1) the period during gestation and infancy when the cortical connections are initially being organized and (2) adolescence when the brain reorganizes itself. Understanding when brain changes take place in development or whether specific genetic factors prevent normal pathways from being developed is crucial to understanding the nature of developmental psychopathologies. Mental health professionals have a difficult task in determining what might just be delayed development in certain skills and what represents a developmental disorder. Treatment can influence greatly the course of development of the individual. In general, the criteria for diagnosis of a developmental disorder are in terms of severity, duration, pervasiveness, and degree of impairment.

The brain's mirror neuron system offers a basis of imitation learning and understanding of another's actions. This network helps the organism understand not only "what" others are doing but also "why" they are doing it. By having my brain work similarly to another's brain, I have some understanding of what he or she is experiencing. It has also been suggested that the mirror neurons lead not only to an understanding of another's actions but also to empathy. The mirror neuron system can be seen as part of a larger cortical network that relates to person perception and feelings toward another. This, in turn, could form the basis of interpersonal relationships and more complex social interactions. Theory of mind is the study of one's ability to understand one's own or another person's mental state. Delays in the development of theory of mind are seen in children with autism spectrum disorder.

Adolescence is a time of great change. It also marks the peak onset of many psychopathologies including anxiety and mood disorders, eating disorders, personality disorders, substance abuse, and psychosis. Research suggests that from childhood to adulthood, the brain goes from a largely undifferentiated system to one composed of specialized neural networks. Adolescence has been characterized as a time in which an individual moves from a more family oriented frame of reference to one of peer relations. Risk taking can play both direct and indirect roles in adolescence in relation to psychopathology. In addition, one of the hallmarks of adolescence risk is that it is more likely to occur in the presence of peers. Our present-day emotionality has largely evolved within a social context. Brain structures involved in social interactions can be organized in terms of three processes: (1) higher-level neocortical regions process sensory information; (2) our affective system helps us predict what people will do socially; and (3) higher cortical regions of the neocortex are involved in cognitive understanding and regulation and let us construct an inner model of our social world and are most likely associated with theory of mind.

DSM–5 describes disorders of childhood in a number of separate categories. This chapter emphasizes three: (1) trauma- and stressor-related disorders, including disorders of attachment; (2) neurodevelopmental disorders, including the autism spectrum disorders, ADHD, disorders of learning, intelligence, and communication, as well as motor disorders such as tics and Tourette's disorder; (3) disruptive, impulse control, and conduct disorders. There are two attachment disorders: (1) RAD, in which the child does not seek comfort or support from a traditional attachment figure when distressed and will not accept comfort when offered; and (2) disinhibited social engagement disorder, in which the child is willing to accept strangers who are not attachment figures. These two disorders have not been studied empirically in terms of treatment procedures, which typically have focused on helping the child develop a relationship with a caregiver.

Autism spectrum disorders are a group of neurodevelopmental disorders in which individuals have difficulty in three separate areas: (1) social interactions, (2) communication, and (3) behavioral processes. *DSM–5* includes what were previously separate disorders—autistic disorder, Asperger's disorder, and a general pervasive developmental disorder—as part of autism spectrum disorders. Individuals with Asperger's syndrome tend to be more intelligent and display higher functioning in terms of social processes than those diagnosed with autism. Developmentally, symptoms of autism are generally not seen until 8 to 12 months of age. Infants with autism show a non-normal pattern of growth of the head. Autism has been shown to have a strong genetic component. Environmental factors such as the age of the mother and father show a complex relationship to autism. Current neuroscience studies show that by the time of full brain development, a person with autism shows deficits in the areas that make up the social brain. Current estimates suggest that around 1 in every 100 children have the disorder with it being more common in boys than in girls. It is estimated that about 10% of individuals with autism spectrum disorder have special abilities in terms of music, art, calculation, or memory called the savant syndrome. An empirically supported treatment for autism, first developed by Lovaas and his colleagues at UCLA, has five stages of treatment lasting for a total of about 3 years: (1) establishing a teaching relationship, (2) teaching foundational skills, (3) focusing on beginning communication, (4) continuing communication processes, and (5) helping the child adjust to school situations. Research has found a number of characteristics associated with successful treatment outcomes: (1) earlier age at which treatment was begun; (2) higher IQ; (3) early intervention in language skills, communication, and peer relationships; and (4) reduction in negative behaviors. In addition to psychosocial treatment approaches, medications have been used to address specific disruptive behaviors seen in autism, but typically only in older children.

ADHD is a disorder of childhood that includes two major dimensions: (1) inattention and (2) hyperactivity and impulsivity. Individuals with ADHD can also show characteristics of both inattention and hyperactivity. ADHD is reported to be the most common emotional/behavioral disorder treated in youth. Epidemiological studies have also shown a comorbidity of ADHD with a variety of other disorders. Children and adolescents with ADHD showed problems in a variety of cognitive processes, including verbal working memory, spatial working memory, response inhibition, cognitive flexibility, vigilance, and planning. There is evidence to suggest that ADHD is influenced by genetic components. The major treatment for ADHD is stimulant medications. Psychosocial treatments, particularly involving parents, are often used in combination with medication with the best treatment results seen with a combination of both.

Children and adolescents with CD display extreme behaviors that reflect little regard for those around them and violate the rules of society. The behaviors associated with CD also lead to problems in other areas such as academic achievement and interpersonal relationships. Children who mainly show anger and defiance but do not act aggressively toward other people or animals or destroy property are described as having ODD. The *DSM–5* diagnostic criteria for both CD and ODD are based on observed behaviors rather than internal processes. Similar treatments have been developed for the treatment of CD and ODD. Empirically supported interventions and treatment for young children with oppositional behavior patterns are largely family based; one approach is PRIDE. Treatment approaches with older children and adolescents may also be conducted in clinic, inpatient, or correctional facilities. Empirically supported approaches include MST and PSST.

Learning disabilities (called specific learning disorder in *DSM–5*) refer to the situation in which a child's achievement is lower than that expected from his or her scores on achievement or intelligence tests. An IDD is defined by three aspects: (1) a deficit in mental abilities, (2) a lack of adaptive functioning in relation to one's age and sociocultural background, and (3) onset of the disabilities prior to adolescence. Problems with intellectual development are considered to occur on a continuum described in terms of mild, moderate, and severe levels of disability. Most types of IDD can be traced to biological causes although the variation is large. One way to organize these disorders is in terms of those directly related to chromosomes, those related to metabolism, and those related to gestation. The most common form of IDD is Down syndrome, which occurs during pregnancy from a chromosomal abnormality. Treatment for individuals with IDD takes place on a number of levels and varies by age and level of functioning.

STUDY RESOURCES

Review Questions

1. Unlike some other species, humans are born into a world in which they cannot survive alone. What implications does this have for normal psychological development as well as for the impact of early disruptions in the developmental process?
2. Given that adolescence marks the peak onset of many psychopathologies, what specific education or treatment programs would you recommend to target adolescent audiences?
3. What is the significance of "spectrum" in the term *autism spectrum disorders*? Why did *DSM–5* group previously separate disorders under this one characterization? How does it help us better understand the disorders in terms of causes, diagnostic criteria, and treatments? What are the disadvantages of grouping the disorders as a spectrum?
4. Childhood disorders have been grouped into externalizing and internalizing disorders. What characterizes these two groupings and how does that help us understand the disorders presented in this chapter?
5. What are the primary differences between specific learning disorders and IDDs in terms of causes, diagnostic criteria, and treatments?

For Further Reading

Grandin, T. (2002, May 6). Myself. *Time, 159*(18), 56.
Robison, J. (2007). *Look me in the eye: My life with Asperger's.* New York: Crown Publishers.

Key Terms and Concepts

anxious/ambivalent attachment pattern
Asperger's syndrome
attachment
attention deficit/hyperactivity disorder (ADHD)
autism spectrum disorders
avoidant attachment pattern
conduct disorder (CD)
disinhibited social engagement disorder

- disorganized/controlling attachment pattern
- disruptive, impulse control, and conduct disorders
- Down syndrome
- empathizing-systemizing theory of autism
- externalizing disorders
- fragile X syndrome
- imitation learning
- Individuals with Disabilities Education Act (IDEA)
- intellectual developmental disorder (IDD)
- internalizing disorders
- learning disabilities
- mental retardation
- mirror neurons
- neurodevelopmental disorders
- oppositional defiant disorder (ODD)
- reactive attachment disorder (RAD)
- secure attachment pattern
- specific learning disorder
- theory of mind
- trauma- and stressor-related disorders

CHAPTER

7

Schizophrenia

CHAPTER OUTLINE

- EXPERIENCE 232
- SCHIZOPHRENIA 234
- POSITIVE AND NEGATIVE SYMPTOMS 234
- COURSE OF SCHIZOPHRENIA 237
- HISTORICAL PERSPECTIVE 238
- SUBTYPES OF SCHIZOPHRENIA? 239
- SCHIZOPHRENIA FROM AN EVOLUTIONARY PERSPECTIVE 242
- FACTORS IN THE DEVELOPMENT OF SCHIZOPHRENIA 244
- GENETIC FACTORS IN SCHIZOPHRENIA 245
- ENDOPHENOTYPES ASSOCIATED WITH SCHIZOPHRENIA 247
- SCHIZOPHRENIA AND BRAIN FUNCTION 249
- WHAT BRAIN CHANGES ARE SEEN IN SCHIZOPHRENIA? 252
- SCHIZOPHRENIA AND BRAIN NETWORKS 255
- NEUROTRANSMITTERS INVOLVED IN SCHIZOPHRENIA 257
- HOW ARE COGNITIVE PROCESSES CHANGED IN SCHIZOPHRENIA? 258
- SCHIZOPHRENIA AND THE EXPERIENCE OF EMOTIONS 259
- FACTS OF SCHIZOPHRENIA 259
- TREATING INDIVIDUALS WITH SCHIZOPHRENIA 260
- ANTIPSYCHOTIC MEDICATIONS 262
- PSYCHOSOCIAL INTERVENTIONS FOR SCHIZOPHRENIA 263
- SUMMARY 266
- STUDY RESOURCES 268

EXPERIENCE

An excellent Indian film titled 15 Park Avenue *is a good way to introduce to the reader what happens to a person with schizophrenia. The film begins with two sisters, Anjali and Mitali, affectionately called Mithi, searching for an address, 15 Park Avenue. Soon the viewer becomes aware that no such place exists, or if it does, it is only in somebody's imaginary world.*

This is indeed Mithi's life.... A strange world within worlds, containing a smattering of facts that truly exist and some that exist only in her head. Mithi's reality is that she has a husband and five children. The whole family, she reiterates, lives happily at 15 Park Avenue. Her "real" family, that is, Anjali and their ageing mother, looks after Mithi, assisted by a maidservant. Most others merely tolerate her.

Anjali's life as caregiver is also difficult. She is divorced, a professor and writer, and never gets a break from her fulltime job as caregiver to her younger sister. The latter may have a psychiatric ailment, but she is intelligent, and counters her sister's arguments with quick repartee. With a typical belief in black magic being the only solution, the maidservant gets a local healer to "cure" Mithi and Mithi gets cruelly beaten. "How would you like it if I told you, you're not a professor, only imagining it?" Mithi asks her, rendering Anjali speechless.

Mithi was to marry but was viciously gang raped and this stressor precipitated her schizophrenia. Her fiancé cannot deal with the illness and leaves her, only to resurface later with a wife and children. Mithi, of course, believes she is married to him all along, in her private reality, and blithely takes him along to "search for 15 Park Avenue."

The ending of the film is moving and yet gracefully open to interpretation because the director is content to let Mithi get off the car in search for her home and "disappear," lost to our world and that of her companion. She is perhaps happy where she is, but no one can know.

Another, more "happy ending" local language film called Devrai *(Marathi, the state language of Maharashtra) is nevertheless more layered, more sensory and abstract, and less narrative in style. This is the story of a young man called Shesh Shahi a brilliant science scholar whose premorbid personality has been turbulent. Shesh lives in a village in the Konkan region of Maharashtra, India, and grows increasingly obsessed with a sacred grove which is to be destroyed to widen the road. There is an abstract parallel between the peace and harmony of the Devrai and the turbulent commotion of the real world that finds an echo in his disturbed mind. To add to the symbolism of the rape of the forest is the marriage of a beautiful village girl to a rough laborer.*

Shesh begins to hallucinate and build delusions around these themes and breaks down, becoming dependent on his rather clueless caregiver, younger sister, Seena, her husband who too is reluctantly dragged into caregiving, and a team of mental health professionals. The facile end sees an unmarried cousin becoming his caregiver back in the less complex village setting. The film is memorable for the seamless segues from city to forest, blending with the protagonist's visual and auditory hallucinations, and the sheer beauty of nature which becomes his sanctuary in the end.

In my fog of isolation and silence, I began to feel I was receiving commands to do things—such as walk all by myself through the old abandoned tunnels that lay underneath the hospital. The origin of the commands was unclear. In my mind, they were issued by some sort of beings. Not real people with names or faces, but shapeless, powerful beings that controlled me with thoughts (not voices) that had been placed in my head. Walk through the tunnels and repent. Now lie down and don't move. You must be still. You are evil.

From *The Center Cannot Hold: My Journey Through Madness* by Elyn Saks.

At the beginning of that summer, I felt well, a happy healthy girl—I thought—with a normal head and heart. By summer's end, I was sick, without any clear idea of what was happening to me or why. And as the Voices evolved into a full-scale illness, one that I only later learned was called schizophrenia, it snatched from me my tranquility, sometimes my self-possession, and very nearly my life.

Along the way I have lost many things: the career I might have pursued, the husband I might have married, the children I might have had. During the years when my friends were marrying, having their babies and moving into houses I once dreamed of living in, I have been behind locked doors, battling the Voices who took over my life without even asking my permission.

Sometimes these Voices have been dormant. Sometimes they have been overwhelming. At times over the years they have nearly destroyed me. Many times over the years I was ready to give up, believing they had won.

Today this illness, these Voices, are still part of my life. But it is I who have won, not they. A wonderful new drug, caring therapists, the support and love of my family and my own fierce battle—that I know now will never end—have all combined in a nearly miraculous way to enable me to master the illness that once mastered me.

Today, nearly eighteen years after that terrifying summer, I have a job, a car, an apartment of my own. I am making friends and dating. I am teaching classes at the very hospital at which I was once a patient.

I began to feel that my friends hated me. That's what the Voices said. I felt they regarded me as scum. That's what the Voices said too.

One weekend, Tara threw a big birthday party for Lori Winters, and invited a lot of her own friends from home. As they began arriving, I began feeling pressured. These people didn't like me. They were talking about me. They were going to start making fun of me. I didn't want to be around, so I jumped into my car and drove four hours home to New York. Then, I turned right around and drove back to Boston.

I spent my junior year abroad. While I was in Spain my first semester, the Voices were softer, but I was so revved up, my motor seemed to be working overtime. When the Voices did speak to me, sometimes they did so in Spanish: "Puta! Puta!" they yelled. "Vaya con el diablo." Go to hell, whore.

From THE QUIET ROOM by Lori Schiller and Amanda Bennett. By permissions of Grand Central Publishing.

Schizophrenia is one of the most debilitating of the mental disorders. It is part of a broad category of disorders referred to as **psychotic disorders.** Psychotic disorders involve a loss of being in touch with reality and are characterized by abnormal thinking and sensory processes. People who do not have schizophrenia may show psychotic symptoms for a brief period of time or for a longer duration. They may also show **delusions,** affective problems outside the normal range, or simply seem odd to those around them. Psychotic symptoms not part of schizophrenia can be induced through drugs and other medical conditions. The *Diagnostic and Statistical Manual of Mental Disorders (DSM)* describes these conditions separately from schizophrenia. This chapter will focus on schizophrenia.

Schizophrenia affects one's ability to express oneself clearly, to have close social relationships, to express positive emotions, and to plan for the future. Not everyone with schizophrenia displays the same symptoms. Individuals with schizophrenia may hear voices, see images not seen by others, believe that others wish to harm or control them, and have bizarre thoughts. The most common set of symptoms seen in individuals with schizophrenia over the past 100 years is a belief that others are out to get them and the hearing of voices that others do not hear (Insel, 2010).

Individuals with schizophrenia can display problems in terms of cognitive processes, emotional processes, and motor processes. Cognitive problems can be seen as a disorganization of thinking and behavior. In listening to a person with schizophrenia, you may note a speech style that although detailed does not seem to have a coherent focus and does seem to constantly change themes. Technically, these are referred to as *circumstantiality* and *tangentiality*. In more severe cases, the speech is actually incoherent and contains a stream of words that are unrelated to one another, which is referred to as *word salad*.

Mood symptoms include impairments in affective experience and expression. Depression is a common experience with schizophrenia along with thoughts of suicide. A number of individuals with schizophrenia hear voices that tell them to kill themselves. Ken Steele's voices told him "Hang yourself. The world will be better off. You're no good, no good at all" (Steele & Berman, 2001). Motor symptoms can range from repetitive behaviors such as rocking to total stiffness or lack of change in posture referred to as *catatonia*.

SCHIZOPHRENIA

Some studies place the incidence closer to 1.4%, cited by Graham Thornicroft (2011) as varying between 0.4% and 1.4%.

Schizophrenia affects about 1% of the population. It is seen throughout the world with similar symptoms regardless of culture or geographical location. Onset of schizophrenia occurs in the late teens or early 20s. Males show an earlier onset than females of about 5 years. Some individuals with schizophrenia display the symptoms throughout their life. However, there is a subgroup of individuals who, a few years after the initial display of symptoms, show a lack of symptoms even without treatment (see Jobe & Harrow, 2010, for an overview). Even with symptoms, some individuals are able to be part of the social and economic world experienced by healthy individuals. In fact, two of the individuals whose self-reports begin this chapter work at major universities in the United States.

The symptoms of schizophrenia are not constantly present. There are examples of individuals with schizophrenia who were able to finish college and maintain jobs. Thus, individuals with schizophrenia may show periods in which they are able to function in terms of external realities. Symptoms for some people tend to appear in times of change or stress. Different individuals with schizophrenia may show very different symptoms. For example, some individuals may hear voices but never see a visual hallucination. Others show a still different presentation of symptoms. This has led some researchers to suggest that there exist a variety of similar disorders that are currently described by the term *schizophrenia*.

POSITIVE AND NEGATIVE SYMPTOMS

Based on initial descriptions used by Hughlings Jackson in the 1800s, symptoms are referred to as positive or negative (Jackson, 1932). The more familiar **positive symptoms** are **hallucinations,** delusions, disorganized thinking, and disorganized behavior. The more familiar **negative symptoms** include lack of affect in situations that call for it, poor motivation, and social withdrawal. Jackson saw positive symptoms as reflecting a lack of high cortical control over more primitive brain processes. Negative symptoms, on the other hand, were the result of loss of function—what today we would refer to as a dysfunctional network of the brain. Positive or negative are not evaluative terms but rather indicate whether the symptom represents the manifestation of a process such as hearing voices or seeing hallucinations, which would be positive symptoms, or the lack of a normal human process such as poor motivation or social withdrawal, which would be negative symptoms.

Positive Symptoms

Hallucinations are sensory experiences that can involve any of the senses although auditory hallucinations are the ones most commonly reported by individuals with schizophrenia. The two examples of hallucinations presented at the beginning of this chapter illustrate the unusual experiences that individuals with schizophrenia can have. Ken Steele, while listening to music on the radio, heard it tell him to kill himself. Richard McLean picked up a phone to hear voices tell him that they were following his every move. These auditory hallucinations were experienced as coming from outside the person. Other individuals experience the voices or thoughts as coming from within their head. Individuals with schizophrenia report that they may hear voices throughout the day and on more than one day.

Of course, it is common for people to mistakenly believe that they heard someone call their name or that the phone rang while they were taking a shower. It is also common to mistake a stick on a path in the woods for a snake or to imagine an experience while falling asleep. These experiences are different from true hallucinations in that we check to see what the reality of the situation is or whether we are mistaken. Individuals with schizophrenia treat their hallucinations as real. In hallucinations in which individuals are instructed to perform an act, it is suggested that the instructions are obeyed by some 40% of people (Junginger, 1990). It should be noted that hallucinations can be produced by other disorders, such as Charles Bonnet syndrome, or the medications used to treat Parkinson's disease. In these situations, the person experiences the hallucination but generally knows that it is not real.

Delusions are beliefs without support for their occurrence and which are at odds with the individual's current environment. One hospitalized patient believed that the CIA had cameras in the drawer pulls of her dresser. Elyn Saks, whose story was presented at the beginning of this chapter, believed that powerful individuals could put thoughts in her head. John Hinckley, who tried to kill President Ronald Reagan, believed that Jodie Foster, the actress, would be impressed by this event. Another patient believed that God spoke to her when the dogs outside her house barked.

The most common delusions can be organized into categories. The first is persecution. This is the belief that other people or groups such as the CIA are plotting against the individual. John Nash wrote letters to the U.S. government describing attempts of others to take over the world. The second category is grandeur. This is the belief that one is really a very famous person. The individual with schizophrenia may tell everyone that he is Jesus or some other famous figure. The third delusion is control. As in the case of Elyn Saks, the delusion is that someone or some entity such as aliens can put thoughts into one's mind. A related delusion is that others can hear or understand your thoughts

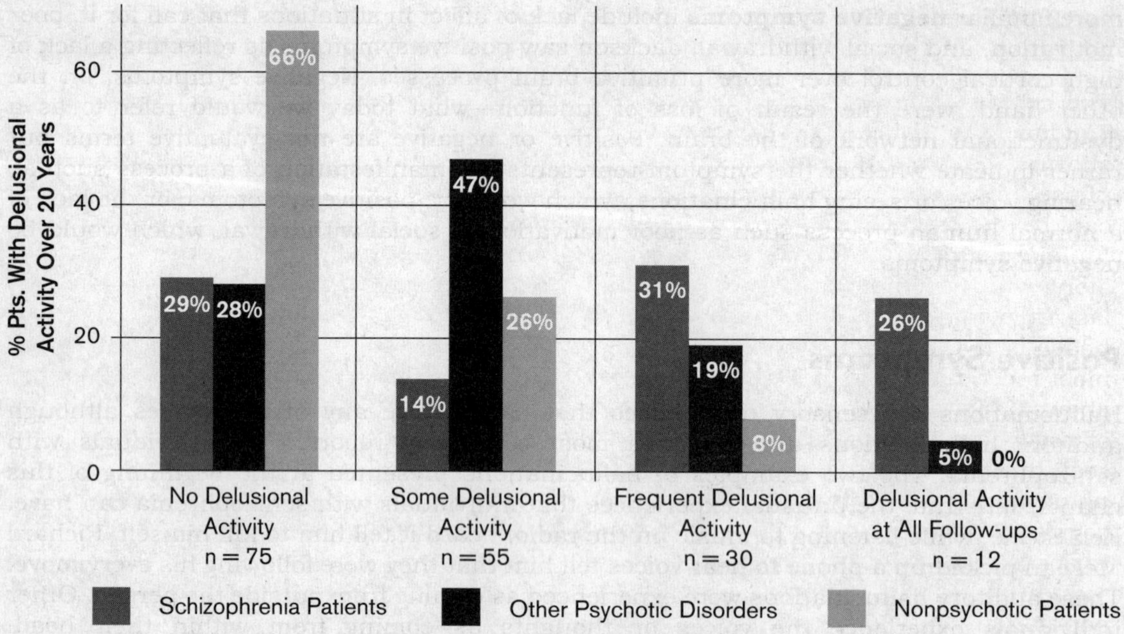

FIGURE 7-1 Presence of Delusional Activity Over a 20-Year Period

Source: Martin Harrow and Thomas H. Jobe, "How Frequent is Chronic Multiyear Delusional Activity and Recovery in Schizophrenia: A 20-Year Multi–follow-up," *Schizophrenia Bulletin* (2010) 36(1): 192–204, by permission of Oxford University Press.

without being told what they are. Finally, one common delusion is that one is special and that god or important individuals are speaking directly to the person.

Long-term delusional activity varies with the individual. In one study, individuals with schizophrenia were assessed 6 times over a 20-year period (Harrow & Jobe, 2010). Twenty-nine percent of those 43 individuals had no delusional activity over the 20 years, another 26% displayed delusions at each of the six assessments, and the remaining individuals had some delusions (see *Figure 7-1*).

Negative Symptoms

Negative symptoms seen in schizophrenia tend to be more constant and stable than positive symptoms. Several studies have linked negative symptoms with a poorer prognosis (see Foussias & Remington, 2010, for a review). Whereas it is usually the positive symptoms that result in a diagnosis of schizophrenia, it is the negative symptoms that tend to persist over time. Many individuals with schizophrenia have little interest in doing simple day-to-day activities such as taking a bath or shopping for food. This lack of will or volition is technically referred to as **avolition.** Individuals with schizophrenia also show a lack of interest in talking with others or answering questions with more than a one- or two-word answer. This is referred to as **alogia.** They also show a flattening of affect or difficulty expressing emotion. Another symptom is referred to as **anhedonia** or the inability to experience pleasure.

COURSE OF SCHIZOPHRENIA

The course of schizophrenia generally begins in adolescence or young adulthood (see Tandon, Nasrallah, & Keshavan, 2009, for an overview). The course of the disorder is shown in *Figure 7-2*. The initial phase is referred to as the *premorbid phase*. During this phase, only subtle or nonspecific problems with cognition, motor, or social functioning can be detected. These are accompanied by poor academic achievement and social functioning. This is followed by a *prodromal phase* in which initial positive symptoms along with declining functioning can be seen. From prospective studies, this phase can last from a few months to years with the mean duration being about 5 years. The next phase is the *psychotic phase,* where the positive psychotic symptoms are apparent. For most individuals, this phase occurs between 15 and 45 years of age with the onset being about 5 years earlier in males than females. This phase is marked by repeated episodes of psychosis with remission in between. The greatest decline in functioning is generally seen during the first 5 years after the initial episode. This phase is followed by a *stable phase* characterized by fewer positive symptoms and an increase in negative ones. Stable cognitive and social deficits also characterize this phase. The actual course of the disorder varies greatly across individuals.

Individuals with schizophrenia tend to die earlier than those their age in the general population. These higher age standardized mortality rates are approximately double those of the general population. The life span of individuals with schizophrenia is abbreviated by 15 to 20 years. Of this abbreviated life span, approximately 25% can be attributed to suicide and 10% to accidents. The remainder is related to medical conditions with cardiovascular disease contributing the most.

One of the major differences in schizophrenia care between the Western world and India is the managed care provided in the West vs institutionalized care that is still provided in India through large residential care institutions run by the government.

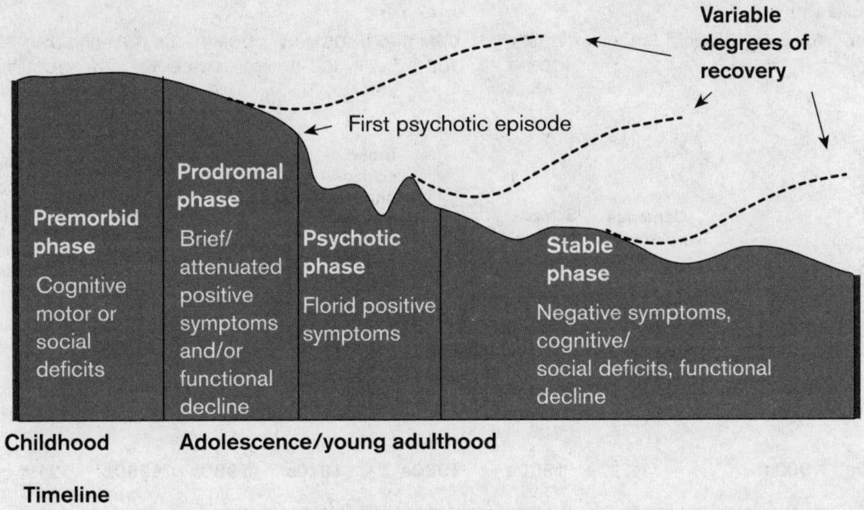

FIGURE 7-2 Natural History and Course of Schizophrenia

Source: Tandon et al. (2009, p. 8), with permission from Elsevier.

HISTORICAL PERSPECTIVE

Disorders with psychotic-like symptoms have been described for at least 4,000 years (see Tandon et al., 2009; Woo & Keatinge, 2008, for overviews). In addition, medical texts have been found throughout the ancient world that suggest that psychosis was present in all cultures. By the 1800s, the present-day terms of schizophrenia were being introduced. The German physician Ewald Hecker in the 1870s referred to a silly, undisciplined mind as "Hebephrenia," named after the Greek goddess of youth and frivolity, Hebe. *Figure 7-3* shows the evolution of the concept of schizophrenia.

In 1874, the German physician Karl Ludwig Kahlbaum used the terms *paranoid* and *catatonic.* Paranoid referred to the idea that someone felt him- or herself to be in danger. Catatonic referred to the mannequin-like muscle stiffness associated with unusual postures. In 1878, Emil Kraepelin combined these various disorders into a single disease entity, which he termed *dementia praecox* or *dementia of early onset.* The term *early* referred to the fact that schizophrenia developed early in life rather than the deterioration of mental functions associated with the dementias of old age. Overall, Kraepelin established what we now refer to as schizophrenia as a disorder with an onset in early

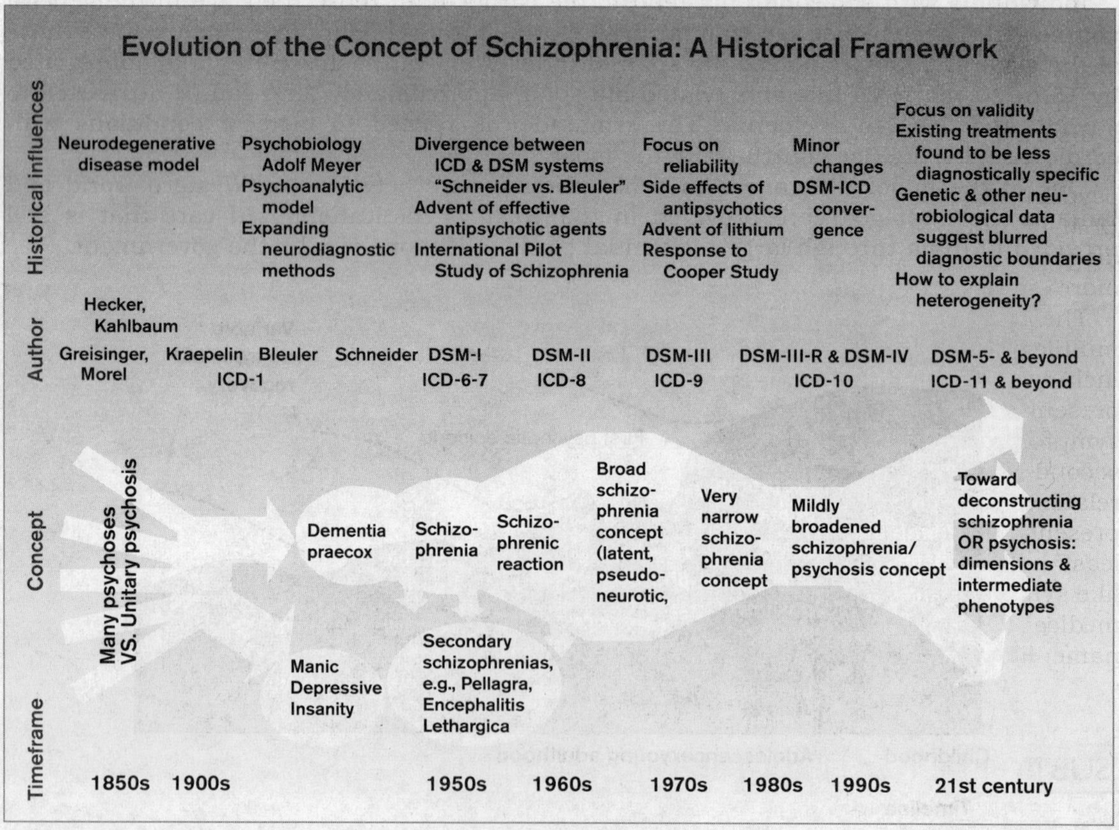

FIGURE 7-3 Evolution of the Concept of Schizophrenia

Source: Tandon et al. (2009, p. 3), with permission from Elsevier.

adulthood that shows chronic and deteriorating progression and results in pervasive impairments in mental functions over the life span.

Kraepelin suggested there were four subtypes of dementia praecox. The first was the simple type, which was characterized by a slow decline along with social withdrawal and apathy. The second type was paranoid characterized by fear of persecution. The third type was hebephrenic characterized by a mania-like presentation. The fourth type was catatonia characterized by a lack of movement. Kraepelin differentiated dementia praecox from what Falret in 1854 referred to as *folie circulaire*. Kraepelin referred to *folie circulaire* as manic-depressive insanity. Thus, Kraepelin established manic depression, which we refer to today as bipolar disorder, as a separate category from schizophrenia.

In 1911, Eugene Bleuler introduced the term *schizophrenia* from the Greek meaning to split the mind. Bleuler was critical of the term *dementia praecox* and suggested that there was not a single schizophrenia but a number of different disorders or schizophrenias with different etiologies and prognoses. There were, however, a series of characteristics described by Bleuler often referred to as the four *A*s.

1. *Affect*—Blunted or diminished emotional response
2. *Associations*—Loosening or inability to think in a logical manner
3. *Ambivalence*—Inability to make decisions
4. *Autism*—Social aloofness and an inability to remain in contact with the external world

In the 1950s, the *DSM* was introduced and described psychosis in broad terms as a disorder resulting in serious functional impairment. Schizophrenia was differentiated from organic disorders such as neurocognitive disorders (dementia), which may produce psychotic behaviors. By *DSM–III*, schizophrenia was defined by more explicit criteria. In *DSM–IV* and *DSM–IV–TR*, the criteria for schizophrenia were broadened. This made the diagnostic criteria used in the United States with *DSM* and Europe with the *ICD* system more similar, thus reducing the differential diagnosis rates in the two continents.

The text revision of the fourth edition of *DSM* (*DSM–IV–TR*) and *DSM–5* set forth a multilevel process for diagnosing schizophrenia. The first level is symptoms, which includes delusions, hallucinations, or disorganized speech. At least one of these must be present. In addition, abnormal psychomotor behaviors, such as catatonia, and negative symptoms, such as a lack of volition or social processing, may also be present. The second level is functioning. A reduction in functioning in the areas of work, interpersonal relations, and/or self-care should be present. The third level is duration in which the presence of the positive or negative symptoms should have existed for 6 months with at least 1 month of positive symptoms. The final levels are designed to rule out psychotic-like symptoms found in other disorders such as mania or depression or related to specific medical conditions such as drug abuse. The following case of James Stern (not his real name) illustrates difficulties in all three areas of functioning.

SUBTYPES OF SCHIZOPHRENIA?

Individuals with schizophrenia have a variety of different symptoms and show an inconsistent picture of the disorder. This has led some to suggest that there is not a single schizophrenia disorder but rather a variety of syndromes. Historically, one approach to

CASE OF JAMES STERN
Schizophrenia

James Stern is a 20-year-old, single, Caucasian male who is a full-time student at a nearby university where he also works part-time to offset living expenses. He resides off campus with three roommates, and has been in an off-again, on-again relationship with his girlfriend since high school. He first sought treatment at a local student counseling center for anxiety, depression, and general distress at the urging of his family, but was then referred for longer-term individual psychotherapy due to the increasing severity of symptoms that were described by his therapist as paranoid ideation, ideas of reference, increasing distress, and dysphoric affect. Mr. Stern confirmed that he began to experience symptoms that "others described as sounding paranoid" since high school, although he also reported that throughout his developmental years he felt a lack of connection with his family, and had few, if any close friends throughout his primary and secondary school years. While he noted that he was always somewhat suspicious and guarded, he also reported that these feelings became much more intense after he relocated to the current local university from a much smaller college near his hometown. During this same time period, James also reported that he became increasingly reliant on the daily use of marijuana to ease/cope with associated symptoms of anxiety and distress. He was eventually "forced" to eliminate his usage because of his growing realization that the marijuana magnified feelings of paranoia that resulted in isolating himself alone in his room for days amidst a growing suspiciousness that his roommates and classmates had been infiltrated by "dark forces" that posed an increasing threat to mankind. Following his cessation of marijuana use, James continued to struggle with perceptions that his professors were dropping surreptitious clues for him to decipher regarding the "dark forces" he still feared were infiltrating society and began to believe that those forces may have already "taken over" at least two of his roommates. At this point, his paranoia and fears about "evil forces" escalated rapidly, and he began to intermittently see "demons" moving among people. His distress elevated to the point he refused to leave his apartment bedroom, which forced his withdrawal from school and termination of employment. Mr. Stern has been diagnosed with Schizophrenia. Since beginning psychotherapy and pharmacotherapy, James has reported moderate to marked reductions in paranoia and distress although he continues to report intermittent suspiciousness and ongoing uncertainty about his future in multiple domains (e.g., relationship, academic, and career goals).

Clinical vignette provided by Sandra Testa Michelson, PhD

the variety of presentations seen in individuals with schizophrenia was to look for subtypes. As noted previously, Kraepelin suggested four subtypes. The fourth edition of *DSM* divided schizophrenia into five subtypes. These are paranoid, disorganized, catatonic, undifferentiated, and residual subtypes.

The **paranoid subtype** is characterized by delusions whose themes generally center on ideas of grandiosity or persecution. Individuals with this subtype might tell stories of how the FBI or CIA is out to get them and they must be constantly vigilant. Normal everyday activities such as a person with a camera or problems running a computer program would be interpreted as proof of the persecution. Others with the disorder might tell of how they have special powers, such as the ability to read someone's mind. The criterion for being diagnosed with this subtype excludes disorganized speech, disorganized or catatonic behavior, or flat or inappropriate affect. Overall, these individuals show the greatest possibility of improvement.

The **disorganized subtype,** which was previously referred to as *hebephrenic schizophrenia,* is characterized by disorganized speech patterns and behavior. Individuals with this subtype display odd speech patterns often referred to as word salad in which a variety of words are put together in incoherent ways. Affective responses also appear odd to others in that little affect is shown to what should be significant events. Instead, silly or childlike responses are shown almost randomly. Whereas individuals with the paranoid subtype tend to have a consistent theme to their delusions, individuals with the disorganized subtype do not.

The **catatonic subtype** is characterized by non-normal activity of the motor system. One classic symptom is referred to as *waxy flexibility* in that the individual will remain in a fixed position. If someone moves the individual's arms or legs, he or she will then remain in this new position. Motor movement can also be characterized by the opposite condition in which the individual shows excessive, purposeless activity of his or her motor system. Other possible manifestations of this subtype include the repeating of someone else's speech, referred to as *echolalia,* and the repeating of someone else's movements, referred to as *echopraxia.* Although these individuals may copy the speech or movements of others, they may not follow instructions and even refuse to speak.

Some researchers have suggested that catatonia should be considered a separate disorder and not part of the schizophrenia group (Fink, Shorter, & Taylor, 2010). Part of the support for this position is that these individuals do not respond as frequently to antipsychotic medication and about 70% respond to the drug lorazepam alone. Lorazepam is a benzodiazepine associated with relaxation and often given for treatment of anxiety disorders.

If an individual shows signs of schizophrenia but does not fit in any of the three major subtypes—paranoid, disorganized, or catatonic—then he or she would be diagnosed with *undifferentiated subtype.*

A final subtype is referred to as the *residual subtype.* These are individuals who have had schizophrenic episodes but no longer display the traditional positive symptoms of delusions and hallucinations. They may still display strange ideas or odd behaviors.

There has been considerable debate as to the value of using the five subtypes for diagnosis and treatment. Part of this debate is a larger question of whether schizophrenia should be considered in terms of discrete categories or existing along a dimension. If schizophrenia exists along a dimension, then it would be meaningless to consider categories or subtypes (Linscott, Allardyce, & van Os, 2010). An additional question is whether the subtype information is actually used in making diagnoses and designing treatment.

Although *ICD-10* uses subtypes, *DSM–5* removed the classification of subtypes but left the diagnostic criteria for schizophrenia almost identical to *DSM–IV–TR. DSM–5* also uses the subtype descriptions in classifying other psychotic disorders. The *DSM–5* criteria are shown in *Table 7-1.*

TABLE 7-1 *DSM–5* **Diagnostic Criteria for Schizophrenia**

A.	Characteristic symptoms: Two (or more) of the following, each present for a significant portion of time during a 1-month period (or less if successfully treated). At least one of these should include 1–3 1. Delusions. 2. Hallucinations. 3. Disorganized speech (e.g., frequent derailment or incoherence). 4. Grossly disorganized or catatonic behavior. 5. Negative symptoms (i.e., diminished emotional expression or avolition).
B.	Social/occupational dysfunction: For a significant portion of the time since the onset of the disturbance, levels of functioning in one or more major areas, such as work, interpersonal relations, or self-care is markedly below the level achieved prior to the onset (or when the onset is in childhood or adolescence, there is failure to achieve expected level of interpersonal, academic, or occupational functioning).
C.	Duration: Continuous signs of the disturbance persist for at least 6 months. This 6-month period must include at least 1 month of symptoms (or less if successfully treated) that meet Criterion A (i.e., active-phase symptoms) and may include periods of prodromal or residual symptoms. During these prodromal or residual periods, the signs of the disturbance may be manifested by only negative symptoms or two or more symptoms listed in Criterion A present in an attenuated form (e.g., odd beliefs, unusual perceptual experiences).
D.	Schizoaffective and mood disorder exclusion: Schizoaffective Disorder and Mood Disorder With Psychotic Features have been ruled out because either (1) no Major Depressive or Manic Episodes have occurred concurrently with the active phase symptoms; or (2) if mood episodes have occurred during active-phase symptoms, their total duration has been brief relative to the duration of the active and residual periods.
E.	Substance/general medical condition exclusion: The disturbance is not due to the direct physiological effects of a substance (e.g., a drug of abuse, a medication) or a general medical condition.
F.	Relationship to a pervasive developmental disorder: If there is a history of Autistic Disorder or another Pervasive Developmental Disorder or other communication disorder of childhood onset, the additional diagnosis of Schizophrenia is made only if prominent delusions or hallucinations are also present for at least a month (or less if successfully treated).

Source: Reprinted with permission from the *Diagnostic and Statistical Manual of Mental Disorders, Fifth Edition*, (Copyright 2013). American Psychiatric Association.

SCHIZOPHRENIA FROM AN EVOLUTIONARY PERSPECTIVE

There is an evolutionary paradox with schizophrenia (Huxley, Mayr, Osmond, & Hoffer, 1964)—individuals with schizophrenia have fewer children than others, and males with schizophrenia have even fewer children than females with schizophrenia. Given this situation, one would expect that the disorder would disappear over evolutionary time and the genes of individuals with schizophrenia would not be passed on to the next generation. This, however, is not the case. How can the disorder exist without a reproductive advantage? A number of suggestions have been made. One is that the genes associated with schizophrenia are also associated with positive traits such as creativity.

It has been noted that highly gifted and creative individuals manifest schizophrenic-like traits, referred to as **schizotypal traits,** without having the disorder. However, it is not uncommon for these individuals to have a first-degree relative with schizophrenia, suggesting a genetic component. Andreasen (2005) suggested there may be a connection with scientific creativity and schizophrenia within one's family. She noted that a number of Nobel laureates had family members who were thought to have schizophrenia, including Albert Einstein, Bertrand Russell, and John Nash himself. (As you may remember, John Nash's story was described in the film *A Beautiful Mind.*) But this still leaves open the question of how schizophrenia came about.

Two separate theories related to the evolutionary existence of schizophrenia were proposed by Tim Crow (2000) and Jonathan Burns (2004). Both of these theories note that schizophrenia is found throughout the world in approximately the same prevalence, and it is found in populations that have been separate from one another for at least 50,000 years. Since similar rates are seen in both industrialized and agrarian societies, this suggests that schizophrenia has existed as a part of the human experience since at least the time humans left Africa some 100,000 years ago. If it were a newer disorder, then one would expect to find different rates in populations of humans in different parts of the world.

Concept Check

- The symptoms of schizophrenia are characterized as positive symptoms and negative symptoms.
  - What is the definition of each symptom type?
  - What are primary examples of each type?
  - What role does each type play in the course of schizophrenia?
- How are the four stages of the course of schizophrenia defined, and when do they typically occur? Is the course the same for each individual? If not, how does it differ?
- What can we say about the prevalence of schizophrenia: Across history? Across the world? Across the life span? Across genders?
- *DSM* has set forth a multilevel process for diagnosing schizophrenia. What are the characteristics of each of the levels?
- What are the five subtypes of schizophrenia as defined by the previous edition of *DSM–IV*, and how are they characterized? How are they used in the current edition of *DSM–5*, and what led to the change?

Tim Crow (2000) suggested that the development of language and the genetic changes required for producing and understanding speech were associated with the development of schizophrenia. Since the time of both Broca and Hughlings Jackson in the 1800s, it has been known that the brain is lateralized with linguistic functions associated with left hemispheric networks. In 1879, Crichton-Browne (1879) suggested that since language processes evolved more recently than many other brain processes, these might be the first involved with mental disorders. Crow noted how one common positive symptom in schizophrenia around the world is the experience of hearing voices, which are experienced as separate from one's normal thought processes. This suggests a disruption in normal language processes resulting from incomplete differentiation of the hemispheres leading to a loss of the ability to differentiate thought and speech. Crow and his colleagues (Angrilli et al., 2009), using electroencephalography (EEG), showed that individuals with schizophrenia compared with normal controls failed to show a left hemispheric dominance when processing phonological information.

Jonathan Burns (2004) suggested that schizophrenia is better understood as a disorder of the social brain rather than language. For Burns, schizophrenia results from disordered connections from the frontal to temporal areas and the frontal to parietal areas, which are critical brain connections related to social functioning. Historically, schizophrenia for Burns exists as the result of a trade-off at two separate stages of cognitive evolution in humans.

The first trade-off occurred between 2 and 16 million years ago. It was during this period that our species evolved specialized neural processing and complex interconnections of the brain required to respond to group living. To perform the tasks required for social living, a higher level of cognitive functioning was required. In order for the brain to develop the circuits required, brain maturation was lengthened. That is, given the physical constraints of the developing brain in the human fetus, brain development needed to be lengthened. This trade-off meant that the developing brain experienced a long period of time in which complex gene interactions or accidents could happen.

The second trade-off for Burns happened more recently, about 100,000 to 150,000 years ago. This date is important. Since schizophrenia is seen in all cultures with similar symptoms, it is assumed that the genes involved in its manifestation would have evolved before humans migrated out of Africa. What happened at this point was that some individuals experienced non-normal connections in the frontal areas of the brain. These connections resulted in some individuals being especially creative and thinking in different ways. These individuals may have been able to make important contributions to culture much as our present-day artists and creative thinkers do. However, some individuals demonstrated a more severe version of these connections, which resulted in psychopathological experiences. Burns further suggested that this different way of experiencing the world in either its mild or severe form did not have any reproductive advantage. However, since the genes that controlled these experiences evolved as a part of the larger cortical networks needed for the cognitive and intellectual demands of social life, these genes continued to be passed on through their connections with adaptive mechanisms. Thus, according to Burns, schizophrenia represents one of the prices paid for evolving complex cognitive and social abilities. Further, it should be noted that ancient burial sites have bones of older individuals with various deformities. Since these individuals could not have survived without care from others, this suggests to some that individuals with schizophrenia-like symptoms may also have been cared for and made part of the community.

Interestingly, both these hypotheses point to two interesting and brain-based aspects of schizophrenia, namely, language production and comprehension and social behavior. It is these aspects of the condition that are complex to understand and decode, and those which require active and continuous rehabilitation and retraining as well as caregiver training to cope with abnormalities that persist in both these areas of functioning.

FACTORS IN THE DEVELOPMENT OF SCHIZOPHRENIA

Schizophrenia typically is first noted during the transition from late adolescence to adulthood. However, theories related to its development generally see its onset at this time as the manifestation of a process that may have begun before the individual was born (see Uhlhaas, 2011, for an overview). In a review of birth cohort studies in which individuals are followed from birth, there is evidence to suggest that children who later develop schizophrenia show different profiles from those who do not (Welham, Isohanni, Jones, & McGrath, 2009). These data from seven different countries show subtle deficits in terms of behavioral disturbances, intellectual and language deficits, and early motor delays.

The current research literature suggests that schizophrenia is a disorder that begins early in life. This has led some researchers to suggest that we consider schizophrenia as a neurodevelopmental disorder (Insel, 2010). A variety of negative events can happen to a fetus including infections and malnutrition. It has been shown, for example, that vitamin D deficiency during pregnancy can be seen as a risk for developing schizophrenia (see McGrath, Burne, Féron, Mackay-Sim, & Eyles, 2010, for a review). Likewise, maternal infection is now being seen as a potential risk factor for schizophrenia (see Brown & Patterson, 2011, for an overview).

Overall, the theory that development of schizophrenia involves events experienced during pregnancy is referred to as the *neurodevelopmental hypothesis*. The basic idea is that during the time the fetus is in utero an insult happens that influences the changes to the brain that take place during adolescence.

Weinberger (1987) was one of the originators of the neurodevelopmental view and suggested that problems during the second trimester lead to an incomplete development of frontal lobe networks in the brain during adolescence. Currently, the neurodevelopmental hypothesis is not completely developed. However, it has clearly been noted as an important period in brain development.

What can be described about the reorganization of brain processes during adolescence in relation to schizophrenia? Adolescence is a time of great reorganization of cortical networks. Gogtay, Vyas, Testa, Wood, and Pantelis (2011) reviewed two longitudinal studies with this question in mind. The first data set is composed of individuals who developed schizophrenia before puberty and has been studied at the National Institute of Mental Health (NIMH). The second data set is from Melbourne, Australia, and includes adolescents who are ultra-high risk for schizophrenia. Imaging studies showed larger ventricles and greater gray matter loss in the parietal and frontal areas in children who developed schizophrenia before puberty as compared with those who developed schizophrenia in adulthood. The data set from Australia showed that those adolescents who developed schizophrenia showed greater gray matter loss especially in the prefrontal cortex (PFC) as compared with those who did not develop the disorder.

Environmental factors can also play a role in the development of schizophrenia (see van Os, Kenis, & Rutten, 2010, for an overview). The basic idea is that environmental factors can influence the developing social brain and lead to the development of schizophrenia in those at risk. Such factors as early life adversity, growing up in an urban environment, and cannabis use have been associated with the development of schizophrenia. Being part of an ethnic group is not associated with schizophrenia per se if the ethnic group lives together, but if one is a minority in a larger ethnic group, then there is an association. Also, if one moves from an urban environment to a rural one, then the chance of having schizophrenia goes down. Overall, greater amounts of stress are associated with greater chances of developing schizophrenia.

GENETIC FACTORS IN SCHIZOPHRENIA

Since schizophrenia tends to run in families and is seen throughout the world, it is assumed to have a genetic component. That is to say, the risk of developing schizophrenia is much higher if someone else in your family also has the disorder. As can be seen in *Figure 7-4*, schizophrenia has a strong genetic component. The more similar the genes between two individuals, one of whom has schizophrenia, the more likely the other person will also develop its characteristics. However, the genetic underpinnings of schizophrenia

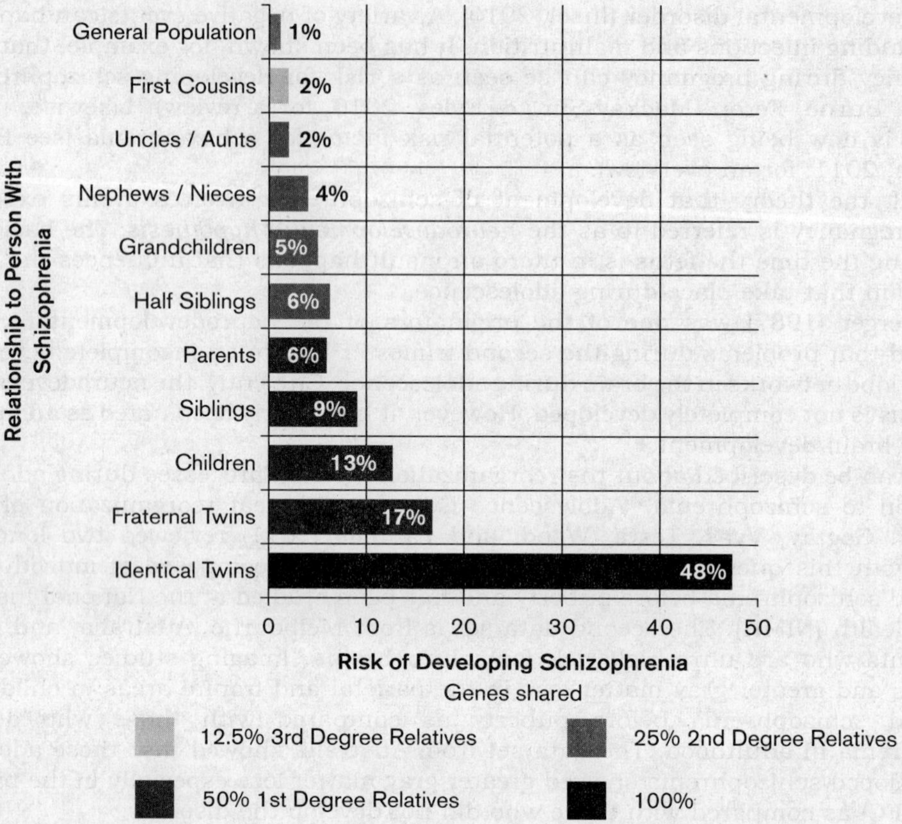

FIGURE 7-4 Graph Showing Strong Genetic Component of Schizophrenia

Source: From Figure 7-10 Graph from the book SCHIZOPHRENIA GENESIS: THE ORIGINS OF MADNESS by Irving I. Gottesman. Copyright 9c0 1990 by Irving I. Gottesman. Reprint by permission of Henry Holt and Company, LLC.

are not simple. It is clearly not the result of a single gene as with some other neurological disorders such as Huntington's disorder.

Research suggests that the number of genetic variants seen in individuals with schizophrenia is very large. There may be 1,000 different genes contributing to the disorder (Walker, Shapiro, Esterberg, & Trotman, 2010; Wray & Visscher, 2010). These genes may act in an additive or interactive manner to produce the disorder. That is to say, there may be a variety of genetic combinations that are associated with schizophrenia. In addition, individuals with schizophrenia compared with healthy controls show more abnormalities in their deoxyribonucleic acid (DNA) in the form of deletions or duplications of DNA sequences. Surprisingly, these gene abnormalities are even seen in the monozygotic (MZ) twin who develops schizophrenia as compared with the one who does not. This suggests that these abnormalities are the result of both inherited and non-inherited factors.

If schizophrenia were a totally inherited disorder, then if one MZ twin developed the disorder, the other would also. However, this is not the case. There are three factors that may be playing a role in this situation. First, as genes are reproduced during fetal and later development, there may be slight changes in one twin as compared with the other. These are referred to as *copy number variations.* Maiti, Kumar, Castellani, O'Reilly, and

Singh (2011) studied copy number variations in MZ twins from families with schizophrenia and found genetic differences in the twins. Second, differences in twins may not result from differences in the DNA itself but from the results of epigenetic factors in which genes of an affected individual may be turned on differently from those of a non-affected individual, suggesting that internal and external environmental factors play a role (King, St-Hilaire, & Heidkamp, 2010). And third, environmental factors may play a role that did not involve genetic changes.

Given the initial 48% concordance rate for MZ twins found in the 1990s, the obvious suggestion would be to consider the environment. Although environmental stress is known to exacerbate the disorder, there is little evidence that psychological stress can actually cause schizophrenia. Further, adopted children from families with schizophrenia show a similar rate to those raised with their natural families. This suggests that the manner in which individuals are reared is not directly related to the development of schizophrenia.

More recent work has suggested a role for poor maternal nutrition or infections during fetal periods. However, this work is also inconclusive. A recent review of the genetics of schizophrenia suggest a higher concordance rate for MZ twins and schizophrenia—82% (Rutter, 2006). Recent speculation suggests that epigenetics (see Chapter 3) may offer a more viable mechanism for the development of schizophrenia (Petronis, 2004). Another way to examine the genetic factor is to look at adolescents whose parents had schizophrenia. When compared with healthy controls, adolescents who did not have schizophrenia but whose parents did were shown to have dysfunctional interactions within cortical networks involved in emotional processing (Diwadkar et al., 2012).

ENDOPHENOTYPES ASSOCIATED WITH SCHIZOPHRENIA

Presently there is no one biomarker that can identify a person with schizophrenia. A number of researchers have sought to find endophenotypes (see Chapter 3) related to schizophrenia. These stable internal physiological or psychological markers associated with schizophrenia have been found in a variety of areas. In a review of the literature, which compared individuals with schizophrenia, their relatives, and healthy control individuals, endophenotypes were found in five major areas (Allen, Griss, Folley, Hawkins, & Pearlson, 2009).

- The first area is minor physical anomalies, which include differences in head or body size or motor movements.
- The second area of physiologic abnormalities is based on the membrane theory of schizophrenia. This theory suggests that normal metabolism in the brain is disturbed in individuals with schizophrenia.
- The third area is neuropsychological measures. Studies reviewed in this area include such measures as the Wisconsin Card Sorting Test (WCST), in which the person must respond to changing demands, and the Continuous Performance Task, which measures attentional abilities.
- The fourth area involves neuromotor abnormalities. One task is of smooth pursuit eye movement. Individuals with schizophrenia show a different pattern of eye movement if asked to follow a person's finger moving from right to left in front of them. Rather than showing a smooth motion of eye movement, they show periods of quick pursuit in which they attempt to catch up with the finger movement.

- The fifth area is sensory processing and event-related potentials. Numerous studies have shown EEG differences between individuals with schizophrenia and others. In response to cognitive tasks, the evoked potential waveform of P50, P300, and N400 were chosen for this review.

Neurocognitive endophenotype markers in unaffected first-degree relatives of schizophrenia are discussed in a study published by researchers from Rajasthan (Solanki et al., 2016). The study concluded that there is a significant difference between first-degree relatives of persons with schizophrenia and control subjects along parameters, including short-term memory, verbal auditory memory, verbal working memory, visuospatial working memory, and executive functions. Many studies also indicate that several neurological soft signs may be implicated, but a more conclusive research is needed.

Another interesting domain for research is the difficulties faced by persons with schizophrenia in tasks involving facial emotion recognition, which may emerge as a possible trait marker for the condition (Behere, 2015).

This finding also ties in well with the known social processing deficits in patients with schizophrenia.

As can be seen in *Figure 7-5*, individuals with schizophrenia and their first-degree relatives without schizophrenia show similar responses to tasks in the five areas. This suggests an endophenotype related to schizophrenia but not a definitive biomarker of the disorder.

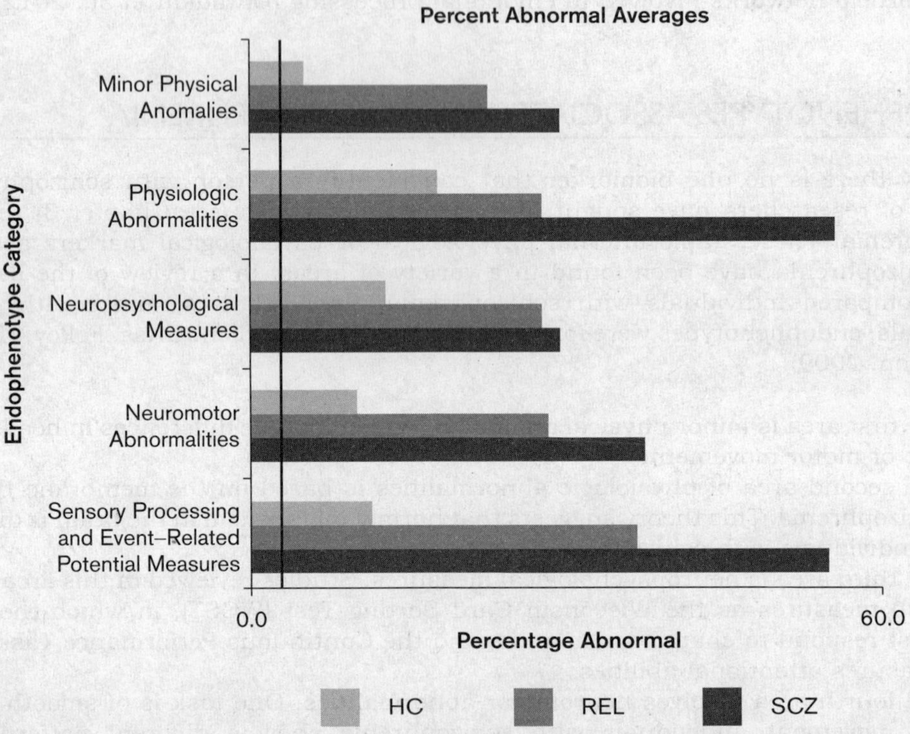

FIGURE 7-5 Average Percentage Abnormal for Each Endophenotype Category

Source: Allen et al. (2009, p. 31), with permission from Elsevier.
Note: HC = normal control; REL = relative; SCZ = schizophrenia.

Ventricle Changes in Schizophrenia

There are four ventricles in the brain (see *Figure 7-6*). These ventricles contain cerebrospinal fluid. From a number of studies, individuals with schizophrenia show larger ventricles (see Vita, de Peri, Silenzi, & Dieci, 2006, for a meta-analysis). Since the walls of the ventricles are not rigid, it is assumed that larger ventricles result from a decrease in volume in other areas of the brain. Some of the other areas that have been shown to be smaller in individuals with schizophrenia are the frontotemporal cortices, the anterior cingulate cortex (ACC), and the right insular cortex. One question is whether this reduction could be related to the medications that individuals with schizophrenia take. To answer this question, one study examined individuals with first episode schizophrenia and compared their brain structure with that of matched healthy controls (Rais et al., 2012). These researchers found brain volume loss in the individuals with schizophrenia. This suggests that the brain volume loss is present when symptoms begin. They found reduced volume in the temporal and insular cortex. *Figure 7-7* shows a larger ventricle in a twin who had schizophrenia and a smaller one in the one who did not.

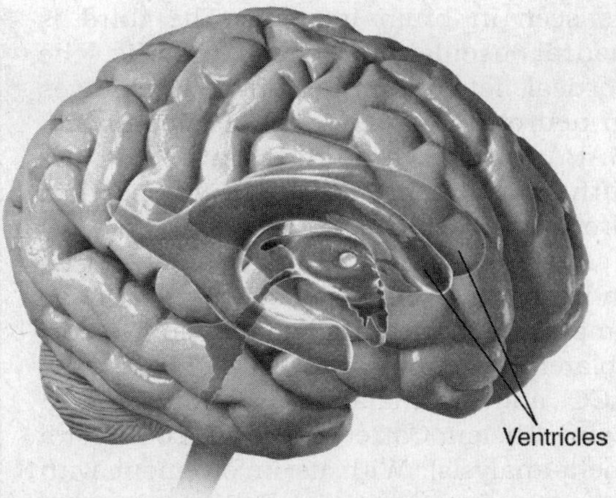

FIGURE 7-6 Location of Ventricles in the Brain

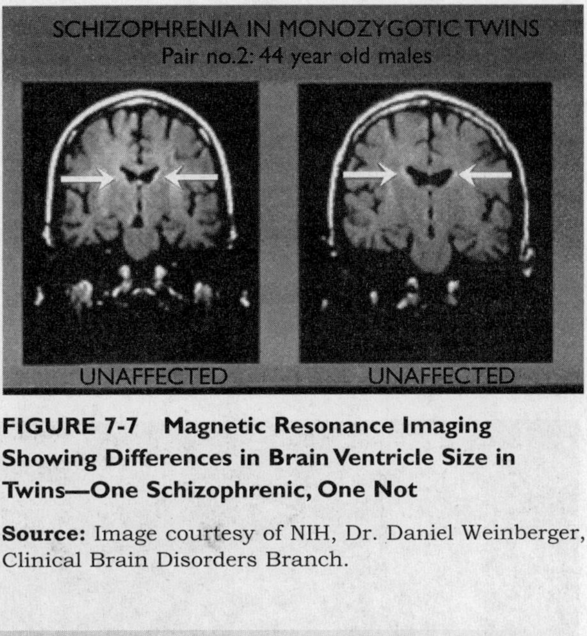

FIGURE 7-7 Magnetic Resonance Imaging Showing Differences in Brain Ventricle Size in Twins—One Schizophrenic, One Not

Source: Image courtesy of NIH, Dr. Daniel Weinberger, Clinical Brain Disorders Branch.

SCHIZOPHRENIA AND BRAIN FUNCTION

Schizophrenia manifests on a variety of levels including abnormal sensory experiences such as hallucinations, problems in cognitive processes such as delusions and disordered thought, changes in affect such as lack of expression, and in some cases problems with language and future directed planning. This presents a challenge to describe the manner in which brain processes relate to the disorder.

Current research examining individuals with schizophrenia has emphasized five different levels of analysis from a neuroscience perspective. The first is anatomical changes such as the loss of brain volume in particular areas. The second is functional processes such as the manner in which cortical areas and networks process information as seen in brain imaging. The third is neural oscillations that underlie the cortical networks. The fourth is changes in neurotransmitters such as **dopamine,** GABA, glycine, and **glutamate.** And the fifth is the development of cortical processes beginning in utero.

A variety of studies have shown that individuals with schizophrenia have emphasized differential activity in the dorsolateral prefrontal cortex (DLPFC), the ACC, and the thalamus (see Minzenberg, Laird, Thelen, Carter, & Glahn, 2009, for a meta-analysis). With its involvement with executive function tasks such as planning and social tasks, the frontal lobes have been extensively studied. When examining the entire brain and schizophrenia, other reviews point to enlargement of the ventricles and abnormalities of the medial temporal lobe structures, including the amygdala, hippocampus, and neocortical temporal lobe functions (see Shenton, Dickey, Frumin, & McCarley, 2001, for a review). More recent reviews point to a connection between the DLPFC and disorganized symptoms (Goghari, Sponheim, & MacDonald, 2009). Additionally, the ventrolateral prefrontal cortex (VLPFC) was associated with negative symptoms and medial prefrontal activity with positive symptoms (see *Figure 7-8*).

EEG reflects the electrical activity of the brain at the level of the synapse (Nunez & Srinivasan, 2006). It is the product of the changing excitatory and inhibitory currents at

Concept Check

- Describe the evolutionary paradox that schizophrenia presents. What different theories did Crow and Burns present to explain the paradox?
- Schizophrenia typically is first noted during the transition from late adolescence to adulthood, but current research suggests that the disorder begins early in life. What evidence points to this characterization?
- There is currently no one biomarker to identify an individual with schizophrenia. However, what internal physiological or psychological markers associated with schizophrenia suggest an endophenotype related to schizophrenia?
- Individuals with schizophrenia show larger ventricles in the brain. What do larger ventricles represent? When do they appear?

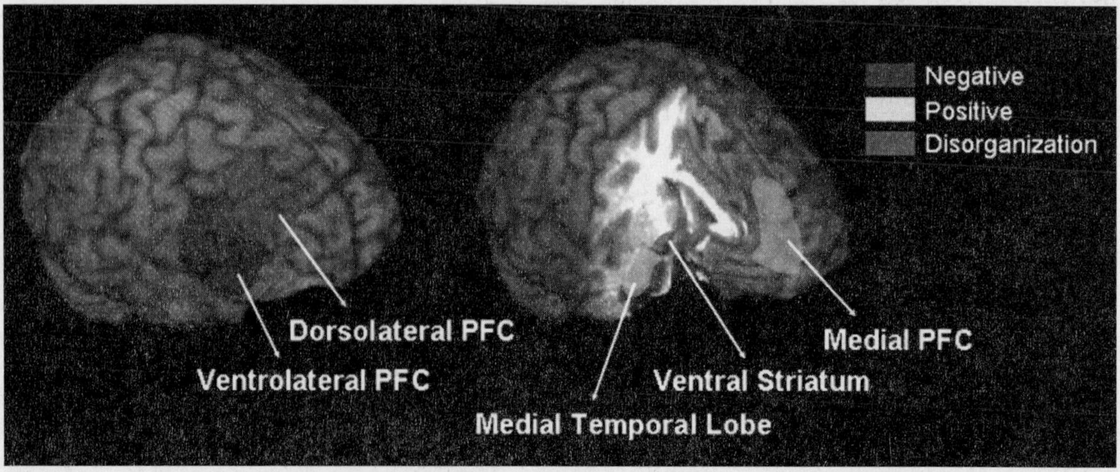

FIGURE 7-8 Differential Brain Activity Exhibited in Schizophrenia

Source: Goghari et al. (2009, p. 481), with permission from Elsevier.

TABLE 7-2 Electroencephalography Frequency Bands, Cognitive Processes, and Their Location in the Brain

Frequency band	*Anatomy*	*Function*
Theta (4–7 Hz)	Hippocampus, sensory cortex, and prefrontal cortex	Memory, synaptic plasticity, top-down control, and long-range synchronization
Alpha (8–12 Hz)	Thalamus, hippocampus, reticular formation, sensory cortex, and motor cortex	Inhibition, attention, consciousness, top-down control, and long-range synchronization
Beta (13–30 Hz)	All cortical structures, subthalamic nucleus, basal ganglia, and olfactory bulb	Sensory gating, attention, motor control, and long-range synchronization
Gamma (30–200 Hz)	All brain structures, retina, and olfactory bulb	Perception, attention, memory, consciousness, and synaptic plasticity

Source: Uhlhaas and Singer (2011).

the synapse. The neural oscillations seen in the EEG offer a window for understanding how brain processes influence cortical networks, which can reflect normal cognitive, emotional, and motor processes. More low frequency oscillations seen in the theta (4–7 Hz) and alpha (8–12 Hz) ranges reflect longer distant relationships in the brain whereas higher frequency oscillations in the beta (13–30 Hz) and gamma (30–200 Hz) ranges reflect more local cortical networks (see Uhlhaas & Singer, 2011, 2012, for an overview).

Activity in the four frequency bands has been associated with a variety of cognitive processes in normal functioning (see *Table 7-2*). Since individuals with schizophrenia may show deficits in these cognitive processes, the study of cortical oscillations offers important insights into how schizophrenic processes affect the brain.

Cortical networks in the brain begin in utero and the period following birth. However, the development of these networks is not perfectly continuous. There is also a fundamental reorganization of these networks in adolescence (see Uhlhaas et al., 2009; Uhlhaas & Singer, 2011, 2012). The reorganization during adolescence is reflected in both cognitive performance and EEG synchrony (Uhlhaas et al., 2009). Prior to adolescence, there is a period of increase over the years in both cognitive performance and EEG synchrony. This synchrony is reflected in similar EEG activity displayed in a variety of sites throughout the head. However, during adolescence there is a decrease in both. After this period, there is a reorganization of EEG activity such that the synchrony is more focused at specific EEG sites, especially parietal and occipital electrodes.

Figure 7-9 depicts three critical periods in which changes in the physiology and anatomy of cortical processes would show changes consistent with the neurodevelopmental hypothesis of schizophrenia. The first period is fetal development in which genetic and epigenetic factors impair the electrical activity of the brain and with that the rhythmical activity associated with the formation of cortical circuits. The second stage involves the reorganization of cortical networks seen in adolescence. Along with this come changes in white and gray matter as well as neurotransmitters. Although all adolescents show gray matter declines in the PFC during this period of synaptic pruning, declines are higher in individuals with schizophrenia (see Karlsgodt, Sun, & Cannon, 2010, for an overview). The third stage describes the situation in which individuals with schizophrenia fail to develop the coordinated networks necessary for normal cognitive processes.

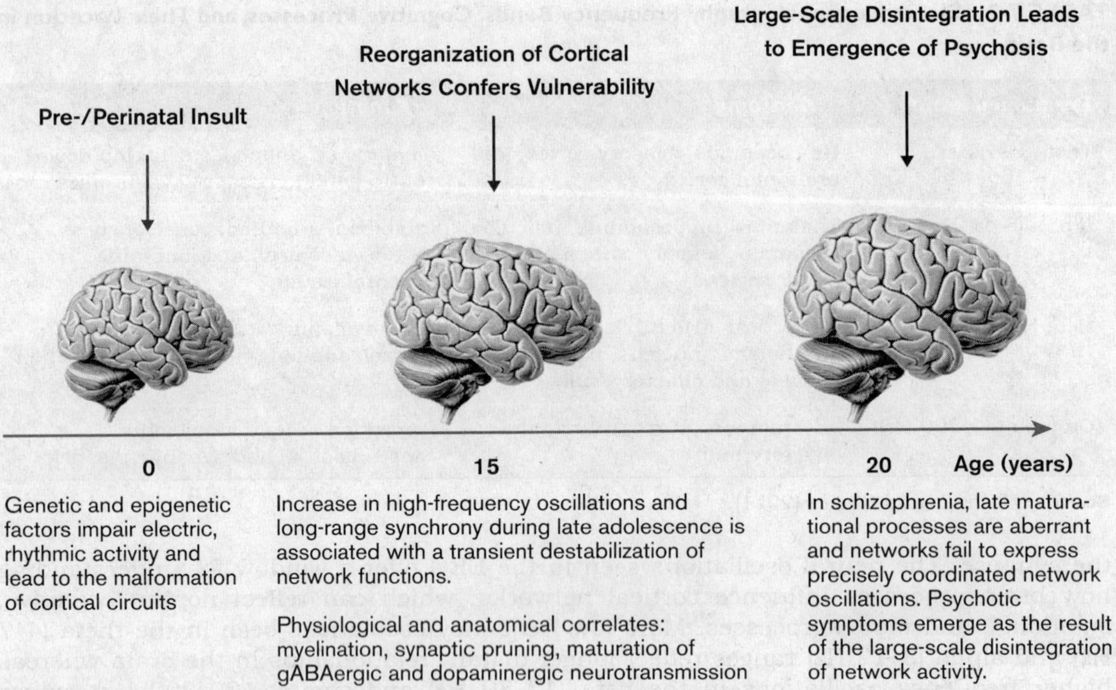

FIGURE 7-9 Three Critical Periods and Changes in the Physiology and Anatomy of Cortical Processes

Source: From Peter J. Uhlhaas and Wolf Singer. "The Development of Neural Synchrony and Large-Scale Cortical Networks During Adolescence: Relevance for the Pathophysiology of Schizophrenia and Neurodevelopmental Hypothesis." Schizophrenia Bulletin, 2011 May; 37(3): 514–523, by permission of Oxford University Press.

WHAT BRAIN CHANGES ARE SEEN IN SCHIZOPHRENIA?

When brain changes take place in those with schizophrenia is an important question. In order to better understand the role of timing in terms of brain structure, John Gilmore and his colleagues (2010) performed imaging studies before and after birth. These researchers used ultrasound scans prior to birth and magnetic resonance imaging (MRI) scans after birth while the babies slept. They compared children whose mothers had schizophrenia with a matched control group whose mothers did not have the disorder. Using ultrasound prior to birth, they found no differences between the two groups. After birth, males whose mothers had schizophrenia showed more gray matter in the brain, increased cerebrospinal fluid, and larger ventricles. Female infants did not show any differences. This suggests that at least the endophenotype for schizophrenia can be seen early in life.

Neuroimaging studies of those with schizophrenia have included both structural and functional approaches (see Karlsgodt et al., 2010; Shenton & Turetsky, 2011, for overviews). Structural approaches have focused on gray matter and white matter differences as well as the size of the ventricles (Thompson et al., 2001). In a variety of reviews, both general and specific reductions in gray matter have been reported for individuals with schizophrenia. Specifically, reductions have been in the temporal cortex, especially the

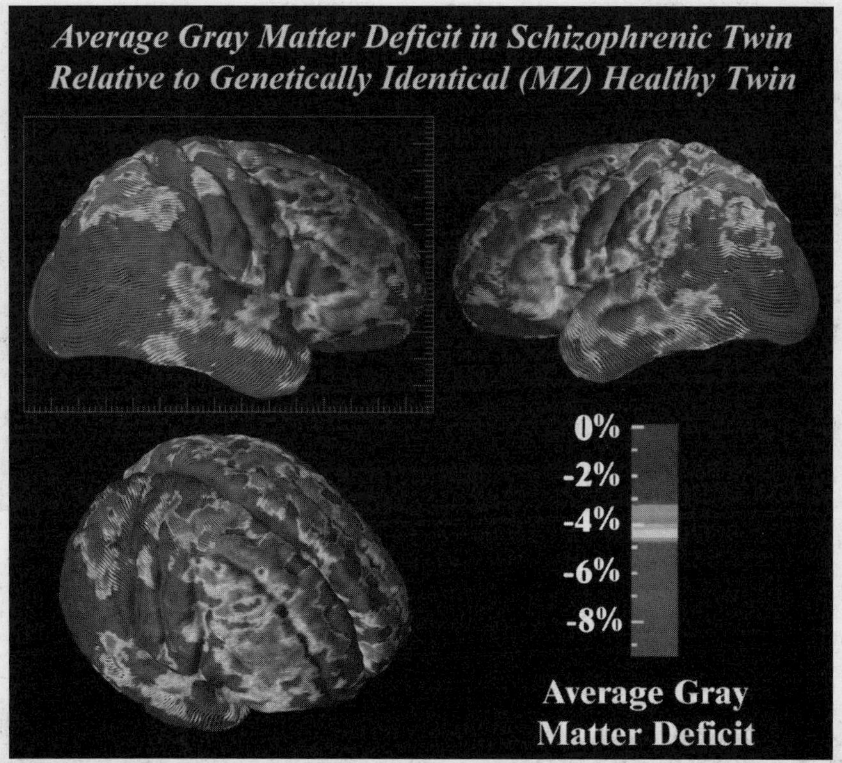

FIGURE 7-10 Average Gray Matter Deficit

Source: Cannon et al. (2001).

hippocampus, the frontal lobe, and the parietal lobe. Additionally, the striatum part of the basal ganglia has been shown to be reduced (Shenton et al., 2001). Gray matter reductions have also been seen in cases when one identical twin has schizophrenia and the other does not (see *Figure 7-10*).

Since brain changes in chronic schizophrenia can be influenced by both the disorder itself and the medications that the individual has taken over a number of years, researchers have sought to determine gray matter changes in individuals who display their first episode of schizophrenia. These studies also suggest a reduction in gray matter in schizophrenia (see Whitford, Kubicki, & Shenton, 2011, for an overview). Overall, these studies rule out the possibility that brain volume results from medication alone.

What might be at the heart of this gray matter reduction? One possibility is that the neurons actually die. However, a number of studies suggest this is not the case. What has been found is that the neurons in the brains of individuals with schizophrenia are more densely packed. This suggests that the substance found between neurons, neuropil, was reduced resulting in a greater density of neurons. Further, gray matter abnormalities have been shown to be partly hereditary and also related to trauma during pregnancy (see Karlsgodt et al., 2010, for an overview). *Figure 7-11* shows the reduction of gray matter in the same set of individuals with schizophrenia over a 5-year period (Thompson et al., 2001). *Figure 7-12* shows the differences in gray matter between individuals with schizophrenia and normal controls.

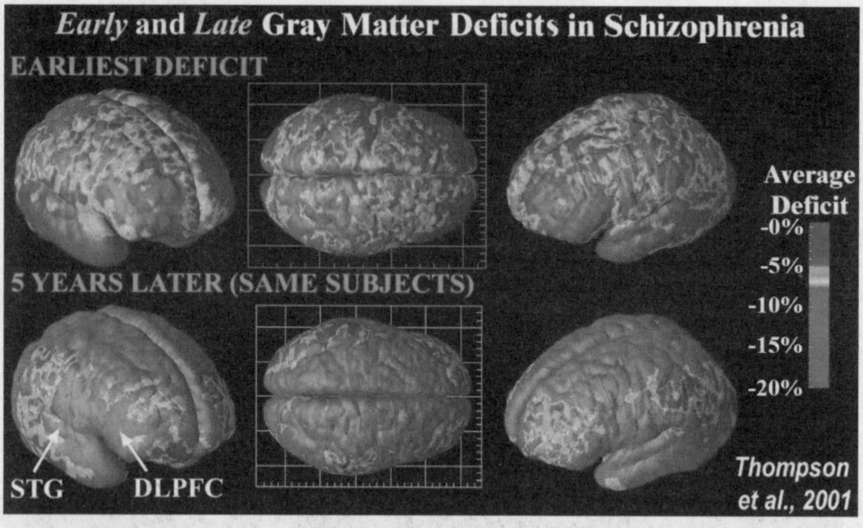

FIGURE 7-11 Early and Late Gray Matter Deficits in Schizophrenia

Source: From Paul M. Thompson, et al. "Mapping adolescent brain change reveals dynamic wave of accelerated gray matter loss in very early-onset schizophrenia." Proceedings of the National Academy of Sciences of the United States of America. 2001 September 25; 98(20). © 2001 National Academy of Sciences, U.S.A.

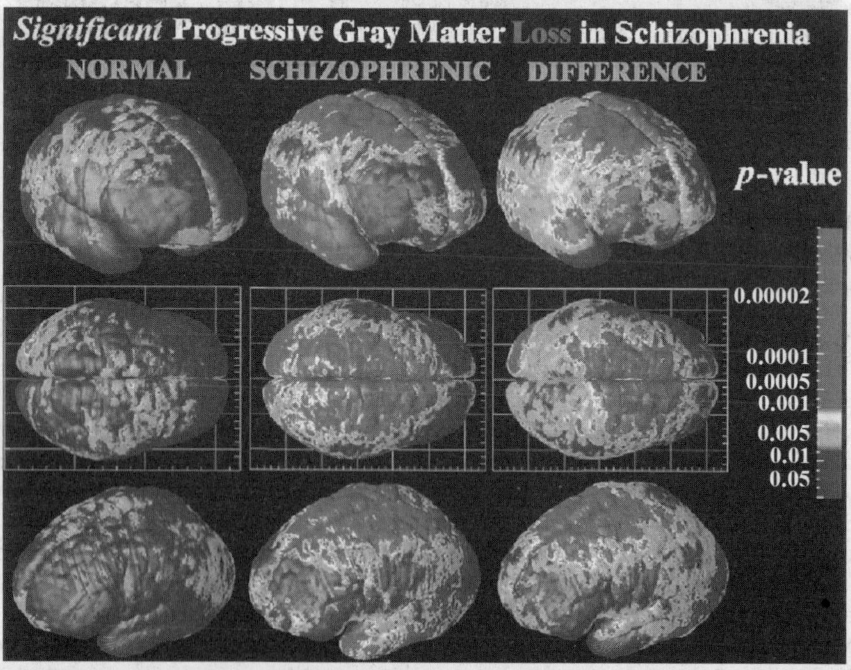

FIGURE 7-12 Significant Progressive Gray Matter Loss in Schizophrenia

Source: From Paul M. Thompson, et al. "Mapping adolescent brain change reveals dynamic wave of accelerated gray matter loss in very early-onset schizophrenia." Proceedings of the National Academy of Sciences of the United States of America. 2001 September 25; 98(20). © 2001 National Academy of Sciences, U.S.A.

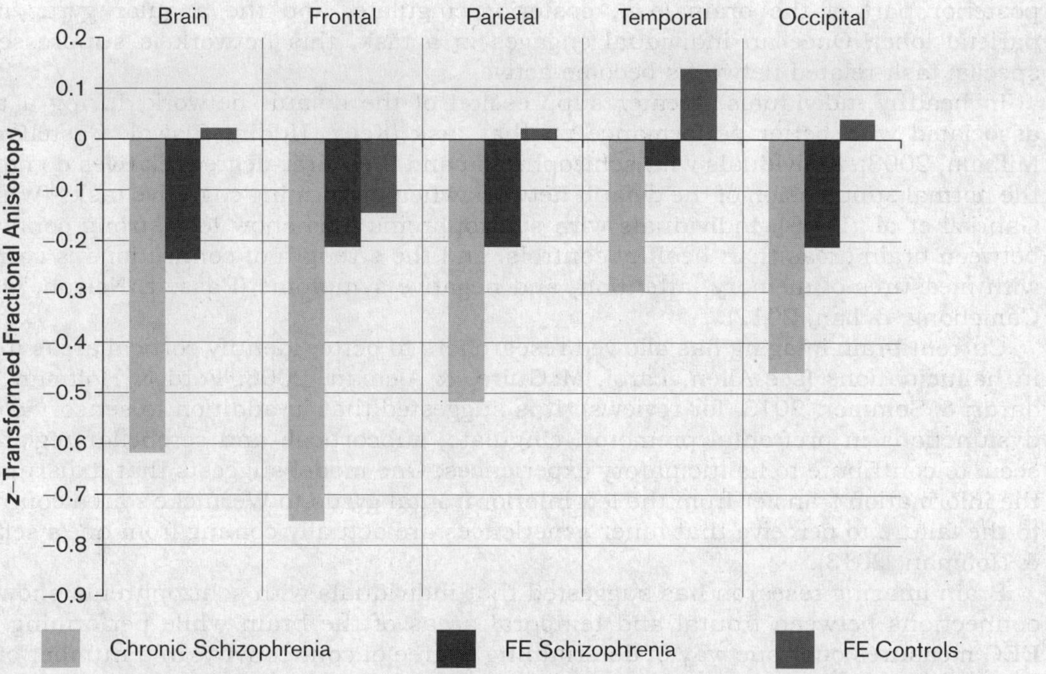

FIGURE 7-13 Differences in z-Transformed Fractional Anisotropy Measures on Cortical White Matter Between FE and Chronic Patients With Schizophrenia and Controls

Source: White et al. (2011, p. 228), by permission of Oxford University Press.
Note: The *z* score for the chronic control group was set to zero; FE= first episode.

White matter changes have also been observed in individuals with schizophrenia. One study compared 114 individuals with schizophrenia with 138 matched controls in terms of white matter (White et al., 2011). Using a brain imaging technique—diffusion tensor imaging (DTI)—sensitive to white matter, individuals with chronic schizophrenia, individuals with first episode schizophrenia, and matched controls were compared. *Figure 7-13* shows an example of tracking white matter through DTI. Measures of white matter were lower for individuals with chronic schizophrenia in the four lobes of the brain but not in the cerebellum or brain stem. Individuals experiencing their first episode of schizophrenia did not show significant differences from controls, which suggests that white matter reduction is part of the progression of the disorder over time.

In addition to white matter and gray matter changes in the brains of individuals with schizophrenia, researchers have sought to study cortical networks in schizophrenia.

SCHIZOPHRENIA AND BRAIN NETWORKS

One common network studied in functional magnetic resonance imaging (fMRI) research is the default mode network (Raichle et al., 2001). This network is activated when individuals are not performing a task and letting their mind wander. The network involves both the frontal part of the brain (i.e., ventromedial prefrontal cortex [vmPFC]) and the posterior part of the brain (e.g., posterior cingulate, and the angular gyrus/inferior parietal lobe). Once an individual engages in a task, this network is suppressed and specific task-related networks become active.

In healthy individuals, greater suppression of the default network during a task is associated with better performance on that task (Kelly, Uddin, Biswal, Castellanos, & Milham, 2008). Individuals with schizophrenia and their first-degree relatives do not show the normal suppression of the default network when performing cognitive tasks (Whitfield-Gabrieli et al., 2009). Individuals with schizophrenia also show less strong connections between brain areas than healthy controls, and the strength of connections is correlated with measures of memory, attention, and negative symptoms (Bassett, Nelson, Mueller, Camchong, & Lim, 2012).

Current brain imaging has allowed researchers to better identify cortical areas involved in hallucinations (see Allen, Larøi, McGuire, & Aleman, 2008; Ford & Hoffman, 2013; Jardri & Sommer, 2013, for reviews). It is suggested that in addition to sensory cortices, dysfunctions in prefrontal premotor, cingulate, subcortical, and cerebellar regions also seem to contribute to hallucinatory experiences. One model suggests that a disruption in the information transfer from the left inferior frontal gyrus to Wernicke's area contributes to the failure to perceive that inner experiences are actually coming from one's self (Ford & Hoffman, 2013).

Brain imaging research has suggested that individuals with schizophrenia show fewer connections between frontal and temporal areas of the brain while performing tasks. EEG measures offer one way of determining degree of connectivity. In a number of studies, Ford and her colleagues have shown that individuals without schizophrenia show a cortical reduction of responsiveness to hearing their own voice talking whereas those with schizophrenia do not (e.g., Ford, Roach, Faustman, & Mathalon, 2007). These researchers also reported that less connectivity between the frontal and temporal regions of the brain was seen when people with schizophrenia were talking versus individuals without schizophrenia (see *Figure 7-14*; Ford, Mathalon, Whitfield, Faustman, & Roth, 2002). Since there was even less connectivity in those individuals prone to hallucinate, this may be one mechanism involved in the mistaken experience that internal voices are produced externally (see also Fletcher & Frith, 2009).

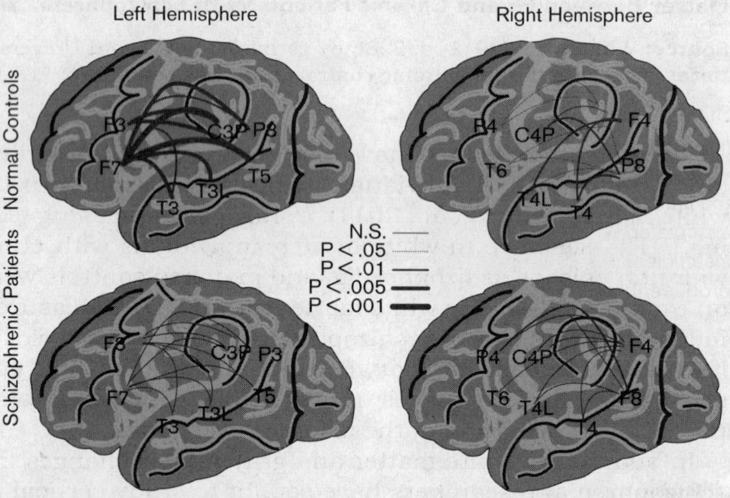

FIGURE 7-14 Differential Connectivity Between the Frontal and Temporal Regions of the Brain for Normal Controls and Schizophrenic Patients

Source: Ford et al. (2002, p. 489), with permission from Elsevier.
Note: Probability levels for *t* tests showing greater frontotemporal EEG coherence during Talking than during Listening superimposed on lateral view of right and left hemispheres for normal controls and schizophrenic patients.

NEUROTRANSMITTERS INVOLVED IN SCHIZOPHRENIA

There are different neurotransmitters that are discussed in relation to schizophrenia (see *Figure 7-15*). The first is dopamine. It has been suggested that dopamine neurons are overactive in schizophrenia in midbrain areas and underactive in higher cortical areas (Abi-Dargham & Grace, 2011). These activations can in turn influence other brain areas with dopamine projections. This is referred to as the dopamine imbalance hypothesis. Supporting this hypothesis is the finding that there is a direct relationship between drugs that treat schizophrenia and their ability to bind to dopamine receptors in the brain. Further, stress not only increases symptoms in schizophrenia but also causes an activation of the hippocampus and an increase in dopamine activity.

On a broader level, creative ability in humans has been associated with dopamine functioning—especially in the thalamus. Specifically, decreased dopamine D2 receptor densities in the thalamus resulted in a lower gating threshold and thus increased information flow. This, in turn, could result in more creative thinking (Manzano, Cervenka, Karabanov, Farde, & Ullén, 2010).

Other researchers have suggested it is not the dopamine system per se that is involved in schizophrenia but that it is the result of other transmitters that regulate the dopamine system (see Grace, 2010, for an overview). This is supported by the fact that dopamine levels are not strongly elevated in schizophrenia. What is greater in individuals with schizophrenia is the induced release of dopamine by amphetamines. Further, the increased release is proportional to the ability of amphetamines to exacerbate psychosis.

The second neurotransmitter involved in schizophrenia is glutamate (see Krystal & Moghaddam, 2011, for an overview). Glutamate is an excitatory neurotransmitter in the

DIFFERENT NEUROTRANSMITTERS, SAME RESULTS

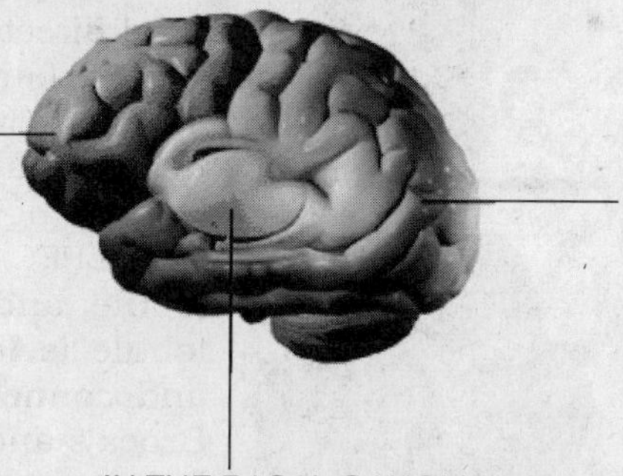

FIGURE 7-15 Two Neurotransmitters, Dopamine and Glutamate, Operate Differently in Schizophrenia

Source: From Daniel C. Javitt and Joseph T. Coyle. Decoding Schizophrenia. *The Scientific American*. January 2004. Volume 290. Number 1.

brain. Further, another neurotransmitter, GABA (γ-aminobutyric acid), is involved in nearly all neuronal processes that engage the glutamate system. If the glutamate receptors in the brain are blocked in normal individuals, those individuals display psychotic-like symptoms.

At one time, the dopamine hypothesis and the glutamate hypothesis were seen as competing explanations involving the mechanisms of schizophrenia. More recent work (Krystal et al., 2005) has shown that giving substances that modify the activity of dopamine or glutamate could produce psychotic-like symptoms in healthy humans; however, the type of psychotic presentation differed in terms of whether dopamine or glutamate receptors were affected.

HOW ARE COGNITIVE PROCESSES CHANGED IN SCHIZOPHRENIA?

Since cognitive tasks utilize specific cognitive networks, one approach to understanding the brains of individuals with schizophrenia is to note deficits in solving cognitive problems (see Barch & Ceaser, 2012; Pearlson, 2011, for overviews). Individuals with schizophrenia show cognitive deficits in a variety of cognitive domains, including executive function, working memory, and episodic memory. Overall, these cognitive processes all involve the DLPFC and its connections to other brain areas.

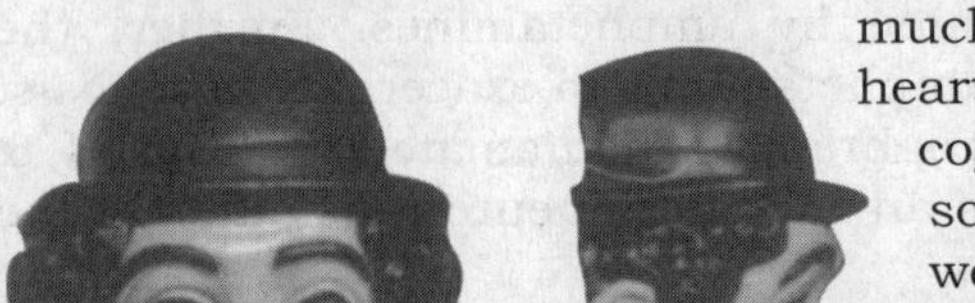

Charlie Chaplin Illusion

One suggestion is to develop a cognitive stress test much like it is possible to determine the integrity of the heart through physical stress tests. Two types of cognitive tasks that distinguish individuals with schizophrenia from healthy controls are those using working memory and attention. Working memory is the ability to keep information available for a short period of time, including its manipulation in planning and goal-directed behaviors. Disturbances in working memory are found in individuals with both acute and chronic schizophrenia as well as in their first-degree relatives without the disorder.

Imaging studies suggest the involvement of the DLPFC as well as the ACC, inferior parietal lobule, and hippocampus. The inferior parietal lobule is located just behind Wernicke's area and connected with large fiber tracts to both Broca's and Wernicke's areas. Overall this area is associated with processing and integrating auditory, visual, and sensorimotor information. As suggested by DTI, the problems seen with schizophrenia are probably better thought of as network problems rather than a deficit in a particular brain area.

One classic example of differential brain processing in individuals with schizophrenia is the Charlie Chaplin illusion. If healthy individuals look at a mask of Charlie Chaplin as it rotates, they will see the reverse side of the mask not as hollow but as convex. A video of the mask rotating can be seen at www.richardgregory.org/experiments. As you can see in the video, as the mask turns, an individual initially sees the hollow mask, but this changes into a normal face. Individuals with schizophrenia do not see the illusion and view the reverse side of the mask as hollow.

Concept Check

- According to current neuroscience research, what are the five different levels of analysis related to individuals with schizophrenia?
- What are the three critical periods of neurological changes in the development of schizophrenia?
- What structural brain changes in white matter and gray matter are characteristic of those with schizophrenia?
- What are the impacts of deficits in the brain's default network and connectivity within and across networks in individuals with schizophrenia?
- "At one time, the dopamine hypothesis and the glutamate hypothesis were seen as competing explanations involving the mechanisms of schizophrenia." What is the support for each hypothesis? What evidence suggests a more complex relationship?
- What is a cognitive stress test? What are three cognitive domains that show deficits in individuals with schizophrenia that would be the focus of the stress test?

The Charlie Chaplin illusion has been studied with fMRI (Dima et al., 2009). What these researchers found was that individuals with schizophrenia and those without showed different types of connectivity in the brain. Specifically, individuals without schizophrenia showed more top-down processing when perceiving the illusion. This suggests that part of the illusion is the sensory expectation of how a face should appear. Thus, in healthy individuals the brain creates the face as it should appear and not hollow as it actually is. Individuals with schizophrenia, on the other hand, show weakened top-down processes and stronger bottom-up ones. In doing so, they see the sensory stimuli as they are without expectation. Overall, this is consistent with other research that suggests that individuals with schizophrenia lack the top-down expectations necessary to predict future events (e.g., Allen et al., 2008).

SCHIZOPHRENIA AND THE EXPERIENCE OF EMOTIONS

Individuals with schizophrenia may describe complex emotional processes when writing in a journal while at the same time show limited emotional expression when interacting with others (see Kring & Elis, 2013, for an overview). Further, people with schizophrenia report similar emotional experiences as do those without schizophrenia. However, individuals with schizophrenia do appear to have problems connecting emotions of others in a social situation with the context in which they occur. Further, they tend to experience positive and neutral situations as more negative than those who do not have schizophrenia.

FACTS OF SCHIZOPHRENIA

In a series of papers, Rajiv Tandon and his colleagues (2009) reviewed the literature to determine what aspects of schizophrenia have been shown to be stable through a number of replications. These are presented in *Table 7-3*. These researchers also suggested that a

TABLE 7-3 Clinical "Facts" of Schizophrenia

• Schizophrenia is generally diagnosed on the basis of the presence of positive symptoms in conjunction with impaired social function in the absence of significant mood symptoms, other recognizable neurological illness, or substance use that can account for the psychotic symptoms.
• The nosological boundaries between schizophrenia and other psychiatric disorders are indistinct.
• There is significant heterogeneity in neurobiology, clinical manifestations, course, and treatment response across patients.
• Schizophrenia is characterized by an admixture of positive, negative, disorganization, cognitive, psychomotor, and mood symptoms.
• The severity of different symptom clusters varies across patients and through the course of the illness.
• There is a generalized but highly variable cognitive impairment.
• There may be additional specific impairment in a range of cognitive functions (such as executive functions, memory, psychomotor speed, attention, and social cognition).
• Cognitive impairments are present prior to onset of psychosis and persist during the course of the illness.
• There is a higher occurrence of obesity and cardiovascular disease.
• There is increased prevalence of cigarette smoking and other substance use disorders.
• There is increased suicidality.
• There is some phase-specific increase in violent behavior.
• There are significant premorbid impairments in a substantial proportion of patients.
• Onset of psychotic symptoms is usually during adolescence or early adulthood.
• The age of onset is earlier in males.
• There is an approximate doubling of age-standardized mortality.
• Schizophrenia is frequently a chronic and relapsing disorder with generally incomplete remissions.
• Social outcomes include reduced rates of employment and financial independence, and increased likelihood of homelessness and incarceration.
• Poor outcome is predicted by male gender, early age of onset, prolonged period of untreated illness, and severity of cognitive and negative symptoms.

Source: Adapted from Tandon et al. (2009).

dimensional approach including the study of endophenotypes will be important in future conceptualizations of schizophrenia.

TREATING INDIVIDUALS WITH SCHIZOPHRENIA

Until about the 1960s, individuals with schizophrenia were placed in mental hospitals, often with little real treatment other than controlling them. With the advent of medications in the middle of the past century, it became possible for individuals with schizophrenia to live within community or home settings. In fact, individuals with schizophrenia tend to show more positive mental health behaviors when living within a community. In some cultures, small towns saw it as their duty to take care of these individuals. Today, after initial hospitalizations to gain control over symptoms, many individuals with schizophrenia return to their family. Other individuals continue their education or work. Some individuals, such as the ones noted at the beginning of this chapter, are able to be productive and have high-level jobs with appropriate support. However, some individuals with schizophrenia become homeless and are at the mercy of their community. The following LENS describes how police around the country try to protect these individuals.

Over the past 100 years, there has been a shift in viewing schizophrenia as a disorder with inevitable deterioration to one in which recovery is possible (see Frese, Knight, &

7-1 LENS
Mercy Bookings of Mental Patients

During the 1800s, individuals with mental disorders would be placed in jails and prisons. Dorothea Dix and others pushed for more humane treatment and state mental hospitals began to be built. During the 1950s, another movement began to overcome the lack of adequate treatment found in many state hospitals. This community mental health movement sought to give individuals with mental disorders more freedom and dignity by moving their care and treatment to the community. However, the lack of funding for community facilities has left many of these individuals without treatment and literally on the streets of many cities. This has involved the police in dealing with those with mental illness.

Traditionally, law enforcement is there to protect the public and the mental health system is there to treat the individual. However, these roles become more ambiguous in what is referred to as mercy booking. As mental hospitals were closed in the last half of the last century, many of the individuals who would previously have been hospitalized found themselves in the community or literally on the streets. Mental hospitals or wards currently give priority to those who are a danger to themselves or others. Others with mental disorders find themselves released to the community, their family, or the streets. This leaves some of these individuals, especially women, open to becoming a victim of robbery or even rape. Mercy booking is the situation in which police create a charge to enable jailing the person in order to protect him or her.

Police from around the United States have described their involvement in mercy booking (see Torrey, 1997, for an overview). One police officer in Los Angeles, California, described mercy booking as crisis intervention in that the individuals arrested were malnourished, in need of medical care, and often hallucinating. By arresting the individuals, they were able to obtain shelter and food and the necessary medications.

Sometimes, it is the person with a mental disorder himself that creates the arrest situation. In this situation, he commits a minor crime near a police station so that he can be arrested and live in the protected context of a jail. There are also cases of families who are unable to care for an individual who refuses her medications and shows disruptive behaviors. The family will often use the police to protect the individual through having her arrested.

It is a critical question for society to determine who should be responsible for treating individuals with mental disorders and how that should be done. In the 1800s, jails were shown not to be the best solution. In the 1900s, mental hospitals offered an alternative that came to have a number of problems in terms of humane treatment. In the 2000s, those with mental disorders experience a patchwork of agencies including the police that determine their treatment. A consistent approach is needed.

Saks, 2009, for an overview). Recovery includes having a career. Living with schizophrenia depends on the resources of the individual in terms of intellectual abilities, coping techniques, and willingness to accept advice of professionals.

The Internet offers access to local and national groups that offer support for those with schizophrenia as well as the caregivers who offer support. In order to help individuals with schizophrenia cope in the community, a number of support procedures have been developed. These include antipsychotic medications as well as educational procedures to help the individual with schizophrenia and his or her family understand the course of the illness and the types of support necessary. As with other mental health disorders, specific psychotherapies for the person himself have been developed. Research suggests that the most effective treatment of schizophrenia should involve both medication and psychosocial approaches (Beck & Rector, 2005).

ANTIPSYCHOTIC MEDICATIONS

A variety of medications have been used in the treatment of schizophrenia (see Hyman & Cohen, 2013; Kutscher, 2008; Minzenberg, Yoon, & Carter, 2010, for overviews). The treatment of schizophrenia changed drastically in 1954 with the discovery of chlorpromazine (brand name Thorazine). When effective, this drug would reduce agitation, hostility, and aggression. It also reduced the positive symptoms such as hallucinations and delusions and increased the time between hospitalizations associated with schizophrenia. However, negative symptoms and cognitive deficits were not changed by the drug.

One problem of this and other initial drugs were side effects such as *tardive dyskinesia,* which is a movement disorder that results in involuntary movement of the lower face and at times the limbs. These purposeless movements include sucking, smacking the lips, and making tongue movements. These and other movement side effects are difficult to reverse if the medication was given over a period of time. Weight gain is also seen with antipsychotic medications. Since the initial drugs were developed for the treatment of schizophrenia, new and different classes of *neuroleptic* medications have been developed with different or fewer side effects. These newer drugs tend to reduce the positive symptoms of schizophrenia such as hallucinations and delusions. They also help the individual think more clearly and remain calmer. Not all medications work for all individuals. There is also some suggestion that different ethnic groups respond differently to neuroleptics although it is less clear whether it is genetic factors or diet that influences these differences.

Overall, medications for schizophrenia have been referred to as first-generation or second-generation antipsychotics. Second-generation antipsychotics are also known as *atypical antipsychotics.* First-generation antipsychotics influence dopamine receptors (D_2) although the exact mechanism by which they work is still being studied. One example of a first-generation antipsychotic medication is haloperidol, which has a number of trade names worldwide. Second-generation or atypical antipsychotic medications influence the dopamine receptors differently. Both first- and second-generation antipsychotics are successful in treating the positive symptoms seen in schizophrenia. One advantage of the second-generation antipsychotics is that they are also able to treat the negative symptoms. Initially, it was thought that the second-generation antipsychotics had fewer motor side effects although this has not always been shown to be the case (Peluso, Lewis, Barnes, &

Jones, 2012). In fact, large-scale studies suggest that second-generation drugs are no more effective than the older ones (Hyman & Cohen, 2013).

One large-scale study of effectiveness of antipsychotic medication was conducted at 57 clinical sites in the United States in the early 2000s involving almost 1,500 individuals with schizophrenia (see Lieberman & Stroup, 2011, for an overview and update). This is referred to as the CATIE (Clinical Antipsychotic Trials of Intervention Effectiveness) study. Individuals with schizophrenia were randomly assigned to one of five antipsychotic medications (olanzapine [Zyprexa], quetiapine [Seroquel], risperidone [Risperdal], ziprasidone [Geodon], and perphenazine) and followed for 18 months. One important aspect of the study was to compare first- and second-generation antipsychotic medications. One surprising result was that the second-generation medications did not show greater effectiveness from the first-generation medication, perphenazine. This included greater effectiveness in terms of negative symptoms and cognitive impairment. These results had implications not only for treatment effectiveness, but also for economic considerations since first-generation medications are less expensive.

PSYCHOSOCIAL INTERVENTIONS FOR SCHIZOPHRENIA

Psychosocial factors play an important role in the overall treatment of individuals with schizophrenia. It has been estimated that over 60% of people with a first episode of a major mental illness return to live with relatives. Thus, families play an important role in supporting these individuals. In fact, family interventions for schizophrenia reduce relapse and hospitalizations. A number of meta-analyses looked at evidence supporting family interventions (see Barrowclough & Lobban, 2008, for an overview). In general, family interventions involve the following key components:

1. Provide practical emotional support to family members.
2. Provide information about schizophrenia, what mental health services are available in the community and nationwide support services (such as the Internet).
3. Help the family develop a model of schizophrenia (including not blaming themselves).
4. Modify beliefs about schizophrenia that are unhelpful or inaccurate.
5. Increase coping for all family members.
6. Enhance problem-solving skills.
7. Enhance positive communications.
8. Involve everyone in a relapse prevention plan.

A number of manuals involving cognitive behavioral therapy (CBT) approaches to schizophrenia are available (e.g., Kingdon & Turkington, 1994; Smith, Nathan, Juniper, Kingsep, & Lim, 2003). The basic model suggests that what is important is the manner in which individuals interpret psychotic phenomena (see Beck & Rector, 2005; A. Morrison, 2008, for overviews). The overall model suggests that neurocognitive impairment in the premorbid state makes the individual vulnerable to difficulties in school or work which lead to nonfunctional beliefs such as "I am inferior," maladaptive cognitive appraisals, and in turn nonfunctional behavior such as social withdrawal (Beck & Rector, 2005). The cognitive approach is aimed at helping the client understand the psychotic experience as well as cope with the experience and reduce distress. One key feature of schizophrenia is the disruption of thought processes, and one part of the treatment is directed at these illogical associations. Another focus of the treatment is directed at interpersonal relationships and success at work. This approach may also involve skills training such as self-monitoring and activity scheduling. Since individuals with schizophrenia may also show mood and anxiety problems, CBT aimed at these processes can also be utilized. The key features of CBT for schizophrenia can be summarized as follows (Beck & Rector, 2005; Turkington, Kingdon, & Weiden, 2006):

1. Develop a therapeutic alliance based on the client's perspective.
2. Understand the client's interpretation of past and present events.
3. Develop alternative explanations of schizophrenia symptoms.
4. Normalize and reduce the impact of positive and negative symptoms.
5. Educate the client in terms of the role of stress.
6. Teach the client about the cognitive model including the role between thoughts, feelings, and behaviors.
7. Offer alternatives to the medical model to address medication adherence.

Developing a therapeutic alliance, that is, a relationship between the therapist and client that helps the work of therapy, is an initial task of therapy. Part of this may include talking with the client about his delusional beliefs. For example, if a client says that he invented a machine to solve the world's problems, then the therapist might ask when the person had this idea and what he has done to create the machine. The therapist might also ask him about others who had helped him with his ideas. As with CBT for other disorders, the basic idea is to look for inconsistent thoughts and conclusions that do not follow logically. For example, if no one would help the person with his machine, it does not follow logically that everyone is out to get him.

Another major task of therapy is helping the individual develop an alternative understanding of his or her symptoms. For example, some individuals with schizophrenia experience the voices that they hear as coming from outside of them. One goal of therapy would be to help the client reinterpret the source of the voices. Part of this may also include a cognitive assessment of alternatives to obeying the voices.

The role of stress in increasing symptoms of schizophrenia is an important concept for clients to understand. It is also important for them to understand the problems associated with not taking medication to control the symptoms of

Concept Check

- What are some of the problems in emotional processing experienced by individuals with schizophrenia?
- Tandon and colleagues have compiled a list of "facts" about schizophrenia after reviewing the research literature. What are some of these facts? How does this compilation help us move forward in our understanding of schizophrenia?
- What are three critical shifts in the past 60 years that have transformed the treatment of schizophrenia from one that was institution-based to one that is community-based?
- A variety of classes of medications have been used in the treatment of schizophrenia. What are they, and what are the advantages and disadvantages of each?
- What three psychosocial approaches are currently used in the treatment of individuals with schizophrenia, and what is the primary focus of each approach?

schizophrenia. Keeping individuals with schizophrenia on their medications is a difficult problem. In studies involving active medication alone versus a placebo alone, the relapse rates are about one half with medication compared with a placebo (32% vs. 72%) (Hogarty & Goldberg, 1973). At this point, CBT for individuals with schizophrenia along with psychotropic medication appears to be an important treatment procedure (see Beck & Rector, 2005, for outcome studies).

A new approach is being tried in the treatment of schizophrenia—early intervention (see Fisher, Loewy, Hardy, Schlosser, & Vinogradov, 2013, for an overview). This approach seeks those who are at high risk for developing schizophrenia. The basic approach is to help these individuals develop cognitive skills as a way to increase attention, memory, executive control, and other cognitive processes. In addition, cognitive therapy is being used to reduce the reactivity to stress seen in the period prior to the development of psychosis and to better understand their thoughts and feelings. Although some success has been reported, this approach for the prevention of schizophrenia is still early in its development.

In India, in the past couple of decades, A marked amount of work has emerged in this area of work for persons with schizophrenia. Considerable research as well a program contribution has come from SCARF, Chennai, pioneered by Sharada Menon (http://scarfindia.org/), and IPH (www.healthymind.org) has conducted six editions of Recovery Awards, *Dwij Puraskars*, for persons recovering from schizophrenia and their caregivers, and the seventh edition was set for October 2017. The institute has also launched a successful partnership with the state-run Regional Mental Hospital to scale up rehabilitation efforts under the umbrella of *Saptasopaan*. Work done at the institute by researchers such as Sovani, Thatte, Apte, Kadaba, and others, some of which were UGC funded, have highlighted several aspects surrounding cognitive processing in schizophrenia, burden and burnout in caregivers and remediation of the same, mismatches between strategies worked out by caregivers and those required by persons with schizophrenia, and contributions of high functioning persons recovering from schizophrenia to the rehabilitation process of those functioning at a lower level.

Writing to any of these researchers at the IPH email or visiting website, or visiting the institute in person would help, if you wish to have them share some of the key findings.

Many other India-based organizations, such as, Banyan, Chennai (www.thebanyan.org); ACMI India (Action for Mental Illness), Bangalore; Shraddha Rehabilitation Foundation, Karjat, among others (www.shraddharehabilitationfoundation.org), also assist rehabilitation of homeless mentally ill.

The thrust of recent work coming out of India emphasizes the process of public awareness and de-stigmatization of schizophrenia. Much research has emerged tracing the roles of cognitive remediation and rehabilitation, sheltered workshops and activity centers for schizophrenia (Tridal at IPH, Thane, being one such), and structured programs aiming at getting persons with schizophrenia back into the social mainstream to the degree possible.

Interesting work on customizing informed consent procedures for people with schizophrenia in India has been published by researchers such as Vikram Patel, who has authored work in *The Lancet* and has won the Brain and Behavior Research Foundation Prize for 2017 for his work in advancing mental healthcare in resource-poor countries (also touching upon traditional, complementary, and alternative medicine approaches to mental healthcare) R. Thara and Graham Thornicroft. Michelle Weiss, a health social scientist and his research group at the Swiss Tropical and Public Health have worked on schizophrenia and the cultural epidemiology of stigma in Bangalore, India. He also hosts an interesting program on Films for Health at Basel, Switzerland. He has partnered on multiple program panels with psychiatrist and actor Mohan Agashe to discuss the destigmatizing impact of films.

Sensitive media efforts, such as, the two films discussed at the beginning of this chapter, help to bring such discussions into the popular social fabric. The film *Devrai* was followed by two more beautifully narrated and visualized films, respectively called *Astu* (focused on dementia) and *Kaasav* (focused on depression). This trilogy by the director duo, Sunil Sukthankar and Sumitra Bhave, has made a mark in the journey towards public awareness about mental illness and mental health.

SUMMARY

Schizophrenia is one of the most debilitating of the mental disorders. It is part of a broad category of disorders referred to as psychotic disorders which involve a loss of being in touch with reality and are characterized by problems in terms of cognitive processes, emotional processes, and motor processes. Schizophrenia affects about 1% of the population. It is seen throughout the world with similar symptoms regardless of culture or geographical location. Onset of schizophrenia occurs in the late teens or early 20s. Males show an earlier onset than females of about 5 years. Symptoms are referred to as positive or negative. The more familiar positive symptoms are hallucinations, delusions, disorganized thinking, and disorganized behavior. The more familiar negative symptoms include lack of affect in situations that call for it, poor motivation, and social withdrawal. Not everyone with schizophrenia displays the same symptoms. This has led some researchers to suggest that there exist a variety of similar disorders that are currently described by the term *schizophrenia*.

Disorders with psychotic-like symptoms have been described for at least 4,000 years, and ancient medical texts suggest that psychosis was present in all cultures. The present-day concept of schizophrenia began to evolve in the middle of the 1800s. Beginning in the 1950s, *DSM* was introduced and described psychosis in broad terms. By *DSM–III*, schizophrenia was defined by more explicit criteria, and in *DSM–IV* and *DSM–IV–TR*, the criteria for schizophrenia were broadened to become similar to the diagnostic criteria used by *ICD*. Most recently, the text revision of the fourth edition of *DSM* (*DSM–IV–TR*) and *DSM–5* set forth a multilevel process for diagnosing schizophrenia: (1) symptoms, (2) functioning, and (3) duration; the final levels are designed to rule out psychotic-like symptoms found in other disorders. Since individuals with schizophrenia have a variety of different symptoms and show an inconsistent picture of the disorder, some have suggested that there is not a single schizophrenia disorder but rather a variety of syndromes. *DSM–IV* divided schizophrenia into five subtypes: paranoid, disorganized, catatonic, undifferentiated, and residual. There has been considerable debate as to the value of using the five subtypes due to the larger question of whether schizophrenia should be considered in terms of discrete categories or existing along a dimension. Although *ICD-10* uses subtypes, *DSM–5* removed the classification of subtypes but left the diagnostic criteria.

There is an evolutionary paradox with schizophrenia: How can the disorder exist without a reproductive advantage? One possible answer is that the genes associated with schizophrenia are also associated with positive traits such as creativity, since it has been noted that highly gifted and creative individuals manifest schizophrenic-like traits referred to as schizotypal traits without having the disorder. Other scientists propose different evolutionary paths: Crow theorizes that the development of language and the genetic changes required for producing and understanding speech were associated with the development of schizophrenia, while Burns suggests that schizophrenia is better understood as a disorder of the social brain rather than language.

Schizophrenia typically is first manifested during the transition from late adolescence to adulthood at a time of great reorganization of cortical networks. However, current research literature suggests that we consider schizophrenia as a neurodevelopmental disorder that begins early in life. The basic idea is that during the time the fetus is in utero an insult happens which influences the changes to the brain that take place during adolescence. Schizophrenia has a strong genetic component; however, the genetic underpinnings of schizophrenia are not simple. The number of genetic variants seen in individuals with schizophrenia is very large, and these genes may act in an additive or interactive manner leading to a variety of genetic combinations associated with schizophrenia. Genetic differences may result not from differences in the DNA itself but from epigenetic factors, suggesting internal and external environmental factors play a role. Finally, environmental factors that do not involve genetic changes may play a role. Presently there is no one biomarker that can identify a person with schizophrenia. However, in comparing individuals with schizophrenia, their relatives, and healthy control individuals, endophenotypes have been found in five major areas: (1) minor physical anomalies; (2) physiologic abnormalities due to normal metabolism in the brain being disturbed; (3) neuropsychological measures; (4) neuromotor abnormalities; and (5) sensory processing and event-related potentials. Another physiological marker that distinguishes individuals with schizophrenia is larger ventricles in the brain resulting from a decrease in volume in other areas of the brain.

Schizophrenia manifests on a variety of levels including abnormal sensory experiences such as hallucinations, problems in cognitive processes such as delusions and disordered thought, changes in affect such as lack of expression, and in some cases problems with language and future directed planning. This presents a challenge to describe the manner in which brain processes relate to the disorder. Current research examining individuals with schizophrenia has emphasized five different levels of analysis from a neuroscience perspective. The first is anatomical changes such as the loss of brain volume in particular areas. The second is functional processes such as the manner in which cortical areas and networks process information as seen in brain imaging. The third is neural oscillations that underlie the cortical networks. The fourth is changes in neurotransmitters such as dopamine and glutamate. And the fifth is the development of cortical processes beginning in utero.

Until about the 1960s, individuals with schizophrenia were placed in mental hospitals, often with little real treatment other than controlling them. With the advent of medications in the middle of the last century, it became possible for individuals with schizophrenia to live within community or home settings. In fact, they tend to show more positive mental health behaviors when living within a community. In addition, over the past 100 years, there has been a shift in viewing schizophrenia as a disorder with inevitable deterioration to one in which recovery is possible. In order to help individuals with schizophrenia cope in the community, a number of support procedures have been developed. These include antipsychotic medications, educational procedures to help the individual with schizophrenia and his or her family understand the course of the illness and the types of support necessary, and specific psychotherapies, particularly CBT approaches. Research suggests that the most effective treatment of schizophrenia should involve both medication and psychosocial approaches.

STUDY RESOURCES

Review Questions

1. This chapter states that "individuals with schizophrenia have a variety of different symptoms and show an inconsistent picture of the disorder. This has led some to suggest that there is not a single schizophrenia disorder but rather a variety of syndromes." What do you think: Is schizophrenia one disorder? What evidence would you cite to support your position?
2. What are the environmental and genetic factors that play a role in the development of schizophrenia?
3. "Current research examining individuals with schizophrenia has emphasized five different levels of analysis from a neuroscience perspective." For each level, what has been the focus of the research and what brain changes have been found in schizophrenia?
   a. Anatomical changes?
   b. Functional processes?
   c. Neural oscillations?
   d. Neurotransmitters?
   e. Development of cortical processes?
4. "Psychosocial factors play an important role in the overall treatment of individuals with schizophrenia." What are the characteristics of each factor and what role does each play in treatment?
   a. Family interventions?
   b. CBT approach?
   c. Early intervention?

For Further Reading

McLean, R. (2003). *Recovered, not cured: A journey through schizophrenia.* Australia: Allen Unwin.
Nasar, S. (1998). *A beautiful mind.* New York: Simon & Schuster.
Schiller, L., & Bennett, A. (1994). *The quiet room.* New York: Warner Books.

Key Terms and Concepts

alogia
anhedonia
avolition
catatonic subtype
delusions
disorganized subtype
dopamine
glutamate
hallucinations
negative symptoms
paranoid subtype
positive symptoms
psychotic disorders
schizophrenia
schizotypal traits

CHAPTER

8

Mood Disorders

CHAPTER OUTLINE

- DEPRESSIVE DISORDERS 270
- BIPOLAR DISORDER 289
- SUICIDE 302
- SUMMARY 305
- STUDY RESOURCES 308

Background

Pesticide suicides are considered the single most important means of suicide worldwide. Centralized pesticide storage facilities have the possible advantage of delaying access to pesticides thereby reducing suicides. We undertook this study to examine the feasibility and acceptability of a centralized pesticide storage facility as a preventive intervention strategy in reducing pesticide suicides.

Methods

A community randomized controlled feasibility study using a mixed methods approach involving a household survey; focus group discussions (FGDs) and surveillance were undertaken. The study was carried out in a district in southern India. Eight villages that engaged in floriculture were identified. Using the lottery method two were randomized to be the intervention sites and two villages constituted the control site. Two centralized storage facilities were constructed with local involvement and lockable storage boxes were constructed. The household survey conducted at baseline and one and a half years later documented information on sociodemographic data, pesticide usage, storage and suicides.

Results

At baseline 4,446 individuals (1,097 households) in the intervention and 3,307 individuals (782 households) in the control sites were recruited while at follow up there were 4308 individuals (1,063 households) in the intervention and 2,673 individuals (632 households) in the control sites. There were differences in baseline characteristics and imbalances in the prevalence of suicides between intervention and control sites as this was a small feasibility study.

The results from the FGDs revealed that most participants found the storage facility to be both useful and acceptable. In addition to protecting against wastage, they felt that it had also helped prevent pesticide suicides as the pesticides stored here were not as easily and readily accessible. The primary analyses were done on an Intention to Treat basis. Following the intervention, the differences between sites in changes in combined, completed and attempted suicide rates per 100,000 person-years were 295 (95% CI: 154.7, 434.8; $p < 0.001$) for pesticide suicide and 339 (95% CI: 165.3, 513.2, $p < 0.001$) for suicide of all methods.

Source: Dr. Lakshmi Vijaykumar et al. (2013).

DEPRESSIVE DISORDERS

Emotional experiences and moods are an important part of our world as humans. Sometimes we feel happy; other times we feel sad. We have all experienced ourselves as having different moods. Our thoughts are often consistent with our moods as when we feel sad and think we are not doing things well. Likewise our behaviors match our moods. To want to stay in bed in the morning or not to want to be with others is often the outcome of feeling blue. Other times we go in the opposite direction and feel full of energy. Our thoughts when we are in a positive mood influence what activities we can engage in or what accomplishments we can achieve. Behaviorally, we tend to seek social interactions and start new projects.

Neither positive nor negative moods as most of us experience them interfere with our daily life or separate us from ourselves or others. However, the mood disorders that I discuss with you in this chapter do. Not only do these disorders separate us; they also last for a long time and in some cases are experienced throughout one's life. The first part of the chapter will focus on depression. The second part will discuss those who experience both depression and mania, previously referred to as **manic depression.** Mania is the experience of tremendous energy and euphoria. Today we call these periods of depression and mania **bipolar disorder.** This is in contrast to **unipolar depression,** which is the experience of depression without mania. Following this coverage of depression and bipolar disorder, the chapter concludes with a section on **suicide,** which is often tied to underlying mood disorders.

Both depression and mania have been described for more than 2,000 years. The ancient Greek writers Hippocrates, Aretaeus, and Galen each described a condition they referred to as **melancholia,** which today we call depression. Melancholia was described in terms of despondency, dissatisfaction with life, problems sleeping, restlessness, irritability, difficulties in decision making, and a desire to die. Mania, on the other hand, was described in terms of euphoria, excitement, cheerfulness, grandiosity, and at times anger. There was also a realization that mania and melancholia could exist in the same person.

Depression is characterized by depressed mood in which one feels sad or empty without any sense of pleasure in one's activities. All individuals experience depressed mood for brief periods, which is usually accompanied by feelings of sadness, loss of energy, social withdrawal, and often negative thoughts about one's self. With a depressive disorder, the individual may also experience sleep problems and weight changes. Included with the disorder is a sense of worthlessness and self-blame. Clinical depression is seen when the majority of these symptoms last for an extended period of time. There is a gender difference in that over the course of a lifetime about 1 in 4 females and 1 in 10 males experiences a major depressive episode (Rutter, 2006). Genetic studies suggest that depression is equally influenced by genetic and environmental factors (Rutter, 2006). In one set of studies, monkeys with a genetic risk for depression were raised by either highly responsive or less responsive foster mothers (Suomi, 1997). In this situation, the mothers influenced the outcome with more responsive mothers having less depressed infants.

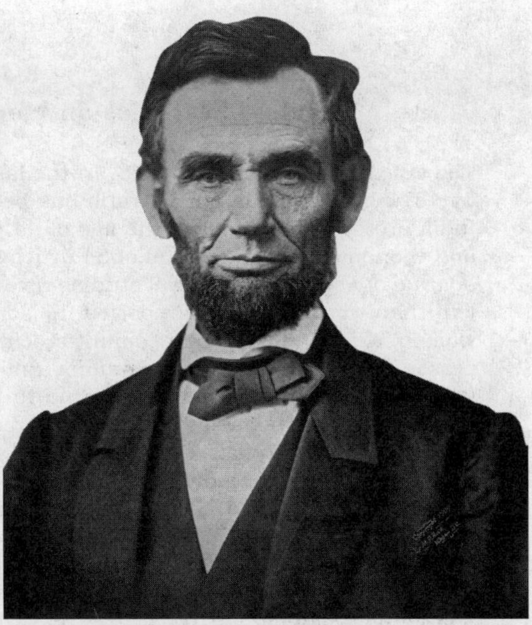

Lincoln is described as suffering from depression

Today, **major depressive disorder (MDD)** is one of the most commonly diagnosed mental disorders among adults and is estimated to be found in about 13 million adult Americans during the preceding 12 months (see Kessler & Wang, 2009). Lifetime estimates are approximately 33 million Americans. For all Americans over the age of 13, the lifetime prevalence for a major depressive episode is 29.9% and 8.6% for a 12-month prevalence (see Kessler, Petukhova, Sampson, Zaslavsky, & Wittchen, 2012, for an overview). It should be noted that three fourths of those with MDD would also meet criteria for an additional *Diagnostic and Statistical Manual of Mental Disorders* (*DSM*) disorder. Anxiety disorder (59%), obsessive-compulsive disorder (OCD) (31.9%), and substance abuse (24%) are all frequently comorbid with MDD.

Depression has been related to a variety of physiological, psychological, family, and social components. It is also estimated to be one of the most economically costly mental disorders worldwide. MDD has been shown to take individuals out of their normal roles or jobs in a number equal to medical disorders. In fact, it is second only to chronic back or neck pain in terms of disability days lost. Part of this is related to the fact that only one third of those with depression seek help in the first year of onset. The median delay for seeking treatment among those who did not seek treatment in the first year was 5 years. Even with treatment, the chance of another episode of depression is high. Most patients experience a recurrence within 5 years (see Boland & Keller, 2009, for an overview). Historical figures such as President Abraham Lincoln have described their own experiences of mood disorders. The singer Sheryl Crow has also documented her own experiences of depression.

Mood Disorders Around the World

In the following LENS, you can see lifetime and prevalence data for any mood disorder by country. Although rates may vary by country, the overall data show that mood disorders are a common occurrence.

8-1 LENS
Indian Statistics on Mental Health Mood Disorders

The suicide rate in India is 10.3. In the last three decades, the suicide rate has increased by 43%, but the male–female ratio has been stable at 1.4:1. Majority (71%) of suicides in India are by persons below the age of 44 years, which imposes a huge social, emotional, and economic burden. A total of 54 articles on suicides have been published in the *Indian Journal of Psychiatry*. Several studies reveal that suicidal behaviors are much more prevalent than what is officially reported. Poisoning, hanging, and self-immolation (particularly women) are the methods to commit suicide. Physical and mental illness, disturbed interpersonal relationships, and economic difficulties are the major reasons for suicides. The vulnerable population has been found to be women, students, farmers, etc. A social and public health response in addition to a mental health response is crucial to prevent suicidal behavior in India.

In India, more than one lakh lives are lost every year due to suicides. In the last three decades (from 1975 to 2005), the suicide rate increased by 43%. The rates were approximately the same in 1975 and 1985, but from 1985 to 1995, there was an increase of 35% and from 1995 to 2005, there was an increase of 5%.

Source: Vijayakumar (2010).

Research suggests that the initial episode of depression has a strong environmental component whereas later episodes are thought to be related to internal physiological changes. Using the Virginia Twin Registry, it has been shown that the initial episode has a stronger relationship with environmental factors than later episodes (Kendler, Thornton, & Gardner, 2000). Thus, major life stress such as loss of a close relationship is highly associated with the development of depression. Individuals with depression are 2.5 to 10 times more likely to have experienced a recent major life event than nondepressive individuals (see Slavich, O'Donovan, Epel, & Kemeny, 2010, for an overview).

A distinction is made between short-term brief stress that has a motivational effect and long-term chronic stress that leads to depression (Lemos et al., 2012). Stress and trauma will be discussed in greater detail in Chapter 9. The pathway from chronic stress to depression includes a reduction in size of brain regions that regulate mood and cognition, such as the prefrontal cortex (PFC) and the hippocampus. Animals under chronic stress also show fewer synapses in these areas (Duman & Aghajanian, 2012). *Figure 8-1* shows the effects of chronic stress over 7 days on dendrite length and branching. Notice the difference between the neurons of the animal that was not stressed compared with the one that was.

Studies in animals show that short-term stress activates the corticotropin-releasing factor (CRF), which acts in the nucleus accumbens to release dopamine. In healthy organisms, including humans, the nucleus accumbens is involved in signaling acts of pleasure. In short-term stress, the nucleus accumbens also facilitates motivational factors and social bonding. Julia Lemos and her colleagues (2012) subjected mice to long-term stress. Following long-term stress, CRF no longer produced dopamine release associated with pleasure but rather a negative state. Further, this state lasted for more than 90 days, including non-reactions to acute stress. These authors suggested that chronic stress acts like a switch that reduces positive motivational responses to aversive ones in the nucleus accumbens. This switch from active coping to lack of motivation may lie at the basis of the development of depression.

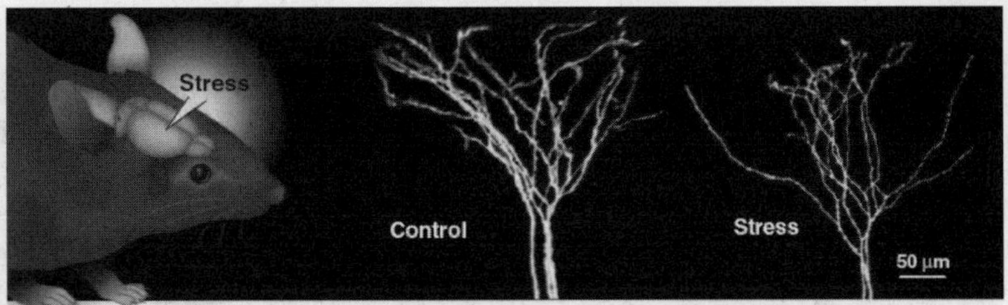

FIGURE 8-1 Effects of Restraint Stress (~30 Minutes per Day, 7 Days) on Dendrite Length and Branching

Source: From Ronald S. Duman and George K. Aghajanian, "Synaptic Dysfunction in Depression: Potential Therapeutic Targets", Science, 5 October 2012: 68–72. Reprinted with permission from AAAS.

An intriguing question is whether genetic factors make some individuals more reactive to environmental stresses. Environmental stress produces the release of **cortisol** in the adrenal cortex. Cortisol is a glucocorticoid hormone. More cortisol is produced in response to stress by those with a depressive disorder. In fact, some individuals with depression show elevated levels of cortisol throughout the day, even without acute stress. Further, a link has been established between gene coding for these stress responses and depression (Liu et al., 2006).

A further set of studies that show the complex nature of the development of depression deal with the **intergenerational transmission of depression** (see Hammen, 2009, for an overview). These studies focus on the manner in which having one or more parents who are depressed leads to a child becoming depressed. If one's parent was depressed, it would change the nature of the emotional and social interactions during childhood. In general, studies have shown that individuals with a depressive parent experience depression 2 to 3 times more frequently by age 15 or 20 than those without a depressive parent. When these individuals develop depression, it is also more severe and recurrent.

DSM–5 distinguishes between a single depressive episode and the case in which there are recurrent depressive episodes punctuated by at least 2-month periods without depression. The *DSM–5* criteria for the MDD episode itself are the same. These criteria note that significant losses such as bereavement, financial ruin, and natural disaster may resemble a depressive episode including feelings of intense sadness, rumination about the loss, insomnia, poor appetite, and weight loss. However, these do not represent MDD. For MDD, *DSM–5* follows closely on the *DSM–IV* diagnostic scheme based on the presence of five or more symptoms with a precise duration (see *Table 8-2*).

Developmental Aspects of Depression

Adolescence is a period of life where drastic changes take place. Social, emotional, hormonal, and brain changes are critical during this period of development. Mood disorders related to anxiety and depression are common, and research is still attempting to articulate a clear picture of the nature of depression in adolescents (see Pine, 2009; Rudolf, 2009, for overviews). It is estimated that clinical depression occurs in around 3% to 5% of the population of adolescents. Prior to this age, the rates are 1% to 2%. Gender

TABLE 8-1 Major Depressive Disorder

A.	Five (or more) of the following criteria have been present during the same 2-week period and represent a change from previous functioning; at least one of the symptoms is either (1) depressed mood or (2) loss of interest or pleasure.
Note: Do not include symptoms that are clearly due to a medical condition.	
	1. Depressed mood most of the day, nearly every day, as indicated by either subjective report (e.g., feels sad, empty, or hopeless) or observation made by others (e.g., appears tearful). Note: In children and adolescents, can be irritable mood. 2. Markedly diminished interest or pleasure in all, or almost all, activities most of the day, nearly every day (as indicated by either subjective account or observation) 3. Significant weight loss when not dieting or weight gain (e.g., a change of more than 5% of body weight in a month), or decrease or increase in appetite nearly every day. Note: In children, consider failure to make expected weight gain. 4. Insomnia or hypersomnia nearly every day 5. Psychomotor agitation or retardation nearly every day (observable by others, not merely subjective feelings of restlessness or being slowed down) 6. Fatigue or loss of energy nearly every day 7. Feelings of worthlessness or excessive or inappropriate guilt (which may be delusional) nearly every day (not merely self-reproach or guilt about being sick) 8. Diminished ability to think or concentrate, or indecisiveness, nearly every day (either by subjective account or as observed by others) 9. Recurrent thoughts of death (not just fear of dying), recurrent suicidal ideation without a specific plan, or a suicide attempt or a specific plan for committing suicide
B.	The symptoms cause clinically significant distress or impairment in social, occupational, or other important areas of functioning.
C.	The episode is not attributable to the direct physiological effects of a substance or another medical condition.
D.	The Major Depressive Episode is not better accounted for by Schizoaffective Disorder and is not superimposed on Schizophrenia, Schizophreniform Disorder, Delusional Disorder, or Psychotic Disorder Not Elsewhere Classified.
E.	There has never been a Manic Episode or a Hypomanic Episode.

Reprinted with permission from the *Diagnostic and Statistical Manual of Mental Disorders,* Fifth Edition (Copyright 2013). American Psychiatric Association.

differences in depression emerge by age 13 or 14. By age 18, females show a 2 to 1 prevalence that remains stable throughout adulthood.

Although diagnostic symptoms for adolescents are similar to adults, depressed children are more likely to describe physical symptoms such as headache or stomach pains whereas adults describe hopelessness, helplessness, and suicidal thinking. The rates of depression are very low prior to puberty, with equal numbers of boys and girls. After puberty, the rates of depression increase and more females than males are affected. There is some suggestion that females of this age cognitively process social stress differently than males, which places them at risk for depression (Pine, 2009).

Environmental factors appear to be a critical factor in the development of depression. One study reported that over 90% of the episodes of depression were related to stressful events. These events included negative experiences with parents such as marital discord, neglect, and abuse and also having a parent with a mental disorder (Goodyer, 2001). Attachment relationships have also been linked to a cognitive vulnerability to depression (see Morley & Moran, 2011, for an overview). If there is a positive relationship, even in children who have been maltreated, there is less depression (Kaufman et al., 2006).

Depression and suicide among adolescents and youth has reached daunting levels in India and major interventions are being planned to avert more tragedies.

In a paper published in the *Indian Journal of Psychiatry*, Radhakrishnan and Andrade (2012) from NIMHANS have eruditely outlined an Indian perspective on suicide. They write, "The rates of suicide have greatly increased among youth, and youth are now the group at highest risk in one-third of the developed and developing countries (including India)." The emerging phenomenon of "cyber-suicide" in the Internet era is a further cause for concern, also because the use of the new methods of suicide are associated with epidemic increases in overall suicide rates. Suicide prevention is now brought into focus by 10 September being celebrated as World Suicide Prevention Day, and much work is done on educational campuses including NIMHANS, Bangalore by, among others, Dr. Seema Mehrotra and team, and on SNDT WU Mumbai campus by Dr. Anuradha Sovani and team.; and IIT Mumbai to name a few. Suicide is the leading cause of death among youngsters aged 10–24 in India, with 62,960 such deaths reported in 2013 (according to the findings of the Lancet Commission on Adolescent Health and Well-being). The "Let's talk" campaign is being run at community-based sites and on educational campuses, and many NGOs too are working hard to stem the epidemic of deaths by suicide.

Cognitive Model of Depression

The **cognitive model of depression** was developed by Aaron Beck (1967) to describe the manner in which individuals with depression maintain the disorder. It also became the basis for a therapeutic approach, which has been studied in a variety of empirical treatment studies (see Beck, 2011). The basic model suggests that individuals with depression display a bias in the way they search for information and process this information. These biases take place out of awareness and represent internal schemas that influence what a person sees, how he organizes information, and what he remembers related to his life. These biases generally result in the person seeing himself as worthless in a world with little support. If asked to remember their past, unlike healthy individuals, individuals with depression tend to remember more negative than positive events. Research with emotional stimuli also suggests that it is difficult for those with depression to disengage from negative stimuli. Additionally, negative rumination in which the individual thinks repetitively about how a negative event came about is also characteristic of depression.

The cognitive model is basically a learning theory model that suggests adverse events that occur early in life can lead to the development of depressive schemas. These depressive schemas are characterized by negative self-referential beliefs. Further, when a new stressor appears, it can activate the prior negative schemas. These negative schemas involve three aspects: the self, the personal world, and the future. This is referred to as the **negative cognitive triad.** In terms of the self, the individual with depression will attribute unpleasant experiences encountered in the world to his or her own mental, physical, and moral defects. The second component involves the person's tendency to tailor the facts to fit the negative schema. The third component involves the person seeing the future as only containing hardship and failure.

Over the 40 years since the original cognitive model of depression was developed, brain imaging techniques have progressed greatly. Researchers now suggest that the underlying neural mechanisms for the cognitive model of depression can be described (see Disner, Beevers, Haigh, & Beck, 2011, for an overview). The neural model begins with the observation that attention in healthy individuals involves a number of brain areas, including the PFC. The ability to switch attention involves a top-down process that includes three different processes. The first involves choosing what to pay attention to (the ventrolateral prefrontal cortex [VLPFC]). The second is executive control (the dorsolateral prefrontal cortex [DLPFC]). And the third involves moving the eyes (the superior parietal cortex).

Attention requires effort when focusing on information that does not normally attract your attention. When normal individuals are asked not to focus on positive information, the anterior cingulate cortex (ACC) shows activity whereas ACC activity is seen in individuals with depression when asked to divert attention from negative stimuli. This suggests that healthy and depressed individuals require cognitive effort to accomplish emotional switching in opposite directions. Further, from a bottom-up process, amygdala reactivity to negative stimuli in individuals with depression is more intense and lasts longer than that seen in healthy individuals. *Figure 8-2* summarizes the cognitive model from a cortical perspective.

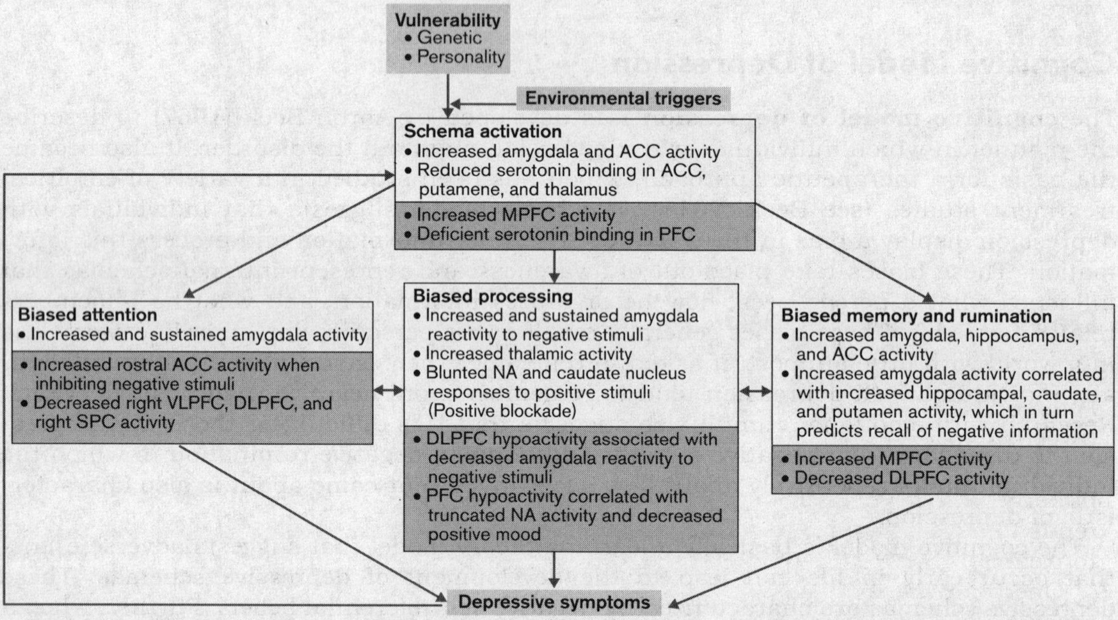

FIGURE 8-2 Summary of an Integrated Cognitive Neurobiological Model of Depression

Source: From Seth G. Disner, Christopher G. Beevers, Emily A. P. Haigh & Aaron T. Beck. "Neural mechanisms of the cognitive model of depression." *Nature Reviews Neuroscience* 12, 467–477 (August 2011).
Note: The brain regions in this flowchart are divided into two groups: regions associated with bottom-up, limbic system influences (shown by the white boxes) and regions that maintain bottom-up influences through altered top-down, cognitive control (shown by the gray boxes).

Are Depression and Inflammation Related?

It has been only recently that researchers have begun to determine a relationship between depression and inflammation (Dantzer, 2012; Dantzer et al., 2008). This work has noted the similarity between the symptoms of physical sickness involving the immune system and depression. In physical sickness involving pathogens, immune system cytokines influence the local and systemic responses. It is these cytokines that act on the brain to produce the experience of sickness. What has been noted is that with both the response to pathogens and depression, there are similar experiences. In both situations, there is a withdrawal from the physical and social environment, which can be accompanied by pain. There is also a general malaise and decreased interest in activities that produce positive rewards. One difference, however, is that once the pathogens have been removed the sickness experience is eliminated, which does not happen with depression. This has led some to suggest that cytokines malfunction may be involved in depression. This has come to be known as the **macrophage theory of depression** (Smith, 1991). Research supporting this idea shows that individuals with depression have increased blood concentration of inflammatory biomarkers.

One of the first studies in the area showed that hospitalized individuals with depression displayed signs of immunosuppression (Stein, Keller, & Schleifer, 1985). Since that time, several meta-analyses have shown an association between depression and biomarkers of inflammation. These studies concluded that individuals with depression were physically healthy, and thus, the presence of the biomarkers was not the result of underlying pathology. At this point, some studies support the link of inflammation with depression while others do not. A recent prospective study involving adolescents who were followed until age 21 suggested that immune responses do not predict depression (Copeland, Shanahan, Worthman, Angold, & Costello, 2012). They used the measure of C-reactive protein (CRP), which reflects the immune system response to inflammation. Whereas CRP did not predict depression by age 21, depression did predict later CRP responses. This is an important health finding since CRP is associated with cardiovascular disease and type 2 diabetes.

Does Depression Run in Families?

From a variety of studies, chronic severe depression has been shown to be familial (see Peterson & Weissman, 2011, for an overview). Offspring of individuals with MDD have a threefold to fivefold increased risk of developing MDD themselves. From longitudinal studies over three generations, individuals initially show elevated anxiety disorders before puberty, which then become MDD in mid to late adolescence. Further, familial MDD tends to have an earlier onset and to be more severe, more recurrent, and less responsive to treatment than is nonfamilial MDD.

One brain imaging study compared individuals at high risk for developing MDD in the second and third generations of a longitudinal MDD study (Peterson & Weissman, 2011). These high-risk individuals were compared with the children of the original nondepressed control group in the study. What these researchers found is that individuals with MDD as well as their unaffected family members showed cortical thinning of the lateral aspect of the right hemisphere and the medial aspect of the left hemisphere along with the bilateral hypoplasia of the frontal and parietal white matter. The unaffected family members also showed signs of inattention and poor visual memory for social stimuli. Further, there was a direct relationship between the deficits and the magnitude of cortical thinning and white matter hypoplasia. Likewise, symptom severity also correlated inversely with cortical thickness and with white matter measures (see *Figure 8-3*).

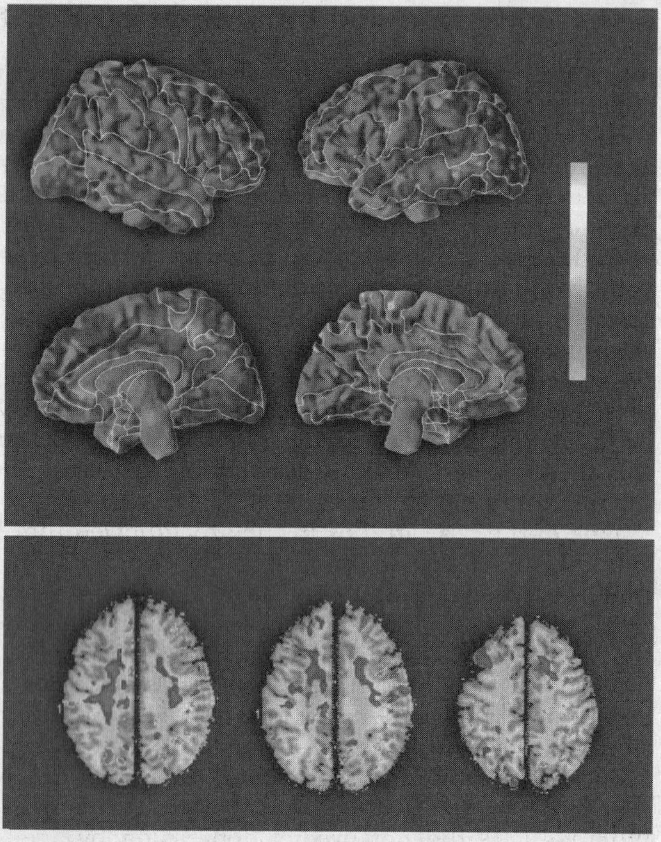

FIGURE 8-3 The Top and Bottom Graphs Show That the Less the Cortical Thickness or Volume (Purple Is Less—Red Is More), the Greater the Symptoms of Major Depressive Disorder

Source: From Bradley S. Peterson and Myrna M. Weissman, "A Brain-Based Endophenotype for Major Depressive Disorder." *Annual Reviews Med.* 2011 February 18; 62: 461–474.

The Evolutionary Perspective Concerning Depression

In terms of an evolutionary perspective, Andrews (2007) suggested that there are only a limited number of hypotheses that might explain the existence of depression. One hypothesis views depression as resulting from a mismatch between the current demands of our society and our brain and nervous system, which evolved in terms of different demands. Thus, depression results from a novel reaction of the nervous system to the modern environment. This hypothesis suggests that our environment has changed quickly whereas our nervous system has not. However, Andrews rejected this hypothesis since depression is seen in a variety of animals such as rats, cats, and primates whose environment has not changed drastically in recent times. Another hypothesis views depression as a process that evolved because it was connected to another trait that was extremely adaptive. This connection has yet to be found.

Gilbert (2005) asked if depression might have evolved because it serves a useful function. Such an advantage would be found in situations in which positive affect and drive should be toned down. One simple answer is that a reduction of positive affect could make one more sensitive to threat. Gilbert then took this question a step further and asked at what point the increase in depressive mood would be adaptive. Sickness or hurt would be one such example. Withdrawing from active life would give the body time to recover health and strength. Likewise, stress, which can result in a variety of depression-like symptoms including reduction of positive affect, activity, and motivational factors such as hunger, may be reduced with a removal from the situation.

Allen and Badcock (2003) considered the role of depressed mood in our social evolutionary history. They saw depressed mood as having evolved in relation to social processes. As with other researchers, they suggested that a depressed state represents a risk management strategy in response to a situation that has a low probability of success and high probability of risk. The emphasis is on social situations in which an individual would be at risk for being excluded from groups or a relationship with another individual. Basically they saw depressed mood as the result of a computational problem on the part of the organism. That is to say, on some level the organism evaluates the situation. In a situation in which there is high risk of being excluded, this evaluation leads to depressed mood. Intrinsic to this way of thinking is the assumption that depressed mood was adaptive in our evolutionary history. That is to say, feeling depressed would help the organism to solve a problem faced by humans from the earliest times. Overall, there are three questions that need to be approached from an evolutionary perspective in relation to depression (Nesse, 1990):

1. What are the situations that occur over and over again in our environment of evolutionary adaptiveness (EEA) responsible for depressive states?
2. What are the selection pressures in these situations? Said in other terms, what reproductive goals would have been threatened?
3. What are the characteristics of depressed mood that would have enabled the organism to cope with these threats?

These questions have been answered by evolutionary psychologists in terms of three broad models. These are (1) **depression in terms of resource conservation,** (2) **depression in terms of social competition,** and (3) **depression in terms of attachment.** Attachment has been discussed previously and would relate to depression in terms of the experience of loss.

Concept Check

- What is the impact of depression from a number of perspectives:
  - o Worldwide prevalence?
  - o Lifetime prevalence?
  - o Gender prevalence?
  - o Costs to economy, society, family, and individual?
  - o Other psychological disorders?
- What are some of the factors related to depression in adolescents? How are they the same or different in children?
- What is the "negative cognitive triad"? What is its role in the cognitive model of depression?
- What evidence would you cite to answer the question of whether depression runs in families?
- What three questions does any theory that takes an evolutionary perspective to why depression exists need to address?

Theories of Resource Conservation

Theories of resource conservation suggest that depressive mood protects the organism by conserving energy. By reducing energy expenditure, the organism can both protect itself in the present situation and conserve energy that can be used in future productive situations. Stress and especially uncontrollable events can affect the organism and produce a depressed-like state. Clinical depression in these theories results when an individual does not move on to the next situation but rather continues in a situation in which there are few positive payoffs.

Theories of Social Competition

In discussing dominance hierarchies across species, it was noted that the most powerful individual has a greater chance of mating and passing on his genes. Typically two males fight to determine which will be higher in power. It has also been observed that when one of the animals loses the competition, this animal begins to make submissive gestures. David Buss (2005), in his writing, has extended this type of thinking to humans and suggested that there exists a powerful motivation to acquire rank and status especially among human males. Price (1996) suggested that there is a connection between depressive mood and losing a fight for status and resources. In particular, he suggested that the losing organism adopts a strategy in which he signals a desire to not continue the competition and withdraw. The winner, on the other hand, tends to escalate the competition and increasingly displays threatening behaviors. Depression from this viewpoint is seen as an involuntary de-escalating strategy that signals to the other individual that he has won.

Social Risk Hypothesis

Allen and Badcock began to integrate the three previous broad models of depression with the social risk hypothesis. This hypothesis suggests that when significant interpersonal relationships are disrupted including social humiliation or defeat, depressed mood is the outcome. In this sense, it is a protective mechanism that prevents further critical losses. It is protective in two ways. First, depressed mood reduces the desire of the individual to immediately enter a social relationship in which there could be an adverse outcome. And second, the outward signs of depressed mood including changes in voice tone, reaction time, eye contact, and facial expression signal to others signs of submission and helplessness.

Prevention and Treatment of Depression

Given that the WHO identifies depression as the leading cause of disability in the world, there have been worldwide movements to develop programs directed toward prevention (see Muñoz, Le, Clarke, Barrera, & Torres, 2009, for an overview). Another aspect of focusing on prevention is that members of certain groups often do not seek treatment for depression. For example, African American and Latino adults are less likely than white adults in the United States to use mental health outpatient services. At this point, prevention programs have been directed at adults, at children during the school years, and at mothers during the period following childbirth. These programs typically follow a cognitive behavioral approach emphasizing skills training in mood regulation and interpersonal relationships. Although not every study showed a reduction in the prevention of MDDs, taken together, the results appear promising.

Much interesting work on depression has emerged in recent years from India.

Grover, Dutt, and Avasthi (2010), in the *Indian Journal of Psychiatry*, review a number of large studies from India and estimate the prevalence of depression in India to be about 15.1%. The same research group has also evaluated the efficacy of antidepressants in India.

Dr. Vikram Patel (2003) and his research group have reported in the *Archives of Disease in Childhood* that postnatal maternal depression is linked to low birth weight in newborns in India and other developing countries. Showing how infant growth is adversely affected by maternal depression, an article by the same group (2002) asserts that gender, poverty, and postnatal depression are closely interlinked. In the same journal, Anoop, Saravanan, Joseph, Cherian, and Jacob (2004) assert that maternal depression and low maternal intelligence are risk factors for malnutrition in children. All these studies thus clearly bring in evidence from Indian studies that maternal depression can have far-reaching morbid effects on child health.

Dr. Patel and his research group have also published an interesting qualitative study in this domain (Rodrigues, Patel, Jaswal, & De Souza, 2003), titling it "Listening to Mothers."

> The study provides validity for the construct of PND in an Indian setting, but also shows that the emotional distress is interpreted from the context of social adversity, poor marital relationships and cultural attitudes towards gender rather than a biomedical psychiatric category. Contrary to the assumption that sociocultural contexts associated with childbirth in non-Western societies protect mothers from depression, factors unique to the culture such as gender preference and the low involvement of husbands in child-care are major causes of stress to mothers. (Rodrigues et al., 2003)

A series of interesting studies pertaining to depression has also emerged from NIMHANS, Bangalore, India. Some of these researches have included animal studies and point to enriched environments helping to ameliorate depression (Veena, Srikumar, Raju, & Rao, 2009). An older paper by Murthy, Gangadhar, Janakiramaiah, and Subbakrishna (1997) reports the normalization of the P300 amplitude following treatment in dysthymia.

Studies also point to pathways to care for depression, focusing on the efficacy of EEG neuro feedback training on verbal and visual learning and memory in patients with depression (Lal, Rajeshwaran, & John, 2015).

Finally, a community-based intervention has been reviewed in a paper by Paudel et al. (2014) wherein they point to the impact of mental health training on village health workers regarding clinical depression in rural India.

Treatment of Depression

Many forms of treatment are available for reducing the problems associated with mood disorders. First, there are techniques for direct manipulation of brain activity. This can be accomplished through electrical or magnetic stimulation of the brain itself. A second technique is to use psychotropic medications to influence neurotransmitters, which in turn may inhibit or facilitate brain processes. Third, the brain may be influenced indirectly through cognitive, emotional, or motor changes. Traditional psychotherapy allows a person to explore how she interprets her world through thoughts or reacts to it through emotions and to consider alternative ways of experiencing her world. Other techniques such as exercise or meditation are also designed with the goal of learning alternative ways of modifying internal processes.

One problem in the treatment of depression is that even in situations in which symptoms are reduced, individuals are at risk for a relapse of the symptoms. For this reason, professionals have searched for a combination of treatments that might help to prevent relapse by involving more than one underlying depressive mechanism. For example, antidepressant medication and a form of psychotherapy such as cognitive behavioral therapy (CBT) have been shown to each be effective in comparison to a placebo treatment (DeRubeis, Siegle, & Hollon, 2008). In *Figure 8-4*, you can see that both CBT and an anti-

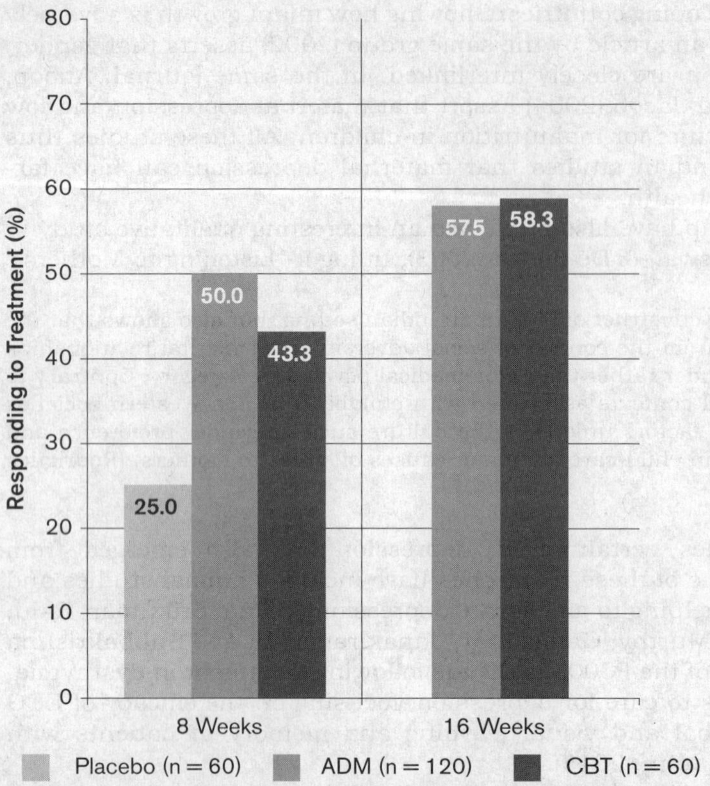

FIGURE 8-4 Cognitive Behavioral Therapy (CBT) and Antidepressant Medication (ADM) Have Comparable Short-Term Effects

Source: DeRubeis et al. (2008, p. 781).

depressant medication show greater progress in reducing symptoms of depression at 8 weeks of therapy as compared with a placebo pill. After 16 weeks of treatment, CBT and medication show equal effectiveness.

With equal effectiveness of CBT and an antidepressant medication, what do you think would happen if they were both discontinued? What happened was that in both groups symptoms of depression began to reappear. However, there were fewer symptoms of depression in the CBT condition than in the drug condition. Thus, what was learned in CBT could continue to be effective although the therapy itself had been stopped. The medication on the other hand showed no lingering positive effects when it was no longer given. Other studies have shown that the combination of CBT with an antidepressant medication is more effective than either alone.

One possibility is that cognitive therapy and medication work through different pathways in the brain (DeRubeis et al., 2008). As noted previously, brain imaging studies show greater amygdala activity and less PFC activity in those with depression compared with healthy controls. After treatment, amygdala activity is decreased and prefrontal activity increases. DeRubeis and his colleagues (2008) suggested that cognitive therapy, with its focus on cognitive processing, may increase prefrontal activity which in turn is able to inhibit amygdala activity. Antidepressant medication, on the other hand, decreases amygdala activation directly. Thus, neuroscience techniques and findings may help to explain the mechanisms of action as well as the value of utilizing more than one treatment approach (see *Figure 8-5*).

Medications for Depression

The first effective medications for depression were introduced in the 1950s and 1960s (see Gitlin, 2009, for an overview). Two of these were imipramine, a tricyclic antidepressant, and iproniazid, a monoamine oxidase (MAO) inhibitor. The term *tricyclic* refers to the three-ring chemical structure of the drug. *MAO inhibitor* refers to the focus of action at the synapse. One problem with these initial medications was side effects such as weight gain, sleep problems, and cardiovascular functioning. Additionally, MAO inhibitors can interact with certain foods, such as cheese, that contain the amino acid tyramine to increase blood pressure to dangerous levels.

In the late 1980s, a second generation of medications was released with fewer side effects. One of the most well known was Prozac (fluoxetine). Prozac became an instant hit and was given to a large number of individuals worldwide, although the popular press suggested it was overprescribed. One problem with Prozac is that it is connected with thoughts of suicide in those under 18 years of age. It has also been associated with less sexual desire and symptoms such as headache and joint pain. Prozac is one of a number of drugs referred to as selective serotonin reuptake inhibitors (SSRIs) because of their effects at the synapse. SSRIs prevent the presynaptic reuptake of serotonin, which in turn increases the level of serotonin at the synapse. Newer antidepressant medications alter the central nervous system by influencing serotonin or norepinephrine or both. These are referred to as SNRIs. It general, it takes more than 4 weeks for antidepressant medications to have an effect.

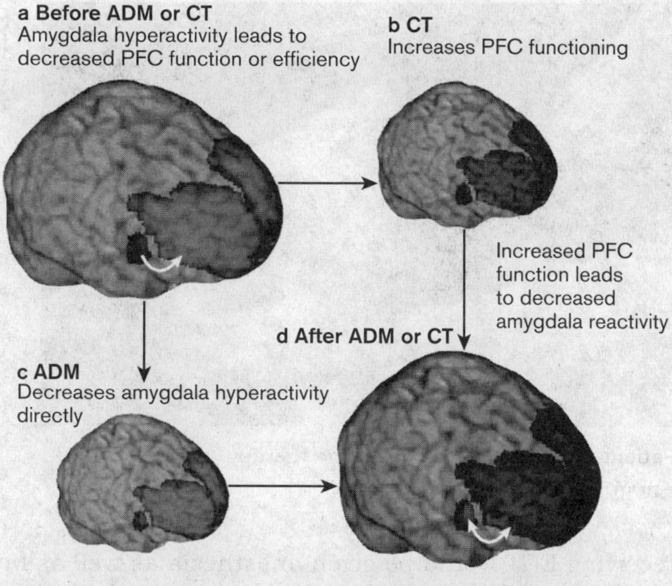

FIGURE 8-5 Hypothetical Time Course of the Changes to Amygdala and Prefrontal Function That Are Associated With Antidepressant Medication and Cognitive Therapy
Source: DeRubeis et al. (2008, p. 793).

Overall, the effectiveness of antidepressant medication is found to be about 50% in clinical trials with adults (Fava, 2003). There have been a number of concerns when antidepressant medication is used with children and adolescents. In particular, some studies have suggested a risk for increased suicide among adolescents on these medications. In children, these drugs may interact with normal processes such as exercise to lead to problems.

Electroconvulsive Therapy

Electroconvulsive therapy (ECT) is a procedure in which electrical current is passed through the brain for a brief period (see Holtzheimer, Kosel, & Schlaepfer, 2012, for an overview). This electrical activity triggers a brief seizure of less than a minute, which most likely influences changes in brain chemistry and specific networks of the cortex. A series of these treatments has been shown to be effective in treating depression—especially in those individuals for whom other treatments do not work. This is referred to as treatment resistant depression. Typically, ECT is only recommended for those individuals with

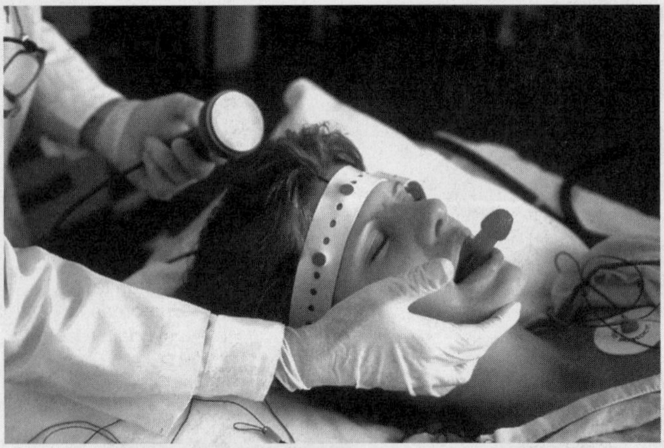

Patient receiving electroconvulsive therapy

© Will McIntyre / Science Source

depression who have not shown improvement with antidepressant medication or psychotherapy treatment.

ECT was introduced in the beginning of the last century as a potential treatment for schizophrenia. Although it was not shown to be effective for schizophrenia, it was shown to have an influence on depression. Because of its initial techniques as well as its portrayal in the popular press and movies, it was seen as a barbaric and dangerous procedure. In the last century, discomfort, broken bones, and severe memory loss were not uncommon. Today, an individual receiving ECT would be given anesthesia as well as muscle relaxing drugs to prevent discomfort and the possibility of broken bones during the seizure itself. Further, the electrical current is often introduced on only one side of the brain, which is thought to reduce memory loss. The current typical treatment procedure is to give ECT 2 to 3 times a week for a total of 6 to 12 treatments. One advantage of ECT is that results in symptom reduction can be shown at a more rapid rate than with medications. This would be beneficial in cases of severe **suicidal ideation.**

With the advent of brain imaging techniques, it is possible to better describe the effects of ECT on the brain. As noted previously, different types of connections are seen in the brain between the frontal areas and the limbic areas—especially the ACC in individuals with depression as compared with healthy controls. Likewise, those taking antidepressant medication have a reduced connectivity between the frontal areas and the amygdala compared with those on a placebo. This has led to a hypothesis that suggests those with depression show more connectivity between the frontal and limbic areas of the brain. Jennifer Perrin and her colleagues (2012) examined the effects of ECT on these fontal limbic connections. What they found was that connections were reduced after ECT as compared with before ECT. This decrease in functional connectivity was also associated with a decrease in depressive symptoms.

Vagal Nerve Stimulation

The vagus nerve is a major cranial nerve. It conveys information concerning the organs of the body to the brain. It is also involved in parasympathetic regulation of the heart and the intestines. With **vagal nerve stimulation (VNS)** treatments, an electrical stimulator is surgically implanted next to the vagus. This stimulator is connected to a pulse generator in the person's chest. Like a pacemaker in the heart, the pulse generator can be programmed to deliver electrical pulses at desirable frequencies and currents. In 1997, VNS was approved by the Food and Drug Administration (FDA) to treat epilepsy. VNS was also found to improve moods in these individuals. This led to the treatment of depression in individuals without epilepsy, which was approved in 2005. A variety of studies have suggested that for individuals whose depression does not respond to antidepressant medication, VNS is a relatively safe alternative (see Holtzheimer et al., 2012, for an overview). However, the effectiveness of the treatment has ranged from 31% to no effect in treating depression.

Transcranial Magnetic Stimulation

It has been known for a long time that electromagnetic activity can induce electrical changes in various materials. In **transcranial magnetic stimulation (TMS),** an electromagnetic coil is placed on the scalp (see Holtzheimer et al., 2012, for an overview). From the coil, a magnetic field induces a small electrical current in the first few centimeters of the brain, which depolarizes the neurons. One advantage is that TMS is a noninvasive method for stimulating cortical cells in fully awake and responsive individuals.

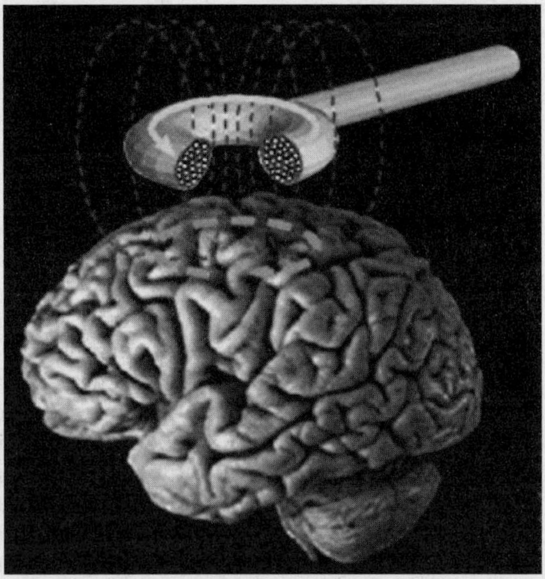

Transcranial magnetic stimulation

© National Institute of Neurological Disorders and Stroke

Initial research used single pulse TMS to study underlying motor processes by placing the TMS coil above the motor cortex. One of these studies showed a relationship between motor responses and a measure of depression (Oathes & Ray, 2006). More recently, it was found that repetitive TMS (rTMS) where multiple pulses are generated in rapid succession is effective in the treatment of depression (cf. Loo & Mitchell, 2005). A study from 42 different locations in the United States with 307 outpatients showed significant changes in depression scores following rTMS treatment (Carpenter et al., 2012). Treatment for depression generally places the coil above the DLPFC, an area of the brain shown to be involved in depression. Animal studies have shown rTMS to have similar effects to ECT. In humans who do not respond to antidepressant medication, rTMS has shown similar results to ECT. The advantage of rTMS in comparison with ECT is that no anesthetic is required and no side effects such as memory loss have been reported. Like ECT, rTMS is recommended for those who do not show changes in depression from medication.

Deep Brain Stimulation

Deep brain stimulation (DBS) involves placing an electrode in the brain (Blumberger, Mulsant, & Daskalakis, 2013). A pulse generator and battery are implanted in the person's chest and connected through wires to the brain electrode. DBS was initially used as a treatment for disorders of movement. More recently, it has been used with those who do not respond to any other treatment of depression. Brain imaging studies have shown that one area of the brain, Brodmann area 25, which is located below the corpus callosum, shows differences in activity between those who respond to treatment of depression and those who do not. In DBS for depression, the electrode is placed in this area. Current research suggests that 18% to 60% of individuals with treatment resistant depression show improvement with DBS (Blumberger et al., 2013). At this point, research in the use of DBS for depression is just beginning in terms of empirical validation.

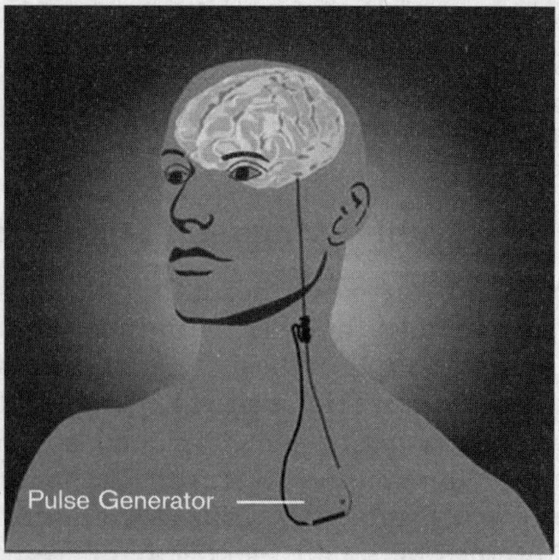

Deep brain stimulation

© The National Institute of Mental Health (NIMH)

Psychological Treatments for Depression

All of the three psychological therapy approaches—dynamic, cognitive behavioral, and existential-humanistic—described in Chapter 2 have empirically supported therapies for the treatment of depression. Emotion-focused therapy for depression, which is based on existential-humanistic techniques, has been shown to be useful for someone with mild to moderate depression (Greenberg & Watson, 2006). As noted previously, whereas the dynamic approach focuses on insight, the cognitive behavioral approach emphasizes the importance of action. That is to say, in dynamic approaches interpersonal difficulties are examined, with some focus on where thoughts and behaviors that did not work in the past came from. This often leads to discussion of early and significant relationships. Cognitive behavioral approaches, on the other hand, spend less time on past relationships and more on how to deal effectively with events in the future. The session itself is more of an educational process in which the client is helped to consider alternative explanations and learn how to cope. In CBT, there is little discussion of the relationship between the therapist and the client as there would be in dynamic approaches. Both approaches examine the manner in which individuals with depression distort and misperceive events in their lives. A number of studies have shown similar changes in depressive symptoms with either a dynamic or CBT approach (Goldfried et al., 1997; Shapiro et al., 1994).

Cognitive Therapy for Depression

Aaron Beck created a cognitive therapy for depression in the early 1960s (Beck, 1967; Beck & Alford, 2009; Hollon & Beck, 2013; see also Judith Beck, 2011, for an overview and update). The cognitive therapy model suggests that dysfunctional thinking and negative information processing maintain depression. Cognitive therapy for depression is structured and problem focused. By learning in therapy how to understand one's thinking, it is possible to change the way one thinks as well as one's emotional state and behaviors. Thus, the therapy process helps the individual with depression to evaluate the validity and utility of her thoughts. For example, if a person says "it is all my fault" or "no one will ever hire me," the therapist would help the client consider ways to test these ideas empirically. Having a person fill out a log of her activities would help someone who says "I never do anything" determine the validity of the statement. The client might also be assigned homework to move beyond inertia and create potentially positive experiences.

The cognitive model is described in terms of a cognitive triad related to depression. The first component of the triad is the individual's negative view of self. This is when the individual attributes unpleasant experiences to her own mental, physical, and moral defects. When something negative happens, the person says this is my fault. In therapy, clients can become aware of the content of their thinking. The second component is the individual's tendency to interpret experiences in a negative manner. That is, the person tailors the facts to fit negative conclusions. The basic idea is that thinking influences emotion and behavior. The third component is that the person regards the future in a negative way. She envisions a life of only hardships and anticipates failure in all tasks. In therapy, the basic idea is that individuals can modify their cognitive and behavioral responses. Overall, the therapy is directed at the automatic thoughts in relation to catastrophizing—believing that nothing will work out; personalization—believing that everything relates to you; overgeneralizaton—believing that one event is how it always is; and dichotomous thinking—believing that things are either good or bad.

A number of researchers and clinicians have further developed the classic approaches of Aaron Beck and others. These cognitive behavioral treatments are referred to as "new wave" or "third wave" approaches (Cristea, Montgomery, Szamoskozi, & David, 2013; Hayes, 2004). These new wave approaches focus less on changing the contents of a person's thoughts and more on the person's relationship to them and how they influence the person's functioning. The goals of these new wave therapies include creating flexibility and a willingness to experience one's thoughts and emotions rather than avoiding them. It is assumed that this experiential avoidance lies at the heart of psychological difficulties. Some examples of these new wave treatment approaches are *acceptance and commitment therapy* (ACT) and *mindfulness-based cognitive therapy* (MBCT), which have been shown to be effective for the treatment of depression (see *Table 8-2*).

TABLE 8-2 Empirically Supported Resources That Apply a Cognitive Approach to Depression

The Society of Clinical Psychology describes a number of empirically supported resources that apply a cognitive approach to depression as follows:
Maintenance of treatment gains is enhanced by booster sessions during the first year after termination. Several variants of cognitive therapy have been developed as more structured relapse prevention programs.
Cognitive Therapy-Continuation (Jarrett & Kraft, 1997) provides 8 to 10 monthly sessions. Patients learn to use emotional distress and depressive symptoms to practice the coping and other skills learned in the acute phase of therapy and to enhance generalization of these skills.
Well-Being Therapy (Fava & Riuni, 2003) provides 8 to 12 sessions designed to facilitate well-being after recovery from depression and reduce the risk of relapse. This therapy is not symptom-focused but rather focuses on building the components of mental health in Ryff's (1989) model: autonomy, personal growth, environmental mastery, purpose, positive relations, self-acceptance. Cognitive restructuring, activity scheduling, assertiveness training, and problem solving skills are used.
Mindfulness-Based Cognitive Therapy (MBCT; Segal, Williams, & Teasdale, 2001) is an eight-session relapse prevention program that combines mindfulness meditation with cognitive therapy techniques. Patients learn to recognize the negative thought processes associated with depression and to change their relationship with these thoughts. By unhooking from these thoughts and recognizing their transient nature, patients can learn to prevent the downward spiral from negative mood to rumination to depression. MBCT is especially helpful to reduce the risk of relapse in those with chronic depression.

Source: from www.div12.org/PsychologicalTreatments/treatments/depression_cognitive.html

Emotion Focused Therapy for Depression

Emotion focused therapy (EFT) for depression is an empirically supported therapy developed by Leslie Greenberg and his colleagues (Greenberg & Watson, 2006). As described in Chapter 2, EFT promotes the individual experiencing and processing emotional aspects of his experience. This may involve bringing past emotional experiences and memories into the present. As part of therapy, the client is able to identify his maladaptive emotions and understand emotional needs in the present. This, in turn, allows the person to discover new ways of satisfying his current needs.

In terms of depression, the treatment begins with the person experiencing the weak or bad sense of self, which lies at the core of depression. Often a sense of shame and fear is associated with this maladaptive sense of self. In EFT, the client must do more than just name the maladaptive sense of self. He or she must fully experience it so change can take place. The role of the therapist is to empathetically be with the person and help the person regulate these negatively emotional states without the fear of being overwhelmed. Thus, EFT works on the level of emotionality rather than the cognitive level as seen in CBT, although they both emphasize the meaning a client gives to his or her experiences. Like dynamic therapy, EFT would also consider the relationship between the therapist and the client on an emotional level. Further, where CBT may be seen as helping the person develop a logic and intelligence for dealing with his thoughts, EFT seeks to develop emotional intelligence.

In their empirical research to study the efficacy of EFT (see Greenberg & Watson, 2006, for an overview), Greenberg and his colleagues found that it worked best in individuals with depression who were not completely immobile. The clients that it worked best with were those who were able to parent, work, or go to school although all of these individuals reported difficulty and found little satisfaction in their activities. EFT emphasizes tailoring the therapy to the client since depression can manifest on a number of levels. Although all of the clients in the study were diagnosed with depression according to *DSM,* their depression symptoms differed. Some were highly critical and felt like failures while others had lost relationships and felt abandoned and sad. Still others felt empty, confused, and aimless. Their interpersonal relationships with the therapist also differed greatly. In testing the effects of EFT against itself and other therapies, EFT was shown to be effective in reducing the symptoms of depression.

Psychodynamic Therapy for Depression

One important aspect of dynamic therapy is the search for insight. One focus would be an understanding of how the depressive symptoms developed. Do they relate to the experience of losses in one's life? Do they relate to previous negative relationships, including critical parents who leave the child with little ability to accomplish life's goals? Do they relate to confusions concerning one's role in a job or relationship? Most short-term psychodynamic therapy would then focus on this theme.

In addition to past experiences, an additional focus would be on current relationships, including the relationship with the therapist. Like the Strupp and Binder (1984) approach described previously, most psychodynamic approaches in relation to depression would begin with an understanding of the client's behavior and relationships and how these contribute to the continuation of the depressive symptoms. Some common themes with depression include a feeling of being helpless and the dependent feeling associated with this, an overdeveloped sense of responsibility, and a feeling of anger for one's situation, which becomes internalized.

The therapeutic relationship between the client and the therapist offers an opportunity to see disturbed relationships in a safe environment. Transference is an important mechanism in which the client tends to see the therapist in terms of significant others in his life. As the client talks with the therapist, he will replay prior conflicts and enact maladaptive patterns. For example, if one of his parents was very critical of his ideas, then he may initially find it difficult to tell the therapist feelings or thoughts that are very important to him or related to how he sees himself. Another situation would be one in which a parent never allowed him to engage in tasks that he could fail at or would save him whenever he encountered problems. These past situations would leave him with unrealistic expectations as to what to expect from the world and others. In these situations, the person has never really learned what the world has to offer and may act as a child expecting someone to protect him and thus miss out on new experiences and learning. By understanding one's life, it is possible to gain insight into how to avoid moving into old patterns in new situations, which would maintain depressive symptoms.

Concept Check

- Relapse of symptoms is a serious problem in the treatment of individuals with depression. What are three specific approaches that have been taken to try to reduce the risk of relapse?
- Currently, what are the primary classes of antidepressant medications? How does each work? What are the advantages and disadvantages of each?
- In what situations is each of the following techniques most effective in treating depression? What are the advantages and disadvantages of each?
  - ECT?
  - VNS?
  - TMS?
- All of the three psychological therapy approaches—dynamic, cognitive behavioral, and existential-humanistic—described previously have empirically supported therapies for the treatment of depression. Considering each of these approaches, what is the primary focus of the therapy in regard to depression and what course does the therapy typically follow in providing an effective treatment?

In the first part of this chapter, I discussed unipolar depression, a disorder that has been described for thousands of years. We know that depression is a common disorder seen worldwide. The disorder has both environmental and genetic components. With its presence, there is a change in cognition to see the future as not being productive or pleasant. In the next section of this chapter, I will describe bipolar disorder including the manic processes seen in that disorder.

BIPOLAR DISORDER

The mania came in four-day spurts. Four days of not eating, not sleeping, barely sitting in one place for than a few minutes at a time. Four days of constant shopping. . . . And four days of indiscriminate, nonstop talking: first to everyone I knew on the West Coast, then to anyone still awake on the East Coast, then to Santa Fe itself, whoever would listen. The truth was, I didn't just need to talk. I was afraid to be alone. There were things hovering in the air around me that didn't want to be remembered: the expression on my father's face when I told him it was stage IV cancer, already metastasized; the bewildered look in his eyes when I couldn't take away the pain; and the way those eyes kept watching me at the end, trailing my every move, fixed on me, begging for the comfort I wasn't able to give. I never thought I could be haunted by anything so familiar, so beloved, as my father's eyes.

Mostly, however, I talked to men. Canyon Road [in Santa FE] has a number of extremely lively, extremely friendly bars and clubs, all of which were in walking distance of my hacienda. It wasn't hard for a redhead with a ready smile and a feverish glow in her eyes to strike up a conversation and then continue that conversation well into the early-morning hours, his place or mine. The only word I couldn't seem to say was "no." I eased my conscience by reminding myself that manic sex isn't really intercourse. It's discourse, just another way to ease the insatiable need for contact and communication. In place of words, I simply spoke with my skin.

I was a senior in high school when I had my first attack of manic-depressive illness; once the siege began, I lost my mind rather rapidly. At first, everything seemed so easy. I raced about like a crazed weasel, bubbling with plans and enthusiasms, immersed in sports, and staying up all night, night after night, out with friends, reading everything that wasn't nailed down, filling manuscript books with poems and fragments of plays, and making expansive, completely unrealistic, plan for my future. The world was filled with pleasure and promise; I felt great. Not just great, I felt really great. I felt I could do anything, that no task was too difficult.

Every day I awoke deeply tired, a feeling as foreign to my natural self as being bored or indifferent to life. Those were next. Then a gray, bleak preoccupation with death, dying, decaying, that everything was born but to die, best to die now and save the pain while waiting. I dragged exhausted mind and body around a local cemetery, ruminating about how long each of its inhabitants had lived before the final moment. I sat on the graves writing long dreary, morbid poems, convinced that my brain and body were rotting, that everyone knew and no one would say. Laced into the exhaustion were periods of frenetic and horrible restlessness; no amount of running brought relief. For several weeks, I drank vodka in my orange juice before setting off for school in the mornings, and I thought obsessively about killing myself.

Bipolar Disorders

Bipolar disorder was previously referred to as manic-depressive disorder. In reading the experiences by Terri Cheney and Kay Jamison, we quickly see both the mania and the depression. By the way, Kay Jamison received her PhD in clinical psychology from UCLA and is a professor of psychiatry at Johns Hopkins University. She has written significant books describing the scientific and clinical aspects of bipolar disorders (e.g., Goodwin & Jamison, 2007) as well as her own experiences in *An Unquiet Mind.*

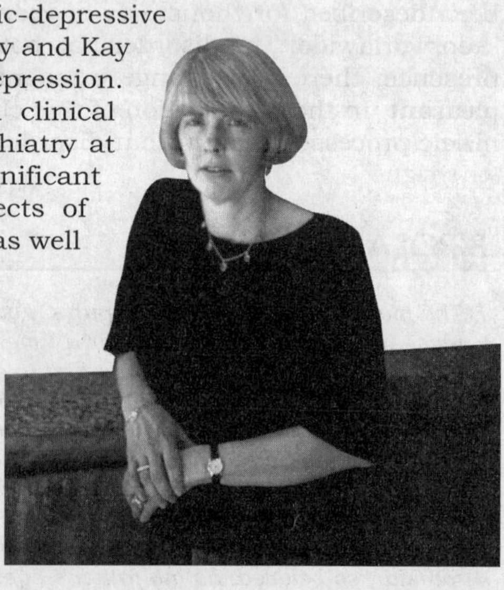

Changes in mood are an important aspect of bipolar disorders. These include the intense sense of well-being along with high energy seen in mania and its opposite seen in depression. Changes in cognition and perception also accompany these states. In mania, thoughts seem to flow easily, and many individuals find themselves very productive during mania. Perceptions and sensations may also be heightened. However, mania can also increase a feeling of pressure with racing thoughts and ideas that do not make sense. Sometimes, this includes a feeling of "I can do anything" and the sense that nothing will not work out. Individuals in a manic state may buy expensive items they cannot afford, place large bets, and engage in all types of risky sexual behavior. It is as if there is nothing to worry about. The depressive episodes show the opposite picture with the person experiencing a bleak outlook, low energy in a world of black-and-white and a wish to do little. One characteristic experienced in both mania and depression by many individuals is a sense of irritability.

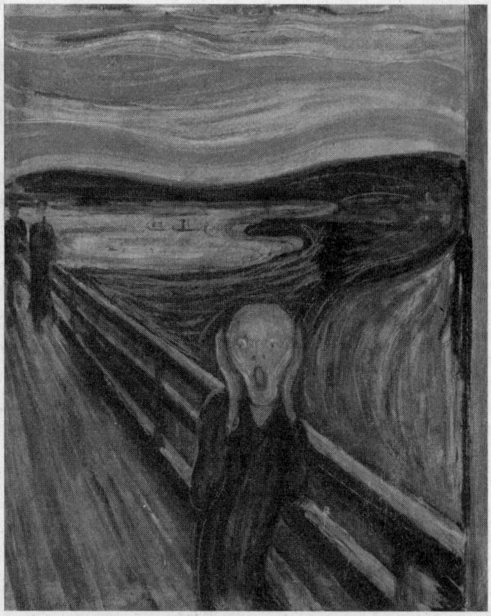

The Scream by Edvard Munch—Munch suffered from bipolar disorder

Descriptions of mania and depression have been with us for more than 2,000 years. Hippocrates (460–377 BC) described both mania and melancholia. He saw these disorders as separate produced by underlying conditions related to an imbalance in the four humors. Today, we would refer to this as a hormonal imbalance. In 150 AD, Aretaeus of Cappadocia linked mania and melancholia as one disorder. He described individuals who after displaying melancholia show fits of mania and vice versa. From this time till the present, mania and depression were considered as different parts of one disorder. For example, in 1854 Falret in France described a circular disorder (La folie circulaire) and Bailarger described "double insanity" (La folie à double forme) to denote the manner in which depressive and mania episodes are part of one disorder. Kraepelin, in the late 1800s and early 1900s, established in his textbooks the idea that manic depression and schizophrenia are two separate disorders, a perspective that has continued to this day. Further, in 1957 Leonhard made a distinction between unipolar and bipolar disorders, and this was adopted in *DSM* in 1980. Unipolar was depression without mania whereas bipolar disorder encompassed both (see Goodwin & Jamison, 2007, for both historical and current perspectives). The artist Edvard Munch, who painted the well-known painting *The Scream,* suffered from bipolar disorder. This painting can be seen in the photo to the right.

Diagnosis of Bipolar Disorder

DSM–5 classifies the disorder in terms of the manic and the depressive symptoms. Bipolar I disorder requires the presence of one or more manic episodes (see *Table 8-5*). Bipolar I does not require any depressive symptoms for the diagnosis. In fact, some individuals with bipolar disorder never report depression (see Johnson, Cuellar, & Miller, 2009, for an overview). However, the majority of individuals with bipolar disorder do experience depression during their lifetime. Bipolar II, on the other hand, requires an episode of a MDD along with a hypomanic episode. A hypomanic episode is similar to mania but shorter in duration and less severe (see *Table 8-3*). Further, an individual with bipolar II disorder cannot have had a manic episode, as described in *Table 8.3.*

TABLE 8-3 Bipolar I Disorder

For a diagnosis of bipolar I disorder, it is necessary to meet the following criteria for a manic episode. The manic episode may have been preceded by and may be followed by hypomanic or major depressive episodes.

Manic Episode

A. A distinct period of abnormally and persistently elevated, expansive, or irritable mood and abnormally and persistently increased goal-directed activity or energy, lasting at least 1 week and present most of the day, nearly every day (or any duration if hospitalization is necessary).

B. During the period of mood disturbance and increased energy or activity, three (or more) of the following symptoms (four if the mood is only irritable) are present to a significant degree, and represent a noticeable change from usual behavior:

1. Inflated self-esteem or grandiosity
2. Decreased need for sleep (e.g., feels rested after only 3 hours of sleep)
3. More talkative than usual or pressure to keep talking
4. Flight of ideas or subjective experience that thoughts are racing
5. Distractibility (i.e., attention too easily drawn to unimportant or irrelevant external stimuli), as reported or observed
6. Increase in goal-directed activity (either socially, at work or school, or sexually) or psychomotor agitation (i.e., purposeless non-goal directed activity)
7. Excessive involvement in activities that have a high potential for painful consequences (e.g., engaging in unrestrained buying sprees, sexual indiscretions, or foolish business investments)

C. The mood disturbance is sufficiently severe to cause marked impairment in social or occupational functioning or to necessitate hospitalization to prevent harm to self or others, or there are psychotic features.

D. The episode is not attributable to the direct physiological effects of a substance (e.g., a drug of abuse, a medication, or other treatment). Note: A full Manic Episode emerging during antidepressant treatment (medication, electroconvulsive therapy, etc.), but persisting beyond the physiological effect of that treatment is sufficient evidence for a Manic Episode and, therefore, a Bipolar I diagnosis. However, caution is indicated so that one or two symptoms (particularly increased irritability, edginess or agitation following antidepressant use) are not taken as sufficient for diagnosis of a Manic Episode, nor necessarily an indication of a Bipolar Disorder diathesis.

Hypomanic Episode

A. A distinct period of abnormally and persistently elevated, expansive, or irritable mood and abnormally and persistently increased activity or energy, lasting at least 4 consecutive days and present most of the day, nearly every day (or any duration if hospitalization is necessary).

B. During the period of mood disturbance and increased energy and activity, three (or more) of the following symptoms have persisted (four if the mood is only irritable), represent a noticeable change from usual behavior, and have been present to a significant degree:

1. Inflated self-esteem or grandiosity
2. Decreased need for sleep (e.g., feels rested after only 3 hours of sleep)
3. More talkative than usual or pressure to keep talking
4. Flight of ideas or subjective experience that thoughts are racing
5. Distractibility (i.e., attention too easily drawn to unimportant or irrelevant external stimuli), as reported or observed
6. Increase in goal-directed activity (either socially, at work or school, or sexually) or psychomotor agitation
7. Excessive involvement in pleasurable activities that have a high potential for painful consequences (e.g., the person engages in unrestrained buying sprees, sexual indiscretions, or foolish business investments)

C.	The episode is associated with an unequivocal change in functioning that is uncharacteristic of the person when not symptomatic.
D.	The disturbance in mood and the change in functioning are observable by others.
E.	The episode is not severe enough to cause marked impairment in social or occupational functioning, or to necessitate hospitalization. If there are psychotic features, the episode is, by definition, manic.
F.	The episode is not due to the direct physiological effects of a substance (e.g., a drug of abuse, a medication, or other treatment).
	Note: A full Hypomanic Episode emerging during antidepressant treatment (medication, electroconvulsive therapy, etc.) and persisting beyond the physiological effect of that treatment is sufficient evidence for a Hypomanic Episode diagnosis. However, caution is indicated so that one or two symptoms (particularly increased irritability, edginess or agitation following antidepressant use) are not taken as sufficient for diagnosis of a Hypomanic Episode, nor necessarily indicative of a bipolar diathesis.
Major Depressive Episode	
A.	Five (or more) of the following symptoms have been present during the same 2-week period and represent a change from previous function, at least one of the symptoms is either (1) depressed mood or (2) loss of interest or pleasure. 1. Depressed mood most of the day, nearly every day, as indicated by either subjective report (e.g., feels sad, empty, or hopeless) or observation made by others (e.g., appears tearful). (Note: In children and adolescents, can be irritable mood.) 2. Markedly diminished interest or pleasure in all, or almost all, activities most of the day, nearly every day (as indicated by either subjective account or observation). 3. Significant weight loss when not dieting or weight gain (e.g., a change of more than 5% of body weight in a month), or decrease or increase in appetite nearly every day. (Note: In children, consider failure to make expected weight gain.) 4. Insomnia or hypersomnia nearly every day. 5. Psychomotor agitation or retardation nearly every day (observable by others; not merely subjective feelings of restlessness or being slowed down). 6. Fatigue or loss of energy nearly every day. 7. Feelings of worthlessness or excessive or inappropriate guilt (which may be delusional) nearly every day (not merely self-reproach or guilt about being sick). 8. Diminished ability to think or concentrate or indecisiveness, nearly every day (either by subjective account or as observed by others). 9. Recurrent thoughts of death (not just fear of dying), recurrent suicidal ideation without a specific plan, or a suicide attempt or a specific plan for committing suicide.
B.	The symptoms cause clinically significant distress or impairment in social, occupational, or other important areas of functioning.
C.	The episode is not attributable to the physiological effects of a substance or another medical condition.
Bipolar I Disorder	
A.	Criteria have been met for at least one manic episode (criteria A–D under "manic episode" above).
B.	The occurrence of the manic and major depressive episode(s) is not better explained by schizoaffective disorder, schizophrenia, schizophreniform disorder, delusional disorder, or other specified or unspecified schizophrenia spectrum and other psychotic disorder.

Source: Reprinted with permission from the *Diagnostic and Statistical Manual of Mental Disorders, Fifth Edition*, (Copyright 2013). American Psychiatric Association.

The major distinctions in *DSM–5* between bipolar I and bipolar II are related to the severity and duration of the manic phase. Bipolar I is the category in which mania is present and although not required may also show symptoms of depression. In this classification, the mania needs to last a week unless medication was given. In bipolar II, the elevated mood is more than that seen in normal mood swings but less than that of bipolar I. In this case, the mania lasts for less than 4 days and has less social impairment than bipolar I. These are referred to as hypomanic episodes. Bipolar II also includes a depressive episode. In fact, individuals with bipolar II, compared with bipolar I, show a greater propensity toward depressive episodes. Only 11% of those with bipolar II develop bipolar I over the following 10 years (Coryell et al., 1995). An additional diagnostic category is cyclothymia, which shows an affective temperament that is less severe than bipolar I or bipolar II. Lifetime prevalence estimates for bipolar I are 1%, bipolar II 1.1%, and cyclothymia 2.4% (Kessler, Merikangas, & Wang, 2007). Using statistical models, it is suggested that the occurrence of bipolar I can be grouped as early, immediate, or late onset (Bellivier, et. al. 2003). These data are shown in Figure 8-6.

Although only one manic episode is required for a diagnosis of bipolar disorder, almost all individuals with bipolar disorder show recurring experiences (see Miklowitz & Johnson, 2006, for an overview). For example, approximately 20% of individuals who enter outpatient treatment have had four or more mania and depression episodes the preceding year. Examining bipolar I individuals, 37% showed recurrences of mania or depression. This increased to 60% when examined for 2 years and 73% for 5 years. Overall, the depressive symptoms last longer than the ones involving mania.

Bipolar I Disorder

For a diagnosis of bipolar I, an individual needs to display three of the following seven characteristics. These are as follows:

1. Inflated self-esteem or grandiosity
2. Decreased need for sleep (e.g., feels rested after only 3 hours of sleep)
3. More talkative than usual or pressure to keep talking
4. Flight of ideas or subjective experience that thoughts are racing
5. Distractibility (i.e., attention too easily drawn to unimportant or irrelevant external stimuli), as reported or observed
6. Increase in goal-directed activity (either socially, at work or school, or sexually) or psychomotor agitation (i.e., purposeless non–goal directed activity)
7. Excessive involvement in activities that have a high potential for painful consequences (e.g., engaging in unrestrained buying sprees, sexual indiscretions, or foolish business investments)

As you read in the personal descriptions of Terri Cheney and also Kay Jamison, you can see examples of some of these seven characteristics—especially the greatly increased energy and a reduced need for sleep. There were also examples of high paced discussions and a willingness to enter into high risk activities such as sex. It is often the sense of "I can do anything" that leads individuals with mania to enter into all sorts of activities without thinking. Other reports describe situations in which people think they will never fail so they place large bets or buy expensive products.

Bipolar II Disorder

Bipolar II disorder includes the presence of a major depressive episode as required for the diagnosis of depression. The diagnosis also requires at least one hypomanic episode. The observable symptoms of hypomania and mania are the same. The difference is that hypomania does not cause as much impairment in social and occupational functioning. Further, hypomanic episodes last for 4 days rather than 1 week. Also, individuals with bipolar II disorder are less likely to be hospitalized for the disorder than those with bipolar I.

Cyclothymic Disorder

Cyclothymic disorder is characterized by mood changes that are not as severe as would be required in the criteria for manic or depressive episodes.

A number of epidemiological studies have examined the 1-year and lifetime prevalence (see Goodwin & Jamison, 2007, for an overview). Overall, the lifetime prevalence for bipolar I is about 1% and not that different from those with the disorder in the last year. Further, the gender differences are not large. Similar prevalence rates have been found around the world. When the spectrum of bipolar disorders are included, the lifetime prevalence increases to between 3% and 8.3%.

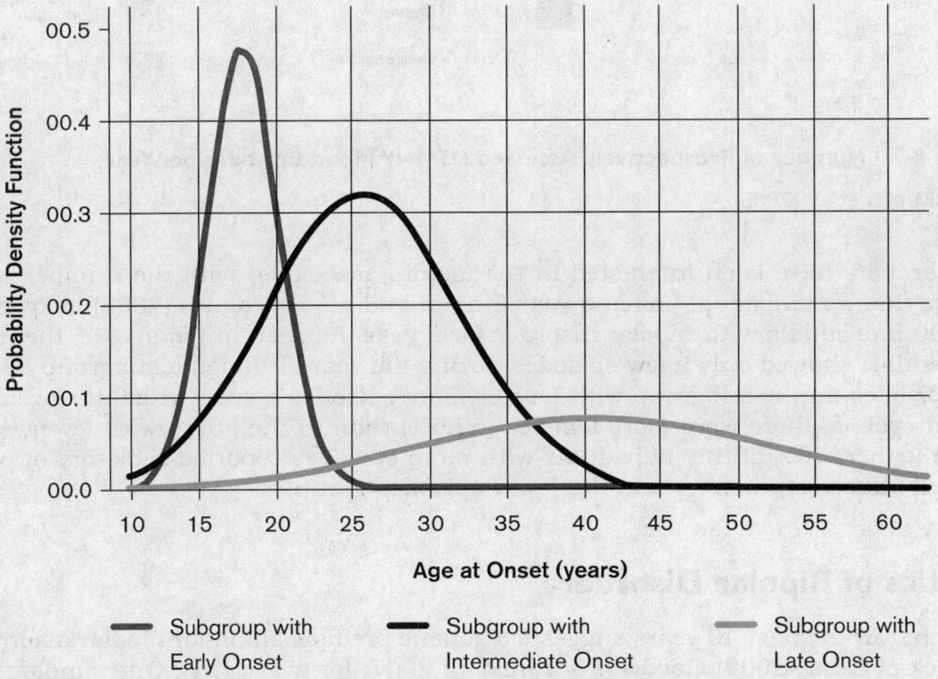

FIGURE 8-6 Theoretical Distributions of Ages at Onset for 579 Patients With Bipolar I Disorder in Subgroups With Early Onset, Intermediate Onset, and Late Onset

Source: From Bellivier et al. (2003, p. 1000). Reprinted with permission from the American Journal of Psychiatry, (Copyright © 2003). American Psychiatric Association.

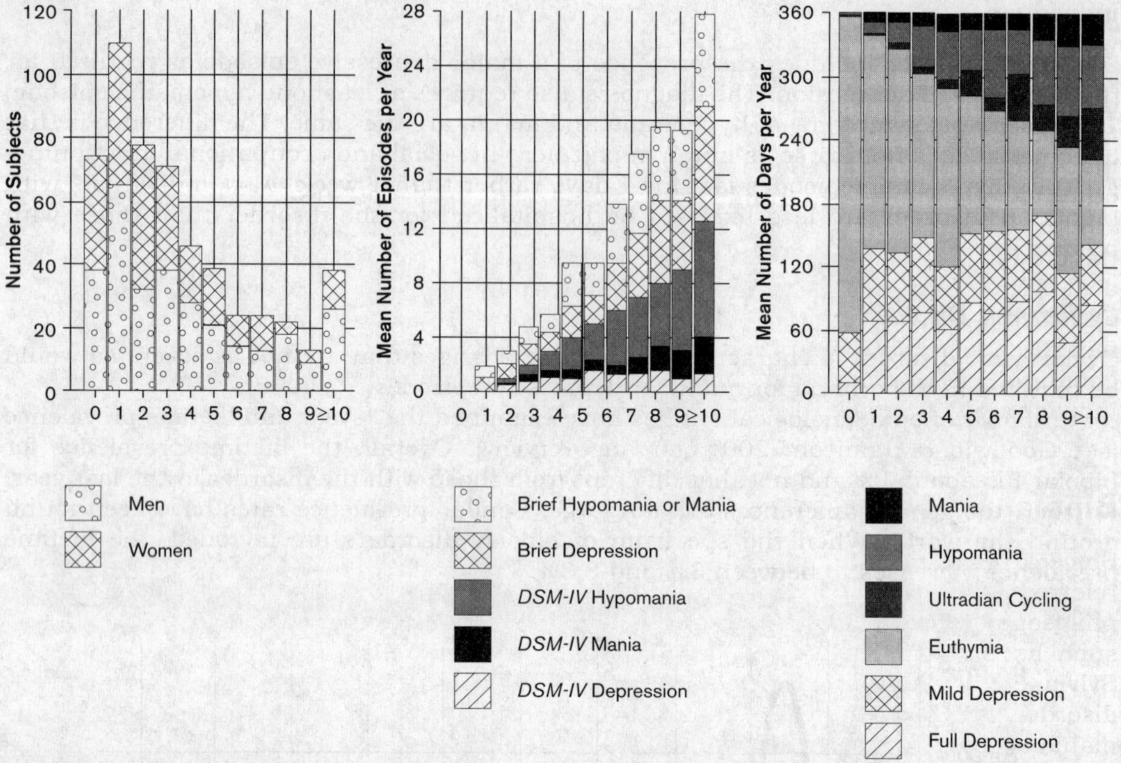

FIGURE 8-7 Number of Prospectively Assessed *DSM–IV* Mood Episodes per Year

Source: Kupka et al. (2005).

Researchers have been interested in the factors associated with the number of mood episodes that an individual has in a year. Kupka and his colleagues (2005) followed more than 500 individuals with bipolar disorder for a year. As seen in *Figure 8-7*, the majority of individuals showed only a few episodes during the year although a subgroup had 10 or more episodes. In the subgroup with four or more episodes a year, which they referred to as rapid cycling, there were more females (62.6%) than in the group with fewer episodes (52%). Further, 40% of the individuals with more episodes reported a history of physical or sexual abuse versus 24.1% in the fewer episodes group.

Genetics of Bipolar Disorder

Research over the past 40 years suggests a genetic predisposition for bipolar disorder (see Craddock & Sklar, 2009; Goodwin & Jamison, 2007, for overviews). One simple test of a genetic predisposition is to see if the disorder runs in families. For bipolar disorders, heritability is about 5% to 10% for first-degree relatives and 40% to 70% for monozygotic (MZ) twins compared with only 14% for fraternal twins. That is to say, a first-degree relative of someone with bipolar disorder has approximately 10 times the risk of having the disorder compared with a random person. This is much higher than first-degree relatives of a person with depression, which is about 3 times higher. Further, relatives of individuals with MDD do not appear to be at risk for mania whereas relatives of those with bipolar disorder are at risk for depression.

Recent research has shown a partial overlap between the genes involved in bipolar disorder and schizophrenia. In an MZ twin with schizophrenia, there is an increased risk for both schizophrenia (40.8%) and mania (8.2%) in the other twin. In an MZ twin with mania, there is an increased risk for mania (36.4%) and for schizophrenia (13.6%) in the other twin.

As noted in Chapter 3, mitochondria are structures within a cell that are involved in the production of energy. These cells evolved separately from traditional deoxyribonucleic acid (DNA). Thus, a given cell in your body contains both nuclear DNA and mitochondria and their DNA. Since mitochondria are involved with energy production, it is possible to measure glucose concentration in cerebrospinal fluid and the blood as related to mitochondrial energy production. Mitochondrial functioning has been shown to be different in individuals with bipolar disorder (Regenold et al., 2009).

Bipolar Disorder and Creativity

Since at least the time of Plato and Aristotle, *divine madness*, as the ancient Greeks referred to it, has been associated with creativity. Aristotle asked why people who excel in philosophy, poetry, or the arts are melancholic. Numerous writers, poets, and artists, such as Ernest Hemingway, Virginia Woolf, Sergei Rachmaninoff, Peter Tchaikovsky, Sylvia Plath, Jackson Pollock, and Mark Rothko, have been associated with bipolar disorder. This has resulted in a link between creativity and bipolar disorder, especially the mania aspect. However, most of this has been of an anecdotal nature.

Recently, Sheri Johnson and her colleagues (2012) sought to determine if there existed a scientific basis for the association between creativity and bipolar disorder. One line that supports this is that above-average accomplishments are seen among the family members of those with the disorder (Johnson, 2005). However, Johnson and her colleagues concluded that at this point a direct relationship between creativity and bipolar disorder is difficult to make. Likewise, Frederick Goodwin and Kay Jamison (2007) reviewed a number of studies examining the relationship between bipolar disorders and creativity. They concluded that most individuals with bipolar disorders are not unusually creative. However, there are specific individuals in whom the extremes of mood may have contributed to their artistic insights and productivity. Thus, a variety of underlying personality and mood traits that would lead one into creative occupations may be similar to those found in bipolar disorders.

Brain Imaging of Bipolar Disorder

In *Figure 8-8*, you can see the inferior frontal cortex in light blue and yellow, the orbitofrontal cortices in light green and purple, the middle frontal cortex in dark blue and purple, and the superior frontal cortices in green and red. Differences in activation have been found in functional magnetic resonance imaging (fMRI) studies between the depression phase of bipolar disorder and the mania phase (Ballmaier, 2004). During the depression phase, there are decreases in prefrontal activation. During the mania phase, there are increases in activation in the ACC and the anterior limbic network, which includes the striatum, thalamus, and amygdala.

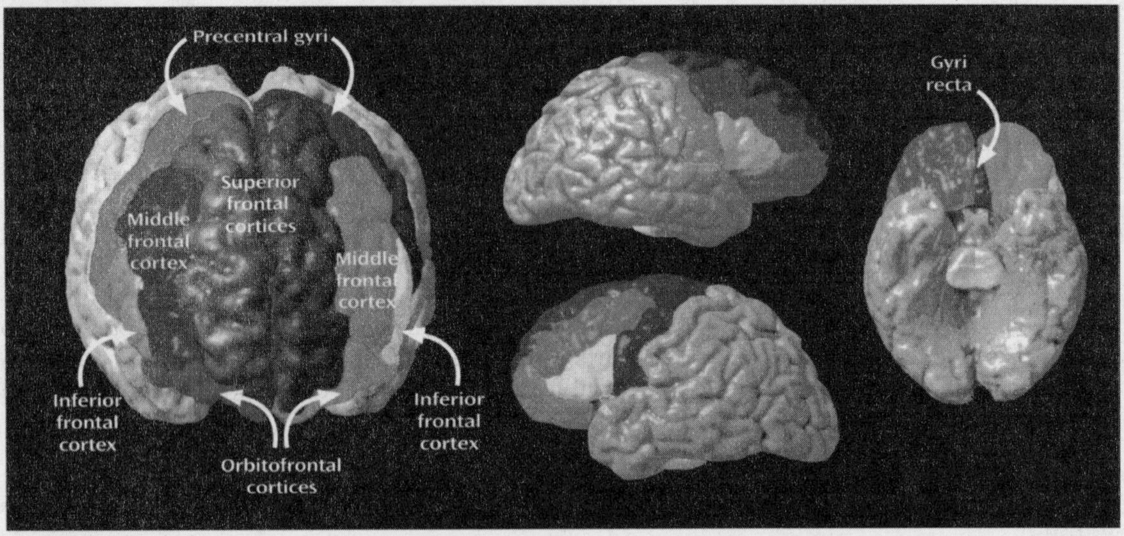

FIGURE 8-8 Brain Areas Involved in Bipolar Disorder

Source: Ballmaier (2004, p. 101).

Overall, a variety of studies have suggested that the brain processes underlying the symptoms seen in bipolar disorder involve the anterior limbic brain networks (see Marchand & Yurgelum-Todd, 2011; Savitz & Drevets, 2009; Strakowski, 2011, for overviews). The first network includes the ventral prefrontal network and its connections to the thalamus, globus pallidus, striatum, and their modification by the amygdala and ACC. This system is seen to be responsible for three important aspects. These are (1) the perception of emotional stimuli, (2) the generation of an emotional state, and (3) the production of autonomic responses associated with the emotional state. A second network involving the DLPFC, medial PFC, dorsal ACC, and hippocampus is seen to regulate affective state. It has been speculated that mood dysregulation in bipolar disorder may involve either or both of these systems.

Researchers have also examined brain differences when bipolar episodes are not present. In one study, unmedicated individuals with bipolar disorder and matched controls performed a cognitive task in the fMRI scanner (Strakowski, Adler, Holland, Mills, & DelBello, 2004). Although both groups performed the task equally well, they displayed different patterns of brain activation. The bipolar group showed more activation in the limbic, paralimbic, and ventrolateral prefrontal areas as well as visual association areas. The healthy control group showed greater activation in the fusiform gyrus and medial PFC. These researchers suggested that individuals with bipolar disorder process cognitive tasks in a manner more consistent with processing emotional tasks whereas healthy controls show inhibition of emotion networks in the brain while they perform cognitive tasks.

Neurotransmitter Dysregulation

The three neurotransmitters studied in relation to bipolar disorder have been norepinephrine, dopamine, and serotonin (see Miklowitz & Johnson, 2006, for an overview). Original perspectives took a simple formulation that mania was associated with high levels of norepinephrine and dopamine and depression with low levels. However, a variety of studies suggest that rather than absolute amount of the neurotransmitters, it is the sensitivity at the postsynaptic receptor site that plays the important role. In particular, it has been noted that organisms exposed to repeated doses of stimulants become more responsive to their effects (Sax & Strakowski, 2001).

Environmental Factors

The environment in which one lives plays an important role in the course of bipolar disorders. For example, Ellicott, Hammen, Gitlin, Brown, and Jamison (1990) studied the stressful events in the lives of individuals with a bipolar disorder. Individuals who experienced more stressful events were at a 4.5 times greater risk for relapse within a 2-year period than those who did not. Miklowitz and his colleagues found that if an individual with a bipolar disorder returned from a hospitalization to a family situation in which criticism, hostility, or emotional overinvolvement were present, they were more likely to have a relapse (Miklowitz, Goldstein, Nuechterlein, Snyder, & Mintz, 1988). Specifically, 94% of those in a negative emotional environment showed relapse within 9 months compared with 17% of those without a negative emotional family situation. A number of politicians, including Winston Churchill, have been thought to experience mania.

Concept Check

- Changes in mood are an important aspect of bipolar disorders. How would you describe these changes?
- What are the important diagnostic criteria for bipolar I, bipolar II, and cyclothymic disorder?
- What evidence can you cite for the role that the following factors play in the development of bipolar disorder?
    - Genetic factors?
    - Brain processes?
    - Neurotransmitter dysregulation?
    - Environmental factors?
- As is true with most disorders, a combination of psychological therapy and medication is recommended for treating bipolar disorders. Specifically, what is recommended in terms of
    - Psychological therapy?
    - Medication?

Indian studies focusing on neuropsychology and Bipolar disorder.

A study from India reported in the *British Journal of Psychiatry* reports neuropsychological dysfunction, soft neurological signs, and social disability in euthymic patients with bipolar disorder (Goswami et al., 2006). Performances on tests reflecting executive function and verbal memory (but not attention) were significantly poorer in the bipolar disorder group.

In another study reported in the *East Asian Archives of Psychiatry* (Soni, Singh, Shah, & Bagotia, 2017), executive dysfunction was found to be the strongest predictor of psychosocial outcome in euthymic bipolar patients. A total of 61 euthymic patients with bipolar disorder and 30 healthy individuals were included in this study. The patients were divided into low-functioning (n = 30) or high-functioning (n = 31) subgroups based on the functioning level measured by the Global Assessment of Functioning Scale score. All three groups differed significantly in the digit span backward test, verbal learning, and memory test, Trail Making Test, and Stroop Color Test. Digit span backward test, Trail Making Test, and Stroop Color Test were significantly correlated with the Global Assessment of Functioning Scale score.

In an Indian study conducted at the Central Institute of Psychiatry (CIP) Ranchi and reported in the *Indian Journal of Health and Well Being*, it was found that cognitive remediation training is effective in improving the overall quality of life among patients with bipolar disorder in remission, specifically in improving their physical health and psychological domains of quality of life.

Another interesting work from the same institute has found temperamental underpinnings to bipolar spectrum disorder, since they found that bipolar probands were significantly more hyperthymic as compared to controls (Gandotra, Ram, Kour, & Praharaj, 2011). The study thus supported the view that affective temperaments could be proximate determinants in the heritability of bipolar disorders.

Goswami et al. (2006) have reported their work on neuropsychological dysfunction, soft neurological signs, and social disability in euthymic patients with bipolar disorder in the *British Journal of Psychiatry*. They state that performance on tests reflecting executive function and verbal memory (but not attention) were significantly poorer in the bipolar disorder group as compared to controls. Working from a large center in New Delhi, the capital of India, they found that the bipolar group was significantly more impaired than normal subjects on a number of standardized neuropsychological tools, even after controlling for residual symptoms.

Treatment of Bipolar Disorder

Until the middle of the last century, there was no effective treatment for bipolar disorder. Even today, bipolar disorder is a complex disorder to treat. There is no accepted treatment for bipolar disorder that does not involve some form of medication. Because its symptoms may vary from depression to mania and this occurs in an irregular manner, there are fewer medications available for bipolar disorder. Further, a large number of individuals with bipolar disorder report a history of being misdiagnosed. This is partly because it is difficult to diagnose bipolar disorder without a clear picture of its course. Young adults who first show the symptoms in college, for example, may experience the symptoms as part of their lifestyle. It is often during a treatment for a depressive episode when mania appears that it is realized that bipolar disorder is the correct diagnosis.

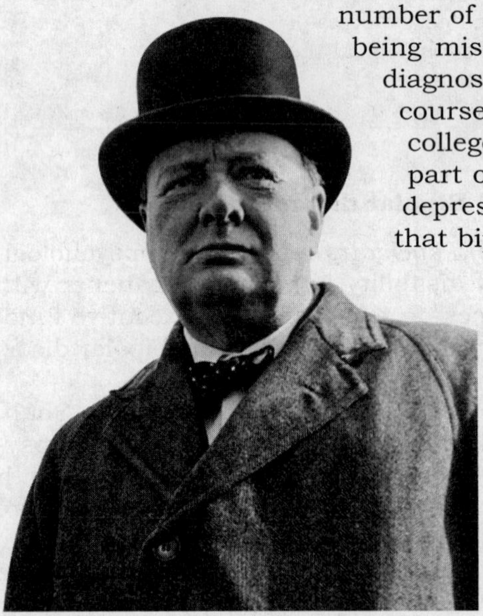

Winston Churchill Is described as experiencing mania

Even with treatment, as just noted, those individuals with bipolar disorder who live in a negative emotional environment are more likely to relapse. Further, some people with bipolar disorder will discontinue their medication on their own, which leads to relapse. They may discontinue the medication because they miss their "highs" or want a wider range of emotional experience. Thus, most professionals recommend a combination of medication and psychotherapy and other types of support including family involvement for those with bipolar disorder. The nature of the disorder and the various psychosocial factors experienced by the person with bipolar disorder make performing research on a single medication or psychotherapy difficult.

Most psychological therapies that have been used with bipolar disorders focus on both an educational and a psychological perspective. Specifically, techniques related to stress reduction and ways to reduce negative interactions with others are emphasized. Additionally, the client is also taught about bipolar disorder, its symptoms, the manner in which it may occur over time, and the importance of the use of medication. Family members and significant others in the client's life may also be involved in the education and stress reduction aspects of therapy.

Monica Basco and John Rush (2005) have developed a 20-session CBT for use with individuals with bipolar disorder. The initial sessions focus on the symptoms of bipolar disorder and the medications that are used to treat them. The next sessions focus on the client's particular symptoms, how to systematically monitor them, and factors related to treatment compliance. Following this, sessions are devoted to understanding one's cognitions including biased thinking and acting in both mania and depression. The final sessions emphasize an understanding of social relationships and ways to problem solve and resolve difficult situations.

Medications for Bipolar Disorder

It is important to keep in mind that there are different stages of treatment that require different processes (Goodwin & Jamison, 2007). These can be described as acute treatment, continuation treatment, and maintenance treatment. Acute treatment refers to the period from the beginning of a manic or depressive episode to remission of the symptoms. This period usually lasts from 6 to 12 weeks. Continuation treatment is the period from the remission of the symptoms to the time that they would not be expected to recur. This time has been determined from noting spontaneous recovery times in individuals who have not been treated. This period is around 6 months for a depressive episode and 4 months for a manic episode. Maintenance treatment is designed to prevent or reduce future episodes of mania and depression.

Psychopharmacological treatments for bipolar disorder involve a treatment for episodes of depression, a treatment for episodes of mania, and drugs to reduce relapse (see Thase & Denko, 2008, for an overview). Lithium is the most common treatment for bipolar disorder. Lithium is a salt found in nature. It was first used in the 1800s to treat mental disorders although real interest in its use for the treatment of bipolar disorder began in the 1950s (Malhi, 2009). Lithium is more effective for the mania aspect of bipolar than the depressive aspects, and it is seen as a mood stabilizer. Although lithium has been used for a number of years, current reviews suggest it is not as effective as commonly believed (Geddes, Burgess, Hawton, Jamison, & Goodwin, 2004). However, this review suggests its use is warranted in those individuals who respond to the drug. One group of individuals who do not respond to lithium are those who show rapid cycling.

Because lithium is not useful with certain groups, drugs referred to as anticonvulsants have been tried and shown to be effective. Two of these anticonvulsants are sodium valproate and carbamazepine. Other classes of drugs such as antipsychotics discussed in the chapter on schizophrenia have also been used in the treatment of bipolar disorder. One might think that antidepressants might work, but in some individuals these cause a switch to mania and rapid cycling.

Bipolar disorder has been seen for thousands of years and in a number of famous individuals. It can represent both a manic phase and a depressive phase. In the manic phase, bipolar individuals are at risk for suicide since they tend to be impulsive. In the next section, I will describe suicide in more detail.

SUICIDE

The term *suicide* has been dated to 1642 in a work *Religio Medici* written by Sir Thomas Browne. It comes from the Latin meaning to kill oneself. Suicidal behaviors can be seen as existing on a continuum ranging from thinking about suicide to attempting suicide to an act that leads to death. However, some individuals think often about suicide—referred to as *suicidal ideation*—without actually attempting to harm themselves. Surprisingly, in the United States the rate of suicide attempts did not change between 1990 and 2000, but the actual number of suicides declined by 15%.

Mental illness has a strong connection with suicide (see Goldsmith, 2001, for an overview). Of those suicide attempts that led to death, it is estimated that 90% of adults and 67% of youth would meet diagnostic criteria for a mental disorder. The most common disorders associated with suicide are depression, bipolar disorder, substance use disorders, personality disorders, and schizophrenia, in that order. In bipolar and personality disorders, suicide is often associated with impulsiveness. With schizophrenia, it is more associated with active manifestation of the disorder. In older adults, mental disorders are often comorbid with physical disorders. However, a physical disorder alone is not highly associated with suicide. In older adults, hopelessness along with depression was associated with suicidal ideation.

To put suicide in perspective, more people die from suicide than from homicide and even war. In 2000, there were 815,000 people from around the world who died from suicide (WHO, 2002). This represents a 1-year prevalence rate of 14.5 per 100,000. This makes suicide the 13th leading cause of death worldwide. It becomes the fourth leading cause of death among those 15 to 44 years of age. In all age-groups, worldwide suicide rates increase with age (see *Figure 8-9*). This graph also shows that males commit suicide more often than females.

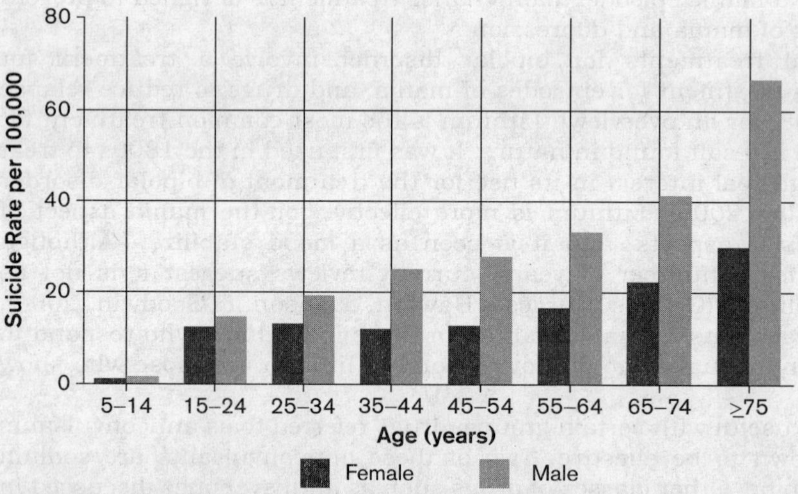

FIGURE 8-9 Worldwide Suicide by Age and Gender

Source: WHO (2002, p. 188).

Cultural Differences in Suicide

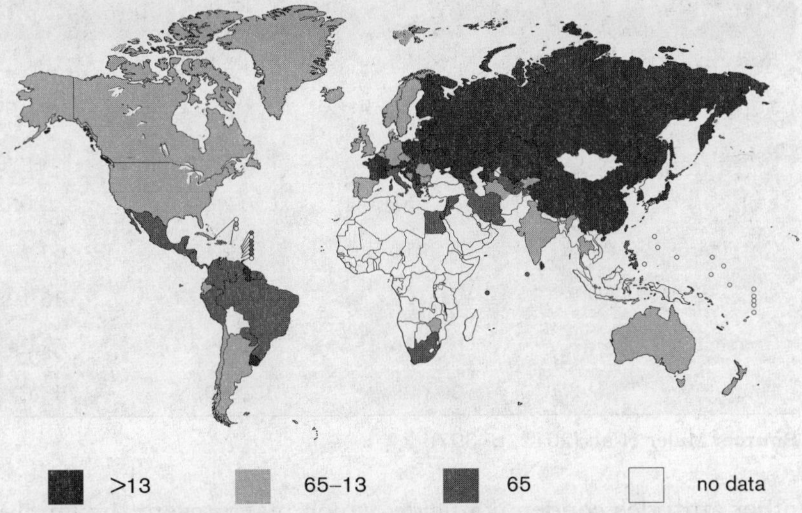

FIGURE 8-10 Map of Suicide Rates Worldwide

Source: from www.who.int/mental_health/prevention/suicide/suicideprevent/en/index.html

Disclaimer: This figure is not to scale. It does not represent any authentic national or international boundaries and is used for illustrative purposes only.

As shown in *Figure 8-10*, there are cultural differences in the rate of suicide. Hungary has the highest national suicide rate in the world followed by Finland and Austria. Their rates are 66, 43, and 42 per 100,000 compared with 11.3 in the United States. Countries with low rates of suicide such as Mexico tend to be predominantly Catholic or Muslim, have strong family ties, and have a younger population. There are also psychological differences related to suicide worldwide. In the United States and Europe, suicide is associated with depression and alcohol use disorder whereas in Asia, impulsiveness plays an important role. There are also cultural differences in gender ratios. The rate is more similar in Asia but higher for males in Chile and Puerto Rico. Further, the suicide rate of Caucasians is approximately twice that observed in other races.

In the United States, the suicide rate is about in the middle of all countries (Miller, Azrael, & Barber, 2012). The U.S. rate is about 11.3 people per 100,000. However, for children under 15 years of age, the suicide rate is higher than in other industrialized countries. In the United States, firearm-related suicide for those under 15 is some 11 times higher. A strong risk factor for attempting suicide is the presence of a mental illness or substance use disorder. Data suggest that more than 8 million Americans report having serious thoughts of suicide, 2.5 million report making a suicide plan, and 1.1 million report a suicide attempt (Substance Abuse and Mental Health Services Administration, 2011).

Gender Differences in Suicide and the Type of Attempts

Although females attempt suicide more often than males, males are 3 to 4 times more likely to die because the methods they use are more lethal (see Miller et al., 2012, for an overview). For example, men are more likely to use firearms or hanging as opposed to overdose. Among men, firearms account for about 62% of all suicide deaths. As seen in *Table 8-4*, firearms and hanging are more likely to lead to death than overdose or cutting oneself.

Suicide attempts and rates may be underestimated since not all attempts result in a hospital visit. Likewise, not all actual suicides are reported. In some cultures, religious or

TABLE 8-4 Suicide Statistics by Type of Attempt as Measured by Emergency Room Visits

Method	*Fatal*	*Nonfatal*	*Total*	*Case fatality ratio*
Firearm	16,869	2,980	19,849	85
Suffocation/hanging	6,198	2,761	8,959	69
Poisoning/overdose	5,191	215,814	221,005	2
Fall	651	1,434	2,085	31
Cut/Pierce	458	62,817	63,275	1
Other	1,109	35,089	36,198	3
Unspecified	146	2,097	2,243	7
Total	30,622	322,992	353,614	9

Source: Miller et al. (2012, p. 397).

other attitudes condemn suicide, which may prevent the family from reporting the event. There is some suggestion that individuals may use automobile accidents or other accidents as a means of committing suicide without it being apparent. Police report provocative situations in which an individual causes the police to use force, which may be attempts to be killed by another. Also, there is very little data on those who attempted suicide but did not succeed. What data there is suggests that in old age more attempts lead to actual suicide than in those under the age of 25.

Endophenotypes and Suicide

Traits associated with suicide might serve as endophenotypes (see Courtet, Gottesman, Jollant, & Gould, 2011, for an overview). That is, there may be characteristics related to one's genetics that increase the probability of suicidal ideation and attempts. Two of these traits are aggression and impulsivity. These two factors have been found to be associated with suicidal behaviors. An additional factor found in studies of those who have engaged in suicidal behavior is making disadvantageous choices in tasks unrelated to suicide. This is consistent with the suggestion that frontal lobe dysfunction is associated with suicidal behaviors. Researchers are currently attempting to describe the complicated interaction between genes, neurotransmitters, and environmental conditions. For example, in those who consider suicide, the serotonin system in the PFC may not function normally. Further, hopelessness has been shown to be influenced by the TPH2 gene variants (Lazary et al., 2012). Finally, two HPA axis genes (CRHBP and FKBP5) have also been shown to interact with childhood trauma and increase suicidal behavior (Roy, Hodgkinson, Deluca, Goldman, & Enoch, 2012).

Short-Term and Long-Term Factors Related to Suicide

There are both long-term and short-term factors related to suicide (see Turecki, Ernst, Jollant, Labonté, & Mechawar, 2012, for an overview). The long-term factors include a family history of suicide. This suggests that genetics may play a role. This is seen to be separate from mental disorders that run in families. Personality traits as described in terms of endophenotypes play a role. Children who received negative feedback or abuse are also more likely to engage in suicidal behaviors. If the abuse was performed by a family member, this has been shown to be associated with greater risk of suicidal behaviors. This suggests that it is the trauma related to a family member rather than the actual abuse that is important. This trauma may be involved in epigenetic change, which influences the stress response. The short-term factors include recent life events, current mental illness, and the feeling of hopelessness. Also prior suicidal behavior and substance abuse are predictive of future suicidal behavior.

Preventing Suicide

Suicide prevention programs seek to reduce the factors that increase the risk for suicidal thoughts and behaviors (see *Table 8-5*). These programs seek to work on at least four levels: the individual, the individual's relationships, the community, and the society. This can be diagrammed as seen in *Figure 8-11.* Suicide prevention began in the United States in the 1950s and has continued through to the present day. Many communities have hotlines for people to call 24 hours a day. There has also been a national focus on groups that are at higher risk for suicide including Native Americans and members of the armed forces and veterans.

TABLE 8-5 The Warning Signs of Suicide

Talking about wanting to die
Looking for a way to kill oneself
Talking about feeling hopeless or having no purpose
Talking about feeling trapped or being in unbearable pain
Talking about being a burden to others
Increasing the use of alcohol or drugs
Acting anxious, agitated, or reckless
Sleeping too little or too much
Withdrawing or feeling isolated
Showing rage or talking about seeking revenge
Displaying extreme mood swings

Source: "Suicide Warning Signs" (n.d.).

Friends and relatives of individuals who show these signs should help them find a mental health professional or suicide prevention center in their community. Interestingly, those who tried to commit suicide but did not succeed tend to feel relieved. This makes it possible for those individuals to receive help.

SUMMARY

Depression has been described for more than 2,000 years. It is characterized by depressed mood in which one feels sad or empty without any sense of pleasure in one's activities. With a depressive disorder, the individual may also experience sleep problems and weight changes, as well as a sense of worthlessness and self-blame. Clinical depression is seen when the majority of these symptoms last for an extended period of time. There is a gender difference in that over the course of a lifetime about 1 in 4 females and 1 in 10 males experience a major depressive episode. Genetic studies suggest that

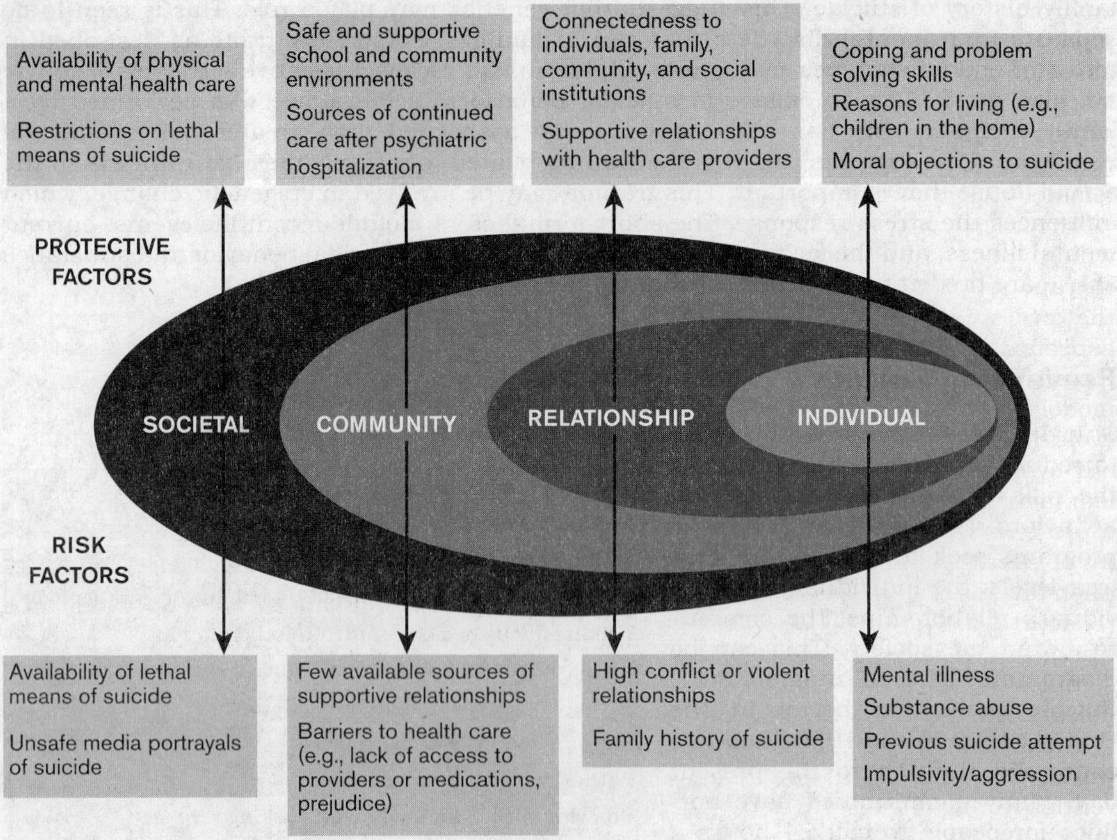

FIGURE 8-11 Examples of Risk Factors Across Four Levels

Source: Office of the U.S. Surgeon General (2012).

depression is equally influenced by genetic and environmental factors. Today, MDD is one of the most commonly diagnosed mental disorders among adults and is estimated to be found in about 13 million adult Americans during the preceding 12 months. Lifetime estimates are approximately 33 million Americans. Three fourths of those with MDD would also meet criteria for an additional DSM disorder. Depression has been related to a variety of physiological, psychological, family, and social components. It is also estimated to be one of the most economically costly mental disorders worldwide. Research suggests that the initial episode of depression has a strong

Concept Check

- What evidence would you cite to show that mental illness is related to suicide?
- What cultural differences are associated with suicide?
- What gender differences are associated with suicide?
- What four endophenotypes have been suggested as markers for suicide?
- What short-term and long-term factors are related to suicide?
- What warning signs would you look for in a friend if you were concerned about suicide? What kinds of programs are available to help an individual at risk for suicide?

environmental component whereas later episodes are thought to be related to internal physiological changes. Major life stress such as loss of a close relationship is highly associated with the development of depression. Although diagnostic symptoms for adolescents are similar to those for adults, depressed children are more likely to describe physical symptoms. The rates of depression are very low prior to puberty with equal numbers of boys and girls. After puberty, the rates of depression increase and more females than males are affected.

The cognitive model of depression was developed by Beck to describe the manner in which individuals with depression maintain the disorder. It also became the basis for a therapeutic approach. It is basically a learning theory model that suggests adverse events that occur early in life can lead to the development of depressive schemas involving three aspects referred to as the negative cognitive triad: the self, the personal world, and the future. Researchers now suggest that the underlying neural mechanisms for the cognitive model of depression can be described. Explaining the existence of depression from an evolutionary perspective includes the assumption that depressed mood was adaptive in our evolutionary history—that feeling depressed would help the individual solve a problem faced by humans from the earliest times. Researchers suggest that a depressed state represents a risk management strategy in response to a situation that has a low probability of success and high probability of risk. The social risk hypothesis was developed by Allen and Badcock (2003) as an integration of three previous broad models of depression: (1) depression in terms of resource conservation, (2) depression in terms of social competition, and (3) depression in terms of attachment. This hypothesis suggests that when significant interpersonal relationships are disrupted including social humiliation or defeat, depressed mood is the outcome.

Given that the WHO identifies depression as the leading cause of disability in the world, there have been worldwide movements to develop programs directed toward prevention. Many forms of treatment are available for reducing the problems associated with mood disorders. First, there are techniques for direct manipulation of brain activity. This can be accomplished through electrical or magnetic stimulation of the brain itself through techniques such as ECT, VNS, and TMS. A second technique is to use psychotropic medications to influence neurotransmitters, which in turn may inhibit or facilitate brain processes. Third, the brain may be influenced indirectly through cognitive, emotional, or motor changes. Traditional psychotherapy—from the dynamic, cognitive behavioral, and existential-humanistic perspectives—allows a person to explore how she interprets her world through thoughts or reacts to it through emotions and to consider alternative ways of experiencing her world. Other techniques, such as exercise or meditation, are also designed with the goal of learning alternative ways of modifying internal processes. One problem in the treatment of depression is that even in situations in which symptoms are reduced, individuals are at risk for a relapse of the symptoms. For this reason, professionals have searched for a combination of treatments that might help to prevent relapse by involving more than one underlying depressive mechanism—for example, antidepressant medication and a form of psychotherapy such as CBT.

Descriptions of mania and depression have been with us for more than 2,000 years. From this time till the present, mania and depression were considered as different parts of one disorder. Changes in mood are an important aspect of bipolar disorders. These include the intense sense of well-being along with high energy seen in mania and its opposite seen in depression. Changes in cognition and perception also accompany these states. *DSM–5* classifies the disorder in terms of the manic and the depressive symptoms.

The major distinctions in *DSM–5* between bipolar I and bipolar II are related to the severity and duration of the manic phase. An additional diagnostic category is cyclothymia, which shows an affective temperament less severe than bipolar I and bipolar II. Overall, across the spectrum of bipolar disorders, the lifetime prevalence is estimated to be between 3% and 8.3%. Gender differences are not large, and similar prevalence rates have been found around the world. Research over the past 40 years suggests a genetic predisposition for bipolar disorder since it has been found to run in families. Other genetic research has shown a partial overlap between the genes involved in bipolar disorder and schizophrenia. A variety of brain imaging studies have suggested that individuals with bipolar disorder show differences in brain processes, as well as a complex pattern of neurotransmitter dysregulation. Environmental factors, particularly stress, play an important role in the course of bipolar disorders.

Suicidal behaviors can be seen as existing on a continuum ranging from thinking about suicide to attempting suicide to an act that leads to death, as well as thinking often about suicide—suicidal ideation—without actually attempting it. Mental illness—particularly depression, bipolar disorder, substance use disorders, personality disorders, and schizophrenia—has a strong connection with suicide. More people die from suicide than from homicide and even war, making it the 13th leading cause of death worldwide. There are cultural, psychological, and gender differences related to suicide worldwide. Although females attempt suicide more often than males, males are 3 to 4 times more likely to die because the methods they use are more lethal. There are both long-term and short-term factors related to suicide. Long-term factors include personality traits, particularly aggressiveness and impulsivity; a family history of suicide suggesting that genetics may play a role; and children who received negative feedback or abuse suggesting epigenetic change, which influences the stress response. Short-term factors include recent life events, current mental illness, and the feeling of hopelessness. Prior suicidal behavior and substance abuse is also predictive of future suicidal behavior. Suicide prevention programs seek to reduce the factors that increase the risk for suicidal thoughts and behaviors and work on at least four levels: the individual, the individual's relationships, the community, and the society. Knowing the warning signs of suicide can help friends and relatives of individuals who show these signs find a mental health professional or suicide prevention center in their community to receive help.

STUDY RESOURCES

Review Questions

1. How would each of the following perspectives answer the question of why depression exists from an evolutionary perspective:
   a. Depression in terms of resource conservation?
   b. Depression in terms of social competition?
   c. Depression in terms of attachment?
   d. Social risk hypothesis?
   e. Your theory of why depression exists from an evolutionary perspective?

2. The WHO identifies depression as the leading cause of disability in the world. We know that cost-effectiveness is a critical factor in designing programs for developing countries. Given that, what proposal would you offer for a comprehensive program for the reduction of depression in developing countries that addresses the following aspects:
   a. Prevention?
   b. Psychotropic medications?
   c. Techniques for direct manipulation of brain activity?
   d. Psychological therapy?
   e. Relapse of symptoms?
3. Bipolar disorder is a complex disorder. How has that complexity impacted the following aspects of bipolar disorder:
   a. Definition and the development of diagnostic criteria?
   b. An individual's experience with bipolar disorder?
   c. Research on biomarkers and the development of endophenotypes for bipolar disorder?
   d. Treatment of bipolar disorder?
4. Mental illness has a strong connection with suicide. This is especially true of depression and bipolar disorder. With what you've learned in this chapter, design a suicide prevention program that targets a specific population of individuals with depression or bipolar disorder.
   a. What cultural, gender, and age factors would you consider?
   b. How would your program focus on the following levels: the individual, the individual's relationships, the community, and the society?
   c. How would your program incorporate the recommended treatment approaches for the disorder you're focusing on?

For Further Reading

Jamison, K. R. (1993). *Touched with fire: Manic-depressive illness and the artistic temperament.* New York: Free Press (Macmillan).

Solomon, A. (2003). *The noonday demon: An atlas of depression.* New York: Scribner.

Key Terms and Concepts

bipolar disorder
cognitive model of depression
cortisol
depression in terms of attachment
depression in terms of resource conservation
depression in terms of social competition
electroconvulsive therapy (ECT)
intergenerational transmission of depression
macrophage theory of depression
major depressive disorder (MDD)
manic depression
melancholia
negative cognitive triad
suicidal ideation
suicide
transcranial magnetic stimulation (TMS)
unipolar depression
vagal nerve stimulation (VNS)

CHAPTER

9

Stress, Trauma, and Psychopathology

CHAPTER OUTLINE

- PSYCHOLOGICAL STRESS AND PSYCHOPATHOLOGY 315
- DOES TRAUMA PRODUCE MENTAL ILLNESS? 316
- IS SOCIAL PAIN LIKE PHYSICAL PAIN? 317
- THE PHYSIOLOGICAL MECHANISMS RELATED TO STRESS AND TRAUMA 318
- TRAUMA CHANGES OUR GENES THROUGH TAGGING (EPIGENETICS) 318
- PHYSICAL ILLNESS AND CONCOMITANT PSYCHOLOGICAL STRESS 320
- PSYCHOLOGICAL STRESS AND THE IMMUNE SYSTEM 321
- WHAT MAKES YOU RUN FROM BEARS? STRESS AND THE HYPOTHALAMIC-PITUITARY-ADRENAL AXIS 323
- THE AUTONOMIC NERVOUS SYSTEM 325
- THE STUDY OF STRESS 327
- TRAUMA- AND STRESSOR-RELATED DISORDERS IN *DSM–5* 331
- SPIRITUALITY AND RESILIENCE, VOLUNTEERING, AND WELLBEING 343
- SUMMARY 343
- STUDY RESOURCES 345

As a journalist, I am used to writing about death and destruction. Natural disasters that rip through homes and lives, leaving tattered and torn pieces of towns in their paths. The tsunami, floods in California, earthquakes in Japan. I have become accustomed, even calloused to these horrors as I write about them and survey the video from a distance. I will never do that again. Hurricane Katrina brought all of us down from our ivory towers. It opened our eyes to the frailty of human life, and man-made structures. We are so small compared to Mother Nature.

My TV station sits about four blocks from the beach, just behind the railroad tracks. I guess we thought we were invincible, because no one there evacuated. As the storm got closer I started to get nervous. Not because of the warnings we were giving to the community, or the projections on the Weather Channel, but because I could hear the fear in our own meteorologists' voices. Professionals who have lived through hundreds of storms were shaking.

As Katrina hit land, the wind sounded like the ocean was in pain, and angry. In awe, we stepped out into our courtyard. I watched as the rain that was falling in sideways circles, ripped the roof off of our newsroom. I ran back inside, only to see a hole above my desk and rain pouring onto my computer. In a frantic rush we grabbed equipment, mainly weather computers, and raced to the other, "safer," side of the building. Pieces of insulation began falling, and metal shards flew past, it felt like a combat zone with enemy fire coming from all directions.

The lights in our studio began pulsating, threating to become hundred pound projectiles. We rushed to the cinder block section of building which had been dubbed "hurricane proof" and set up makeshift operations, only to hear a crash above us. A piece of concrete had slammed through the roof and into the second floor. Water began seeping in the front and back doors. Then one of transmitting towers, weighing hundreds of pounds, collapsed. It looked like a twist tie that had been hastily discarded just inches from where we were huddled. If the storm had been any stronger, or lasted even an hour more, I don't know that we would have made it.

As scary as it was at the station, that wasn't the part that frightened me most. As we were rushing out of our crumbling newsroom the phones were still ringing, with frantic viewers on the other end of the line. The sound of the phone crying made my heart ache. I had talked to dozens of people who were stranded, trapped, and scared just minutes before. I still wonder what happened to the woman who called sobbing, climbing to her attic with her baby. There was a man stuck in his house, trying to punch his way to the roof. One of my coworkers called as she jumped out her bedroom window, and her house was sucked into the murky waters. I can only imagine the horror of seeing a 30 foot wave coming towards you and making what might be your last phone call.

Shilo Groover is a graduate of GW's School of Media and Public Affairs (BA, 2003). She now works as a television producer at WLOX (ABC 13) in Biloxi, Mississippi.

From Shilo Groover. (2005, October 19). The storm: A first-hand account of Katrina [Letter to the editor]. By George! Retrieved from www.gwu.edu/~bygeorge/oct1905/letter.html

I came home from Iraq in March 2004, yet I'm still fighting a war, a war here at home. It's a war of shadows, one that no one seems to really understand. A war of anger and anxiety, fought in the recesses of my mind.Just like in the two wars I fought in Iraq and Afghanistan, I don't know who the enemy is. There, insurgents take potshots at you, then go back into hiding. Combating post-traumatic stress disorder, PTSD, is the same. Some days I feel as if I have the enemy on the run; other days it has me pinned down.

I am a former military policeman. I was among the first soldiers to move into Afghanistan after the Sept. 11 attacks. For nine months, my company provided support for Rangers and special operations forces. We returned home in September 2002. Four months later, in January 2003, we were in Kuwait preparing for another war.

I remember the day we moved into Iraq. It was about a week after D-Day. As soon as we crossed the border, we saw cratered highways, dead bodies and burning vehicles. For the next year, my company provided security for main supply routes and patrolled the streets of Mosul. There was never a firefight, just constant, low-level violence. Sniper fire, RPGs, IEDs and mortar attacks kept us on edge at every moment. We were hypervigilant. We couldn't shut it off. It reached the point when we thought that anything could be a bomb, that anything on the road could blow up.

Now, the war is on my home front. I often ask myself, why am I still fighting? I'm safe now, aren't I? But PTSD, like an insurgency, is elusive. It attacks from all angles, almost invisibly. The enemy is out there, but you don't know when or from where an attack will come. As a soldier, I saw things no one ever should. I once responded to a call from a field artillery unit that had shot an Iraqi who tried to flee a checkpoint. Have you ever seen what a .50-caliber round does to a person's head? Imagine a large wooden mallet smashing a watermelon. The .50-cal. does the same. Brain matter was splattered all over the inside of the Iraqi's truck. At the time, I didn't feel anything. I felt numb. It was as if nothing had happened. No emotion at all.

Once I came home, once my mind wasn't racing at 100 miles an hour, I had time to think and to detox from the military. And as I processed my memories, I wondered if something was wrong with me. In truth, my family and my wife knew before I did.

Before I deployed, I was very laid-back, an easygoing guy. I joked around a lot. When I returned from Iraq, I was edgy and short-tempered. The smallest thing could trigger an outburst. I viewed everything from a life-or-death perspective. I would get ticked off if my wife and I left five minutes late for an appointment. On a mission, "five minutes late" can get someone killed. You can't be "five minutes late" to a firefight.

I couldn't get out of The Zone.

In Iraq and Afghanistan, I was constantly telling soldiers what to do to stay alive. I did the same at home. In the evening, when my wife would tell me what she did or where she went that day, I might bark at her. "What the hell's wrong with you? You could have gotten hurt."

I couldn't focus on any one particular task. I had to juggle several jobs at once to relax. That's why I thrived in the chaos at my workplace, at a job I hated. I had trouble sticking to a conversation, and I had no patience. I couldn't sit still for more than five or 10 minutes before I had to walk around the house. I couldn't sit through a movie with my wife unless it was full of action. I played war-based video games to put me in my comfort zone. They soothed me.

At my Vet Center, the staff told me what benefits I was eligible for and walked me through enrollment. They helped me with my job hunt. They gave me their personal phone numbers and told me to call if I needed anything.

And they got me the help I needed. A Vet Center counselor had me tested for traumatic brain injury and PTSD, and got me into group and individual therapy. It's still a struggle, but I'm taking back control of my life and my feelings. Each day I'm one step closer.

The author deployed to Afghanistan from January to September 2002 and to Iraq from March 2003 to March 2004. He is now studying sociology at a college in Northern California, and plans to pursue a career assisting fellow vets.

From Jeremy P. (2010, February 21). Fighting the war at home. New America Media. Retrieved from newamericamedia.org/2010/02/fighting-the-war-at-home.php

First Person Account of the Floods in Chennai in 2015

"Once the bullfrogs start, it's a sign that the rains are over," my Mum always said.

It is day three of the North East monsoon attack on Tamil Nadu. The trains have stopped. The drains have stopped. In most parts of the city, the current has stopped. Trees have dropped. They lie in obscene tangles: their branches outstretched, catching at passersby, asking for help. The rivers are rising. Life as we know it has come to a standstill.

Only the bullfrogs of Chennai are rocking. They begin with a chorus of hoarse calls to their mates. For months, they have been lying dormant under the earth. The rain sets them free to perform their mating rituals. They perform their Louis Armstrong imitations. They get ready to march. Just like the Saints, the bullfrogs of Chennai are marching in. And boy, do they get their number! When it is that time, the trumpets sound and that City, gateway to the South, pride of the Dravidians, comes floating by.

By Sunday, November 15, Chennai is too waterlogged to march.

A new situation

I am sending silent e-mails to my mother complaining that her theories no longer hold good. Even the bullfrogs have wizened up. They are no longer croaking. There are rumors that there are snakes now. They are attacking the frogs. We don't dare go out into our own garden.

After three days of intermittent Chennai rainstorms, records 245 mm of rain. The Chennai Meteorological Department warns that there is more rain to come. They have been forecasting the onset of a harsh monsoon for the last two months. When it arrives no one quite believes it is happening. We have had six months of water starvation. For months, water lorries and tankers supply water from the outlying areas to the city in buckets. We have deepened our wells and employed water diviners to tell us where we might find the aquifers to sink our bore wells. We learn to sip water that has been drawn deep from the earth and spit it out.

"Too brackish. Too metallic. It will rust your guts." But everywhere there is the sound of pounding. It's not just the bore wells that drill holes into the flat cityscape, but the foundations for the pylons that will string a network of flyovers across the city.

We can't believe that it's raining. It's actually been raining for the past ten days. It's only when the rivers start rising that it dawns on us that we are in the midst of a major natural calamity.

We've seen it before...

We've had our tsunami moment in 2004. Since then, the repeat performance of floods due to the monsoon in 2005, 2010, 2013, and now 2015 have left us almost waiting for the dark. We are disaster freaks. We are so immune to disaster that until we hear about it on the media, or read about it from the morning newspapers we don't notice that the flood waters are creeping into our homes. We ignore the cars that are wallowing in dirty water like water buffaloes. We stand along the ocean's edge on Marina beach, one known as the second-longest sandy beach in the world and look at the urchins swimming in pools of water formed by the rain-water filling the sand in waist-deep stretches. Even the beach is inundated.

"No one has announced that there's going to be a cyclone," my neighbor informs me. "Why are you stocking up on vegetables and bread?"

"It's part of the Gujarati side of my inheritance," I tell her. "Gujaratis always prepare for the worst, either drought or flood by stocking up on essentials. It's called a frontier mentality."

It gets heavier

On Sunday night, the rain takes on the form of a bombardment. The telephone lines are still working. I am on the line with a young family that has moved into a house one street away from the main road. They tell me that they have moved into a ground floor house from the 17th-floor of an apartment in a newly built area called Chemmencherry, close to the electronic highway that now defines Chennai at OMR, or Old Mahabalipuram. They have a young child. The locals tell them that the Cooum River is rising. The river will soon be in their house.

"You better move in with us," I tell them. We wait till midnight. That's when I know that the tide will turn. The waters will subside. And yes, the bullfrogs know it too. They start croaking again in the early hours of the morning. We have survived the night. The schools are filling up with displaced people. Others just lie in the open under blue plastic sheets. Bus stops provide a temporary shelter. In one of the neighborhood autorickshaws I notice that a family of kittens has made a home. There's still a sense of community amongst the ordinary folk of the city.

Chennai drowning is the most unreported event. Of course, the timing is also wrong. In the wake of the horrors recorded by and on the international networks about the terror strikes in Paris, the pugilistic fury of the political pundits shadow boxing on the daily Goswami rabble stadium, Chennai's ordeal appears irretrievably local. In a city of five million, or thereabouts, a hundred dead, or thereabouts, does not warrant too much media space.

Another planet

It's not just the timing that has led to Chennai drowning but not waving. Geographically and politically it is too close to the ground, too far south, too mired in the darkness of the Dravidian family discourse, to warrant the attention of the national interest.

There is of course Chennai's famous resilience to natural and humanoid disasters that we citizens can count upon. As environmentalists like to say, a river never forgets its history. In times of crisis it returns to its bed. So also in the case of the two major rivers that define the city, the Cooum and the Adyar, (a third river Kosathalaiyar feeds the life-giving lakes in the north west), and the British-era Buckingham Canal that cuts through in a north-south direction have dictated the deployment of people in clusters along its sides.

Before becoming a booming electronic hub, Chennai used to crawl back at night and revert to a series of villages. Each of these villages used to have a temple with a tank to conserve water, and inlets leading to the tank or lake were kept open. There used to be 650 such water bodies in the city. Now by most accounts, there are just 27. Unlike other coastal cities, Chennai is as flat as a dosa, with an average elevation of 6.7 metres above the mean sea level with many areas that are marshlands. These shallow lakes and man-made tanks were an essential part of the city's natural cycle of self-preservation. As it happened, the areas least affected by the floods were the older parts of the city, where temple tanks remembered their history and culverts and drains constructed in the 19th century managed to find ways to carry the overflow.

Spilling over

On Monday morning, we hear that one of the largest of the water bodies has breached its bank.

"The Chembarambakkam Lake has broken its banks!" The cry is taken up with additional rumors that some miscreants have deliberately allowed the floodwaters to flow into the city.

In the some of the newly developed estates of the feeder communities servicing Chennai's electronic lifeline at Old Mahabalipuram Road, the floodwaters have no memory of where to go. They craw into every subway, underpass and ground floor households bringing in leeches, scorpions, toads, and water snakes.

Even further down the OMR highway at Chemmencherry, where my newly found family of a young couple lived, there is a crisis. There is a clash of lifestyle. Low-rise communities surround the high-rise apartments. Both are now flooded by the opening of the Chembarambakkam Lake. After the fifth day of rain, the inhabitants in the high-rise DLF apartments have no choice but to leave their homes. Not many want to do that. They have children, infants in arms. The only option is to get into the boats deployed hastily by various authorities, the police, the Navy, the fire brigade.

When they get into the boats, the Low-Risers, the people who live in the newly built Tsunami Villages surrounding DLF, stop the boats. "Why should only the affluent be evacuated?" they ask. "Why not us?" Small boys swim across the water and attempt to topple the boats. There are rumors that they have thrown poisonous snakes into some of the boats. "The snakes will bite you!" they scream at the High-Risers. Even snakes, it seems, are well trained to bite only the rich and not those who are swimming in the water. Many of the High-Risers have to get out of the boats and wade through the mud to safety.

New contours

One of the interesting sidelights of this conflict is that the people who live in the Tsunami Villages are not all fisherfolk. They are some of the people displaced from the communities that lived along the Cooum and Buckingham Canal to make way for the plans to convert Chennai into the Singapore of the South. In the haste to create redraw the contours of the city, people living along the rivers' edge have been brutally re-located. Lacking a sense of community, or being forced to live in arid clusters of concrete blocks, far from their original places of work, they have now reverted to a hunter-gatherer phase of existence.

When I go to the riverbank of the Cooum near our house, I notice that at least a hundred people are camping outside of their washed-out homes. They are sleeping in the open next to the heaving black river.

"This is our home," says an old woman who is stirring a pot of rice. "We will not leave."

In Amma country, the Amma Canteens have been providing hot food in vast quantities to the flood affected, as well as a solatium of rice, kerosene, a sari, a dhoti and ₹1,000 in cash for those who have a rice ration card.

"I really enjoyed the last time there was a flood, I was given a splendid sari and enough food for a week," claims one of the lucky winners of the November 2015 Chennai rains.

For some, it is a lottery of rain-bearing gifts. For others the time to listen to the frogs.

When the rain stopped the ducks began their noise,
Hoarse-throated, full-chested, and we heard them
Away in the big house, after dinner, and my niece
Asked, "Are they bullfrogs?" I said yes, or perhaps birds.
But I knew all the time they were only ducks.

From Vijay Nambisan's poem, Dirge.

Source: Doctor (2015).

PSYCHOLOGICAL STRESS AND PSYCHOPATHOLOGY

Psychological stress is experienced when something we do not expect and cannot control happens to us. It can be a building we are in catching on fire. It can be another person robbing us in a big city. Stress can even come from trying to help someone but finding ourselves in a situation we did not expect. The stories that begin this chapter show people doing their job when a hurricane hit and confronting the horrors of war and life-and-death decisions. At times, these experiences lead to strong emotional reactions and at other times to psychological disorders such as post-traumatic stress disorder (PTSD). Further, as we saw in the chapter on depression, the first episode of depression is often connected to a psychologically stressful event happening in someone's life.

Understanding the manner in which stress and trauma are related to health and psychopathology is a

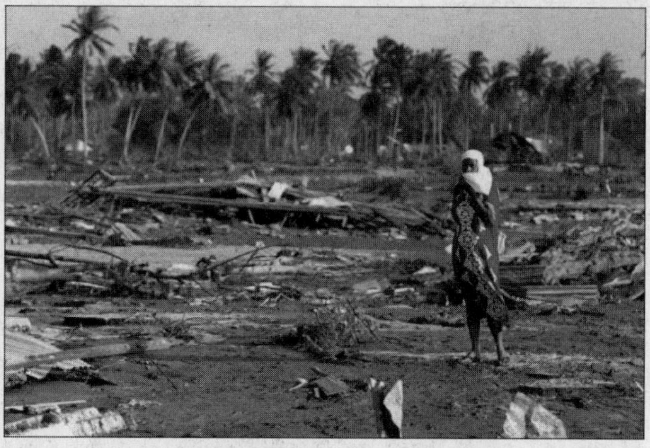

Aftermath of the Indian Ocean Tsunami of 2004. An Indonesian woman stands at the site her home used to be

Source: Remembering the Indian Ocean tsunami. Volume 384, No. 9960, pp. 2095–2098, 13 December 2014. *The Lancet.*

complicated one. Research is beginning to put in place the roles that these factors play in psychopathology. Some disorders have a clear relationship with stress and trauma. PTSD, by definition, is clearly the result of traumatic experiences. Likewise, individuals with depression are 2.5 to 10 times more likely to have experienced a recent negative stressful major life event than nondepressive individuals (see Slavich, O'Donovan, Epel, & Kemeny, 2010, for an overview). Further, severe stress and trauma from childhood abuse and neglect are associated with depression, alcohol abuse, and criminal behavior. In disorders such as schizophrenia and bipolar, stress can increase the symptoms.

Overall, early stress has been associated with later mental and physical health (see Taylor, 2011, for an overview). One pathway to changes in mental and physical health is that stressful experiences change both psychological and physiological reactions to future stressful experiences. These changes can be related to psychological factors, developmental changes in the brain, genetic factors, epigenetic modifications, endocrine factors, and economic and social factors.

DOES TRAUMA PRODUCE MENTAL ILLNESS?

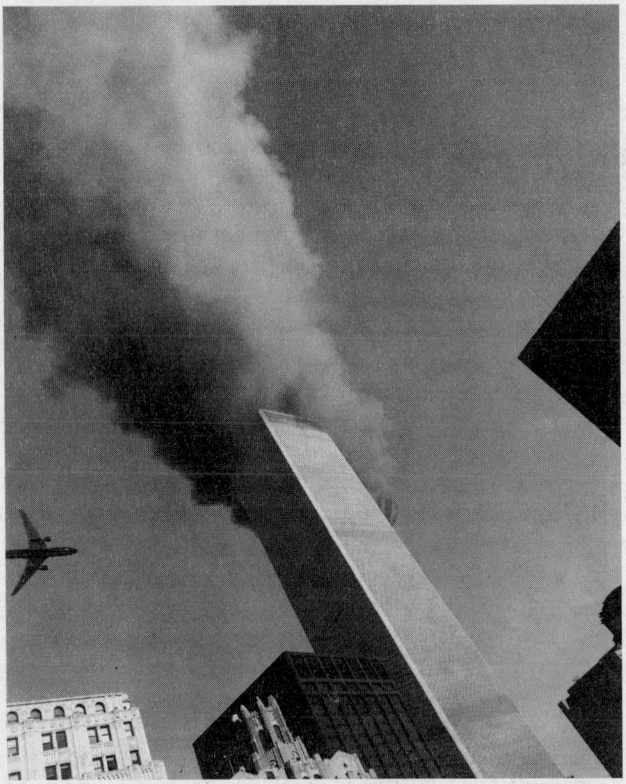

The 9/11 attack on the world trade center in New York changed many people's lives

© Rob Howard/Corbis

Trauma can produce psychological disorders, especially PTSD. However, although various types of trauma show a relationship to psychopathology, this relationship is not found for every individual (see Nikulina, Widom, & Brzustowicz, 2012, for an overview). What researchers have articulated is that children show differential responses to environmental influences, such as maltreatment, which are modulated by genetic factors. Specifically, the monoamine oxidase A (MAO-A) gene located on the X chromosome makes certain neurotransmitters inactive and has been associated with aggression in mice and humans. Specifically, this gene encodes the brain enzyme MAO-A and makes such neurotransmitters as serotonin, norepinephrine, and dopamine inactive.

Following a large number of boys over a long term, Caspi and his colleagues (2002) found that mistreatment as a child influenced some boys differently than others later in adulthood. Those boys who were mistreated in childhood and had a particular form of the MAO-A gene were more likely to be violent and engage in a variety of antisocial behaviors as adults, including problems with law enforcement officials. Those without this particular form of the gene did not display antisocial behaviors, even if they had been mistreated as children. Thus, environmental influences in terms of maltreatment would be modulated by the presence of certain genetic structures. Another type of research support for the idea that children show differential effects to the parental influences is behavioral. Jay Belsky (2005) has reviewed a variety of these studies. What he determined is that the infants who are most inhibited, fearful, and display negative emotions are the ones most affected by positive parenting. Thus, positive interventions can also influence later outcomes for the better.

In this chapter, I begin by noting how evolution adapted the pain system associated with physical pain to be involved in social pain such as rejection and the loss of a close relationship. As you will see in Chapter 15 on personality disorders, some individuals experience rejection as extremely painful and react with thoughts of anger and suicide. As noted in Chapter 6, some individuals experience the loss of an attachment relationship with distress that can be predictive of later negative emotional processing as seen in anxiety. I then turn to the physiological systems that are influenced by stress and trauma. Finally, I describe disorders such as PTSD, which are directly influenced by psychological stress and trauma, from the fifth edition of the *Diagnostic and Statistical Manual of Mental Disorders* (*DSM–5*) (American Psychiatric Association [APA], 2013). One example of a stressful event was the attack on the World Trade Center in New York City on 9/11.

IS SOCIAL PAIN LIKE PHYSICAL PAIN?

Over evolutionary time, our physiological and psychological systems have evolved to protect us in a variety of situations as well as to offer mechanisms for sexual and social encounters. One of the most important of these protections is the pain system, which alerts individuals to tissue or nerve damage or times in which our physiological systems are not functioning normally. Muscle pains and headaches are clear examples of these situations.

What about social pain? Rejection and loss of loved ones, for example, involve some of the most painful experiences for humans. What is interesting is that over evolutionary time the processing of social pain appears to have co-opted the basic brain structures involved in physical pain (see Panksepp, 1998; Eisenberger & Lieberman, 2004, for overviews). Linguistically, to refer to emotional pain we use some of the same phrases as with physical pain. We say we have a broken heart or that our feelings are hurt. The impetus for a system to detect and prevent social separation would have developed in childhood to keep the infant close to his or her mother.

Pain research suggests that there are two separate components to the experience of pain. The first is the sensory experience itself and the second is the felt unpleasantness (Price, 2000). The sensory experience involves the somatosensory cortex and the posterior insula. The experienced unpleasantness is associated with the anterior cingulate cortex (ACC). It is the second system that appears to be altered in psychopathology and is most sensitive to psychological factors.

Research has shown that in both physical and social pain, the ACC plays a critical role (Eisenberger & Lieberman, 2004). An intact ACC is required for young animals to emit distress sounds when separated from their caregivers. It is also the case that an intact

ACC is required for caregivers to show affiliative behaviors. With humans, playing a video game in which the person felt exclusion was associated with ACC activity. Further, the magnitude of the ACC activity correlated with the self-report of social distress. Those with borderline personality disorder experience this rejection greater than other individuals. Additional evidence for the relationship between physical pain and social pain is that an increase in one type of pain also produces an increased sensitivity for the other type of pain. Comforting experiences such as social support will also reduce sensitivity to physical pain. This has implications for the treatment of psychological disorders.

Emotion arousal and control as a factor in Stress v/s Happiness.

Indian neuropsychologist, Professor C. R. Mukundan, who has worked at NIMHANS, Bangalore, and Gujarat Forensic Sciences University, Gujarat, has published a paper titled, "Emotion—Arousal and Control" in the *International Journal of Indian Psychology* (2016). He has interpreted the presence of emotion as a driving force that can harm or help, depending on its usage. He explains, "Response inhibition ability is a critically important aspect of socialization process, which each growing infant needs to acquire during the neurodevelopmental stages." He further adds,

> Emotion comes to exist as a force driving individuals to move and act, and transforms itself into a complex force, propelling positive and negative behavior and their related experiences. We can learn to control our movements and behavior by learning control of the emotional drive. Learning to maintain emotion in its original state as a drive inducing happiness is important. It may be considered the aim of religious or spiritual ways of life.... Several living practices engaged by people for thousands of years help work on emotional arousal as well as happiness. Hence, we have always encouraged practices of these, like meditation, and spiritual attachments, which has been called "Bhakti," and prayers for attaining happiness, as well as drive for living a positive life. If we further work on this state, it may unfold differently, helping further its semantic interpretations.

He ends his brief by saying that response inhibition may start as a forced practice for the cultivation of the ability, which gradually enables the growing child and adult to hold back emotional arousal so that related responses and actions are not automatically initiated. Self-induction of training on emotional arousal also helps cultivate immense control on emotional arousal and related expressions. Meditative practices may be the best way to cultivate such self-controls, so that one can use emotional arousal for self-development.

THE PHYSIOLOGICAL MECHANISMS RELATED TO STRESS AND TRAUMA

Our physiological reactions to stress and trauma occur on a variety of levels. These include the tagging of genes, the reaction of the **immune system,** the endocrine system involving the **hypothalamic-pituitary-adrenal (HPA) axis,** the **autonomic nervous system (ANS),** and changes in cortical processes (see *Figure 9-1*).

TRAUMA CHANGES OUR GENES THROUGH TAGGING (EPIGENETICS)

Let's briefly review the nature of epigenetics as related to stress. Instead of actually changing the gene itself, epigenetic modifications tag a gene. This alters how the gene is turned on and off. Briefly, deoxyribonucleic acid (DNA) is wrapped around clusters of proteins called histones. These are further bundled into structures called chromosomes. Being tightly packed keeps genes in an inactive state by preventing access to processes

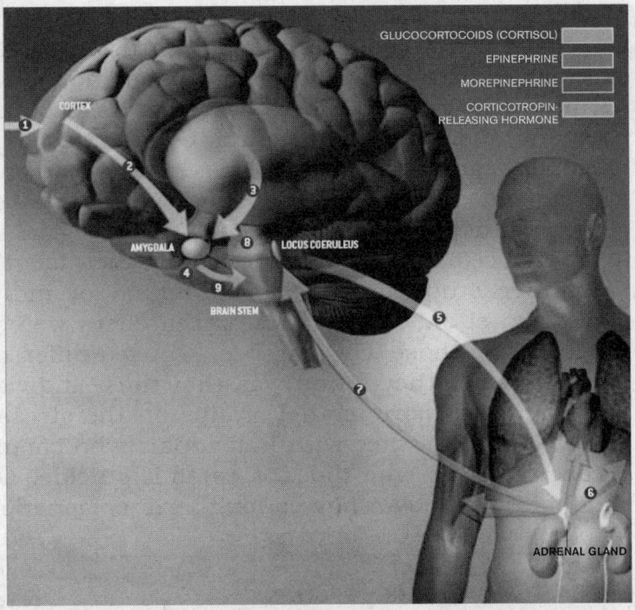

STRESS PATHWAYS are diverse and involve many regions of the brain in feedback loops that can sometimes greatly amplify a response. The process—simplified somewhat in this diagram—begins when an actual or perceived threat activates the sensory and higher reasoning centers in the cortex [1]. The cortex then sends a message to the amygdala, the principal mediator of the stress response [2]. Separately, a preconscious signal may precipitate activity in the amygdala [3]. The amygdala releases corticotropin-releasing hormone, which stimulates the brain stem [4] to activate the sympathetic nervous system via the spinal cord [5]. In response, the adrenal glands produce the stress hormone epinephrine; a different pathway simultaneously triggers the adrenals to release glucocorticoids. The two types of hormones act on the muscle, heart and lungs to prepare the body for "fight or flight" [6]. If the stress becomes chronic, glucocorticoids induce the locus coeruleus [7] to release norepinephrine that communicates with the amygdala [8], leading to the production of more CRH [9]—and to ongoing reactivation of stress pathways.

FIGURE 9-1 Stress

Source: Sapolsky (2003, p. 89).

that turn genes on. When action is needed, a section of DNA unfurls and the gene turns on. Whether a segment is relaxed and able to be activated or condensed, which results in no action, is influenced by epigenetic marks. As a tag, histone acetylation tends to promote gene activity and is called a writer. Histone methylation and DNA methylation tend to inhibit it and are called an eraser.

The environment can influence these writer and eraser tags. Tags help an organism respond to a changing environment. Some tags last a short time whereas others can last a lifetime. In one study introduced previously (see Miller, 2010; Weaver et al., 2004, for an overview), researchers observed that some rat mothers display high levels of nurturing behavior, licking and grooming their pups, whereas others are less diligent. Behaviorally, the offspring of the more active mothers were less anxious and produced less stress hormone when disturbed than pups cared for by more passive mothers. Further, the females raised by nurturing mothers became nurturing mothers themselves.

In terms of stress, those rat pups raised by less nurturing mothers became more sensitive to stress throughout their lives. When confined to a Plexiglas tube, which restricted their movement, they produced more of the stress hormone cortisol. If the mouse mother lacks access to basic needs, then she shows difficulty making nests and spends less time with the young (see Roth & Sweatt, 2011, for an overview). This, in turn, is related to the methylation of the genes, which is passed on to the next generation. Other research found that mice raised by multiple mothers, which is the norm for mice in the wild, show better social adjustment as adults. These mothers also spend more time with their own daughters, and this shows an association with oxytocin receptors (Curley, Davidson, Bateson, & Champagne, 2009).

Although less epigenetic research has been performed with humans, there are suggestions that similar mechanisms may be at work in terms of human stress. In one of the first studies to examine the effects of intimate partner violence during pregnancy on offspring, Radtke et al. (2011) found changes in epigenetic factors. Examining human mothers and their children some 10 to 19 years after birth, DNA methylation of the gene associated with the stress hormone cortisol was seen in the children whose mothers had experienced partner violence during pregnancy. Children whose mothers did not experience partner violence or those whose mothers experienced partner violence before or after pregnancy did not show the effect. Overall, this suggests that mothers' experiences during pregnancy can have long-term epigenetic effects on their children. Although the epigenetic mechanisms were previously unknown, a number of earlier studies have shown that children of mothers who experience psychological stress during pregnancy are more likely to experience anxiety and depression in their life (Huizink, Mulder, & Buitelaar, 2004).

Another study examined the brains of individuals who had committed suicide (McGowan et al., 2009). These researchers were interested in the question of whether the brains of those who had been abused differed in epigenetic factors from those who had not. What they found was that those individuals who had experienced childhood abuse showed more methyl groups on the stress gene receptor involved with cortisol. This was not the case with individuals who committed suicide but were not abused or a control group who did not commit suicide. Overall, initial evidence suggests that childhood abuse can have a long-term epigenetic effect. This illustrates the manner in which action on one level—the behavioral level—can result in changes in other levels such as the molecular one.

Overall, a variety of recent studies have considered the possibility that epigenetic changes such as DNA methylation and histone modification are involved in mental illness (see Iwamoto & Kato, 2009, for a review). At this point, the strongest evidence for epigenetic mechanisms relates to schizophrenia and bipolar disorder although the marital disorder research suggests anxiety and depression can also be related. However, there is still much research to be performed to describe the pathways from psychological stress to psychopathology (Albert, 2010).

Concept Check

- What evidence can you cite to show that stress experienced early in life is associated with later mental and physical health?
- Although various types of trauma show a relationship to psychopathology, what factors can affect that relationship?
- In what respects is social pain like physical pain?
- Our physiological reactions to stress and trauma occur on a variety of levels. What are five important levels?
- Describe an example of how trauma can lead to epigenetic changes.

PHYSICAL ILLNESS AND CONCOMITANT PSYCHOLOGICAL STRESS

Studies from NIMHANS (Mehrotra and Sukumar, 2007; Mehrotra and co-workers, 2010) have explored the stress associated with caring for a relative afflicted with cancer. The findings of a qualitative exploratory study, based on the narratives of female family member caregivers for patients afflicted with cancer, showed self-reported occurrence of positive moments and personal changes experienced during the caregiving process. In another study, exploring illness meanings in the context of cancer, it is reported that "'Challenge', 'value', 'punishment', 'weakness' and 'enemy' were the five categories from the Lipowski's framework that were found to be applicable in the current study sample whereas 'strategy', 'relief' and 'loss' were not applicable in the sample. Five new categories of illness meanings emerged namely; 'burden', 'part of life', 'God's plan', 'fate' and 'low threat'" (Tandon, Mehrotra, & Vallikad, 2010). The authors thus concluded that Lipowski's illness meaning framework requires expansion to capture the breadth of illness experiences in Indian patients.

Several studies have reported other forms of trauma such as road traffic accidents. In a study on trauma care in India and Germany (2013), the authors found that the total number of registered motor vehicles had increased 473-fold in India and 100-fold in Germany from 1951 to 2011. The number of road traffic deaths increased in both countries until 1970, but thereafter decreased in Germany (3606 in 2012) while continuing to increase in India (142,485 in 2011). The authors attribute the differences between Germany and India to the relative sizes and populations of the countries (1:9 and 1:15, respectively), and differences in prevention and prehospital care (nationwide versus big cities) and hospital trauma systems (nationwide versus exceptional).

In a paper from Gujarat, the authors (Joshipura et al., 2004) review trauma care systems in India and report that there is a high mortality rate amongst those with multisystem injuries, which can be attributed to the primitive state of trauma-care systems, lack of prehospital care, and inadequate critical care. They assert that mortality in serious injuries is six times worse in a developing country such as India compared to a developed country, and add that as far back as 1998, nearly 80,000 lives were lost and 330,000 people were injured. Of these, 78% were men in the age group of 20–44 years, causing significant impact on productivity. A trauma-related death occurs in India every 1.9 minutes or perhaps oftener.

With regard to psychological trauma, Thara, Rao, and John (2008) report their work on the post-tsunami psychosocial training programs in Tamil Nadu.

Dr. Srinivasa Murthy (2014) of NIMHANS reports that the survivors of the Bhopal gas tragedy of 1984 still poses mental health challenges. Similar aftermath of trauma is felt by persons who faced the terror attacks in Mumbai, and various floods, cyclones and tsunamis all over the country.

MIMH, Pune, also completed a project post the 6.4 Richter earthquake at Latur in Maharashtra (Pande, 2016) and reported the massive efforts at post-disaster evaluations and relief work accomplished (1993).

PSYCHOLOGICAL STRESS AND THE IMMUNE SYSTEM

Imagine that you are ending your first year in medical school and it is time to take a series of final exams. Clearly, this is a stressor for most students. How do you think taking exams will affect your immune system and your experience of psychological distress? To answer this question, Janice Kiecolt-Glaser and her colleagues (1984) took blood samples and gave psychological inventories a month before the exams and on the day of the exams. What they found was that compared with the previous month, the immune system was more suppressed on the day of the exam. This is consistent with the finding that students often get sick or have mouth or lip sores at the end of the term. They also found that the students reported more anxiety, depression, and bodily concerns on the day of the exam. Overall, this suggests that even milder stress in the form of exams can change immune function and cause psychological distress. Since this classic study was performed, we have learned much about the immune system.

It is the task of the immune system to recognize foreign agents in the body and then destroy them. These agents are traditional pathogens, which are involved in infection.

These pathogens can be either viruses or bacteria. Of course, the basic protection from pathogens is our skin. Basic reflexes such as sneezing, coughing, and crying are additional mechanisms for removing pathogens before they can enter the body. If pathogens do enter the body then there are a number of layers of immune function.

The immune system evolved to help organisms protect themselves from pathogens. These protective mechanisms appear to be some of the earliest to have evolved. One important task of the immune system is to determine what is foreign and what cells are part of the self. These foreign substances include bacteria, viruses, and parasites that enter our system and are detected by the immune system. Antibodies that are produced by our immune system can detect literally millions of different foreign substances and engage in a process that hopefully leads to their destruction. Our immune system has evolved to recognize a variety of pathogens. It is also capable of learning the characteristics of new pathogens and attacking them upon later exposure. This, of course, is the basic mechanism through which immunizations work.

The immune system comes into play both in terms of specific pathogens such as viruses and also in terms of stress. At one time, the immune system was viewed as a separate system that functioned independently. However, since the 1970s a variety of studies have demonstrated that the immune system is influenced by the brain and vice versa. In particular, it has been shown that psychological stress can influence the immune system such that the organism is more likely to become ill. Robert Ader (2007) was also able to show that the immune system could be classically conditioned. These types of studies helped to create the field of **psychoneuroimmunology** (see Kemeny, 2007, for an overview).

Psychoneuroimmunology is the study of how psychological factors can influence the immune system. One meta-analysis of more than 300 studies shows that stress in the form of loss or trauma suppresses the immune system (Segerstrom & Miller, 2004). Current research suggests that negative emotions can change immune responses and delay healing (Kiecolt-Glaser, McGuire, Robles, & Glaser, 2002). Some of the psychological factors that can influence the immune system include loneliness, poor social support, negative mood, disruption of marital relationships, bereavement, and natural disasters (Cohen & Herbert, 1995). Factors such as close friendships, which reduce negative emotions, also enhance immune system functioning (Kiecolt-Glaser, Gouin, & Hantsoo, 2010). It has also become apparent that not only does experience influence the immune system; the immune system can also influence the brain and thus behavior.

A relatively recent finding is that the immune system can be involved in mental illness. We all know that infections can leave us feeling sick and experiencing low energy levels. One type of cell involved in this process is called cytokines. What is striking to some scientists is that the symptoms associated with sickness as well as depression are similar. With both sickness and depression, the person withdraws from interactions with others and does not actively seek new experiences. These individuals also do not respond to positive experiences or rewards.

There is now evidence that cytokines can also lead certain individuals to develop depression (Dantzer, 2012; Dantzer, O'Connor, Freund, Johnson, & Kelley, 2008). What makes this relationship complicated is that in some studies the inflammation precedes depression whereas in others, the opposite is the case. That is, individuals with clinical depression show inflammatory biomarkers in their bloodstream. Other studies have shown that immune cells in the brains of individuals with autism are more active, resulting in increased inflammation (Pardo, Vargas, & Zimmerman, 2005). Clearly, researchers who study psychopathology now must also consider the immune system.

WHAT MAKES YOU RUN FROM BEARS? STRESS AND THE HYPOTHALAMIC-PITUITARY-ADRENAL AXIS

The evolutionary logic of survival is one of the easiest to comprehend. If an organism is not able to successfully respond to threat, it can be hurt or killed. If it is killed, its genes can no longer be passed on. If it is hurt, this may make it a less appealing mate or not allow it to seek mates. Thus, it is expected that organisms will have evolved sophisticated mechanisms that benefit survival. The basic mechanisms include the ANS; a network of hypothalamic, pituitary, and adrenal responses; the cardiovascular system; metabolism; and the immune system. These mechanisms are particularly sensitive to changes in the environment, and repeated stressful events can modify their functioning.

The basic consequence of these pathways is to prepare the body for action. If you see a bear, you will need energy to run. It actually does not need to be a bear. Almost all stressors use the same physiological systems to save your life. These pathways move physiological energy resources to the necessary organs and muscles. They create an overall shift from storing energy to using energy. This is like you pressing on the accelerator of your car to quickly leave a dangerous situation. Temporally, considerations move from a flexibility, including past and future considerations, to focus on immediate circumstances. You no longer store energy, pay attention to sexual matters, or have your immune system worry about long-term disease. Cognitively and emotionally, threat-relevant cues and memories become critical as related to the current situation. As you know, your brain plays an important role in deciding what is stressful whether it is taking an exam or responding to a loud noise. The brain has two mayor pathways in which it influences peripheral physiology.

The first pathway is the ANS, which innervates a variety of organs including the adrenal medulla, which results in the release of catecholamines (norepinephrine and epinephrine) from the terminal of sympathetic nerves (see *Figure 9-2*). Norepinephrine and epinephrine are fast acting, and you are ready to respond within seconds. It can be noted that if these substances are released at the synapse, they are referred to as neurotransmitters. If they are released into the bloodstream, they are referred to as hormones.

The second pathway involves cells in the hypothalamus that are released

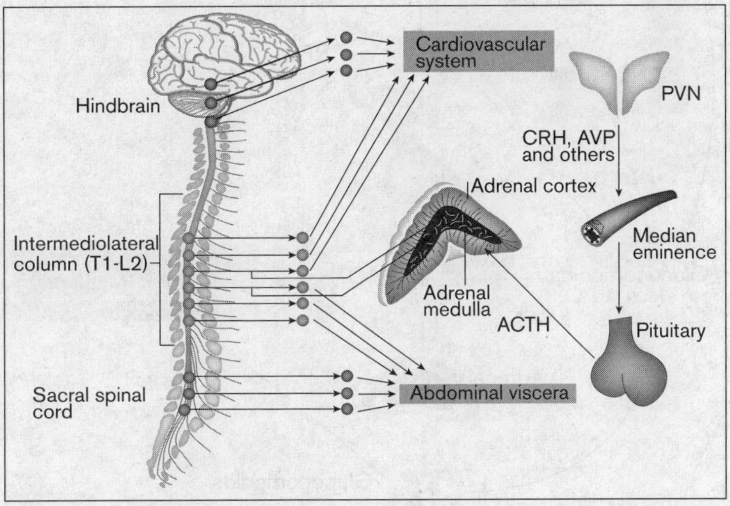

FIGURE 9-2 Physiological Response to Psychology Stress

Source: Ulrich-Lai and Herman (2009).

Note: The HPA axis and sympathetic system have largely complementary actions throughout the body, including energy mobilization and maintenance of blood pressure during stress.

into the bloodstream and go to the pituitary gland. This causes the pituitary to release hormones that influence other hormones, which in turn influence peripheral organs such as the adrenals as well as cells in the immune system. These hormones are referred to as glucocorticoids. Simply said, this system helps to convert stored fats and carbohydrates into energy sources that can be used immediately. Historically, given that survival processes that would have activated this system would have involved conflict and fights, it was important that the immune system also be activated to protect the organism from wounds. This **hypothalamus, pituitary, and adrenal pathway** is called the *HPA axis.* In psychology and physiology, these mechanisms have been studied under the rubric of psychological stress. Further, underactivity or overactivity in the HPA axis is seen in a number of psychopathologies including schizophrenia, autism, and depression (see Roggers, Morgan, Bronson, Revello, & Bale, 2013, for an overview).

The stress response is accomplished by a variety of interacting systems, which include the amygdala and other cortical systems that result in the hypothalamus activating the sympathetic nervous system and the HPA axis. Basically, the brain through the hypothalamus produces a substance referred to as corticotropin-releasing hormone (CRH) (also called corticortropin-releasing factor [CRF]), which in turn produces adrenocorticotropic hormone (ACTH) in the pituitary. ACTH in the blood, in turn, results in the adrenal glands producing glucocorticoids (see *Figure 9-3*). HPA is under excitatory control of the amygdala and inhibitory control of the hippocampus. The hippocampus releases CRF, which is transported to the adrenal cortex that releases *cortisol.* Research studies will often take a measure of cortisol to reflect the stressfulness of the situation. Daily cortisol levels are also higher in individuals with depression. Further, variants in the gene related to CRH can influence the individual's reactivity to stress. Research suggests that this variation influences brain processes before childhood trauma takes place and leaves the individual at risk for greater negative effects from childhood trauma (Rogers et al., 2013).

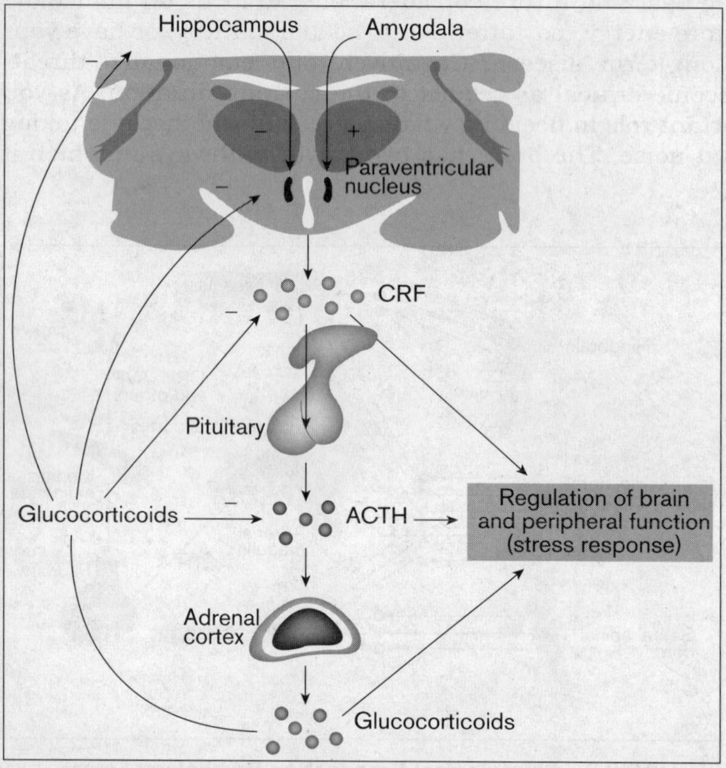

FIGURE 9-3 Hypothalamic-Pituitary-Adrenal Axis Is Under Excitatory Control of the Amygdala and Inhibitory Control of the Hippocampus

Source: Hyman (2009).

The stress response was initially described by Walter

Cannon in 1932 as a bodily response to danger. Although Cannon originally studied animals, research since his time has shown the basic stress response also applies to humans. The overall stress reaction has been referred to as the **fight-or-flight response** (Cannon, 1932). What happens when faced with a potential threat? According to Cannon, the body prepares you either to fight or to leave the scene. Cannon's work emphasized the sympathetic nervous system and the role of epinephrine and norepinephrine in the stress response.

Since that original work, we have come to see that the stress response is accomplished by a variety of interacting systems that include the amygdala and other cortical systems, which results in the hypothalamus activating the sympathetic nervous system and the HPA axis.

In terms of psychopathology, the HPA axis has been linked to anxiety and depression (Lamers et al., 2013). HPA axis overactivity was seen in individuals with more severe forms of depression. As shown in *Figure 9.3,* the response to short-term stress results in the production of cortisol and the secretion of CRF and ACTH. Short-term stress also suppresses the immune system and makes energy available. With depression, the mechanisms involved in the HPA axis are disrupted and the normal stress response is not present.

The HPA axis has also been associated with the development of psychosis in adolescence (see Walker, McMillan, & Mittal, 2005, for an overview). These researchers noted that four lines of research exist showing that HPA dysregulation is involved in the vulnerability for psychosis. First, behavioral studies have shown that clinical symptoms can be exacerbated by exposure to stress. Second, medical disorders such as Cushing's, which involve elevated levels of cortisol, are associated with increased risk for psychosis. Third, unmedicated patients with psychosis show abnormalities in the HPA axis and a positive correlation between cortisol levels and symptoms. And fourth, the hippocampus, which plays a role in regulating the HPA axis, is shown to be smaller in patients with psychosis. Reduced hippocampal volume is seen early in the development of psychosis.

THE AUTONOMIC NERVOUS SYSTEM

The function of the ANS is threefold. The first task is to maintain homeostatic conditions within the body. This keeps the processing of internal functions, such as heart rate and blood pressure, in balance. The second function is to coordinate the body's response to exercise and stress, which is the function I will emphasize in this chapter. The third function is the manner in which the ANS helps the endocrine system regulate reproduction.

The ANS is generally discussed in terms of the **sympathetic division** and the **parasympathetic division.** As can be seen in *Figure 9-4,* the sympathetic division connects with its target organs through the middle part of the spinal cord. The sympathetic division is responsible for the fight-or-flight response. This emergency response produces resources for the body to energize. As such, its connections are *adrenergic,* which produce the adrenaline reaction of energizing the body. In general, the sympathetic system produces a continuous influence on the organ it innervates. This is referred to as sympathetic tone.

The parasympathetic system, on the other hand, is involved in the restoration of bodily reserves and the elimination of bodily waste. It connects through the upper and lower

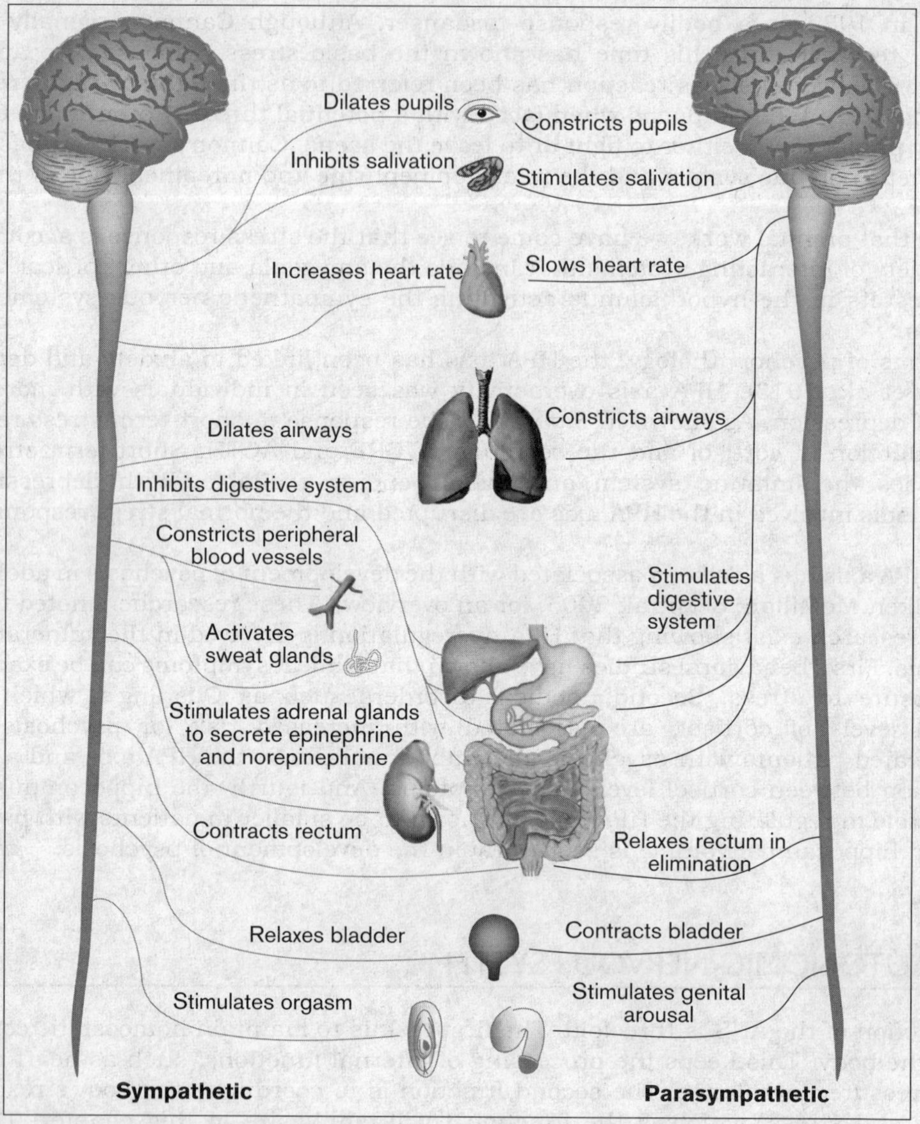

FIGURE 9-4 Sympathetic and Parasympathetic Branches of the Autonomic Nervous System and the Internal Organs Targeted

Source: Garrett (2010, Figure 3.21, p. 73).

parts of the spinal cord. As such, its connections are *cholinergic,* which involves acetylcholine. These reactions are generally a reduction of activity and a process of bringing the body back to a state of *homeostasis*. It should be noted that although the sympathetic and parasympathetic systems are often seen to function in the opposite manner, the actual relationship between the two is much more complicated (Berntson, Cacioppo, & Quigley, 1991, 1993).

What we have seen thus far are the various systems that have evolved to help the body manage changes within the environment. We make predictions about what to expect. When we see something we did not expect such as a bear in the woods, our body through these systems prepares us to protect ourselves by leaving the situation. If the unexpected continues to occur, we experience it as psychological stress. This can result in negative reactions in these systems that can lead to psychological disorders. In the next section, I will describe some of the ways that psychological stress has been studied and move the discussion to the level of the person.

THE STUDY OF STRESS

One of the major figures in stress research was the Hungarian endocrinologist Hans Selye, who worked at the University of Montreal. It was actually Selye who borrowed the term *stress* from physics. In that case, stress refers to the strain placed on a material. Selye used the term as a way of organizing physiological responses to a variety of challenges including heat, cold, pain, noise, hard work, and so forth. One of Selye's early findings was that the body reacts similarly to a variety of these different stressors. Selye called this response the **general adaptation syndrome (GAS).** The GAS was seen to involve three stages. The first was the alarm stage. The alarm stage was an initial reaction to the stress that involved an increase in adrenal activity as well as sympathetic nervous system reactions such as increased heart rate. The second stage was the resistance stage. This stage represents an adjustment to the stress that includes the availability of additional energy resources and mechanisms for fighting infection and tissue damage. The third stage was the exhaustion stage in which bodily resources are depleted. One of the paradoxes that Selye recognized was that the physiological stress responses that protect and restore the body can also damage it. However, Selye also reported that repeated exposure to a particular stress situation could also increase the organism's ability to withstand that same stress in greater amounts.

More recently, Bruce McEwen (2010) has begun to address the paradoxical nature of the stress response. He began by suggesting part of the problem in understanding stress is the ambiguous meaning of the term *stress*. He suggested that the term *stress* be replaced with the term **allostasis.** Allostasis refers to the body's ability to achieve stability through change. Brain processes can achieve stability in a number of different ways.

Allostatic systems are thus systems designed to adapt to change. Change traditionally related to stress for humans takes on a broad range of possibilities, including dangerous situations, being in crowded and unpleasant environments, getting an infection, and performing in front of others. Some researchers even suggest that stress may be greater for humans than other animals since we are also able to use our cognitive abilities to increase the experience of stress through imagination. The overall stress response involves two tasks for the body. The first is to turn on the allostatic response that initiates a complex adaptive pathway. Some examples of this turning on are the fight-or-flight response and the **tend-and-befriend response.** Once the danger has passed then the second task needs to be initiated—turning off these responses. A variety of research suggests that prolonged exposure to stress may not allow these two mechanisms to function correctly and in turn leads to a variety of physiological problems. This cumulative wear and tear on the body by responding to stressful conditions is called **allostatic load.**

Allostatic load has been discussed by McEwen (1998) in terms of four particular situations. The first situation reflects the fact that allostatic load can be increased by frequent exposure to stressors. These stressors can be both physical and psychological in nature. A variety of psychological studies have shown an association between worry, daily hassles, and negative health outcomes. One of the most studied areas is cardiovascular risk factors with stress showing a strong association with heart attacks and the development of atherosclerosis. The second condition for the increase in allostatic load is where an individual does not adapt or habituate to the repeated occurrence of a particular stressor. Some people for example continue to show larger physiological responses to everyday situations like driving a long distance or taking an airline flight even though the data suggest there is limited risk in these situations. Asking individuals to talk before a group also induces stress-like responses in many individuals. The third situation reflects the fact that not all individuals respond the same to changing situations. In particular some individuals show a slower return to a nonchallenge physiological condition once the initial threat is removed. These individuals appear to be more at risk for developing health-related conditions. Some researchers suggest that high blood pressure is associated with a normal stress response not being turned off. The fourth and final condition discussed by McEwen reflects the situation in which a nonresponse to stress produces an overreaction in another system. That is, if one system does not respond adequately to stress then activation of another system would be required to provide the necessary counterregulation and return the system to homeostasis. Overall, McEwen emphasized the important question of individual differences and the variety of ways in which perceived stress can influence future health. His graphic depiction of the allostatic system is seen in *Figure 9-5*.

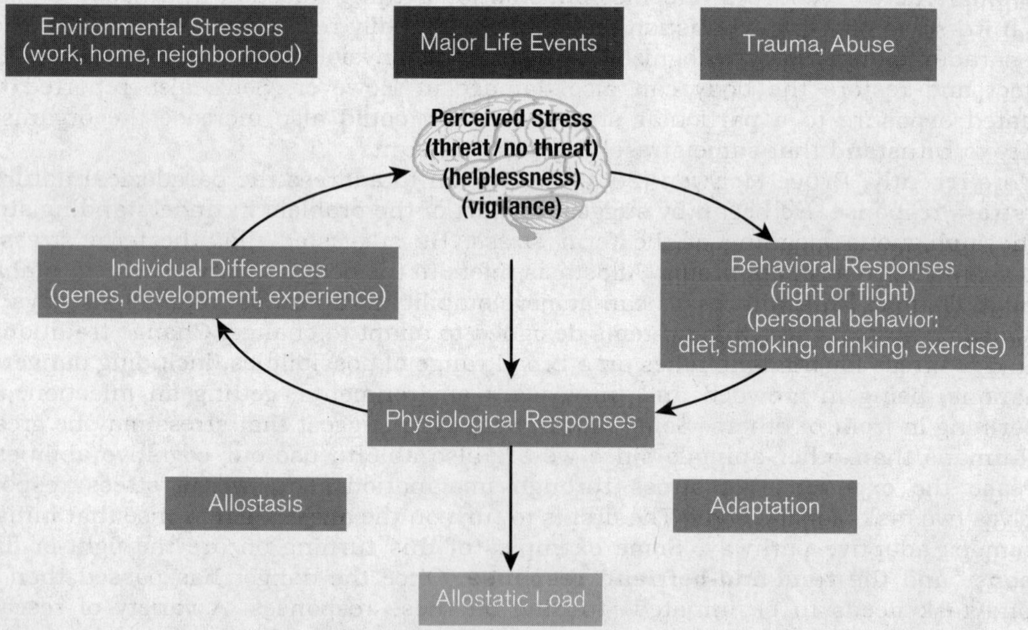

FIGURE 9-5 The Brain Interprets Experience and Determines What Is Threatening and Therefore Stressful

Source: Bruce McEwen, The Rockefeller University Laboratory of Neuroendocrinology.

Does Fight or Flight Apply Equally to Males and Females?

The fight-or-flight response is seen as a critical mechanism for responding to stress. The problem for current-day humans is that many of the stressors we face do not require a fighting or fleeing response. For example, imagine that you are working in a large company where there are rumors that a number of people are being laid off. Your boss calls you into the office. Your initial response is probably to feel stress as you could be the next to be fired. As you go in, you can feel your heart pounding. At this point, your boss says, "You have been doing a great job, and I want to ask your opinion on another project." The threat is gone, but your body is still reacting. This fight-or-flight reaction has been critical throughout our evolutionary history, but today, in our different social structure, it may lead to stress-related disorders.

In many ways, males and females have had different evolutionary pressures on them including the manner in which they respond to various challenges. After examining a variety of studies, Shelley Taylor and her colleagues (2000) suggested that the fight-or-flight response better describes a human male's response to stress and not a female's. For females, they suggested a better descriptor is tend and befriend. What do they mean by this? First, they suggested that, over evolutionary time, females have evolved behaviors that maximize the survival of both themselves and their offspring. Second, when stressed, females respond by nurturing offspring as well as displaying behaviors that protect them from harm. These tending behaviors have also been shown to reduce the presence of stress hormones in the infants. Third, like fight or flight, these behaviors are associated with particular neuroendocrine responses although different hormones are involved. These responses make up the *tending response*. The tending response activated by stress is seen as part of the larger attachment process. The *befriending response* involves a large social group. Females under stress seek contact with their social group, which is also protective in survival terms.

What is intriguing is that the basic neuroendocrine responses to stress appear to be similar in both males and females (Taylor, Dickerson, & Klein, 2002). It is initially a sympathetic response, as described previously. What is different is that these hormones affect males and females differently. Human males show the sympathetic response of activation and increased arousal, which can lead to aggression—the fight part of fight or flight. The male brain appears to be organized to give aggressive responses in the presence of substances such as testosterone that are less present in the female brain. What is present in the female brain is the hormone *oxytocin*, which is released in larger amounts in females compared with males. Oxytocin has been found in a variety of animal studies to reduce anxiety and calm the organism. According to Shelly Taylor and her colleagues, oxytocin leads females to quiet and calm down offspring in response to stress. Thus, whereas males are seen to produce more sympathetic-like responses to stress, females show more parasympathetic-like responses. Oxytocin is seen to lie at the basis of these responses for females—the tend-and-befriend response.

Additional support for the presence of gender differences in response to stress has come from the work of Repetti (1989). She examined the behaviors of fathers and mothers following a stressful workday. Whereas fathers tended to isolate themselves at home following stress, mothers tended to be more nurturing and caring toward their children. Further, similar differences also are found in the larger social networks where stressed females tend to seek out other women for comfort and support. Compared with females, males seek support from same-sex friends less often. A variety of anthropological studies suggest that males and females form groups for different purposes. Male groups tend to be larger and directed at well-defined tasks such as defense. Female groups tend to be smaller and carry with them social and emotional connections to a greater degree.

Why did researchers initially not see differences in male and female responses to stress? The answer is simple. During most of the 20th century, females were not studied in this research. Even the animal studies typically used males. Once females were studied more intensely, these differences emerged. If you think about it, you can see that these stress response differences are consistent with mating differences and investment in the care of offspring. That is to say, given that the female typically has a greater role in caring for offspring, her response to stress should not jeopardize herself or her offspring as might be the case with fleeing or fighting.

What is less well known is that stressful events activate the same immune and brain circuits as do infections (Watkins & Maier, 2002). Why is this so? What Maier and Watkins suggested is that the immune system first evolved to be sensitive to pathogens such as those associated with disease or the common cold for example. In evolutionary time, the immune system is seen to have evolved before such responses as fight or flight since all organisms have mechanisms for dealing with pathogens.

Does Social Stress Produce a Similar Reaction to Physical Stress?

Not only does our stress system respond when we are faced with threatening situations from our environment; it also responds to challenges to our social world (see Flinn, 2008, for an overview). Just being asked to stand up and talk in front of a group of people will produce characteristic stress responses along with the experience of anxiety. Given the social nature of human beings, it is not unreasonable to assume threats to our social system would be important. However, the evolutionary link that connects social challenges with the stress system for life-and-death situations is less well understood. One would assume that as with many other evolutionary processes, nature used systems already available. Flinn (2008) reviews the idea that the adaptive value of the social stress response begins in childhood. A variety of studies across a variety of species have shown that early exposure to stress will modify how the stress response is expressed in later life. It appears that children who experience trauma in the form of abuse, or a death of a parent, or divorce,

Concept Check

- There is evidence that the immune system is influenced by the brain and vice versa. What is an example where the brain influences the immune system? What is an example where the immune system influences the brain?
- What are the two pathways of the stress response that we have evolved to save us from threats such as bears? What are some of the effects of the stress response for psychopathology?
- What are the functions and structure of the ANS?
- According to McEwen, the overall stress response involves two tasks for the body. What are they? What are the impacts of prolonged stress on these mechanisms?
- How is the tend-and-befriend response different from the fight-or-flight response?
- Does social stress produce a similar reaction to physical stress? What factors would you cite in support of your answer?

show larger stress responses to social stress later in life. Depression is one disorder that can be modified by these prior experiences. PTSD and dissociative disorders result from a more direct pathway with psychological stress and trauma. It is not the case, however, that early physical stress such as experiencing hurricanes or political upheaval in one's country results in a differential stress response. In the next section, I will describe stress-related disorders.

TRAUMA- AND STRESSOR-RELATED DISORDERS IN *DSM–5*

There are several disorders in *DSM–5* that result from the experience of stress. The three most significant of these are **adjustment disorders, acute stress disorder,** and PTSD. The severity of the stressor is the least in adjustment disorder and the greatest in PTSD. In fact, an adjustment disorder does not require the experience of a traumatic event but only an event experienced as distressing. An acute stress disorder was originally conceived as a shorter-term reaction to a stress, and the stress may be nontraumatic in nature. In PTSD, symptoms must exist for more than a month whereas an adjustment disorder or acute stress disorder can be diagnosed immediately following a distressing experience. An adjustment reaction does not require specific symptoms but more global distress within 3 months after a stressful event. The requirement for an adjustment disorder is that the reaction to the event is out of proportion to the severity of the stressor. Acute stress disorder and PTSD do require specific symptoms. These specific symptoms are shown in *Tables 9-1 and 9-2*. Loss of property as shown in the photo to the left can lead to stress-related disorders.

TABLE 9-1 Acute Stress Disorder

A. Exposure to actual or threatened: a) death, b) serious injury, c) sexual violation, in one or more of the following ways:
   1. Directly experiencing the traumatic event(s)
   2. Witnessing, in person, the event(s) as they occurred to others
   3. Learning that the event(s) occurred to a close family member or close friend; cases of actual or threatened death must have been violent or accidental
   4. Experiencing repeated or extreme exposure to aversive details of the traumatic event(s) (e.g., first responders collecting human remains, police officers repeatedly exposed to details of child abuse)

B. Presence of nine (or more) of the following symptoms in any of the four categories of intrusion, dissociation, avoidance, and arousal, beginning or worsening after the traumatic events occurred:

Intrusion Symptoms

1. Recurrent, involuntary, and intrusive distressing memories of the traumatic event(s) (Note: In children, repetitive play may occur in which themes or aspects of the traumatic event(s) are expressed.)
2. Recurrent distressing dreams in which the content and/or affect of the dream is related to the event(s) (Note: In children, there may be frightening dreams without recognizable content.)
3. Dissociative reactions (e.g., flashbacks) in which the individual feels or acts as if the traumatic event(s) were recurring. (Such reactions may occur on a continuum, with the most extreme expression being a complete loss of awareness of present surroundings) (Note: In children, trauma-specific reenactment may occur in play.)
4. Intense or prolonged psychological distress or marked physiological reactions in response to internal or external cues that symbolize or resemble an aspect of the traumatic event(s)

(Continued)

(Continued)

Negative Mood

5. Persistent inability to experience positive emotions (e.g., inability to experience happiness, satisfaction, or loving feelings)

Dissociative Symptoms

6. An altered sense of the reality of one's surroundings or oneself (e.g., seeing oneself from another's perspective, being in a daze, time slowing)
7. Inability to remember an important aspect of the traumatic event(s) (typically due to dissociative amnesia, and not to other factors such as head injury, alcohol, or drugs)

Avoidance Symptoms

8. Efforts to avoid distressing memories, thoughts, or feelings about or closely associated with the traumatic event(s).
9. Efforts to avoid external reminders (people, places, conversations, activities, objects, situations) that arouse distressing memories, thoughts, or feelings about or closely associated with the traumatic event(s).

Arousal Symptoms

10. Sleep disturbance (e.g., difficulty falling or staying asleep, or restless sleep)
11. Irritable behavior and angry outbursts (with little or no provocatin), typically expressed as verbal or physical aggression toward people or objects.
12. Hypervigilance
13. Problems with concentration
14. Exaggerated startle response

C. Duration of the disturbance (symptoms in Criteria B) is 3 days to 1 month after trauma exposure.

Note: Symptoms typically begin immediately after the trauma, but persistence of at least 3 days and up to a month is needed to meet disorder criteria

D. The disturbance causes clinically significant distress or impairment in social, occupational, or other important areas of functioning.

E. The disturbance is not attributable to the direct physiological effects of a substance (e.g., medication or alcohol) or another medical condition (e.g., mild traumatic brain injury), and the symptoms are not better accounted for by those of Brief Psychotic Disorder.

Source: Reprinted with permission from the *Diagnostic and Statistical Manual of Mental Disorders, Fifth Edition*, (Copyright 2013). American Psychiatric Association.

TABLE 9-2 Post-Traumatic Stress Disorder

A. Exposure to actual or threatened death, serious injury, or actual or sexual violence in one or more of the following ways:
   1. Directly experiencing the traumatic event(s).
   2. Witnessing, in person, the event(s) as it occurred to others.
   3. Learning that traumatic event(s) occurred to a close family member or close friend. In cases of actual or threatened death must have been violent or accidental.
   4. Experiencing repeated or extreme exposure to aversive details of the traumatic event(s) (e.g., first responders collecting human remains; police officers repeatedly exposed to details of child abuse).

Note: Criterion A4 does not apply to exposure through electronic media, television, movies, or pictures, unless this exposure is work related.

B. Presence of one (or more) of the following Intrusion symptoms associated with the traumatic event(s) beginning after the traumatic event(s) occurred.

1. Recurrent, involuntary, and intrusive distressing memories of the traumatic event(s).

Note: In children, repetitive play may occur in which themes or aspects of the traumatic event(s) are expressed.

2. Recurrent distressing dreams in which the content and/or affect of the dream is related to the event(s).

Note: In children, there may be frightening dreams without recognizable content.

3. Dissociative reactions (e.g., flashbacks) in which the individual feels or acts as if the traumatic event(s) were recurring. (Such reactions may occur on a continuum, with the most extreme expression being a complete loss of awareness of present surroundings.)

Note: In children, trauma-specific reenactment may occur in play.

4. Intense or prolonged psychological distress at exposure to internal or external cues that symbolize or resemble an aspect of the traumatic event(s).
5. Marked physiological reactions to internal or external cues that symbolize or resemble an aspect of the traumatic event(s).

C. Persistent avoidance of stimuli associated with the traumatic event(s), beginning after the traumatic event(s), as evidenced by efforts to avoid 1 or more of the following:
   1. Avoidance of or efforts to avoid distressing memories, thoughts, or feelings about or closely associated with the traumatic event(s).
   2. Avoidance of or efforts to avoid external reminders (people, places, conversations, activities, objects, situations) that arouse distressing memories, thoughts, or feelings about or closely associated with the traumatic event(s).

D. Negative alterations in cognitions and mood associated with the traumatic event(s), beginning or worsening after the traumatic event(s) occurred, as evidenced by two or more of the following:
   1. Inability to remember an important aspect of the traumatic event(s) (typically dissociative amnesia; not due to head injury, alcohol, or drugs).
   2. Persistent and exaggerated negative expectations about one's self, others, or the world (e.g., "I am bad," "no one can be trusted," "my whole nervous system is permanently ruined," "the world is completely dangerous").
   3. Persistent distorted cognitions about the cause or consequences of the traumatic event(s) that lead the individual to blame himself/herself or others.
   4. Pervasive negative emotional state – (e.g., fear, horror, anger, guilt, or shame).
   5. Markedly diminished interest or participation in significant activities.
   6. Feeling of detachment or estrangement from others.
   7. Persistent inability to experience positive emotions (e.g., inability to experience happiness, satisfaction, or loving feelings).

E. Marked alterations in arousal and reactivity associated with the traumatic event(s), beginning or worsening after the traumatic event(s), as evidenced by two (or more) of the following:
   1. Irritable behavior and angry outburst (with little or no provocation) typically expressed as verbal or physical aggression toward people or objects.
   2. Reckless or self-destructive behavior
   3. Hypervigilance
   4. Exaggerated startle response
   5. Problems with concentration
   6. Sleep disturbance (e.g., difficulty falling or staying asleep, or restless sleep).

F. Duration of the disturbance (Criteria B, C, D and E) is more than one month.

G. The disturbance causes clinically significant distress or impairment in social, occupational, or other important areas of functioning.

H. The disturbance is not due to the direct physiological effects of a substance (e.g., medication or alcohol) or another medical condition.

Source: Reprinted with permission from the *Diagnostic and Statistical Manual of Mental Disorders, Fifth Edition*, (Copyright 2013). American Psychiatric Association.

Although the stress-related disorders other than PTSD have not been studied extensively in terms of treatment, there is data to suggest that psychotherapy presented early can reduce the development of PTSD (see Bryant, Friedman, Spiegel, Ursano, & Strain, 2011, for an overview). One difficult question is the way to distinguish a normal stress reaction from an acute stress disorder. In terms of treatment, it should be noted that stress reaction should be treated only in those asking for treatment. In studies looking at trauma, requiring workers to be part of a treatment session actually made matters worse (Ehlers & Clark, 2003). This suggests that timing of treatment is important.

Post-Traumatic Growth

Although post-traumatic stress disorder and acute stress disorder are commonly seen, it is not unusual for subjects to report post-traumatic growth. A study from NIMHANS (Tandon & Mehrotra, 2016) aimed at exploring the extent and nature of self-reported posttraumatic growth following cancer diagnosis in a heterogeneous sample of Indians undergoing treatment for cancer. Post traumatic growth refers to "positive psychological changes experienced as a result of the struggle with highly challenging life circumstances" (Calhoun & Tedeschi, 2001).

The paper shows that among the psychosocial resources of respondents, self-efficacy, social support, and emotional processing and adaptive coping strategies, namely, information seeking and support seeking, were positively related with PTG. Patients with positive and fate illness appraisals also reported higher PTG as did those with lower depression and higher quality of life.

Adjustment Disorders

Everyone reacts when things do not go as expected. Someone loses a job, their boyfriend or girlfriend breaks up with them, they lose money in a business relationship. Natural disasters such as a tree falling on your house or your basement flooding from strong rains create an emotional reaction. Emotional reactions can also be more long term, such as living in a difficult neighborhood or living with a physical disability. These are examples that are upsetting. However, when the reactions to such events are out of proportion to the severity of the event, it can be considered an *adjustment disorder.* The reaction to the event may also interfere with social functioning and job performance. A diagnosis of adjustment disorder requires that the reaction to the stressful event occur within 3 months of its occurrence and not last for longer than 6 months.

Although formal epidemiological studies for adjustment disorders are rarer than for other disorders such as anxiety or depression, these disorders are thought to be common within the mental health system. They are estimated to represent up to 20% of those seeking mental health treatment and about 7.1% for inpatients (Jones, Yates, & Zhou, 2002). They are slightly higher in females than males (approximately 60% to 40%). Although fairly prevalent, there is little research concerning empirically supported therapies. In general, the same treatments used for anxiety as well as PTSD are used with adjustment disorders. These include both psychosocial therapy and antianxiety medications. These will be described in more depth in the section concerning PTSD in this chapter and in Chapter 10, which focuses on anxiety.

Acute Stress Disorder

Acute stress disorder is a short-term reaction to traumatic events that lasts from 3 days to 1 month. If the clinical symptoms continue past this period, the disorder would be described as PTSD, which I will describe in the next section. Like PTSD, the trauma can include events such as war experiences; physical attack; muggings; terrorist attacks; torture; physical and sexual abuse; transportation accidents; and natural disasters such as hurricanes, fires, and earthquakes. Acute stress disorder can also occur from watching traumatic events happen to another.

Clinical symptoms following the trauma are described in terms of five categories. The first category is that of intrusion and can include such symptoms as involuntary distressing memories, distressing dreams, and flashbacks. The second category is that of negative mood and includes the inability to experience happiness. The third category is dissociative symptoms such as feeling in a fog or the inability to remember important aspects of the trauma. The fourth category is that of avoidance symptoms. These symptoms include avoiding situations, people, and places that remind one of the trauma. The fifth category is that of arousal symptoms. These include sleep disturbance, angry outbursts, showing extreme vigilance, problems with concentration, and a sensitivity to events that cause a startle. A given individual may show symptoms in a limited number or all of these five categories.

The prevalence of acute stress disorder varies in terms of type of assault (APA, 2013). Highest rates (20%–50%) are seen when the traumatic event involves being assaulted, being raped, and witnessing a mass shooting. Other prevalence rates are lower. These include being part of a motor vehicle accident (13%–21%), being burned severely (10%), being assaulted (19%), and being involved in industrial accidents (6%–12%). Overall, the prevalence is higher for females than males. On an individual level, a number of factors including negative appraisals of the trauma, high trait anxiety, showing signs of depression, suicide risk, and not being married or employed have been associated with greater severity of acute stress symptoms. However, when these are considered using regression analysis, only trait anxiety, suicide risk, and trauma appraisal significantly predicted severity of symptoms (Suliman, Troeman, Stein, & Seedat, 2013).

Post-Traumatic Stress Disorder

I am a middle-aged woman, married with two children. I was diagnosed with posttraumatic stress disorder (PTSD) at age 25. I am grateful to say that I have had tremendous support, terrific professional help, a strong will to recover, and a resolve to do whatever work necessary to overcome all of my trauma. Other miraculous help has been my spiritual beliefs and practices.

As a child I suffered numerous traumatic events that began when I was just two years old. I was physically abused, sexually abused, emotionally abused, and spiritually abused. I was terrorized, tortured, neglected, and abandoned. Unfortunately, there were multiple perpetrators; that has made the healing and confusion about what pieces of the puzzle fit together tiresome at times.

The good news is that it's gotten better! One tremendous step in the right direction was putting myself in therapy at age 21 years. Another was quitting drinking alcohol with the help of Alcoholics Anonymous. I abused alcohol to escape reality. I am grateful to say I have been sober for almost two decades.

It was just after my first AA anniversary that I began having persistent, terrifying flashbacks that came in many forms, including flashes of images in my mind (like a movie, only skipping some parts), body memories, and loss of time due to dissociation. I admitted myself into a psychiatric hospital, and the journey to recovery began. It was while there I was diagnosed with PTSD.

I'd like to say I no longer suffer from flashbacks, but even at the time of this writing, I am in the middle of recovering another memory from my childhood. This has become routine after all these years, but unfortunately it does include horrible flashbacks—and that is the frustrating part. I have learned they won't kill me or make my head explode, which is something I used to believe.

From K. Waheed. (n.d.). *Honoring the person I am.* Retrieved from Anxiety and Depression Association of America website: www.adaa.org/living-with-anxiety/personal-stories/honoring-person-i-am

Since at least the American Civil War, there have been studies of long-term health problems related to combat (see Levy & Sidel, 2009, for an overview). These experiences have been referred to as "shell shock," "combat fatigue," and "war neurosis." During World War I, it was believed that the pressure of exploding shells produced changes in the brain, thus shell shock. However, after the Vietnam War, the nature of the trauma became apparent. The most commonly reported experience involved the intense experience of threat, which is currently referred to as PTSD.

PTSD results from an experienced threat that produces intense fear, helplessness, or horror (see Keane, Marshall, & Taft, 2006; Vermetten & Lanius, 2012, for overviews). In addition to war, these experiences can involve family and social violence, rape and assaults, and accidents (see *Table 9-3*). The highest risk for PTSD is assaultive violence.

TABLE 9-3 Stressors Related to Developing Post-Traumatic Stress Disorder

Type of stressor	*Examples*
Serious accident	Car, plane, boating, or industrial accident
Natural disaster	Tornado, hurricane, flood, or earthquake
Criminal assault	Being physically attacked, mugged, shot, stabbed, or held at gunpoint
Military	Serving in an active combat theater
Sexual assault	Rape or attempted rape
Child sexual abuse	Incest, rape, or sexual contact with an adult or much older child
Child physical abuse or severe neglect	Beating, burning, restraints, starvation
Hostage/imprisonment/torture	Being kidnapped or taken hostage, terrorist attack, torture, incarceration as a prisoner of war or in a concentration camp, displacement as a refugee
Witnessing or learning about traumatic events	Witnessing a shooting or devastating accident, sudden unexpected death of a loved one

Source: Vermetten and Lanius (2012, p. 293).

Cumulative stress also can lead to PTSD. Whereas acute stress disorder is a short-term reaction to trauma, PTSD is present when the reaction lasts more than 6 months.

It has been estimated that 60% of all men and 50% of all women will experience a threat to their life or that of another close to them during their lifetime. Of these, 8.7% will develop PTSD during their lifetime. Twelve-month prevalence is 3.5% in the United States (APA, 2013). The occurrence of PTSD is twice as common in women as men. Females also experience PTSD for a longer period than males. Although PTSD is found in a variety of cultures, its prevalence is less in Europe, Asia, Africa, and Latin America. In these cultures, it is estimated to be around 1% although New Zealand shows a rate of 6.1% (World Health Organization [WHO], 2005). Additionally, *DSM–5* reflects the possibility that PTSD can develop in childhood as illustrated by the first person account at the beginning of this section.

PTSD has been an important focus of the U.S. Department of Veterans Affairs in that PTSD shows in greater numbers in the military than in the general population. Part of this results from the nature of current military actions in war in which small groups of soldiers go out from the base and cannot predict when there will be an attack. In this situation, there is not a traditional front line. Further, roadside bombs and suicide bombers present additional dangers. Thus, soldiers find their lives under constant threat. Among the Vietnam veterans, lifetime prevalence of PTSD is estimated to be 30.9% for men and 26.9% for women (www.ptsd.va.gov/professional/pages/epidemiological-facts-ptsd.asp). For Gulf War veterans, the lifetime prevalence was lower and estimated to be around 10% to 12%. The Iraq War estimates are around 13.8%. Soldiers who were in recent war zones have not only experienced PTSD but also mild traumatic brain injuries (TBIs) usually in the form of concussions. The LENS in this section examines stress-related disorders in the military.

The *DSM–5* diagnostic criteria for PTSD include a variety of traumatic experiences followed by negative reactions (see *Table 9-2*, which was given earlier). First, the individual is exposed to aversive experiences involving the potential for injury or assault. Repeated exposures of first responders collecting body parts or police investigating child abuse are also included in the definition. Second, following the exposure, the individual experiences intrusions related to the exposure. These intrusions can include flashbacks in which the individual relives the experiences, dream content related to the experience, distressing memories of the event, and distress or physiological reactions to reminders of the event. Third, the individual avoids stimuli involved with the traumatic event. These stimuli could include people, places, or things associated with the event as well as internal thoughts or feelings. Fourth, the individual experiences changes in cognitive processes such as an inability to remember important aspects of the event, negative attributions about one's self, blame of others, negative emotions, detachment, lack of interests, and inability to experience positive emotions. Fifth, the individual experiences increased arousal and reactivity including sleep disturbances, irritability, and problems with concentration.

Overall, symptoms should have lasted for more than one month and produced clinically significant distress. The following case of Victoria English (not her real name) illustrates these symptoms in a person who experienced a bomb attack at the World Trade Center in New York City.

The Physiological Aspects of Post-Traumatic Stress Disorder

Animal models of PTSD expose animals to inescapable stress, or repeated stressors. Similar stress responses as seen in humans are reported that include the CRF, which activates the HPA axis to cause release of ACTH and other chemical substances as

CASE OF VICTORIA ENGLISH
Post-Traumatic Stress Disorder

Victoria English is a single woman in her early 30s. She occupied a position of significant authority in a large corporation. She sees herself as efficient and independent and has never sought mental health services in the past. On February 25, 1993, she was working in her office at the World Trade Center when a bomb exploded. In the initial interview, she showed little emotion when she described being blown into the air and landing on her arm. This resulted in her having a broken arm. During the interview, Ms. English became more tearful and frightened as she described the bombing and how it affected her life. Specifically, she is currently feeling vulnerable and reported difficulties with the demands of her job. When she returned to work 2 weeks after the bombing, she reported being anxious on the subway. She began to work from home. The company physician, after consulting with her, suggested that she obtain a temporary disability and discontinue working.

During Ms. English's assessment, she was administered a Structured Clinical Interview for *DSM* Disorders (SCID) and met criteria for PTSD. Her symptoms included nightmares and intrusive daytime recollections. These could bring her to tears. She also had intrusive fantasies of catastrophic events, such as buildings falling on people, as she went about her daily life. Ms. English also avoided situations such as riding the subway or going to the World Trade Center, which would make her feel vulnerable or remind her of the bombing. She also found herself cut off from others even when they reached out to her. She began cognitive processing therapy with cognitive behavioral components. By the end of therapy, her level of functioning had greatly improved. At the 1-year follow-up, she reported that she was doing well and had moved to a new city and become romantically involved with someone who would become her husband. She also reconsidered her priorities and according to her began to live a more balanced life. At the 2.5-year follow-up, she no longer met criteria for PTSD although she reported minor types of psychological distress.

From "Cognitive Processing Therapy for PTSD in a Survivor of the World Trade Center Bombing: A Case Study," Difede, J., & Eskra, D, *Journal of Trauma Practice*, (2002) 1, 155–165. Reprinted by permission of Taylor & Francis Ltd, http://www.tandf.co.uk/journals.

described previously. This generally results in a lessened stress response to additional stimuli and an avoidance of novel situations.

In terms of brain structures, animal models of stress and trauma have shown that exposure to severe and chronic stress can damage hippocampal formation. This is seen to be mediated by elevated corticosteroids, which are thought to damage cells, diminish neuronal regeneration, and reduce dendritic branching. This has resulted in a variety of human studies examining the hippocampus in individuals with PTSD (see Gilbertson, 2011; Shin et al., 2011, for overviews).

In addition, an improved understanding of the cortical networks involved in the acquisition and extinction of fear have pinpointed specific brain regions connected with PTSD. These include the hippocampus, the amygdala, and the medial prefrontal cortex (PFC). The hippocampus is important because of its role in the encoding of memories including emotional ones. The amygdala is involved in the assessment of threat and plays a role in

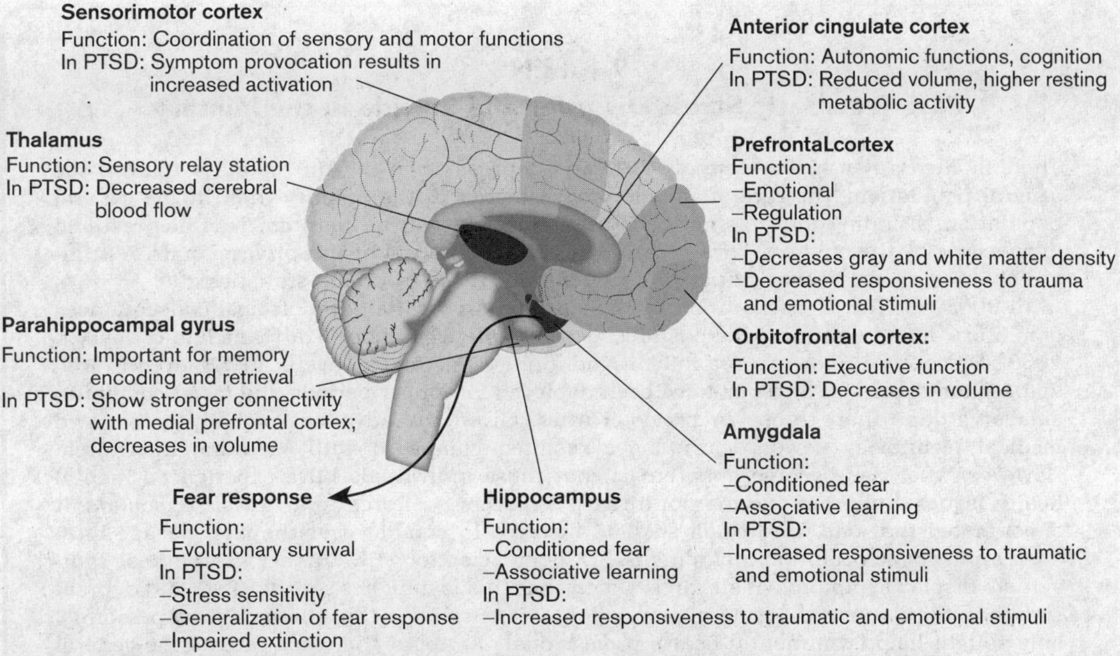

FIGURE 9-6 Areas of the Brain Related in Psychological Stress and Trauma

Source: Mahan and Ressler (2012), with permission from Elsevier.

fear conditioning. The medial PFC, including the ACC, is involved in the inhibition of emotional information during task performance. These are the same brain areas involved in anxiety and fear processes. The brain areas involved in PTSD are shown in *Figure 9-6.*

In general, there is clear support that individuals with PTSD have smaller hippocampal volume than those without PTSD. In one meta-analysis (Smith, 2005), individuals with PTSD had, on average, a 6.9% smaller left hippocampus and a 6.6% smaller right hippocampus by volume. An intriguing idea is that stress limits the normal regeneration of new neurons in the hippocampus (Lucassen et al., 2013). ACC differences have also been noted in PTSD as well as reduced connectivity between the ACC and the amygdala. Although an important part of the fear network, consistent reductions have not been observed in the amygdala.

It is suggested that the hyperresponsiveness of the amygdala is related to the exaggerated fear response (Rauch, Shin, & Phelps, 2006). This may result from a lack of inhibition from the frontal areas to the amygdala. This would also be associated with the inability to inhibit or extinguish fear-related stimuli.

Post-Traumatic Stress Disorder Treatment

One way to consider the physiological changes associated with trauma is to consider the networks involved on both an associative and cortical level. On an associative level, it has been suggested that some associations become more potent or "hot" than others that remain "cold" (Rockstroh & Elbert, 2010). It has been shown that repeated experiences of

9-1 LENS
Post-Traumatic Stress Disorder and Suicide in the Military

There is currently a higher rate of PTSD and depression in the U.S. military than in the general population. The rate of suicide is also higher in the military than in the general population, a finding that has not been seen since the war in Vietnam. This has resulted in concerns by the military, government officials, and mental health professionals. A number of studies have been conducted to understand these troubling statistics.

In 2008, the RAND Corporation published a report on the psychological consequences of military deployment over the past decade, *Invisible Wounds of War* (Tanielian & Jaycox, 2008). Since 2001, more than a million and a half U.S. troops have been deployed in Iraq and Afghanistan. These troops have been deployed for longer periods and faced combat in smaller groups than troops in previous wars. Given the advances in body armor and medical technology, fewer deaths have resulted compared with Vietnam and Korea. However, what has become apparent is that these individuals have experienced mental health issues and brain trauma not initially apparent—referred to as *invisible wounds*. It is estimated that one third of all soldiers involved in combat over the past decade have such an invisible condition including PTSD, depression, or TBI. Further, 5% of these individuals display symptoms of all three. Given that this is a higher rate of PTSD and depression than that seen in the general population, it is surprising that these military personnel only sought help from mental health professionals at about the same rate as the general population. Roughly half of those who met the criteria for PTSD, depression, or TBI had sought help in the year preceding the RAND study. An important reason given for not seeking help was that the soldiers were concerned that the information would not be kept confidential and would hurt future job searches or military advancement.

Not seeking help for a mental condition not only has consequences for the individual himself but also for society in general. Often individuals with stress-related disorders show other problems such as substance abuse as well as experiencing problems in their marriage and social relationships. For society, these conditions can lead to missed days at work, lower productivity, and even homelessness and suicide. However, there is potential to deal with these problems. The RAND report estimates that evidence-based treatments for depression and PTSD would pay for themselves within 2 years and save the country as much as $1.7 billion in lost productivity. For both the individual and society, there is great value in not having the person become homeless or commit suicide. There is also increased quality of life that results from effective treatments of these disorders.

Based on their research, the RAND Corporation made four recommendations:

1. Increase the cadre of providers who are trained and certified to deliver proven (evidence-based) care, so that capacity is adequate for current and future needs.
2. Change policies to encourage active duty personnel and veterans to seek needed care.
3. Deliver proven, evidence-based care to service members and veterans whenever and wherever services are provided.
4. Invest in research to close information gaps and plan effectively.

trauma will make it more difficult to integrate the experiences into less emotional or cold autobiographical memories. *Figure 9-7* illustrates such a network in which being on a dark street results in a cognitive proposition such as "there is no way out" and the following emotional and physiological responses. One goal of therapy is to help the individual move the hot trauma associations to a more cold, or nonreactive, memory process.

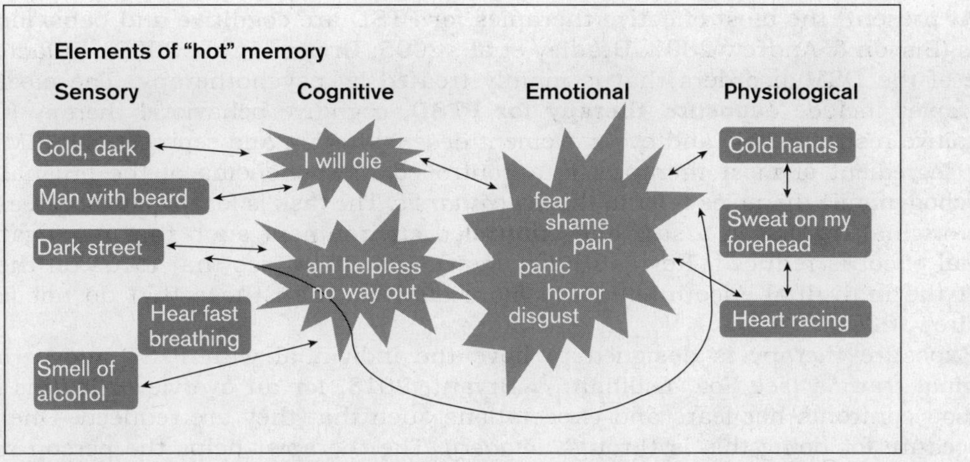

FIGURE 9-7 Schematic Outline of an Exemplary Network of Propositions Implemented as "Trauma Network"

Source: Rockstroh and Ebert (2010, p. 15), with permission from Elsevier.
Note: In PTSD, the border between "hot" and "cold" memory elements (thick black line) is firm and prevents the integration of emotional and autobiographical memories. Additional experiences add to the "hot" elements but not to the context, thereby strengthening the separation of the two memories.

PTSD is frequently comorbid with other disorders such as depression, substance abuse, and anxiety disorders such as obsessive-compulsive disorder (OCD), panic disorder, agoraphobia, and social anxiety. For example, the National Vietnam Veterans Readjustment Study shows that 98% of individuals with combat-related PTSD have a comorbid lifetime mental disorder (Kulka et al., 1990). They also reported more physical health problems. This suggests that the treatment of PTSD requires more than a single strategy.

Given the plethora of symptoms seen in PTSD, pharmacological treatments have been varied and have used antidepressants, anxiolytics, adrenergic inhibitors, mood stabilizers, and anticonvulsants. Overall, drug treatments were shown to be superior to placebos in reducing symptoms of PTSD (Davidson et al., 2006). New drugs are also being tested that influence the ability to remember traumatic events. For example, animal work has shown that the dopamine D_1 receptor is involved in processing emotional information in the PFC. If these receptors are manipulated, it is possible to block the experiencing of emotional memories (Lauzon, Bechard, Ahmad, & Laviolette, 2013).

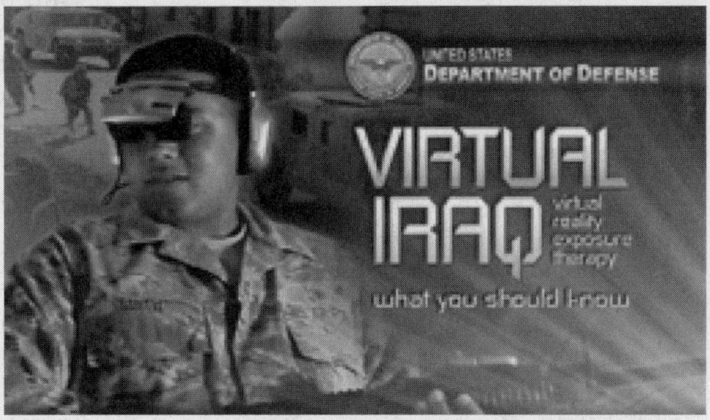

The U.S. department of defense is using virtual reality techniques as means of treating post-traumatic stress disorder for those who served in Iraq and other Combat locations

Source: From www.health.mil/MHSCIO/news_resources/portal/june2010/ptsd.aspx

At present, the most effective therapies for PTSD are cognitive and behavioral therapies (Bisson & Andrew 2007; Bradley et al., 2005; Ursano et al., 2008). In fact, PTSD is one of the *DSM* disorders that is mainly treated by psychotherapy. The most studied therapies include **exposure therapy for PTSD,** cognitive behavioral therapy (CBT) and cognitive restructuring, and eye movement desensitization and reprocessing (EMDR). One key ingredient of most therapies is a controlled reexperiencing of the original trauma. Psychodynamic therapies refer to this as *catharsis.* The task is for the client to reexperience the original trauma in a safe and controlled environment such that its negative emotional effect is reduced. Reviews have shown that therapies that focus on the trauma that the individual encountered are more effective than those that do not (Bisson & Andrew, 2007).

Exposure therapy is designed to have the individual with PTSD reexperience the original trauma (see Foa, Gillihan, & Bryant, 2013, for an overview). In this way, the person confronts her fears and expectations such that they are reduced. One common procedure for doing this is through *imagery.* The therapist helps the person remember and image the details of the experience, including the factors that led up to the event. In some situations such as a car accident, the therapist and the client may actually go to the location of the event and reexperience in detail the situation. One goal of the therapy is to have the person develop a sense of mastery over the situation.

EMDR is a form of therapy in which a person imagines the traumatic situation while moving his or her eyes (Shapiro, 2001, 2013). The basic idea is that PTSD is related to unprocessed memories in the brain. The purpose of therapy is to reactivate these stored memories through direct processing. The person is told to keep his head still and follow the therapist's finger (or a light panel) with his eyes while imagining the trauma. The procedure is repeated until the person no longer experiences distress. Although the procedure has been shown to be effective, there are no psychological or neuroscience perspectives that can explain the results; thus, it remains controversial (Russell, 2008).

Cognitive behavioral approaches as described previously seek to modify dysfunctional thoughts and consider new ways to interpret the situation. One important focus is to help the person restructure her way of thinking and feeling. One way of doing this is to have the person identify the thoughts such as "I am going to be hurt" that precede the negative emotions experienced in PTSD. Likewise, if a woman had been raped, she might blame herself for being in the situation and say, "It is all my fault." The therapist would help this person to reconsider this belief and replace it. Overall, the CBT process is one of identifying dysfunctional thoughts, evaluating their validity, and replacing them with more productive ones.

New and improved treatment approaches are being developed within the context of modern technology and more sophisticated treatment research. Since many types of trauma-related disorders are largely environmentally determined, this

Concept Check

- When a negative event occurs, what criteria would you use to distinguish between a normal emotional reaction and an adjustment disorder?
- What are the five categories of clinical symptoms that describe acute stress disorder?
- PTSD results from an experienced threat. What are some of the common stressors?
- How are specific areas of the brain involved in PTSD?
- What are the most effective therapies for PTSD? Give three examples, and explain the focus of each related to treating PTSD.

allows for prevention programs. One aspects of prevention can include bringing the psychological situation that led to trauma to light. Currently, sexual assault in the military is one example in which prevention programs have been developed. Another aspect of prevention is helping those who have experienced trauma to recognize the signs and symptoms of psychological distress and learn how to seek help. Assaults against children have also been focused on by many communities and states with the goal of prevention and treatment.

SPIRITUALITY AND RESILIENCE, VOLUNTEERING, AND WELLBEING

In an interesting endnote, and in the spirit of the drift in psychological research from illness to wellness and health, some Indian studies have underlined the apparent utility of positive activities such as volunteering and their contribution to Psychological wellbeing.

Elias, Sudhir, and Mehrotra (2016) report, in a study published in *Behavioral Science*, that long-term volunteers experienced higher levels of psychological well-being (sense of mastery and competence, self-acceptance, and sense of engagement and growth) than a matched group of short-term volunteers. Development of volunteering as a public health intervention has been discussed as a potential measure to promote mental health and survival. The authors believe that it is likely to influence not merely mental health but also social wellbeing in those who sustain their volunteering engagement.

Further, Mehrotra and Tripathi (2016) have contributed a book chapter that focuses on spirituality and resilience and end by saying that "an as yet underexplored mechanism that could explain the links between spirituality and resilience in the Indian context is generation and a steady experience of positive emotions such as contentment and peace in individuals leading spiritually oriented lives."

Dr. Srinivasa Murthy (2014) has reviewed the mental health status of survivors of the 1984 Bhopal tragedy. He stresses on the need for more longitudinal health studies. He ends the paper by saying, "Using a public health approach in priority setting, identification of interventions and training of existing personnel, utilizing the community resources the needs of the population can be addressed."

Dr. Murthy has also written some seminal articles on caregiving and the stress faced by caregivers, and also on the need for mental health professionals to look after their own mental health. He has also written a well-researched epidemiological paper (Murthy, 2007) on mass violence and mental health, quoting examples from Vietnam, Afghanistan, Iraq, Iran, Israel, Lebanon, Palestine, Sri Lanka, Somalia and Sudan.

SUMMARY

Psychological stress is experienced when something we do not expect and cannot control happens to us. At times, these experiences lead to strong emotional reactions and at other times to psychological disorders such as PTSD. Understanding the manner in which stress and trauma are related to health and psychopathology is a complicated one. Overall, early stress has been associated with both later mental and physical health. One pathway to changes in mental and physical health is that stressful experiences change both psychological and physiological reactions to future stressful experiences. Our physiological reactions to stress and trauma occur on a variety of levels including the tagging of genes (epigenetics), the reaction of the immune system, the endocrine system involving the HPA axis, the ANS, and changes in cortical processes. Over evolutionary time the processing of social pain appears to have co-opted the basic brain structures involved in physical pain. Pain research suggests that there are two separate components to the experience of pain: (1) the sensory experience itself and (2) the felt unpleasantness. It is the second system that appears to be altered in psychopathology and is most sensitive to psychological factors.

Our immune system has evolved to recognize a variety of pathogens. It comes into play both in terms of specific pathogens such as viruses and also in terms of stress. The immune system is influenced by the brain and vice versa. It is expected that organisms will have evolved sophisticated mechanisms, which benefit survival. The basic mechanism is to prepare the body for action through two pathways: (1) the ANS and (2) the HPA axis. The overall stress reaction has been referred to as the fight-or-flight response. This reaction has been critical throughout our evolutionary history, but today, in our different social structure, it may lead to stress-related disorders. Given the different evolutionary pressures on males and females, it has been suggested that the fight-or-flight response better describes a human male's response to stress, while the tend-and-befriend response better describes the female's. However, the basic neuroendocrine responses to stress appear to be similar in both males and females.

Early stress research by Selye found that the body reacts similarly to a variety of different stressors. Selye called this response the GAS. One of the paradoxes was that the physiological stress responses that protect and restore the body can also damage it. However, repeated exposure to a particular stress situation could also increase the organism's ability to withstand that same stress in greater amounts. McEwen suggested that the term *stress* be replaced with the term *allostasis,* which refers to the body's ability to achieve stability through change. The overall stress response involves two tasks for the body: (1) turning on the allostatic response that initiates a complex adaptive pathway—for example, the fight-or-flight or tend-and-befriend response—and (2) turning off these responses once the danger has passed. Research suggests that prolonged exposure to stress may not allow these two mechanisms to function correctly and in turn leads to a variety of physiological problems. Overall, McEwen emphasized the important question of individual differences and the variety of ways in which perceived stress can influence future health.

There are several disorders in *DSM–5* that result from the experience of stress. The most significant are adjustment disorders, acute stress disorder, and PTSD. The severity of the stressor is the least in adjustment disorder and the greatest in PTSD. An adjustment reaction does not require specific symptoms but more global distress whereas acute stress disorder and PTSD do require specific symptoms. Whereas acute stress disorder is a short-term reaction to trauma, PTSD is present when the reaction lasts more than 6 months. PTSD is frequently comorbid with other disorders such as depression, substance abuse, and anxiety disorders such as OCD, panic disorder, agoraphobia, and social anxiety. This suggests that the treatment of PTSD requires more than a single strategy. Drug treatments reduce symptoms of PTSD; however, at present, the most effective therapies for PTSD are cognitive and behavioral therapies. The most studied therapies include exposure therapy, CBT and cognitive restructuring, and EMDR. One key ingredient of most therapies is a controlled re-experiencing of the original trauma, referred to as catharsis. New programs related to prevention are also being developed by both communities and the military.

STUDY RESOURCES

Review Questions

1. What are specific examples of how past stressful experiences change both our psychological and physiological reactions to future stressful situations in relation to the following:
   a. Psychological factors?
   b. Developmental changes in the brain?
   c. Genetic factors?
   d. Epigenetic modifications?
   e. Endocrine factors?
   f. Economic and social factors?
2. In the study of stress, researchers Selye and McEwen both referred to the paradox that the same physiological stress responses that protect and restore the body can also damage it. In terms of that paradox, please answer the following questions:
   a. How did our stress responses evolve, and what led to the paradox?
   b. How do our stress responses protect and restore our body and mind?
   c. How can our stress responses damage our body and mind?
3. *DSM–5* includes three psychological disorders that result from the experience of stress—adjustment disorder, acute stress disorder, and PTSD. For each disorder, please answer the following questions:
   a. What are examples of triggering events and common symptoms?
   b. What are the diagnostic criteria?
   c. What is the prevalence?
   d. What are effective treatments?

For Further Reading

Sapolsky, R. (2004). *Why zebras don't get ulcers* (3rd ed.). New York: St Martin's Griffin.

Key Terms and Concepts

acute stress disorder
adjustment disorders
allostasis
allostatic load
autonomic nervous system (ANS)
exposure therapy for PTSD
fight-or-flight response
general adaptation syndrome (GAS)
hypothalamic-pituitary-adrenal (HPA) axis
hypothalamus, pituitary, and adrenal pathway
immune system
parasympathetic division
psychological stress
psychoneuroimmunology
sympathetic division
tend-and-befriend response

CHAPTER

10

Anxiety Disorders and Obsessive-Compulsive Disorder

CHAPTER OUTLINE

- ANXIETY DISORDERS 346
- OVERVIEW OF ANXIETY DISORDERS 348
- MAJOR TYPES OF ANXIETY DISORDERS 359
- OBSESSIVE-COMPULSIVE DISORDER 373
- SUMMARY 379
- STUDY RESOURCES 381

ANXIETY DISORDERS

Donny Osmond has been performing in public since he was 5 years old.

"I grew up in front of a television camera," said Osmond, the former child star who in recent times has hosted a daytime talk show.

"Once that camera turned on, once I got on stage, once I heard the roar of the crowd, and I heard the music, whew! I was on Cloud Nine," he remembered.

But the stage also terrified him. About four years ago, he was diagnosed with social anxiety disorder, a condition that causes an irrational fear of social or performance situations.

"There are times I remember before I walked on stage," he said, "where if I had the choice of walking on stage or dying, I would have chosen death."

Osmond's problem has its origins in his childhood stardom. He first began feeling anxious when he was 11. Being a star at such a young age "took its toll," he said.

"Ever since I started in the business, I knew at least somebody in that audience is looking at me all the time," he said. "So I've got to be perfect."

His sister Marie, who had coped with her own marital crisis—a separation—remembered seeing her brother struggle with his fear.

"When we worked together on the previous show in the '70s, there would be times he would be in his dressing room, and he would just, you know, have really really difficult times," she said. "I just thought he was over-stressed."

Like many child celebrities, Donny had trouble making it as an adult star. When he finally had another hit as the star of the musical Joseph and the Amazing Technicolor Dreamcoat, he felt even more stress than he had as a child.

"Now the pressure was even greater to be perfect," he said.

The pressure triggered a full-blown panic attack. "I thought I was actually going crazy in my mind," he said. "I remember shaking in bed, and I just, I couldn't get out of bed. Something was wrong, and my wife took me to the hospital."

"I felt like he was having a nervous breakdown," said his wife Debbie. "He kept saying, 'I can't stop shaking; there's something wrong with me.'"

At one point, he was having trouble performing. The musical's producers brought in therapist Jerilyn Ross to work with their star.

Ross, who runs the Anxiety Disorders Association of America, diagnosed Osmond with social anxiety disorder.

She believes that the problem started when Osmond was a child performer. Said Ross: "He was judged as a tiny child—if he missed a step when he was dancing or he didn't hit a note or he wasn't funny enough. I mean these are incredible pressures for anybody."

To help him overcome it, she showed Osmond how to confront his fear. "I kind of taught him to play with the fear, instead of running from it," said Ross, who herself has suffered from panic attacks. "He was telling me he gets butterflies in his stomach. I said, 'OK, let's let the butterflies fly in formation. Let's give them a color, even a name.'"

The exercises worked. After three days of therapy, Osmond learned to deal with his problem. He sometimes still struggles with fear, but says he now knows how to work through these moments.

"I know when I walk out there, I'm not going to give the best performance," he said. "I'll make a mistake. I'll trip. I'll do something stupid. But it's OK; you pick up and just move on."

From CBS News. (2009, February 11). Donny Osmond confronts panic. Retrieved from www.cbsnews.com/8301-18559_162-164444.html

I felt incredibly awkward and out of place. It seemed everyone's eyes were on me and that they could see how uncomfortable I was. While my brother and the neighborhood kids talked and carried on with the others, I sat there rigid, looking straight ahead and not saying a word—immobilized. I did not fit in here. I did not belong here. I felt like an alien. My throat and chest tightened and my mouth went dry.

From Grazia, D. (2010). On the outside looking in: My life with social anxiety disorder. Bradenton, FL: BookLocker.com, Inc.

OVERVIEW OF ANXIETY DISORDERS

We all feel anxious at times. We worry that things may not work out the way we want them to. Sometimes, we have bodily symptoms such as a dry mouth or gastrointestinal (GI) problems consistent with the stress responses described in the last chapter. We may have problems sleeping. At times, our anxiety may have the positive effect of alerting us to something that we need to pay attention to. This lets us be more vigilant. The experience of anxiety in itself is part of the human situation. However, when this experience becomes chronic, creates distress, and interferes with our life, we see it as an anxiety disorder.

As you will see in this chapter, there are a number of different conditions that are classified as anxiety disorders. One of the most common is referred to as **generalized anxiety disorder (GAD)** in which the person worries about something that could happen in the future, such as losing a job or a partner. There are also specific situations that bring forth anxiety, such as giving a speech in public or being with others. This is referred to as a **social anxiety disorder (SAD).** There are also phobias to other specific objects, such as snakes or spiders, or situations, such as being in a high place or swimming in the ocean. Another anxiety disorder is *panic disorder.* A **panic attack** comes quickly and carries with it an intense feeling of apprehension, anxiety, or fear and usually happens without an actual situation that would suggest danger. In the fifth edition of the *Diagnostic and Statistical Manual of Mental Disorders (DSM–5)* (American Psychiatric Association [APA], 2013), **separation anxiety disorder** has been moved from the childhood disorders section and is now included as one of the anxiety disorders. Also, **obsessive-compulsive disorder (OCD)** is considered separately from anxiety disorders in *DSM–5,* but I will cover it at the end of this chapter.

Anxiety is to be afraid of what might happen. What if I don't do well when I give a presentation to a room full of important people? Will I get the job I want? What if a snake bites me when I am in the woods? What if the plane I am on crashes? What if I get germs on my hands when I go into a public restroom? What if others do not like me? In this sense, anxiety is about the future whereas fear typically has a stimulus in the present. With fear, we see a snake and become apprehensive. We look down from a tall building and feel unease. With anxiety, there is often no stimulus in front of us. With anxiety, the stimulus is in our mind. However, our cognitive and emotional consideration of a negative possibility does not make it any less real. Our body, mind, and emotions experience our ideas as real possibilities. In anxiety, we increase the probability in our mind that an event will happen.

DSM–5 Anxiety Disorders

- Separation Anxiety Disorder
- Panic Disorder
- Agoraphobia
- Specific Phobia
- Social Anxiety Disorder (Social Phobia)
- Generalized Anxiety Disorder
- Substance-Induced Anxiety Disorder
- Anxiety Disorder Attributable to Another Medical Condition
- Anxiety Disorder Not Elsewhere Classified

Some of these reactions appear to be built into our system. Most individuals feel apprehensive when looking down from a high building. Infants of about 9 months of age cry when a stranger takes them from their mothers. Other fears appear to be learned in a complex set of processes. Currently, what constitutes the fear and anxiety system in not clearly worked out. Post-traumatic stress disorder (PTSD), for example, which I discussed in the last chapter, is thought to use different cortical networks than anxiety. Panic attacks, which I will discuss in this chapter, may also be under a different set of cortical processes than our general feeling of anxiety.

What we do know is that fear and anxiety involve high-level as well as more primitive brain processes. Cognitively, we can make ourselves feel more anxious by thinking of all the terrible things that can happen in a given situation. We get on an airplane feeling somewhat anxious. We then hear a sound from the engine that we interpret to be a problem. This, in turn, results in our being even more vigilant and listening for every sound. The plane begins to move down the runway, and we tell ourselves it is not going to make it. This allows for emotional reactions that our body normally keeps in check to increase and we feel anxious.

Limbic system processes can also respond to stimuli on their own. For example, our amygdala can respond to an angry face in a manner that begins an autonomic nervous system reaction. In research with rats, Joseph LeDoux has shown that there are two pathways for the processing of fear (see *Figure 10-1*) (LeDoux, 2000, 2003). The higher

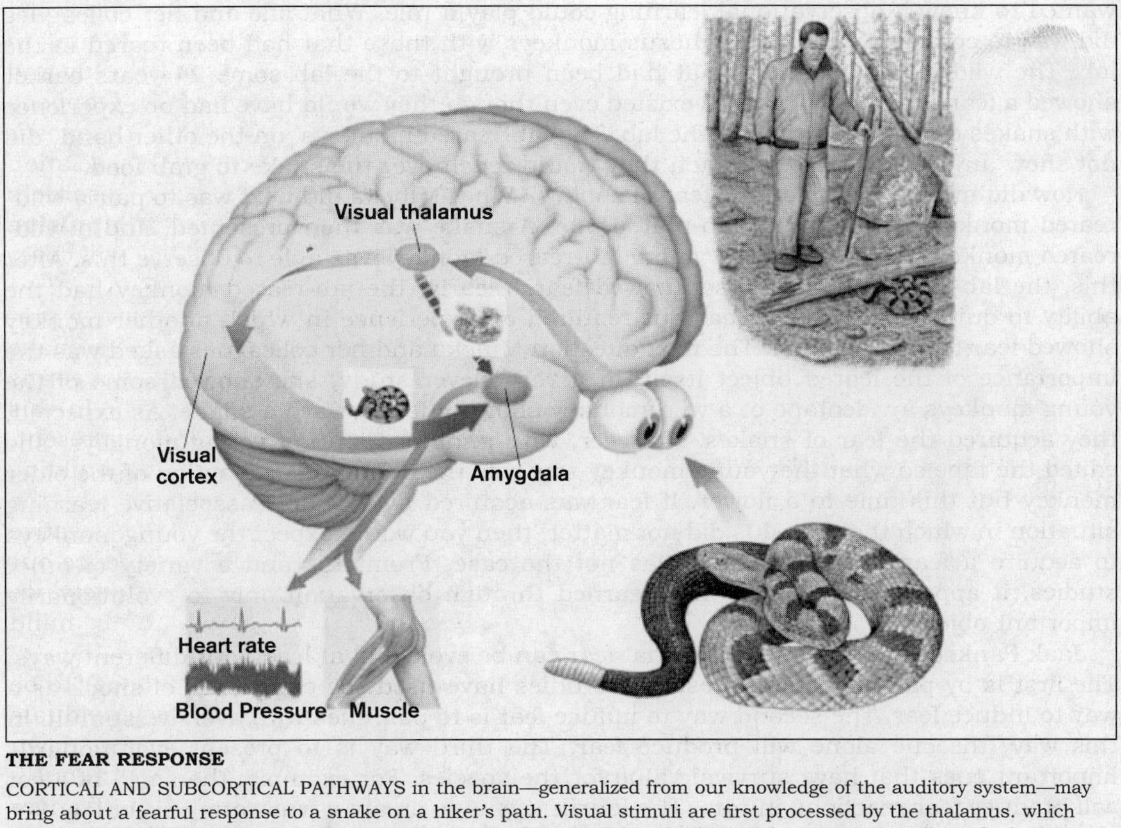

THE FEAR RESPONSE

CORTICAL AND SUBCORTICAL PATHWAYS in the brain—generalized from our knowledge of the auditory system—may bring about a fearful response to a snake on a hiker's path. Visual stimuli are first processed by the thalamus. which passes rough, almost archetypal information directly to the amygdal (*red*). This quick transmission allows the brain to respond to the possible danger (*green*). Meanwhile the visual cortex also received information from the thalamus and, with more perceptual sophistication and more time, determines that there is a snake on the path (*blue*). This information is relayed to the amygdala, causing heart rate and blood pressure to increase and muscles to contract. If, however, the cortex had determined that the object was not a snake, the message to the amygdala would quell the fear response.

FIGURE 10-1 The Fear Response

Source: LeDoux (1994).

pathway goes through the cerebral cortex and has high spatial resolution. The lower pathway goes more directly through the amygdala and is very fast but with less conscious experience. This suggests that the organism has a way to respond quickly to potential danger—even if its initial reaction is not correct. Simultaneously, the slow pathway is able to make a conscious appraisal of the situation. Thus, there is both a cortical and subcortical pathway to respond to dangerous situations. As such, there is great survival value to be wrong in responding to a stick as if it is a snake when a snake could be dangerous.

From an evolutionary perspective, to be fearful in the presence of dangerous situations would be adaptive. One scientific aspect of this is the question of how fixed or plastic these fears are. From research, we know that certain phobias run in families, suggesting a genetic component. However, not everyone has exactly the same fears, suggesting that fears can be learned during development. One classic study in fear development is that of Susan Mineka and her colleagues (see Öhman & Mineka, 2001, for an overview). It had been observed that primates in the wild show a fear of snakes. Since a similar fear was seen in lab monkeys, it was assumed that the fear was somehow innate. However, Mineka asked the question of whether early experience could influence this. In particular, she wanted to know if observational learning could play a role. What she and her colleagues did was to compare wild-reared rhesus monkeys with those that had been reared in the lab. The wild-reared monkeys that had been brought to the lab some 24 years earlier showed a fear of snakes. This fear existed even though they would have had no experience with snakes during their time in the lab. The lab-reared monkeys, on the other hand, did not show any fear of snakes. If fact, they would reach over the snake to grab food.

How did monkeys develop the fear of snakes? What Mineka did next was to pair a wild-reared monkey with a young lab-reared one. A snake was then presented, and a wild-reared monkey showed fear. The young lab-reared monkey was able to observe this. After this, the lab-reared monkey also showed fear. Clearly, the lab-reared monkey had the ability to quickly acquire the fear but required an experience in which another monkey showed fear for it to happen. The next question Mineka and her colleagues asked was the importance of the feared object itself. In a very clever study, she showed some of the young monkeys a videotape of a wild monkey showing fear toward a snake. As expected, they acquired the fear of snakes. However, with another group of young monkeys, she edited the tape so what the young monkey saw was the original fear reaction of the older monkey but this time to a flower. If fear was acquired by a simple associative learning situation in which the stimulus did not matter, then you would expect the young monkeys to acquire a fear of flowers. This was not the case. From this and a variety of other studies, it appears that fear can be learned through observation only to evolutionarily important objects.

Jaak Panksepp (2004) suggested that fear can be evoked in at least four different ways. The first is by painful stimuli. Research studies have used the experience of shock as a way to induce fear. The second way to induce fear is to pair cues with aversive stimuli. In this way, the cue alone will produce fear. The third way is to present evolutionarily important cues that have survival value for the species. For example, the smell of a cat will produce fear reactions in rats. The fourth way is to create a frustrating situation. For example, if an organism is expecting a reward that is delayed, fear and apprehension will result. This model suggests that anxiety can be produced by expectations that either negative events will happen or that positive events will not happen.

Thus, the brain predicts the future. Part of the way we predict the future is based on past information. As we listen to a person speak or drive down the road, we are constantly predicting what will happen next. This prediction is demonstrated by the research that shows that if something happens different from what we expect, then we show electroencephalogram (EEG) changes in the brain. Generally, we predict that our drive down the road will be fine. However, individuals with anxiety disorders see negative alternatives and worry that things will not work out.

Cognitive Processes in Anxiety

In our evolutionary history, it has been suggested that fear mechanisms evolved to aid our ability to disengage from the task at hand to pay attention to threats or potential danger. An unexpected loud noise will cause us to jump and focus our attention in its direction. Although this process occurs with all individuals, what is becoming apparent is that individuals with anxiety are even more sensitive than others to the possibility of potential threat (see Bishop, 2007; MacLeod & Mathews, 2012, for overviews). This sensitivity is referred to as **cognitive bias.**

Cognitive bias has been studied in a number of ways. One is to use a modified **Stroop test.** The traditional Stroop test has color names in ink of a different color. That is, the word *green* would be shown in red ink. When asked to name the color of the ink, individuals are slower when the name and color do not match as compared with when the ink and color name are the same (see *Figure 10-2*). When using a "threat" Stroop, the name of the color is replaced by a threat word (see *Figure 10-3*). Another research procedure is to use a dot-probe task. One version of the task asks individuals to focus on an X in the middle of the computer screen. On each side of the X are words. The person is to press a computer key whenever a word is replaced by a dot. In anxiety studies, both words can be neutral, represent different types of threat, or one neutral and one threat.

BLUE	GREEN	YELLOW
PINK	RED	ORANGE
GREY	BLACK	PURPLE
TAN	WHITE	BROWN

FIGURE 10-2 Stroop Effect—Individuals Are Slower When Asked to Name the Color of the Ink

FAILURE
REJECTION
INFERIOR
USELESS

FIGURE 10-3 Stroop Using Threat Words. Neutral Words Would Also Be Added to Compare Differences in Reaction Time.

The basic question is as follows: Does an individual who is anxious show differential reaction times when threat or negative emotional words are present? Overall, the answer is yes. Individuals with anxiety disorders show a selective attentional bias toward threat-related words. When a threat-related word is present, individuals with anxiety show slower reaction times and increased error rates. Even if stimuli are presented in a manner that the individual could not detect, anxious individuals will display this cognitive bias. This suggests that attention to threat involves more primitive brain processes such as the amygdala rather than just being under higher cortical control (MacLeod & Mathews, 2012).

Individuals with anxiety disorders show a tendency to focus on information that is negative and to expect more negative things to actually happen. They also interpret ambiguous information in a negative manner. Overall, anxious individuals have a difficult time not paying attention to potential threats in their environment. This, in turn, supports the experience of negative internal emotional states. This type of cognitive bias leads to both the development and maintenance of the condition of anxiety.

Neurobiology of Anxiety Disorders

Although fear and anxiety are often studied together, research suggests that different brain areas are involved. Specifically, those areas involved in anxiety are not those directly responsible for the expression of fear. Rather, anxiety is related to those areas of the brain that regulate the fear system. These include the prefrontal cortex (PFC), the amygdala, and the hippocampus. These are systems involved in cognitions, emotional reactivity, and memory—all important components in the social and cognitive aspects of anxiety. These systems are also seen in humans to be the ones involved in increased vigilance and attention to threat. The amygdala is also involved in fear conditioning.

One of the major neurotransmitters involved in anxiety is **gamma-aminobutyric acid (GABA)** (see Millan, 2003, for an overview). GABA is the major inhibitory neurotransmitter in the brain. Although GABA is involved in a variety of processes, it is thought to play a major role in anxiety. The basic idea is that individuals with anxiety have reduced GABA activity, which in turn results in less inhibition of those brain structures that are involved in threat responses. It should also be noted that GABA receptors are located densely in the PFC, the amygdala, and the hippocampus. Benzodiazepines, which are common drugs used in the treatment of anxiety disorders, influence the GABA system, which in turn increases its inhibitory effects. Further, animal models of anxiety have shown increased GABA activity in the amygdala and a reduction of fear with the introduction of serotonin in the hippocampus and amygdala. An adult rat that was nurtured and licked as an infant will have great expression of GABA activity in the amygdala with fewer signs of fearfulness and stress responses (Fries, Moragues, Caldji, Hellhammer, & Meaney, 2004).

In reviewing studies with both humans and other animals, Gross and Hen (2004) suggested that anxiety should be seen as a developmental problem involving both environmental and genetic factors. From twin studies, it is apparent that the genetic contribution to anxiety is moderate (30%–40%). Genetic studies of individuals with anxiety disorders show the highest concordance for monozygotic (MZ) versus dizygotic (DZ) twin pairs as would be expected if there were a genetic component. Panic disorder was associated with a heritability of 48% (Hettema, Neale, & Kendler, 2001). Similar heritability numbers were found for specific phobias, such as animal (47%), blood injury (59%), and situational (46%). Social phobia was found to be 51%. In studies examining twins with GAD, modest relationships ranging from 15% to 30% have been reported (Kendler & Baker, 2007). Family interviews also suggest the presence of GAD in first-degree relatives. Overall, this suggests genetic contributions to the development of anxiety disorders.

With the discovery of functional networks in the brain, psychopathology can be mapped in terms of which cortical networks differ from normal functioning. Chad Sylvester and his colleagues (2012) have performed this analysis in relation to anxiety. They described anxiety disorders in relation to four functional networks (see *Figure 10-4*). The first network is the salience or cingulo-opercular network, which is seen to be important in detecting errors or conflicts. Error detection would result in the need for changes in cognitive control. The second network is the executive control or frontoparietal network. This is the network that implements increased cognitive control. The third network is the ventral attentional network and is involved in detecting new stimuli rather than the task at hand. The fourth network is the default network, which is involved in internal processing including self-inspection, future planning, and emotional regulation. Overall, these researchers suggest that anxiety disorders display a particular pattern of action in the four networks. This pattern includes overactivity in the salience network and underactivity in the executive and default networks. This is consistent with seeing individuals with anxiety disorders as being oversensitive to threat.

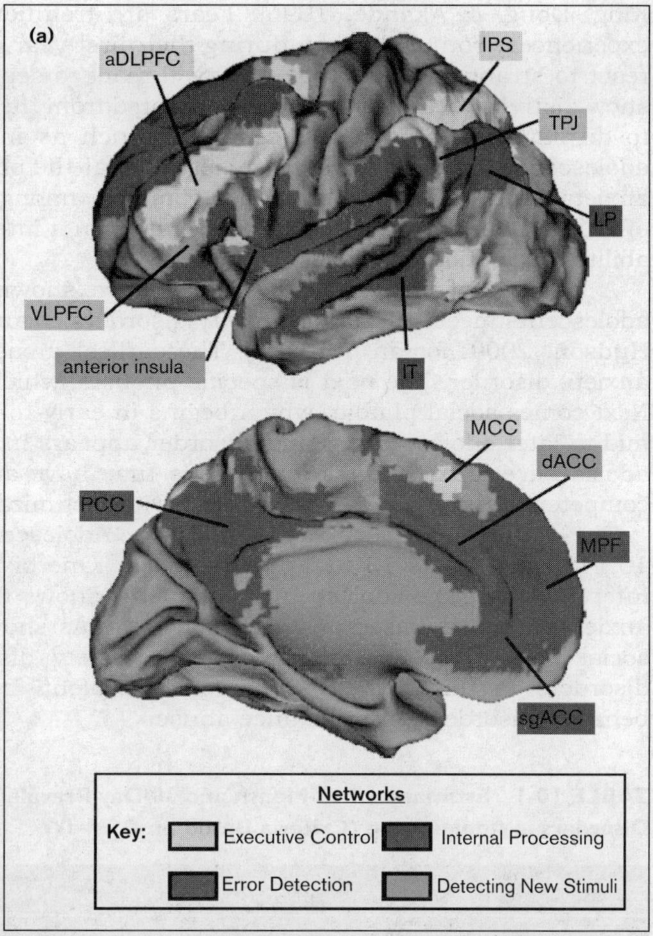

FIGURE 10-4 Four Networks Involved in Anxiety That Are Involved in Error Detection, Executive Control, Detecting New Stimuli, and Internal Processing

Source: From Sylvester, et al. "Functional network dysfunction in anxiety and anxiety disorders." *Trends in Neuroscience.* Volume 35, Issue 9, September 2012. With permission from Elsevier.

Abbreviations: PFC, prefrontal cortex; aDLPFC, anterior dorsolateral PFC; dACC, dorsal anterior cingulate cortex; IPS, intraparietal sulcus; IT, inferior temporal cortex; LP, lateral parietal cortex; MCC, middle cingulate cortex; PCC, posterior cingulate cortex; sgACC, subgenual anterior cingulate cortex;; STG, superior temporal gyrus; TPJ, temporal-parietal junction; VLPFC, ventrolateral PFC

Developmental Aspects of Anxiety

The development of anxiety and fear follows a trajectory that is part of the human condition. Children and adolescents show similar profiles of anxiety and fear across cultures; however, cultures that favor inhibition, compliance, and obedience also show increased levels of fear (Ollendick, Yang,

King, Dong, & Akande, 1996). Fears are traditionally seen in relation to immediate experiences. Young children during their first year of life, usually around 9 months, will react to strangers. After that, they will react to separation. Infants of other species also show distress vocalizations when separated from their mothers. Human infants also begin to display distress to specific stimuli, such as insects or flying bees or animals. By adolescence, the fear turns to anxiety in that the object of concern is not present. Social anxiety about a future situation is common among adolescents. The normal expression of fear and anxiety becomes pathological when it interferes with the child's or adolescent's ability to function or causes distress.

A number of epidemiology studies have shown that 2.5% to 5% of children and adolescents meet criteria for anxiety disorders at any one time (see Rapee, Schniering, & Hudson, 2009, for an overview). The earliest anxiety disorder to develop is separation anxiety disorder. The next is specific phobias, which begin in early to middle childhood. Next comes social phobia, which begins in early to middle adolescence. OCD appears in mid to later adolescence. Panic disorder appears in early adulthood. Given the nature of adolescence, anxiety disorders at this time have an influence on popularity and social competence. They are also associated with victimization.

The National Comorbidity Replication Adolescent Supplement is a U.S. survey of 10,148 adolescents 13 to 17 years of age. One of its advantages is that it is based on interviews with the adolescents. *Table 10-1* shows the 12-month prevalence rates for the anxiety disorders based on *DSM–IV* criteria. As shown in the table, specific phobias and social phobia are the most common anxiety disorders among adolescents. Anxiety disorders in this survey were more prevalent in adolescents than mood disorders, behavior disorders, or substance abuse.

TABLE 10-1 Estimates of 12-Month and 30-Day Prevalence Rates for Anxiety and Other Disorders in Adolescence (Criteria Based on *DSM–IV*)

	Prevalence	
Disorder	***12-mO***	***30-d***
Mood disorder		
Major depressive disorder or dysthymia	8.2 (0.8)	2.6 (0.3)
Bipolar I or II disorder	2.1 (0.2)	0.7 (0.1)
Any mood disorder	10.0 (0.8)	3.1 (0.4)
Anxiety disorder		
Agoraphobia	1.8 (0.2)	0.8 (0.1)
Generalized anxiety disorder	1.1 (0.2)	0.4 (0.1)
Social phobia	8.2 (0.4)	4.6 (0.3)
Specific phobia	15.8 (0.8)	9.5 (0.6)
Panic disorder	1.9 (0.2)	0.8 (0.1)
Posttraumatic stress disorder	3.9 (0.4)	1.6 (0.2)

	Prevalence	
Disorder	***12-mO***	***30-d***
Separation anxiety disorder	1.6 (0.2)	0.6 (0.1)
Any anxiety disorder	24.9 (0.9)	14.9 (0.6)
Behavior disorder		
Attention-deficit/hyperactivity disorder	6.5 (0.5)	4.5 (0.3)
Oppositional-defiant disorder	8.3 (0.7)	2.9 (0.3)
Conduct disorder	5.4 (0.8)	1.5 (0.3)
Eating disorder	2.8 (02.)	1.1 (0.1)
Any behavior disorder	16.3 (1.1)	7.6 (0.7)
Substance disorder		
Alcohol abuse with or without dependence	4.7 (0.3)	1.3 (0.1)
Drug abuse with or without dependence	5.7 (0.5)	1.6 (0.3)
Any substance disorder	8.3 (0.5)	2.6 (0.3)
Total disorders, No.		
Any	40.3 (1.2)	23.4 (1.0)
Exactly 1	21.9 (0.8)	16.4 (0.8)
Exactly 2	8.7 (0.6)	4.8 (0.5)
≥3	9.8 (0.7)	2.2 (0.3)

Source: Kessler et al. (2012, p. 375).
Note: 12-MO = 12 month; 30-D = 30 day; numbers represent % prevalence and standard error.

It is not always the case that if a person has an anxiety disorder in childhood, it will continue into adulthood. This is especially true for specific phobias. These prevalence rates for those over 18 years of age can be seen in *Table 10-2*. As with adolescence, in adulthood, rates for anxiety disorders are higher than mood disorders. One anxiety disorder that shows increases in prevalence is GAD.

Anxiety Disorders Around the World

In LENS 10.1, you can see lifetime and prevalence data for any anxiety disorder by country. Although rates may vary by country, the overall data show that anxiety disorders are a common occurrence.

These data show that anxiety disorders are common throughout the world. Although not shown here, Kessler et al. (2009) reported additional data to suggest that only a small number of those individuals with a mental disorder receive treatment and even fewer receive high quality treatment. This, in turn, results in impaired functioning, which has real costs to a society in terms of productivity, financial resources, and quality of life.

TABLE 10-2 Twelve-Month Prevalence of Mental Disorders From 9,282 Adults Above the Age of 18 Based on *DSM–IV* Criteria

	Total
Anxiety disorders	
Panic disorder	2.7 (0.2)
Agoraphobia without panic	0.8 (0.1)
Specific phobia	8.7 (0.4)
Social phobia	6.8 (0.3)
Generalized anxiety disorder	3.1 (0.2)
Posttraumatic stress disorder	3.5 (0.3)
Obsessive-compulsive disorder	1.0 (0.3)
Separation anxiety disorder	0.9 (0.2)
Any anxiety disorder[||]	18.1 (0.7)
Mood disorders	
Major depressive disorder	6.7 (0.3)
Dysthymia	1.5 (0.1)
Bipolar I and II disorders	2.6 (0.2)
Any mood disorder	9.5 (0.4)
Impulse control disorders	
Oppositional defiant disorder	1.0 (0.2)
Conduct disorder	1.0 (0.2)
Attention-deficit/hyperactivity disorder	4.1 (0.3)
Intermittent explosive disorder	2.6 (0.2)
Any impulse control disorder	8.9 (0.5)
Substance disorders	
Alcohol abuse	3.1(0.3)
Alcohol dependence	1.3 (0.2)
Drug abuse	1.4 (0.1)
Drug dependence	0.4 (0.1)
Any substance disorder	3.8 (0.3)

Source: Kessler et al. (2005, p. 610).

10-1 LENS
Global Mental Health Anxiety Disorders

The World Health Organization (WHO), as part of its mission, has collected data on mental health from countries around the world. Face-to-face household surveys were undertaken with community adult respondents in low-income or middle-income countries (Colombia, Lebanon, Mexico, Nigeria, China, South Africa, Ukraine) and high-income countries (Belgium, France, Germany, Israel, Italy, Japan, the Netherlands, New Zealand, Spain, the United States). Prevalence data were assessed with the WHO composite international diagnostic interview.

Lifetime and 12-month prevalence data in relation to anxiety disorders has been compiled (see *Tables 10-3 and 10-4*).

TABLE 10-3 Lifetime Prevalence

	Any Anxiety Disorder	
	%	*(sE)*
I. WHO Region: Pan American Health		
Colombia	25.3	(1.4)
Mexico	14.3	(0.9)
United States	31.0	(1.0)
II. WHO Region: African Regional Office		
Nigeria	6.5	(0.9)
South Africa	15.8	(0.8)
III. WHO Region: Eastern Mediterran		
Lebanon	16.7	(1.6)
IV. WHO Region: European Regional		
Belgium	13.1	(1.9)
France	22.3	(1.4)
Germany	14.6	(1.5)
Israel	5.2	(0.3)
Italy	11.0	(0.9)
Netherlands	15.9	(1.1)
Spain	9.9	(1.1)
Ukraine	10.9	(0.8)
V. WHO Region: Western Pacific Region		
PRC	4.8	(0.7)
Japan	6.9	(0.6)
New Zealand	24.6	(0.7)

Source: Kessler et al. (2009).

TABLE 10-4 Twelve-Month Prevalence for Anxiety Disorders Worldwide

	Any Anxiety Disorder		*Any Mood Disorder*	
	%	(sE)	%	(sE)
I. WHO Region: Pan American Health Organization (PAHO)				
Colombia	14.4	(1.0)	7.0	(0.5)
Mexico	8.4	(0.6)	4.7	(0.3)
United States	19.0	(0.7)	9.7	(0.4)
II. WHO Region: African Regional Office (AFRO)				
Nigeria	4.2	(0.5)	1.1	(0.2)
South Africa	8.2	(0.6)	4.9	(0.4)
III. WHO Region: Eastern Mediterranean Regional Office (EMRO)				
Lebanon	12.2	(1.2)	6.8	(0.7)
IV. WHO Region: European Regional Office (EURO)				
Belgium	8.4	(1.4)	5.4	(0.5)
France	13.7	(1.1)	6.5	(0.6)
Germany	8.3	(1.1)	3.3	(0.3)
Israel	3.6	(0.3)	6.4	(0.4)
Italy	6.5	(0.6)	3.4	(0.3)
Netherlands	8.9	(1.0)	5.1	(0.5)
Spain	6.6	(0.9)	4.4	(0.3)
Ukraine	6.8	(0.7)	9.0	(0.6)
V. WHO Region: Western Pacific Regional Office (WPRO)				
PRC	3.0	(0.5)	1.9	(0.3)
Japan	4.2	(0.6)	2.5	(0.4)
New Zealand	15.0	(0.5)	8.0	(0.4)

Source: Kessler et al. (2009).

Indian Work on Anxiety Disorders

A paper in the *Indian Journal of Psychiatry* provides an overview of work done in India in this realm (Trivedi & Gupta, 2010). Rural occurrences are naturally harder to trace and document than urban. Also, prevalence rates would change across the vast landmass of India and across age group ranging from pediatric to geriatric. Many of the studies are the evaluations of different molecules and their efficacy in the treatment of anxiety, and are conducted at large teaching hospitals and public health centers in the country. Some work has been done on PTSD and GAD (Khambaty, 2017). Vahia et al. (1993) have carried out studies comparing meditation with pharmacotherapy and interestingly found the former as effective as the latter, with meditation in fact being superior in the management of trait anxiety.

Bodas, Ollendick, and Sovani, and also Sovani, Thatte, and Nadkarni (2000) have carried out interesting cross-cultural work on test anxiety, comparing students across the United States of America and India on the stress they experience while facing examinations. The phenomenon of examination stress is certainly more pervasive in India due to the competitive examination system. Some interesting modules have been developed by the IPH, Maharashtra, to teach children rational emotive methods to handle their own test anxiety that is likely to interfere with their examination performance.

Khambaty and Parikh (2017) have reviewed cultural aspects of anxiety disorders in India and observe that while patients from the Western world present with more psychological symptoms in GAD, Indians present with more somatic symptoms. Further, Indians with panic disorder present with fewer cognitive and vestibular symptoms. The Dhat syndrome that is peculiar to India and a few other cultures is described with the associated hypochondriacal fear of loss of vitality.

Faith healers and Ayurveda, Unani medicine and homeopathy, naturopathy, and yoga are some of the commonly used therapeutic remedies for anxiety disorders in the Indian setting.

Herzog, Lele, et al. (1990) found that transcendental meditation has been linked to the increased regional cerebral metabolic rate of glucose consumption (rCMRG1c) in the frontal lobe of the brain and reduction in the primary and secondary visual centers. Vipassana meditation and mindfulness are also found effective by a number of studies.

MAJOR TYPES OF ANXIETY DISORDERS

Separation Anxiety Disorder

Human infants, as well as the infants of most other mammal species, show distress when separated from their caregivers.

Concept Check

- What are the two pathways in the brain for processing fear, and how do they work? From an evolutionary perspective, what is the advantage of the two pathways?
- What are some of the ways cognitive bias leads to both the development and maintenance of anxiety?
- How is the brain involved in anxiety in terms of brain areas, neurotransmitters, and networks?
- How does the developmental trajectory of anxiety and fear map onto normal human developmental stages?
- What do we know about the prevalence rates of anxiety disorders across the life span and around the world?

Human infants will generally cry. As the infants develop and learn that their caregivers are available, even when they cannot see them, the distress is reduced. You can watch children at times checking to see if their parents are around as they play on a playground for example. You can notice that some preschool children are hesitant to go to a birthday party or other event. However, once they are with other children, they forget the initial hesitation and enjoy themselves. These are all normal developmental processes as children develop independence and the ability to function on their own.

Some children—even as they develop—do not show this sense of independence and continue to feel distress when not with their caregivers. These children may not want to go to school and even follow their caregivers around. They become concerned that something could happen to their caregivers and worry about the caregiver's health. They may have nightmares involving fears of separation. They will not want to leave the house unless their caregiver is with them. This sense of concern and distress can continue into elementary school years, adolescence, and even adulthood. Such children, adolescents, and adults would be diagnosed with separation anxiety disorder.

Separation anxiety disorder in *DSM–5* requires that the symptoms last for at least 4 weeks in children and adolescents. Further, three of eight different types of symptoms must be present. The first category of symptoms is that the person experiences distress when he or she is not at home or with major attachment figures. The second is that the person worries about the well-being of the attachment figure. The third is that the person worries that an event such as being kidnapped or getting lost could happen to himself or herself. The fourth is an unwillingness to leave home for fear of separation. The fifth is a fear of being alone. The sixth is an unwillingness to sleep alone or outside the house. The seventh is having nightmares related to separation. And the eighth is to have complaints of physical symptoms such as headaches or stomachaches.

Separation anxiety disorder is the most prevalent anxiety disorder for those under 12 years of age. The 12-month prevalence of separation anxiety disorder is approximately 4% in children and drops to 1.6% in adolescents (*DSM–5*). In adults, the 12-month prevalence is between 0.9% and 1.9%. In community samples, it is more commonly seen in girls than boys.

Generalized Anxiety Disorder

In *DSM–5,* GAD is characterized by excessive anxiety and worry that has been present for more than 3 months (see *Table 10-5*). Bodily symptoms such as feeling on edge and muscle tension must also accompany the worry. In fact, one of the more consistent physiological patterns seen in GAD is high muscle tension. Finally, the anxiety must lead to one or more of the following four behaviors. These are (1) avoiding activities that can have negative outcomes; (2) overpreparation for activities that can have negative outcomes; (3) marked procrastination in behaviors due to worries; and (4) repeatedly seeking reassurance due to worries.

GAD, along with depression, is the most frequently diagnosed mental disorder in the United States. GAD prevalence rates are 3.1% for a given year with lifetime rates being 5.7% for those over 18 years of age (Kessler et al., 2005). However, these have changed over the years with changing *DSM* criteria. Prevalence rates are twice as high for women as compared with men. GAD occurrence peaks in middle age and declines after that. Most individuals (86%) with GAD also meet criteria for another disorder, mainly major depressive disorder, social phobia, or panic disorder (Brown et al., 2001). In those with

TABLE 10-5 Generalized Anxiety Disorder

A. Excessive anxiety and worry (apprehensive expectation) occurring more days than not for at least 6 months, about a number of events or activities (such as work or school performance).

B. The individual finds it difficult to control the worry.

C. The anxiety and worry are associated with three (or more) of the following six symptoms (with at least some symptoms having been present for more days that not for the past 6 months):

Note: Only one item is required in children.

1. Restlessness or feeling keyed up or on edge.
2. Being easily fatigued.
3. Difficulty concentrating or mind going blank.
4. Irritability.
5. Muscle tension.
6. Sleep disturbance (difficulty failing or staying asleep, or restless, unsatisfying sleep).

D. The anxiety, worry, or physical symptoms cause clinically significant distress or impairment in social, occupational, or other important areas of functioning.

E. The disturbance is not attributable to the physiological effects of a substance (e.g., a drug of abuse, a medication) or another medical condition (e.g., hyperthyroidism).

F. The disturbance is not better explained by another mental disorder (e.g., anxiety or worry about having panic attacks in panic disorder, negative evaluation in social anxiety disorder [social phobia], contamination or other obsessions in obsessive-compulsive disorder, separation from attachment figures in separation anxiety disorder, reminders of traumatic events in posttraumatic stress disorder, gaining weight in anorexia nervosa, physical complaints in somatic symptom disorder, perceived appearance flaws in body dysmorphic disorder, having a serious illness in illness anxiety disorder, or the content of delusional beliefs in schizophrenia or delusional disorder).

Source: Reprinted with permission from the *Diagnostic and Statistical Manual of Mental Disorders, Fifth Edition*, (Copyright 2013). American Psychiatric Association.

both GAD and a major depressive disorder, the GAD was seen in individuals some 7 years before the onset of depression. This has suggested to some that a period of significant worry may lead to the onset of depression.

Research has analyzed worry in terms of both content and one's ability to control it. In one study comparing those with GAD and non-anxious controls, non-anxious controls reported they were able to control their worrying to a greater degree than those with GAD. Whereas 100% of those with GAD reported problems controlling their worries, only 5.6% of controls reported problems of control (Abel & Borkovec, 1995). There is also some suggestion that those with GAD are not able to move from a process of worry to active problem solving or coping. Those with GAD also reported that they worry about minor things (100%) versus those with other types of anxiety disorders (50%) (Barlow, 2002). In terms of frequency, those with GAD also reported that they worry a larger percentage of each day and tend to have a larger set of domains such as family, money, and friends that they worry about than those without GAD.

What is the role of worry? One answer is that worry is the manner in which an individual with GAD attempts to reduce the negative emotional experiences associated with GAD (Borkovec, 1994). This is referred to as the **cognitive avoidance model** of GAD (see Borkovec, Alcaine, & Behar, 2004, for an overview). Worry, in this case, serves two functions. The first function is to use worry as a way to prepare for bad events—or even to prevent them from occurring. The second function is to use worry as a way to reduce the person's emotional response. Although a consistent physiological picture of worry has

CASE OF ADAM CALDWELL
Generalized Anxiety Disorder

Adam Caldwell is a 50-year-old European American. He came to the clinic to seek treatment to address his GAD symptoms. At the onset of therapy he was also experiencing marital difficulties and stress at work. He had previously been divorced and was remarried, living with his second wife at the time of treatment. He had several children from his first marriage as well as several stepchildren. He had a doctoral degree and was employed in an applied science field.

Adam Caldwell defined himself as a man with integrity (trustworthy, honest) and deep commitment to his religion and the contract of marriage. In terms of coping style, he revealed himself to be a logical and analytical thinker, frequently providing detailed and intellectual responses and at first rarely expressing emotions even when directly prompted. His problem-solving style was such that in stressful situations he reportedly tended to deny ("stuff away") his painful feelings and act in a manner that was impulsive and hostile.

At the beginning of therapy, Adam reported a high level of GAD symptoms. These symptoms included worry and somatic distress across a broad range of situations. He reported that he was also experiencing stress at work and was having marital conflict.

Adam reported a difficult interpersonal history. His father was authoritarian, distant, and physically abusive. His mother was kind but submissive to his father and did not protect him from the father's abuse. He reported being a rebellious child who had no close friends. His divorce from his first wife was traumatic, and his children were removed from his care.

Early in treatment, Adam had difficulty implementing and benefiting from techniques prescribed in the cognitive behavioral therapy (CBT) protocol in response to the stressful events. At the end of a guided relaxation exercise in Session 4, the client reported a substantial reduction in anxiety and stated to the therapist, "That's the impact you have on me." In Session 5, Adam reported having experienced a shift in his average mood from anxious to relaxed. He also stated that he was able to make this shift by monitoring his anxiety during the day and challenging the associated thoughts. As therapy progressed Adam appeared to become confident, forthright, active, and even happy.

Based on Louis Castonguay, Dana Nelson, James Boswell, Samuel Nordberg, Andrew McAleavey, Michelle Newman, and Thomas Borkovec. (2012). Corrective Experiences in Cognitive Behavior and Interpersonal–Emotional Processing Therapies: A Qualitative Analysis of a Single Case. In Louis Castonguay and Clara Hill (Eds.), *Transformation in Psychotherapy: Corrective Experiences Across Cognitive Behavioral, Humanistic, and Psychodynamic Approaches* (pp. 245–279). Washington, DC: American Psychological Association.

yet to appear, research does suggest that worry does produce short-term relief from physiological responses to stress. The following case study of Adam Caldwell (not his real name) describes an individual with GAD.

Treatment of Generalized Anxiety Disorder

Anxiety is a common experience of many individuals that they may report to many types of health professionals including psychologists, psychiatrists, and even their family physician. These individuals are often given medications such as benzodiazepines or offered one of the types of psychotherapy described in Chapter 2. Studies using psychodynamic, existential-humanistic, and cognitive behavioral approaches have all reported reductions in anxiety. At this point, both medications and psychological treatments show similar reductions in GAD in the short term. However, only about 40% to 60% of those treated with either medication or psychological treatments show full improvement. This is in comparison with other anxiety disorders such as phobias, which show higher rates of improvement after treatment.

The best-studied psychological interventions have involved cognitive behavioral approaches and behavioral approaches with GAD although dynamic approaches have also been shown to be effective (Barber, Muran, McCarthy, & Keefe, 2013). The behavioral approaches include relaxation training and other such techniques. The cognitive behavioral techniques focus on automatic thinking. Typical approaches train clients to detect internal and external anxiety cues and to apply new coping skills that focus on both psychic and somatic symptoms (Borkovec & Ruscio, 2001). Initially, clients are asked to pay close attention to those factors in their daily life that trigger anxiety responses. They are also asked to pay attention to physiological and cognitive responses experienced as anxiety develops. In the therapy itself, the client is asked to imagine a situation that would increase stress or anxiety or choose a topic that he or she would worry about and notice the associated thoughts, feelings, and images. Overall, the major cognitive behavioral approaches are designed to be offered for a specific period of time. These techniques help the client learn how to reduce anxiety and worry, which is a major component of GAD.

Some important components of a cognitive behavioral therapy (CBT) approach are as follows:

1. Identifying the anxiety-associated thoughts, images, beliefs, etc.
2. Discussing these to bring out their causal role
3. Leading clients to question the validity of thoughts or beliefs, and to search for evidence
4. Helping clients develop alternative, less anxiety-arousing assumptions or interpretations
5. Testing alternative viewpoints in homework assignments or experiments
6. Teaching the above methods as self-helping coping devices to be used in real life

These components were developed by Tom Borkovec and his colleagues. They have tested the effectiveness of therapy components in a variety of outcome studies. Additionally, Borkovec and Ruscio (2001) reviewed outcome research from 13 randomized controlled GAD studies that involved a CBT component. As a whole, these CBT studies showed decreases in anxiety and depression following treatment, which was maintained in a 6- to 12-month follow-up. This suggests that CBT is effective not only for GAD but also for some of the comorbid conditions. Successful treatment was also associated with psychophysiological changes such as EEG gamma activity (Oathes et al., 2008).

Another effective treatment for GAD is that of mindfulness (Hoge et al., 2013). Mindfulness-based treatments have the person with GAD focus on the present moment. This attention to the present is performed with openness and a nonjudgmental manner. This allows for better emotional regulation and reduction of anxiety symptoms. In randomized control trials for the treatment of GAD, mindfulness-based treatment has been shown to be more effective than one involving stress reduction techniques (Hoge et al., 2013). Further, functional magnetic resonance imaging (fMRI) changes were seen following mindfulness training in those with GAD in the amygdala and the connections between the frontal areas and the amygdala (Hölzel et al., 2013). These cortical changes were also associated with symptom reduction.

Since the 1970s, benzodiazepines have been used to treat anxiety. Benzodiazepines are thought to influence GABA activity. Individuals with anxiety have reduced GABA activity, which in turn results in less inhibition of those brain structures that are involved in threat responses. Unlike antidepressant medications, benzodiazepines show their effect within a week. A large number of studies have shown anxiety reductions in approximately 65% to 70% of GAD clients when given benzodiazepines (see Roemer, Orsillo, & Barlow, 2002, for an overview). A smaller percentage shows a full remission of anxiety symptoms. However, when a person discontinues benzodiazepines, GAD symptoms will reappear.

A second class of medication referred to as azapirones were introduced in the 1990s. Buspirone is a common azapirone that influences serotonin receptors in the brain. This drug influences more of the cognitive components of GAD and has fewer side effects than benzodiazepines. A third class of drugs for GAD is antidepressants. Both tricyclic antidepressants, such as imipramine, and serotonin reuptake inhibitors (SSRIs), such as paroxetine, have been shown to be effective with GAD.

Social Anxiety Disorder

Most individuals can think of a time that they were concerned about meeting someone or giving a talk in front of a group. *Perhaps I will say the wrong thing. Perhaps others will think I am foolish. Perhaps I will spill my food on my shirt when I am eating.* These are all common reactions and are part of our human condition. However, when these feelings are severe and last for more than 6 months, it would be considered an SAD. SAD is characterized by marked fear or anxiety about one or more social situations in which the individual is exposed to possible scrutiny by others. Approximately 8% of U.S. citizens will experience an SAD during their lifetime (Kessler et al., 2010). It is suggested to be more common in women than men. The disorder is also associated with later mood disorders and substance abuse.

SAD, which was referred to as social phobia in *DSM–IV,* is characterized by persistent and severe fear of social situations. One key feature of the social setting is that it can involve evaluation. Evaluation can take many forms and can involve any of three different types of situations. The first is social interactions, such as having a conversation with others. The second type of situation is one in which the person could be observed, such as eating or drinking. The third type of situation is one in which the person is performing in front of others, such as giving a talk to a group. When in these situations, the individual with social anxiety will experience anxiety symptoms similar to those seen with GAD.

The individual with social anxiety will fear that he could be humiliated, embarrassed, or rejected. He may also be concerned that others could be offended. He imagines that the outcome of social encounters will be negative and tries to prevent the experience of anxiety by not putting himself in social situations. This, in turn, results in the person living a less than full life with discomfort and distress.

Previous experiences appear to be more important in individuals with social anxiety as compared with other anxiety disorders. Some 92% of adults with social anxiety report having experienced negative social events in childhood prior to becoming socially anxious (McCabe, Antony, Summerfeldt, Liss, & Swinson, 2003). This is in comparison with 35% of those with panic disorder and 50% of those with OCD.

Neuroscience Aspects of Social Anxiety

Previously, I introduced you to the concept of the social brain (Adolphs, 2003, 2009), which involves such areas of the brain as the PFC, the amygdala, the anterior cingulate cortex (ACC), and the insula. These regions are particularly important in social and emotional processing in normal and anxiety processing (see Hahn et al., 2011, for an overview). The amygdala is involved in the initial processing of emotional memory and arousal, fast evaluation of novel stimuli, and threat perception. Electrical stimulation of the amygdala will elicit fear, anxiety, and social withdrawal.

The social brain regions are also involved in social anxiety, especially the amygdala and insula areas (see Miskovic & Schmidt, 2011, for an overview). It may be the case that the insula as part of the salience network is overactive. This, in turn, would lead to neutral signals receiving excessive reactivity in which the person with social anxiety pays more attention than should be required. Likewise, higher cognitive processes may not inhibit amygdala responses in those with social anxiety, which would result in greater emotional responses than would be required by the situation. In one study examining brain activation during public versus private speaking, exaggerated amygdala activation was found in individuals with social anxiety compared with non-anxious individuals (Tillfors et al., 2001).

Theoretically, it has been suggested that individuals with social anxiety process social situations with evolutionarily older alarm systems such as the amygdala whereas non-anxious individuals process the same situations with newer cognitive–analytic processes using the PFC. It has also been suggested that social anxiety can be seen as part of the larger dominance and submissive system seen across primate species (Öhman, 1986, 2009). This view is supported by research that shows that individuals with social anxiety show enhanced amygdala activation to images of hostile faces. Further, the degree of amygdala activity is positively correlated with the severity of social anxiety but not general anxiety (Phan, Fitzgerald, Nathan, & Tancer, 2006). Another similar study using faces also found greater activation of the amygdala as well as fewer connections between the frontal areas and the ACC (Hahn et al., 2011).

Treatment of Social Anxiety Disorder

There are a number of psychological therapies that have been developed for treating SAD (see Hofmann & Barlow, 2002; Rodebaugh, Holaway, & Heimberg, 2004; Weiss, Hope, & Cohn, 2010, for overviews). These therapies include CBT, exposure therapy, social skills training, and group CBT. These different approaches may also be combined in different ways. Both CBT type therapies and medication have been shown to be effective with SAD. Medications appear to show a faster reduction in anxiety initially. However, following treatment when no additional medication or psychotherapy is offered, there is a greater relapse with medication treatment than with CBT therapy.

Exposure therapy places a client in a feared situation despite the experience of distress. One technique is for clients to create a hierarchy of situations that they would fear or avoid. They can rank this hierarchy in terms of the level of anxiety they would expect to experience. These situations can then be used in the therapy. Typically, the person

Concept Check

- What are the eight different categories of diagnostic symptoms describing separation anxiety disorder? How many must be present before an individual receives a diagnosis of separation anxiety disorder?
- What evidence would you cite to show that GAD has a significant impact on the U.S. population?
- What medications and psychological therapies are recommended for treating GAD? What aspects of GAD does each type of treatment target?
- What characteristics might make an individual more at risk for developing SAD?
- How is the social brain involved in SAD?

begins with the least anxiety-producing situation and moves over time to the most feared. The situation can be experienced by either role-playing or actually being in the feared environment. Although the underlying mechanisms leading to change have not been determined precisely, exposure therapy has been shown to reduce anxiety in social situations for individuals with SAD (see Abramowitz, Deacon, & Whiteside, 2011, for an overview).

Social skills training is based on the idea that individuals with social anxiety have inadequate social interaction skills. Social skills training teaches the individual practical social skills through modeling, corrective feedback, reinforcement, and other such techniques. Since this type of training involves trying out new behaviors, it is difficult to separate it completely from exposure therapy in outcome studies.

CBT, as described previously, assumes that social anxiety is produced by the person's automatic thoughts in the social situation or the expectation of a social situation. The task is to help the person detect and restructure these thoughts and expectations. In the treatment of social anxiety, it has been offered in both individual and group therapy.

Psychopharmacological approaches have been shown to be useful in the treatment of social anxiety. One of the earliest drugs used was a monoamine oxidase (MAO) inhibitor, phenelzine sulfate, which was seen as the drug of choice. More recent medications have included the SSRIs, paroxetine and sertraline. The norepinephrine-SSRI venlafaxine has also been used. The choice of medication is often left with the individual health professional based on a specific person's side effects.

Agoraphobia

Agoraphobia is the condition in which a person experiences fear or anxiety when in public. These situations can involve public transportation, open spaces such as parking lots or marketplaces, or places with a number of individuals such as theaters or shops, as well as being in a crowd or just being outside the home. One characteristic of agoraphobia is that the person is concerned that escape from the situation would be difficult. Prior to *DSM–5,* agoraphobia was diagnosed in relation to panic disorder (see Wittchen et al., 2010, for a review). In some individuals, panic disorder and agoraphobia go together and in others they do not. Age of onset in both agoraphobia and panic disorder is around 21 to 23 years of age. Agoraphobia is seen more frequently in women than men. Some studies have shown that negative experiences in childhood, such as the death of a parent, are associated with both agoraphobia and panic disorder. With *DSM–5,* agoraphobia is considered a separate disorder although it may occur with any other disorder, especially the anxiety disorders. Both CBT approaches and antidepressants are effective in treating agoraphobia.

Specific Phobia

A **specific phobia** is a condition in which an individual experiences fear or anxiety to a particular condition or object. Common phobias are fear of snakes, spiders, flying, height, blood, injections, and the dark. Although almost all individuals have experiences such as driving in bad weather in which they feel concern from time to time, these fears tend not to be long lasting or result in major changes in lifestyle. To be diagnosed with a specific phobia, the individual must actively avoid the condition or object and the fear or anxiety must have lasted for 6 months or more. Further, the fear or anxiety causes distress and is out of proportion to the actual danger posed by the situation.

As a background for classifying specific phobias in *DSM–5*, a review of the literature was conducted (LeBeau et al., 2010). These researchers found that prevalence rates in the United States differed by type of phobia (see *Table 10-6*). Animal phobias were a common phobia and showed a lifetime prevalence of 3.3% to 7%. Natural phobias, such as fear of heights, storms, or water, show lifetime prevalence rates of 8.9% to 11.6%, collectively. Of the natural phobias, height phobia is the most common with a 3.1% to 5.3% prevalence rate. Situational phobias, such as fear of flying, enclosed places, or driving, show prevalence rates of 5.2% to 8.4%. Except for height phobia, large gender differences have been found with more females than males displaying phobias. These include 91% of those with animal phobias being female, as well as 87% to 90% with situational phobias whereas height phobia was 60%. Further, over 50% of people with one phobia were found to also have three or more additional phobias during their lifetime. European rates for specific phobias were similar to those in the United States (APA, 2013). Rates in Latin America, Africa, and Asia were lower.

Table 10-6 summarizes the clinical features of three types of phobias. As can be noted, animal and natural event phobias are seen earlier than situational phobias. In terms of focus of fear, individuals were asked, "What are you most concerned will happen?" For the natural environment and situational phobias, the concern was around danger. For the animal phobias, such as spiders or snakes, the concern was one of disgust or revulsion. For the blood, injection, or injury phobias, the concern was fainting or disgust but not physical harm. The physiological pattern of individuals with blood-injection-injury (B-I-I) phobias was different from the other types. It involved an initial heart rate acceleration followed by a deceleration that increased the likelihood of fainting. All other phobias showed heart rate acceleration alone. Although the research is limited, individuals with spider phobia showed a different pattern of brain activation than those with B-I-I phobias.

Neuroscience Aspects of Specific Phobias

There are a variety of mechanisms that have been associated with developing a phobia. As with lab-reared monkeys, seeing another individual being afraid of an object or condition could lead to the development of the phobia through observational learning (see *Table 10-7*). Consistent with the observational learning perspective is the finding that individuals with animal phobias were likely to have relatives with an animal phobia. Likewise, those with situational phobias or B-I-I phobias were likely to have relatives who had similar phobias. Although this could also suggest a genetic factor, the genetic relationship has not been shown to be that strong.

Other types of traditional conditioning processes could also be possible. In the classic case study of Little Albert, John Watson, in the 1930s, showed that animals that a child

TABLE 10-6 Clinical Features of Specific Phobia Types

	Types			
Phobia Features	***Animal Phobia***	***Natural Environment***	***Situation Phobia***	***B-I-I Phobia***
Prevalence	3.3–5.7%	4.9–11.6%	5.2–8.4%	3.2–4.5%
Onset	6.3–9.2 years	6.5–13.6 years	13.4–21.8 years	5.5–9.4 years
Gender ratio	Female > male	Female > male, most common type among males	Female > male	Mixed findings
Impairment			Seeking professional help, medication, interference with daily and social life	
Focus of fear	Disgust, revulsion	Danger of harm	Danger of harm	Physical symptoms (fainting), disgust, revulsion
Physiological fear response	Activation of dorsal anterior cingulated cortex, anterior insula			Vasovagal fainting, activation of bilateral occipito-parietal cortex and thalamus
Comorbidity	Depression	Depression, heights phobia in women → anxiety disorders	Affective disorders, childhood-onset disorders, substance use disorders, panic attacks	Marijuana abuse, depression, panic disorder, OCD, AG, SAD, Among diabeties → peripheral vascular disease, cardiovascular disease
Risk factors	Experiential, genetic			Women, low education

Source: LeBeau et al. (2010, p. 151).
Note: B-I-I = blood-injection-injury.

had previously played with happily could, through classical conditioning, come to be feared. In this case, a loud sound was made when the animal, such as a rabbit or white rat, was with the child. Although initially the child would play with the animal, after the pairing with a loud sound, the child would withdraw. As a result, Little Albert showed fear when in the presence of these animals. Watson's demonstrations with Little Albert appear in many introductory textbooks. However, what is left out is the finding that fear conditioning worked better with evolutionally relevant objects such as animals but less so with a bag of wool or with person-made objects such as a wooden toy (cf. English, 1929; Watson & Rayner, 1920).

In reviewing the literature related to fear conditioning in humans, those brain areas involved relate to the social brain processes. These include the ACC, the insula, the medial PFC, the orbitofrontal cortex (OFC), and the thalamus (see Sehlmeyer et al., 2009, for a review). When fear objects such as snakes or spiders are shown to individuals with

TABLE 10-7 Lifetime Prevalence and Standard Error of Specific Fears

	*Lifetime Fears**		*Lifetime Phobia Given Fear†*		*Lifetime Phobia With Specific Fear in Total Sample††*	
Specific Fear	*%*	*(se)*	*%*	*(se)*	*%*	*(se)*
Height	20.4	0.7	26.2	1.8	5.3	0.5
Flying	13.2	0.7	26.9	2.4	3.5	0.3
Closed spaces	11.9	0.6	35.1	2.5	4.2	0.4
Being alone	7.3	0.6	40.7	3.3	3.1	0.4
Storms	8.7	0.5	33.1	3.4	2.9	0.4
Animals	22.2	1.1	25.8	1.2	5.7	0.4
Blood	13.9	0.7	32.8	2.1	4.5	0.3
Water	9.4	0.6	35.8	2.8	3.4	0.3
Any	49.5	1.2	22.7	1.1	11.3	0.6

*Prevalence of lifetime fears in the total sample.
†Probability of specific phobia diagnosis in people endorsing each fear.
††Percentage of people in total sample with specific phobia and each lifetime fear (i.e., 5.3 % of total sample have lifetime-specific phobia and a height fear).

Source: Curtis et al. (1998). Specific fears and phobias: Epidemiology and classification. British Journal of Psychiatry, 173, 212–217. Reproduced with permission from The Royal College of Psychiatrists.

phobias, exaggerated activity is seen in the amygdala, the insula, and the cingulate cortex (see Etkin & Wager, 2007, for a meta-analysis). Jan Schweckendiek and his colleagues (2010) studied individuals with spider phobia in an fMRI scanner. In this study, neutral pictures were paired with three types of pictures—pictures of spiders, pictures of aversive scenes (e.g., mutilations), or neutral pictures. In comparison with a non-phobia group, those with spider phobias showed enhanced brain activity within the fear network (medial PFC, ACC, amygdala, insula, and thalamus) in response to the phobia-related conditioned stimulus. Further, spider phobic subjects displayed higher amygdala activation in response to the phobia-related conditioned stimulus than to the non-phobia-related conditioned stimulus. This supports the idea that once a phobia is developed, those conditions or objects that evoke it are associated with greater brain activity in the network of structures associated with fear.

Treatment of Specific Phobias

It is commonly accepted that phobias are best treated by exposure to the feared object (see Antony & Barlow, 2002, for an overview). Lars Öst has shown in a number of studies that a phobia such as fear of snakes or spiders can be significantly reduced after a single 3-hour session although similar results are found in a larger number of shorter sessions (Öst, 1989, 1996). The basic procedure would be for the client to describe her fears as well as catastrophic expectations and the situations that evoke these in a session with her therapist. This would be followed by the therapist slowly introducing the feared object such as a snake from a distance. The therapist checks with the client as this is happening to determine the magnitude of fear. In general, it is the client who directs the speed of the

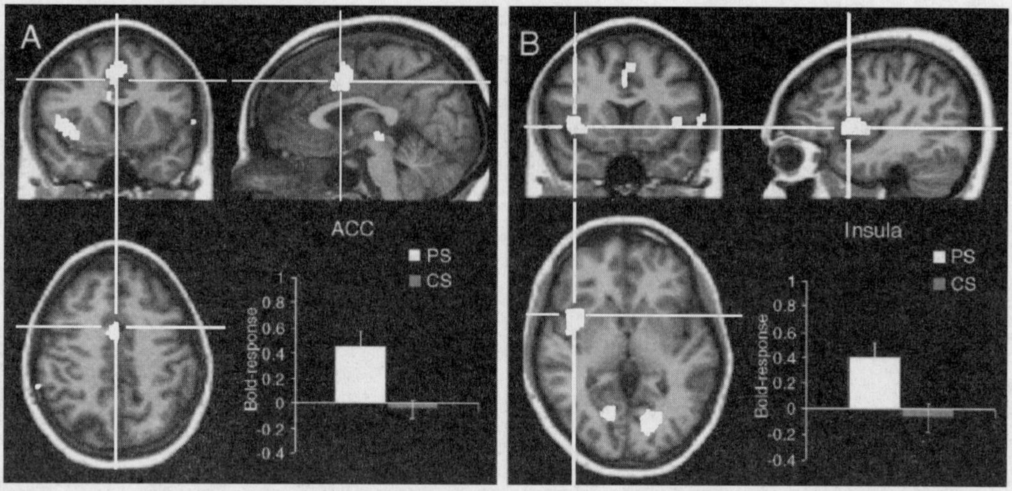

FIGURE 10-5 Increased Activation in Anterior Cingulate Cortex and Insula to Spider Versus Neutral Images in Individuals With Spider Phobia Compared With Control Individuals

Source: Straube et al. (2006, p. 129), with permission from Elsevier.

introduction of the feared object. During the session, the therapist would bring the feared object closer to the person until she was able to touch it with reduced fear.

Using the rapid gradual exposure techniques of Lars Öst, Thomas Straube and his colleagues measured brain changes prior to and following therapy (Straube, Glauer, Dilger, Mentzel, & Miltner, 2006). They studied a group of individuals with spider phobia. These individuals received two sessions of therapy with a duration of 4 to 5 hours. Gradual exposure started with the presentation of spider pictures. Then, the individuals were shown the skin of a tarantula, followed by an actual tarantula. The goals of the therapy were fourfold. These are (1) to hold a living tarantula for about 10 minutes, (2) to catch moving and nonmoving spiders at least 10 times with a glass at different locations within the therapy room, (3) to catch any species of spider in the basement of the institute at least 3 times, and (4) to touch a rapidly moving house spider. By the completion of the therapy, all of the individuals with spider phobia were able to fulfill the four treatment goals without strong feelings of anxiety.

An fMRI session was conducted prior to the beginning of any therapy in which the individuals with spider phobia and a control group were shown pictures of spiders as well as neutral pictures. As expected, individuals with spider phobia showed greater activation in the insula and ACC, which is part of the fear network (see *Figure 10-5*). Following therapy, this activation was reduced.

Panic Disorder

A panic attack comes quickly and carries with it an intense feeling of apprehension, anxiety, or fear (see Craske et al., 2010; Fava & Morton, 2009, for overviews). It happens without an actual situation that would suggest danger. Physiological symptoms can include shortness of breath, trembling, heart palpitations, dizziness, faintness, and hot or cold flashes. The person can also experience the world as if it were not real and be concerned about dying. The symptoms usually peak within the first 10 minutes of the attack. The experience of one's heart pounding (97%) and dizziness (96%) are reported by almost all individuals who experience panic attacks. It is a frequent cause of individuals going to a hospital emergency room. There is some suggestion that panic is more common during periods of stress. Although many individuals experience an episode of panic-like symptoms at some point in their lives, it is necessary for these symptoms to be recurrent and followed by a month of concern or change in lifestyle to be diagnosed with a panic disorder (see *Table 10-8*).

Once individuals experience a panic attack, they often become concerned about having another attack. They may also try to change their behavior as a way to prevent panic attacks. For example, some individuals will not exercise or do other tasks that would raise their heart rates. Although presented as a separate anxiety disorder, panic attacks can occur within the context of any of the other anxiety disorders. Lifetime prevalence rates are 4.7% for panic disorder (Kessler et al., 2006). The modal age of onset for panic disorder is between 21 and 23 years of age although children and adolescents may

TABLE 10-8 ***DSM–5* Panic Disorder**

A. Recurrent unexpected panic attacks. A panic attack is an abrupt surge of intense fear or intense discomfort that reaches a peak within minutes, and during which time four (or more) of the following symptoms occur: Note: The abrupt surge can occur from a calm state or an anxious state.

1. Palpitations, pounding heart, or accelerated heart rate.
2. Sweating.
3. Trembling or shaking.
4. Sensations of shortness of breath or smothering.
5. Feelings of choking.
6. Chest pain or discomfort.
7. Nausea or abdominal distress.
8. Feeling dizzy, unsteady, light-headed, or faint.
9. Chills or heat sensations.
10. Paresthesias (numbness or tingling sensations).
11. Derealizaton (feelings of unreality) or depersonalization (being detached from oneself).
12. Fear of losing control or "going crazy."
13. Fear of dying.

Note: Culture-specific symptoms (e.g., tinnitus, neck soreness, headache, uncontrollable screaming or crying) may be seen. Such symptoms should not count as one of the four required symptoms.

B. At least one of the attacks has been followed by 1 month (or more) of one or both of the following:

1. Persistent concern or worry about additional Panic Attacks or their consequences (e.g., losing control, having a heart attack, "going crazy")
2. A significant maladaptive change in behavior related to the attacks (e.g., behaviors designed to avoid having panic attacks, such as avoidance of exercise or unfamiliar situations)

C. The disturbance is not attributable to the direct physiological effects of a substance (e.g., a drug of abuse, a medication) or another medical condition (e.g., hyperthyroidism, cardiopulmonary disorders).

D. The disturbance is not better accounted for by another mental disorder (e.g., the Panic Attacks do not occur only in response to feared social situations in Social Anxiety Disorder, circumscribed phobic objects or situations in Specific Phobia, obsessions in Obsessive-Compulsive Disorder, reminders of traumatic events in Posttraumatic Stress Disorder, or separation from attachment figures in Separation Anxiety Disorder).

Source: Reprinted with permission from the *Diagnostic and Statistical Manual of Mental Disorders, Fifth Edition*, (Copyright 2013). American Psychiatric Association.

experience panic attacks along with other anxiety disorders. Studies have shown that twice as many women as men have panic disorder.

On a brain level, it is suggested that panic and anxiety involve different areas of the brain (Graeff & Del-Ben, 2008). Anxiety is integrated in the forebrain whereas panic is organized in the mid-brain, especially the basal ganglia and limbic structures. Decreased gray matter in individuals with panic disorder has also been reported in these areas (Lai, 2011). The idea of different areas for anxiety and panic is consistent with the suggestion that there are two defense systems in the brain (Gray & McNaughton, 2000; McNaughton & Corr, 2004). The basic model suggests that fear and anxiety are involved in different approach-and-avoidance systems that utilize distinct brain networks.

Concept Check

- What characteristics would you expect to read in a case study of an individual with agoraphobia in terms of symptoms, prior history, and treatment protocols?
- What are examples of specific phobias? Are the prevalence rates the same for different kinds of phobias? If not, how are they different?
- What do we know about how specific phobias are developed, as well as how they are treated? What is the common thread between development (initiation) and treatment (extinction)?
- What are the characteristics of a panic attack? How is it different from a panic disorder?

As described previously, the stress response involves the hypothalamic-pituitary-adrenal (HPA) axis and the hormone cortisol. HPA is under excitatory control of the amygdala and inhibitory control of the hippocampus. The hippocampus releases corticotropin-releasing factor (CRF), which is transported to the adrenal cortex that releases cortisol. When confronted with situations that evoke anticipatory or generalized anxiety, cortisol is released. However, cortisol is not released during panic attacks. Overall, this suggests that anxiety and panic reflect different brain and hormonal processes. Specifically, anxiety involves limbic forebrain structures such as the PFC, the amygdala, and the hippocampus. Panic attacks, on the other hand, involve more primitive structures of the hindbrain such as the hypothalamus and periaqueductal gray (PAG). It has been shown that electrical stimulation of the PAG in surgical patients results in panic-like symptoms (Nashold, Wilson, & Slaughter, 1974). It also suggests that a panic attack does not involve the traditional stress reaction in the same way that generalized anxiety does.

The currently preferred medication treatments for panic disorder are SSRIs, which have been shown to be more effective than placebo treatments. Benzodiazepines have also been shown to be effective. The best-studied psychological treatment for panic disorder is CBT, which has been shown to be effective. In general, CBT approaches educate the individual concerning the nature of panic symptoms and reduce misconceptions. Internal exposure techniques can also be employed. For example, the person could be asked to exercise to increase his or her heart rate or spin around in a chair to feel dizzy. In this way, the person is exposed to the internal situation associated with a panic attack. More global aspects of CBT, such as cognitive restructuring in terms of distortions in thinking, are also used. This helps to reduce the catastrophic expectations such as thinking that one is going to die when one's heart rate increases. Meta-analyses have shown that combining CBT and antidepressant medication is more effective than either one alone (Mitte, 2005; Watanabe, Churchill, & Furukawa, 2009).

OBSESSIVE-COMPULSIVE DISORDER

I like to make stars in my head, or trace them with my finger. Just like you doodle with a pencil on the side of a piece of paper. Someone will be talking to me and I look like I'm listening, but really all I'm doing is drawing one line of the star for every one word that person says. Our conversation has to end on a multiple of 5, a complete star. My husband might say to me, "What do you want for dinner?" I'm looking him straight in the eyes so I guess he believes I'm deciding, but in fact I'm drawing and thinking 1 and 1/5 stars. He says, "How about pizza?" I still just stare at him, but think 1 and 4/5 stars. He continues, "Do you have any idea?" 2 and 4/5. Finally he'll conclude, "Why don't we just make pasta?" 4 stars.

OCD is characterized by repetitive thoughts and feelings usually followed by behaviors in response to them. The thoughts are usually perceived as unpleasant and not wanted. A distinction is made between **obsessions** and **compulsions.** Obsessions are generally unwelcome thoughts that come into one's head. In studies examining these thoughts in patients with OCD, they involve avoiding contamination, aggressive impulses, sexual content, somatic concerns, and the need for order. Compulsions are the behaviors that one uses to respond to these thoughts. Some behaviors, like cleaning or placing objects in order, reflect a desire to respond to the obsessions. Other compulsions, such as hand washing, are more avoidant in nature for fear of what one might say, do, or experience in a particular situation. Often individuals with OCD will constantly check to see if they performed a particular behavior such as turning off the stove or unplugging an iron. Interestingly, individuals with OCD may be aware that their thoughts and actions may seem bizarre to others, but they cannot dismiss the thoughts or need for action.

OCD has traditionally been considered an anxiety disorder in *DSM* history. Some experts have suggested this is not the best way to view OCD, and it is considered as a separate disorder in *DSM–5* (see *Table 10-9*; see Leckman et al., 2010, for an overview). One way to inform this question is to examine individuals with OCD and determine which other disorders are seen in these individuals and their first-degree relatives as compared with individuals without OCD. In one large-scale study, OCD was found to have a relationship with anxiety disorders such as GAD and agoraphobia as well as depression, grooming disorders (e.g., skin picking), and hypochondriasis (Bienvenu et al., 2012). However, OCD did show differences with control individuals in terms of eating disorders, impulse control, and substance abuse.

OCD is characterized by two types of symptoms (see Franklin & Foa, 2008, 2011, for overviews). The first type is obsessions in which unwanted, intrusive, and recurrent thoughts enter the person's mind. The themes of these thoughts may be person specific. In general, the obsessions involve such themes as contamination with a concern about germs, a mistake, aggression, sex, religion, or serious illness such as cancer. The second type is compulsions or behavioral rituals. These may include excessive checking of everyday activities such as turning off a stove or other appliance as well as repetitive behaviors such as washing hands, checking locks, checking the stove, or counting or repeating routine actions. Traditionally, compulsions have been seen as a mechanism for reducing the anxiety or distress caused by the obsession. Not being allowed to engage in these behaviors results in distress and anxiety. Over 90% of those with OCD show both obsessions and

TABLE 10-9 Obsessive-Compulsive Disorder

A. Presence of obsessions, compulsions, or both:

Obsessions are defined by (1) and (2):

1. Recurrent and persistent thoughts, urges, or images that are experienced, at some time during the disturbance, as intrusive and unwanted and that in most individuals cause marked anxiety or distress
2. The individual attempts to ignore or suppress such thoughts, urges, or images, or to neutralize them with some other thought or action (i.e., by performing a compulsion)

Compulsions are defined by (1) and (2):

1. Repetitive behaviors (e.g., hand washing, ordering, checking) or mental acts (e.g., praying, counting, repeating words silently) that the individual feels driven to perform in response to an obsession, or according to rules that must be applied rigidly
2. The behaviors or mental acts are aimed at preventing or reducing anxiety or distress, or preventing some dreaded event or situation; however, these behaviors or mental acts are not connected in a realistic way with what they are designed to neutralize or prevent or are clearly excessive

B. The obsessions or compulsions are time-consuming (for example, take more than 1 hour a day) or cause clinically significant distress or impairment in social, occupational, or other important areas of functioning.

C. The obsessive-compulsive symptoms are not attributable to the direct physiological effects of a substance (e.g., a drug of abuse, a medication) or another medical condition.

D. The disturbance is not better explained by the symptoms of another mental disorder (e.g., excessive worries, as in generalized anxiety disorder; preoccupation with appearance, as in body dysmorphic disorder; difficulty discarding or parting with possessions, as in hoarding disorder; hair pulling, as in trichotillomania [hair-pulling] disorder; skin picking, as in excoriation [skin-picking] disorder; stereotypies, as in stereotypic movement disorder; ritualized eating behavior, as in eating disorder; preoccupation with substances or gambling, as in substance-related and addictive disorder; preoccupation with having an illness, as in illness anxiety disorder; sexual urges or fantasies as in paraphilia disorders; impulses, as in disruptive, impulse-control, and conduct disorders; guilty ruminations, as in major depressive disorder; thought insertion or delusional preoccupations, as in schizophrenia spectrum and other psychotic disorders; or repetitive patterns of behavior, as in autism spectrum disorder).

Indicate whether OCD beliefs are currently characterized by:

Good or fair insight: The individual recognizes that OCD beliefs are definitely or probably not true, or that they may or may not be true

Poor insight: The individual thinks OCD beliefs are probably true

Absent insight: The individual is completely convinced OCD beliefs are true

Specify if:

Tic-related OCD: The individual has a lifetime history of a chronic tic disorder

Source: Reprinted with permission from the *Diagnostic and Statistical Manual of Mental Disorders, Fifth Edition*, (Copyright 2013). American Psychiatric Association.

behavioral rituals. OCD has an adulthood prevalence of 2% to 3% and a child and adolescence prevalence of 1% to 2%. Approximately 40% of those with childhood OCD report continuing symptoms into adulthood. There is not a gender difference in rates.

There is clearly a parallel between the themes found in OCD and concerns expressed by those without the disorder. Most individuals naturally avoid contamination or express concern when they experience unusual bodily sensations. On a society level, there are often rituals concerned with health and success in the world. Tribal cultures would perform rituals to dispel evil spirits or bring in the good ones. Most modern societies have a variety of rituals including not walking under a ladder, not stepping on sidewalk cracks, or not partaking in other behaviors as ways of avoiding bad luck. Sports teams also have rituals for how to prepare for an important game. Not performing any of these rituals may result in a feeling of anxiety for many individuals.

A variety of studies have suggested that OCD is found throughout the world in similar rates (see Feygin, Swain, & Leckman, 2006, for an overview). Feygin and colleagues (2006) suggested that OCD results from the exaggeration of normal traits that can be mapped onto a developmental trajectory. In particular, they discussed four developmental themes as a response to stress. The first theme is loss similar to anxious attachment disorder. The obsession is that someone could be lost to the person. There are a large variety of situations in which this could happen. A friend, lover, or child could be killed in an accident, for example. To prevent this, the compulsion is to check on the person to make sure that he or she is still okay or to create situations in which the person will not be able to be in a situation with risk. The second theme is physical security in one's own environment. A common manifestation is that the person checks to make sure everything is in its place. The third theme is environmental cleanliness. The fear is that objects or the person himself are dirty and that this will result in disease or other negative events. The behavior of course is to clean obsessively. The fourth theme is that the person will be deprived of resources or objects that are important to him. A person who experiences these obsessions will either hoard objects or resources or try to prevent any situation in which he could come in contact with loss. Each of these themes could be tied to a normal development stage in which fear or threatening situations were overemphasized.

In looking at the types of thoughts specified by those with OCD, consistent groupings have been found (see Leckman et al., 2010, for an overview). The first grouping includes thoughts and images concerning aggressive, sexual, and religious content and related checking compulsions. This factor may be experienced by the person as forbidden thoughts that they would not want to share with another person. The second grouping concerns symmetry and ordering, such as placing objects in a regular pattern or making sure pictures are straight. The third grouping centers on contamination and cleaning. The fourth grouping relates to **hoarding.** Meta-analyses including individuals from non-English-speaking countries show similar groupings suggesting a universal nature to these groupings across cultures (Bloch, Landeros-Weisenberger, Rosario, Pittenger, & Leckman, 2008).

Other studies have sought to determine if these four groups are related to different comorbid disorders (see Leckman et al., 2010, for an overview). The answer is yes. Those with OCD centered on aggressive, sexual, and religious content were more likely to also have anxiety or depressive disorders. Individuals with OCD centered on symmetry and ordering were more likely to also have tic disorders, bipolar disorder, panic disorder, or agoraphobia. A contamination and cleaning focus was associated with comorbid eating disorders. The fourth grouping of hoarding was associated with comorbid personality disorders. *Figure 10-6* shows the compulsions seen in one group of individuals as they were initially evaluated, referred to as admission.

Historically, hoarding has been seen as a specific type of OCD. In *DSM–5*, hoarding is considered a separate disorder. It is defined in terms of an excessive acquisition of objects

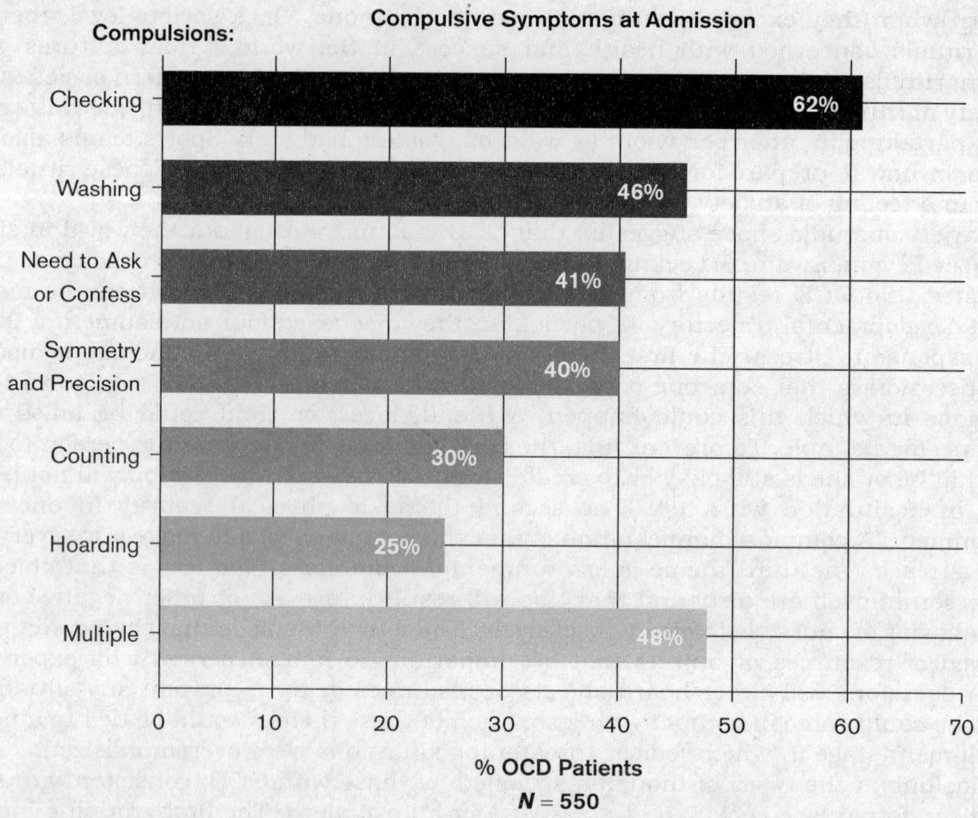

FIGURE 10-6 Compulsions Found in an Initial Evaluation of 555 Patients

Source: Pato, Fanous, Eisen, and Phillips (2008, p. 1445).

and an inability to discard these objects. Cognitive deficits, including difficulties in making decisions about possessions and avoidance of such decisions, are seen in individuals with hoarding disorder. These individuals also show resistance to family members and others who try to intervene in their behavior. Overall, it is suggested that areas of the brain related to executive decision and control, such as the frontal lobes and the ACC, are involved in the disorder.

Brain Processes Associated with Obsessive-Compulsive Disorder

Researchers have asked what the problems of thinking are that are found in those with OCD. Individuals with OCD have problems in shifting from one idea to another. They also have difficulty not thinking about a certain idea. Overall, specific cognitive dysfunction associated with OCD, such as response inhibition, set shifting, working memory, and planning, suggest involvement of the dorsolateral prefrontal cortex (DLPFC), insula, the temporal and parietal lobes, and the cerebellum (see Gilbert,

Gilbert, de Almeida, & Szeszko, 2011; Gu, Kang, & Kwon, 2011; Menzies et al., 2008, for overviews). In addition to cognitive dysfunction, motor responses have been related to networks connecting the basal ganglia with the OFC. Individuals with OCD show less volume in the OFC than normal controls. This is also true of the ACC, basal ganglia, and thalamus. Imaging studies suggest overactivation of these circuits in individuals with OCD.

OCD appears to run in families with first-degree relatives of a person with OCD having an eightfold chance of developing OCD themselves. This would lead one to expect the existence of a genetic relationship. However, this has been difficult to demonstrate. Another line of research involves searching for underlying similarities in brain processing that is associated with OCD. In one study, individuals with OCD, their first-degree relatives without OCD, and a matched control group were given a task that required the individual to reverse what was learned previously (Chamberlain et al., 2008). On each side of a screen, the participant was shown a face superimposed on top of a building. One of the images was considered the target. The faces and buildings were different, and the person had to guess which image was considered correct. After each guess, feedback was given as to whether the person was correct or not. Thus, after a few trials the person could learn the "correct" image. Once an individual was correct on six trials, either the "correct" image was changed or a new set of images was presented. Either way, new learning was required. Using brain imaging techniques (fMRI), it was shown that individuals with OCD and their unaffected relatives had similar patterns of brain activation as compared with controls. In particular, controls showed greater brain activation in the OFC than the OCD individuals and their relatives. Other studies have shown this area of the frontal cortex to be related to reversal learning and flexibility.

Using fMRI techniques, David Tolin and his colleagues (2012) compared individuals with hoarding disorder, individuals with OCD, and healthy controls. These individuals were requested to bring 50 unsorted items, such as junk mail and newspapers, to the scanner. The researchers also had a second set of similar items that did not belong to the participants. When the individuals were at the scanner, they performed a practice trial in which they were asked to determine whether the item shown to them should be discarded or not. If they said discard, they saw it placed in a shredder. During the actual scanning section, the participants were shown pictures of either the items they brought or those from the researchers. They were allowed 6 seconds to make a decision. If no decision was made, the next item was shown.

The behavioral data showed that those with hoarding disorder discarded fewer of their own items (29) versus the healthy controls (40) and those with OCD (37). All three groups were equally willing to discard items from the researchers (over 40). There were also differences in self-reported anxiety rating between those with hoarding disorder (35), OCD (20), and healthy controls (10). The individuals with hoarding behavior also reported "not feeling right" during the task. In terms of brain imaging, differences were found in the ACC, which is involved in error detection, and the insula, which reflects internal processes including a sense of self and self-feeling. When dealing with items that belonged to the researchers, there was less activity in these two areas. However, when deciding about their own possessions, they showed greater activity than the other groups. It may be that this overactivity reflects an experience that things are not right, and they may make a mistake that, in turn, interferes with the cognitive task of making a decision.

Indian Studies on Obsessive-Compulsive Disorder

As far back as 1988, studies on OCD emerged from the National Institute of Mental health and Neurosciences, Bangalore, an institute of national importance. These studies focused on the phenomenology of OCD and attempted to categorize obsessions into six categories of form and twelve categories of content, and compulsions into four categories of form and eight categories of content. Four reliable clusters were derived using variables present in 10–90% of the subjects—washing, checking, thoughts of past, and embarrassing behavior. Some studies have also reported more sot neurological signs among OCD patients as compared to age matched neurotypical people. NIMHANS has an active OCD clinic with close to a hundred publications that have emerged from their work (http://www.ocdclinic-nimhans.com/publications.html). Studies of neuropsychological functions in OCD have documented deficits in several cognitive domains, particularly with regard to visuo-spatial abilities, executive functioning, motor speed, and memory. Agarwal et al. (2013) report deficient activation of bilateral anterior prefrontal, dorsolateral prefrontal, orbitofrontal, anterior cingulate, insular and parietal cortices, precuneus, and caudate areas in persons with OCD. A study by Kashyap, Kumar, Kandavel, and Reddy (2013) reports deficits in scanning, planning time, concept formation, decision making, and encoding of non-verbal memory in persons suffering from OCD, after controlling for the effects of age, gender, and education. The authors opine that this profile is suggestive of a predominantly executive dysfunction, with difficulties in strategizing and organizing stimuli and cognitive resources for maximum efficiency. Interestingly, these findings implicate dorsolateral prefrontal, superior medial prefrontal, and anterior cingulate cortices. Thus, perhaps OCD may not prove to be a purely orbitofronto-striatal disorder as was previously conceptualized.

Concept Check

- What are obsessions? What are compulsions? What is their relationship in OCD?
- How is hoarding different from OCD in terms of both observable behaviors and brain processing?
- If a friend or family member asked you for a recommendation of the best treatment for OCD, what would you include in your answer?

Treatment of Obsessive-Compulsive Disorder

Both psychopharmacological and behavioral therapies have been shown to be effective for OCD. The most common medications are SSRIs and the tricyclic antidepressant clomipramine. These have been shown to be effective for about 60% of people with the disorder.

The psychosocial treatment that has the best empirical support is exposure and response prevention (EX/RP), which is largely based on the work of Foa and Kozak (1986; see also Franklin & Foa, 2008, 2011, for overviews). One component includes discussions with the client concerning beliefs related to the outcome of feared behaviors. For example, the client may think that he or she would get germs from being in public bathrooms. Discussions can also be focused on what the person needs to do to prevent the expected negative outcome. Another component of this approach includes prolonged exposure to obsessional cues. For example, if the person finds it distressing to go into public restrooms, then he or she would be exposed to that actual situation. By prolonged exposure, rituals can be blocked. In addition to the actual situation, imagery can be used to repeat the situation without the ritual until the anxiety is lessened. Thus, the initial inability to conduct rituals produces distress. The basic idea, according to Foa and Kozak, is that repeated, prolonged exposure to feared thoughts and situations will provide information to the person concerning his or her mistaken beliefs and in turn allow for habituation.

In February 2009, the U.S. Food and Drug Administration (FDA) approved the use of a device for deep brain stimulation to treat OCD. As with deep brain stimulation for severe depression, an electrode is implanted in the brain along with a generator and battery placed under the person's skin. Currently, there are a number of clinical trials examining this treatment.

SUMMARY

The experience of anxiety in itself is part of the human situation. However, when this experience becomes chronic, creates distress, and interferes with our life, we see it as an anxiety disorder. Anxiety is to be afraid of what might happen. With anxiety, there is often no stimulus in front of us—the stimulus is in our mind. However, our cognitive and emotional consideration of a negative possibility does not make it any less real. Our body, mind, and emotions experience our ideas as real possibilities. In anxiety, we increase the probability in our mind that an event will happen. Some of these reactions appear to be built into our system. We know that fear and anxiety involve high-level as well as more primitive brain processes. From an evolutionary perspective, to be fearful in the presence of dangerous situations would be adaptive. And, in fact, it appears that fear can be learned through observation only to evolutionarily important objects. In our evolutionary history, it has been suggested that fear mechanisms evolved to aid our ability to disengage from the task at hand to pay attention to threats or potential danger. One model suggests that anxiety can be produced by expectations that either negative events will happen or that positive events will not happen. Individuals with anxiety are even more sensitive than others to the possibility of potential threat. This sensitivity is referred to as cognitive bias. Although fear and anxiety are often studied together, research suggests that different brain areas are involved. Specifically, those areas involved in anxiety are not those directly responsible for the expression of fear but for the regulation of the fear system. Research suggests that anxiety should be seen as a developmental problem involving both environmental and genetic factors. The development of anxiety and fear follows a trajectory that is part of the human condition. Children and adolescents show similar profiles of anxiety and fear across cultures although cultures that favor inhibition, compliance, and obedience also show increased levels of fear.

In *DSM–5,* GAD is characterized by excessive anxiety and worry that leads to one or more of the following: (1) avoiding activities that can have negative outcomes, (2) overpreparation for activities that can have negative outcomes, (3) marked procrastination in behaviors due to worries, and (4) repeatedly seeking reassurance due to worries. GAD, along with depression, is the most frequently diagnosed mental disorder in the United States. Although a consistent physiological picture of worry has yet to appear, research does suggest that worry does produce short-term relief from physiological responses to stress. Both medications and psychological treatments show similar reductions in GAD in the short term. However, only about 40% to 60% of those treated with either medication or psychological treatments show full improvement. SAD is characterized by a persistent and severe fear or anxiety about one or more social situations in which the individual is exposed to possible scrutiny by others. Previous experiences appear to be more important in individuals with SAD as compared with other anxiety disorders. It has been suggested that individuals with SAD process social situations with evolutionarily older alarm systems such as the amygdala whereas non-anxious individuals process the same situation with newer cognitive–analytic processes using the PFC. Both CBT type therapies and medication have been shown to be effective with SAD. Therapies including CBT, exposure therapy, social skills training, and group CBT may also be combined in different ways to provide treatment.

Human infants, as well as the infants of most other mammal species, show distress when separated from their caregivers. However, when this persists and negatively impacts daily activities, individuals would be diagnosed with separation anxiety disorder. *DSM–5* describes eight different categories of symptoms, of which three must be present for an individual diagnosis of the disorder. Separation anxiety disorder is the most prevalent anxiety disorder for those under 12 years of age and is more commonly seen in girls than boys. Agoraphobia is the condition in which a person experiences fear or anxiety when in public. With *DSM–5,* agoraphobia is considered a separate disorder although it may occur with any other disorder, especially the anxiety disorders. Both CBT approaches and antidepressants are effective in treating agoraphobia. A specific phobia is the condition in which an individual experiences fear or anxiety to a particular condition or object and the fear or anxiety causes distress and is out of proportion to the actual danger posed by the situation. It is commonly accepted that phobias are best treated by exposure to the feared object. A panic attack comes quickly and carries with it an intense feeling of apprehension, anxiety, or fear and happens without an actual situation that would suggest danger. It is necessary for symptoms to be recurrent and followed by a month of concern or change in lifestyle to be diagnosed with a panic disorder. Although presented as a separate anxiety disorder, panic attacks can occur within the context of any of the other anxiety disorders. On a brain level, it is suggested that panic and anxiety reflect different brain and hormonal processes. The currently preferred medication treatments for panic disorder are SSRIs. The best studied psychological treatment for panic disorder is CBT, which has been shown to be effective. Combining CBT and antidepressant medication is more effective than either one alone.

In OCD, a distinction is made between obsessions and compulsions: (1) obsessions are generally unwelcome thoughts that come into one's head and (2) compulsions are the behaviors one uses to respond to these thoughts. Research suggests that OCD results from the exaggeration of normal traits that can be mapped onto a developmental trajectory. In looking at the types of thoughts specified by those with OCD, consistent groupings have been found that are related to different comorbid disorders. Hoarding is considered as a separate disorder in *DSM–5* and is defined in terms of an excessive acquisition of objects and an inability to discard these objects. Specific cognitive dysfunction associated with OCD includes response inhibition, set shifting, working memory, and planning that suggest involvement of the DLPFC, the insula, the temporal and parietal lobes, and the cerebellum. OCD appears to run in families; however, the existence of a genetic relationship has been difficult to demonstrate. Both psychopharmacological and behavioral therapies have been shown to be effective for OCD. The most common medications are SSRIs and the tricyclic antidepressant clomipramine. The psychosocial treatment that has the best empirical support is EX/RP.

STUDY RESOURCES

Review Questions

1. How are anxiety and fear related? When is our experience of anxiety and fear a normal part of the human condition? What turns it into a psychopathology?
2. How are GAD and worry related?
3. In what ways are agoraphobia, specific phobias, and panic disorder similar in terms of their causes, symptoms, treatment, and prevalence? How are they different?
4. How would you show graphically the relationships in OCD among stressors, developmental stages, symptoms, and comorbid disorders?

For Further Reading

Barlow, D. (2004). *Anxiety and its disorders* (2nd ed.). New York: Guilford Press.

Craske, M. (1999). *Anxiety disorders: Psychological approaches to theory and treatment.* Boulder, CO: Westview Press.

Hazlett-Stevens, H. (2005). *Women who worry too much: How to stop worry and anxiety from ruining relationships, work, and fun.* Oakland, CA: New Harbinger Publications.

Key Terms and Concepts

agoraphobia
cognitive avoidance model
cognitive bias
compulsions
gamma-aminobutyric acid (GABA)
generalized anxiety disorder (GAD)
hoarding
obsessions
obsessive-compulsive disorder (OCD)
panic attack
separation anxiety disorder
social anxiety disorder (SAD)
specific phobia
Stroop test

CHAPTER

11

Dissociative Disorders and Somatic Symptom Disorders

CHAPTER OUTLINE

- DISSOCIATIVE DISORDERS 383
- SOMATIC SYMPTOM AND RELATED DISORDERS 393
- SUMMARY 404
- STUDY RESOURCES 405

Describing her experience when the Federal Building in Oklahoma City was blown up by a bomb in 1995, a 28-year-old woman said the following:

I felt that what was happening around me was like a scene from a war movie. I was observing it, but I wasn't participating in it. It all seemed so strange and unreal. I saw my burns and the blood pouring out from a deep gash on my arm, but I didn't feel any pain. I was numb, and everything around me was a blur—the noise, the screaming, the smoke. My thoughts started moving a mile a minute, thoughts like where was the nearest exit, how could I get there, how much time did I have before the whole building collapsed. I felt myself moving automatically, almost like a robot walking through a fog, and the next thing I knew, I was outside.

Most of us have had the experience of sitting in a lecture and realizing that we have not been listening for a period of time. Most of us also have had the experience of driving down a highway and all of a sudden realizing that 30 minutes had passed with no awareness of what we had been doing. Sometimes while watching a movie, people become so absorbed in the film that they forget they are in a theater. These are common experiences of **dissociation,** or "spacing out," shared by most people. Overall, this is the situation in which there is a disruption in our normal ability to integrate information from our sensory and psychological processes such as memory and awareness.

Many researchers see dissociation as a normal experience. In times of stress, it is a mechanism that protects the individual and allows her to survive (see Steinberg & Schnall, 2000, for an overview). The example previously presented of the woman who was working when a bomb went off at the Federal Building in Oklahoma is one such example.

In one study using a community sample of 1,055 individuals from Winnipeg, Canada, it was suggested that over 25% of the individuals reported dissociative experiences, and some 5% showed symptoms consistent with a clinical diagnosis (Ross, Joshi, & Currie, 1990). Overall, Ross and colleagues concluded that dissociative experiences are common in the general population; do not differ in terms of socioeconomic status, gender, education, or religion of the respondent; and are reported less by older respondents.

Pathological dissociative symptoms are generally experienced as involuntary disruption of the normal integration of consciousness, memory, identity, or perception. These can range from not having a sense of who one is or not remembering large parts of one's past to having no memory of one's personal history or to experiencing a lack of a developmental self. *DSM–5* describes four dissociative disorders. These are depersonalization–derealization disorder, **dissociative amnesia, dissociative identity disorder (DID),** and dissociative disorder not elsewhere classified. *DSM–5* combines **depersonalization** and **derealization,** which *DSM–IV* did not.

DISSOCIATIVE DISORDERS

> ***DSM–5* Dissociative Disorders**
>
> Depersonalization-Derealization Disorder
> Dissociative Amnesia
> Dissociative Identity Disorder
> Dissociative Disorder Not Elsewhere Classified

Historically, the term *dissociation* (*désaggregation* in French) was introduced by Janet in 1889 to describe symptoms such as repetitive behaviors triggered by distressful memory, presentation of different incongruous personality characteristics (e.g., shy, flirtatious) after a triggering event, and limb paralysis under hypnosis. Janet saw these as representing amnesic processes (memory loss from shock or trauma) where patients "forgot" the ability to receive external stimulation, their own personality, and the ability to move limbs. The common thread in these experiences according to Janet was a traumatic event. That is, a traumatic event or talk of a traumatic event preceded the dissociative experiences. For Janet, dissociation resulted from a weak ego that could not tolerate the overwhelming trauma. Freud, on the other hand, saw dissociation resulting from a strong ego that sought to wall off the experience of trauma as something separate and not part of the self.

Another study examined 658 individuals in a longitudinal community sample in upstate New York (Johnson, Cohen, Kasen, & Brook, 2006). Individuals were assessed for dissociative disorders at age 33. In this nonclinical sample, 9.1% of the individuals had a dissociative disorder. As can be seen in *Figure 11-1*, depersonalization disorder was seen in less than 1% of the sample, dissociative amnesia in less than 2%, and dissociative

Dissociative disorder	Prevalence of disorder in the past year[b] Males ($N = 309$) n (%)	Females ($N = 349$) n (%)	Total sample ($N = 658$) n (%)
Depersonalization disorder[a]	2 (0.6)	3 (0.9)	5 (0.8)
Dissociative amnesia	3 (1.0)	9 (2.6)	12 (1.8)
Dissociative identity disorder (DID)	5 (1.6)	5 (1.4)	10 (1.5)
Dissociative disorder not otherwise specified (DDNOS)	21 (6.8)	15 (4.3)	36 (5.5)
Any dissociative disorder	30 (9.7)	30 (8.6)	60 (9.1)

FIGURE 11-1 Prevalence of Dissociative Disorders at Mean Age

Source: Johnson et al. (2006, p. 135), with permission from Elsevier.

[a]One individual met the diagnostic criteria for both depersonalization disorder and dissociative amnesia. Two individuals met the criteria for both depersonalization disorder and DID.

[b]The differences in the prevalence of dissociative disorders among males females were not statistically significant.

identify disorder in 1.5%. This study did not find gender differences. However, other studies have found that females seek help for dissociative disorders more than males. Further, Johnson and his colleagues found that dissociative disorders co-occur with anxiety, mood, and personality disorders among the adults in this New York sample.

In order to better understand dissociative experiences as seen in normal populations, Lukens and Ray (1995) interviewed college students who scored high on a common measure of dissociation. These young adults reported a variety of dissociative experiences. Three of these are presented here:

- One person reported that she would walk through town and the next moment she would "wake up" standing in line at a store's cash register with unfamiliar store items in her hands. She also reported feeling embarrassed at having no explanation for her actions.
- Another individual reported, "While I was sitting in my room, I zoned out, and then as a third person or camera, I watched myself, my body, leave the room to visit a friend. I then returned to my room whereupon I snapped out of it. An hour had passed."
- Another person said, "I have episodes where I see everything differently, everything starts blending . . . things look more fluid. I snap out of it on purpose because it is a disturbing experience. I can't tell what is real and what is not."

Dissociative experiences can last for a few minutes or hours but reoccur. They can also last for a longer period of time. Some of these experiences are severe and represent significant disruptions in the organization of identity, memory, perception, or consciousness (see Maldonado & Spiegel, 2008; Spiegel et al., 2013, for overviews). More pathological symptoms of dissociation are often connected with trauma and experiences greatly beyond the individual's control such as torture (Ray et al., 2006). In this study, all of the individuals who had been tortured showed signs of post-traumatic stress disorder (PTSD) but varied in terms of their level of dissociation. This suggests that dissociation is a separate process from PTSD. Additionally, the number of dissociative experiences in these individuals directly and positively correlated with magnetoencephalography (MEG) activity in the left frontal cortex and negatively correlated with MEG activity in the right frontal cortex. This suggests that brain changes associated with not experiencing the overwhelming nature of torture become permanent and result in a disruption of networks involved in integrating emotional experience with the language features and executive control associated with the left hemisphere.

Verbatim histories and family reports were the basic methodologies used to study dissociation early on. At the beginning of the 1900s, a number of dissociation studies were published in the United States in the *Journal of Abnormal Psychology*. These case histories led to the view that dissociation was the narrowing of the field of one's consciousness. Trauma was seen as critical and the cause of dissociation since one's mind could not integrate traumatic experiences and memories of trauma in a coherent manner.

Dissociation and hypnosis have been connected in a variety of theoretical discussions of the underlying processes since at least the 1880s. However, in a nonclinical population of more than 800 individuals, the relationship between hypnosis and dissociation has been shown to be orthogonal (Faith & Ray, 1994). That is to say, the two factors are not correlated with one another. Although dissociation and the hypnotic experience both represent an incomplete integration of sensory and other experiences, they are brought forth in different ways. Dissociation happens to a person without voluntary awareness whereas one allows oneself to enter a hypnotic trance.

Depersonalization–Derealization Disorder

Depersonalization is the experience of not experiencing the reality of one's self. This experience can include feeling detached or observing one's self as if you were an outside observer. Derealization, on the other hand, is the experience that the external world is not solid. One's world is experienced with a sense of detachment or as if in a fog or a dream, or in other ways distorted or unreal. It is estimated that at least 50% of all adults in the United States have experienced depersonalization–derealization symptoms sometime in their life (American Psychiatric Association [APA], 2013). However, the lifetime prevalence for the disorder is around 2%. There are no gender differences with this disorder.

In order to better understand depersonalization, 30 individuals with the disorder were interviewed (Simeon et al., 1997). These individuals ranged in age from 18 to 56 years. The age at onset of the disorder was on average during adolescence with no one having an onset after age 25. The mean duration of the illness was 15.7 years. Half of the individuals reported a sudden onset of the experience of depersonalization whereas the other half reported a gradual onset over weeks to months. In comparison with a healthy control group, these individuals reported more traumatization. Also, comorbid mood, anxiety, and personality disorders were common among those with depersonalization disorder. The following case studies are based on this research.

Depersonalization and derealization are seen as normal responses to many types of acute stress. However, when they cause distress or impairment in important areas of

TWO CASE STUDIES
Depersonalization

The first case study describes a 43-year-old woman who was living with her mother and worked at a clerical job. She reports a trauma history of her mother fondling her and frequently giving her enemas until the time she was 10 years old. From the earliest times, this person reported having depersonalization experiences. She explains them this way: "It is as if the real me is taken out and put on a shelf or stored somewhere inside of me. Whatever makes me me is not there. It is like an opaque curtain . . . like going through the motions and having to exert discipline to keep the unit together." Each year, she experiences several such depersonalization experiences.

The second case study is that of a 37-year-old married professional man who had suffered from depersonalization disorder. He described his life as a child as one with little human contact. His parents gave him food and clothing but rarely touched or kissed him. His parents also rarely showed emotions. At the age of 10, he was playing football when he was tackled by another boy. As he was tackled, he felt his body disappear. Initially, similar experiences of depersonalization would happen from time to time. By age 14, he described a more continuous experience. He described it as "not being in this world . . . I am disconnected from my body. It is as if my body is not there."

Based on Daphne Simeon, Shira Gross, Orna Guralnik, Dan Stein, James Schmeidler, and Eric Hollander. (1997). Feeling unreal: 30 cases of DSM-III-R depersonalization disorder. *American Journal of Psychiatry, 154,* 1107–1113.

one's life, they qualify as a *DSM* disorder. Depersonalization refers to experience of unreality, detachment, or feeling as if one is an outside observer of one's own experiences. Derealization, on the other hand, refers to experiences of detachment in relation to one's environment. Immediately following an automobile accident, for example, many individuals report feeling as if the world and what is occurring is not real. Unlike psychotic experiences, reality testing is still available to individuals experiencing depersonalization and derealization.

Some researchers have even suggested that these experiences are a hardwired inhibitory response to acute stress that increases survival by reducing arousal and anxiety (Sierra, 2008). One study examined skin conductance response, which is a direct measure of autonomic nervous system activity to unpleasant, pleasant, and neutral stimuli (Sierra et al., 2002). These researchers compared individuals with depersonalization disorder, anxiety disorders, and healthy controls. As seen in *Figure 11-2,* individuals with depersonalization disorder showed reduced autonomic responses to unpleasant stimuli in comparison with the other groups. This suggests that individuals with depersonalization disorder show inhibitory responses to negative emotional information. The factors that allow these responses to stress to move to a pathological state are still being determined.

Brain imaging studies with depersonalization disorder have been limited. One of the first studies used positron emission testing (PET) measures to compare individuals with depersonalization disorder and a matched set of controls (Simeon et al., 2000; see *Figure 11-3*). Overall, these researchers reported differences in terms of lower metabolic activity in sensory areas as well as brain areas responsible for integrated body schema for individuals with depersonalization disorder.

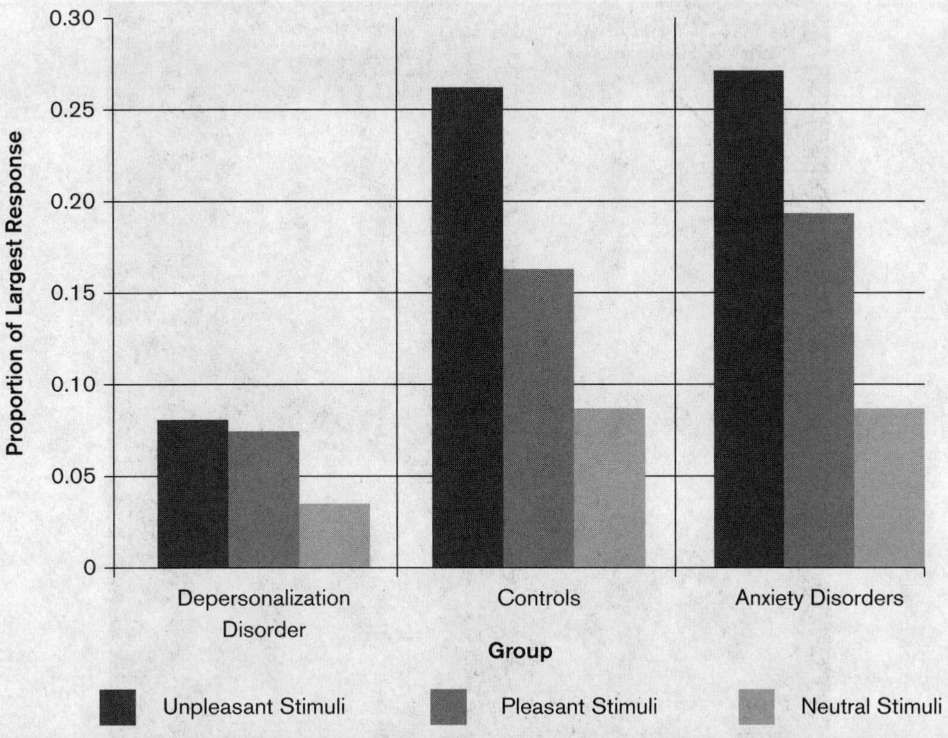

FIGURE 11-2 Skin Conductance Response Magnitude to Stimuli Groups. Because the Range of Skin Conductance Response Amplitudes Can Vary Across Participants, Responses Are Standardized as Range-Corrected Scores (for Each Participant, Skin Conductance Response Magnitudes Were Computed as a Proportion of That Participant's Largest Response).

Source: Sierra et al. (2002, p. 835).

Dissociative Amnesia

The main diagnostic element of dissociative amnesia is an inability to recall important autobiographical information. In *DSM–5,* dissociative amnesia and **dissociative fugue** fall under the diagnosis of dissociative amnesia. Dissociative fugue is a sudden, unexpected travel away from one's home or place of work with an inability to recall one's past. Memory loss in terms of dissociative amnesia appears to be of a particular first-person nature rather than a global memory disorder. In fact, interacting with these individuals would seem like nothing out of the ordinary until they are asked about personal history. At that point, they are unable to remember any of their historical experiences. It should be noted that procedural memory, for example, is not lost nor is the ability to create new long-term memories. Dissociative amnesia may last for a few days to years. Unlike the other dissociative disorders, dissociative amnesia occurs most often when someone is in his 30s or 40s. Twelve-month prevalence is estimated to be about 1.8% with a 2.6 to 1 female to male ratio (APA, 2013).

In the psychological literature, fugue has been discussed for at least the past 100 years. William James described the case of Reverend Ansel Bourne, who reported leaving

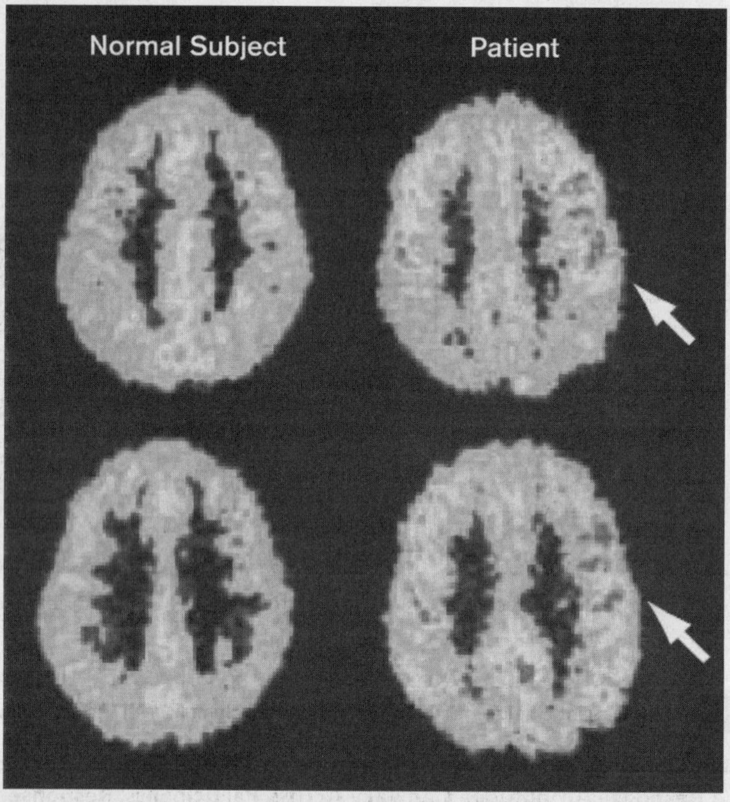

FIGURE 11-3 PET Images of the Brains of a Healthy Comparison Subject and a Patient With Depersonalization Disorder at Two Consecutive Levels in the Parietal Lobe[a]

Source: From Simeon, Guralnik, Hazlett et al. "Feeling Unreal: A PET Study of Depersonalization Disorder." *American Journal of Psychiatry*. 2000;157:1782–1788. Reprinted with permission from the American Journal of Psychiatry, (Copyright ©2000). American Psychiatric Association.

[a] Higher relative metabolic activity (region/whole brain) in the patient with depersonalization disorder occurred in the parietal association areas in more dorsal (Brodmann's area 7B) and ventral (Brodmann's area 39) regions.

his home and adopting a new identity after he had become amnesic for his previous life. However, most individuals with dissociative amnesia do not show the adoption of a new identity but just the forgetting of their past. During World War II and other states of conflict, fugue states were frequently documented. Cases of dissociative amnesia continue to be seen and are often reported in the newspapers as medical staff seek to obtain information about the person. The following case study took place in 2013.

Unless a mental health or medical professional suspects that dissociation is involved, documentation that would lead to a diagnosis of dissociative amnesia is often lacking. For example, dissociation information is rarely asked for even in those who would be at risk for dissociative processes, such as adolescent runways from abusive homes or the homeless.

CASE OF MICHAEL BOATWRIGHT
Dissociative Amnesia

Michael Boatwright was taken to the emergency room of the Desert Regional Medical Center in Palm Springs, California. He had been found unconscious in his motel room. When he awoke in the hospital, he said his name was Johan Ek and he only spoke Swedish. He had with him five tennis rackets, two cell phones, a duffel bag filled with casual athletic clothes, some money, photos, and identification cards. Each of the cards—including a passport, a VA card, and a social security card—said he was Michael Boatwright. When asked by a translator about the identification cards, the man reported that he was Johan and did not know Michael. The hospital determined it would be unsafe to release this person without any memory who only spoke Swedish. He remained in a nursing facility for a few weeks to evaluate his condition. He had nightmares almost every night. During this time hospital personnel sought to determine his past through his ID cards. They discovered that he recently flew in from China where he had taught English and was a graphic designer for the previous 4 years. Before that, he had worked in Japan for 10 years. The hospital staff also found that he did live in Sweden when he was younger. Through contacts in these countries, they were able to obtain some pictures of him with others. He reported that although he did not recognize the pictures, they give him a sense of comfort and security. The hospital staff also sought to determine if he showed any signs of faking, which he did not. He was diagnosed with dissociative amnesia.

Based on Pelham, V. (2013, July 7). Michael Boatwright awakes in Palm Springs with apparent amnesia. The Desert Sun. Retrieved from www.mydesert.com/article/20130706/LIFESTYLES03/307060025/Michael-Boatwright-awakes-Palm-Springs-apparent-amnesia?nclick_check=1

Dissociative Identity Disorder

DID has received considerable attention from the media and popular press. Previously referred to as *multiple personality disorder*, there is a large amount of misinformation concerning its existence. Most popular press or movie versions of DID are not true to life. Current views suggest it is less multiple personalities than it is a developmental disorder where one consistent sense of self does not occur—that is, the person does not experience her thoughts, feelings, or actions in terms of a well-developed "I" or sense of self. Rather, the person experiences different "personalities" at different times. DID is seen as a complex disorder related to the experience of trauma occurring before the age of 5 or 6. This is the time at which a sense of self is in development.

Epidemiological studies suggest the prevalence to be between 1% and 3% with slightly more males than females showing the disorder (see Vermetten, Schmahl, Lindner, Loewenstein, & Bremner, 2006, for an overview). Although the prevalence is similar in males and females, the manner of presentation is different (APA, 2013). Females with DID are more likely to be seen in adult clinical settings. Males, on the other hand, tend to deny their symptoms and trauma history. However, the symptoms can be seen following combat conditions or acts of physical or sexual assault. Cultural differences are also seen. In developing countries or rural communities, the fragmented identities can become part

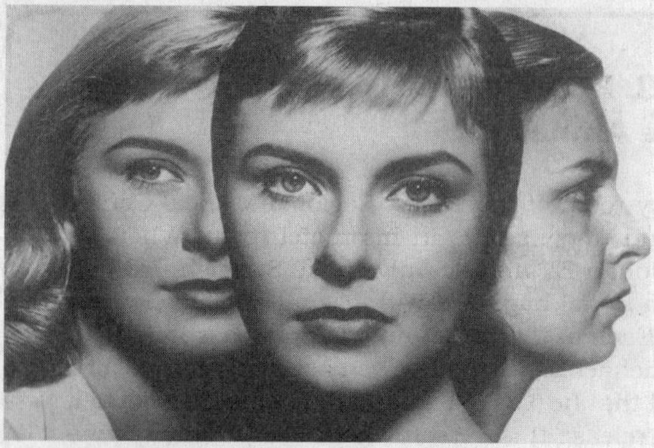

The 1957 film *three faces of eve* brought the existence of dissociative identify disorder to the public consciousness

© Moviestore collection Ltd / Alamy

of religious or other experiences. For example, possessions by gods or spirits are seen in a number of cultures.

Marlene Steinberg developed a screening device for dissociative disorders, the *Structured Clinical Interview for DSM–IV Dissociative Disorders* ***(SCID-D)*** (Steinberg, 1994). She described DID as the situation in which a person shifts between distinct personality states that take control of his behavior and thoughts (Steinberg & Schnall, 2000). These alter personalities, or *alters,* are clearly defined, and each may have its own name, memories, traits, and behavioral patterns. However, it is possible for one alter not to know of the existence or experiences of another. At times, the "host" personality may experience the alters as arguing with one another. One of her patients described one such situation:

> "I was about to walk into a meeting that I needed to attend, and the only chair that was available was between two men. I didn't turn around and walk out, but my body turned around and walked out. And I couldn't talk to save my soul because there was this battle going on about whether or not I should go into the meeting, and someone wanting some memory to come up and someone else suppressing it. I tried to walk into that meeting, but I couldn't do it."
>
> Brief excerpt from pp. 109 from *The Stranger in the Mirror* by Marlene Steinberg and Maxine Schnall. Copyright © 2000 by Marlene Schnall, M.D. Reprinted by permission of HarperCollins Publishers.

At other times, an alter may take control of the host without the host's awareness of the situation. This amnesia may lead to the person being told by others of events, conversations, or agreements that took place out of awareness. Likewise, the person may find notes or items that he or she did not remember writing or buying. This can lead to difficulties with friends and employers.

Historically, DID was described in terms of possession in which an individual loses his or her identity to become another person. Possession by outside forces was a common understanding of DID. Descriptions seen as early as 1787 referred to an "umgetauschte Personlichkeit," or exchanged personality. Likewise, Benjamin Rush described such patients in the early 1800s followed by Charcot, Janet, and Morton Prince in the early 1900s. However, Bleuler included DID under the rubric of schizophrenia with the resultant disuse of the DID diagnosis during the middle of the last century.

Gleaves, May, & Cardeña (2001) reviewed a variety of studies that examined DID populations and their core features. As seen in *Table 11-1*, amnesia was reported in almost 100% of all individuals studied. Further, previous child abuse was present on average in over 90% of the individuals with DID.

Neuroscience research related to DID has been limited compared with other disorders. In one study, the volume of the hippocampus and amygdala was studied using

TABLE 11-1 Frequency of Core Features of Dissociative Identity Disorder From Large-Scale Investigations

Core Feature	*PutnAm et al., 1986 (n = 100)*	*Coons et al., 1988 (n = 50)*	*Ross et al., 1989 (n = 236)*	*Ross et al., 1990a,b (n = 102)*	*Boon & Draijer, 1993a,b (n = 71)*
Amnesia	98.0	100.0	94.9	100.0	99.0
Identity alteration	–	–		81.4	100.1
Depersonalization	55.0	38.0	–	–	100.0
Derealization	–	–	–	56.9	73.1
Auditory hallucinations	29.0	72.0	71.7	82.4	94.0
Childhood abuse	97.0	96.0	88.5	95.1	94.4

Source: Gleaves et al. (2001, p. 579), with permission from Elsevier.
Note: All values are percentages of persons reportedly experiencing the symptom.

magnetic resonance imaging (MRI) (Vermetten et al., 2006; see *Figure 11-4*). Those with DID had hippocampal volume that was 19.2% smaller and amygdala volume that was 31.6% smaller compared with a healthy control group. Less volume of the hippocampus and amygdala has also been reported in stress-related disorders, including PTSD (see *Table 11-2*).

Relative Paucity of Work in India, Yet Plethora of Cultural Factors

As mentioned previously and much like the world over, there is not a great deal of research work done in India on dissociative disorders. Some estimates place the occurrence of these disorders at around 0.15/1000 patients per year. Some interesting cultural manifestations of dissociation, however, are tied to various religious and festive occasions in India, a large patchwork quilt if customs, beliefs and rituals. A common manifestation is the

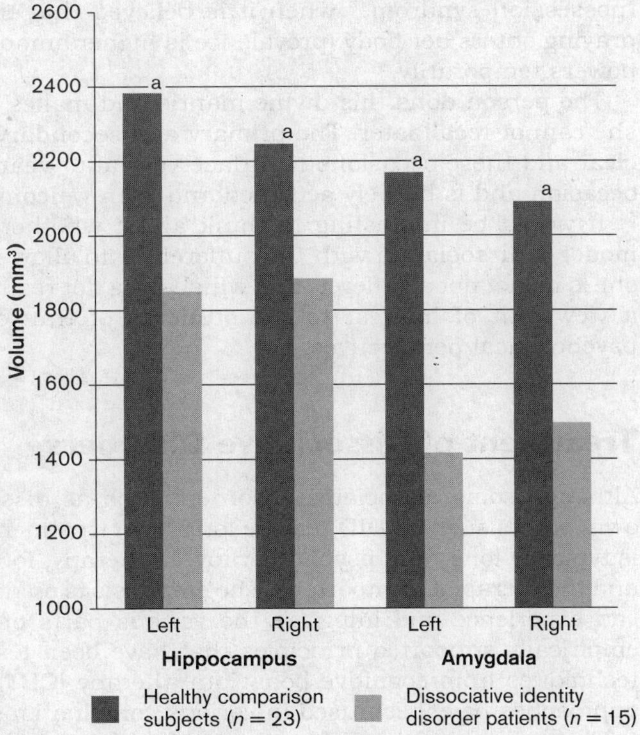

FIGURE 11-4 Significant Difference Between Groups

Source: Vermetten et al. (2006, p. 633).
[a]Significant difference between groups ($p < 0.05$, t test for nonpaired samples).

TABLE 11-2 Dissociative Identity Disorder

A. Disruption of identity characterized by two or more distinct personality states, which may be described in some cultures as an experience of possession. This disruption in identity involves marked discontinuity in sense of self and sense of agency, accompanied by related alterations in affect, behavior, consciousness, memory, perception, cognition, and/or sensory-motor functioning. These signs and symptoms may be observed by others or reported by the individual.

B. Recurrent gaps in the recall of everyday events, important personal information, and/or traumatic events that are inconsistent with ordinary forgetting.

C. The symptoms cause clinically significant distress or impairment in social, occupational, or other important areas of functioning.

D. The disturbance is not a normal part of a broadly accepted cultural or religious practice. Note: In children, the symptoms are not better explained by imaginary playmates or other fantasy play.

E. The symptoms are not attributable to the physiological effects of a substance (e.g., blackouts or chaotic behavior during alcohol intoxication) or another medical condition (e.g., complex partial seizures).

Source: Reprinted with permission from the *Diagnostic and Statistical Manual of Mental Disorders, Fifth Edition*, (Copyright 2013). American Psychiatric Association.

"possession syndrome" when it is believed that the deity to whom the pious has been praying enters her body (prevalence is higher among women) and endows her with special powers temporarily.

The person dons this divine mantle and makes pronouncements and predictions that she cannot recall later. The primary and secondary gain involved in the process is amply clear and these occasions resurface year after year with every recurrence of the religious occasion and is blithely accepted and even welcomed by the patient the world around.

It would be interesting to think about whether it is healthier to share the scientific model of dissociation with the sufferer, or to allow her the moment in the limelight where she is in fact not a sufferer, and which does not really hamper social emotional functioning, a viewpoint of interest to the students of transcultural psychiatry and multicultural psychological perspectives.

Treatment of Dissociative Disorders

Although some dissociative disorders such as dissociative amnesia may resolve on their own, others such as DID require long-term treatment. The basic procedure for treating DID is typically long-term psychotherapy. In therapy, focus on a relationship between the client and the therapist is important. The emphasis is on developing a safe place where individuals can experience and integrate the various parts of themselves. At present, there are no empirically supported principles that have been tested in terms of dissociation. However, techniques from cognitive behavioral therapy (CBT), humanistic-existential, and dynamic approaches have been used in various combinations (see Ross, 1997).

The common theme seen in all of the dissociative disorders is a loss of the normal integration of cognitive functioning. This includes the person's sense of self, autobiographical memory, sense of control and agency, and an integrated awareness of functioning. Historically, dissociative disorders have been a way to avoid the distress of trauma and other psychologically changing events. In the next section of this chapter, I focus on those disorders that focus on a person's reaction to bodily symptoms referred to as somatic symptom disorders.

> **Concept Check**
>
> - In what ways are dissociative disorders similar to the types of dissociative experiences common to most people? In what ways are they different?
> - What can we say about when and how the following dissociative disorders occur and their prevalence in the general population:
>   - Depersonalization–derealization?
>   - Dissociative amnesia?
>   - DID?
> - What is currently available for the assessment and treatment of individuals with dissociative disorders?

Most of us experience some sort of somatic, or bodily, symptom regularly. We may feel tired, feel a pain in our leg, or have a stomachache. In fact, it is estimated that 60% to 80% of the general population experiences some sort of somatic symptom in a given week (Kellner, 1985). The most common symptoms include chest pain, headache, fatigue, and dizziness. Most of us consider these experiences as part of life and assume they will go away. If they don't or if the symptoms concern us, we may go see our physician. He may do an examination, run some tests, or do other procedures. The physician may diagnose a possible cause or say that he can find nothing wrong. If he says that nothing is wrong, most of us will feel relieved.

Some people, however, do not feel relieved. They may continue to search for organic problems by going to other physicians or request more tests be done. They are certain something is wrong with them. Others may feel anxiety that the simple symptoms they have are really something serious, perhaps cancer or the beginning of a heart attack. These are two aspects of what are referred to as **somatic symptom and related disorders.** Another aspect is the situation in which a person shows the signs of a disorder but the disorder does not follow what we know to be the underlying physiology. These disorders were previously referred to as *hysteria* and are now called **conversion disorders.**

Before *DSM–5,* these disorders were referred to as *somatoform disorders*. Somatoform was a confusing term to many clinicians and researchers. For some, there was confusion with psychosomatic illness or somatization. A *psychosomatic disorder* is an actual physical illness in which psychological factors play an important role. *Somatoform* was also a difficult term to translate into different languages, and this made cross-cultural studies difficult. Because of these and other reasons, the specific diagnosis of somatoform disorder was changed to somatic symptoms and related disorders in *DSM–5. DSM–5* also removed the category of pain disorder.

SOMATIC SYMPTOM AND RELATED DISORDERS

> ***DSM–5* Somatic Symptom and Related Disorders**
>
> Somatic Symptom Disorder
> Illness Anxiety Disorder
> Conversion Disorder (Functional Neurological Symptom Disorder)
> Psychological Factors Affecting Medical Condition
> Factitious Disorder
> Somatic Symptom Disorder Not Elsewhere Classified

Somatic symptom disorders represent an interface between psychological processes and medical ones. Individuals with these disorders do not seek mental health professionals. Thus, it is one set of disorders in which the professional doing the diagnosis, typically a physician, is a person who does not specialize in the treatment of mental disorders. This will influence the estimates of the prevalence of these disorders since few physicians will use this diagnosis. For example, if one went to an emergency room, the physician would perform an examination and then release the person if she found no physical problems. She would not make a diagnosis since she did not see a physical disorder. It is only when the person's behavior is seen in a larger context—such as going to a series of different physicians—that the possibility of somatic symptom disorders becomes apparent.

Physicians in emergency rooms will also describe cases in which individuals fake medical disorders for other types of gain. In some cases, they may be trying to avoid going to work or do other activities that they do not want to do. This is referred to as *malingering.* Some individuals may actually take substances to create a disorder. This is referred to as a **factitious disorder.**

Somatic Symptom Disorder

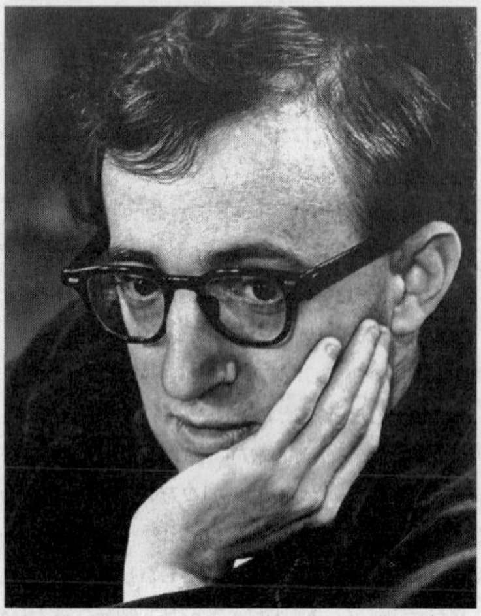

Woody Allen in his movies often plays the role of someone who Is overconcerned about his health

Somatic symptom disorder is the condition in which a person's somatic or bodily symptoms cause distress or disruption in physical health that is not consistent with a medical disorder. For a diagnosis of the disorder, the person must do one of the following: have persistent thoughts about the seriousness of her symptoms, have a high level of anxiety about her health or symptoms, or spend excessive time and energy on her health. Further, these characteristics must have lasted for longer than 6 months.

These individuals may go from physician to physician or emergency room to emergency room seeking to be told that they have a medical disorder. They are not satisfied when the professional cannot find the cause of their symptoms. This leads to inconsistent statistics concerning the disorder and a lack of research compared with other disorders. One estimate suggests the prevalence of somatic symptom disorder is around 5% to 7% (APA, 2013). Since females seek medical advice more often than males and are more willing to report symptoms, a gender difference would be expected.

Indian Studies on Somatic Symptom Disorder

It is interesting to note that the Indian cases of dissociation mentioned previously are also often conceptualized as functional somatic symptoms and a manifestation of "hysterical neurosis." Even in studies involving children and adolescents, somatoform and dissociative disorders are closely linked.

Kallivayalil and Punnoose (2010), in a paper, suggest that much of Indian understanding finds it difficult to accept a body–mind duality. They thus urge that giving an explanatory model for the patient for the symptoms is very important. Thus,

> A model which focuses on dysfunctional neurotransmission and brain circuits which are influenced by external stressors and internal conflicts leading on to symptoms may be appropriate... Abnormal signal transmission and processing in the nervous system may also be brought in as legitimate explanations for these conditions. When pharmacological agents are prescribed, they should be explained as agents to correct these irregularities and not as tranquillizers. (Kallivayalil & Punnoose, 2010)

The paper uses the acronym FuSS for functional somatic patients.

Illness Anxiety Disorder

Illness anxiety disorder is when a person is preoccupied with the possibility of having a serious illness. However, unlike somatic symptom disorders, the person experiences few, if any, symptoms. This disorder was previously referred to as *hypochondriasis* but was renamed in *DSM–5.* In illness anxiety disorder, the anxiety is focused on health issues; the person may become alarmed at any suggestion or thought that he may have a health problem. For example, the person might read an article about symptoms of cancer or have a sensation in his body and decide that he has cancer. In addition to anxiety, behavioral components such as checking one's body for changes may be present. Although it would be reasonable to be concerned if a particular disorder was part of one's family history, illness anxiety disorder takes this to the extreme. Generally, reassurance from the health care worker will not reduce the anxiety. Paradoxically, some individuals with this disorder actually avoid seeing a health professional since this would increase their anxiety, fearing that the doctor might confirm a serious condition.

In many ways, it is not the symptom itself but the person's reaction to the symptom that is the critical feature of illness anxiety disorder. *DSM–5* makes a distinction between those whose major concern is the symptoms versus those whose concern is the possibility of having a disorder. Those whose concern is with the symptom itself would be diagnosed with somatic symptom disorder. Those whose concern is with the possibility of developing a particular disorder would be diagnosed with illness anxiety disorder.

As you think about illness anxiety disorder, you might wonder if it is just an anxiety disorder with a different focus: the body. A number of studies have suggested that individuals with illness anxiety disorder are different than those with other disorders in the manner in which they conceptualize bodily processes. For example, in one study, those with illness anxiety disorder reported that they believed bodily complaints are always a sign of disease, which was not the case of those with other disorders such as depression (Rief, Hiller, & Margraf, 1998). Individuals with illness anxiety disorder, in comparison with those with anxiety disorders and healthy controls, were shown to have a different concept of what good health means (Weck, Neng, Richtberg, & Stangier, 2012). Those with illness anxiety disorder were shown to have a more restrictive concept in that they saw bodily symptoms as incompatible with good health. This was not true of those with anxiety disorders. Further, if asked to compare symptoms in other people or themselves, those with illness anxiety disorder saw symptoms in themselves as more severe than those in others. Other studies have shown that those with illness anxiety disorder can be distinguished from those with panic disorder (Hiller, Leibbrand, Rief, & Fichter, 2005).

Conversion Disorder

Conversion disorder refers to what historically has been called hysteria. This is the situation in which a person reports sensory or motor symptoms such as not being able to hear or see or feel pain or move a part of the body. However, the symptoms do not follow known physiological or neurological patterns. **Glove anesthesia,** for example, refers to the phenomenon when a person says, "I cannot feel anything in my hand." The pattern of insensitivity is that of a glove. However, the touch receptors in our hand do not follow this pattern. The ulnar nerve is involved in sensitivity beginning in the ring finger and little finger and continuing up the wrist. The area of sensitivity is shown in *Figure 11-5*. The radial nerve is involved with sensitivity on the other side of the hand. Thus, if there was damage to the nerves, we would see a very different pattern of insensitivity.

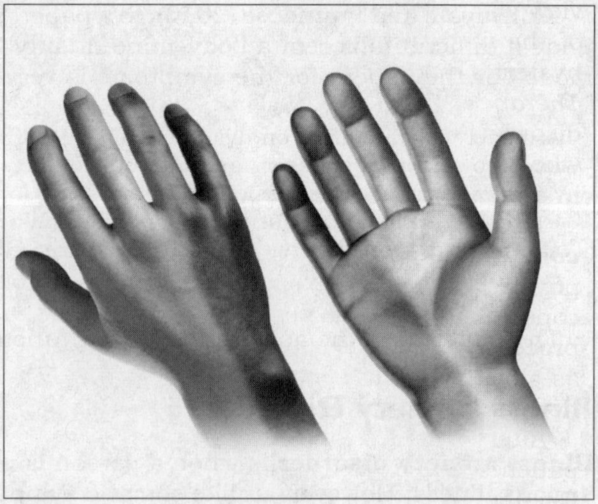

FIGURE 11-5 Figure Region of Skin Innervation of the Ulnar Nerve

Source: From Tandon et al. (2009, p. 8).

In comparison to malingering and factitious disorder in which a person voluntarily creates the symptoms, conversion disorder is seen to take place in an involuntary manner outside of the person's consciousness. Common symptoms include paralysis, seizures, tremor, blindness, anesthesia, and problems with movement. In the clinical literature, conversion disorders show a high comorbidity with anxiety, depression, and personality disorders. In some cases, the conversion symptoms develop after an emotional stress or trauma. Some individuals show what is referred to as *la belle indifférence* (the beautiful indifference) and seem unconcerned about their symptoms.

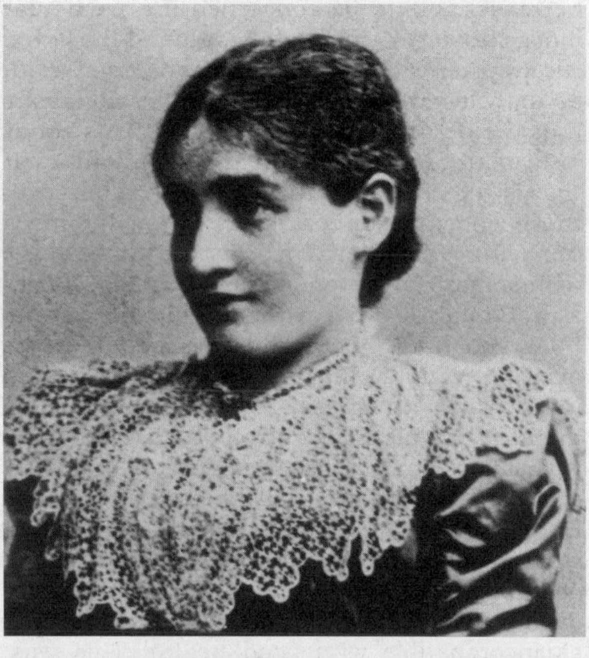

Bertha Pappenheim (Anna O.)

A form of conversion disorder has been recorded for at least 2,000 years as one seen in women. The unfounded view was that the disorder resulted from movement of the uterus. The medical literature of the fifth century CE took the Greek word for uterus and described the disorder as hysteria. In 1859 in France, Paul Briquet wrote a landmark monograph, *Traité Clinique et Thérapeutique de L'hystérie,* which influenced the conceptualization of conversion disorder until the present day. He used the term *hysteria* in describing a series of patients who showed medical symptoms without a known cause. They described their symptoms in a dramatic and excessive manner.

These were the type of patients that Freud did his early work with. In fact, the term ***conversion reaction*** refers to Freud's idea that psychic energy was converted into physical symptoms. The basic concept is that painful memories or trauma are not consciously experienced in an emotional manner but rather converted into physical processes. Freud learned from Charcot that individuals with a conversion disorder, such as glove anesthesia, would under hypnosis be able to recall painful memories and have normal feeling in their hands.

After Freud left Paris, he went to Vienna and worked with Josef Breuer. One of Breuer's patients was referred to as Anna O, who we now know was Bertha Pappenheim (see Ellenberger, 1970; Sulloway, 1979, for overviews). At the age of 21, Bertha Pappenheim developed a variety of medical symptoms. During this time, her father became ill and eventually died. Prior to this time, she had led the life of a young woman raised in a wealthy family. Breuer described her as attractive, intelligent, and with much imagination. Freud described her in terms of her treatment with Breuer as a woman "whose numerous hysterical symptoms disappeared one by one, as Breuer was able to make her evoke the specific circumstances that had led to their appearance" (Ellenberger, 1970, p. 480). Many historians see this case as one that led Freud to view treatments for conversion disorder to include a reintroduction of the original trauma.

Today, the term *conversion disorder* is used in *DSM–5* without reference to psychoanalytic theory. *DSM–5* also refers to conversion disorder as **functional neurological symptom disorder** since this is a common term in neurology. In the medical literature conversion reactions are also called **psychogenic disorders or functional disorders.** There has been a resurgence of interest in conversion disorders with recent conferences and books (see Hallett, Lang, Jankovic, Fahn, Halligan, Voon, & Cloninger, 2011, for an overview). One focus has been psychogenic movement disorders and psychogenic seizures.

The specific neuroscience mechanisms that underlie conversion disorder are still to be fully understood. Pavlov (1941) suggested that an overexcitation of the subcortical centers due to strong emotions could in turn produce cortical inhibition. This inhibition of the frontal lobes could affect sensory and motor areas and functionally turn them off. These basic ideas continue in current hypotheses, which suggest that activation of motor pathways might be suppressed by inhibitory processes related to emotional experiences. Others have suggested that rather than inhibitory cognitive processes, conversion symptoms are related to midline brain regions associated with representations of the self and emotional regulation (see Cojan, Waber, Carruzzo, & Vuilleumier, 2009; Nowak & Fink, 2009, for overviews). Beginning in the late 1990s, brain imaging studies began to examine individuals with various types of conversion reaction. Let's look at three of these studies.

Ghaffar, Staines, and Feinstein (2006) examined three individuals with conversion disorder using functional magnetic resonance imaging (fMRI). The first person was a 34-year-old woman with an 8-month history of numbness and tingling on her left side—mainly her left hand. The second person was a 44-year-old woman with left-sided numbness, most prominently in her foot. This had existed for 9 years. The third person was a 35-year-old woman who had a left-sided numbness on her foot. When the normal limb was stimulated, as expected you would see brain activity on the contralateral side of the brain in the sensory area related to that limb. When the limb that was experienced as numb was stimulated, there was no brain activity. However, if both sides were stimulated, then brain activity was seen on both sides of the brain (see *Figure 11-6*). The exact mechanism that makes this happen is not fully understood.

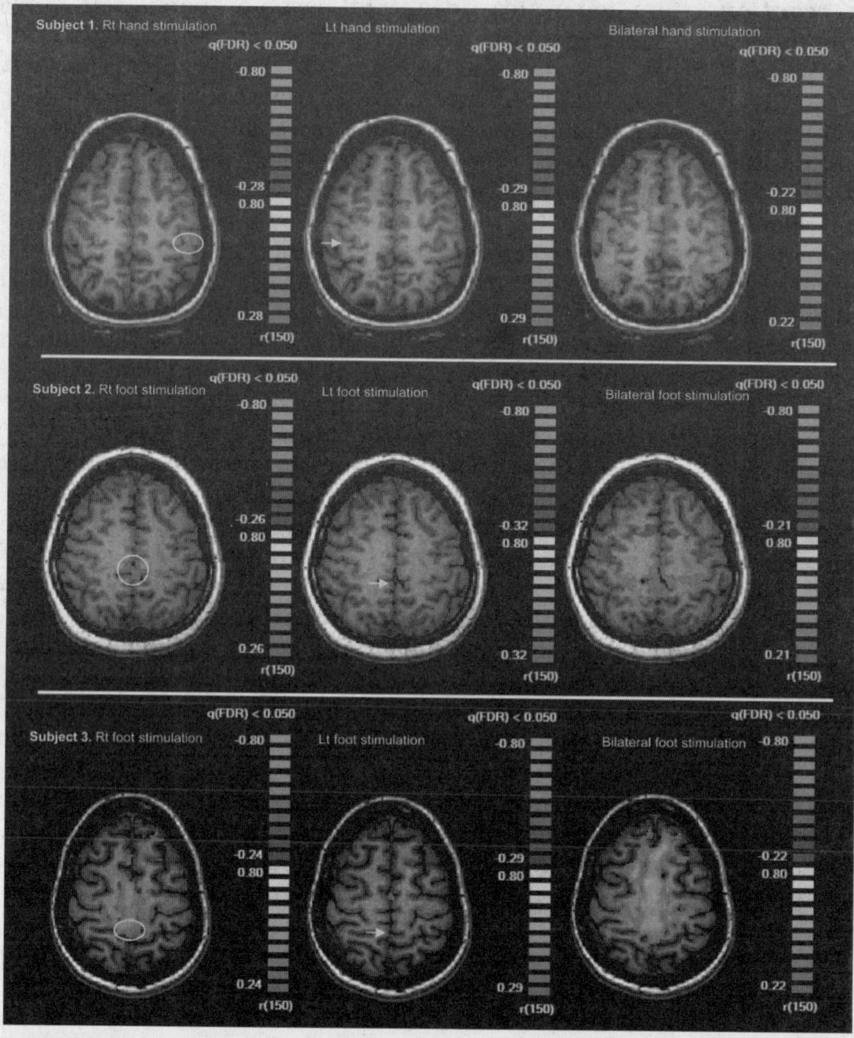

FIGURE 11-6 Unexplained Neurologic Symptoms

Source: From Omar Ghaffar et al. "Unexplained neurologic symptoms: An fMRI study of sensory conversion disorder." *Neurology Online*. http://www.neurology.org/content/67/11/2036.short © 2012 American Academy of Neurology.

Note: Left panel: As expected, stimulation of the limb in which stimulation is felt is shown on the contralateral side. Middle panel: No stimulation influences the brain response on the side of the conversion reaction. Right panel: When both sides were stimulated, the brain showed as if both were normal.

Mirror neurons in our brain are active when we observe movement in others—that is, if we watch someone move her left hand then we see activity in the parts of our brain as if we made the same movement. Markus Burgmer and his colleagues (2006) wondered if they would see mirror neuron activity in a functional motor paralysis. In order to answer this question, they performed brain imaging on seven healthy individuals and four individuals with a functional paralysis. These results are shown in *Figure 11-7*. The top

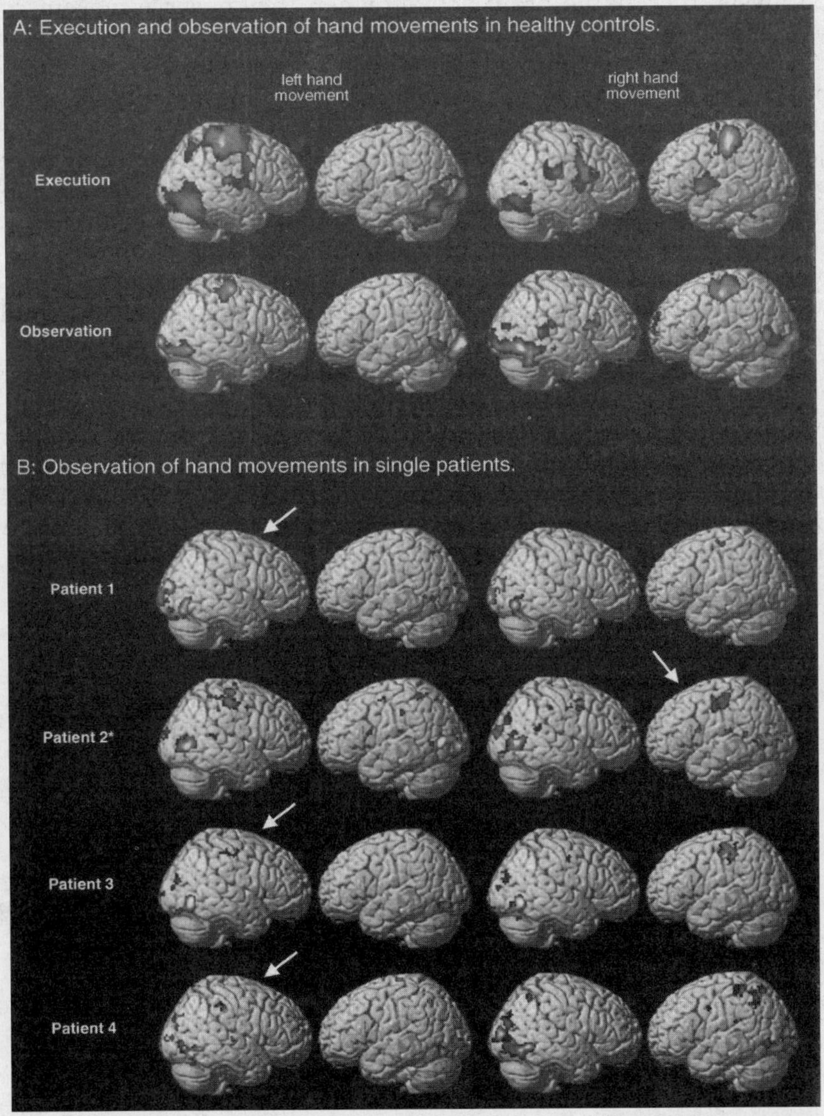

FIGURE 11-7 Top Two Rows Show Brain Activation for Healthy Controls While They Move or Watch Movement

Source: Burgmer et al. (2006), with permission from Elsevier.

Note: The bottom four rows show the observation of movement for each of the four patients. The arrow represents where activation was expected. Patient 2 showed paralysis on the right side rather than the left.

two rows show brain activation for healthy controls while they move or watch movement. As expected, moving the left hand shows greater activation in the right motor strip. Right-hand movement shows greater activation in the left motor area. Also, making a movement results in greater activation than just watching the movement. The bottom four rows show the observation of movement for each of the four patients. The arrows in the figure represent where activation was expected. Patient 2 showed paralysis on the right side whereas the other three patients showed it on the left. As you can see, in individuals with functional paralysis, there is no brain activity when they observe movement on the side of their paralysis. However, brain activity was seen in healthy controls while they observed movement. This suggests that individuals with a conversion disorder do not create an internal representation or motor map while watching movement, as is the case with healthy controls.

Yann Cojan and his colleagues (2009) used a go-nogo task to study a person with a single-sided conversion paralysis in comparison with healthy controls. In the brain scanner, she was given a cue to prepare to make a movement. This was followed by a gray image of a hand that conveyed to her which of her hands she was to move. The hand either became a green hand, which meant she was to make a movement (go), or a red hand, which meant she was not to make a movement (nogo). The ratio of green to red hands was 3 to 1 (see *Figure 11-8*).

The fMRI data showed that the patient's right motor cortex was suppressed when she was instructed to make a movement. However, it did show activation when she saw the gray hand and prepared to make a movement. This suggests that the functional paralysis did not influence motor preparation in the brain but only the actual movement. When examining the difference between preparation of left-hand movement and right-hand movement in this patient, these researchers discovered different areas of the brain being activated in the patient as compared with the healthy controls. In the preparatory

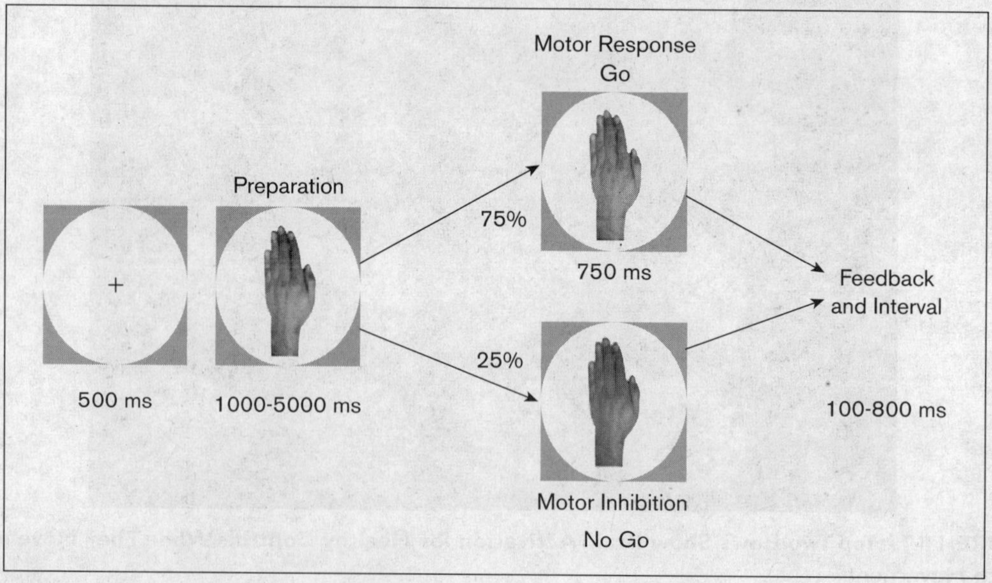

FIGURE 11-8 Illustration of the Paradigm

Source: Cojan et al. (2009, p. 1028), with permission from Elsevier.

movement stage, the patient showed increases in the left orbitofrontal cortex (OFC), the ventromedial prefrontal cortex (vmPFC), and the posterior cingulate cortex. These are areas involved in the default network and suggest that conversion disorder may include an inability to turn off the default network and remain in a more internally focused state. This fMRI activity was not seen in the healthy controls.

Overall, the brain imaging data suggest individuals with conversion disorder show differences in their cortical networks from healthy controls. As you can see from the three fMRI studies, there is a clear difference when the person is asked to make a response. However, the mechanisms that create these differences are still to be discovered. In the following LENS, the manner in which our brains give us our sense of our bodies is explored.

11-1 LENS
Awareness of the Body and the Brain

Tom was driving home from soccer practice when a car crossed over into his lane. The car went out of control, and he was thrown out of the car. He looked up to see that his hand was still in the car. Tom lost his left arm, but strangely, he could still feel it as if it were there. He had the sense of moving each finger and being able to grab an object. Tom is not alone in his sensation of a lost limb. This phenomenon has been reported since antiquity, and following the U.S. Civil War, it came to be known as "phantom limb." Not only do individuals with a lost limb experience its presence, but over 70% of them also experience pain in the limb, which can last for years after the amputation.

An intriguing way to treat the pain, which may involve the mirror neuron system, is referred to as a mirror box. It is literally a box with a mirror that divides it in half. On each side of the mirror is a hole in the box such that a person could put a hand in each side. A person who had lost their left arm could put their right arm through the hole. Looking at the right hand and arm, the person would see both it and its reflection, creating the illusion of having two hands. What is amazing is that the person has the sensation of moving not only the right hand but also the left one as well. Not only does the person have the experience of moving the phantom limb, but for some the pain can also be modified.

As scientists have examined phantom limb with neuroscience techniques, it turns out that our sense of our body is all in our heads—just not in the way that most people think. It is not "made up"; it is real. Wilder Penfield in the 1940s and 1950s was able to map how the body is represented in the brain (see *Figure 11-9*). What became clear is that the body is represented on a thin strip in the brain. Some areas such as the hands and lips have more brain areas devoted to them than do other body parts. However, the body's representation is not how it appears in real life. The hands—not the neck—are next to the face in the brain.

Experiences such as learning a new skill can change the connections in the brain. Losing a body part can do the same. If a person lost his middle finger, for example, then the area represented by it in the brain could be taken over by the fingers on each side of it. If the individual loses his arm, then the brain area that represents the arm can be taken over by the face. Now when the person touches his face not only does he experience his face; he also experiences the sensation of the arm being touched. What if someone lost his leg? As Penfield's map suggests, both males and females have reported sensations in their lost leg when they are having sex. This may also help to explain why it is more common to have a foot fetish than a hand fetish.

Based on V. S. Ramachandran and Sandra Blakeslee. (1998). *Phantoms in the brain.* New York: William Morrow and Company.

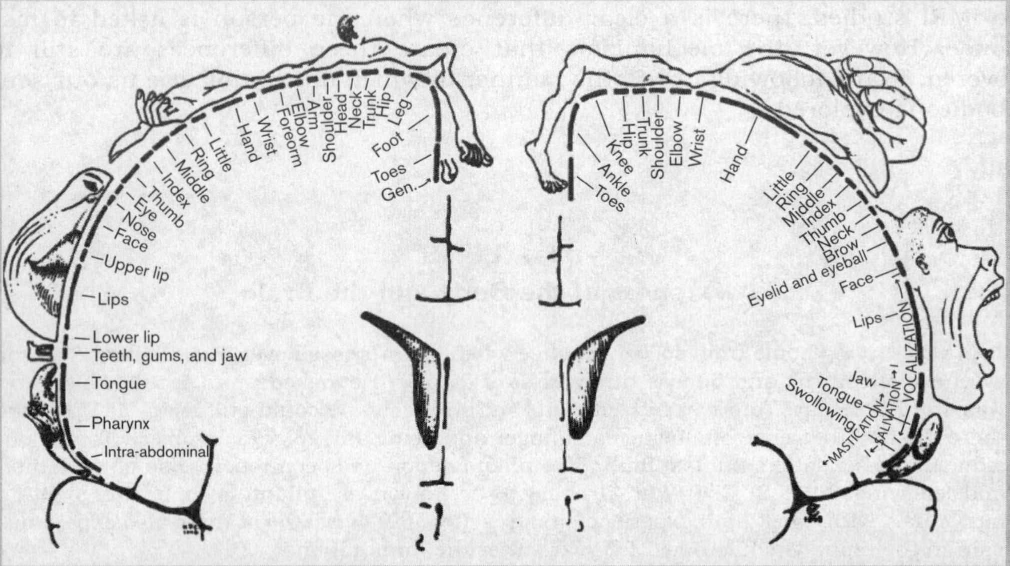

FIGURE 11-9 Penfield's Homunculus Showing the Representation of the Body in the Brain

Source: From The cerebral cortex of man by Wilder Penfield and Theodore Rasmussen. Copyright 1950 Macmillan Publishing Company; copyright renewed 1978 Theodore Rasmussen.

Factitious Disorder

Medical records describe a man who went to the emergency room with a history of fever and bilateral pain (Turner & Reid, 2002). He had a tender abdomen, and blood tests and images were taken. While waiting for the test results, a nurse realized she had seen the man at another hospital. In fact, he had gone to the other hospital three times over 6 months with the same symptoms. At no time was any pathology found. When confronted after a number of these trips to the hospital, the man admitted that he had falsified his condition.

A factitious disorder is the situation in which a person creates the symptoms seen by the health care professional. Such an individual may take laxatives or even inject insulin to mimic an actual physical disorder such as a stomach flu or low blood sugar. Although it seems strange that someone would actually hurt herself or himself for only the gain of receiving medical attention, this is indeed the case. The person with a factitious disorder will attempt to manipulate the health care system by seeking extra medical tests or even medical procedures such as surgery. It can be initially difficult to determine when the person has medical training, since he or she can describe accurately and produce known symptoms. When the person does not receive the attention she or he seeks, he or she may become angry and claim mistreatment. There is some suggestion that it is seen more often in women than men.

DSM–5 makes a distinction between **factitious disorder imposed on self** and **factitious disorder imposed on another.** In a factitious disorder imposed on another, typically a caregiver such as a parent would produce symptoms in her child. She then seeks medical attention and procedures for the child. She may even be seen as a devoted parent who cares for her child whereas she is actually the one causing the symptoms. Historically, those with a factitious disorder imposed on self have also been referred to in terms of *Munchausen syndrome*. The disorder is named after a German baron who liked to embellish his stories of military adventures and came to be known as the "Baron of Lying." Those who produce the symptoms in another have been referred to as *Munchausen syndrome by proxy*. Munchausen by proxy is seen almost exclusively in women (Sheridan, 2003).

Concept Check

- What is the difference between a somatic symptom disorder and a psychosomatic disorder? How are they the same?
- What are the primary diagnostic criteria for each of the following somatic symptom and related disorders:
    - Somatic symptom disorder?
    - Illness anxiety disorder?
    - Conversion disorder?
    - Factitious disorder?
- What are important implications for the diagnosis and treatment of somatic symptom disorders due to the fact that many individuals seek help from medical professionals instead of mental health professionals?

One classic case study describes more than 400 pages of medical records in which a child beginning at age 2 was brought to the hospital for treatment of conditions brought on by the mother (Bryk & Siegel, 1997). As a 2-year-old girl, the patient was initially brought to the hospital for a trivial injury to the right ankle, which had not healed. It was reported that the infant had fallen down the stairs. What was not known by the medical professional at the time was that the injury was that the mother had inflicted repeated blows to the foot with a hammer. Over the next 8 years, the patient experienced 28 hospitalizations, 24 surgeries, and a number of other medical procedures related to swelling and bone problems as well as high temperature. Not only did the mother cause the damage; she also added soil or coffee grounds to infected wounds to prevent healing. What complicated the situation even more was that the mother was a nurse. Thus, hospital personnel assumed she was giving correct care to her own daughter.

In the period of more than half a century since this case occurred, medical personnel have been better trained to determine potential child abuse and look for alternative explanations for continuing unexplained medical conditions. However, short-term cases of factitious disorder imposed on another continue to be seen. Some examples include altering a child's diet to produce medical conditions and use of fecal or other material to induce infections or describing symptoms of the child only seen by the mother.

Factitious disorder should be differentiated from malingering in that malingering involves deceiving to obtain external rewards such as not going to work, obtaining financial compensation through an insurance claim, receiving paid sick leave, or avoiding undesired activities. Also, some individuals fake symptoms as a means of obtaining drugs that they can use or sell.

Treatment of Somatic Symptom Disorders

Since individuals with somatic symptom disorders are generally seen in a medical setting, the most common approach for treatment is an educational one. With conversion disorder, the health care professional will discuss aspects of the patient's stress and suggest that his or her symptoms will improve. This is consistent with reports that about 50% of these individuals will not have symptoms by time of discharge from a general hospital (Folks, Ford, & Regan, 1984). It is common for individuals with somatic symptom disorder not to seek therapy.

In one review of treatments for somatic symptom disorders, it was noted that three approaches exist (Sumathipala, 2007). These are antidepressant medication, CBT, and other nonspecific interventions. Although there is little empirical research related to the treatment of somatic symptom disorders, CBT shows the best effects for reducing physical symptoms, psychological distress, and disability (see Woolfolk, Allen, & Tiu, 2007, for an overview). CBT treatments for illness anxiety disorder are typically modeled after those for panic disorder and have been shown to be effective (Hollon & Beck, 2013). However, treatment research in this area of somatic symptom disorders overall is somewhat limited.

Overall, somatic symptom disorders (previously referred to as somatoform disorders) represent an interface between psychological and medical processes. Individuals with these disorders do not seek mental health professionals. Thus, it is one set of disorders in which the professional doing the diagnosis, typically a physician, is a person who does not specialize in the treatment of mental disorders. This will influence the estimates of the prevalence of these disorders since few physicians will use this diagnosis. The major somatic symptom disorders described in this section were somatic symptom disorder, illness anxiety disorder, conversion disorder, and factitious disorder.

SUMMARY

Many researchers see dissociation as a normal experience. Dissociative experiences can last for a few minutes or hours but reoccur, but they can also last for a longer period of time. In times of stress, it is a mechanism that protects the individual and allows her to survive. Pathological dissociative symptoms are generally experienced as involuntary disruption of the normal integration of consciousness, memory, identity, or perception. *DSM–5* describes four dissociative disorders: (1) depersonalization–derealization disorder, (2) dissociative amnesia, (3) DID, and (4) dissociative disorder not elsewhere classified. Depersonalization is the experience of not experiencing the reality of one's self; derealization, on the other hand, is the experience that the external world is not solid. The main diagnostic element of dissociative amnesia is an inability to recall important autobiographical information. Dissociative fugue—a sudden, unexpected travel away from one's home or place of work with an inability to recall one's past—also falls under the diagnosis of dissociative amnesia. DID is less a case of multiple personalities than it is a developmental disorder where one consistent sense of self does not occur. Although some dissociative disorders, such as dissociative amnesia, may resolve on their own, others, such as DID, require long-term psychotherapy.

Most of us experience some sort of somatic, or bodily, symptom regularly, consider these experiences as part of life, and assume they will go away. Some people, however, do not feel relieved. They may continue to search for organic problems—certain that something is wrong with them—or may feel anxiety that the simple symptoms they have are really something serious. These are two aspects of somatic symptom and related disorders. Another aspect is the situation in which a person shows the signs of a disorder but the disorder does not follow the underlying physiology. Some individuals may actually take substances to create a disorder. Somatic symptom disorders represent an interface between psychological processes and medical ones in that it is one set of disorders in which the professional doing the diagnosis, typically a physician, does not specialize in the treatment of mental disorders.

Major somatic symptom and related disorders described in *DSM–5* include (1) somatic symptom disorder, (2) illness anxiety disorder, (3) conversion disorder, and (4) factitious disorder. Somatic symptom disorder is the condition in which a person's somatic or bodily symptoms cause distress or disruption in physical health that are not consistent with a medical disorder. Illness anxiety disorder is when a person is preoccupied with the possibility of having a serious illness. However, unlike somatic symptom disorders, the person experiences few, if any, symptoms. Conversion disorder, or functional neurological symptom disorder, refers to the situation in which the person reports sensory or motor symptoms such as not being able to hear or see or feel pain or move a part of the body; however, the symptoms do not follow known physiological or neurological patterns. A factitious disorder is the situation in which a person creates the symptoms seen by the health care professional. *DSM–5* makes a distinction between factitious disorder imposed on self and factitious disorder imposed on another, where a caregiver such as a parent would produce symptoms in her child. Since individuals with somatic symptom disorders are generally seen in a medical setting, the most common approach for treatment is an educational one.

STUDY RESOURCES

Review Questions

1. "In times of stress, dissociation is a mechanism that protects the individual and allows her to survive." Considering all of the dissociative disorders, how do they protect the individual? What are they protecting her from? What are some of the costs of that protection?
2. Most of us have had experiences of dissociation including "spacing out." Does that mean that dissociative disorders are just at the extreme end of normal processes? In what ways are psychopathologies an extension of normal human functioning? In what ways are they categorically different?
3. Somatic symptom disorders represent a set of disorders in which the professional doing the diagnosis, typically a physician, does not specialize in the treatment of mental disorders. As an expert on somatic symptom disorders, you are called on to create a program to educate physicians about the characteristics, diagnosis, and treatment of these disorders. What are the critical areas of information you include in your program?

4. "Somatic symptom disorders represent an interface between psychological processes and medical ones." What evidence can you cite from neuropsychological research that shows disordered brain functioning in individuals with somatic symptom disorder? How might medical professionals use this information in diagnosis and treatment in the future?

For Further Reading

Dell, P., & O'Neil, J. (Eds.). (2009). *Dissociation and the dissociative disorders: DSM–V and beyond.* New York: Taylor & Francis.

Hyman, J. (2007). *I am more than one.* New York: McGraw-Hill.

Walker, M., & Antony-Black, J. (Eds.). (1999). *Hidden selves: An exploration of multiple personality.* Buckingham, UK: Open University Press.

Key Terms and Concepts

conversion disorders
conversion reaction
depersonalization
derealization
dissociation
dissociative amnesia
dissociative fugue
dissociative identity disorder (DID)
factitious disorder
factitious disorder imposed on another
factitious disorder imposed on self
functional neurological symptom disorder
glove anesthesia
illness anxiety disorder
psychogenic disorders or functional disorders
SCID-D
somatic symptom and related disorders

CHAPTER

12

Eating Disorders

CHAPTER OUTLINE

- OVERVIEW: FEEDING DISORDERS, OBESITY, AND EATING DISORDERS 408
- FEEDING DISORDERS 409
- THE PROBLEM OF OBESITY 410
- THE MAJOR EATING DISORDERS 418
- SUMMARY 432
- STUDY RESOURCES 433

It was that simple: One minute I was your average nine-year-old, shorts and a T-shirt and long brown braids, sitting in the yellow kitchen, watching Brady Bunch reruns, munching on a bag of Fritos, scratching the dog with my foot. The next minute I was walking, in a surreal haze I would later compare to the hum induced by speed, out of the kitchen, down the stairs, into the bathroom, shutting the door, putting the toilet seat up, pulling my braids back with one hand, sticking my first two fingers down my throat, and throwing up until I spat blood.

I started losing weight in the spring of my freshman year in college, but in some miracle of denial, I didn't initially see it as a problem. Nor did I see it as intentional; it was merely a side effect of discovering how much I loved being hungry. . . . I didn't even notice I'd lost weight until it was pointed out to me by my roommate's boyfriend. . . . In any case, I continued my new eating habits, which involved fasting until I was light-headed and then rewarding myself with a big meal. In my view, I didn't really eat less than other people, just differently. But I continued to lose weight. . . . By the end of my sophomore year, though, I could no longer convince myself I was okay. The telltale symptom was back: namely, that even when I knew I should eat more, I often couldn't make myself do it.

OVERVIEW: FEEDING DISORDERS, OBESITY, AND EATING DISORDERS

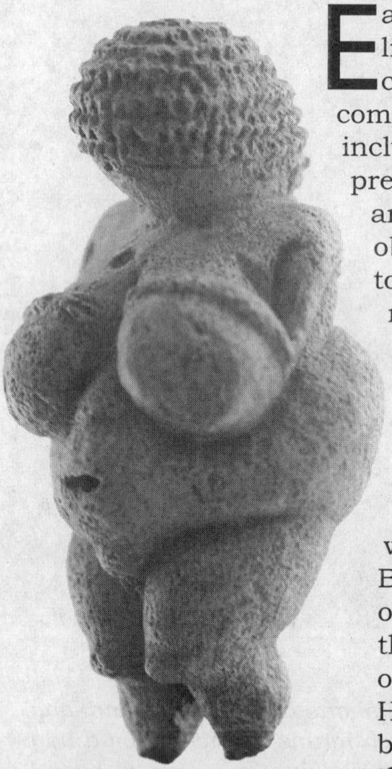

One of the earliest figures of a human was created around 25,000 BCE, referred to as the venus of willendorf

© MatthiasKabel

Eating seems simple. We eat to give ourselves energy and live life. However, as you will see in this chapter, it is extremely complicated. What we eat and how we eat represents a complex relationship between all levels of human functioning including culture, evolutionary history, genetics, our physiology, preferences, and psychological attitudes toward our appearance and that of others. Some people eat substances that have no obvious nutritional value, such as dirt. Some people continue to eat food long after they have consumed sufficient calories necessary for their daily needs. Others starve themselves because they believe they are fat when they are actually extremely underweight.

Although we often suggest that our view of ideal appearance is related to the media and movies, humans have had ideas of ideal appearance for thousands of years. In fact, one of the earliest known human figures is that of an obese woman estimated to be craved from limestone around 25,000 BCE. Besides this figure found in southern Austria, there are other figures of obese females with large breasts found throughout Europe. With recorded history came the possibility of knowing attitudes toward appearance and **obesity.** Both Hippocrates and Galen in ancient Greece saw a connection between being obese and physical disorders and wrote that those who are overweight die early. They also understood how food intake and exercise were related to weight and used exercise and diet as a treatment for being overweight (Christopoulou-Aletra & Papavramidou, 2004). Many of the concerns they had concerning obesity continue to this day.

Although upper-class women in ancient Rome starved themselves to look thin, it was not until the Middle Ages that medical texts began to describe what we now call anorexia. During the period, there were also a number of references to women who starved themselves for religious and other purposes. By the late 1800s, **eating disorders** were considered part of medical diagnosis and treatment. This history will be continued later in the chapter.

In this chapter, I will introduce you to three separate areas related to eating. The first is **feeding disorders,** which includes eating substances that do not have nutritional value. The second topic examines obesity. And the third is a presentation of eating disorders. Unlike the fourth edition of the *Diagnostic and Statistical Manual of Mental Disorders (DSM–IV), DSM–5* combines **feeding and eating disorders** into one category.

FEEDING DISORDERS

Previously, feeding disorders were considered part of a category of disorders usually first diagnosed in infancy, childhood, and adolescence (see Bryant-Waugh, Markham, Kreipe, & Walsh, 2010, for an overview). Even normally developing children show changes in eating patterns and preferences for particular foods. It has been estimated that 25% to 45% of normally developing children and up to 80% of those who are developmentally delayed show such changes.

According to Bryant-Waugh et al. (2010), some of the types of problems seen in clinical settings include the following:

- Delayed or absent development of feeding or eating skills
- Difficulty managing or tolerating fluids or foodstuffs
- Reluctance or refusal to eat based on taste, texture, and other sensory factors
- Lack of appetite or interest in food
- Utilizing feeding behaviors to comfort, self-soothe, or self-stimulate

However, since feeding disorders can be seen in individuals of all ages, it was made part of a larger feeding and eating disorders category in *DSM–5.* The three major feeding disorders are **pica, rumination disorder,** and **avoidant/restrictive food intake disorder** (see *Table 12-1*).

TABLE 12-1 Table of *DSM–5* Feeding Disorders

Pica—Persistent eating of nonnutritive substances
Rumination Disorder—Repeated regurgitation of food
Avoidant/restrictive food intake disorder—Lack of interest in certain food which can lead to weight loss and/or nutritional deficiency

Pica

Pica is a feeding disorder in which the person eats something that would not be considered food. Some common substances include clay, cornstarch, charcoal, paste, newspaper, coffee grounds, paint chips, and blackboard chalk. The process of eating nonnutritive substances has been described historically for more than 2,500 years using various terms (see Young, 2010, 2011, for an overview). The onset of eating nonnutritive substances can begin in childhood, adolescence, or adulthood. Prevalence rates for pica are unknown.

In terms of a disorder, historically, pica has generally been described as part of another disorder such as obsessive-compulsive disorder (OCD) or

Concept Check

- "With recorded history came the possibility of knowing attitudes toward appearance and obesity." What are some historical examples described in this chapter? How are they different from, and similar to, current views?
- What do we know about the prevalence of feeding disorders? What are some of the common examples of feeding disorders seen in clinical settings?
- What is the defining characteristic of each of the following feeding disorders, and what is a negative consequence of each:
  - Pica?
  - Rumination disorder?
  - Avoidant/restrictive food intake disorder?

developmental disorder or the normal condition of being pregnant. In the 1970s, the medical journal *Lancet* suggested that pica is a worldwide practice found more commonly in underdeveloped countries in comparison with developed ones (see Lacey, 1990, for an overview). Additionally, it was seen more often in individuals who were poor compared with those who were well-off, blacks than whites, pregnant than not pregnant, and children than adults. Some researchers have tried to determine if there is any positive value to eating nonnutritive substances (see Stokes, 2006, for an overview). Indeed, there is some suggestion that clay, for example, may bind to trace elements in the stomach and thus help to clean the intestinal tracks.

The nutritional problem with pica is that it leads to health problems, including vitamin deficiency and visits to the emergency room. *DSM–5* restricts the conditions of pica and states that pica should not be part of another disorder, cultural practice, or pregnancy. It also requires that the eating behavior has lasted for longer than a month.

Rumination Disorder

A rumination disorder is the condition in which a person regurgitates his food. This swallowed food is then re-chewed, re-swallowed, or spit out. The choice of what to do with the food is often determined by whether the person is in a social situation or not. To be diagnosed as a rumination disorder, the condition must occur for more than a month and not be part of any of any other medical or eating disorder.

Avoidant/Restrictive Food Intake Disorder

Avoidant/restrictive food intake disorder is, as the name implies, the condition in which an individual does not eat certain foods, which leads to such conditions as weight loss or nutritional deficiency. A person may avoid certain foods because of the sensory characteristics of the food. It could be taste, hardness, color, or any other characteristic. Although most people have foods they like and dislike, their avoidance of certain foods does not lead to significant weight loss or nutritional deficiency. Likewise, if someone has eaten a food that made them sick, they will normally avoid it for at least 2 or 3 years. This is referred to as the Garcia effect or one-trial learning. However, these individuals will eat other foods to obtain the energy and nutrition necessary for a healthy life.

THE PROBLEM OF OBESITY

Everyone has certain foods that they love and foods that they hate. Some of us have comfort foods that give us a good feeling. Some of our food choices are cultural and related to the foods that we grew up with. Some of our choices are genetic, such as the ability to drink milk into adulthood, which was described in Chapter 1. As humans, we have an evolutionary history in which not having enough food was a more frequent event than having too much. One theory referred to as the *thrifty gene hypothesis* suggests that times of scarce food sources helped to shape our genetic makeup (Neel, 1962).

Current conditions of food abundance and lack of exercise do not match our evolutionary history and can lead to obesity. Everywhere you look in a city, there are restaurants, cafes, and food stores. In the United States, bookstores have cafes as do many other shops. Fast-food snacks with high calorie content are everywhere. Most of these fast foods are designed to engage our physiological and psychological mechanisms that compel us to seek food and experience it as rewarding. Just looking at a piece of chocolate cake can lead to our seeking it even when we are not hungry.

Our evolutionary history may have us seeking substances that do not lead to a healthy lifestyle. For example, in our early history thousands of years ago, sugar was not easy to come by. It was only found in foods that were not constantly available, such as fruits. Since sugar gives us a pleasant feeling, we came to seek it. In fact, we consume sugars even when full. One study showed that rodents are more likely to work for sweet rewards, even when not hungry, than to work for cocaine (Lenoir, Serre, Cantin, & Ahmed, 2007). The constant availability of sugars and other such substances today plays a critical role in obesity and some eating disorders although other factors also play a role (Drewnowski, 1997).

Overall, obesity is seen to result from a mismatch between the amount of calories that we eat and the amount of energy that we expend. However, the factors that influence these two variables are complicated. Some of these other factors related to obesity are the environment in which we live, psychological factors, and biological factors (Bouchard, 2010). These factors can influence both the intake of calories and their expenditure through exercise. Environmental factors can include our family and our culture, which influence the foods we cook as well as how much we eat. The environment of our towns and cities can also influence our ability to walk or ride bikes or require us to drive a car. Psychological factors such as self-esteem or need for comfort can also determine how we eat and when we eat. Some people love eating with others and the association of food and friends. Others are always worried about being or becoming fat. Denying certain types of foods as some diets do will actually increase our desire for that food. Biological factors such as genetic makeup have also been shown to be an important factor in terms of the risk to become obese.

Twin studies have shown that a child's weight tends to be more like his or her natural parents, even when they are adopted (see Moustafa & Froguel, 2013, for an overview). It is also the case that genetics can influence the amount and distribution of body fat. This is greatly influenced by environmental factors. In Finnish twins who have low physical activity, the heritability of body fat has been estimated to be 90%. However, if the twins engage in high levels of physical activity, the heritability is reduced to 20%. This suggests that environmental factors such as exercise can influence the manner in which genetic influences are related to body fat. Further, if you overeat for a period of time, you will develop additional fat cells in your body. If you then lose weight, your fat cells can become smaller, but the number will not decrease. This is thought to make losing weight more difficult for someone who was heavier as a child. In summary, the more common form of obesity is the result of the combined effects of multiple genes acting in relation to environmental factors. However, it should be noted that there is a rare form of obesity that results from the action of a single gene.

In terms of the brain, a homeostatic system regulates body weight. Its basic task is to produce energy for the body. This system involves the hypothalamus, which has been seen as important for appetite and weight regulation. Fat is deposited in adipose tissue so that we can store energy that is available during times of famine. When nutrients are easily accessible, humans and other animals tend to overload with nutrients and become obese. Research points to brain processes involving the limbic system that encode the rewarding aspect of food intake along with emotional and cognitive aspects. These brain processes lead to an overconsumption of food even when the person feels full.

Since humans and other animals will continue to eat even when they feel full and do not need additional energy, researchers have asked if similar mechanisms are involved in both obesity and drug addiction (see Volkow, Wang, Tomasi, & Baler, 2013, for an overview). Both drug addiction and obesity involve disruptions in the dopamine pathways of the brain. These pathways modulate behavioral responses to environmental cues. With both food and drugs, psychological processes interact in a complex manner. For example, when we see a food or drug we like, there is memory (hippocampus), emotional reactivity (amygdala), arousal (thalamus), and cognitive control (prefrontal cortex [PFC] and cingulate) as well as autonomic nervous system reactions related to consuming the substance. In the case of food, there are a number of peripheral mechanisms involving such organs as the stomach, pancreas, intestine, and hypothalamus that signal when food is needed. With food our bodies also make a computation in terms of energy needs and the feelings of hunger and satiety. Drugs, on the other hand, mainly influence the reward pathways of the brain (see *Figure 12-1*). I will describe these pathways in greater detail in Chapter 14.

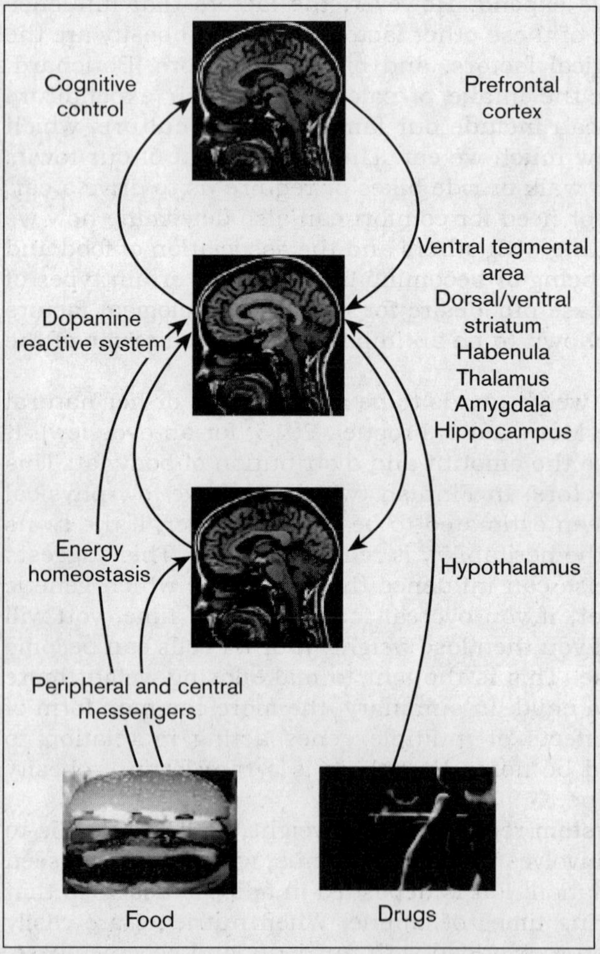

FIGURE 12-1 Figure Showing the Interconnected Systems Involved in the Intake of Food and of Drugs

Source: Volkow et al. (2013, p. 6).

Although our bodies tell us when we are hungry, environmental factors can lead to cravings and obesity. These environmental factors can be how attractive the food is, how expensive it is, what kind of deal we get with super-sizing, and so forth. We also have a memory of eating the food previously and the associations connected with it. In addition, psychological stress increases our consumption of food and thus weight gain. One important new finding is that brain mechanisms related to these systems are changeable even in adulthood (Dietrich & Horvath, 2013). That is, as environmental conditions change, metabolic brain circuits change in relation to eating.

Based on brain imaging studies, obese adolescent girls process the anticipation and consumption of food differently than lean adolescent girls (Stice, Spoor, Bohon, Veldhuizen, & Small, 2008). Individuals who are obese show less activation of reward circuits in the brain when they consume food than lean individuals. However, they show greater activation of somatosensory brain areas when they anticipate consumption. Further, amount of activation was related to body mass index (BMI) in terms of anticipation but inversely related in terms of consumption. Less activation of the dopamine reward circuits in obese individuals may be one mechanism that leads to greater consumption of food.

According to the World Health Organization (WHO), obesity worldwide has doubled since 1980. In 2008, approximately 1.4 billon adults (age 20 and over) were overweight and 200 million men and 300 million women obese (www.who.int/mediacentre/factsheets/fs311/en/index.html). That works out to 30% of the world population being overweight and 11% obese. In 2011, more than 40 million children under the age of 5 were overweight. These overweight children are found not only in high-income countries but also in low- and medium-income countries. As described in the following LENS, many countries around the world are beginning to focus on obesity in the same way they previously focused on tobacco smoking.

12-1 LENS
Reducing Obesity Worldwide

Nations around the world are now examining obesity as a public health problem. The current approach is similar to how tobacco use was previously approached—that is, to consider it as an epidemic with the goal of reducing its use. The developed countries have the best statistics concerning obesity (see *Figure 12-2*). Besides the United States, current

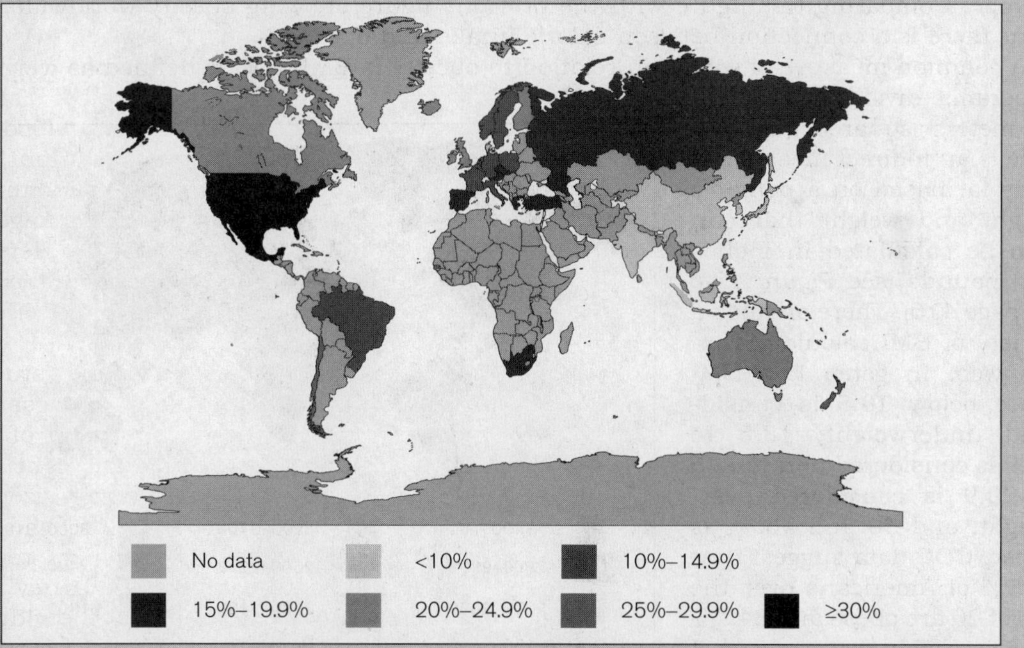

FIGURE 12-2 Worldwide Obesity Rates, 2009

Source: Elder and Arredondo (2013, p. 527), with permission from Elsevier.
Disclaimer: This figure is not to scale. It does not represent any authentic national or international boundaries and is used for illustrative purposes only.

(Continued)

(Continued)

approaches to reducing obesity are also under way in Mexico and South America (Elder & Arredondo, 2013; Holub et al., 2013). Mexico is second only to the United States in terms of an obesity epidemic. In the United States, obesity is present in all ethnic groups but it is higher in adult Latinos (38.7%) compared with white/Anglo (25.6%) individuals. This relationship is also seen in adolescence.

At this point, a number of intervention programs have been implemented and evaluated in terms of outcomes (Holub et al., 2013). School-based programs to increase physical activity have occurred in Mexico, Brazil, and Chile. Other studies in Latin America also were directed at teaching individuals how to eat in a healthy manner. Currently, the best evidence has been with programs that target obese individuals rather than prevention programs.

The Centers for Disease Control and Prevention (CDC) has a number of resources to help individuals eat well (www.cdc.gov/nutrition/everyone/index.html). Likewise, the U.S. Department of Health and Human Services has a series of dietary guidelines for healthy eating (health.gov/dietaryguidelines/). However, Americans consume more calories than do people in many other places in the world. Daily calorie intake for various countries in the world is shown in *Figure 12-3*. As can be seen in this figure, people living in Africa and China consume fewer calories than those in America, Canada, and Western Europe. Comparing this figure with the previous figure showing obesity worldwide, it is clear there is a connection between calorie intake and obesity.

A common measure of weight in relation to obesity is BMI. BMI is defined as weight in kilograms divided by height in meters squared (kg/m^2). This is an indirect measure of body fat based on a person's height and weight that can also be calculated in inches and pounds (see *Figure 12-6* on page 416). There are also a variety of BMI calculators on the web. In general, a BMI score below 18.5 is considered underweight; 18.5 to 24.9 is considered normal; 25 to 29.9 is considered overweight; and 30 and above is obese. CDC data suggest that 33.9% of Americans over the age of 20 are obese and 34.4% are overweight (www.cdc.gov/nchs/fastats/overwt.htm). There is a difference in these statistics by states in the United States. All states show an increase in obesity over

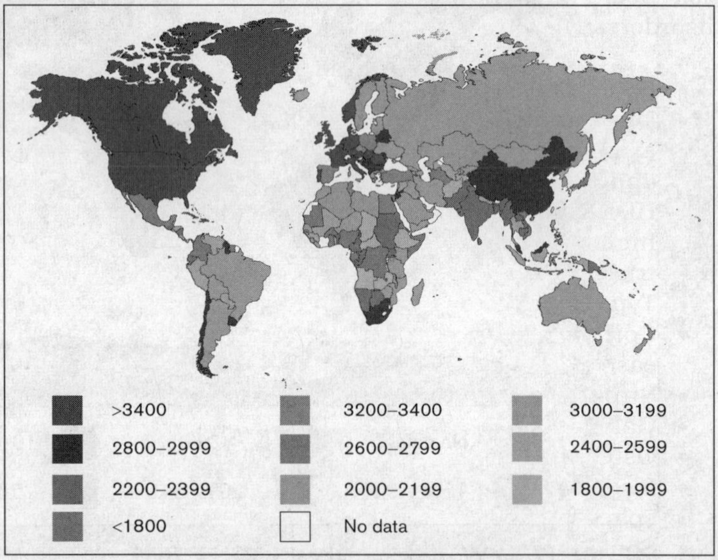

FIGURE 12-3 Daily Calorie Intake 2003–2005

Source: Reuters Staff (2009).
Disclaimer: This figure is not to scale. It does not represent any authentic national or international boundaries and is used for illustrative purposes only.

the past 20 years (see *Figure 12-4*).

There is currently a debate in terms of whether this increase in obesity results from lack of activity, supersizing foods, or a combination of factors. In terms of adolescents, there has also been an increase in obesity for both boys and girls in the latest data over 20 years. Data also show that from 1971 to 2006, BMI ratios in the United States have increased no matter when the person was born (see *Figure 12-5*). This suggests it is not a cohort or age effect.

According to the CDC, overweight and obese individuals are at higher risk for the following disorders:

- Hypertension
- Dyslipidemia (for example, high LDL cholesterol, low HDL cholesterol, or high levels of triglycerides)
- Type 2 diabetes
- Coronary heart disease
- Stroke
- Gallbladder disease
- Osteoarthritis
- Sleep apnea and respiratory problems
- Some cancers (endometrial, breast, and colon)

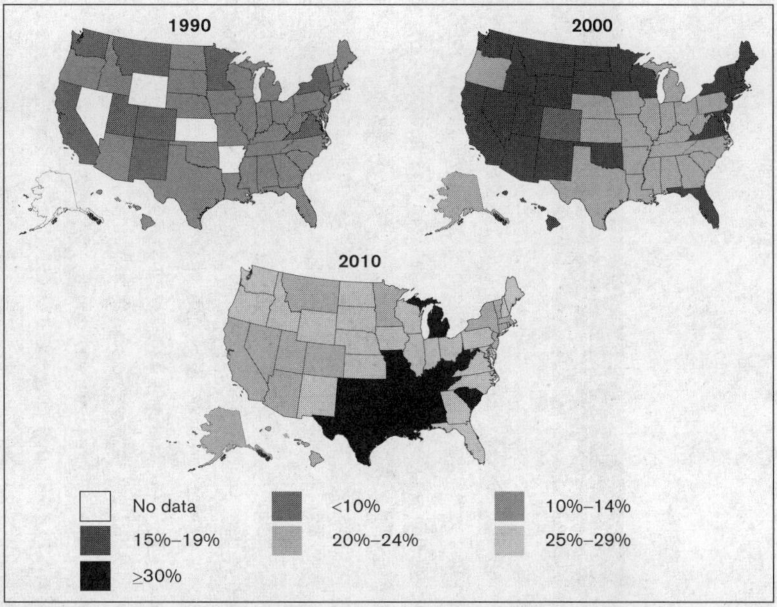

FIGURE 12-4 Obesity Trends by State in the United States

Source: CDC (2013).

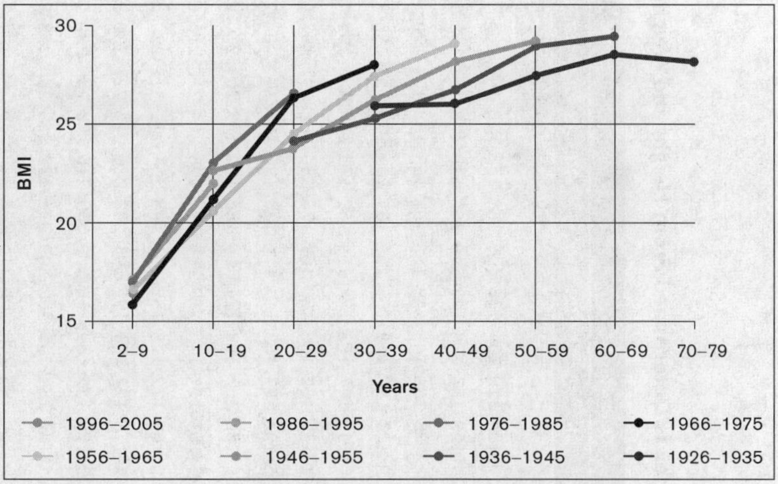

FIGURE 12-5 Age Trend in Body Mass Index by When a Person Was Born (Data From 1971 to 2006)

Source: Lee et al. (2010, p. 619).

In addition to physical disorders, depression has also been linked to obesity (Roberts, Deleger, Strawbridge, & Kaplan, 2003). More than 2,000 individuals age 50 or older were

FIGURE 12-6 Body Mass Index Is Determined From Height and Weight

	Normal						*Overweight*					*Obese*										*Extreme Obesity*														
BMI	***19***	***20***	***21***	***22***	***23***	***24***	***25***	***26***	***27***	***28***	***29***	***30***	***31***	***32***	***33***	***34***	***35***	***36***	***37***	***38***	***39***	***40***	***41***	***42***	***43***	***44***	***45***	***46***	***47***	***48***	***49***	***50***	***51***	***52***	***53***	***54***
Height (Inches)														Body Weight					(Pounds)																	
58	91	96	100	105	110	115	119	124	129	134	138	143	148	153	158	162	167	172	177	181	186	191	196	201	205	210	215	220	224	229	234	239	244	248	253	258
59	94	99	104	109	114	119	124	128	133	138	143	148	153	158	163	168	173	178	183	188	193	198	203	208	212	217	222	227	232	237	242	247	252	257	262	267
60	97	102	107	112	118	123	128	133	138	143	148	153	158	163	168	174	179	184	189	194	199	204	209	215	220	225	230	235	240	245	250	255	261	266	271	276
61	100	106	111	116	122	127	132	137	143	148	153	158	164	169	174	180	185	190	195	201	206	211	217	222	227	232	238	243	248	254	259	264	269	275	280	285
62	104	109	115	120	126	131	136	142	147	153	158	164	169	175	180	186	191	196	202	207	213	218	224	229	235	240	246	251	256	262	267	273	278	284	289	295
63	107	113	118	124	130	135	141	146	152	158	163	169	175	180	186	191	197	203	208	214	220	225	231	237	242	248	254	259	265	270	278	282	287	293	299	304
64	110	116	122	128	134	140	145	151	157	163	169	174	180	186	192	197	204	209	215	221	227	232	238	244	250	256	262	267	273	279	285	291	296	302	308	315
65	114	120	126	132	138	144	150	156	162	168	174	180	186	192	198	204	210	216	222	228	234	240	246	252	258	264	270	276	282	288	294	300	306	312	318	324
66	118	124	130	136	142	148	155	161	167	173	179	186	192	198	204	210	216	223	229	235	241	247	253	260	266	272	278	284	291	297	303	309	315	322	328	334
67	121	127	134	140	146	153	159	166	172	178	185	191	198	204	211	217	223	230	236	242	249	255	261	268	274	280	287	293	299	306	312	319	325	331	338	344
68	125	131	138	144	151	158	164	171	177	184	190	197	203	210	216	223	230	236	243	249	256	262	269	276	282	289	295	302	308	315	322	328	335	341	348	354
69	128	135	142	149	155	162	169	176	182	189	196	203	209	216	223	230	236	243	250	257	263	270	277	284	291	297	304	311	318	324	331	338	345	351	358	365
70	132	139	146	153	160	167	174	181	188	195	202	209	216	222	229	236	243	250	257	264	271	278	285	292	299	306	313	320	327	334	341	348	355	362	369	376
71	136	143	150	157	165	172	179	186	193	200	208	215	222	229	236	243	250	257	265	272	279	286	293	301	308	315	322	329	338	343	351	358	365	372	379	386
72	140	147	154	162	169	177	184	191	199	206	213	221	228	235	242	250	258	265	272	279	287	294	302	309	316	324	331	338	346	353	361	368	375	383	390	397
73	144	151	159	166	174	182	189	197	204	212	219	227	235	242	250	257	265	272	280	288	295	302	310	318	325	333	340	348	355	363	371	378	386	393	401	408
74	148	155	163	171	179	186	194	202	210	218	225	233	241	249	256	264	272	280	287	295	303	311	319	326	334	342	350	358	365	373	381	389	396	404	412	420
75	152	160	168	176	184	192	200	208	216	224	232	240	248	256	264	272	279	287	295	303	311	319	327	335	343	351	359	367	375	383	391	399	407	415	423	431
76	156	164	172	180	189	197	205	213	221	230	238	246	254	263	271	279	287	295	304	312	320	328	336	344	353	361	369	377	385	394	402	410	418	426	435	443

Source: Adapted from *Clinical Guidelines on the Identification, Evaluation, and Treatment of Overweight and Obesity in Adults: The Evidence Report.*

followed for 5 years. At the beginning of the study, both BMI and depression were measured. Obesity, as measured by a BMI over 30, was associated with increased risk for depression 5 years later. Depression at baseline, however, was not related to obesity some 5 years later.

Differences in the View of Ideal Weights Between Males and Females

In addition to an individual's actual weight, there is also the person's attitude toward his or her weight. In some cultures, being heavier in weight is seen as positive whereas in others, it is thinness that is sought. Currently, in the United States, as shown by the popular press including books, dieting is a topic of great interest. However, there are times in which attitudes and behaviors related to eating go to the extreme. These situations may involve eating disorders. Even when the individual does not experience an eating disorder, there are gender and cultural factors that play a role in a person's attitude.

Males and females think about their weight differently. Studies have shown that females tend to overestimate their weight whereas males tend to underestimate their weight (see Fallon & Rozin, 1985). In one study, females were asked to rate female figures in terms of their ideal weight, what would be considered attractive to males their own current weight, and the attractive weight of males. Males were asked to do the same task. *Figure 12-7* shows the results of this study. As can be seen in the figures, males rated a higher weight for females to be seen as attractive than females considered attractive or ideal. Males, on the other hand, rated all three categories (attractive, current, and ideal) as very similar. Overall, this suggests that females are more dissatisfied with their current weight than males.

Similar findings were also seen in 22 countries around the world (Wardle, Haase, & Steptoe, 2006). In this study, BMI was calculated from 18,512 university students. No matter what their BMI, more women than men felt overweight. The perception of being overweight was similar in all of the regions of the world. One difference between regions was that in Asian countries where body weight tends to be lower, most individuals were attempting to lose weight. Overall,

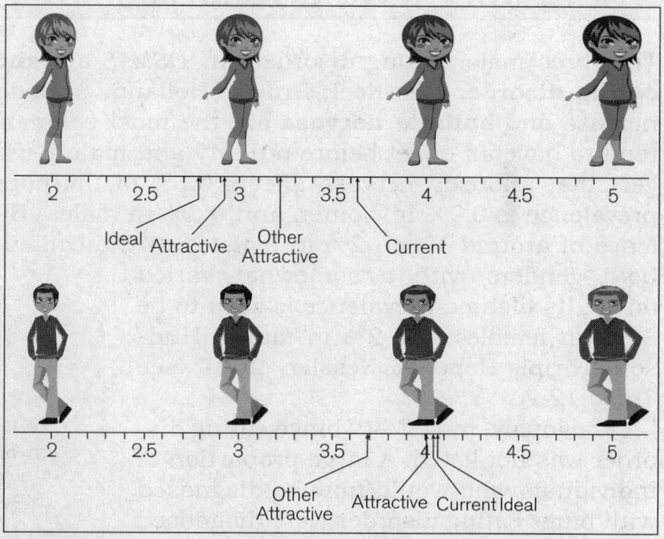

FIGURE 12-7 Mean Rating by Women (Top) and Men (Bottom) of Their Current Figure, Ideal Figure, and the Figure Most Attractive to the Opposite Sex

Source: Fallon and Rozin (1985, p. 183).

Note: Participants were shown four figures varying in size and asked to make a mark along the arbitrary scale in terms of ideal, attractive, current and opposite sex.

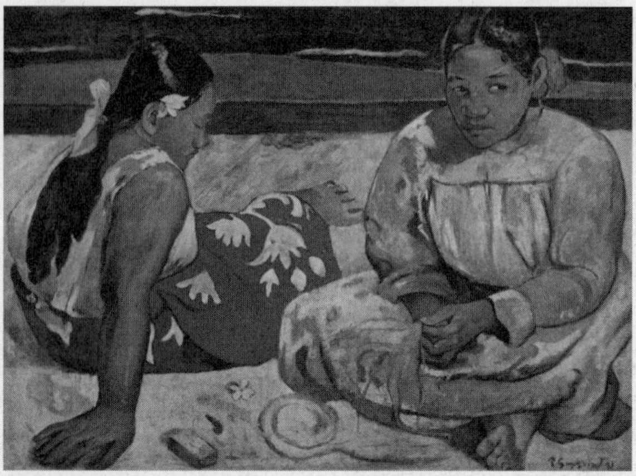

Some Cultures See Heavier Females as More Attractive Than Less Heavy Women (Gauguin)

Source: P. Gauguin (1891).

this study showed that young adult females around the world tend to overestimate weight whereas males tend to underestimate their weight if they themselves are heavier.

Culture also plays a role in the perception of ideal body size. Pacific Island people, for example, find a fuller figured body more attractive as seen in the art of Gauguin. One study examined 433 Maori individuals in New Zealand, 657 Pacific Islanders, and 4,464 Europeans in terms of their perceptions of body size (Metcalf, Scragg, Willoughby, Finau, & Tipene-Leach, 2000). Although both the Maori and Pacific people had an actual larger BMI than the Europeans, they perceived themselves as having a smaller body size compared with Europeans. Thus, culture plays a role in what individuals see as overweight.

THE MAJOR EATING DISORDERS

The three major eating disorders in *DSM–5* are **anorexia nervosa,** bulimia, and **binge eating disorder** (see Keel, Brown, Holland, & Bodell, 2012, for an overview). Anorexia nervosa and **bulimia nervosa** are the most commonly discussed eating disorders. They tend to have an onset before puberty and mainly influence women. Various studies suggest that anorexia nervosa affects 0.5% of the population at any one time. Its lifetime prevalence is 0.9% in women and 0.3% in males. Bulimia is seen to have lifetime prevalence of around 1% to 2% in females in the United States. Binge eating tends to affect both genders with a somewhat varied onset. Its lifetime prevalence is seen to be 3.5% in females and 2% in males (Hudson, Hiripi, Hope, & Kessler, 2007; see *Table 12-2*).

Previously, in *DSM–IV* binge eating disorder was not listed. A large proportion of individuals who would now be diagnosed with binge eating disorder were diagnosed in *DSM–IV* with an *eating disorder not otherwise specified.* It was the goal of *DSM–5* to minimize the use of this category by adding binge eating disorder. *DSM–5* also includes a category of *other specified feeding or eating disorder.* The *other specified feeding or eating disorder* category

Concept Check

- How do our evolutionary history and current conditions of food abundance interact to promote obesity?
- What are some of the environmental, psychological, and biological factors involved in obesity?
- How is the brain involved in obesity?
- What are some of the physical and psychological disorders for which obese individuals are at higher risk?
- What are some of the factors at different levels that influence views of ideal weight?

TABLE 12-2 Prevalence and Its Standard Error for Eating Disorder by Gender

	Male		*Female*		*Total*	
	%	*(se)*	*%*	*(se)*	*%*	*(se)*
I. Lifetime prevalence						
Anorexia nervosa	.3*	(.1)	.9*	(.3)	.6	(.2)
Bulimia nervosa	.5*	(.3)	1.5*	(.3)	1.0	(.2)
Binge eating disorder	2.0*	(.5)	3.5*	(.5)	2.8	(.4)
Subthreshold binge eating disorder	1.9*	(.5)	.6*	(.1)	1.2	(.2)
Any binge eating	4.0	(.7)	4.9	(.6)	4.5	(.4)
II. Twelve-month prevalence†						
Bulimia nervosa	.1*	(.1)	.5*	(.2)	.3	(.1)
Binge eating disorder	.8*	(.3)	1.6*	(.2)	1.2	(.2)
Subthreshold binge eating disorder	.8	(.3)	.4	(.1)	.6	(.2)
Any binge eating	1.7	(.4)	2.5	(.3)	2.1	(.2)
(*n*)	(1,220)		(1,760)		(2,980)	

Abbreviations: SE, standard error.
*Significant sex difference based on a 0.05 level, 2-sided test.
†None of the respondents met criteria for 12-month anorexia nervosa.
Source: Hudson et al. (2007, p. 350), with permission from Elsevier.

includes atypical anorexia nervosa in which all criteria except weight loss are met, bulimia nervosa of low frequency or limited duration, binge eating disorder of low frequency or limited duration, purging disorder without binge eating, and night eating disorder in which excessive food is consumed after the evening meal.

In order to determine the effects of eating disorder changes in *DSM–5,* Eric Stice and his colleagues reclassified the female participants of an 8-year prospective community sample (Stice, Marti, & Rohde, 2012). This study annually assessed 496 adolescents for 8 years beginning at age 13. Overall, they found that the changes in *DSM–5* eating disorders resulted in higher prevalence as compared with *DSM–IV.* These results are shown in *Table 12-3.* Overall, these findings suggest 1 in 8 young women experience some type of eating disorder before they are 21.

There is good evidence that eating disorders have a partial genetic

TABLE 12-3 Lifetime Prevalence Rates for *DSM–5* Eating Disorders

Eating Disorder	*Lifetime Prevalence*
Anorexia nervosa	.8%
Bulimia nervosa	2.6%
Binge eating disorder	30.0%
Feeding or eating disorder–not elsewhere classified	11.5%
Atypical anorexia nervosa	2.8%
Subthreshold bulimia nervosa	4.4%
Subthreshold binge eating disorder	3.6%
Purging disorder	3.4%

Source: Stice et al. (2012, p. 450).

component (Rankinen & Bouchard, 2006). As you will see, this genetic component may influence temperament, which sets the stage for an eating disorder. There is also a cultural component. When eating disorders are examined in terms of ethnic diversity within the United States, ethnic differences are seen. One common finding with adolescent girls is that there is a higher prevalence of disordered eating in Hispanic and Native American females and a lower prevalence in white, black, and Asian females (see Lynch, Crosby, Wonderlich, & Striegel-Moore, 2011, for an overview).

Those with eating disorders experience a number of serious medical conditions related to reducing body weight or **purging.** They also show a higher death rate, including suicide rates of between 4% and 5% (Crow et al., 2009). Often, those with eating disorders conceal their symptoms and do not seek treatment. Even when they seek help for medical disorders related to purging, such as problems with their teeth and gastrointestinal system, they continue to hide the underlying eating disorder.

Anorexia Nervosa

Historically, anorexia nervosa has been described in the medical literature since the 1600s. Richard Morton, an English physician, in 1689 described an adolescent boy and girl who suffered from "want of appetite" and "nervous consumption" (Gordon, 1990). These adolescents lost weight but did not appear to have any medical disorder. Sir William Gull is credited with first using the term *anorexia nervosa* in his description in 1870. He described a condition affecting young adolescent females who starved themselves (Gull, 1874). In France, Charles Lasègue described young women with significant weight loss as *anorexie hystérique*.

From the 1600s till the present, the disorder was commonly described in terms of three characteristics:

1. Food refusal
2. Onset in adolescence
3. Lack of concern of the consequences of not eating

The age of onset with anorexia nervosa takes place in a narrow range in adolescence. There is a consistency in symptoms. These include a preoccupation with food while at the same time showing a resistance to eating. Body image is also distorted. Even when significantly underweight, individuals with anorexia nervosa see themselves as fat. They also show a lack of concern for their lack of weight. This lack of concern also results in these individuals not seeking treatment for their anorexia nervosa. The following describes the experience of a daughter with anorexia nervosa as seen from the perspective of the mother.

DSM–5 criteria for a diagnosis of anorexia nervosa include a restriction of food, which results in a weight that is below normal; a fear of gaining weight; and a lack of recognition of the seriousness of current body weight and a distortion of how body weight is experienced. Unlike other mental disorders such as depression in which different types of symptoms can lead to the overall diagnosis, individuals with anorexia nervosa show a similar pattern in their behavior and attitudes. This consistency has led some researchers to suggest that anorexia nervosa has the most homogeneous presentation of any psychiatric disorder (Kaye, Fudge, & Paulus, 2009).

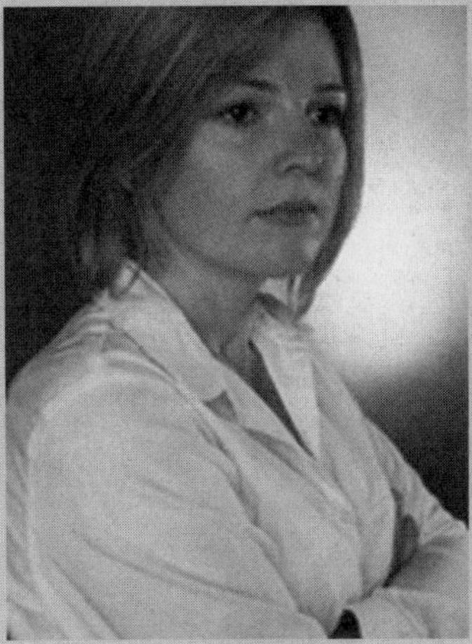

The story of a daughter named Jen with anorexia nervosa

Source: Office on Women's Health (2009a).

Jen's Story

It was 6 months ago when I realized my daughter, Jen, had an eating disorder. Jen has always been a picky eater. But I started to see that she moved food around her plate. And she never ate very much. She exercised all the time–even when she was sick. And she was sick a lot. She became very skinny and pale. Her hair thinned. Jen became moody and seemed sad–I thought that's what teens act like. But once I put the signs together, I talked to Jen about anorexia. She denied she had a problem. But I knew she needed help. I took her to our doctor, and she asked me to put Jen in the hospital. Jen's treatment helped her return to a normal weight. It's been a tough road since then for all of us, but Jen is back home now. She is still seeing her doctors, and may need help for some time. But she's doing much better.

Within this consistency, *DSM–5* describes two subtypes. The first subtype is referred to *restricting type*. As the name implies, individuals of this subtype accomplish weight loss through dieting, fasting, and/or excessive exercise. The second subtype is referred to as *binge-eating/purging type*. Low-weight individuals with this subtype display episodes of binge eating or purging through self-induced vomiting or the use of laxatives, diuretics, or enemas. The photo to the right shows the image of a young woman with anorexia nervosa. She may not actually see herself to be as thin as she is.

Although adolescents are often concerned about their body image, only about 1% of females go on to develop anorexia nervosa. What can we say about these individuals? One thing is that they tend to have certain personality characteristics that can be thought of as an endophenotype (see Kaye, Wierenga, Bailer, Simmons, & Bischoff-Grethe, 2013, for an overview). They tend to be anxious, and this anxiety exists before the onset of anorexia nervosa and will continue even after treatment, which includes weight gain. They also tend to be perfectionistic with an overemphasis on self-imposed standards. Perfectionism is also seen prior to the onset and continues after treatment. The higher the level of perfectionism, the poorer the recovery from treatment and the shorter the duration before relapse. There is also a difficulty in flexibility and changing rule structures. This is also seen in terms of an obsessiveness around order, exactness, and symmetry. *Figure 12-8* shows a pathway by which these characteristics become part of the development of anorexia nervosa.

In addition to the outward signs of anorexia nervosa, there are also distortions in body image (see Gaudio & Quattrocchi, 2012, for an overview). One common characteristic is for the person to see both specific body parts and overall weight as being heavier than they are. The body image distortion has been described as having a perceptual, an emotional, and a cognitive component. The perception consists of whether one's self or others are underweight, normal, or overweight. The affective component involves whether

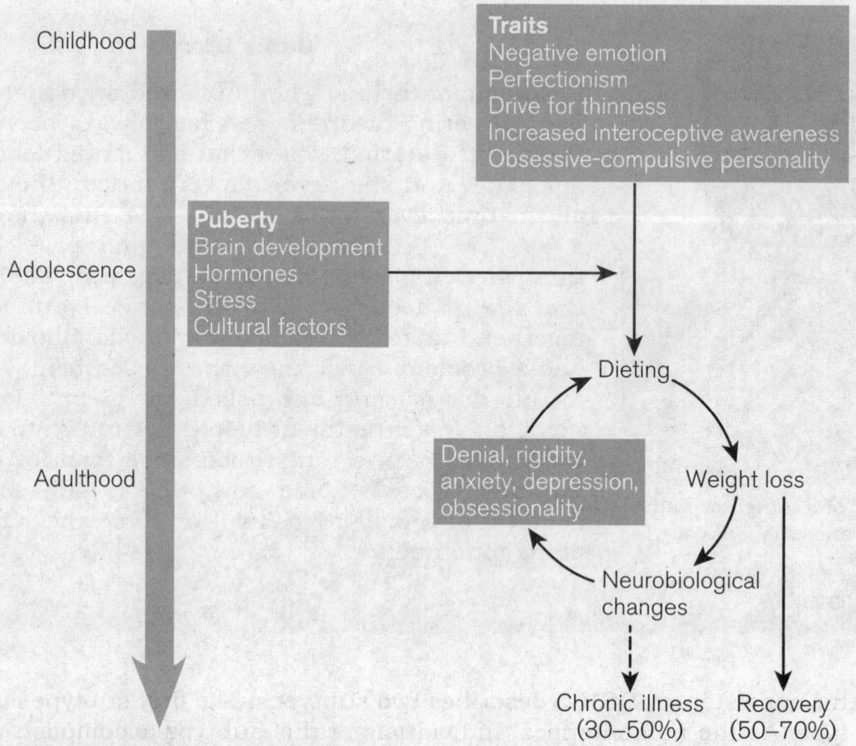

FIGURE 12-8 The Time Course and Phenomenology of Anorexia Nervosa
Source: Kaye et al. (2009, p. 575).

the person is satisfied or dissatisfied with his or her own body. The cognitive component consists of beliefs concerning one's body image as well as the mental representation of one's body. These beliefs exist separately without actually viewing body types. The figure to the right portrays the manner in which a thin person sees herself as overweight.

In a review of brain imaging studies concerning differences in these three components between those with anorexia nervosa and healthy controls, it was found that each involves different areas of the brain (Gaudio & Quattrocchi, 2012). As can be seen in *Figure 12-9*, the perception component showed differences in the precuneus and the inferior parietal lobe. The affective component involved the PFC, the insula, and the amygdala. One task of the insula is to process internal information that gives rise to a sense of self. Those individuals with anorexia nervosa may experience different internal information that leads to a distorted body image, lack of response to hunger, and lack of motivation to change.

In previous studies, the cognitive component was often combined with a negative affective component. This made it impossible to study beliefs concerning body image alone. However, when the cognitive network is considered to modulate selective attention, planning, and effortful regulation of affective states, it is possible to see changes in the hippocampus, anterior cingulate cortex (ACC), dorsolateral prefrontal cortex (DLPFC), and parietal areas (Kaye et al., 2009).

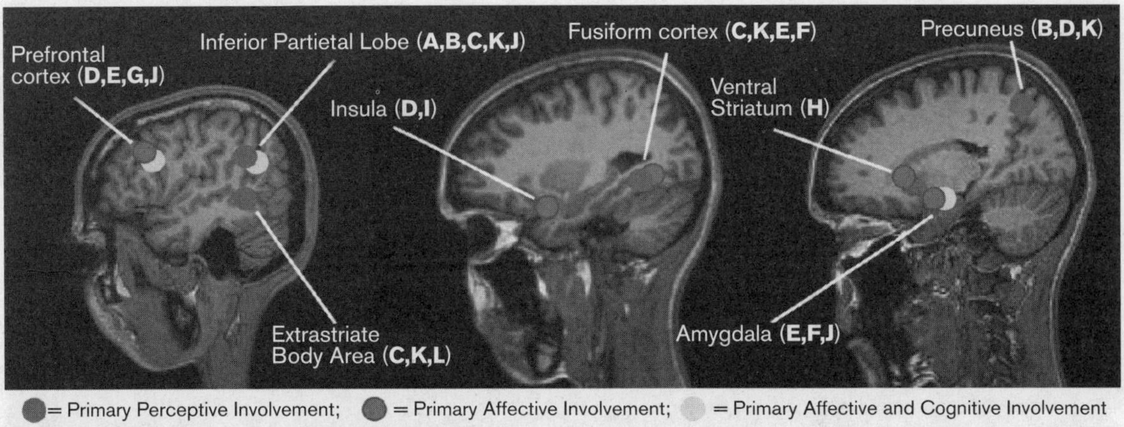

FIGURE 12-9 Scheme of the Main Findings of Functional Magnetic Resonance Imaging Studies

Source: Gaudio and Quattrocchi (2012, p. 1844), with permission from Elsevier.

On a neurotransmitter level, both serotonin and dopamine systems have been shown to be different in those with eating disorders (see Kaye et al., 2009, for an overview). The serotonin system is thought to play a role in eating disorders by influencing the feeling of being full, impulse control, and mood. The binding potential of the serotonin (5-HT) receptor is increased in individuals with eating disorders whereas it is decreased in those with depression, social phobia, and panic disorder. Research also suggests that the dopamine system and its relationship to reward is different in those with eating disorders (Kaye et al., 2013). That is, individuals with anorexia nervosa do not show signs of reward in the dopamine system in relation to eating. Thus, individuals with anorexia nervosa do think about food but do not find satisfaction or reward from this or even other activities.

Individuals with anorexia nervosa develop a variety of medical problems that may be related to lack of nutrition and changes in hormones such as lower levels of estrogen and higher levels of cortisol. The most serious medical outcome of anorexia is death although a number of other medical conditions are also seen. One of these is a decreased level of bone density, which increases the chances of fracture. Other problems related to cardiovascular functioning and reduced motility of the gastrointestinal tract are also seen in individuals with anorexia nervosa. It is possible to reverse these disorders when the individual returns to a normal weight.

The specific causes of anorexia nervosa are still being researched. However, there appear to be a variety of factors involved (see Kaye et al., 2009, for an overview). *Figure 12-10* lists a variety of these factors that have been shown to be related to the development of anorexia nervosa although not every person will have each of these factors.

One factor is genetics. Twin studies suggest that 50% to 80% of the variance in both anorexia nervosa and bulimia can be accounted for by genetics (see Kaye et al., 2009, for an overview). However, the identification of specific genes has been difficult to determine. As noted, most studies look for endophenotypes that include psychological personality factors and food intake. Overall, these genetic influences appear to show heritability of global attitudes toward food and dieting including the restriction of eating, binge eating, and self-induced vomiting.

A. Familial
   1. A family member or relative with anorexia nervosa, bulimia nervosa
   2. A family member or relative with depression or alcohol/drug abuse/dependence

B. Individual Biological Factors
   1. Early menarche
   2. Mildly overweight

C. Individual Psychological Factors
   1. Perfectionistic—obsessional personality
   2. Sense of ineffectiveness, lack of confidence, low self-esteem
   3. Affective disorders (depression)

D. Individual Behaviors
   1. Dieting
   2. Involvement in activities or professions that emphasize weight control: gymnastics, ballet, wrestling, jockeys, actors, and models

E. Cultural
   1. Living in an industrialized country
   2. Emphasis on thinness as beauty
   3. General significant weight increase in the general population in the U.S. over the past 40 years

F. Stressful life events
   1. Death of a close relative or friend
   2. Sexual abuse

FIGURE 12-10 Suggestive Risk Factors in Anorexia Nervosa

Source: Halmi (2005, p. S21).

Another factor involved in the development of anorexia nervosa results from restricting the intake of food. For example, brain volume is less in individuals with anorexia nervosa. There is also a reduction in brain metabolism in specific areas of the brain, including the frontal, cingulate, temporal, and parietal areas. Also, even when puberty has been achieved, individuals with anorexia nervosa show characteristics of prepubertal functioning. As a way of conserving energy, these and other physiological changes may actually lead the person to increase his or her desire to reduce food intake. As such, it becomes a dangerously self-perpetuating situation. As with other medical conditions, these characteristics tend to return to normal after the individual gains weight in treatment.

Cultural factors also play an important role. For example, individuals with anorexia nervosa in Hong Kong, Japan, Singapore, and Malaysia do not show the same phobic response to fat that is seen in Western cultures (see Becker, 2011, for an overview). This has led to some professionals questioning the diagnostic criteria in *DSM* since one requirement of anorexia nervosa is a fear of becoming fat. Likewise, screenings in those countries with large amounts of poverty will identify individuals who are preoccupied with food as the result of hunger rather than an eating disorder. In general, anorexia is seen more in developed economies. Paradoxically, anorexia nervosa is higher in cultures where food is abundant. As a country develops, there is an increase in the occurrence of anorexia. It has been suggested that with economic development come changing roles for women, a shift in eating patterns, and an emphasis on thinness (Nasser, Katzman, & Gordon, 2001).

It is interesting to note that starvation in itself may lead to similar psychological characteristics in non-anorexic individuals. In a classic study performed during World War II, there were 36 men who were conscientious objectors who volunteered to be part of a study of starvation (Franklin, Schiele, Brozek, & Keys, 1948). During the first 3 months of the study, these men ate a good diet of some 3,492 calories a day. This is actually higher than the recommendation today that males should consume roughly 2,500 calories a day based on physical size for a healthy lifestyle (see *Table 12-4*). For the next 6 months, these men began a semi-starvation diet of 1,570 calories a day. This was followed by 3 months of rehabilitation when calorie intake was increased. The photo on the next page shows some of the men in this study.

By the end of the semi-starvation period, the men had lost about 24% of their previous weight. Physically, their faces and bodies showed emaciation. Also, they lost muscle and adipose tissue such that sitting on hard surfaces was uncomfortable. They experienced some of their hair falling out. They reported feeling cold, even in the summer. They played with the food they ate. Food also became part of their conversations, reading, and day-dreams. They showed periods of emotional instability and depression. Overall, they became

TABLE 12-4 Daily Calorie Allowance Table

Women Weight	*Super Active*	*Very Active*	*Active*	*Moderate Active*	*Low Active*	*Sedentary*
80	1600	1440	1280	1120	960	800
90	1800	1620	1440	1260	1080	900
100	2000	1800	1600	1400	1200	1000
110	2200	1980	1760	1540	1320	1100
120	2400	2160	1920	1680	1440	1200
130	2600	2340	2080	1820	1560	1300
140	2800	2520	2240	1960	1680	1400
150	3000	2700	2400	2100	1800	1500
160	3200	2880	2560	2240	1920	1600
170	3400	3060	2720	2380	2040	1700
180	3600	3240	2880	2520	2160	1800
Men Weight	*Super Active*	*Very Active*	*Active*	*Moderate Active*	*Low Active*	*Sedentary*
100	2600	2350	2100	1850	1600	1350
110	2800	2530	2260	1990	1720	1450
120	3000	2710	2420	2130	1840	1550
130	3200	2890	2580	2270	1960	1650
140	3400	3070	2740	2410	2080	1750
150	3600	3250	2900	2550	2200	1850
160	3800	3430	3060	2690	2320	1950
170	4000	3610	3220	2830	2440	2050
180	4200	3790	3380	2970	2560	2150
190	4400	3970	3540	3110	2680	2250
200	4600	4150	3700	3250	2800	2350

Source: From Reuters Staff. "Future of Food: Daily calorie intake." Reuters. November 9, 2009.

indecisive, unable to make personal plans, and unwilling to participate in group activities. These men showed a narrowing of focus and mainly stayed alone. During the rehabilitation phase, recovery to normal as seen before the start of the experiment was very slow. Although these men did not begin with an eating disorder, their experiences parallel the cognitive and emotional changes seen in anorexia nervosa.

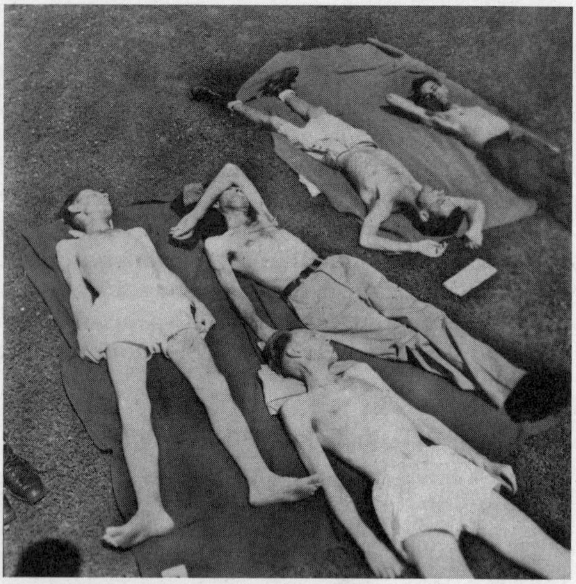

Minnesota volunteers after weight loss

Treating Anorexia Nervosa

Anorexia nervosa is seen as one of the most difficult disorders to treat (see Halmi, 2005, for an overview). Many individuals with anorexia do not want to be treated. In fact, there are some websites in which those with anorexia nervosa share with one another techniques for remaining underweight and avoiding recognition that they have the disorder. The disorder itself has resulted in psychological and physiological changes, and many individuals deny that they actually have a disorder when they have agreed to treatment, or with adolescents it is often the family that pushes for treatment.

One of the first tasks for someone with anorexia nervosa is to gain weight. This often requires a hospital stay in which the individual's consumption of food is gradually increased. This also includes nutritional analysis as to the needs of the person. Following this, psychological or family therapy is typically the next step. Family therapy has strong support with adolescents. A critical component is the person's willingness to be involved in treatment and experience change, such as bodily and psychological feelings.

One family-based treatment approach for adolescents with anorexia nervosa is referred to as the Maudsley approach (Lock, Le Grange, Agras, & Dare, 2001; see also www.maudsleyparents.org/whatismaudsley.html). The Maudsley approach is based on treatment research of anorexia nervosa at the Maudsley Hospital in the United Kingdom and is used by a number of university-based medical centers in the United States. The approach is designed to take place in the family rather than a hospital. There are three basic phases to the approach. The first phase is that of weight restoration. In this phase, the mental health professional works with the parents to encourage their child to eat during family meals without blaming the adolescent for having the eating disorder. The second phase focuses on having the adolescent taking more control over his or her eating problems. This phase takes place after the adolescent has begun to gain weight associated with increased food intake. Once the individual approaches a normal body weight, the third phase begins. This phase emphasizes developing a healthy adolescent identity as well as developing personal autonomy. The current limited research suggests that this approach is effective, especially for those adolescents who have experienced anorexia nervosa for less than 3 years (Le Gange & Eisler, 2009).

With adults, cognitive behavioral therapy (CBT) has been shown to be an effective approach. The basic approach is to help the person develop productive thoughts and feelings around his or her eating and view of self. As with the treatment of other disorders, CBT focuses on the irrational thoughts and conclusions that an individual with anorexia nervosa has. Some of these irrational thoughts can include the need to follow strict rules and the belief that self-control can only be achieved through dieting.

There are currently two versions of CBT for use with any eating disorder, including anorexia and bulimia (Fairburn, 2008; Fairburn, Cooper, & Shafran, 2003, 2008, 2009). The first version focuses on pathology related to eating disorders exclusively. The second form is more complex and also addresses mood intolerance, clinical perfectionism, low self-esteem, and interpersonal difficulties. Both of these approaches have been shown to be effective in reducing symptoms in about 50% of those with eating disorders (Fairburn et al., 2009).

A number of medications have been tried with anorexia nervosa (Walsh, 2008). Generally, the medications that have been tried are neuroleptics, for which the main focus is in treating psychosis. The basic idea is that these medications are associated with weight gain and the reduction of disordered thinking and might help those with anorexia nervosa. Tricyclic antidepressants have also been tried without any apparent benefits. Currently, there is no good evidence to suggest a critical role for medication in the treatment of anorexia nervosa (Walsh, 2008).

There are a limited number of studies evaluating treatment approaches for anorexia nervosa. The dropout rates for adults in treatment are high. In one treatment outcome study comparing CBT with a medication and the combination of the two, the dropout rate was 46% (Halmi et al., 2005). Only 27% of those in the medication group completed treatment whereas 38% in the combination group and 43% in the CBT group completed treatment. In another study that compared nutritional counseling with CBT, all of the individuals in the nutritional counseling group dropped out whereas 8% of the CBT condition dropped out. In another similar study, the numbers were 73% dropout rate for nutritional counseling and 22% for CBT. Although this suggests that individuals are more willing to be part of CBT treatments than other types, the dropout rates made it difficult to know the effectiveness of therapy.

Also, individuals—especially adults with anorexia nervosa—may refuse treatment. At the beginning of another study for the treatment of anorexia nervosa with a particular drug, there were 139 individuals who met criteria for the study (Bissada, Tasca, Barber, & Bradwejn, 2008). Of these, 63 individuals refused day hospital treatment. Out of the remaining 76 individuals, 42 declined to be part of the study, leaving only 14 individuals in the drug treatment group and 14 in the placebo group. With adolescents, parental pressure increases the involvement in treatment and treatment studies.

Individuals with anorexia nervosa show a great variety in the outcomes of the disorder (see Zerwas et al., 2013, for an overview). Previous research showed that about one third of individuals recover about 4 years after the onset of anorexia nervosa. By year 10 after onset, about 50% recover. Past this time it increases to 73%. The other individuals either experience medical complications from the disorder or die of suicide. Given these data, researchers have sought to determine the factors associated with successful outcomes (Zerwas et al., 2013). These researchers looked at eating disorder features, personality traits, and comorbid psychological disorders. Presence of vomiting and higher levels of trait anxiety were associated with less positive levels of recovery. Impulsivity on the other hand was associated with recovery.

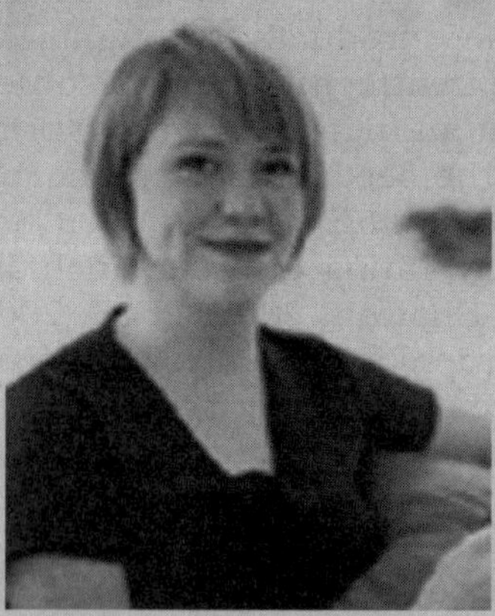

The story of another person named Jen who suffers from bulimia nervosa

Source: Office on Women's Health (2009b).

Jen's Story

It was ten years ago when I became bulimic. I had always worried about my weight and how I looked. I thought I looked fat, no matter what the scale showed or anyone said. But I had never made myself throw up–not until after college. I felt stressed out after graduating from college. I was very overwhelmed with my new job and turned to food to feel more in control of my life. Sometimes, I'd eat a lot of food and throw it up. Other times, I'd throw up a normal meal. At the time, it seemed like the only way I could cope with my stress. Luckily, I got help from a doctor, after a friend talked to me about the problem. It took a lot of work, but I am better now.

Bulimia Nervosa

Although overeating followed by purging has been described since Roman times more than 2,000 years ago, the eating disorder bulimia nervosa was not introduced into the medical literature until 1979 (Russell, 1979). The main characteristics are periods of overeating in which the person feels out of control followed by purging. In general, individuals with bulimia nervosa report that once they begin eating, they are unable to stop until a large amount of food has been consumed. In order to prevent weight gain associated with excessive eating, the person self-induces vomiting or takes laxatives or other medication to eliminate the food. The person may also overexercise or fast to prevent weight gain.

This disorder is generally reported in women and associated with an overconcern related to weight and appearance. Twelve-month prevalence in females is around 1% to 1.5% (American Psychiatric Association [APA], 2013). Although it is seen to have a 10 to 1 female to male ratio, it may be missed in men such as those involved in sports where they are required to "make weight." The prevalence of bulimia nervosa is low in developing countries. In developed countries such as the United States, Canada, Japan, Australia, and countries of Europe, the prevalence is similar.

The typical onset is described as one in which a young woman who sees herself overweight begins to diet (Walsh, 2008). After some initial success, she begins to overeat. Fearing that she will become fat and not having a sense of control in her eating, the person then looks for ways to overeat and not be fat at the same time. She then learns techniques from friends, the media, or the Internet. Initially, these techniques may work and give her a sense of control. However, afterward she will find herself using these techniques more often and feeling guilty and not wanting to be discovered. The binge eating tends to occur in the late afternoon or evening when the person is alone. The eating often involves sweet foods such as ice cream or cake. Some individuals describe themselves as "numb" when they are engaging in binge eating episodes. Purging usually follows shortly after the eating.

Bulimia nervosa can also lead to secondary medical problems related to vomiting and the overuse of medications such as laxatives. These can include menstrual disturbances, dental erosion—especially of the upper front teeth—and electrolyte imbalances.

Overall, there are three major aspects of bulimia nervosa in terms of *DSM–5.* The first is binge eating in which the person consumes large amounts of food. Typically, the individual consumes 2,000 calories in one sitting, which is equal to the amount of calories recommended for a female's daily intake for a healthy lifestyle. The person also experiences a lack of control over her eating. The second aspect is the purging. Purging is where a person eliminates food from the body by such means as vomiting, taking laxatives, diuretics, or enemas. The third aspect is a psychological one in which one's self-worth is seen in relation to one's weight or body shape.

In *DSM–5,* the binging and purging need to occur at least once a week for 3 months. The following case study of Anne Hart (not her real name) shows these characteristics.

CASE OF ANNE HART
Bulimia Nervosa

Anne Hart is an 18-year-old, single, Caucasian female, who is in her junior year at a local university. She is majoring in Theatre. She lives in an off-campus apartment with two female roommates and works part-time as a waitress in a local restaurant. She is very involved in athletics and is on the collegiate gymnastics team, through which she received a college scholarship that has enabled her to pursue her goal of attending college. Anne Hart initially reported that she had a largely "uneventful childhood" where she grew up in an intact family along with three older siblings, although she did acknowledge that her parents "didn't like each other." She also reported that her parents frequently engaged in loud verbal arguments for "as long as she can remember." As a result, she noted that her home environment was stressful and chaotic, where minor disagreements tended to result in "shouting matches" between family members. As a result, Ms. Hart reported that she tended to spend most of her time alone in her room or outside the home with friends. She also reported that although she was never without basic necessities while growing up, she was also aware that her parents often struggled to make ends meet, which she believes also intensified their arguments and tensions within the home. Although Ms. Hart described herself as high functioning throughout her primary and secondary school years, she also noted that she has always been somewhat shy and reserved, with a tendency to be perfectionistic about her academics and unassertive in social relationships. Anne Hart was initially referred for therapy by her collegiate coach when Ms. Hart was observed to appear increasingly more dysphoric at which time she also started to voice greater ambivalence about her future in collegiate athletics. When presenting for therapy, Ms. Hart acknowledged that she has been feeling increasingly distressed by her problems, which has been compounded by her strong reluctance to openly share her concerns with her coach or any of her friends, especially in relation to worsening problems with her body image and concerns about maintaining the "right weight" in order to successfully compete alongside her teammates, as well as feeling trapped in remaining on the team given her financial

(Continued)

reliance on her collegiate athletic scholarship. She indicated that her preoccupation with weight began when she was initially encouraged to lose 8 pounds in order to optimize her physical performance in athletics approximately 2 years ago. Although Ms. Hart was successful with that goal, she noted that since then she has become increasing more preoccupied with her body weight and eating habits, which she believes were further intensified given her major in Theatre, where she believes there is also an emphasis on physical appearance. Although Ms. Hart reported that purging, in particular, was initially limited to times when she was actively focused on losing weight, she reported that the frequency of binge/purge cycles has progressively increased within the past year, where she now reports that she has purged several times per week in the last few months. Perhaps most distressing to Ms. Hart., she has noticed that the binge/purge cycles have been increasingly triggered at times when she is experiencing general feelings of pressure or distress, such as when dealing with academic pressures, relationship difficulties, and uncertainties related to prioritizing responsibilities and goals. Ms. Hart was diagnosed with bulimia nervosa and accepted recommendations to participate in therapy focused on eating-related issues.

Clinical Vignette provided by Sandra Testa Michelson, PhD

Treating Bulimia Nervosa

CBT is the best-evaluated treatment for bulimia (see Anderson & Maloney, 2001, for an overview). Outcome research suggests that about 40% to 50% of those treated with CBT recover from bulimia in terms of binging and purging. Therapy is most effective in those individuals who are willing to keep a food diary and self-monitor their feelings and thoughts concerning earing and binge–purge episodes. In two studies, those who were able to reduce purging by Session 6 showed the best outcomes (Agras, Walsh, Fairburn, Wilson, & Kraemer, 2000; Fairburn, Agras, Walsh, Wilson, & Stice, 2004).

CBT typically begins with a psychoeducational and monitoring phase including discussions of regular eating. This is followed by a more cognitive phase that emphasizes techniques to eliminate binge eating and challenge obstacles to normal eating behavior. The final sessions discuss ways to cope with relapse, which is experienced by a number of individuals with bulimia. Antidepressant medications such as fluoxetine (Prozac) have been used to treat the depressive aspects of bulimia and shown to be more effective than a placebo. However, CBT is more effective than medication in the treatment of bulimia nervosa.

Binge Eating Disorder

Jane Brody, who writes health books and columns for the New York Times, has described her own experience with binge eating. She begins by telling of her first newspaper job in which she felt bored and had a difficult boss. Her answer to this was to eat since food was associated with love and happiness for her. This started a pattern of gaining weight and going on a diet. Feeling desperate when she could not stop eating, she would fast during the day and binge eat at night. She would spend the night eating and could go through 3,000 calories at a sitting. Something sweet and then something salty—she could eat a half-gallon of ice and go on from there. Jane Brody continued to gain weight till her weight was 1/3 more than her normal weight. She became suicidal. Calling a psychologist she knew at 2:00 AM got her into treatment. She said, "Just talking about my behavior and learning from the psychologist that I was not the only person with this problem helped relieve my despair. Still, he was not able to help me stop bingeing. That was something I would have to do on my own."

Adapted from Jane Brody. (2007, February 20). Out of Control: A True Story of Binge Eating. *New York Times.*

Binge eating was described by Stunkard in 1959 in obese individuals in terms of recurrent episodes of eating excessive amounts without purging (Stunkard, 1959). It was not categorized as a separate disorder until *DSM–5* (see Striegel-Moore & Franko, 2008, for an overview). Binge eating disorder is characterized in *DSM–5* by the consumption of large amounts of food and the sense that one cannot control his or her eating behavior. Although the amount of food varies from person to person, it can go as high as 10,000 calories. Binge eating is higher in those who are overweight than those who are normal weight. The prevalence is 2.9% in overweight individuals and 1.5% in normal weight individuals. Also, obese individuals take in a larger number of calories during binge eating and non-binge eating episodes.

There is evidence to suggest that binge eating runs in families and is not related to obesity per se. Thus, it should be considered to be different from familial obesity. It is estimated to have a lifetime prevalence rate of 3.5% in women and 2% in men (Hudson et al., 2007). Similar frequency of the disorder is seen in developed countries around the world (APA, 2013). In the United States, there are few ethnic differences found between Latinos, Asians, African Americans, and Caucasians.

In addition to binge eating and a lack of control, *DSM–5* requires three of the following five: (1) eating much more rapidly than normal; (2) eating until feeling uncomfortably full; (3) eating large amounts of food when not feeling physically hungry; (4) eating alone because of feeling embarrassed by how much one is eating; and (5) feeling disgusted with oneself, depressed, or very guilty after overeating.

Overall, the goals of treatment are to cease binge eating, to reduce negative emotions and cognitions, and to lose weight. Psychosocial treatments, especially CBT, have been shown to be effective for treating binge eating disorder. At times, other approaches such as exercise have been added to CBT treatments. Drug treatments such as the use of antidepressant medication show limited evidence of success.

Concept Check

- What are some of the negative consequences of eating disorders?
- How are the following factors implicated in "causing" anorexia nervosa:
  - Genetics?
  - Physiological changes?
  - Cultural factors?
- Considering the three eating disorders described in this section—anorexia nervosa, bulimia nervosa, and binge eating disorder—answer the following questions:
  - What are the primary diagnostic criteria for each?
  - What are the prevalence rates of each in terms of lifetime and gender differences?
  - Is there a genetic component to the disorder?
  - What is the treatment of choice for each, and what do we know about the effectiveness of treatment?

SUMMARY

Eating seems simple; however, it is extremely complicated. What we eat and how we eat represent a complex relationship between all levels of human functioning including culture, evolutionary history, genetics, our physiology, preferences, and psychological attitudes toward our appearance and that of others. Humans have had ideas of ideal appearance for thousands of years, and many of the concerns they had concerning obesity continue to this day.

Previously, feeding disorders were considered part of a category of disorders usually first diagnosed in infancy, childhood, and adolescence. However, since feeding disorders can be seen in individuals of all ages, they were made part of a larger feeding and eating disorders category in *DSM–5*. The three major feeding disorders are (1) pica, in which the person eats something that would not be considered food; (2) rumination disorder, in which a person regurgitates his food; and (3) avoidant/restrictive food intake disorder, in which an individual does not eat certain foods, which leads to such conditions as weight loss or nutritional deficiency.

Current conditions of food abundance and lack of exercise do not match our evolutionary history and can lead to obesity. Our evolutionary history may have us seeking substances that do not lead to a healthy lifestyle. Overall, obesity is seen to result from a mismatch between the amount of calories that we eat and the amount of energy that we expend complicated by other factors, including (1) environmental factors including family and culture, (2) psychological factors such as self-esteem or need for comfort, and (3) biological factors such as genetic makeup. In terms of the brain, a homeostatic system regulates body weight. Its basic task is to produce energy for the body. When nutrients are easily accessible, humans and other animals tend to overload with nutrients and become obese. Research points to brain processes involving the limbic system encoding the rewarding aspect of food intake along with emotional and cognitive aspects. These brain processes lead to an overconsumption of food even when the person feels full. Obesity, like drug addiction, involves disruptions in the dopamine pathways of the brain, which modulate behavioral responses to environmental cues.

According to WHO, obesity worldwide has doubled since 1980. Data also show that from 1971 to 2006, BMI ratios in the United States have increased no matter when the person was born. This suggests it is not a cohort or age effect. According to the CDC, overweight and obese individuals are at higher risk for a number of physical disorders. Depression has also been linked to obesity. In addition to an individual's actual weight, there is also the person's attitude toward his or her weight. In some cultures, being heavier in weight is seen as positive whereas in others, it is thinness that is sought. Males and females think about their weight differently. Studies around the world have shown that females tend to overestimate their weight whereas males tend to underestimate their weight.

The three major eating disorders in *DSM–5* are anorexia nervosa, bulimia, and binge eating disorder. There is good evidence that eating disorders have a partial genetic component. Those with eating disorders experience a number of serious medical conditions related to reducing body weight or purging.

DSM–5 criteria for a diagnosis of anorexia nervosa include a restriction of food that results in a weight that is below normal, a fear of gaining weight, and a lack of recognition of the seriousness of current body weight and a distortion of how body weight is experienced. The body image distortion has been described as having a perceptual, an emotional, and a cognitive component, and research shows that each component involves different areas of the brain. *DSM–5* describes two subtypes of anorexia: (1) the restricting type and (2) the binge-eating or purging type. Individuals with anorexia tend to have certain personality characteristics that can be thought of as an endophenotype: (1) anxious with anxiety that exists before the onset of anorexia nervosa and continues even after treatment; (2) perfectionistic with an overemphasis on self-imposed standards; (3) difficulty in flexibility and changing rule structures; and (4) obsessiveness around order, exactness, and symmetry. Individuals with anorexia nervosa develop a variety of medical problems that may be related to lack of nutrition and changes in hormones. The specific causes of anorexia nervosa are still being researched. However, there appear to be a variety of factors involved including (1) genetics, (2) physiological factors resulting from restricting the intake of food, and (3) cultural factors. Anorexia nervosa is seen as one of the most difficult disorders to treat. Many individuals with anorexia do not want to be treated. The disorder itself results in psychological and physiological changes, and many individuals deny that they actually have a disorder. One of the first tasks for someone with anorexia nervosa is to gain weight. This often requires a hospital stay. Psychological or family therapy is typically the next step. Family therapy has strong support with adolescents. With adults, CBT has been shown to be an effective approach. Currently, there is no good evidence to suggest a critical role for medication in the treatment of anorexia nervosa.

There are three major characteristics of bulimia nervosa: (1) binge eating in which the person consumes large amounts of food; (2) purging where a person eliminates food from the body by such means as vomiting, taking laxatives, diuretics, or enemas; and (3) a psychological aspect in which one's self-worth is seen in relation to one's weight or body shape. Bulimia nervosa can also lead to secondary medical problems related to vomiting and the overuse of medications such as laxatives. CBT is more effective than medication in the treatment of bulimia nervosa.

Binge eating disorder is characterized by the consumption of large amounts of food and the sense that one cannot control his or her eating behavior. It is more prevalent in those who are overweight than those who are of normal weight. There is evidence to suggest that binge eating runs in families and is not related to obesity per se. Overall, the goals of treatment are to cease binge eating, to reduce negative emotions and cognitions, and to lose weight. Psychosocial treatments, especially CBT, have been shown to be effective. At times, other approaches such as exercise have been added to CBT treatments. Drug treatments such as the use of antidepressant medication show limited evidence of success.

STUDY RESOURCES

Review Questions

1. What we eat and how we eat represent a complex relationship between all levels of human functioning including culture, evolutionary history, genetics, our physiology, preferences, and psychological attitudes toward our appearance and that of others. What is an example of each of these levels?

2. Historically, feeding disorders were categorized with other childhood disorders; now they are part of a more general feeding and eating disorders grouping. What are some of the advantages of this change? Are there any disadvantages?
3. "Researchers have asked if similar mechanisms are involved in both obesity and drug addiction." What evidence can you cite to support the position that obesity is like drug addiction? Does the evidence convince you? Why or why not?
4. What is it about eating disorders that makes them so difficult to treat? If you were asked to put together an awareness program about eating disorders targeting a college-age audience, what information would you include, and what approach would you take?

For Further Reading

Le Grange, D., & Lock, J. (Eds.). (2011). *Eating disorders in children and adolescents: A clinical handbook.* New York: Guilford Press.

Key Terms and Concepts

anorexia nervosa	bulimia nervosa	obesity
avoidant/restrictive food intake disorder	eating disorders	pica
	feeding and eating disorders	purging
binge eating disorder	feeding disorders	rumination disorder

CHAPTER

13

Sexuality Disorders and Gender Dysphoria

CHAPTER OUTLINE

- HISTORICAL PERSPECTIVES 436
- SEXUAL ACTIVITIES OF AMERICANS 438
- SEXUAL AROUSAL AND SEXUAL DRIVE 439
- SEXUAL AROUSAL 444
- NORMAL SEXUAL FUNCTIONING 445
- SEXUAL DYSFUNCTION DISORDERS 450
- TREATMENT APPROACHES FOR SEXUAL DYSFUNCTION DISORDERS 454
- PARAPHILIC DISORDERS 457
- TREATMENT APPROACHES FOR PARAPHILIC DISORDERS 464
- GENDER DYSPHORIA 465
- OTHER INDIAN WORK ON GENDER DYSPHORIA, GENDER IDENTITY ISSUES AND THEIR MANAGEMENT 469
- SUMMARY 470
- STUDY RESOURCES 473

I am not talking about my many—indeed many thousands—instances of lusting after girls' and women's bodies while giving little thought to relating to them as persons. As I noted before, frotteurism was a ubiquitous part of my life from my fifteenth year to my nineteenth year—during which time I bestrode the New York subways (and many of my female fellow passengers) with vim, vigor, and vitality. Lusting after women's fore and aft parts is only moderately reprehensible. Debatably, it can be viewed as minimally harassing as long as one keeps one's big mouth shut—which I invariably did.

Many people may not understand how, being born female, I can state with total clarity and certainty that as a child I felt like a boy. That's mainly because most people don't know the difference between gender and gender identity. Gender is the sex that one is born as, and for most of us that sex is either female or male. Your gender identity, however, is based on feelings and not biology. I like to say that your gender identity is between your ears, not between your legs. I am here to attest to the fact that you can be born one sex and yet feel with every fiber of your being that you really are the opposite. And as a kid, it was no more complicated to me than this: I felt like a little boy.

The World Health Organization (WHO) estimates that more than 100 million acts of sexual intercourse between humans take place each day around the world. Thus, sexuality is a driving force in humans as well as other species. Unlike most other species, humans are one of the few species that engages in sexual intercourse while looking at one another. This suggests that sexual activity has an important pair bonding and social component for humans beyond that of procreation. Humans also spend more time in the sex act itself than other species. For example, unlike male chimpanzees who go from penile penetration to ejaculation in only 90 seconds, humans take around 7 minutes preceded by 12 minutes of foreplay (Miller & Byers, 2004). Seven out of 10 American adults questioned reported spending 15 minutes to 1 hour overall making love. Other species such as some primates only engage in sexual activity when there is a high probability of producing offspring. Humans, on the other hand, can and do engage in sexual activity at any time. Overall, humans use the internal experience of sexual arousal and the external experience of sexual activity for a variety of purposes (see Levay & Baldwin, 2012, for an overview). Some of these experiences enhance people and their relationships with themselves and others. Other sexual experiences, on the other hand, can lead to distress. In this chapter, I want to discuss with you sexual experiences of both types.

HISTORICAL PERSPECTIVES

Humans have depicted sexual activities in painting and carving for thousands of years. Some of the more famous are the Etruscan ceramic plates showing a variety of sexual positions dating from some 2,500 years ago in Italy. With the excavation of Pompeii and Herculaneum near Naples, Italy, a variety of scenes were discovered on the walls in the cities that graphically depicted sexual activities. These towns were covered by volcanic ash when Mount Vesuvius erupted in 79 CE. Similar sexual illustrations have been found throughout the world.

India—The Land of the Kamasutra

Although a large part of Indian society is traditional and does not encourage discussion of sex and sexuality, it is also credited with the Kamasutra, an ancient Indian text written by sage Vatsyayana. This Sanskrit text contains discussions about sexuality, choice of sexual partner, and practical information such as positions for sexual intercourse. It also discusses the nature of love and connects pleasure and spirituality.

Indian philosophy is also enriched with concepts such as *Ardhanaareeswara*, a symbolic representation of male and female as one, of a combination of constructive and generative power. The concept derives from *Samkhya* philosophy which talks of *Purusha* (the male energy) and *Prakriti* (the female energy) within humanity. A combination of the two is thought to create cosmic energy. The concept may also be linked with the biological fact that the male and female reproductive organs and genitals both develop from same tissue in the fetus.

At another level, India is also credited with the origin of the Dhat syndrome, often construed as a culture-bound sexual neurosis that has now been reported from other Asian countries as well. Patients complaining of Dhat syndrome commonly present with depression, anxiety, and multiple non-specific somatic symptoms. They complain of sexual dysfunction and easy fatigability. Cognitive symptoms, such as, lack of concentration, are reported too, and all of this is attributed to semen loss due to masturbation. Once patients are helped deal with the myths and misconceptions about masturbation, there is some symptoms of relief. However, depression and anxiety are common comorbidities with Dhat syndrome in particular and sexual dysfunctions in general.

However, at certain times, some cultures have seen sexual activity as a negative force in human life. In the 18th and 19th centuries in Europe and the United States, there were those in the medical profession who suggested that sexual stimulation, especially masturbation, could lead to mental illness. In the 1800s, both graham crackers and unsweetened corn flakes were introduced as an aid for reducing sexual desire. John Kellogg was a physician who ran the Battle Creek Sanitarium in Michigan and crusaded against masturbation. His brother added sugar to the corn flakes and sold them through his Kellogg's company.

In the 1800s, a number of scientists began to approach sexuality from a scientific perspective. Charles Darwin presented the manner in which sexual selection and self-preservation were important instincts seen across many species. Sigmund Freud emphasized the manner in which sexuality was an important driving force in humans. Havelock Ellis in England was one of the first to study human sexuality itself. From 1897 to 1910, Ellis published a series of books entitled *Studies in the Psychology of Sex*. In these books, he suggested variations in sexuality should be viewed statistically in terms of frequency. He also suggested that variations in sexual practices had their roots in normal sexual practices. Ellis also went against a common notion at that time and suggested that females—like males—have sexual desires and seek and enjoy sex. Further, he suggested that a gay or lesbian orientation was a normal variation of human sexuality and should not be viewed as a disorder. He also suggested that homosexual tendencies were present at birth.

In the 1930s, Alfred Kinsey, a zoologist, was asked to teach a course on marriage. In preparing for the course, Kinsey realized that little was known about the sexual behavior of Americans. Further, students found it difficult to obtain factual information free of moral or social perspectives. This led Kinsey to conduct a large-scale survey of some 12,000 individuals across the United States. The results of these surveys were published in two books: *Sexual Behavior in the Human Male* (Kinsey, 1948) and *Sexual Behavior in the Human Female* (Kinsey, 1953). In 1947, the Institute for Sex Research was established at Indiana University with Alfred Kinsey as director. This was later renamed the Kinsey Institute and continues performing research related to sexuality (www.kinseyinstitute.org/about/index.html).

The original Kinsey survey focused on six different outlets to sexual orgasm. These six were masturbation, petting, nocturnal dreams, heterosexual coitus, homosexual behaviors, and bestiality. These six outlets were related in terms of frequency to various socioeconomic variables such as age, education, marital status, occupation, and religious identification. Prevailing cultural myth was that females merely engaged in sex for procreative purposes or to please their male partners. Many Americans in the 1950s were shocked to learn that females are as capable as males of sexual response. Further, 50% of the females interviewed had engaged in premarital coitus and 25% had engaged in extramarital sex. In addition, 84% of the males and 69% of the females reported being aroused by sexual fantasies. Also, 89% of the males and 64% of the females used fantasy as part of masturbation. Even more shocking to some was the number of males and females who reported they had masturbated (92% for males and 62% for females). Some newspapers and magazines refused to publish stories about this survey and its data. Some lawmakers even suggested it undermined the moral fiber of the nation.

SEXUAL ACTIVITIES OF AMERICANS

To understand sexual disorders, it is important to gain a perspective on sexual activities in the general population. In 2002, the Centers for Disease Control and Prevention (CDC) performed a survey that included face-to-face interviews with a national sample of 12,571 males and females in the United States. In order to obtain more accurate information, the information in this survey related to sexuality was collected using a laptop computer without communicating it directly with the interviewer. As can be seen in *Figure 13-1*, among males and females 25 to 44 years of age, 97% of males and 98% of females have had vaginal intercourse. Further, 90% of males and 88% of females have had oral sex with a member of the opposite sex. Anal sex with the opposite sex was lower: 40% for males and 35% for females. In this survey, same-sex contact was 7% for males and 11% for females. According to the National Survey of Sexual Health and Behavior (NSSHB), about 8% of men and 7% of women identify as gay, lesbian, or bisexual (www.nationalsexstudy.indiana.edu/; see Herbenick et al., 2010, for an overview). More women see themselves as bisexual than men (about 3.6% vs. 2.5%). More men see themselves as gay (approximately 4.2%) than there are women who see themselves as lesbian (approximately 0.9%).

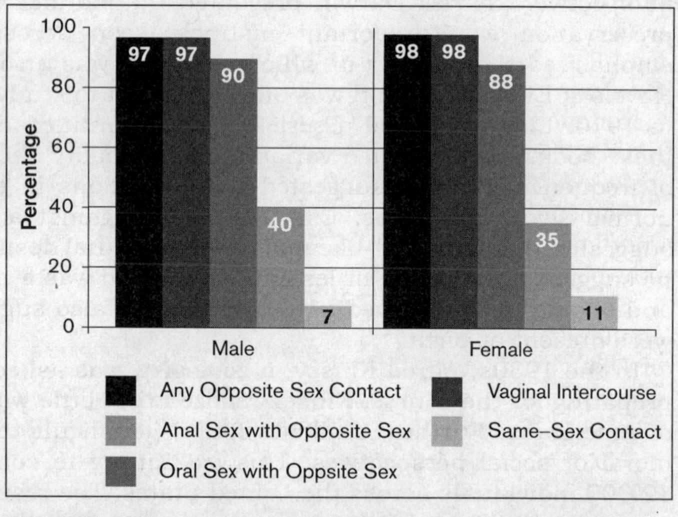

FIGURE 13-1 Percentage of Males and Females 25–44 Years of Age Who Have Had Each Type of Sexual Contact, United States, 2002

Source: Mosher, Chandra, and Jones (2005).

In 2010, the Center for Sexual Health Promotion at Indiana University's School of Health, Physical Education and Recreation published a comprehensive study on sexual attitudes and behaviors. The survey included descriptions of more than 40 combinations of sexual acts that people perform during sexual events, the use of condoms, and the percentage of Americans participating in same-sex encounters. The survey gathered information from 5,865 adolescents and adults ages 14 to 94. This survey (see *Figure 13-2* on page 440) shows that sexual activity continues across the life span and that there is a variety in the types of sexual acts that humans engage in. It should be noted that the CDC study asked if a person had performed a specific sexual act whereas the Center for Sexual Health Promotion study asked if the sexual act had been performed in the past 12 months.

Indian Epidemiological Data

An epidemiological study of sexual disorders (Rao, Darshan, & Tandon, 2015) has been reported in the *Indian Journal of Psychiatry* with data collected from a rural population from South India. India has vast variations from rural to metropolitan, and there will be lot of differences across these various populations. This study by Rao et al. (2015) reports that 21.15% of the male subjects were diagnosed to have one (or more) sexual disorder. "Prevalence of erectile dysfunction was found to be 15.77%, male hypoactive sexual desire disorder (HSDD) 2.56%; premature ejaculation was found to be prevalent in 8.76% of the male subjects" (Rao et al., 2015).

The authors also report that 14% of the female subjects were diagnosed to have female sexual disorders, with female arousal dysfunction seen in 6.65%, and female HSDD 8.87%, female anorgasmia in 5.67%. Female dyspareunia was found in 2.34% and female sexual aversion disorder was found to be prevalent in 0.37% of the female subjects.

The same research group also explored sexual disorders among the elderly in rural South India and found that only 27.4% of the individuals above 60 years were sexually active. Sexual activity dropped as age advanced and none were active after 75 years of age. The study also reports the percentage prevalence of various disorders in the elderly, for example, 43.5% of erectile dysfunction among the sexually active males, premature ejaculation in 10.9%, hypoactive sexual desire disorder (HSSD) in 0.77%, and anorgasmia in 0.38% of the subjects. They report that among females, arousal disorder was prevalent in 28%, HSSD in 16%, anorgasmia in 20%, and dyspareunia in 8%.

Some Indian data is also presented by Varghese et al. in the *International Urogynecological Journal* of 2012 with similar findings. The study was done at CMC Vellore and demonstrated that poorer QOL is associated with sexual dysfunctions in women.

Similar studies from other large tertiary care centers all over India have reported similar frequencies of referral. A common factor that seems to emerge is the occurrence of Dhat syndrome among unmarried males, reflecting a clear psychosocial correlate of sexual disorders and beliefs held about sexually taboo behaviors.

SEXUAL AROUSAL AND SEXUAL DRIVE

The desire for sex has been described in a variety of ways in the scientific literature using words such as *drive, arousal, need, desire, obsession,* and *motivation.* Heiman and Pfaff (2011) have attempted to clarify these terms in terms of sexual activity. Arousal has

Age-Groups																				
Sexual Behaviors	*14–15*		*16–17*		*18–19*		*20–24*		*25–29*		*30–39*		*40–49*		*50–59*		*60–69*		*70+*	
	Men	*Women*	*Men*	*Women*	*Men*	*Women*	*Men*	*Women*	*Men*	*Women*	*Men*	*Women*	*Men*	*Women*	*Men*	*Women*	*Men*	*Women*	*Men*	*Women*
Masturbated Alone	62%	40%	75%	45%	81%	60%	83%	64%	84%	72%	80%	63%	76%	65%	72%	54%	61%	47%	46%	33%
Masturbated With Partner	5%	8%	16%	19%	42%	36%	44%	36%	49%	48%	45%	43%	38%	35%	28%	18%	17%	13%	13%	5%
Received Oral From Women	12%	1%	31%	5%	54%	4%	63%	9%	77%	3%	78%	5%	62%	2%	49%	1%	38%	1%	19%	2%
Received Oral From Men	1%	10%	3%	24%	6%	58%	6%	70%	5%	72%	6%	59%	6%	52%	8%	34%	3%	25%	2%	8%
Gave Oral to Women	8%	2%	18%	7%	51%	2%	55%	9%	74%	3%	69%	4%	57%	3%	44%	1%	34%	1%	24%	2%
Gave Oral to Men	1%	12%	2%	22%	4%	59%	7%	74%	5%	76%	5%	59%	7%	53%	8%	36%	3%	23%	3%	7%
Vaginal Intercourse	9%	11%	30%	30%	53%	62%	63%	80%	86%	87%	85%	74%	74%	70%	58%	51%	54%	42%	43%	22%
Received Penis in Anus	1%	4%	1%	5%	4%	18%	5%	23%	4%	21%	3%	22%	4%	12%	5%	6%	1%	4%	2%	1%
Inserted Penis Into Anus	3%		6%		6%		11%		27%		24%		21%		11%		6%		2%	

FIGURE 13-2 Percentage of Americans Performing Certain Sexual Behaviors in the Past Year

Source: Herbenick et al. (2010).

traditionally been seen as a general term in relation to central nervous system activity. An organism can be aroused without being sexually motivated. However, sexual motivation and arousal go together. Motivation has been described in terms of an organism performing an act that has a positive reward. A related concept is that of drive, which traditionally reflects a state of need. In this sense, hunger or thirst is seen as a drive when the organism lacks food or water, and this is reflected in the internal physiological processes. Freud and Havelock Ellis described sex as a drive although current theories suggest this concept may not explain human sexuality. Human sexuality also carries with it a social or pair-bonding relationship that moves it beyond a simple drive.

Like many human processes, sexual arousal and desire take place on a number of levels in a complex manner. There are cognitive considerations through which an individual may increase desire or choose to inhibit sexual activity. Thoughts, images, and other human cognitive processes can both increase and decrease desire. This level of functioning is only beginning to be understood in terms of sexual disorders. There are also emotional experiences contained within the sexual experience, which may include joy and love. There is also the physical level of functioning, which includes the activities included in sexual encounters. Our experience of these levels also involves our culture, as shown in the following LENS on page 442.

Within the cognitive, emotional, and physical level, one important research question has been the manner in which measurements can be made. With the advent of psychophysiological techniques to measure blood flow in the sexual organs of males and females, a different type of precision is possible. However, as with a number of psychophysiological measures, the relationship between changes in physiology and the experienced cognitions and feelings may not be exact. More recently, measures of brain activity using such brain imaging techniques as electroencephalography (EEG) or functional magnetic resonance imaging (fMRI) allow for an understanding of cortical involvement. Sexual responding in a variety of species is related to specific external signals that are related to the possibility of conception. Humans, on the other hand, can also respond to internal thoughts and continued sexual arousal even without external stimuli.

In the popular media, men are often portrayed as thinking about sex much more often than women. However, clear research has not been available. In order to study the differences between men and women in cognitions, college students were asked to click a small counter every time they thought about sex, food, and sleep (Fisher, Moore, & Pittenger, 2012). These data show that men did indeed think more about sex than women. However, they also thought more about food and about sleep than women did. Statistical analyses did not show that either males or females thought differently about food, sleep, and sex. Thus, the gender differences may relate to appetites in general rather than a specific domain.

In studies of sexual orientation, including heterosexual, homosexual, and bisexual individuals, it has been shown that these different groups are aroused by different types of stimuli. One study examined self-reported arousal in males as well as changes in penis size in relation to videos of explicit sexual interactions (Cerny & Janssen, 2011). Males who identified themselves as heterosexual, homosexual, or bisexual were asked to watch videos of males and females engaging in sex, males engaging in sex, and scenes including both males and females in a bisexual situation. As in previous research, heterosexual males showed the most changes in erections and self-report arousal to the heterosexual videos. They also showed the least changes to the homosexual videos. Both bisexual and homosexual men showed similar changes to the homosexual videos. However, the bisexual males showed the greatest changes to the bisexual videos. Overall, this research suggests that males show both subjective and physiological arousal in a manner that is consistent with their sexual orientation.

Your Brain and Sexual Activity

Brain imaging studies allow for cortical measures of arousal in addition to self-report and blood flow changes in sexual organs. Overall, when both males and females achieve orgasm, there are changes in the brain. In males, areas involved in vigilance shut down. When males experience an ejaculation, positron emission testing (PET) studies show that the same areas of the midbrain (e.g., the ventral tegmental area (VTA) show activity as when a person takes heroin. In females, areas involved in controlling thoughts and emotions become silent (see Portner, 2008, for an overview).

13-1 LENS
Sexuality and the Clashing of Cultures

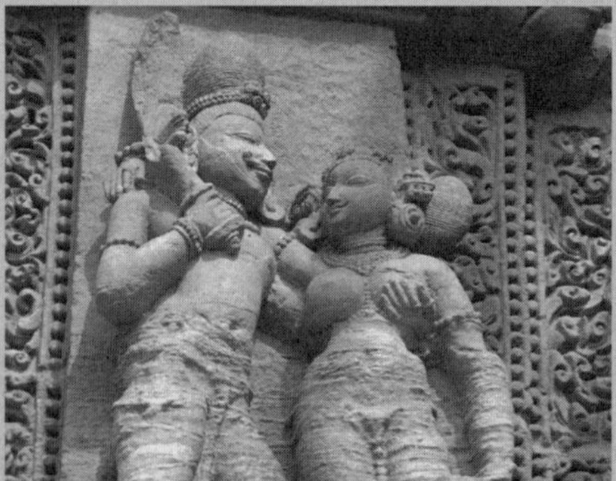

Eleventh century carving on the Rajarani temple, known as the love temple, in Bhubaneshwar, India

From an evolutionary perspective, all humans seek sexual experiences. Let us begin with the culture of the U.S. college student (McAnulty, 2012). Over the past 100 years, relationships between college students in the United States have gone from "dating" to "hooking up." In between were periods of openness and free love in the 1960s. By the 1970s, few colleges tried to "protect" women with required curfews. During the 1970s, coed dorms were set up in many colleges. A similarity of rules and other changes within the culture led to a greater sense of empowerment. Premarital sex for those who were age 20 increased from 48% in the 1950s to 65% in the 1960s to 70+% for the rest of the century (Finer, 2007).

Recent studies on college students suggest that 61% of young women and 70% of young men report having initiated sex within 6 months of a relationship. Although the popular press emphasizes "hooking up" among college students, surveys suggest it is less frequent than suggested and involves sexual activity only about half of the time. Also, it is estimated that 24% of college students are virgins. Similar sexual activity data in terms of gay and lesbian individuals is difficult to determine.

Both the implicit and explicit rules related to sexuality vary greatly from culture to culture. Some nonindustrialized cultures encourage adolescents to experiment with and engage in sex play whereas others discourage any display of public affection. Among the industrial countries, Europe, Australia, and the United States report the greatest satisfaction with sexual experiences and East Asian countries the least (Laumann et al., 2006). There was also a strong association between relationship satisfaction and sexual satisfaction. This is also reflected in the WHO report that a quarter of married couples in Japan had not had sex in the past year whereas the Kinsey Institute reported a 5% to 10% rate for American couples although the rate does go up after age 50. Likewise, in one survey, the average number of times a 16- to 45-year-old in Hong Kong had sex in a year was 57 times compared with 138 times for an American and 141 for a French person ("Durex Global Sex Surveys," 1996, 1998).

Although finding a mate and sexual behaviors are present in all cultures, the ease of migration throughout the world brings together a plethora of attitudes toward sexual relationships. This has resulted, for example, in Germany banning a custom of some of its immigrants: forced marriages. In 2006, the Netherlands introduced a change in its immigration law. One change requires that those seeking to immigrate to the Netherlands watch a 108-minute film that includes nudity at a beach and same-sex couples kissing. The basic idea is that the person who seeks to move to the Netherlands should understand the types of sexual activities that take place in the country. Although all humans share a search for sexuality, it is the culture that shapes the process.

Antonio Ferretti and his colleagues showed males erotic videos in a scanner (Ferretti et al., 2005). By using longer videos, these researchers were able to measure changes in penile tumescence, which led to an erection along with self-reports of arousal and fMRI measures. In comparison with a sports film, the erotic video was associated with brain changes in the inferior parietal lobule and precuneus, cuneus, extrastriatal visual cortices, frontal cortices, hippocampus, and amygdala (see *Figure 13-3*). Further, specific areas of the brain were correlated with the transition from no erection (NE) to the beginning of erection (OE) to a full erection (SE). These areas include anterior cingulate, insula, amygdala, hypothalamus, and secondary somatosensory cortices. Overall, the processing of sexual arousal involves complex brain networks involving cognitive, emotional, and self-processes.

Do men and women look at different aspects of a picture depicting sexual activity? One way to answer this question is to use eye tracking, which measures where a person looks when viewing stimuli in real time. One study suggests that both males and females look at the bodies of opposite sex nudes rather than the faces (Lykins, Meana, & Kambe, 2006). In another study, while viewing sexually explicit photographs of heterosexual couples engaged in intercourse or oral sex, males spent more time looking at the face of the female whereas females spent more time looking at genitals (Rupp & Wallen, 2007). Females who were taking birth control pills spent less time looking at the sexual characteristics of the picture. Females also spent less time looking at sexually related characteristics in nonsexually related pictures (Nielsen & Pernice, 2008). From an evolutionary perspective, this suggests that there is a close relationship between what attracts one's attention and the ability to conceive.

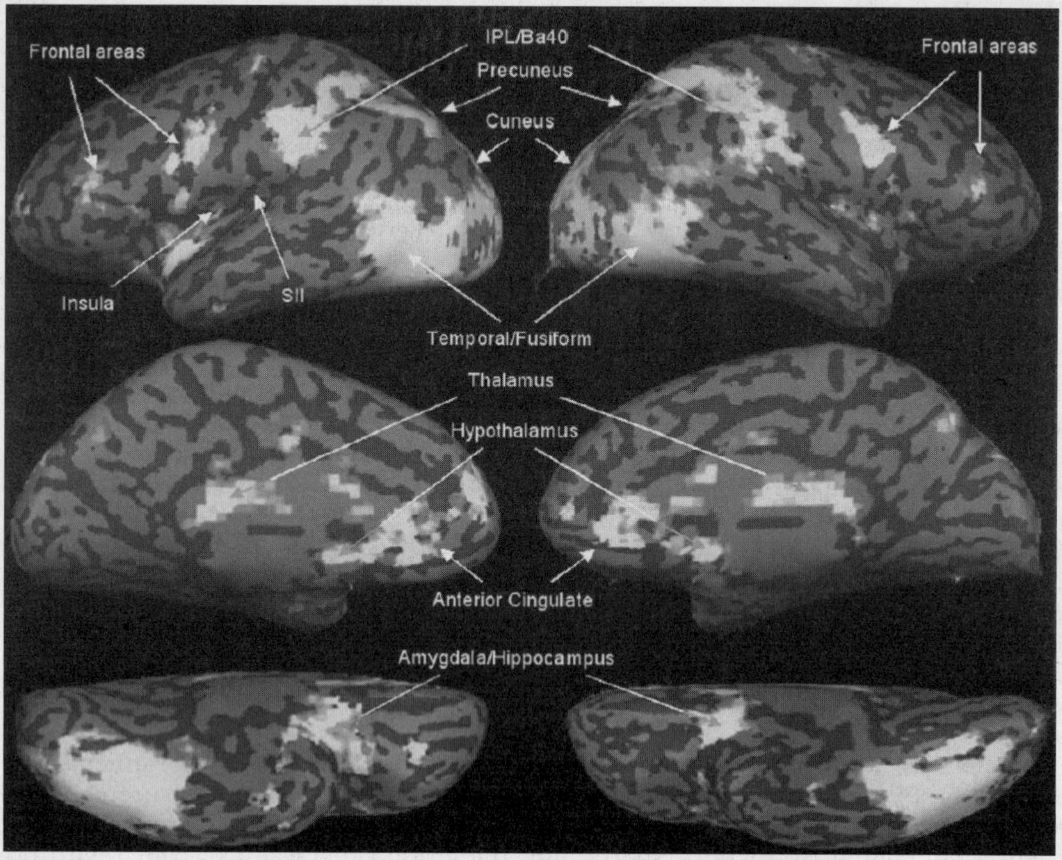

FIGURE 13-3 Group Results: Cortical Areas That Are Significantly More Active (Larger BOLD Signal) During Erotic as Compared With Sport Visual Stimulation With Video Clips

Source: Ferretti et al. (2005, p. 1090), with permission from Elsevier.
Note: Light and dark gray indicate gyri and sulci, respectively.

SEXUAL AROUSAL

Since the term *sexual arousal* was introduced to the scientific literature in the 1930s, it has referred to a number of distinct processes (see Janssen, 2011; Sachs, 2007, for overviews). The term has been used in a psychological sense to refer to the internal experience of both cognitive and emotional processes. It has also been used in a physiological sense to refer to hormonal changes, brain changes, and changes in sexual organs related to blood flow. It is also the case that the subjective experience of arousal and genital physiological responses and arousal may not go together. In terms of gender differences, males show a higher correlation between genital responses and subjective sexual arousal than women (Chivers, Pittini, Grigoriadis, Villegas, & Ross, 2010). This has led some researchers to suggest that females are more sensitive to the situational context in which sexual activity takes place than are males.

NORMAL SEXUAL FUNCTIONING

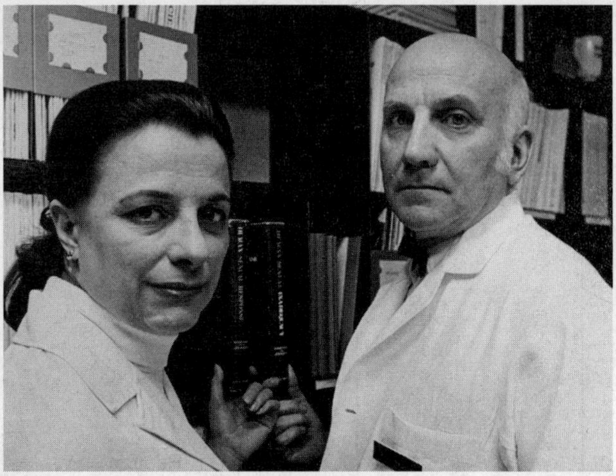

Masters and Johnson
© Bettmann/Corbis

In the 1960s, William Masters and Virginia Johnson began laboratory studies of the human sexual response by observing couples engaging in sexual activities. Although sexual activity has been studied in animals for at least 200 years, human laboratory studies were first reported in the 1960s. Before this time, little was known concerning what happens to our bodies as we become aroused and engage in sexual activity. In order to understand these processes, Masters and Johnson created instruments that were able to film and measure changes in male and female sexual responsiveness during arousal and sex. Masters and Johnson also studied clinical populations to help treat sexual and reproductive problems. Their major books include *Human Sexual Response* (1966), *Human Sexual Inadequacy* (1970), and *Homosexuality in Perspective* (1979). For your information, *Figures 13-4* through *13-6* show the anatomy of males and females in relation to sexual functioning.

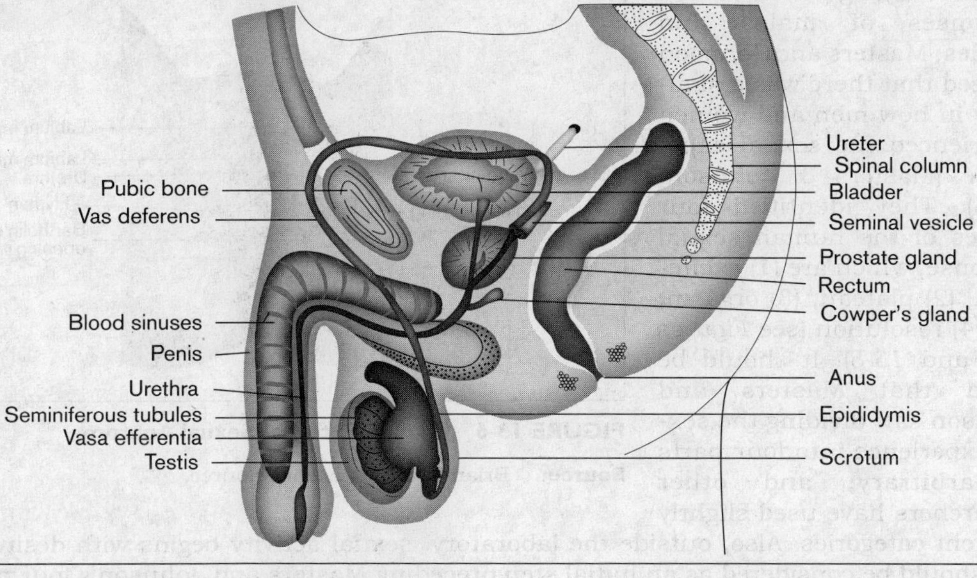

FIGURE 13-4 Male Reproductive System

Source: Kimball's Biology Pages © John W. Kimball.

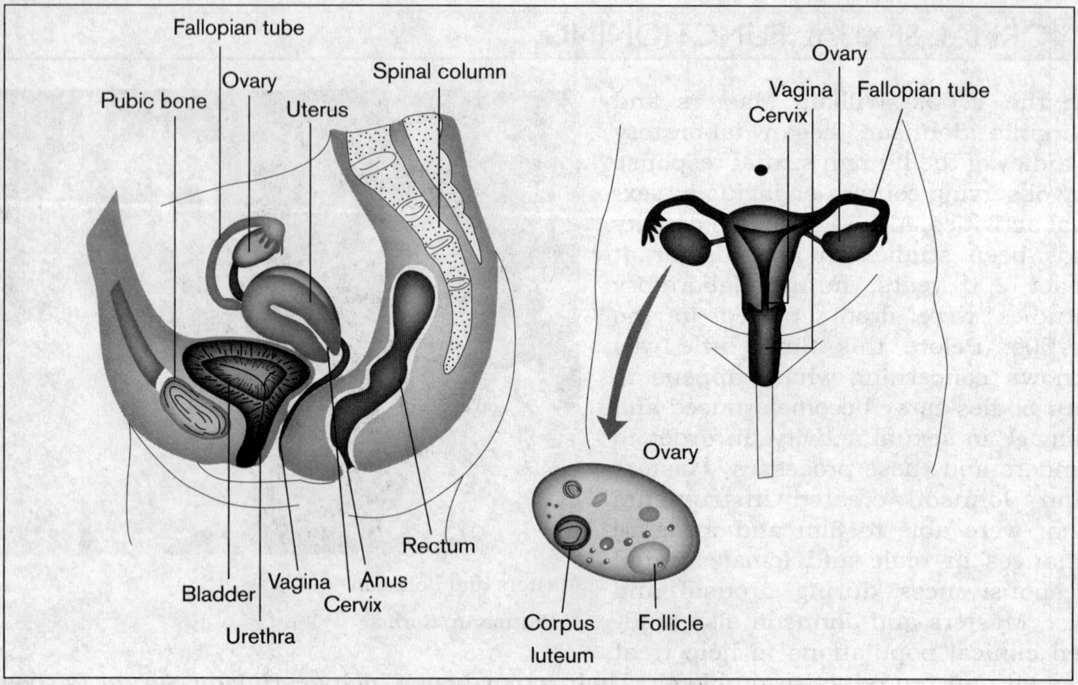

FIGURE 13-5 Female Reproductive System

Source: Kimball's Biology Pages © John W. Kimball.

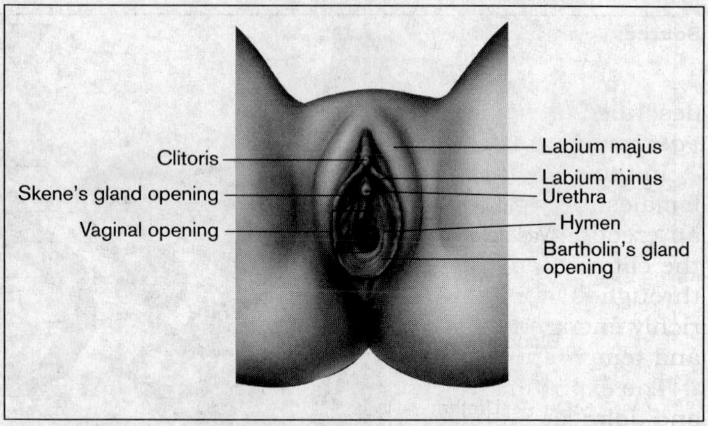

FIGURE 13-6 Female External Sexual Anatomy

Source: © Brian Evans / Science Source.

In studying the sexual responses of males and females, Masters and Johnson realized that there was a similarity in how men and women experienced the sexual experience (Masters & Johnson, 1966). They identified four phases of the human sexual response, which are (1) excitement, (2) plateau, (3) orgasm, and (4) resolution (see *Figures 13-7* and *13-8*). It should be noted that Masters and Johnson saw dividing the sexual experience into four parts as arbitrary, and other researchers have used slightly different categories. Also, outside the laboratory, sexual activity begins with desire, and this should be considered as an initial step preceding Masters and Johnson's four phases (see Wincze & Carey, 2001, for an overview). The four phases of sexual response can be

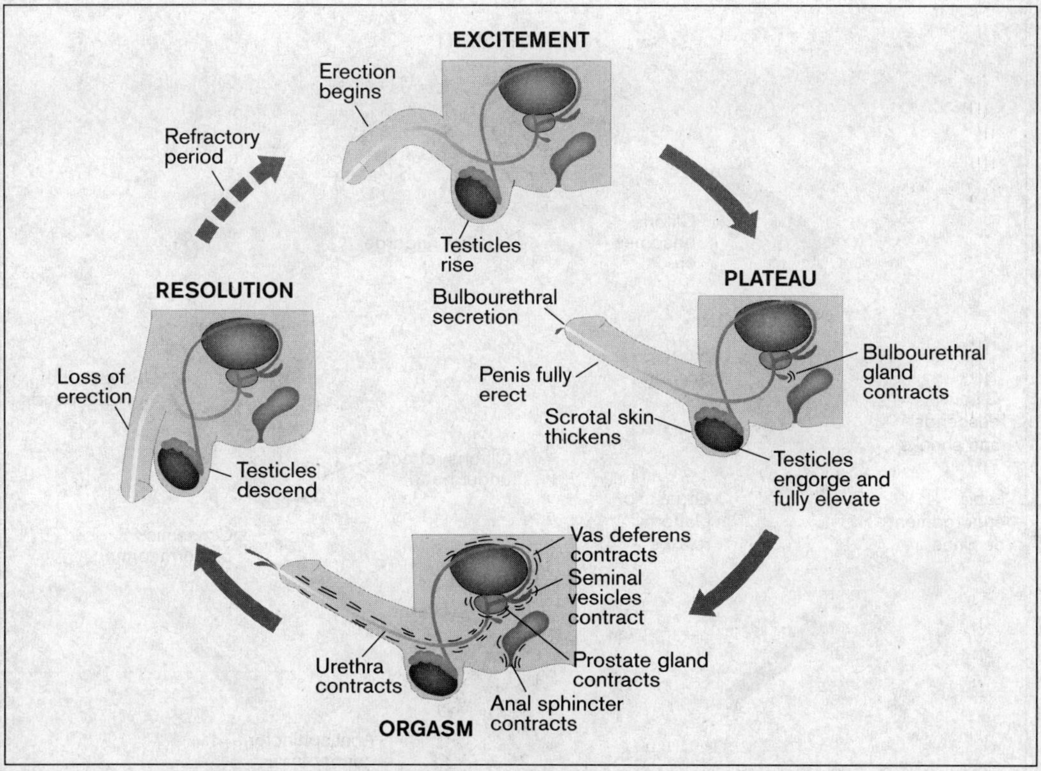

FIGURE 13-7 Genital Changes in Men During the Sexual Response Cycle

Source: Levay and Baldwin (2012, p. 241).

described on a variety of levels. The two main ones are blood flow, which is referred to as *vasocongestion,* and muscular tension, which is referred to as *myotonia.*

In the excitement phase, blood flow is increased in the genital region in both males and females. This is both a physiological and a psychological state. In males, this results in an erection of the penis and the testes becoming elevated. In females, blood flow swells the clitoris and enlarges the labia. Also, the vagina begins to moisten. Excitement is felt throughout the body with increased muscle tension. Both the penis and the clitoris are richly endowed with nerve endings, which make them highly sensitive to touch, pressure, and temperature, which leads to the sensation of pleasure.

The experiences begun in the excitement phase continue during the second of Masters and Johnson's phases: the plateau phase. During this phase, most individuals pay little attention to external stimuli as the pleasurable internal experiences continue. In the male, the Cowper's glands, which are two pea-sized glands, release a substance that changes the pH of the urethra from the acidity of urine to protect the sperm that will be released during orgasm. Since this slippery substance appears between erection and ejaculation, it is colloquially referred to as pre-ejaculate or "pre-cum." During the plateau phase, there is also an increase in heart rate and breathing. Some individuals also show a flush throughout their body.

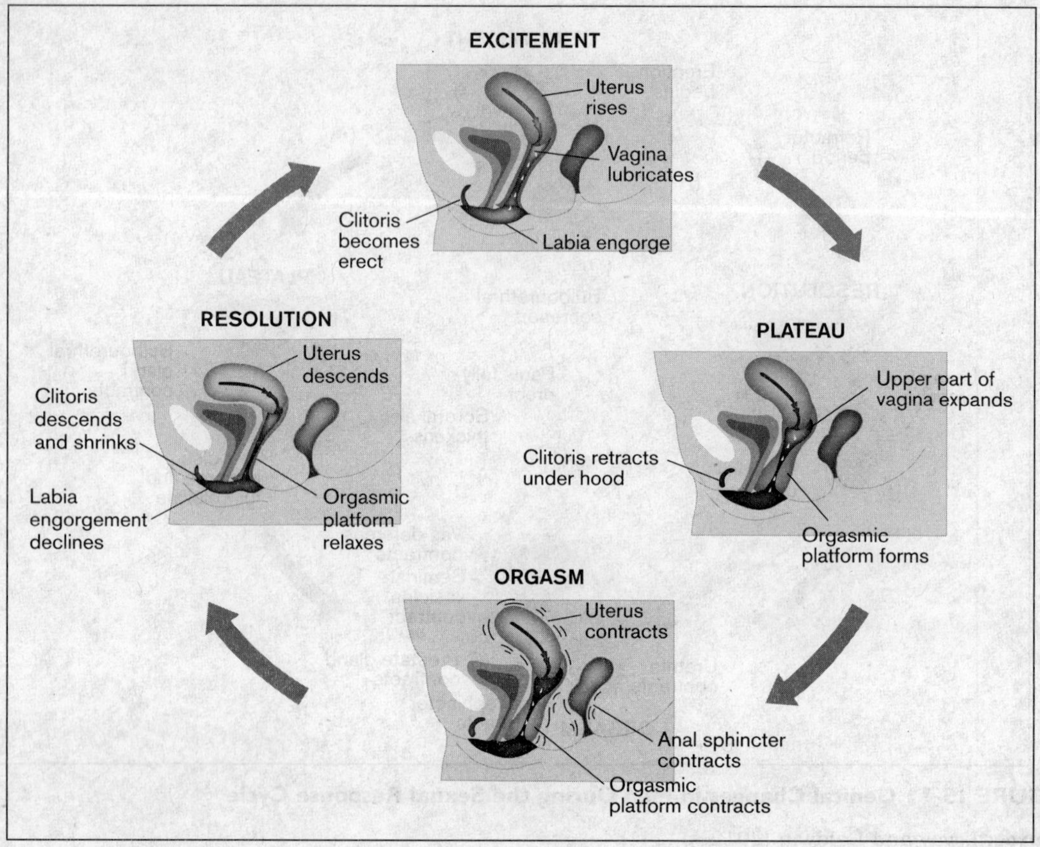

FIGURE 13-8 Genital Changes in Women During the Sexual Response Cycle

Source: Levay and Baldwin (2012, p. 240).

The tension of the plateau stage climaxes in the third phase—orgasm. Muscular contractions in the male cause the sperm from the testes to be released, become part of the seminal fluid from the prostate, and be expelled. This experience lasts only a few seconds. In the process of ejaculation, the internal sphincter of the bladder closes in a manner that both prevents semen under pressure from entering the bladder and urine from the bladder from becoming part of the seminal fluid. In females, pelvic muscles also contract in a somewhat rhythmical manner, which may lead to the experience of a climax. Both men and women show muscular spasms throughout their bodies.

The fourth phase is the resolution phase following orgasm. Both males and females return to pre-arousal levels during the resolution phase. This includes a decrease in blood flow and muscle tension. During resolution, males—unlike females—experience a time period in which they cannot achieve another orgasm. This time period generally increases with age (see *Figure 13-9*).

In the preceding section, you were introduced to a short history of sexuality in America and the types of sexual behaviors that we as humans engage in. Following this, I discussed the manner in which sexual arousal and drive have been scientifically

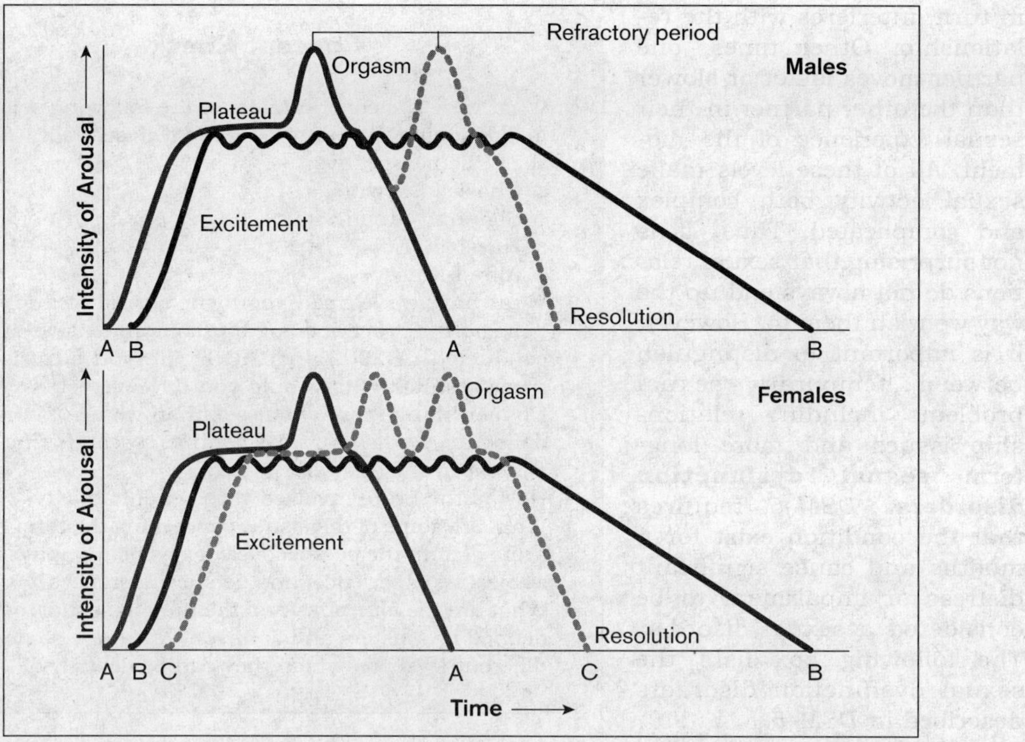

FIGURE 13-9 The Human Sexual Response in Terms of Masters and Johnson's Four Stages

Source: From NAIRNE. Psychology, 2E. © 2000 South-Western, a part of Cengage Learning, Inc. Reproduced by permission, www.cengage.com/permissions.

Note: The letters A, B, and C show different patterns of sexual responses seen in the study. Pattern A in males and females shows an orgasm. Pattern B shows a pattern that does not lead to orgasm. Pattern C shows multiple orgasms.

studied. This included an often-ignored organ of sexual arousal and activity: the brain. Next, the physiology of sexual experience and behavior was discussed. In the next section, I will discuss disorders related to sexual functioning from the fifth edition of the *Diagnostic and Statistical Manual of Mental Disorders* (*DSM–5*) (American Psychiatric Association [APA], 2013).

We all think about sexual activities. As humans, sexual functioning is important to us. We have ideas and fantasies concerning a sexual relationship. We also share our ideas with our partner, which may lead to emotional intimacy. Some couples find the emotional connectedness as critical to a meaningful sex life. There is also a physical aspect to sexuality.

As with any activity, there are times when our sexual functioning is not optimal. At times, individuals may not be in the mood for sexual activity. At other times, there may be a physical problem, such as diabetes, that interferes. Mental disorders such as depression and anxiety have also been shown to interfere with sexuality. At other times, it may be our attitude or desire at the moment that interferes. For example, we may have been trying to impress the other person or concerned about our performance. This, in turn, interferes with the relationship. Other times, one partner moves faster or slower than the other partner in their sexual experience of the moment. All of these levels make sexual activity both complex and complicated. Thus, it is not surprising that sexual relations do not always end up the way we wish them to. However, it is important to distinguish between temporary sexual problems including relationship issues and more long-term **sexual dysfunction disorders.** *DSM–5* requires that the condition exist for 6 months and cause significant distress or impairment to be considered a sexual disorder. The following box lists the sexual dysfunction disorders described in *DSM–5*.

Concept Check

- What were the contributions of the following scientists in advancing our understanding of sexuality from a scientific perspective:
  - Charles Darwin?
  - Sigmund Freud?
  - Havelock Ellis?
  - Alfred Kinsey?
- What have we learned about the sexual attitudes and behaviors of Americans from comprehensive surveys conducted in 2002 and 2010? Are you surprised by these results? What would you have expected?
- Do men think more about sex than women? What evidence do we have from scientific research that adds context to the answer?
- How is the brain involved with sexual activity?
- What are some of the issues concerning the term *sexual arousal* from the perspectives of psychology, physiology, subjective experience, and gender differences?
- What are the four phases of the human sexual response defined by Masters and Johnson? What are some of the different levels on which they can be described?

SEXUAL DYSFUNCTION DISORDERS

***DSM–5* Sexual Dysfunctions**

Erectile Disorder
Female Orgasmic Disorder
Delayed Ejaculation
Early Ejaculation
Female Sexual Interest/Arousal Disorder
Male Hypoactive Sexual Desire Disorder
Genito-Pelvic Pain/Penetration Disorder
Substance/Medication-Induced Sexual Dysfunction
Sexual Dysfunction Not Elsewhere Classified

As with other disorders, it is important to consider three perspectives in order to understand sexual dysfunction. The first includes medical and biological factors. A number of medical disorders, such as diabetes and vascular disease, can interfere with normal sexual functioning. Also, health conditions such as not exercising, not maintaining normal weight, and not limiting alcohol or tobacco can influence sexual responding. Shakespeare, referring to alcohol, noted in Macbeth, "It provoketh desire and taketh away the capacity."

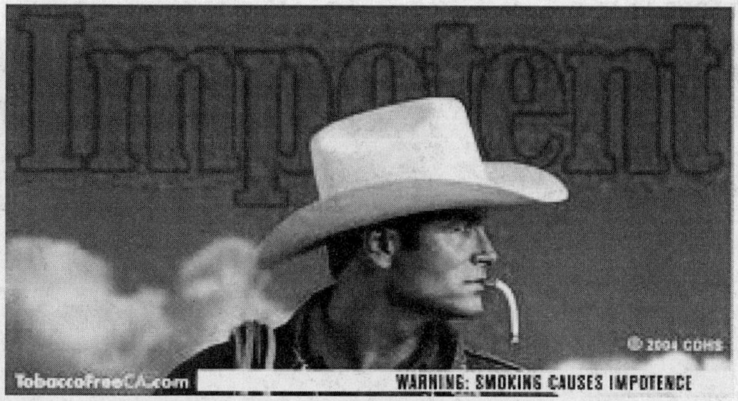

Poster from an antismoking campaign
Source: California Department of Public Health.

The second perspective is the psychological one. This can include previous experiences such as childhood abuse. It can also include such factors as performance anxiety. For example, if a person did not perform in the way he wished in a previous sexual encounter, then he may try too hard at the next one. Psychological conditions such as anxiety and depression have also been shown to influence sexual functioning. Some individuals also carry with them prohibitions they have been given by their parents, their culture, or their religion, which interfere with their sexual activity. The third perspective is the relationship itself. If there is an argument or previous situation in which someone had his or her feelings hurt, then this may inhibit sexual responding. Of course, good communication with a partner including desires and expectations can reduce some problems of sexual functioning.

Epidemiological data collected in the 1990s suggest that sexual dysfunctions are common. In a national sample of 1,749 women and 1,410 men ranging in age from 18 to 59, it was found that 43% of the women and 31% of the men reported sexual dysfunctions (Laumann, Paik, & Rosen, 1999). Specific dysfunctions reported by women were lack of interest in sex (31%), unable to achieve orgasm (approximately 26%), the experience of pain during sex (16%), sex not pleasurable (23%), anxious about performance (12%), and trouble lubricating (21%). Sexual dysfunctions reported by men were lack of interest (15%), unable to achieve orgasm (8%), climax too early (30%), sex not pleasurable (8%), anxious about performance (18%), and trouble maintaining or achieving an erection (10%). Since this was part of a larger health study, it was found that age, health, and stress were associated with sexual dysfunctions. A later study sought to update these data with an older population. *Table 13-1* shows the sexual problems reported by those 57 to 85 years of age. With aging, testosterone levels decline in men and influence sexual desire. Many men also show erectile dysfunction as they age. Women following menopause show a reduction in estrogen, which influences vaginal dryness. This, in turn, influences their desire to engage in sexual acts. Other medical conditions associated with aging can also influence sexual desire and responsiveness.

Sexual dysfunction disorders can be thought of in terms of four categories related to desire, arousal, orgasm, and pain. In *DSM–5,* sexual dysfunction disorders are characterized by changes in sexual desire as well as problems in the experience of the sexual act. These include problems of low interest or desire in both males and females, male erectile dysfunction, delayed or **early ejaculation,** and problems with a woman feeling pain during intercourse or not experiencing an orgasm. There is also a classification related to changes in sexual functioning related to taking a drug or medication.

TABLE 13-1 Prevalence of Sexual Problems by Age and Gender

	Women				*Men*			
	Percentage				*Percentage*			
	Age 57–64	*Age 65–74*	*Age 75–85*	*Trend Test*	*Age 57–64*	*Age 65–74*	*Age 75–85*	*Trend Test*
Lack of sexual interest	44.2 (3.7)	38.4 (4.4)	49.3 (6.2)	0.403	28.2 (3.5)	28.6 (2.9)	24.2 (3.9)	0.920
Erectile problems					30.7 (2.7)	44.6 (2.9)	43.5 (4.5)	<0.001
Vaginal lubrication problems	35.9 (3.2)	43.2 (4.2)	43.6 (7.8)	0.125				
Premature climax	9.2 (1.5)	6.9 (2.1)	8.5 (3.7)	0.874	29.6 (3.0)	28.1 (2.4)	21.3 (4.0)	0.406
Inability to climax	34.0 (3.0)	32.8 (3.9)	38.2 (7.2)	0.129	16.2 (2.1)	22.7 (2.6)	33.2 (4.1)	<0.001
Pain during intercourse	17.8 (2.2)	18.6 (3.9)	11.8 (3.7)	0.450	3.0 (0.9)	3.2 (1.0)	1.0 (0.7)	0.125
Lack of pleasure in sex	24.0 (3.0)	22.0 (3.5)	24.9 (5.0)	0.909	3.8 (0.7)	7.0 (1.7)	5.1 (1.9)	0.075
Performance anxiety	10.4 (2.1)	12.5 (3.2)	9.9 (4.1)	0.850	25.1 (2.0)	28.9 (3.0)	29.3 (4.7)	0.094
Avoided sex due to problems	34.3 (4.7)	30.5 (4.5)	22.7 (6.6)	0.114	22.1 (2.4)	30.1 (3.4)	25.7 (5.4)	0.256

Source: Waite, Laumann, Das, and Schumm (2009, p. i62), by permission of Oxford University Press.
Notes: These questions were asked only of participants reporting sex in the preceding year.

Erectile Disorder

Erectile disorder requires that a male has a problem in one of three areas. The first is that he cannot obtain an erection during sexual activity. The second is that he cannot maintain an erection until the completion of sexual activity. And the third is a decrease in the rigidity of the penis in a way that interferes with sexual activity. Further, the experience of the erectile problem produces significant distress. As noted previously, 10% of the men in one general population survey reported difficulties maintaining or achieving an erection. It should also be noted that with aging the ability to establish and maintain an erection changes. For example, various studies suggest that around 2.3% of 30- to 39-year-olds experience erectile dysfunction; this increases to 11% to 55% in one's 50s, 47% to 53% in the 70s, and 64% to 76% above 80 years of age (see Beutel, Weidner, & Brähler, 2006, for a review of these studies). By middle age, most men require some manual stimulation to achieve an erection.

There are a number of lifestyle factors that can influence erectile dysfunction. For example, smoking can double the risk of erectile dysfunction. Likewise, not exercising, being obese, and abusing alcohol can increase the probability of erectile dysfunction. Medical conditions such as diabetes, hypertension, and atherosclerosis as well as some psychotropic medications have an influence. There are also a large number of psychological factors including stress and relationship problems that influence erectile dysfunction.

Female Orgasmic Disorder

Female orgasmic disorder is the condition in which a woman either does not experience an orgasm or has a reduced intensity of the sensation of the orgasm. Further, this condition causes significant distress. The female orgasm has been a topic of much confusion (see Graham, 2009, for an overview). Unlike males in which orgasm is closely tied to puberty, the initial experience of orgasm in females may follow puberty by a number of years. Also, data suggest that females are more likely to have an orgasm during masturbation than with a partner. Another difference is that females are less likely to complain of having an orgasm too early in the sex act. Studies performed in both the United States and Europe suggest that orgasmic disorder is seen in between 20% and 30% of females (see Palacios, Castaño, & Grazziotin, 2009, for an overview).

Delayed Ejaculation

Delayed ejaculation is the situation (over a 6-month period) in which a male shows a delay in ejaculation or shows a lack of ejaculation and this causes significant distress (see Segraves, 2010, for an overview). Using a definition of ejaculatory problems as occurring on 75% of sexual experiences, the worldwide prevalence is somewhere around 2%. However, there is no clear agreement as to what would be considered delayed.

Early Ejaculation

Early ejaculation is diagnosed when a man experiences an ejaculation within approximately the first minute of sexual activity and this causes significant distress over a 6-month period (see Segraves, 2010, for a *DSM* overview). *Premature ejaculation* (as the disorder has traditionally been called) was first noted in the medical literature in 1887 (see Waldinger, 2008, for an overview). Initially, early ejaculation was seen mainly as a psychological disorder and treated with psychoanalytic techniques. In the middle of the last century, there was a realization that both psychological and biological factors were involved. In the 1990s, it was discovered that selective serotonin reuptake inhibitors (SSRIs) would delay ejaculation.

As noted earlier in this chapter, some 30% of the men in one study reported problems with early ejaculation although other studies show slightly lower numbers. There is little data in terms of the number of males affected using *DSM–5* criteria. In one study of men who had reported experiencing premature ejaculation, their female partners were asked to use a stopwatch at home to time ejaculation over a 4-week period. What was found was that 90% of these men ejaculated within 1 minute, with 40% of these men ejaculating within 15 seconds after penetration (see Waldinger, 2008, for an overview).

Female Sexual Interest/Arousal Disorder

In studies from around the world, approximately 30% of women report a significantly decreased desire to engage in sexual activities (see Palacios et al., 2009, for an overview). In particular, sexual desire decreases with age. In *DSM–5,* **female sexual interest/arousal disorder** requires significant distress or impairment along with at least three specific symptoms. The symptoms include a reduction or absence of interest in sexual activity, sexual fantasies, excitement or pleasure during sex, and internal or external sexual cues or sexual sensations.

Male Hypoactive Sexual Desire Disorder

Male hypoactive sexual desire disorder refers to the situation in which a male has little desire for sexual activity or even erotic thoughts for 6 months. Further, this condition causes significant distress to the man. Overall, lack of sexual desire is reported more frequently by females than by males. As noted previously, some 15% of men in the general population report a lack of interest in sexual activities. Other studies have found similar numbers throughout the world. However, when asked if this is a significant problem lasting for 6 months, the numbers drop to only a few percent.

Genito-pelvic Pain/Penetration Disorder

In females, pain during sexual activity has traditionally been seen as two types. The first is *dyspareunia.* This type of pain is experienced during intercourse. The pain may be experienced initially as the penis is inserted into the vagina. It may also be present once the penis is inserted and associated with thrusting. The causes of dyspareunia can be varied. Dryness of the vagina can result from aging or certain medications. Infections and previous injury such as from childbirth or operations can also cause painful experiences. The second type is *vaginismus.* When penetration of the vagina is attempted the muscles of the vaginal wall or the pelvic floor begin to spasm. This is accompanied by either pain or fear of pain, and penetration is impossible. This condition is not limited to sexual experiences and includes the penetration of any object such as a speculum used by a gynecologist, a tampon, or even a finger. In *DSM–5,* the **genito-pelvic pain/penetration disorder** refers to conditions associated with dyspareunia or vaginismus or the fear or anxiety associated with these conditions. As noted previously, some 16% of women report painful sexual experiences. Unlike with other sexual disorders, younger women report more painful sexual experiences than older women.

TREATMENT APPROACHES FOR SEXUAL DYSFUNCTION DISORDERS

Given the complexity of factors that can be involved in sexual dysfunction disorders, a thorough assessment is critical. It is important to understand the person's attitudes toward sexual behavior and his or her understanding of the presenting problems. Often, during the initial assessment it becomes apparent that the person is missing some critical information regarding sexual activity. Thus, part of successful future treatment may include teaching the individual the basics of sexual activity or filling in gaps in his or her knowledge. This may also include behavioral techniques such as directed masturbation. The second important assessment procedure is to determine if there is a medical problem that contributes to the sexual dysfunction. In addition to specific medical conditions, some medications have side effects that influence sexual desire and responsiveness. The third important assessment procedure is understanding the psychological factors involved. These can include relationship problems or family or cultural prohibitions toward sexual practices. Some individuals may also have expectations concerning how a sexual encounter should progress that are incompatible with the expectations of their partner. Based on a psychological assessment, couples therapy can be directed at helping the couple to communicate with their needs and desires in terms of sexual activity.

Sexual therapy begins with a thorough assessment as described and then uses straightforward techniques to help a couple achieve a more fulfilling sexual life. Many of the techniques were initiated by Masters and Johnson in their clinic and described in their book *Human Sexual Inadequacy* (Masters & Johnson, 1970). Masters and Johnson believed that performance anxiety was a part of a number of sexual dysfunction disorders. That is, the person was worried about being aroused, or having a climax, or not getting an erection. These worries could indeed interfere with satisfying sexual relationships. Also, some individuals had never had the experience of slowly moving through a sexual experience. Thus, part of their treatment was designed reduce worries and help individuals understand how their body functions sexually.

Masters and Johnson's treatment procedure lasted for 2 weeks. In their clinic, Masters and Johnson initially requested that the couple not engage in sexual activity. The couple would initially talk individually with a therapist of the same gender, and a thorough social and sexual assessment was made. The overall approach was to see problems in sexual functioning as an issue for the couple rather than the individual to work on. Beginning on the third day, the couple was to use a "sensate focus," which meant that they were to pleasure each other through kissing, touching, massaging, and doing other such behaviors without attempting sexual intercourse or involving genital areas. Part of this was the opportunity to communicate to the other person what was pleasurable. The next step in the sequence was to include genital stimulation without the goal of having an organism. Part of the technique was to have a time in which the woman directed the activity of the couple and determined the timing of the interaction. In their sessions, both the man and woman learned to listen to the other as well as ask for what they wanted in the sexual encounter. Many couples reported more satisfying intercourse as the result of the treatment.

Scientifically, Masters and Johnson collected data on their 2-week treatment program followed by a 5-year follow-up. They reported complete success with 29 of 29 women with vaginismus and 182 out of 186 of men with premature ejaculation. These high rates of success may have resulted in part from the high motivation of the clients involved. That is, the couple had to agree to take 2 weeks off, fly to St. Louis, and spend this time working on their sexual relationship. More recent work with similar procedures shows positive but lower rates of success.

Since the work of Masters and Johnson, a variety of specific techniques have been used by sex therapists. Some required changes in the sex act. With premature ejaculation, for example, the couple would be instructed to practice foreplay and penile stimulation to the point prior to ejaculation. Stimulation is then paused until the arousal level is decreased. Stimulation is then applied again. This technique is performed at least 3 times before ejaculation. A variant on this technique is referred to as the squeeze technique. In this case, as the man approaches ejaculation, his partner squeezes the penis near the top, which reduces arousal. This is then repeated. For a female with vaginismus, it is important for her to learn to tense and relax the muscles of her vagina. In a comfortable setting, she is instructed to insert her finger in her vagina and practice relaxation. Later, she can insert two fingers or a vaginal dilator. Slowly she learns to insert larger dilators while practicing relaxation. After she is comfortable and feels in control, a partner can be involved with the woman remaining in control.

Pharmacological approaches are also used to treat a number of sexual dysfunction disorders. With painful sexual activity in women, creams that contain antifungal, corticosteroid, or estrogen can be applied to the vaginal area. With male erectile disorder, drugs such as Viagra, Levitra, or Cialis increase blood flow to the penis and nearby areas. This allows for an erection. However, these drugs do not influence sexual desire. It is generally reported that these drugs work in over half of the men although the satisfaction of the sexual experience varies. Best results have been found when pharmacological techniques for a sexual dysfunction are combined with behavioral techniques, psychosocial approaches such as cognitive behavioral therapy, and therapy focused on the interpersonal relationship.

Concept Check

- What factors distinguish temporary sexual problems from sexual dysfunction disorders?
- Sexual dysfunction disorders can be thought of in terms of four categories related to desire, arousal, orgasm, and pain. Into which category would you place each of the sexual dysfunction disorders covered in this chapter?
- What are the diagnostic criteria for each of the sexual dysfunction disorders covered in this chapter?
- What are examples from each of the following categories of factors that influence erectile dysfunction: age, lifestyle, medical, and psychological factors?
- What are the similarities and differences between female sexual interest/arousal disorder and male hypoactive sexual desire disorder?
- What are the two types of genito-pelvic pain/penetration disorder? What are the causes of each?
- Therapy for sexual dysfunction disorders begins with a thorough assessment focusing on three factors. What are these factors and how are they important in successful treatment?

In this section, you have seen problems associated with the act of sex itself. These disorders include lack of desire and inability to initiate or complete the sexual intercourse successfully. You also learned about treatment approaches for these disorders. In this next section, I describe disorders in which the person experiences distress in relation to his or her objects of desire.

As demonstrated by the popularity of sexual themes in novels and on the Internet, humans are attracted to and enjoy reading about and imagining different types of sexual encounters. Sexual surveys also demonstrate that humans engage in a variety of sexual activities. In addition to traditional sexual activities, humans may play games with each other and act out various sexual roles. Some individuals experience sexual arousal in seeing themselves or their partner dress in a particular manner. For example, some people like to wear leather or dress in the traditional clothes of the opposite sex. Imagining oneself in nontraditional sexual activities or actually engaging in them with a consenting partner is not a mental disorder.

Professionals involved with *DSM–5* wanted to distinguish between nontraditional sexual activities and sexual disorders. That is, they wanted to distinguish between

paraphilia and **paraphilic disorders.** The term *philia* is derived from Greek and refers to love. The term *para,* as in paranormal, refers to something that exists alongside of the traditional or normal. Thus, the term *paraphilia* refers to practices that exist alongside the traditional expressions of love. In the same way that short-term experiences of anxiety or depression do not qualify for a mental disorder, nontraditional sexual practices do not qualify as a disorder. However, when sexual desires or behaviors become problematic, they can be classified under the heading of paraphilic disorders. This is analogous to the situation with eating disorders or addictions where individuals no longer have control or can make decisions in terms of their cognitions and behaviors.

For a sexual desire or sexual behavior to qualify as a disorder, it must cause distress to the person or interfere with important areas of the person's life. The acts associated with the disorder may also be illegal when they involve other nonconsenting individuals. Illegal activity such as pedophilia, exhibitionism, and rape has received the most attention in the clinical literature. Further, it should be noted that although rape can be committed by someone with a mental disorder, this is not always the case. Since those who have been convicted of an illegal sexual act are easier to track and study scientifically, much of the current research has focused on these individuals. At present, a scientific understanding of the development of sexual disorders and their treatment in both legal and illegal forms is very incomplete.

In general, the paraphilic disorders included in *DSM–5* are long-term in nature, cause distress to the person involved, and may cause distress or harm to others. Overall, there is a large gender difference with more men than women displaying paraphilic disorders. These disorders can include behaviors such as exposing oneself to others, being sexually aroused by inanimate objects, being aroused by touching or rubbing against others, becoming aroused by children, gaining sexual arousal by seeking humiliation or suffering from others, gaining sexual arousal by making another person suffer, gaining sexual arousal from cross-dressing, and gaining sexual arousal by watching unknowing individuals disrobe or engage in sexual activities. *DSM–5* describes these types of behaviors in terms of the eight paraphilic disorders described next as well as *paraphilic disorders not elsewhere classified.* The following box lists the paraphilic disorders described in *DSM–5.*

PARAPHILIC DISORDERS

***DSM–5* Paraphilic Disorders**

Exhibitionistic Disorder
Fetishistic Disorder
Frotteuristic Disorder
Pedophilic Disorder
Sexual Masochism Disorder
Sexual Sadism Disorder
Transvestic Disorder
Voyeuristic Disorder
Paraphilic Disorders Not Elsewhere Classified

Exhibitionistic Disorder

An **exhibitionistic disorder** is the case in which a person becomes sexually aroused by exposing his genitals to an unsuspecting stranger (see Morin & Levenson, 2008, for an overview). Although *DSM–5* describes the disorder as gender neutral, it is infrequently displayed by women. Often called a *flasher*, a male exhibitionist will find a place where women are expected to be, such as a park. A common scenario is that upon seeing a woman, he will move in front of her and open his coat so that his genitals are exposed. He may use this experience later to be part of his sexual fantasies.

Exhibitionism is also a crime in the United States, referred to as *indecent exposure*. Society has treated exhibitionism as a nuisance crime since there is no physical contact. However, there are reasons to take it seriously (see Firestone, Kingston, Wexler, & Bradford, 2006, for an overview). First, one third to two thirds of all sexual offenses reported are related to exhibitionism—although this is probably an underreported crime. Putting together a variety of studies, research suggests that 32% to 39% of college female students and 40% to 48% of community samples of women have experienced someone exposing themselves (Murphy & Page, 2008). Second, those individuals who engage in exhibitionism tend to perform the act frequently and show high recidivism after treatment. Firestone and his colleagues (2006) studied 208 men diagnosed with exhibitionism. They found over a 19-year period that these men showed recidivism rates of 23.6% for sexual crimes, 31.3% for violent crimes, and 38.9% for criminal offenses. Third, there is a tendency for exhibitionists to move from exhibitionism to more serious sexual assaults. Fourth, an important result is that victims of exposure experience distress and trauma.

Snaith and Collins (1981) described five patients referred to a psychosexual clinic in the United Kingdom. One of these descriptions is as follows:

> Mr. D. was 30 years old when he referred himself to the clinic. He said that he felt that an arrest for his deviant sexual behaviour would be inevitable unless he could gain some degree of self-control. He spent many hours a week prowling around the neighbourhood in the evenings and exposed to adolescent girls, masturbating as he did so. In addition to exhibitionism he indulged in frotteurism in crowded public places. He had been exposing since the age of 17 and in view of the very blatant nature of the behaviour it was remarkable that he had never been arrested.

This person would qualify for an exhibitionistic disorder since he engaged in exhibitionism for more than 6 months and this behavior caused him distress. Unlike with other paraphilic disorders, those who display exhibitionism tend not to have themselves a history of higher rates of physical or sexual abuse.

Few individuals with an exhibitionistic disorder seek treatment on their own. Thus, most of the treatment literature has been related to those who were sent to treatment by the courts. One approach is that of group therapy in which the individual has an opportunity to discuss his exhibitionistic tendencies and receive feedback from others. Whether presented in groups or individually, the majority of treatment programs have a cognitive behavioral orientation. This is often combined with an approach directed at relapse prevention in which they discuss how they will handle future situations in which desires to expose themselves are present. Some approaches also seek to develop empathy in the person so that he can better understand his impact on the victim. Some health care professionals have also used SSRIs as a psychopharmacological approach. This is based on the finding that serotonin has an inhibitory effect on male ejaculatory functioning. SSRIs have been shown to reduce sexual fantasies and impulsivity.

Frotteuristic Disorder

Frotteuristic disorder refers to the condition in which an individual gains sexual arousal from touching or rubbing against another nonconsenting person (see Lussier & Piché, 2008, for an overview). The word *frottage* means rubbing or friction in French. This disorder has only been seen in men. Men with this condition will report that they seek crowded situations, such as a subway, in which they can make contact with others as if by accident. Generally, the contact is from the side or behind with little eye or face-to-face contact. In extremely crowded situations, the actual contact may go unnoticed. Female undercover police officers, seeking to stop theft and other crimes on subways, have discovered frotteurism to be more common than traditional crimes. Some subway systems, such as the one in Tokyo, have established women-only cars during rush hours.

A frotteuristic disorder diagnosis requires two conditions. The first is that the sexual arousal, which results from touching or rubbing against a nonconsenting person, has lasted for at least 6 months. The second is that the condition results in marked distress or impairment in the individual's functioning. As with other paraphilic disorders, few individuals seek treatment on their own as opposed to being court ordered. Treatment approaches for paraphilic disorders in general will be described later in this chapter.

Fetishistic Disorder

A *fetish* is an erotic fixation on an object or body part that is not sexual in nature (see Darcangelo, 2008, for an overview). The word *fetish* comes from the French *fétiche,* which may have come from the Portuguese *fetico,* which means spell or magic charm. In this sense, an object creates a spell over the person. A person with a particular fetish experiences sexual arousal from focusing on the object. Shoes with high heels and the feet are common fetish objects. Although sound epidemiological data are lacking, fetishes appear to be more common with males than females. It is an open question why certain objects or parts of the body take on a sexual connotation.

Masters, Johnson, and Kolodny (1986) described a man who had a fetish for women's high-heeled shoes. He had collected more than 1,000 of these shoes, which he had catalogued and concealed from his wife in his attic. Other fetish objects may involve a particular type of material, such as latex, leather, or silk. A person with a fetish may feel or stroke the object or even masturbate while doing this. Even a picture or drawing of the object may be enough for sexual arousal. Although many couples incorporate clothing such as lingerie or other objects to enhance their sexual experience, a **fetishistic disorder** involves a fixation that lasts for more than 6 months and results in clinically significant distress or impairment in important areas of functioning. Treatment approaches for paraphilic disorders in general will be described later in this chapter.

Pedophilic Disorder

I believe that I was born a pedophile, because I have had feelings of sexual attraction toward children and love for them as long as I can remember. . . . I remember being fascinated by children even during my own childhood. . . . By now, it was clear to me that I loved children, especially boys, and was happiest when I was in their company. What I took pleasure in most was seeing them happy and developing healthily in mind and body. So, I encouraged their interests if I felt these interests were healthy, or I exposed them to experiences that I thought would contribute to their educational or cultural edification. . . . Even in sex, producing pleasure in the children was the most gratifying aspect to me."

From Donald Silva. (1990). Pedophilia: An Autobiography (p. 464). In Jay Feierman (Ed.), *Pedophilia: Biosocial Dimensions.* New York: Springer, reprinted with kind permission from Springer Science+Business Media.

Donald Silva, who wrote the quote you just read, is in prison in Europe. *Pedophilia* is not only a mental disorder but also a crime in most countries. **Pedophilic disorder** involves a persistent sexual interest in prepubescent or early pubescent children. In the popular media, the word *pedophilia* carries with it the connotation of sexual acts with children. However, the clinical definition of pedophilic disorder does not require an actual sexual act although this can be the case. There are some individuals with pedophilic disorder who have not acted on their urges. However, others may pick out a particular child and "groom" the child by giving him or her attention or gifts to make the child feel special. Over a period of time, the child is led into more behaviors that the pedophile finds sexually arousing. As seen in the quote from Donald Silva, many pedophiles claim they are only trying to make the child happy.

As can be seen in the *DSM–5* criteria for pedophilic disorder, there are a number of conditions required. The first is that the person gains more sexual arousal from children than from adults. The second is that the person has acted on these urges or that these urges cause problems in the person's functioning and distress. And third, the condition has lasted for more than 6 months.

The term *pedophile* was coined in 1886 by the German psychiatrist Richard Freiherr von Krafft-Ebing. The term comes from the Greek meaning love of children. In his work, Krafft-Ebing differentiated the attraction to children from the act of sexual abuse. Some pedophiles may use child pornography and have limited contact with children while others seek out child contact. It should be pointed out that not everyone who performs a sexual act with a child is a pedophile. Some adults who abuse children may not gain arousal from thinking of the child as an object. They just abuse the child as a matter of convenience. This, of course, is against the law but may not qualify for a pedophilic disorder. Although both men and women can sexually abuse children, pedophilia appears only in males.

Any type of abuse of children brings out a strong emotional reaction in people hearing about specific situations as portrayed in the media. Part of the emotional reaction to pedophilia is that many of these children are yet to experience their own sexuality. Pedophilic disorder is the most common paraphilia discussed in both the scientific and legal literature.

Pedophilic disorder is seen to develop during adolescence (see Seto, 2008, for an overview). Studies suggest that 40% to 50% of offenders against unrelated boys and 35% to 40% of offenders against unrelated girls reported this attraction before the age of 20. Although solid longitudinal research has yet to be conducted, the general consensus is that a sexual interest in children lasts across the life span for pedophiles. Brain imaging research has shown reduction in the right amygdala in those with pedophilic disorder (Poeppl et al., 2013). In addition, within the pedophilic group, sexual interest in children and sexual recidivism were correlated with gray matter decrease in the left dorsolateral prefrontal cortex ($r = -.64$) and insular cortex ($r = -.45$).

At this point, there is no evidence that an individual with pedophilic disorder can change his sexual attraction to children (Seto, 2008). Treatment approaches tend to focus on teaching the individual how to control his sexual arousal as well as other self-regulation skills. Currently, there is no effective treatment of pedophilic disorder. There are also a number of school-based programs designed to teach children how to protect themselves from pedophilic individuals.

Sexual Masochism Disorder

The blows fell rapidly and powerfully on my back and arms. Each one cut into my flesh and burned there, but the pains enraptured me. They came from her whom I adored, and for whom I was ready at any hour to lay down my life.

From Leopold von Sacher-Masoch. (2013). *Venus in Furs.* New York: Dover Publications. (Original work published 1888)

The term *masochism* is derived from the Austrian author Sacher-Masoch, who in the 1800s described men who derived sexual satisfaction from being whipped or beaten. The previous passage from *Venus in Furs* is from one of his books. Masochism involves deriving sexual pleasure from being subjected to pain or humiliation. This may include being restrained by ropes or other devices, blindfolded, humiliated, or dominated as well as being whipped or beaten. Judging from masochism themes in popular press books and the number of websites devoted to themes or objects involved in masochistic activity, it cannot be a rare fantasy in humans. Fewer individuals act on these fantasies. Some surveys suggest that 5% to 10% of men and women find these activities to be sexually pleasurable on an occasional basis (Masters et al., 1986).

However, masochist fantasies or activities can also become a compulsion, which limits human functioning. **Sexual masochism disorder** is present when the person experiences sexual arousal from the act of being humiliated, beaten, bound, or otherwise made to suffer, as manifested by fantasies, urges, or behaviors for more than 6 months. Further, these urges or behaviors cause distress or impairment in the person's life. This is one of the paraphilic disorders that can be seen in both males and females although the number of females is much less than that of males.

Although there is limited neuroscience research related to masochism, it can be noted that both sexual stimuli and pain stimuli can heighten central nervous system states of arousal and motivation (Bodnar, Commons, & Pfaff, 2002). Further, there is an overlap between the neuroanatomical pathways and mechanisms of pain and sex. Thus, there is the possibility that in some individuals those stimuli that would normally produce an avoidance or withdrawing process would activate approach-like sexual processes.

The criteria for sexual masochism disorder also ask if asphyxiation is present. This is the process by which a person puts a plastic bag over his head or a rope around his neck to cut off oxygen temporarily and enhance the sexual experience, especially during masturbation. A tragic number of individuals who lose consciousness before they can remove the bag or noose and die.

Sexual Sadism Disorder

She stopped. "I am beginning to enjoy it," she said, "but enough for today. I am beginning to feel a demonic curiosity to see how far your strength goes. I take a cruel joy in seeing you tremble and writhe beneath my whip, and I hearing your groans and wails; I want to go on whipping without pity until you beg for mercy, until you lose your senses. You have awakened dangerous elements in my being. But now get up".

From Leopold von Sacher-Masoch. (1888). *Venus in Furs.* New York: Dover Publications. (Original work published 1888)

The term *sadism* is derived from the French author Marquis de Sade, who in the 1700s described sadist features in his novels. Sadism is characterized by the experience of sexual arousal from violent sexual fantasies or by subjecting another to pain or humiliation. This may include restraining, blindfolding, humiliating, or dominating another. This may also include producing physical pain such as whipping another. Although prevalence rates have not been fully determined, it is believed to be more common in males than females.

Sexual sadism disorder involves deriving sexual pleasure from inflicting pain or humiliation on others. To be referred to as a disorder, the occurrence of sexual arousal from the suffering of another must have been present for at least 6 months. It is also required that the person has acted out these impulses with a nonconsenting individual or experienced distress or impairment from these impulses. Some individuals with the disorder require a nonconsenting person to experience the sexual arousal. Sexual sadism does not appear in isolation but is often comorbid with other disorders. These include impulse control disorders, antisocial personality disorder, and borderline personality disorder.

Transvestic Disorder

Transvestism refers to dressing in clothing that is typically used by the opposite sex. This in itself may not produce sexual arousal and would not be considered a fetish. It can become a fetish when this cross-dressing produces sexual arousal. In general, it is males who experience arousal from dressing in women's items of clothing. Most researchers differentiate individuals who are satisfied with their biological sex and cross-dress from those who are dissatisfied and would be commonly referred to as **transsexual** (see Newring, Wheeler, & Draper, 2008, for an overview). Typically, individuals who consider themselves transsexual do not experience sexual arousal from dressing in clothes of the opposite sex.

Early research mainly examined heterosexual males who cross-dressed. Similar patterns were found in both Australia and the United States (Buhrich & Beaumont, 1981). Half of the individuals studied began cross-dressing before puberty, and a majority established cross-dressing by late puberty. Långström and Zucker (2005) examined a random sample of 2,450 individuals in the general population of Sweden. The overall survey was related to health with questions related to sexuality embedded within the larger survey. They found that 2.8% of men and 0.4% of women reported being sexually aroused from cross-dressing. Fifty percent of these individuals reported that they did not find this behavior acceptable to themselves. It is these individuals who would be diagnosed with **transvestic disorder.** The other 50% would not seek treatment unless there occurred relationship or other problems related to the behavior.

Transvestic disorder is characterized by recurrent and intense sexual arousal from cross-dressing, as manifested by fantasies, urges, or behaviors. It also needs to last for a period of at least 6 months and cause distress or impairment.

Voyeuristic Disorder

Voyeurism is the act of watching unsuspecting others engage in nonpublic activities such as undressing, having sexual relations, or engaging in other such behaviors. In some countries such as England, Wales, and the United States, it is an illegal activity. It is seen almost exclusively in men and usually begins before the age of 15. Voyeurs are also called *peeping Toms* after the Lady Godiva story. Lady Godiva rode through the town on her horse nude to protest a tax. She asked the townspeople not to look at her. Tom the tailor was the only person who looked at her and thus became known as "peeping Tom."

It can also be a fetish when the individual gains sexual arousal from watching others. Voyeurs generally are not interested in meeting or having a relationship with the person they are watching. Rather, they use voyeurism as a means for sexual excitement, which may include masturbation. Generally, voyeurs seek a place outside a house or apartment where they can observe the woman without being seen although some use the risk of being caught as an additional source of excitement. In a city, voyeurs may use a telescope or other device to watch others in their apartments. They may also hide Internet cameras in locker rooms or other places where people undress. Hacking into another person's computer can allow someone to turn on the camera without this being noticed. Paradoxically, most voyeurs do not go to places such as nude beaches or nude stage shows where nudity is acceptable.

Voyeuristic disorder involves obtaining sexual arousal from watching unsuspecting people when they are undressing, naked, performing sexual acts, or going to the bathroom. This activity needs to have existed for at least 6 months. It also needs to involve a nonconsenting individual or cause marked distress or impairment.

Other Paraphilic Disorders

There are two additional categories of paraphilic disorders. The first is referred to as *other specified paraphilic disorder*. This category includes symptoms that cause significant distress or impairment in important areas of one's life but do not satisfy the criteria in any of the disorders previously described in this chapter. This can include intense sexual arousal from making obscene phone calls, corpses, animals, feces, urine, enemas, or other such sexually arousing events for the individual. The second disorder is referred to as *unspecified paraphilic disorder*. The requirements for this disorder are the same as the first except that there may be insufficient information to make a more specific diagnosis.

At times, individuals are mandated by the courts to receive treatment for a sexually related crime. Some of these crimes, such as rape, are not seen to have resulted from the person having a mental disorder although there could be a relationship in terms of sexual sadism or a personality disorder. Other crimes, such as child pornography, can be directly related to a paraphilic disorder. The following case study of George Nadel (not his real name) is someone who was mandated for treatment for the crime of possessing child pornography. Although a mental health professional would initially consider a pedophilic disorder, George Nadel, as you will see, reported being more sexually attracted to adults than children and came to have an interest in child pornography later in his life. Thus, the mental health professional might choose *other specified paraphilic disorder* as the *DSM–5* diagnosis.

CASE OF GEORGE NADEL

Court-Mandated Treatment for Child Pornography Possession

George Nadel is a 47-year-old unemployed twice-divorced male who presented to the Rising Sun Center for Treatment of Sexual Offenders with complaints of depressed mood, anxiety, and impulsive behavior. He reports that he is heterosexually oriented. The client reports a history of depression since childhood, which he has managed through what he describes as self-destructive behaviors. In addition to substance abuse and impulsive spending, the client has a recent history of possessing child pornography (depicting boys and girls ages 9–16), which resulted in pending legal charges for possession (and possible distribution) of child pornography. His pending charges cause him a significant amount of anxiety and shame.

George reports behavior that is consistent with a preoccupation with sexual behaviors. He has engaged in anonymous fellatio in the back rooms of bookstores. He also spends significant portions of his income on legal pornography and preparations used to reverse erectile dysfunction. George says that while he feels he can stop downloading child pornography, he claims an addiction to pornography depicting adults. The client said that he became interested in child pornography more than 7 years ago when he heard a television news report that caused him to become curious regarding images of child pornography. Since that time, George has downloaded nearly 20,000 image of child pornography. At his intake, George expressed his concern over his pending legal charges, which have lasted over the past 2 years.

Clinical vignette provided by Clifford Evans, MEd, RN

TREATMENT APPROACHES FOR PARAPHILIC DISORDERS

Since many individuals with paraphilic disorders do not seek treatment, sound studies of treatment efficacy are lacking. What is available is either case studies or research studies in which the paraphilic disorder was treated in terms of other comorbid problems. In some paraphilic disorders, the individuals themselves may have experienced physical, emotional, or sexual trauma in childhood, which would influence the nature of the treatment.

When treatment is sought, it generally has three sources. The first is through the courts. These are individuals who were arrested for paraphilia involving nonconsenting others. The second source is when a partner or spouse encourages the person to seek treatment to improve their relationship. And the third source is when the person himself finds his fantasies or behaviors distressing or is afraid of being caught doing the behavior by another person.

Psychopharmacological treatments have been used to reduce sexual drive in general. SSRIs have been shown to reduce sexual drive and have been used with a number of paraphilic disorders. These have been shown to have the best effects with disorders that have a strong affective component. Other drugs that influence sexual hormones directly have also been tried. Inconsistent results and side effects do not make these the treatment of choice for paraphilic disorders.

Cognitive behavioral orientations make up the majority of treatment approaches to paraphilic disorders. This approach focuses on how the person interprets his thoughts and emotions in relation to others. This is often combined with an approach directed at relapse prevention. This is similar to the approach used with those addicted to drugs in which discussions focus on how to avoid future high-risk situations.

GENDER DYSPHORIA

The truth that was slowly emerging had a hazy beginning. Since I was a child, I'd been aware of a part of me that did not fit. At first, I thought this sense of not fitting in was about me being gay. But as time went on, and I tried different ways of "being a lesbian"—from lipstick to stone butch—I had to admit to myself that the "something" nagging at me was a lot more complicated than just my sexual orientation. Even when I was active in the gay community, I never felt completely at ease. There was something else about me that didn't make sense, something that was much more profound and a lot more threatening. . . .

It would take me almost ten more years before I truly understood the significance of my gender dysphoria, a clinical description that gets to the disconnection between how the body presents its sex and how the brain experiences its sex. In essence, when these two are different (the brain feels itself to be a man but the body is a woman's, and vice versa), the confusion and discomfort is so deep, so disturbing, that most of us try anything to either deny our true feelings or otherwise avoid dealing with ourselves.

The hours I spent as Renée were a very small part of my active life, but they cast a continuing shadow over all the relationships I formed. There was no time as a child or teenager when I could say that anyone really knew me. They knew Dick, but I kept the female component of my personality deeply buried. The idea that it might get out haunted me. Had I been able to talk to someone, it would have decreased my isolation, but I never met anyone to whom I gave even passing consideration to telling my secret. No matter how kind or understanding people seemed, even my good friends, I couldn't imagine that they would forgive me.

From Renée Richards. (1983). *Second Serve* (p. 41). New York: Stein and Day.

There is great variety in the traditional **gender roles** that boys and girls experience. These gender roles are typically defined by one's culture in terms of the kinds of activities boys and girls are expected to engage in. Some girls tend to engage in activities that are seen as more male oriented and are called "tomboys." Some boys may like to do more traditional female activities such as dressing and playing with dolls and are referred to as "sissies." Some individuals stay with their childhood interests and continue in occupations that follow. Females who become construction workers or males who design clothes would be two examples. However, just because their culture would say they were a tomboy or sissy, they continue to see themselves as their biological gender. This is referred to as **gender identity.** Gender identify is the internal experience of knowing that you are male or female. Even if individuals find themselves sexually attracted to members of their same sex, they would describe themselves as male attracted to another male or as female attracted to another female. Being gay or lesbian or bisexual does not change one's gender identity. However, some individuals experience a discrepancy between their physical sexual characteristics and their experience of themselves. For these individuals, their gender identity does not match their sexual anatomy at birth.

As noted by the reports by Chaz Bono, who was born as Chastity Bono to Sonny and Cher, some adults feel that they are in the wrong body. They may have been born as a male in terms of their body, but their internal experience is that they feel like a female. A smaller number of those born in a female body feel that they are really a male. In *DSM–5,* this is referred to as **gender dysphoria.** Dysphoria is defined as a sense of unease or suffering.

Gender dysphoria can be seen in children, adolescents, and adults. In children, the gender dysphoria diagnosis requires that the condition last for at least 6 months and cause the child significant distress or impairment in school, social, or other areas. In order to make the diagnosis, six of eight criteria must be present. These include (1) a strong desire to be the other gender; (2) a strong preference for wearing clothes of the opposite gender; (3) a strong preference for cross-gender roles in make-believe play; (4) a strong preference for toys, games, or activities associated with the opposite gender; (5) a strong preference for playmates of the opposite gender; (6) a strong rejection of toys or games associated with one's physical gender; (7) a strong dislike of one's sexual anatomy; and (8) a strong desire to have the physical sexual anatomy of the opposite gender. There is greater variety in the patterns of behaviors seen in children than adolescents and adults with gender dysphoria. Not all children who show gender dysphoria will continue to show it into adolescence or adulthood. Its continuance has been estimated to range from 2% to 30% in those born as males as opposed to 12% to 50% in those born as females (APA, 2013).

In adolescents and adults, the experience of the situation is seen as more stable. For a diagnosis, it also requires 6 months' duration and significant distress or impairment in social, occupational, or other areas of functioning. Also two of the following six criteria must be present. These are (1) a marked incongruence between one's experienced gender and one's anatomical sex characteristics; (2) a strong desire to be rid of one's primary sex characteristics because of a marked incongruence with one's experience; (3) a strong desire for the sex characteristics of the other gender; (4) a strong desire to be of the other gender; (5) a strong desire to be treated as the other gender; and (6) a strong conviction that one has the typical feelings and reactions of the other gender.

Current estimates of prevalence is around 1 in 10,000 for those who are biologically male and experience themselves as female and slightly lower for those who are biologically female and experience themselves as male (APA, 2013). At present, it is difficult to make these estimates since this information is not generally sought on studies of epidemiology. However, individuals who experience gender dysphoria are found throughout the world.

The common term used for individuals who have the anatomy of one sex and the gender identity of the other is **transgender.** If the transgendered individual has sought medical intervention such as hormone treatment and sexual reassignment surgery to change his or her body into that of the opposite sex, the term used is *transsexual.* Both Chaz Bono and the professional tennis player Renée Richards, who described their experiences at the beginning of this section, underwent medical treatment to change their biological sexual characteristics.

Gender dysphoria is a topic of great debate. One position is that although there exist individuals who exemplify the characteristics of the condition, it should not be considered as a mental health disorder. This would be parallel to the situation with homosexuality.

Until 1973, homosexuality was listed in *DSM* as a sexual disorder. However, mental health professionals believed that this resulted in making a common behavior a pathology. Similarly, the question arises as to whether the clinical and scientific evidence exists for seeing gender dysphoria as a mental disorder.

The task force that created *DSM* criteria reviewed the evidence for including gender dysphoria in *DSM–5* (Byne et al., 2012). One aspect related to childhood diagnosis. It was noted that it was not uncommon for children to show cross-gender behaviors. However, the majority of these children do not show these behaviors as they move through puberty and into adolescence. Further, few studies have been able to identify which children who show cross-gender behaviors will continue these experiences in adolescence. There are also few treatment studies with this population.

The overall question involves what a mental health professional would seek to treat. No treatment to date has shown any effect on gender identity or sexual orientation in young adulthood (Byne et al., 2012). Clearly, if a child is not gaining the support he or she needs for psychological development from those around him or her, then psychological interventions designed to create positive ways of coping and techniques for dealing with negative emotions and self-esteem would be important. These treatments could involve family therapy and child based therapy.

For adolescents and adults, the relatively infrequent occurrence of gender dysphoria has limited the research directed at the topic. As noted, it is a complicated and politically charged topic that brings forth many issues around the meaning of sexuality and gender. When examined in non-dysphoria conditions, neuroscience research suggests that brain differences exist in relation to gender. Using this knowledge, some researchers have sought to determine similarities between non-dysphoric males and females and those who experience gender dysphoria. One study found that white matter fiber pathways in female-to-male transgendered individuals were more similar to those found in males (Rametti et al., 2011). The brain imaging took place before any hormonal treatment was applied and was not influenced by medical intervention. Thus, fiber pathways in those who experienced themselves as male did indeed look similar to those non-dysphoric individuals who were anatomically male.

Another study examined cortical thickness in male-to-female transgendered individuals (Luders et al., 2013). This study compared non-dyphoric males and individuals who experienced male-to-female gender dysphoria before any hormonal treatment had taken place. As seen in *Figure 13-10*, cortical thickness was greater in several cortical regions. There was no area in which the control group showed greater thickness. Previous research had shown great cortical thickness in non-dysphoric women as compared with non-dysphoric men. Previous research has also shown that a cluster of cells in the hypothalamus (bed nucleus of stria terminalis) that is involved in sexual activity. It is not only smaller in women as compared with men but also smaller in men with gender dysphoria (Zhou, Hofman, Gooren, & Swaab, 1995). Thus, individuals with gender dysphoria who experience themselves as female have brain structures that are more similar to those of non-dysphoric females. Overall, these neuroscience studies suggest that the experience of gender is reflected in brain structures.

Some adults with gender dysphoria seek gender transition surgery. This is a complicated procedure that carries with it a variety of mental health concerns along with political and medical issues. Some individuals want to talk with a mental health professional to help them clarify their concerns about engaging in sex change procedures. Sexual transition procedures may include hormonal supplements, which will produce secondary

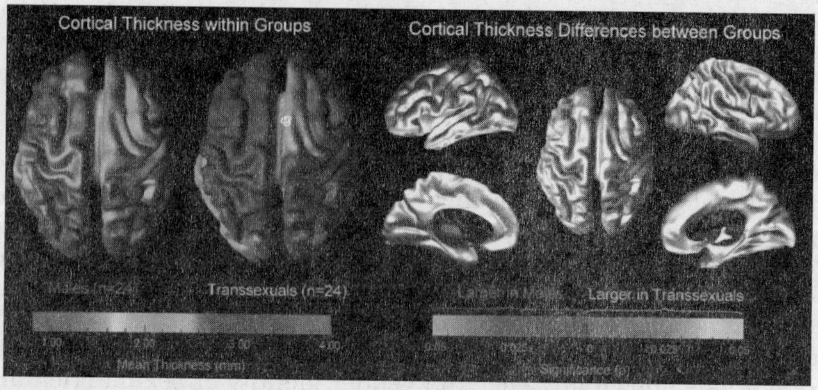

FIGURE 13-10 The Right Side of the Figure Shows Cortical Thickness for the Control and Transgender Groups Separately in Terms of Millimeter Thickness

Source: Luders et al. (2012, p. 359).

Note: The left side of the figure shows brain areas in which cortical thickness significantly differed between the two groups. Note that differences are mainly shown for the transgender group (yellow and red show greater thickness for this group).

sex characteristics such as facial hair or voice deepening for the change to a male or skin softening and fat distribution changes for the change to a female. These are followed by surgical procedures to modify sexual organs and other sexual characteristics.

As with any major life change, a variety of positive and negative experiences have been reported by those who engage in a sex change procedure. One review of the research involving more than 1,000 people who changed from male to female and more than 400 who changed from female to male reported a general reduction of psychological distress (Pfäfflin & Junge, 1998). Overall, there was a general satisfaction and lack of regret for engaging in the sex change procedure. Another review reported that 80% of those who had a sex change procedure experienced improved quality of life and decreased gender dysphoria (Murad et al.,

Concept Check

- What factors distinguish paraphilia from paraphilic disorders?
- What are the diagnostic criteria for each of the paraphilic disorders covered in this chapter?
- Exhibitionism is a crime in the United States as well as a *DSM–5* paraphilic disorder. What are some of the reasons to treat it seriously as a crime?
- Does the clinical definition of pedophilic disorder require an actual sexual act with a child? Is anyone who performs a sexual act with a child a pedophile? Why, or why not?
- In terms of treatment approaches for paraphilic disorders overall, please answer the following questions:
    - What are the three primary sources through which treatment is initiated?
    - What pharmacological approaches are used, and what aspects of the disorder do they target?
    - What psychotherapy approaches are used, and what aspects of the disorder do they target?
- What are the definitions for the following terms, and what relationships exist among them?
    - Gender roles?
    - Gender identity?
    - Gender dysphoria?
    - Transgender?
    - Transsexual?
    - Transvestism?

2010). Strong regrets or ambivalence was estimated to have occurred in less than 2% of the individuals. This is a change from earlier reviews in which a higher proportion of individuals reported regrets. The positive change may have resulted from the number of clinics around the world that have created teams of mental health, medical, and surgical professionals to thoroughly evaluate and offer comprehensive services to individuals with gender dysphoria. Overall, it is not recommended that sex change procedures take place before young adulthood.

At this time, gender dysphoria is not well understood. Most cultures do not offer much support for individuals who experience gender dysphoria. Few states offer the same protections as those offered to homosexual individuals. Many individuals who experience gender dysphoria often find support within the larger lesbian, gay, bisexual, and transgender (LGBT) community. Stigmatization is a common experience of these individuals. Research in relation to gender dysphoria is in the early stages although a research literature search in PubMED (pubmed.gov) shows research on the topic from around the world.

OTHER INDIAN WORK ON GENDER DYSPHORIA, GENDER IDENTITY ISSUES AND THEIR MANAGEMENT

A short paper from NIMHANS (Andrade, 2005) interestingly highlights the need for systematic epidemiological research on sexual dysfunction in India given the rapidly changing biopsychosocial scenario.

A complete section in the last chapter of the book will be reserved for the developments in the POCSO Act that focuses on legal aspects of dealing with child sexual abuse, and hence this is not covered here although pedophilia has already been discussed.

Gender dysphoria needs to be studied in the Indian cultural context due to the strong delineation of gender roles, and several researchers report a dual role adopted by male patients, where they marry a female and play the role of a dutiful husband at home as prescribed by the social delineation of social role for them and outside the home can express their desire to be a woman and play a female gender role. This would be a coping strategy that fits with the sociocultural guidelines and values and an ambiguous legal position, a rift between the gender and the social dichotomy.

Some interesting work is also published regarding female sexuality, another less discussed topic in the cultural context. In a paper, Rao and Nagaraj (2015) underline the fact that longevity would increase years of active sexuality in females and yet this is a much neglected and less studied area.

Many studies have also underlined the fact that social taboo and lack of informative family support lead to delayed medical consultation and have accounted for complexities in the presentation of gender identity issues and dysphoria (Sanyal and Majumdar, 2016).

An interesting study (Karia, Jamsandekar, Alure, De Sousa, & Shah, 2016) reports MMPI 2 profiles of patients seeking sexual reassignment surgery. No marked elevations were seen on the psychopathology scales except for slight elevations on F and 8 due to the distress experienced and scale 6 due to the mistrust they feel towards society at large after being stigmatized. Scale 5 elevations were seen in the expected direction, that is, high scores on the Mf scale with patients attesting to stereotypes of femininity in male to female SRS, and to stereotypes of masculinity in female to male SRS.

Interesting Work on Infertility Treatment in India and the Psychosocial Consequences

On an endnote to the chapter, an associated and interesting area for psychosocial intervention is emerging in India with regard to IVF treatments in pursuit of having a baby. Interesting findings of research conducted with this difficult to study population (due to unwillingness to share personal details and high stigma associated with infertility) include some of the following (Tulsiyan and Sovani, 2017):

When married heterosexual couples who had chosen to undergo infertility treatment were assessed, it was found that female participants had higher scores on anxiety, lower scores on adjustment to infertility, and lower scores on self-esteem as well as subjective wellbeing as compared to their male counterparts.

Couples undergoing treatment for infertility perceive the greatest support to be coming from their significant other, then look towards their family for support, and least of all perceive support coming from friends or peer group.

Marital satisfaction and sexual satisfaction were found to be significantly more negatively affected compared to general life satisfaction by the condition of infertility.

Perceived social support, particularly family support was found to be strongly negatively correlated with anxiety, positively correlated with subjective well-being and marital satisfaction for women in the current sample. Family support could thus be an important factor that healthcare providers and counsellors could tap on, in order to help deal with emotional concerns of infertile women.

Self-esteem among men and women and perceived support from family and from significant other among women were found to be significantly lesser among those who had undergone infertility treatment for more number of years compared to those who had undergone such treatment for lesser number of years (reported with permission from Dr. Tulsiyan since some of the work is as yet unpublished).

SUMMARY

Sexuality is a driving force in many species including humans. Humans use the internal experience of sexual arousal and the external experience of sexual activity for a variety of purposes. Humans have depicted sexual activities in painting and carving for thousands of years. At certain times, some cultures have seen sexual activity as a negative force in human life. In the 1800s, a number of scientists—including Charles Darwin, Sigmund Freud, and Havelock Ellis—began to approach sexuality from a scientific perspective. In the 1930s, Alfred Kinsey, a zoologist, conducted a large-scale survey of some 12,000 individuals across the United States on sexual activities. It is important to gain a perspective on sexual activities in the general population to understand sexual disorders scientifically. It is also important to understand normal sexual functioning. In studying the sexual responses of males and females, Masters and Johnson realized that there was a similarity in how men and women experienced the sexual experience. They identified four phases of the human sexual response: (1) excitement, (2) plateau, (3) orgasm, and (4) resolution. Outside the laboratory, sexual activity begins with desire, and this should be considered as an initial step preceding Masters and Johnson's four phases. The four phases of sexual response can be described on a variety of levels—the two main ones are blood flow (*vasocongestion*) and muscular tension (*myotonia*).

Like many human processes, sexual arousal and desire take place on a number of levels in a complex manner: (1) cognitive considerations, (2) emotional experiences, and (3) physical level of functioning. Within these three levels, one important research question has been the manner in which measurements can be made. With the advent of psychophysiological techniques to measure blood flow in the sexual organs of males and females, a different type of precision is possible. However, as with a number of psychophysiological measures, the relationship between changes in physiology and the experienced cognitions and feelings may not be exact. More recently, measures of brain activity using such brain imaging techniques as EEG or fMRI allow for an understanding of cortical involvement. Research suggests that gender differences between men and women in amount of time spent thinking about sex may relate to appetites in general rather than a specific domain. Research also suggests that males show both subjective and physiological arousal in a manner that is consistent with their sexual orientation. Brain imaging studies allow for cortical measures of arousal in addition to self-report and blood flow changes in sexual organs. Overall, when both males and females achieve orgasm, there are changes in the brain—the processing of sexual arousal involves complex brain networks involving cognitive, emotional, and self-processes.

Sexual functioning is important to humans. Sexual relations encompass all aspects of human behavior—thinking, feeling, and doing all interact to contribute a satisfying sex life. However, there are times when our sexual functioning is not optimal. It is important to distinguish between temporary sexual problems including relationship issues and more long-term sexual dysfunction disorders. As with other disorders, it is important to consider three perspectives in order to understand sexual dysfunction: (1) medical and biological factors, (2) psychological factors, and (3) relationship factors. Epidemiological data suggest that sexual dysfunctions are common. Sexual dysfunction disorders can be thought of in terms of four categories related to desire, arousal, orgasm, and pain.

Erectile disorder requires that a male has a problem in one of three areas—obtaining an erection, maintaining an erection, or having a decrease in rigidity of erection—and the experience of erectile problem produces significant distress. Female orgasmic disorder is the condition in which a woman either does not experience an orgasm or has a reduced intensity of the sensation of the orgasm. Delayed ejaculation is the situation in which a male shows a delay in ejaculation or shows a lack of ejaculation. Early ejaculation is diagnosed when a man experiences an ejaculation within approximately the first minute of sexual activity. Female sexual interest/arousal disorder requires significant distress or impairment along with at least three specific symptoms including a reduction or absence of interest in sexual activity, sexual fantasies, sexual activity, excitement or pleasure during sex, internal or external sexual cues, or sexual sensations. Male hypoactive sexual desire disorder refers to the situation in which a male has little desire for sexual activity or even erotic thoughts. Genito-pelvic pain/penetration disorder refers to conditions associated with dyspareunia or vaginismus or the fear or anxiety associated with these conditions. Sexual therapy begins with a thorough assessment and then uses straightforward techniques to help a couple achieve a more fulfilling sexual life. Assessment includes (1) the individual's attitudes and understanding; (2) any medical problems; and (3) psychological factors. Many of the techniques were initiated by Masters and Johnson in the 1960s in their clinic and described in their book *Human Sexual Inadequacy.* Since the work of Masters and Johnson, a variety of specific techniques have been used by sex therapists. Best results have been found when pharmacological techniques for a sexual dysfunction are combined with behavioral techniques, psychosocial approaches such as cognitive behavioral therapy and therapy, focused on the interpersonal relationship.

Humans are attracted to and enjoy reading about and imagining different types of sexual encounters, and they engage in a variety of sexual activities. *DSM–5* distinguishes between nontraditional sexual activities and sexual disorders—that is, between paraphilia and paraphilic disorders. In general, paraphilic disorders in terms of *DSM–5* are long-term in nature, cause distress to the person involved, and may cause distress or harm to others. The acts associated with the disorder may also be illegal when they involve other nonconsenting individuals. Overall, there is a large gender difference with more men than women displaying paraphilic disorders.

An exhibitionistic disorder is the case in which a person becomes sexually aroused by exposing his genitals to an unsuspecting stranger. Exhibitionism is also a crime in the United States referred to as *indecent exposure.* Frotteuristic disorder refers to the condition in which an individual gains sexual arousal from touching or rubbing against another nonconsenting person. A fetishistic disorder involves a fixation that lasts for more than 6 months and results in clinically significant distress or impairment. Pedophilic disorder involves a persistent sexual interest in prepubescent or early pubescent children. Pedophilia is not only a mental disorder but also a crime in most countries. Sexual masochism disorder is present when the person experiences sexual arousal from the act of being humiliated, beaten, bound, or otherwise made to suffer, as manifested by fantasies, urges, or behaviors. Sexual sadism disorder involves deriving sexual pleasure from inflicting pain or humiliation on others. Transvestic disorder is characterized by recurrent and intense sexual arousal from cross-dressing, as manifested by fantasies, urges, or behaviors. Voyeuristic disorder involves obtaining sexual arousal from watching unsuspecting people when they are undressing, naked, performing sexual acts, or going to the bathroom. Many individuals with paraphilic disorders do not seek treatment. When treatment is sought, it generally has three sources: (1) the courts, (2) a partner or spouse, or (3) the person himself or herself. Psychopharmacological treatments have been used to reduce sexual drive in general. Cognitive behavioral orientations make up the majority of treatment approaches to paraphilic disorders.

There is great variety in the traditional gender roles that boys and girls experience. These gender roles are typically defined by one's culture. Gender identity is the internal experience of knowing that you are male or female. Being gay or lesbian or bisexual does not change one's gender identity. However, some individuals experience a discrepancy between their physical sexual characteristics and their experience of themselves. For these individuals, their gender identity does not match their sexual anatomy at birth. In *DSM–5,* this is referred to as gender dysphoria. Dysphoria is defined as a sense of unease or suffering. Gender dysphoria can be seen in children, adolescents, and adults. Not all children who show gender dysphoria will continue to show it into adolescence or adulthood. In adolescents and adults, the experience of the situation is seen as more stable. Individuals who experience gender dysphoria are found throughout the world. The common term used for individuals who have the anatomy of one sex and the gender identity of the other is *transgender.* If the transgendered individual has sought medical intervention such as hormone treatment and sexual reassignment surgery to change his or her body into that of the opposite sex, the term used is *transsexual.* Gender dysphoria is a topic of great debate. One position is that although there exist individuals who exemplify the characteristics of the condition, it should not be considered as a mental health disorder. This would be parallel to the situation with homosexuality in which mental health professionals believed that this resulted in making a common behavior a pathology. The overall question involves what a mental health professional would seek to treat. No treatment to date has shown any effect on gender identity or sexual orientation in young adulthood. For adolescents and adults, the relatively infrequent occurrence of gender dysphoria has limited the research directed at the topic. However, overall, neuroscience studies suggest that the experience of gender is reflected in brain structures. Some adults with gender dysphoria seek gender transition surgery. As with any major life change, a variety of positive and negative experiences have been reported by those who engage in a sex change procedure. Overall, it is not recommended that sex change procedures take place before young adulthood. At this time, gender dysphoria is not well understood.

STUDY RESOURCES

Review Questions

1. How are sexual arousal and drive described scientifically?
   a. What are the relationships in the scientific literature among the terms *drive*, *arousal*, *need*, *desire*, *obsession*, and *motivation*?
   b. Sexual arousal and desire take place on a number of levels in a complex manner. What are these levels?
   c. What advances have been made in psychophysiological measures to support research?

2. What are the treatment approaches for sexual dysfunction disorders?
   a. How would you describe the complexity of factors that can be involved in sexual dysfunction disorders thus making thorough assessment critical?
   b. What was the procedure Masters and Johnson introduced? What issues were they targeting with their treatment protocol?
   c. What are some of the techniques that have been developed since the period of Masters and Johnson?
   d. What pharmacological techniques are available for treating sexual dysfunction disorders?

3. Please answer the following questions for each of the paraphilic disorders:
   a. What neuroscience research informs our understanding of the disorder?
   b. What are the treatment issues?
   c. What are the legal issues related to this disorder, if any?
   d. What do we know about gender and lifespan prevalence rates?

4. There is a debate in the mental health community as to whether gender dysphoria should be considered a disorder in *DSM*. Choose one side of the debate and provide evidence in support of your position. What questions would you ask of proponents of the other side of the debate?

For Further Reading

Laws, D., & O'Donohue, W. (Eds.). (2008). *Sexual deviance: Theory, assessment, and treatment* (2nd ed.). New York: Guilford Press.
Meana, M. (2012). *Sexual dysfunction in women.* Cambridge, MA: Hogrefe Publishing.
Rowland, D. (2012). *Sexual dysfunction in men.* Cambridge, MA: Hogrefe Publishing.

Key Terms and Concepts

delayed ejaculation
early ejaculation
erectile disorder
exhibitionistic disorder
female orgasmic disorder
female sexual interest/arousal disorder
fetishistic disorder
frotteuristic disorder
gender dysphoria
gender identity
gender roles
genito-pelvic pain/penetration disorder
male hypoactive sexual desire disorder
paraphilia
paraphilic disorders
pedophilic disorder
sexual dysfunction disorders
sexual masochism disorder
sexual sadism disorder
transgender
transsexual
transvestic disorder
voyeuristic disorder

CHAPTER

14

Substance-Related and Addictive Disorders

CHAPTER OUTLINE

- INDIAN STATISTICS ON DRUG USE 478
- DRUG USE IN THE UNITED STATES 479
- SUBSTANCE ABUSE, DEPENDENCE, AND ADDICTION 482
- QUALITATIVE STUDY FROM INDIA ON ONSET AND PROGRESSION OF ALCOHOL USE 485
- ALCOHOL 491
- PUBLICATIONS FROM INDIA, BASED ON THE PREMIUM STUDY 502
- CANNABIS 503
- OPIOIDS 510
- AMPHETAMINES 514
- CAFFEINE AND TOBACCO 516
- GAMBLING 519
- TREATMENT OF SUBSTANCE-RELATED DISORDERS 522
- SUMMARY 529
- STUDY RESOURCES 532

Indian Case: Internet Addiction

P.R., a young, intelligent boy studying in grade seven in a school located in a mid-sized town in Maharashtra, usually very shy and timid in class, had no real friends in his class or in his vicinity because he kept himself quite aloof from others. He did not have a negative attitude towards others; he was just shy.

He did get along to some extent with two older boys in school, studying in a higher grade. He probably hung out with them just because they spoke "his" language – this language was that of online games and the gamer community

To most others he seemed to be an alien since he hardly spoke, and if at all he did, it would sound like Greek and Latin to the rest. He used to mention names of online games which nobody had heard of, and so they would shy away and wonder what he was talking about.

Of late, he had been reaching school late very often, and so was reprimanded for the same. His only reason for the delay was not being able to get up in time for school, since he stayed up late into the night gaming. His parents were called in for parent–teacher meetings several times and threatened by the school but in vain. They said they had no time to come for meetings and that the school should just deal with their son and discipline him.

P.R.'s parents had no clue what the boy was up to every night. He slept in a separate room, away from their bedroom. Since the school complaints had started coming in, they noticed that his room was locked most of the night, for more than ten hours at least, post early dinner which was a norm in the home. So if everybody ate at 8:00 pm, they could not check what he was doing till at least 6 am next morning, and after that they would see he was sleeping and just could not wake up till noon.

Nobody made an attempt to talk to him since he refused to answer, and if they persisted he threw a fit of rage and was extremely aggressive and violent with his parents as well as anyone else who tried to speak to him. The parents did think of drug addiction but found no needles or powder packets when they searched his room in his absence, nor did they see needle marks or tracks on his arms, which is what they had been asked to look out for.

Gradually his grades dropped, he started coming to school unkempt and disoriented and actually looked unhealthy since he was not eating or sleeping well. After a lot of probing, intervention and coaxing by his favorite teacher who incidentally also was a game buff, he admitted that he hated school and home. All he loved were online games. The teacher asked further, and luckily knew the right questions to ask. This probing and investigation revealed that he was hooked on to online gaming with strangers across the world, he had to stay awake to match up to their time lines which lead to lack of sleep and increased dependency.

His condition worsened when he stopped eating and sleeping because he felt these activities were just a waste of time, and took him away from gaming. His hands trembled and he was violent when the gadget on which he was gaming was taken away from him.

By now the teacher had shared with the parents what was really going on and requested that they consult mental health professionals. The parents, still in disbelief, were also extremely superstitious, and invited priests to conduct a "hawan", a sort of prayer and incantation, to deal with "his curse" as they believed it to be, and to bless him and cure him.

Precious time was lost in this as he missed school further. By then he was almost constantly online and gaming for 14 to 15 hours a day. Finally he made an attempt to harm himself which fortunately failed. This finally led the family to consult mental health professionals and the case could be handled in a scientific manner.

P.R. has now dropped out of school and is currently under treatment for de-addiction. The family and school authorities hope he will be back on track soon and get back to studies.

(Thanks is due to Responsible Netism for sharing the case)

Throughout our evolutionary history, we discovered that some plants changed the way we felt. Betel nut has been crewed for its nicotine-like effects for at least 13,000 years in Timor (Saah, 2005). **Cocaine** is naturally available in coca leaves, and morphine is available from poppy plants. Archaeological evidence suggests that Peruvian foraging societies were chewing coca leaves some 8,000 years ago. Actual poppy seeds were recovered from a 4,500-year-old settlement in Switzerland. Other evidence shows that opium was available in Europe in the Neolithic, Copper, and Bronze Ages. We as humans thus discovered naturally occurring psychoactive substances, and we have used them throughout history.

When we began to move away from being hunter–gatherers about 10,000 years ago, we also discovered how to make alcoholic beverages such as beer and wine, although it may have happened earlier. In fact, there is some suggestion that we made beer before we made bread (Hayden, Canuel, & Shanse, 2013). Throughout the world, the natural ingredients are available for making **alcohol** (McGovern, 2009). One of these is honey. Other ingredients are region-specific. In the Middle East, there is barley, wheat, and grapes. In China, there is rice, millet, and hawthorn fruit. In present-day Lebanon, Syria, Jordan, and Israel, there are figs and dates. In Africa, there are grasses and palm sap. In the Americas, there is corn, cacao, cactus fruit, and yucca. Pottery artifacts have been found in China dating from 7000 BCE with residue of fermented beverages. Other pottery has been found in Iran from around 3500 BCE-, which was used to store wine. Thus, the use of psychoactive substances has been part of our history.

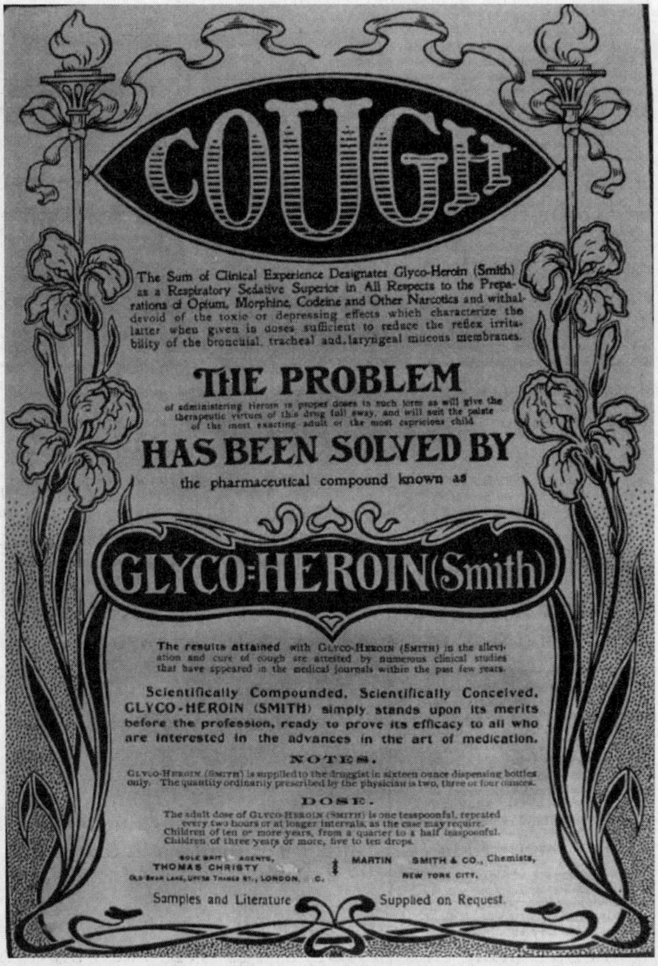

The label from heroin cough syrup dating from the turn of the last century

Source: Musto (1991, p. 40).

In the United States, our attitude toward drug use has changed drastically over the past 200 years (see Musto, 1991, for an overview). Both Benjamin Franklin and the poet Samuel Taylor Coleridge in the United Kingdom often took a substance made of opium and alcohol for medical reasons. During the 1800s, drugs such as cocaine and opiates were seen as everyday compounds to be used by all. In fact, the original formula for Coca-Cola, which was introduced in 1886, included cocaine. In 1898, the Bayer Company was able to synthesize a substance from morphine, which they named heroin. This was the year before they introduced the Bayer aspirin. The photo to the right shows a label for heroin cough syrup. Opium imports rose until the drug was made illegal in 1909 (see *Figure 14-1*).

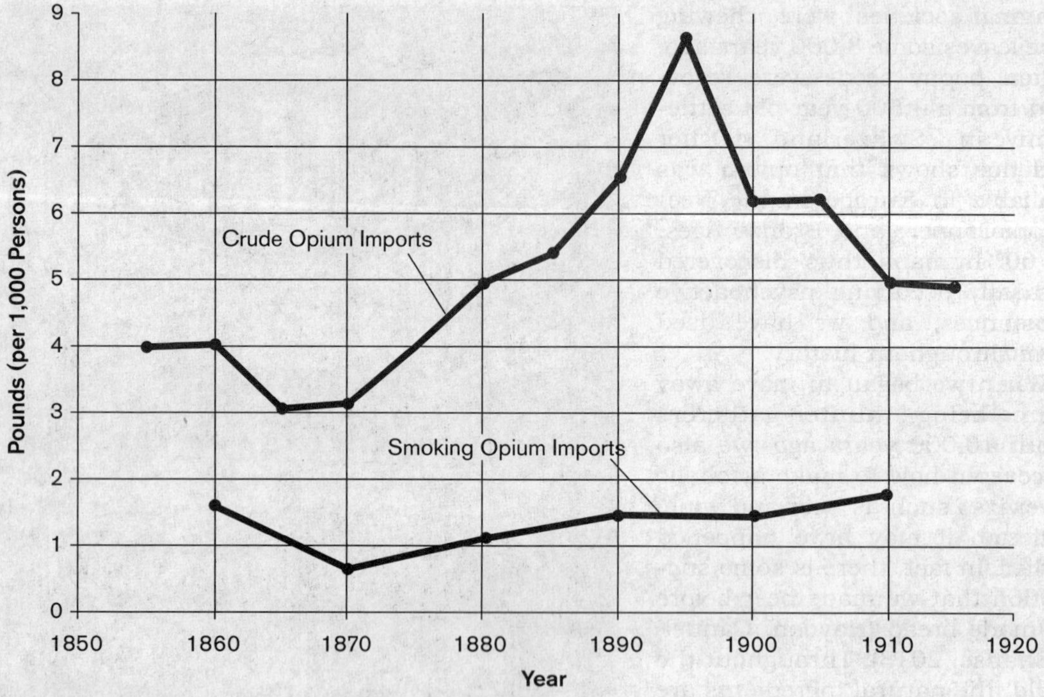

FIGURE 14-1 U.S. Opiate Consumption as Documented by the Treasury and Commerce Departments

Source: Musto (1991, p. 42).
Note: In 1909, the importation of opium for smoking became illegal. Crude opium and its derivatives were severely restricted in 1915. After 1915 the data in the graph reflects medical use.

From the early 1900s through the 1940s, our view of drugs changed in a dramatic fashion. During this period, drugs were seen as dangerous and in need of strict control. During the 1920s, even alcohol was made illegal. This period was followed by the 1960s in which drugs were viewed as a form of recreation and a method for changing consciousness. Marijuana, which was probably introduced to the United States in the 1920s by the Mexican immigrants coming to work in agriculture, was widely used in the 1960s. Opiates and cocaine also showed an increase in use during the 1960s and 1970s. Synthesized substances such as LSD were also freely available in the 1960s. Society's view of drugs in the 1980s began to change with the popular media running stories on a "crisis of addiction."

INDIAN STATISTICS ON DRUG USE

There are lot of work done in India that shows that about 40% of road traffic accidents occur under the influence of alcohol, there is a higher prevalence (3.6%, as compared to rate without influence being 2.1%) of sexually transmitted infections, and that overall prevalence of alcohol use is high (29.6%) (NHP India, 2015).

In an interesting study conducted in Bengaluru, where the researchers conducted a survey on 717 participants using a mall intercept method, it was found that the non-medical use of different prescription medicine classes over the past 12 months was as follows: anti-inflammatories and analgesics (26%), opioids (17%), antibiotics (13%), and sedatives (12%). The majority reported "use without prescription," while "use in ways other than as prescribed" was also reported. Of the 12% reported use of benzodiazepines, 73% reported in ways other than prescribed, compared to 27% use without prescription. For opioids, of the 16% of non-medical use, 40% was used in ways other than prescribed and 60% without prescription (Nattala, Murthy, Kandavel, & Cottler, 2015).

In a study from Jodhpur, published in the *Indian Journal of Medical Research* (2014), it was reported that the records of treatment seekers at the Drug De-addiction and Treatment Centre, over 10 years (2002–2011) were scanned to identify 92 cases reporting inhalant use. Of these, the 87 available case files were reviewed and the relevant data were collected and analyzed.

Authors found that over this 10-year period, the number of cases with inhalant abuse per year rose steadily to peak at 20 cases (4.08% of new cases) in 2006 and then stabilized at 1–3% of new cases annually.

Of the 87 cases studied, all were males with a mean age of 18.9 ± 4.12 years, mean education of 9.8 ± 3.42 years and mean family income of ₹7676 ± 7343.15 (median: ₹5,000).

Most of the users were unmarried (89.7%), urban resident (79.3%), and from a nuclear family (78.2%). About half of the subjects were students (50.6%).

The most common inhalant used was typewriter correction fluid (73.6%) followed by typewriter diluent fluid (19.5%) and glue (6.9%). The most common reason for initiation was curiosity.

The mean age of onset of inhalant use was 16.3 ± 4.22 years. Most of the subjects fulfilled the criteria for inhalant dependence (85.1%).

Hence, it is clear that most of the inhalant users were mostly urban youth belonging to middle socio-economic class families. The principal sources of inhalant abuse were the commonly available substances such as typewriter correction fluids and majority of the subjects initiated it out of curiosity (Gupta, Nebhinani, Basu, & Mattoo, 2014). Studies reported from Manipur, India also show that inhalant use among youngsters and students is on the rise (Bishwalata & Raleng, 2014).

DRUG USE IN THE UNITED STATES

If you look at the current information, it becomes apparent that many of the 315,000,000 U.S. citizens over 18 years of age use a variety of both illegal and legal drugs. In 2011, over 50% of Americans age 18 or older say they regularly use alcohol whereas 18% say they use **tobacco** (www.cdc.gov/nchs/data/series/sr_10/sr10_256.pdf). Tobacco use has steadily decreased from 24.1% in 1997. Those with a mental disorder show double the rate for tobacco use (42.1%), and this rate has not decreased since 1997 (www.samhsa.gov/data/spotlight/spot120-smokingSPD.pdf). For those who are under the legal drinking age of 21, some 13% report drinking alcohol and 10.7% report tobacco use.

Since 1971, the U.S. government through the Department of Health and Human Services has collected data on drug use through the U.S. Substance Abuse and Mental Health Services Administration (SAMHSA; www.samhsa.gov/). In 2011, this agency estimated that approximately 22.5 million Americans age 12 or older used an illicit drug in the past month. Illicit drugs include marijuana/hashish, cocaine (including crack), heroin, **hallucinogens,** inhalants, and prescription-type psychotherapeutics (pain relievers, tranquilizers, stimulants, and sedatives) used nonmedically. Some illicit drugs are not illegal in themselves—prescription drugs, for example—but are used in ways a health professional would not support. *Figure 14-2* shows the total illicit drug use along with the totals by drug used in the last month. This figure shows that marijuana is the most commonly used illicit drug—used by some 18.1 million people or 5.8% of the U.S. population in the past month. Although not shown in the figure, the use of marijuana, cocaine, and **amphetamines** have all decreased significantly since the 1980s. In terms of age-group, college-age individuals (18–20 years of age) currently show the highest percentage of illicit drugs use (see *Figure 14-3*).

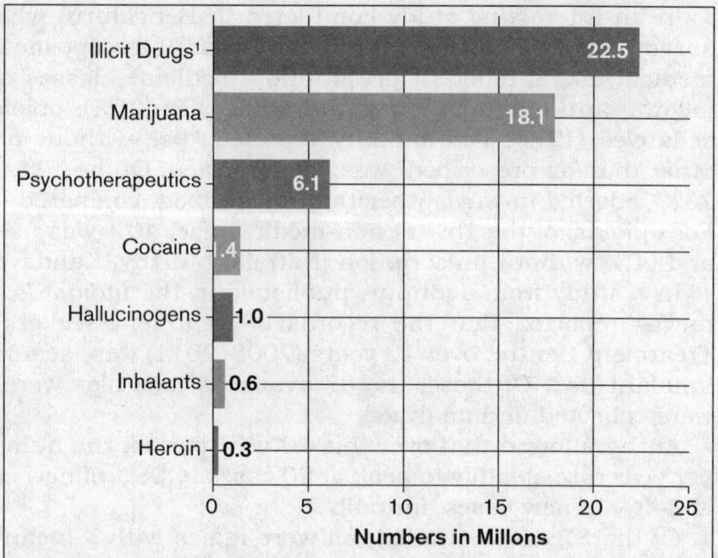

[1]Illicit Drugs include marijuana/hashish, cocaine (including crack), heroin, hallucinogens, inhalants, or prescription-type psychotherapeutics used nonmedically.

FIGURE 14-2 Drug Use Over a 30-Day Period in 2012 for Those 12 and Over

Source: From Substance Abuse and Mental Health Services Administration, Results from the 2011 National Survey on Drug Use and Health: Summary of National Findings, NSDUH Series H-44, HHS Publication No. (SMA) 12-4713. Rockville, MD: Substance Abuse and Mental Health Services Administration, 2012.

The United Nations also collects data on drug use throughout the world. *Figure 14-4* shows the use of illicit drugs throughout the world. From this table and back in *Figure 14-2*, it can be determined that drug use in the United States is higher than it is worldwide. The United States is one of the larger users of illicit drugs such as marijuana, amphetamines, **opioids** such as heroin and opium, and cocaine. Other developed economies such as Australia and the countries of Europe show greater drug use than developing economies. Overall, these drugs are used more by males than females throughout the world. Illicit drugs can have economic consequences for countries in terms of health care costs and the loss of work productivity. They also have personal consequences in terms of social and family relationships. In the next section, I will introduce you to the nature of **addiction** and how drugs can influence and change your brain. Following this, I will discuss particular drugs including alcohol, **cannabis,** opioids, amphetamines, and tobacco. Gambling is now considered an addictive disorder in the fifth edition of the *Diagnostic and Statistical Manual of Mental Disorders* (*DSM–5*) (American

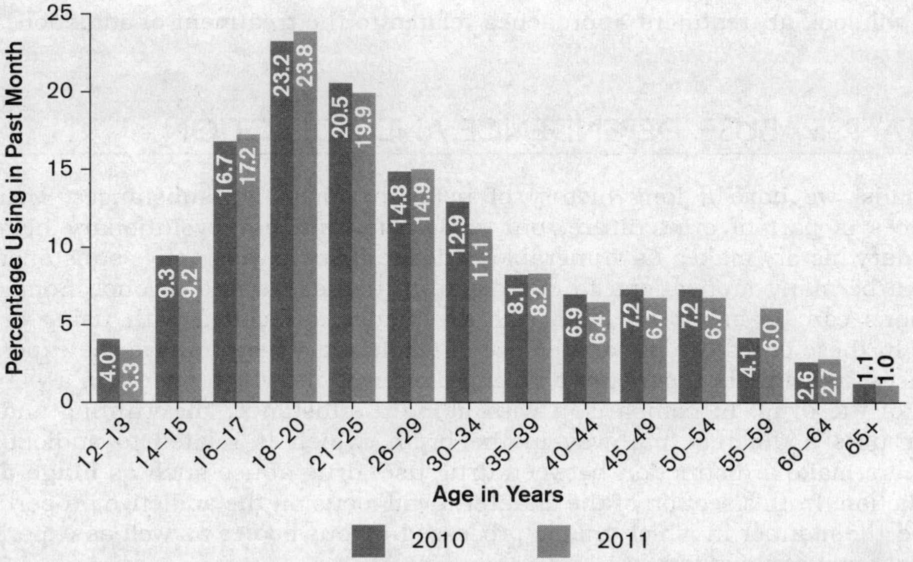

+Difference between this esimate and the 2011 estimate is satistically significant at the 0.05 level.

FIGURE 14-3 Drug Use for the Past Month by Age

Source: From Substance Abuse and Mental Health Services Administration, Results from the 2011 National Survey on Drug Use and Health: Summary of National Findings, NSDUH Series H-44, HHS Publication No. (SMA) 12-4713. Rockville, MD: Substance Abuse and Mental Health Services Administration, 2012.

	Prevalence (Percentage)		Number (Thousands)	
	Low	High	Low	High
Cannabis	2.6	5.0	119,420	224,490
Opioids	0.6	0.8	26,380	36,120
Opiates	0.3	0.5	12,980	20,990
Cocaine	0.3	0.4	13,200	19,510
Amphetamine-type stimulants	0.3	1.2	14,340	52,540
“Ecstasy”	0.2	0.6	10,480	28,120
Any illicit drug	3.4	6.6	153,000	300,000

FIGURE 14-4 Annual Prevalence and Number of Illicit Drug Users at the Global Level for the Year 2010

Source: United Nations Office on Drugs and Crime (2012).

Psychiatric Association [APA], 2013) and will be discussed next. The final section of the chapter will look at treatment approaches related to the treatment of addiction.

SUBSTANCE ABUSE, DEPENDENCE, AND ADDICTION

As humans, we have a long history of using psychoactive substances. Using these substances is part of our culture, our social life, and our evolutionary history. Our evolutionary history makes us vulnerable to desire many psychoactive substances. Thus, there can be many motivations to our desire to use drugs and alcohol. Some of these motivations can be based on liking the experience associated with using drugs and alcohol. In these cases, we make a choice of when and where to have the experience. In other cases, individuals experience a stronger motivation, which results in a wanting and seeking of the drug. In comparison with liking a substance, the wanting and seeking behavior uses a different pathway in the brain, which is related to addiction. Many researchers make a distinction between drug use, drug abuse such as **binge drinking,** and addiction. In this section of the chapter, I will focus on the addictive properties of the drug and the manner in which this is processed by our bodies as well as experienced in emotional and cognitive terms.

Addiction is also described in terms of substance **dependence.** There are three major components to dependence. The first component is the desire to seek and take a certain substance. The second component is the inability to avoid or limit the intake of the substance. And the third component is the experience of negative emotional states when the substance is not available. SAMHSA, of the United States, estimates that some 20.6 million individuals in 2011 could be considered substance dependent or abusing a psychoactive substance.

Substance abuse and addiction is a burden not only to the individual person but to the family and society at large. It is estimated that approximately half a trillion dollars is lost to the U.S. economy from substance abuse and addiction. This includes medical problems, loss of productivity, accidents, and crime. Family relationships are also disturbed including the person's relationship with his or her children and their care.

Substance Disorders in *DSM–5* and *ICD-10*

DSM–5 and *ICD-10* examine a disordered level of involvement with a psychoactive substance in terms of use, **intoxication,** and **withdrawal.** To be considered a disorder, the use of the psychoactive substance must cause distress or cause impairment that interferes with normal functioning. **Disordered use** refers to the condition in which the person experiences significant impairment or distress. Part of this impairment or distress can be related to such factors as the person taking more of the substance than was intended, not being able to reduce the use of the substance, spending time trying to obtain the substance, not being able to do one's work or keep up with other obligations, having the substance interfere with social relationships, reducing one's activities because of the substance, having the substance create medical problems, and engaging in hazardous activities such as driving while on the substance.

Intoxication refers to the effects of the psychoactive substance. These are drug related but typically involve psychological changes and behavioral abilities. Alcohol intoxication, for example, may produce such symptoms as slurred speech, problems with attention and memory, inability to make coordinated motor movements including walking, and passing out. Marijuana intoxication on the other hand may lead to increased appetite, a different experience of time, a withdrawal into inner experience, a cognitive and emotional overvaluation of ideas, and at times anxiety.

Withdrawal refers to the symptoms experienced when a psychoactive substance is no longer used. Withdrawal symptoms can also be seen when the amount of a drug is reduced, especially when this follows a long period of use. Withdrawal symptoms are typically drug-specific. Alcohol withdrawal can produce tremors, problems with sleep, nausea or vomiting, anxiety, and autonomic nervous system (ANS) overactivity such as sweating or a high heart rate. An extreme form of alcohol withdrawal is referred to as delirium tremens. After a long period of heavy drinking, withdrawal of alcohol can produce not only the normal symptoms of withdrawal but also hallucinations, confusion, and seizures. Individuals with delirium tremens (DT) may believe they are picking bugs off their body or see various insects crawling on the walls when there is nothing there. The cultural idea that alcohol causes one to see pink elephants comes from DTs.

DSM–5 and *ICD-10* describe use, intoxication, and withdrawal in terms of a number of psychoactive substances including alcohol, **caffeine,** cannabis, hallucinogens, opioids, sedatives, stimulants, and tobacco. They also include a general category of inhalant-related disorders. Gambling as a disorder is now part of substance use and addictive disorders. The criteria for substance use and addictive disorder for each drug such as alcohol, cannabis, hallucinogens, and so forth are very similar.

Explanatory Models for Alcohol Use

In an interesting study (2013) by a research group led by Dr. Vikram Patel was published in the *Asian Journal of Psychiatry.* Defining explanatory models as notions about a sickness and its treatment adopted by all those involved in the clinical process, the researchers report that a qualitative study based on thematic analysis of semi-structured interviews conducted at two sites in India (Goa and Satara) yielded the finding that alcohol consumption is linked mainly to psychosocial stress, peer influences, availability of disposable income, and drinking for pleasure.

Who Becomes Addicted?

There is no one answer as to what causes addiction (see Volkow & Li, 2005, for an overview). One factor is related to timing of first use. With alcohol, those who began using alcohol before the age of 15 in the United States are 4 times more likely to become addicted in their lifetime in comparison with those who begin at age 20 or older. Current research suggests that drugs affect adolescents in a different manner than they do adults. Further, it has been shown that the attitudes of society at the time you grew up will later influence your drug use (Keyes et al., 2012). It has been suggested that since European youth are introduced to alcohol use, such as wine with meals, earlier than American youth, they have fewer problems with alcohol. Data from the U.S. Department of Justice suggest this is not the case (www.udetc.org/documents/YouthDrinkingRatesAndProblems.pdf; Friese & Grube, n.d.). While 15- and 16-year-olds in Europe do report drinking more than American adolescents, as shown in *Figure 14-5*, European youth in general do not report less intoxication in the past month than American adolescents.

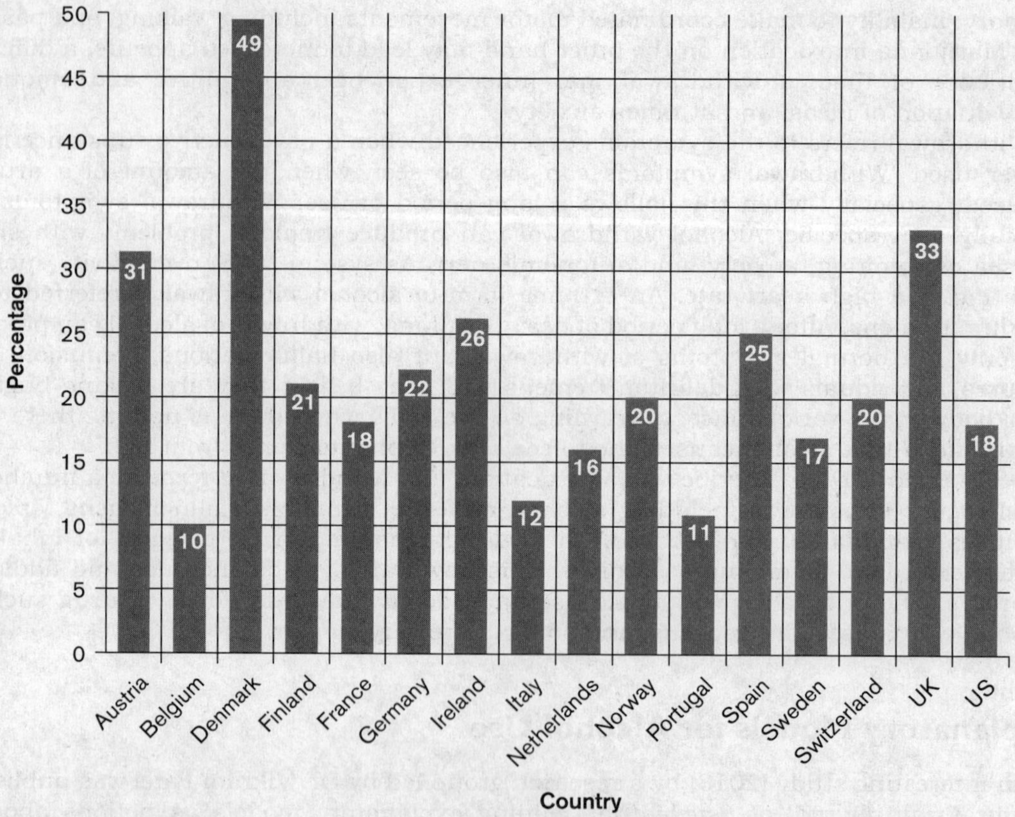

FIGURE 14-5 Percentage of 15- to 16-Year-Olds Reporting Intoxication in the Past 30 Days: Based on 2007 Data

Source: Friese and Grube (n.d.).

As discussed in Chapter 6, adolescence is clearly a time that the brain is reestablishing connections and networks and is sensitive to environmental and internal changes. Related to these brain changes is the development of better impulse control, social understanding, self-awareness, and other executive functioning in the frontal lobes. As you will see, drugs have a direct influence on the frontal lobes in individuals of all ages. Adolescents are particularly at risk for drug use to influence both short-term and long-term brain development (Blakemore, 2013).

Another important factor is genetics. Research has shown that 40% to 60% of vulnerability to addiction can be attributed to genetic factors. These genetic factors and their relationship with the environment can be seen in the manner in which different drugs show different levels of reinforcing factors and influence metabolism. That is, some drugs are more addictive than others. Also, individuals show different sensitivities to particular drugs and thus some people can become addicted to some drugs more quickly than they can to other drugs as well as more quickly than other individuals can become addicted to a particular drug (see Volkow, Wang, Fowler, & Tomasi, 2012, for an overview).

Environmental factors such as stress and/or low socioeconomic level are associated with greater drug use, which can lead to addiction. With adolescents, peer pressure can play an important role in deciding whether or not to try new types of drugs. Adolescence is also a time when individuals take risks and try new things. The environments in which both adults and adolescents live play a crucial role. This is compounded, research shows, by the fact that drugs may disrupt networks of the brain involved in making decisions. Drugs not only influence what people seek for reinforcement but also the ability to inhibit these desires.

Another way in which the environment plays a role is in terms of epigenetics (see Robison & Nestler, 2011, for an overview). Although numerous studies suggest that the genetic contribution to the risk for addiction is about 50%, it is not known which genes are involved. An alternative suggestion is that epigenetic mechanisms relate to addiction by determining how genes are turned on and off.

With the advent of brain imaging and other neuroscience techniques, research has suggested that there is a common underlying process to a variety of disorders including drug addiction, bulimia nervosa, **pathological gambling,** and sexual addiction (see Goodman, 2007, for an overview). These disorders are also associated with affective disorders, anxiety disorders, attention deficit disorder, and personality disorders at frequencies that are higher than their frequencies in the general population.

Addiction to psychoactive substances is not unique to humans. Neuroscience research has shown that other mammals show compulsive behaviors to take in the same addictive substances as humans (Wise, 1998). This supports an evolutionary perspective but also raises some interesting questions as to why a number of species including humans seek these substances. Clearly addiction can cause harm, but is there another side to understanding addiction? Traditionally, from an evolutionary perspective we can ask if taking psychoactive substances helps us protect ourselves, or mate, or engage in social activities.

It can also be noted that psychoactive substances use the same networks in the brain that are associated with a feeling of social well-being. In particular, the opioid system in the brain that is involved in the addiction to morphine and heroin is also involved in the satisfaction derived from social relationships, sexual stimulation, and tasty food. One of the ways these processes may be influenced is through our emotions (see Panksepp, Knutson, & Burgdorf, 2002). We perform activities such as eating, sleeping, and being with others that not only make us feel good but also increase our ability to take care of ourselves and have sexual and social relationships. As infants, feeling taken care of in terms of food, closeness, and attachment are critical for successful development. Research with other mammals such as rats and monkeys shows that isolation in early life leads to a greater sensitivity to psychoactive substances including alcohol. This suggests that early environmental factors can play a role in later drug use.

QUALITATIVE STUDY FROM INDIA ON ONSET AND PROGRESSION OF ALCOHOL USE

In a more recent qualitative study on the onset and progression of alcohol use from the research group from Sangath, Goa, published in the *Journal of Ethnicity in Substance Abuse*, Mackinnon, Bhatia, & Nadkarni (2017) report,

> Reasons to begin drinking included social drinking, functional use of alcohol, stress, and boredom. Progression to problematic drinking patterns was characterized by drinking alone, alternating between abstinent and heavy drinking periods, and drinking based on the availability of finances.

Some enablers to reduce/stop drinking included the consequences of drinking lifestyle and personal resolve; some barriers included availability of alcohol at social events and stress. Some reasons for persisting heavy use of alcohol included lack of family support, physical withdrawal symptoms, peer pressure, stress, and easy availability.

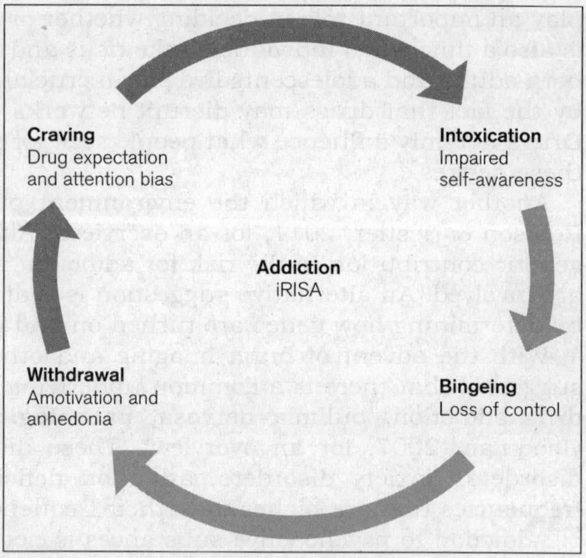

FIGURE 14-6 Pattern of Addiction—iRISA Refers to Impaired Response Inhibition and Salience Attribution

Source: Goldstein and Volkow (2011, p. 653).

Pattern of Addiction

There is a pattern that is seen in addiction (see *Figure 14-6*). Initially, the positive experience of taking the drug leads to a compulsion to seek and take a given substance. It can be experienced as a rush or sense of well-being. This period of intoxication is also associated with impaired cognitive abilities. This is followed by a **craving** in which the individual loses control of the ability to limit intake of the drug. For example, even when the blood alcohol of a person with an alcohol addiction is high, he or she still drinks more. The next condition is the emergence of a negative emotional state when the substance is unavailable or access to it is limited. What once gave a positive feeling now does little. In fact, the person needs the drug to feel normal. There is a paradox in that by this last stage, people who are addicted want their psychoactive substance more than they enjoy it.

A more detailed pattern of addiction is described by Goodman (2007):

Topic	*Details*
Course of illness	The disorder typically begins in adolescence or early adulthood and follows a chronic course with remissions and exacerbations
Behavioral features	Narrowing of behavioral repertoire, continuation of the behavior despite harmful consequences
Individuals' subjective experience of the condition	Sense of craving, preoccupation, excitement during preparatory activity, mood-altering effects of the behavior, sense of loss of control
Progressive development of the condition	Craving, loss of control, narrowing of behavioral repertoire, and harmfulness of consequences all tending to increase as the duration of the condition increases
Experience of tolerance	As the behavior is repeated, its potency to produce reinforcing effects tends to diminish
Experience of withdrawal phenomena	Psychological or physical discomfort when the behavior is discontinued

Topic	Details
Tendency to relapse	That is, to return to harmful patterns of behavior after a period of abstinence or control has been achieved
Propensity for behavioral substitution	When the behavioral symptoms of the disorder have come under control, tendency for addictive engagement in other behaviors to emerge or intensify
Relationship between the condition and other aspects of affected individuals' lives	For example, neglect of other areas of life as the behavior assumes priority
Recurrent themes in the ways individuals with these conditions relate to others and to themselves	Including low self-esteem, self-centeredness, denial, rationalization, and conflicts over dependency and control

Can Drugs Change Your Brain?

The quick answer is yes—drugs change your brain. In fact, for someone addicted to a particular drug, just seeing the paraphernalia associated with it can produce physiological changes before the drug is actually ingested. It does not matter if it is heroin or whiskey. This works in a manner similar to how all learning changes your brain, although drug addiction seems to last longer than simple learning (see Nestler & Malenka, 2004, for an overview). It can last for weeks, months, or even years after the last ingestion of the drug. This sets up the possibility of relapse since a person has a difficult time forgetting the effects of the drug.

On one level, drugs are rewarding to our body and give us experiences we seek. This can result in some amazing situations. For example, if an animal is given the choice of drugs or food, it will choose drugs over food. Catnip is one example of this seen outside of the laboratory. In the lab, the typical procedure is to use a Skinner box in which the animal can press a lever for food or a different lever for the drug. With previous experience with the drug, the animal will ignore the food lever and press the drug lever. If the ratio is set so that the animal will need to press the lever a number of times before the drug is administered, the animal will actually spend much of its waking hours working for the drug. This is not unlike the human who is addicted to a drug who spends considerable energy to obtain it including engaging in illegal activities to acquire the money to purchase it.

Neuroscience studies show the rewarding effect of drugs is their ability to increase *dopamine* (see Hyman, Malenka, & Nestler, 2006; Volkow et al., 2012, for overviews). One important pathway related to addiction is the mesolimbic dopamine system. This system begins in the ventral tegmental area (VTA), which is located near the base of the brain (see *Figure 14-7*).

These pathways connect with the nucleus accumbens, prefrontal cortex (PFC), dorsal striatum, and amygdala. Dopamine is released in these structures. Dopamine was initially thought to be the neurobiological correlate of reward or pleasure. However, more recent research has clarified dopamine's function, which includes signaling the incentive salience of events. That is, it is not so much associated with pleasure as with the expectation of pleasure. In this sense, it is involved in driving motivated behavior including rewarding, aversive, novel, and unexpected stimuli. Thus, it is involved in predicting reward or nonreward as well as in facilitating consolidation of memory for salient events. The important point is that many drugs of addiction increase activity in the VTA and the nucleus accumbens.

Molecular mechanisms of many drugs leave excessive dopamine available in the brain (see *Figure 14-8*). This works by different mechanisms. Cocaine either blocks dopamine uptake in the synapse or increases dopamine released by the terminals of VTA cells, which increases dopamine signaling in the nucleus accumbens. Alcohol and opiates such as

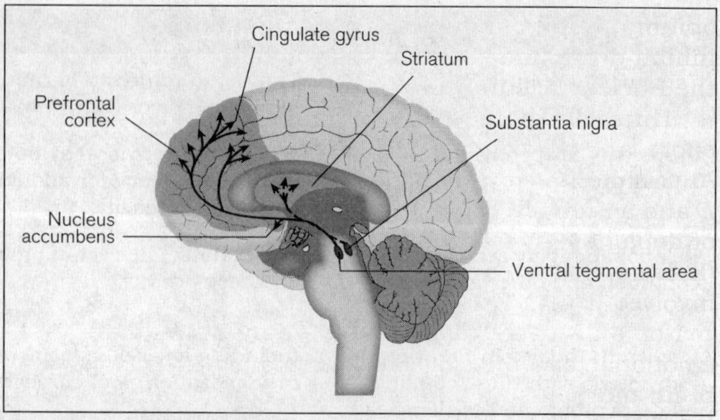

FIGURE 14-7 Brain Reward Circuitry

Source: Hyman et al. (2006, p. 571).

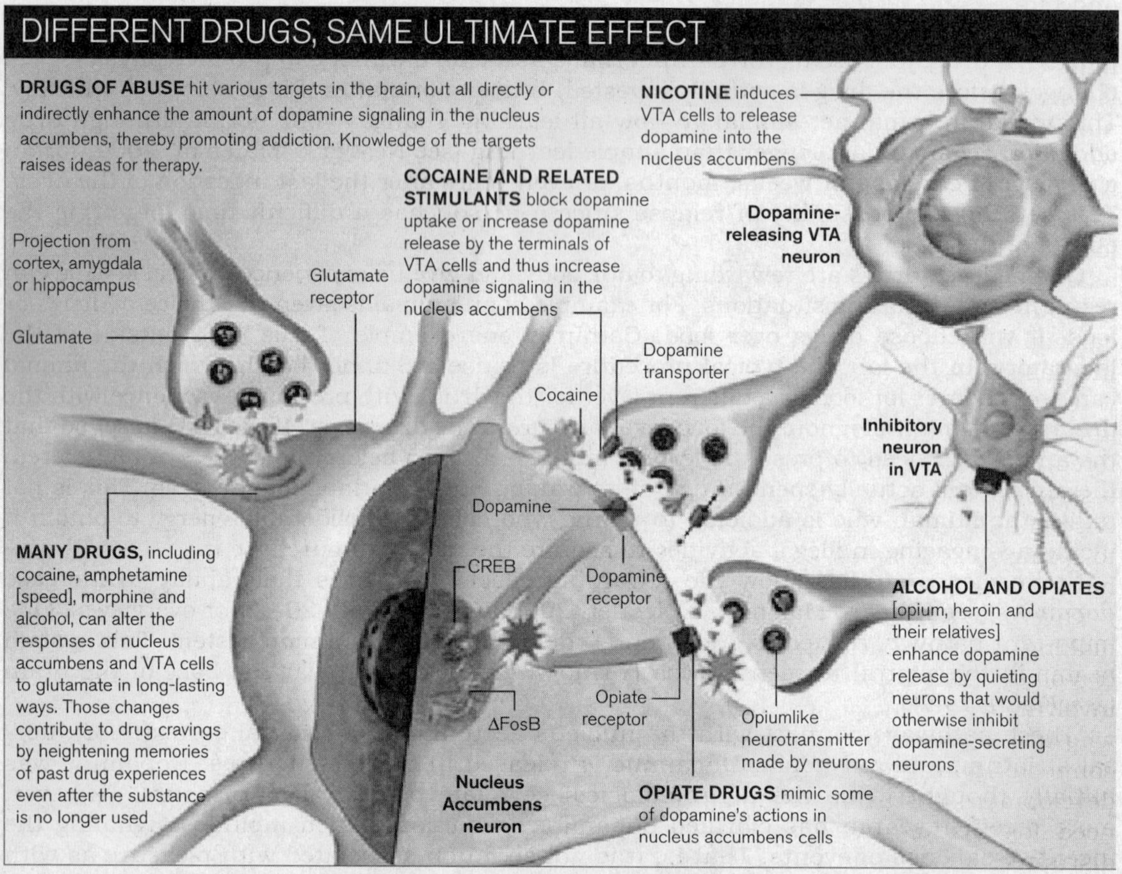

FIGURE 14-8 The Manner in Which Different Drugs Affect the Brain

Source: Nestler and Malenka (2004, p. 84).

opium and heroin enhance dopamine release by quieting neurons that would otherwise inhibit dopamine-secreting neurons. **Nicotine** induces VTA cells to release dopamine into the nucleus accumbens.

Thus, dopamine plays an important role in motivation, which includes activation, effort, and persistence. Drug addiction can be seen as one form of enhanced motivation. At this point, five dopamine receptors have been identified, which are labeled by the letter *D* and a number. Short-term exposure to drugs involves the dopamine system. The release of dopamine in relation to addictive drugs changes drug use into drug-seeking behavior (Kalivas, 2009). Over time, other neurotransmitters such as glutamate and GABA become involved (Uys & Reissner, 2011).

Not only can drugs change your brain but they can also take over the cognitive, emotional, and physiological mechanisms that we use for everyday life. They take over the brain mechanisms that are involved in reward (see Hyman et al., 2006, for an overview). In addiction, compulsive drug use limits our level of human functioning. Our functioning is largely reduced to seeking means for obtaining the drug. This results in a decrease in social functioning as well as personal creativity and productivity. Additionally, brain changes in certain areas such as the frontal lobe lead us to deny we even have a problem and reduce our desire to make changes.

The rewarding mechanisms are seen as the main reason humans and laboratory animals choose to self-administer drugs. The main mechanism for these rewarding effects is the ability of drugs to increase dopamine in the nucleus accumbens (see Volkow et al., 2012, for an overview). Dopamine appears to encode the prediction of reward whereas endogenous opioids and cannabinoids mediate the experience of pleasure. Nicotine, alcohol, stimulants, and marijuana all increase dopamine in the dorsal striatum and ventral striatum (VS). Interestingly, research suggests that individuals with a low dopamine level—as seen in Parkinson's disease, for example—when given dopamine as a treatment may show pathological gambling, hypersexuality, compulsive shopping, compulsive eating, and compulsive medication use (Voon & Fox, 2007). Through classical conditioning, a neutral stimulus that is linked to a drug can by itself produce increased dopamine.

The speed at which specific drugs enter the brain is related to the experience of reward and the nature of the "high" experienced. This can happen with the same drug administered in different ways. For example, cocaine that is snorted through the nose produces a slower and less intense high than if it is given intravenously. Further, the peak experience of different drugs happens at different times. Nicotine has a peak level at around 2 to 3 minutes. Cocaine has a peak level at around 4 to 6 minutes. Methamphetamines have a peak level at around 10 to 15 minutes

Given the role of the PFC in executive functions such as inhibitory control and decision making, it is not surprising to see a disruption of this area with addiction (see Goldstein & Volkow, 2011, for an overview). It appears that the PFC is connected to networks involving the striatum, which are modulated by dopamine. In studies that compare those who use drugs with nonusers, the worst task performance was found on tasks that are connected with the PFC. It is assumed that dysfunction of these areas contributes to the development of craving, compulsive use, and the denial that a problem exists or there is need for treatment. *Figure 14-9* shows processes associated with the PFC that are disrupted in addiction.

With our current understanding of brain mechanisms in addiction, it is possible to redraw *Figure 14-6* and add the brain mechanisms involved (see *Figure 14-10*). Once the

Process	Possible disruption in addiction	Probable PFC region
Self-control and behavioral monitoring: response inhibition, behavioral coordination, conflict and error prediction, detection and resolution	Impulsivity, compulsivity, risk taking and impaired self-monitoring (habitual, automatic, stimulus-driven and inflexible behavioral patterns)	DLPFC, dACC, IFG and vlPFC
Emotion regulation: cognitive and affective suppression of emotion	Enhanced stress reactivity and inability to suppress emotional intensity (for example, anxiety and negative affect)	mOFC, vmPFC and subgenual ACC
Motivation: drive, initiative, persistence and effort towards the pursuit of goals	Enhanced motivation to procure drugs but decreased motivation for other goals, and compromised purposefulness and effort	OFC, ACC, vmPFC and DLPFC
Awareness and interoception: feeling one's own bodily and subjective state, insight	Reduced satiety, "denial" of illness or need for treatment, and externally oriented thinking	rACC and dACC, mPFC, OFC and vlPFC
Attention and flexibility: set formation and maintenance versus set-shifting, and task switching	Attention bias towards drug-related stimuli and away from other stimuli and reinforcers, and inflexibility in goals to procure the drug	DLPFC, ACC, IFC and vlPFC
Working memory: short-term memory enabling the construction of representations and guidance of action	Formation of memory that is biased towards drug-related stimuli and away from alternatives	DLPFC
Learning and memory: stimulus-response associative learning, reversal learning, extinction, reward devaluation, latent inhibition (suppression of information) and long-term memory	Drug conditioning and disrupted ability to update the reward value of non-drug reinforcers	DLPFC, OFC and ACC
Decision making: valuation (coding reinforcers) versus choice, expected outcome, probability estimation, planning and goal formation	Drug-related anticipation, choice of immediate reward over delayed gratification, discounting of future consequences, and inaccurate predictions or action planning	lOFC, mOFC, vmPFC and DLPFC
Salience attribution: affective value appraisal, incentive salience and subjective utility (alternative outcomes)	Drugs and drug cues have a sensitized value, non-drug reinforcers are devalued and gradients are not perceived, and negative prediction error (actual experience worse than expected)	mOFC and vmPFC

FIGURE 14-9 Processes Associated With the Prefrontal Cortex That Are Disrupted in Addiction. Brain Areas Are Prefrontal Cortex, Anterior Cingulate Cortex, Orbitofrontal Cortex, and Interior Frontal Gyrus

Source: Goldstein and Volkow (2011, p. 654).

Note: Orbitofrontal cortex (OFC) includes Brodmann area (BA) 10 -14 and 47 (REF. 216), and inferior and subgenual regions of anterior cingulate cortex (ACC) (BA 24, 25 and 32) in the ventromedial prefrontal cortex (vmPFC)217; ACC includes rostral ACC (rACC) and dorsal ACC (dACC) (BA 24 and 32, respectively), which are included within the medial PFC (mPFC). The mPFC also includes BA 6, 8, 9 and 10 (REF. 218); dorsolateral PFC (DLPFC) includes BA 6, 8, 9 and 46 (REF. 219); and the inferior frontal gyrus (IFG) and ventrolateral PFC (vlPFC) encompass inferior portions of BA 8, 44 and 45 (REF. 220). These various processes and regions participate to a different degree in craving, intoxication, bingeing and withdrawal. lOFC, lateral OFC; mOFC, medial OFC; PFC, prefrontal cortex.

person has taken a drug and experiences the pleasant or euphoric effects, the individual has been reinforced to want more. This reward circuit includes the VTA, nucleus accumbens, amygdala, and hippocampus. This circuit involves the neurotransmitter dopamine and is related to reward and expectation and memory of the drug experience. Following the reinforcing effects of a drug comes the expectation or craving of using the drug again. This is a conscious experience involving the PFC, the orbitofrontal cortex (OFC), and the anterior cingulate cortex (ACC). This is followed by a loss of control or binging in which the VTA and nucleus accumbens reward circuit is increased and the normal inhibition of the frontal cortex is decreased. These areas are also thought to be involved in the experience of withdrawal when an addicted individual does not receive the drug.

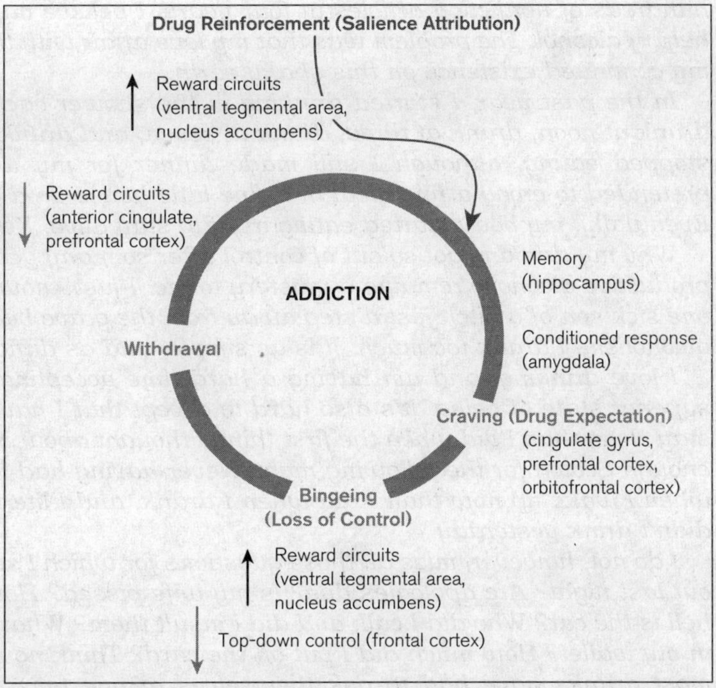

FIGURE 14-10 Model of Brain and Behavior During Addiction

Source: Goldstein and Volkow (2002, p. 1648).

Concept Check

- What can we say about the use of both legal and illegal substances in the United States? What are the worldwide patterns of drug use?
- What is the distinction between drug use, drug abuse such as binge drinking, and addiction? What are the three major components to dependence?
- *DSM–5* and *ICD-10* identify the level of involvement with a psychoactive substance in terms of use, intoxication, and withdrawal. What are the characteristics of each of these levels? Do they apply across the board, or are they substance related or both?
- What factors play a role in who becomes addicted and who doesn't?
- What are the steps in the pattern of addiction? What mechanisms move the process from one step to the next?
- How do drugs change your brain? In what ways can they be said to control it?

ALCOHOL

Until recently, I hadn't gone to bed sober in twenty-five years. I was a drunk when I first met my wife of twenty-three years, and I have been one ever since. I have been a pretty good drunk, as drunks go, without the usual DWIs, abusive behavior, or too dear a price paid for being too honest after my seventh or tenth drink. I am a flirt when drunk but have never been unfaithful.

I worked hard while I drank, and once wrote three novels and hundreds of nonfiction articles in four years. I believe my work was more lyrical with the help of alcohol. The problem was that my love affair with the bottle finally began to threaten my continued existence on this shaky earth.

In the past year, I started drinking in the shower each morning. I was drunk by nine, drunk at noon, drunk at three, drunk at seven, and drunk at ten o'clock. I had pretty much stopped eating, although I still made dinner for my wife, our dogs, and myself, and pretended to enjoy a fine meal in a fine little house on a pretty street in a nice little town. Eventually, my body started eating itself to stay alive. Ketosis is the medical term.

Why my drinking got so out of control after so many years of my being a functioning and productive alcoholic remains a mystery to me. I just know that I had become (and still am) one sick son of a bitch just a step away from the grave because I suffer from the disease of alcoholism. I drank too much. It is as simple, and as difficult, as that.

I love drinking, and am having a hard time accepting that being sober is somehow a superior state of being. It's also hard to accept that I have to expend even more energy to stay clean than I did when the first thing I thought about in the morning was whether I had enough Scotch for the following night. Never having had hangovers, I don't feel any better when I wake up now than I did when I drank, and I literally have to remind myself that I didn't drink yesterday.

I do not, however, miss all those questions for which I seldom found answers: Did I black out last night? Are apologies due? Is my wife pissed? How did I get home, and where the hell is the car? Who did I call, and did I insult them? What happened to all the money I had in my wallet? How much did I put on the card? Think now, Davidson. These are questions most drunks have had to ask themselves at one time or another. After a while, I just stopped asking them.

From Neil Davidson. "Goodbye, Johnnie Walker." Originally published in *The Sun Magazine*. July 1998 Issue 271.

An Older Indian Study on Neuropsychological Rehabilitation for Alcohol

An article in a volume of the *Indian Journal of Psychiatry* by Mathai, Rao, and Gopinath (1998) reflects one of the earliest efforts from India to use neuropsychological rehabilitation for persons with alcohol addiction. The work reports that cognitive retraining given to the treatment group improved attention, information processing, memory, and planning and reasoning.

DSM–5 Alcohol-Related Disorders

Alcohol use disorder is defined in *DSM–5* as a pattern of alcohol use that leads to significant impairment or distress. As seen in *Table 14-1*, the criteria also require two or more of other factors such as the person taking more of the substance than was intended, not being able to reduce the use of the substance, spending time trying to obtain the substance, not being able to do one's work or other obligations, having the substance interfere with social relationships, reducing one's activities because of the substance, having the substance create medical problems, and engaging in hazardous activities such as driving while on the substance.

TABLE 14-1 Alcohol Use Disorder

Alcohol Use Disorder

A. A problematic pattern of alcohol use leading to clinically significant impairment or distress, manifested by at least two of the following, occurring within a 12-month period:
   1. Alcohol is often taken in larger amounts or over a longer period than was intended.
   2. There is a persistent desire or unsuccessful effort to cut down or control alcohol use.
   3. A great deal of time is spent in activities necessary to obtain alcohol, use alcohol, or recover from its effects.
   4. Craving, or a strong desire or urge to use alcohol.
   5. Recurrent alcohol use resulting in a failure to fulfill major role obligations at work, school, or home.
   6. Continued alcohol use despite having persistent or recurrent social or interpersonal problems caused or exacerbated by the effects of the substance.
   7. Important social, occupational, or recreational activities are given up or reduced because of alcohol use.
   8. Recurrent alcohol use in situations in which it is physically hazardous.
   9. Alcohol use is continued despite knowledge of having a persistent or recurrent physical or psychological problem that is likely to have been caused or exacerbated by the substance.
   10. Tolerance, as defined by either or both of the following:
       a. A need for markedly increased amounts of alcohol to achieve intoxication or desired effect.
       b. A markedly diminished effect with continued use of the same amount of the substance.
   11. Withdrawal, as manifested by either of the following:
       a. The characteristic withdrawal syndrome for alcohol (refer to Criteria A and B of the criteria set for Withdrawal).
       b. Alcohol (or a closely related) substance is taken to relieve or avoid withdrawal symptoms.

Specify the following:

In early Remission: After full criteria for alcohol use disorder were previously met, none of the criteria for alcohol use disorder have been met for at least 3 months but for less than 12 months (with the exception that Criterion A4, "Craving, or a strong desire or urge to use alcohol," may be met).

In sustained Remission: After full criteria for alcohol use disorder were previously met, none of the criteria for alcohol use disorder have been met at any time during a period of 12 months or longer (with the exception that Criterion A4, "Craving, or a strong desire or urge to use alcohol," may be met).

***Specify* if:**

In a Controlled Environment: This additional specifier is used if the individual is in an environment where access to alcohol is restricted.

Source: Reprinted with permission from the *Diagnostic and Statistical Manual of Mental Disorders, Fifth Edition*, (Copyright 2013). American Psychiatric Association.

In the United States, about 12.5% of males and 5% of females would meet the criteria for alcohol use disorder in a given year (Hasin, Stinson, Ogburn, & Grant, 2007). Lifetime prevalence is estimated to be 42% for males and 20% for females. This means that almost half of all U.S. males will qualify for a alcohol use disorder at some point in their life.

The second alcohol-related disorder in *DSM–5* is alcohol intoxication disorder (see *Table 14-2*). The criteria for this disorder specify the changes needed for a diagnosis of alcohol intoxication. The third alcohol-related disorder specifies the criteria required for an alcohol withdrawal disorder (see *Table 14-3*).

Alcohol has been available to humans for a large part of our history. For at least 10,000 years, humans have made wine, beer, and other drinks through a process of fermentation. During fermentation, yeast breaks down sugar found in grains, such as barley, and fruits, such as grapes, into ethanol (alcohol) and carbon dioxide. Once carbon dioxide is

TABLE 14-2 Alcohol Intoxication

Alcohol Intoxication
A. Recent ingestion of alcohol.
B. Clinically significant problematic behavioral or psychological changes (e.g., inappropriate sexual or aggressive behavior, mood lability, impaired judgment, impaired social or occupational functioning) that developed during, or shortly after, alcohol ingestion.
C. One (or more) of the following signs, developing during, or shortly after, alcohol use: 1. Slurred speech 2. Incoordination 3. Unsteady gait 4. Nystagmus 5. Impairment in attention or memory 6. Stupor or coma
D. The symptoms are not due to a general medical condition and are not better accounted for by another mental disorder or intoxication with another substance.

Source: Reprinted with permission from the *Diagnostic and Statistical Manual of Mental Disorders, Fifth Edition* (Copyright 2013). American Psychiatric Association.

TABLE 14-3 Alcohol Withdrawal

Alcohol Withdrawal
A. Cessation of (or reduction in) alcohol use that has been heavy and prolonged.
B. Two (or more) of the following, developing within several hours to a few days after the cessation of (or reduction in) alcohol use described in Criterion A: 1. Autonomic hyperactivity (e.g., sweating or pulse rate greater than 100) 2. Increased hand tremor 3. Insomnia 4. Nausea or vomiting 5. Transient visual, tactile, or auditory hallucinations or illusions 6. Psychomotor agitation 7. Anxiety 8. Generalized tonic-clonic seizures
C. The symptoms in Criterion B cause clinically significant distress or impairment in social, occupational, or other important areas of functioning.
D. The symptoms are not due to a general medical condition and are not better accounted for by another mental disorder, or intoxication or withdrawal from another drug.

Source: Reprinted with permission from the *Diagnostic and Statistical Manual of Mental Disorders, Fifth Edition*, (Copyright 2013). American Psychiatric Association.

removed, the ethanol and water remain in the form of wine or beer. Alcohol levels above about 12% will greatly slow down fermentation and above 14% will kill the yeast. Higher alcohol drinks such as gin, vodka, rum, and whiskey are further heated after fermentation in the process of distilling to remove the water. The percentage of alcohol in a substance is measured in terms of *proof,* which is twice the percentage of alcohol (e.g., 20% alcohol equals 40 proof). Researchers consider 12 oz. of beer, 5 oz. of wine, and 1.5 oz. of liquor to contain ½ oz. of pure alcohol.

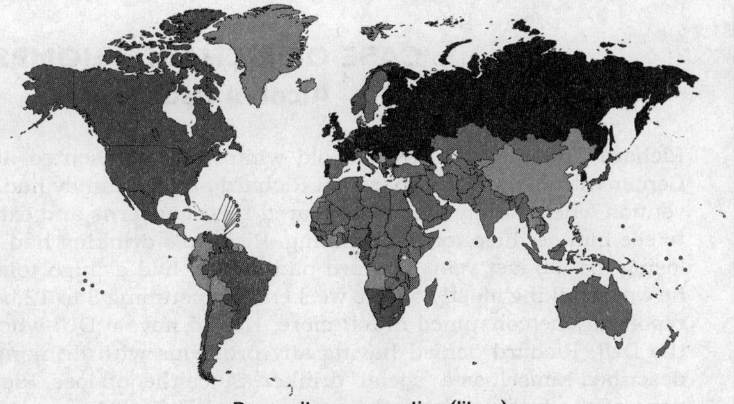

FIGURE 14-11 Total Adult Consumption in Liters of Pure Alcohol per Person in 2005

Source: World Health Organization (WHO) (2011).
Disclaimer: This figure is not to scale. It does not represent any authentic national or international boundaries and is used for illustrative purposes only.

Alcohol is consumed throughout the world (see *Figure 14-11*). This figure shows the amount of alcohol—in liters—consumed by people over 15 years of age. A bottle of wine is three fourths of a liter, and a gallon contains not quite 4 liters. In many cultures around the world, alcohol is used for celebrations such as weddings and parties. In some cultures, alcohol is even part of funerals, such as the traditional Irish wake. In other cultures—Islamic, for example—it is not used and even banned in some places. Some individuals, such as those from Asian countries, have a genetic makeup that causes their faces or body to become flush when drinking alcohol, which results in lower alcohol consumption. Thus, there are both cultural and genetic factors related to the use of or abstinence from alcohol in a given country.

Part of the reason for alcohol's use in celebrations is its effect on our central nervous system. In most humans, the experience of alcohol intake includes pleasant subjective experiences that may lead to increased social interactions. This is partly related to the effects of alcohol on such neurotransmitters as serotonin, endorphins, and dopamine. Alcohol will also decrease inhibition by reducing the effects of the GABA system, which is associated with anxiety. However, if the amount of alcohol intake is increased, it will increase the effects of GABA, which can lead to sedation. This is why alcohol is generally listed as a depressant.

As an addictive substance, it can also lead to social, legal, and medical problems. It often causes problems within the family, as shown in the following case study of Richard (not his real name).

Through loss of productivity, automobile accidents, and medical problems such as alcohol-related cancers, alcohol is estimated to cost the United States $185 billion annually (www.cdc.gov/workplacehealthpromotion/implementation/topics/substance-abuse.html). WHO lists alcohol as the leading risk factor for death in males ages 15 to 59 (www.who.int/substance_abuse/publications/global_alcohol_report/msbgsruprofiles.pdf). This is due to injuries, violence, and cardiovascular disease. Worldwide, they estimate that 6.2% of all male deaths are related to alcohol compared with 1.1% for females. Overall, alcohol consumption is the world's third largest risk factor for disease and disability. It is also the third leading cause of preventable death in the United States.

CASE OF RICHARD THOMPSON
Alcohol Use Disorder

Richard Thompson, a 28-year-old white male, presented at the Serene Oaks Recovery Center with his wife and parents. Richard and his family had just participated in an intervention where family members shared their concerns and expressed their collective desire to see him get help for his drinking. Richard's drinking had escalated quite rapidly since losing his job last year. Richard had always had a "high tolerance." Prior to the job loss, he was drinking mostly on the weekends consuming 8 to 12 beers on occasion, yet at times reportedly he consumed much more. He did have a DUI when he was 21, but other than the DUI, Richard denied having any problems with drinking prior to losing his job and described himself as a "social" drinker. Since the job loss, Richard has been drinking most days of the week and has begun consuming hard liquor in addition to beer, sometimes including a fifth of vodka per day. He has been having trouble remembering events while intoxicated and has been asked by his wife to leave the home on several occasions while drinking due to his belligerent behavior. At one point, the police were called to the home due to Richard's aggressive behavior. This incident prompted the recent family intervention and subsequent admission to Serene Oaks Recovery Center.

Clinical vignette provided by Michael Cameron Wolff, PhD, CADC

Effects of Alcohol on the Human Body

Unlike most of the other foods you eat, alcohol is absorbed directly in the bloodstream without digestion. When you drink a beer or other alcoholic beverage, it goes to your stomach. In your stomach, only a small amount of alcohol is absorbed as most alcohol is absorbed in the small intestine. However, if there is food in your stomach, it is absorbed more slowly. If the alcoholic drink contains food substances as does beer, it is also absorbed more slowly. On the other hand, drinks with carbon dioxide such as champagne or a mixed drink with a carbonated beverage are moved from the stomach to the small intestine more rapidly where most alcohol is absorbed into the blood stream. The experience of feeling the effects of alcohol takes place when alcohol is carried through the bloodstream to the brain. Champagne will give you the experience of alcohol faster than beer since it gets to your brain faster.

Once in the bloodstream, alcohol also goes to the other organs of the body such as the brain, heart, lungs, and liver. In the lungs, it is vaporized and exhaled. This is the basis for breathalyzers used by the police to measure alcohol levels. In the liver, it is broken down into carbon dioxide and water. Alcohol is absorbed into the bloodstream faster than it is metabolized by the liver. The speed at which your body breaks down or metabolizes alcohol is fairly constant although women absorb and metabolize alcohol differently from men. This means that a woman can have a higher blood alcohol concentration (BAC) level than a man even if they both drank the same amount of alcohol. Alcohol can have both positive and negative long-term effects on the body (see *Figure 14-12*).

As seen in *Figure 14-13*, if you have one standard drink, the BAC level peaks within 30 to 45 minutes and then returns to zero after about 2 hours. Thus, having one drink every

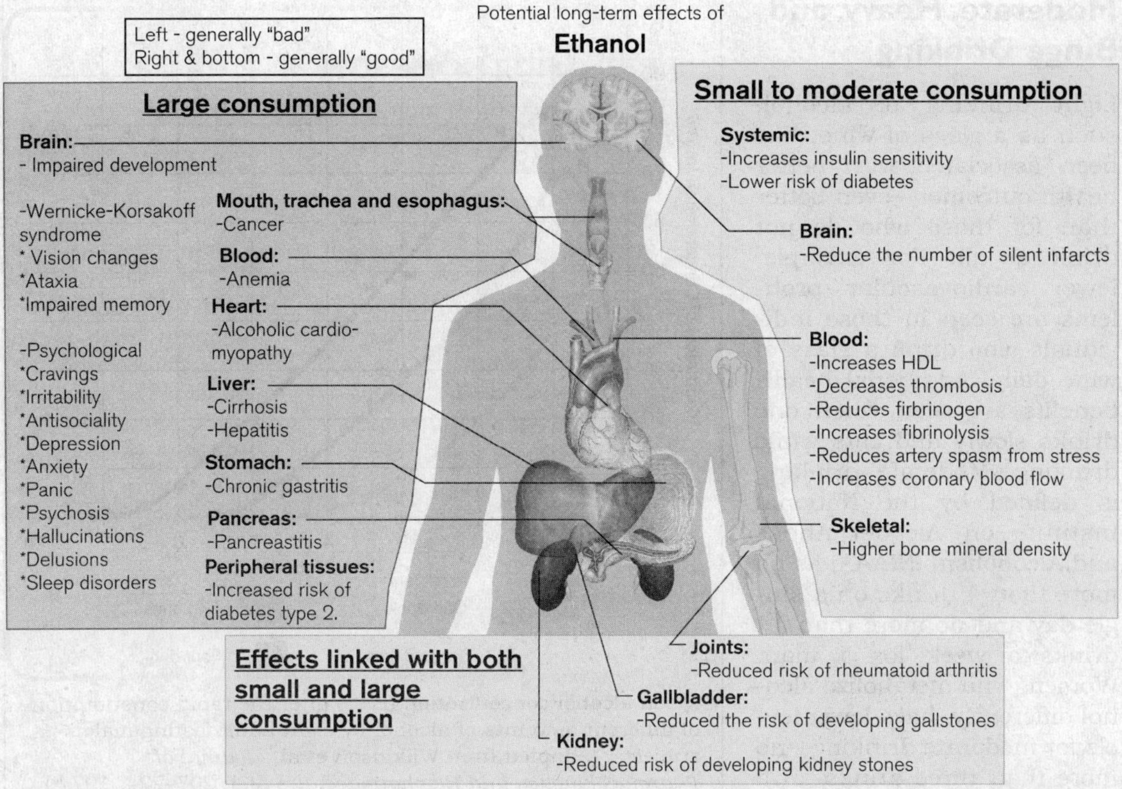

FIGURE 14-12 Alcohol Can Have Both Positive and Negative Long-Term Effects on the Body

Source: Häggström (2009).

couple of hours would not lead to intoxication since the alcohol would be metabolized and removed from the bloodstream. However, since alcohol is absorbed faster than it is metabolized, drinking more than one drink in an hour leads to increased BAC levels. As seen in *Figure 14-13*, drinking two, three, or four drinks in an hour both increases BAC and increases the amount of time for alcohol to be removed from the bloodstream. This graph is from males who have not recently eaten food. Having food in the stomach will delay the absorption of alcohol.

Alcohol dependence runs in families (see Treutlein et al., 2009, for an overview). Twin studies suggest that 40% to 60% of the variance in dependence can be accounted for by genetics. Further, research suggests there is a common genetic component involved in alcohol, tobacco, and cannabis dependence across adolescence and young adulthood (Palmer et al., 2013). What is interesting is that this genetic influence increases from adolescence to your adulthood with a decrease in the influence of the environment. Since dopamine pathways have a large genetic component, this may be the critical dimension that influences alcohol dependence. The overall picture suggests that environmental influences such as friends, peer pressure, and one's culture influence the use of drugs. However, genetics have more influence on the person being drug dependent. These genetic effects appear to be slightly stronger for females than males.

Moderate, Heavy, and Binge Drinking

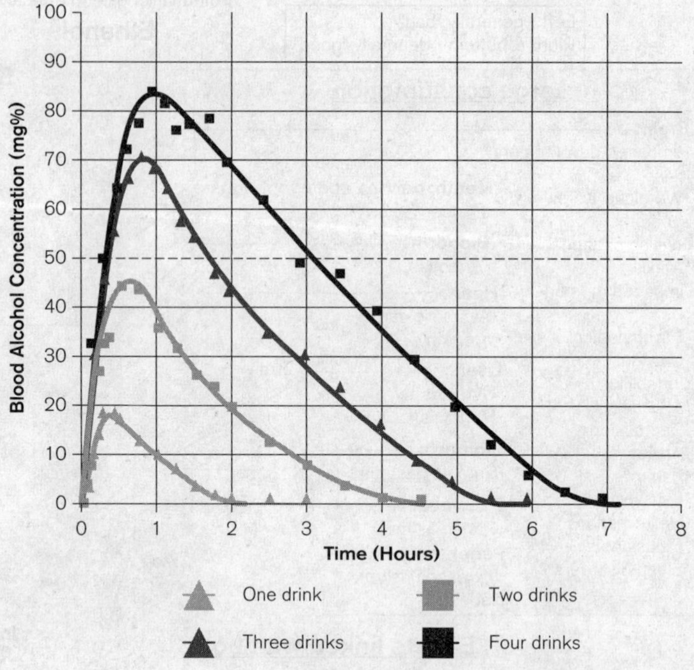

Blood alcohol concentration (BAC) after the rapid consumption of different amounts of alcohol by eight adult fasting male subjects. (Adapted from Wilkinson et al., *Journal of Pharmacokinetics and Biopharmaceutics* 5(3): 207–224, 1977.)

FIGURE 14-13 The Change in Blood Alcohol Concentration Is Related to Both How Much Alcohol Is Consumed and How Fast It Is Consumed

Source: From Wilkinson, Paul K.; Sedman, Allen J.; Sakmar, Ermelinda; Kay, Donald R.; Wagner, John G.; (1977). "Pharmacokinetics of ethanol after oral administration in the fasting state." *Journal of Pharmacokinetics and Biopharmaceutics* 5 (3): 207–224.; with kind permission from Springer Science+Business Media B.V.

Light drinking of alcohol, such as a glass of wine, has been associated with better health outcomes—even better than for those who do not drink at all. For example, fewer cardiovascular problems are seen in those individuals who drink a glass of wine daily. Additional health benefits are seen when one drinks slowly and eats while drinking. Moderate drinking is defined by the National Institute on Alcohol Abuse and Alcoholism (NIAAA) as no more than 4 drinks on a single day and no more than 14 drinks a week for a man. Women, who metabolize alcohol differently, have lower levels for moderate drinking—no more than three drinks on a single day and no more than seven drinks a week.

Those who drink more than these amounts are considered to be heavy or "at risk" drinkers who are susceptible to a number of health and other problems. Binge drinking is defined by NIAAA as consuming enough alcohol in a 2-hour period to have a BAC of 0.08 g/dL. *Figure 14-14* and *Figure 14-15* show BAC levels for men and women. Currently, all 50 states in the United States define 0.08 as the legal definition of being intoxicated. Since BAC levels are often not available, for example in surveys of previous use, NIAAA uses four or more drinks for women and five or more for men as the definition of binge drinking. *Table 14-4* shows changes in psychological and physical functions as BAC increases.

Rates of Drinking

About two thirds of all Americans over 18 have had at least one drink in the past year (see *Table 14-5*). Around 40% of men and 20% of women have at least one drink a week. Results from the 2011 National Survey on Drug Use and Health: Summary of National

Men

Approximate Blood Alcohol Percentage									
Drinks	Body Weight in Pounds								
	100	120	140	160	180	200	220	240	
0	.00	.00	.00	.00	.00	.00	.00	.00	Only Safe Driving Limit
1	.04	.03	.03	.02	.02	.02	.02	.02	Driving Skills Significantly Affected
2	.08	.06	.05	.05	.04	.04	.03	.03	
3	.11	.09	.08	.07	.06	.06	.05	.05	
4	.15	.12	.11	.09	.08	.08	.07	.06	Possible Criminal Penalties
5	.19	.16	.13	.12	.11	.09	.09	.08	
6	.23	.19	.16	.14	.13	.11	.10	.09	Legally Intoxicated
7	.26	.22	.19	.16	.15	.13	.12	.11	
8	.30	.25	.21	.19	.17	.15	.14	.13	Criminal Penalties
9	.34	.28	.24	.21	.19	.17	.15	.14	
10	.38	.31	.27	.23	.21	.19	.17	.16	Death Possible

Subtract 0.01% for each 40 minutes of drinking.

One drink is 1.25 oz. of 80 proof liquor, 12 oz. of beer, or 5 oz. of table wine.

FIGURE 14-14 BAC Chart for Men

Source: Campus Alcohol Abuse Prevention Center, Virginia Tech.

Women

Approximate Blood Alcohol Percentage										
Drinks	Body Weight in Pounds									
	90	100	120	140	160	180	200	220	240	
0	.00	.00	.00	.00	.00	.00	.00	.00		Only Safe Driving Limit
1	.05	.05	.04	.03	.03	.03	.02	.02	.02	Driving Skills Significantly Affected
2	.10	.09	.08	.07	.06	.05	.05	.04	.04	
3	.15	.14	.11	.10	.09	.08	.07	.06	.06	Possible Criminal Penalties
4	.20	.18	.15	.13	.11	.10	.09	.08	.08	
5	.25	.23	.19	.16	.14	.13	.11	.10	.09	

(Continued)

(Continued)

6	.30	.27	.23	.19	.17	.15	.14	.12	.11	Legally Intoxicated
7	.35	.32	.27	.23	.20	.18	.16	.14	.13	
8	.40	.36	.30	.26	.23	.20	.18	.17	.15	Criminal Penalties
9	.45	.41	.34	.29	.26	.23	.20	.19	.17	
10	.51	.45	.38	.32	.28	.25	.23	.21	.19	Death Possible

Subtract 0.01% for each 40 minutes of drinking.

One drink is 1.25 oz. of 80 proof liquor, 12 oz. of beer, or 5 oz. of table wine.

FIGURE 14-15 BAC Chart for Women

Source: Campus Alcohol Abuse Prevention Center, Virginia Tech.

TABLE 14-4 Psychological and Physical Effects at Various Blood Alcohol Levels

Progressive Effects of Alcohol		
Blood Alcohol Concentration	***Changes in Feelings and Personality***	***Physical and Mental Impairments***
0.01–0.06	Relaxation Sense of Well-being Loss of Inhibition Lowered Alertness Joyous	Thought Judgment Coordination Concentration
0.06–0.10	Blunted Feelings Disinhibition Extraversion Impaired Sexual Pleasure	Reflexes Impaired Reasoning Depth Perception Distance Acuity Peripheral Vision Glare Recovery
0.11–0.20	Over-Expression Emotional Swings Angry or Sad Boisterous	Reaction Time Gross Motor Control Staggering Slurred Speech
0.21–0.29	Stupor Lose Understanding Impaired Sensations	Severe Motor Impairment Loss of Consciousness Memory Blackout
0.30–0.39	Severe Depression Unconsciousness Death Possible	Bladder Function Breathing Heart Rate
=> 0.40	Unconsciousness Death	Breathing Heart Rate

Source: Campus Alcohol Abuse Prevention Center, Virginia Tech.

TABLE 14-5 Frequency of Drinking in the United States for Individuals Age 18 and Over

Percentage who drank:	*Women*	*Men*
Daily	2.45%	5.78%
Nearly every day	2.39%	4.98%
3–4 times a week	5.55%	10.00%
2 times a week	5.82%	10.46%
Once a week	6.77%	10.33%
2–3 times a month	8.27%	9.55%
Once a month	7.19%	6.72%
7–11 times in the past year	4.44%	3.51%
3–6 times in the past year	9.26%	5.67%
1–2 times in the past year	8.73%	4.91%
Never in the past year (former drinker or lifetime abstainer)	39.13%	28.09%

Source: National Institute on Alcohol Abuse and Alcoholism.

Findings suggest that 22.6% of the population participated in binge drinking in the past 30 days. They also found that binge drinking was highest in college-age populations (see *Figure 14-16*).

College-age young adults who engage in binge drinking generally believe that they do not have a drinking problem. They also believe that they have no problem driving in these conditions. These types of cognitive distortions and lack of inhibition can lead to problems ranging from passing out to traffic accidents to problematic sexual and physical encounters. In fact, WHO data worldwide show a larger proportion of deaths related to alcohol in this age-group than in any other.

Concept Check

- What are the effects of alcohol on an individual's body and brain?
- What can we say about the prevalence rates of alcohol use disorder in terms of genetics, gender, age, and culture?
- What is considered moderate, heavy, and binge drinking?

Do People Who Drink More Like It More?

Given that people who binge drink take in more alcohol than others, the question arises as to whether they experience more positive effects from drinking than do light drinkers. You might think that those who drink more would like it more. However, some individuals want or crave alcohol even though they might not like it that much.

The role of drinking and its experience was studied by following 104 weekly binge drinkers and 86 light drinkers over 2 years (King, de Wit, McNamara, & Cao, 2011). In the initial part of the study, the researchers used a double-blind design in which the participants did not know if they were receiving a drink with alcohol or a similar tasting placebo. The initial

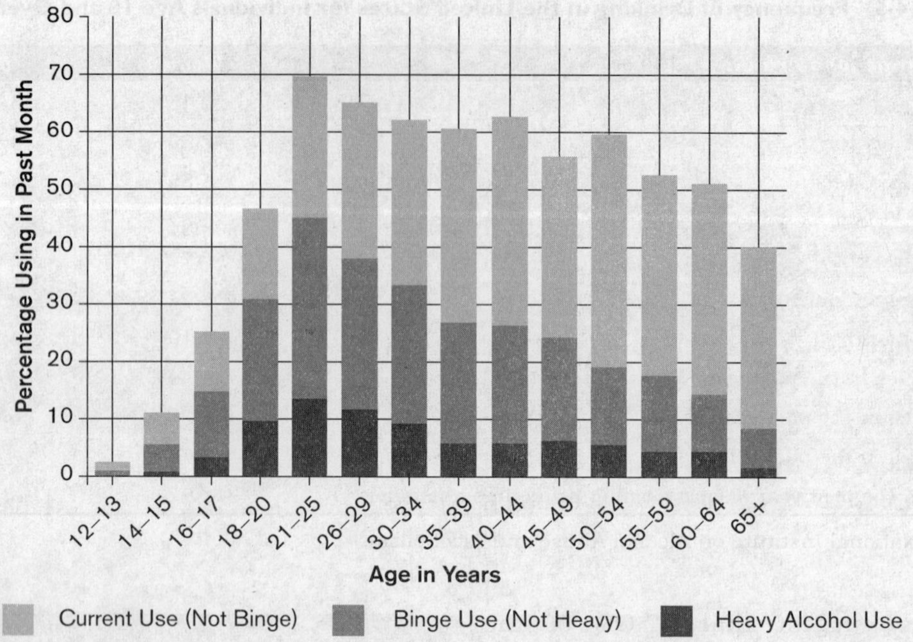

FIGURE 14-16 Current Binge Drinking and Alcohol Use by Age-Group

Source: Substance Abuse and Mental Health Services Administration, Results from the 2011 National Survey on Drug Use and Health: Summary of National Findings, NSDUH Series H-44, HHS Publication No. (SMA) 12-4713. Rockville, MD: Substance Abuse and Mental Health Services Administration, 2012.

sessions during which the participants rated their experience of both alcohol and the placebo were followed during the next 2 years by sessions in which the participants reported their current drinking habits. Heavy drinkers, as compared with light drinkers, reported they wanted alcohol more. Further, light drinkers found less stimulation from alcohol and were more sedated by the effects of alcohol than were heavy drinkers.

PUBLICATIONS FROM INDIA, BASED ON THE PREMIUM STUDY

In a novel research effort from India, several publications highlight the outcomes of the PREMIUM study: A Program for Effective Mental Health Interventions. The aim of the work is to evaluate the effectiveness and cost-effectiveness of psychological treatment developed for the treatment of alcohol use disorders in primary care in India (Patel et al., 2014).

Patel et al. (2014) offers the counselling for alcohol problems (CAP) program for adults with harmful drinking or alcohol dependence.

The goal of PREMIUM is to establish the utility of effective psychological treatments for mental disorders that are culturally appropriate, feasible, acceptable, and affordable in under-resourced settings. "A core element of this methodology is a long-term vision of ultimate scalability of treatments by emphasizing their delivery by the same pool of lay counsellors working in routine primary healthcare settings," write Patel et al. (2014).

Non-specialist health workers are trained to deliver this program. Another interesting element of the material used is an audiovisual aid called *Prakashdoot* (messenger of light), which conveys to the lay viewer that alcohol use disorders are a mental health condition that requires treatment like any other mental illness. This module was developed by the IPH, Thane, Maharashtra, India (Nadkarni and Sovani).

Outcome studies of this work from India are also published in *The Lancet* (Nadkarni et al., 2017) and *Alcoholism: Clinical and Experimental Research* (Nandkarni et al., 2015).

CANNABIS

Cannabis is a plant species also referred to as *marijuana*. Cannabis resin is referred to as *hashish*. The cannabis plant can easily be cultivated both indoors and outdoors. For this reason, it is grown and used throughout the world. The United Nations estimates that 4% of the population of the world uses cannabis. The United States is one of the larger users of cannabis in the world (see *Figure 14-17*).

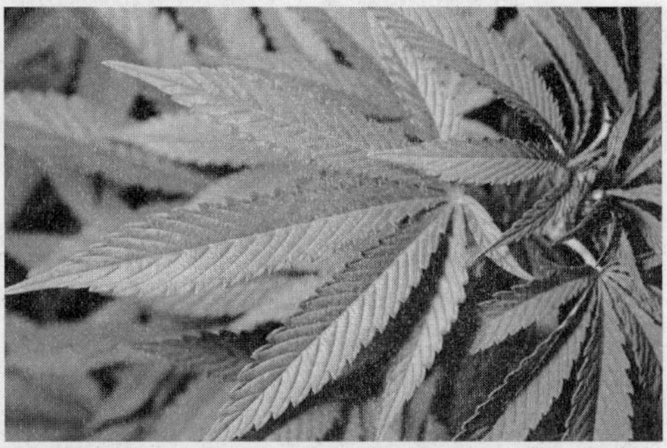

Image of a cannabis plant

Cannabis has been used worldwide for at least 4,000 years for its psychoactive effects. During this period, it has been seen as an important medical compound and as a religious and recreational substance. The physician Galen in AD 200 wrote that it was customary to give cannabis to guests to promote hilarity and enjoyment (Stuart, 2004). It has a history of use in China, India, Europe, and the Middle East. It came to the United States during the 1900s. In the United States during the 1960s, it became a recreational drug of choice for many individuals. Since the 1960s, there have been changing views as to whether the drug should be decriminalized for all adults, made available strictly for medical purposes such as pain relief, or banned completely. *Figure 14-18* (see p. 504) shows a time line related to cultural and scientific views of cannabis.

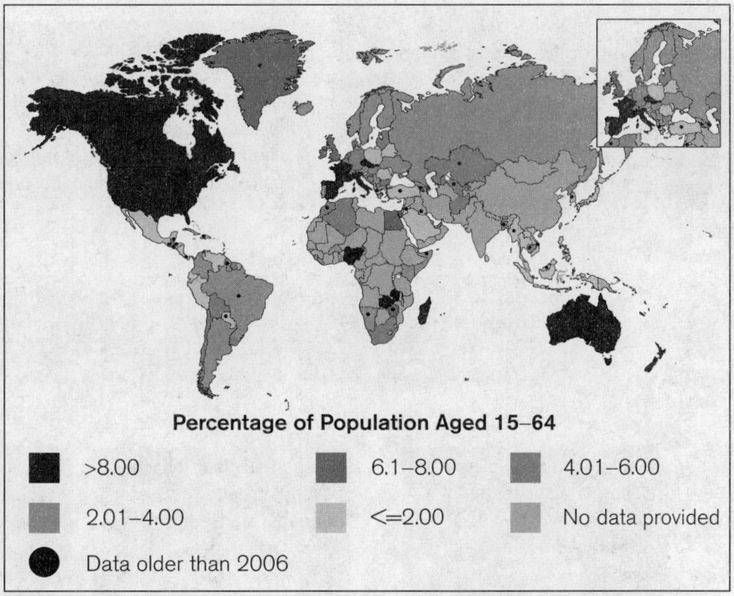

FIGURE 14-17 Prevalence of Cannabis Use in 2010

Source: United Nations Office on Drugs and Crime (2012).
Disclaimer: This figure is not to scale. It does not represent any authentic national or international boundaries and is used for illustrative purposes only.

- **2727 BC** — The Pên–ts'ao Ching, the oldest known pharmacopoeia, describes medicinal properties of cannabis, as well as psychiatric side-effects from excessive use.
- **~1200 BC** — In the Indus Valley civilization, cannabis is regarded as one of five sacred plants: "a source of happiness and bringer of freedom."
- **1894** — The seven-volume Report of the Indian Hemp Drugs Commission concludes that "There is no evidence of any weight regarding mental and moral injuries from moderate use of these drugs."
- **1928** — Recreational use of cannabis is banned in the United Kingdom.
- **1937** — The Marijuana Tax Act effectively prohibits recreational cannabis use in the United States.
- **1942** — Cannabis is removed from the American Pharmacopoeia.
- **1961** — 60 nations sign the Uniform Drug Convention, which pledges to end cannabis use within 25 years.
- **1965** — Mechoulam and colleagues isolate and subsequently synthesize Δ^9-tetrahydrocannabinol (THC).
- **1967** — Groups such as NORML (National Organisation for the Reform of Marijuana Laws), in the United States, and SOMA, in the United Kingdom, lobby for the legalization of cannabis. Over 3,000 people attend a smoke-in in Hyde Park, London.
- **1970** — It becomes clear that the psychological effects of cannabis are attributable to THC.
- **1976** — In the Netherlands, the Opium Act separates cannabis from hard drugs. Subsequently, the sale of cannabis is tolerated under strict conditions. In the United States, government funding for medical research on cannabis is banned.
- **1982** — The National Institutes of Health sponsored Relman study concludes that ". . . there is no evidence that cannabis causes permanent health damage, ... affects brain structure, . . .is addicitive or leads to harder drug [use] . . . ."
- **1987** — The link between cannabis use and the development of schizophrenia is shown for the first time period.

FIGURE 14-18 A Brief History of Cannabis

Source: Murray, Morrison, Henquet, and Di Forti (2007, p. 886).

Individuals who use cannabis report a wide variety of experiences. Small doses produce enjoyable positive feelings associated with a feeling of being "high." This can include states in which time stands still. The person often may see his or her own ideas as exceptionally creative and important. Cannabis can also influence appetite with short-term users reporting increasing hunger or "munchies." Larger doses can produce negative feelings such as anxiety and paranoia. Hallucinations and persecutory delusions have also been reported. Most of these experiences are short-lived but in some cases can last longer. More long-term use is also associated with cognitive impairment in executive functions (Crean, Crane, & Mason, 2011).

The main psychoactive ingredient in cannabis is THC (Δ9-tetrahydrocannabinol) and was first described in the 1960s. THC particularly affects receptors in the hippocampus, the cerebellum, the basal ganglia, and the neocortex. THC affects receptors in the brain that also release GABA, an inhibitory neurotransmitter related to anxiety. The brain also produces substances that are similar to cannabis referred to as cannabinoids. These cannabinoids appear to be related to reducing the negative experiences associated with troubling past experiences, which is similar to the effects of cannabis. Society is currently debating if cannabis should be legalized for its medical benefits, which are discussed in the following LENS on p. 507.

Cannabis and Psychosis

Although a number of reports from governments around the world suggest no negative medical effects from using cannabis, a persistent question relates to its relationship to psychosis (see Murray et al., 2007, for an overview). As noted, larger doses of cannabis can produce hallucinations and delusions. However, it was also reported that individuals with an established psychosis had worse outcomes with continued cannabis use. In particular, a continued use of cannabis by those with a recent onset of psychosis was associated with earlier relapse of the psychotic symptoms, more frequent hospitalization, and poorer social functioning over a 4-year period.

Research that followed about 2,000 individuals for 10 years suggests a more direct relationship between the use of cannabis and symptoms such as hallucinations and delusions (Kuepper et al., 2011). It should be noted that just having these symptoms might not in itself result in a diagnosis of psychosis or schizophrenia. Cannabis use and psychotic symptoms were assessed at baseline, some 3.5 years later, and some 8.4 years later. These researchers first looked at individuals who had not used cannabis at baseline and reported no psychotic symptoms. They then examined those from this group who used cannabis between baseline and the session 3.5 years later. They found that this group showed an increased risk for displaying psychotic symptoms prior to the 8.4 years session.

In reviewing the evidence from a number of studies, Murray et al. (2007) suggested that there is strong evidence to suggest that heavy cannabis use increases the risk of both psychotic symptoms and schizophrenia. These studies were conducted around the world and are presented in *Table 14-6* on p. 506. The odds ratio column reflects the odds that cannabis use is related to psychotic symptoms. If there were no relationship, then the odds would be 1. Thus, odds above 1 suggest that cannabis use is related to having psychotic symptoms. It can be noted that all of the studies reviewed show an odds ratio from 1.5 to 3.1, suggesting a relationship.

TABLE 14-6 Effects of Cannabis Use and Psychosis

Country in which the study was conducted	*Number of participants*	*Follow-up*	*Odds ratio (95% confidence interval)*	*Study design*
United States	4,494	NA	2.4 (1.2, 7.1)	Population based
Sweden	50,053	25 years	2.1 (1.2, 3.7)	Conscript cohort
The Netherlands	4,045	3 years	2.8 (1.2, 6.5)	Population based
Israel	9,724	4–15 years	2.0 (1.3, 3.1)	Population based
New Zealand (Christchurch)	1,265	3 years	1.8 (1.2, 2.6)	Birth cohort
New Zealand (Dunedin)	1,253	15 years	3.1 (0.7, 13.3)	Birth cohort
The Netherlands	1,580	14 years	2.8 (1.79, 4.43)	Population based
Germany	2,436	4 years	1.7 (1.1, 1.5)	Population based
United Kingdom	8,580	18 months	1.5 (0.55, 3.94)	Population based

NA: not applicable.
Source: From Murray, Morrison, Henquet, and Di Forti (2007).

Later research looked at individuals with psychosis and their unaffected siblings (van Winkel, van Bevern, Simons, & Genetic Risk and Outcome of Psychosis [GROUP] Investigators, 2011). These studies suggest that genetic factors may play a role in those individuals who use cannabis and go on to develop psychosis. A later meta-analysis also showed that the use of cannabis was associated with an earlier age of onset of psychotic disorders (Large, Sharma, Compton, Slade, & Nielssen, 2011). This relationship was not found for alcohol.

Hallucinogens

Hallucinogens are drugs that alter perceptual experiences (see Nichols, 2004, for an overview). The word *hallucinate* actually comes from the Latin meaning to wander in the mind. Some of these drugs occur in nature and have been used by various cultures for thousands of years. These include mescaline, which comes from the peyote cactus and psilocybin, which comes from a variety of mushroom. Historians suggest they were often part of religious ceremonies to give experiences not part of everyday life. Other hallucinogens such as LSD (*d*-lysergic acid diethylamide) begin with a grain fungus, ergot. Although the fungus is naturally occurring, LSD was first made in the laboratory. Other laboratory-made drugs include MDMA, commonly known as ecstasy, MDA, sometimes referred to as the love drug, and PCP, also known as angel dust.

Hallucinogens are also called *psychedelics* and are able to alter perception, mood, and cognitive processes in often unpredictable ways (Hollister, 1984). These can be described as follows:

1. Somatic symptoms: dizziness, weakness, tremors, nausea, drowsiness, paresthesias, and blurred vision
2. Perceptual symptoms: altered shapes and colors, difficulty in focusing on objects, sharpened sense of hearing, and at times synesthesias

14-1 LENS
The Legalization of Marijuana

The United States as well as many other countries has gone through periods in which drugs were legal and times in which they were illegal. Alcohol is one classic example of a drug that has been banned completely and then legalized. Currently there is a debate in the United States concerning the legalization of marijuana. Many polls suggest that about one half of all Americans would support legalization. On the other side, the federal government has suggested that legalizing marijuana is "a bad idea" (www.WhiteHouseDrugPolicy.gov).

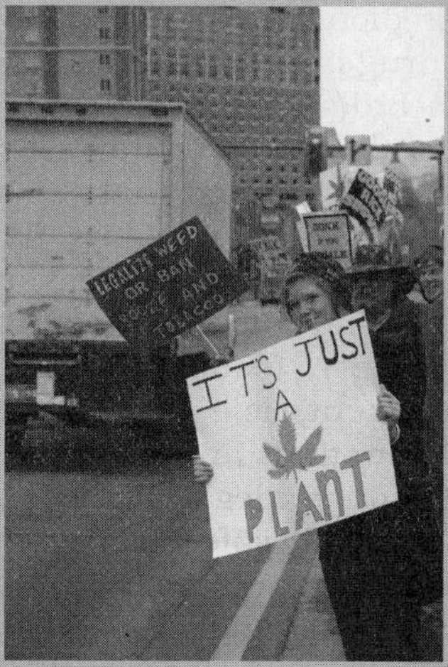

© David R. Frazier Photolibrary, Inc. / Alamy

Those who want to legalize marijuana suggest a number of different reasons that regulating it like alcohol would benefit society. They begin with the fact that it is the most commonly used illegal drug on the planet. This means that a wide variety of government resources are being devoted to police illegal marijuana use. These range from public information campaigns to law enforcement procedures, to spending money on jail terms, and missing out on taxes available from legal drugs. The economic benefits can be seen if you consider all of the businesses related to production, distribution, and sale of such legal drugs as alcohol and coffee including advertising. In any given town, the number of bars and coffeehouses is typically quite large. With marijuana being legal, it is also suggested that the price would decrease and illegal drug dealers would be unnecessary. On another level, it is suggested that marijuana has medical benefits.

Those who are opposed to the legalization of marijuana often begin with the health effects. The U.S. government information arguing against the legalization of marijuana lists the following problems:

- Marijuana use is associated with dependence, respiratory and mental illness, poor motor performance, and impaired cognitive and immune system functioning, among other negative effects.
- Marijuana intoxication can cause distorted perceptions, difficulty in thinking and problem solving, and problems with learning and memory.
- Studies have shown an association between chronic marijuana use and increased rates of anxiety, depression, suicidal thoughts, and schizophrenia.
- Other research has shown marijuana smoke to contain carcinogens and to be an irritant to the lungs. Marijuana smoke, in fact, contains 50% to 70% more carcinogenic hydrocarbons than does tobacco smoke.

As of 2012, 18 states and the District of Columbia have legalized marijuana for medical use. California was the first state to legalize medical marijuana in 1996. Since that time, other states, including Washington (1998), Oregon (1998), Alaska (1998), Maine (1999), Nevada (2000), Hawaii (2000), Colorado (2000), Vermont (2004), Montana (2004), Rhode Island (2007), New Mexico (2007), Michigan (2008), New Jersey (2010), Washington, D.C. (2010), Arizona (2010), Delaware (2011), Massachusetts (2012), and Connecticut (2012), have legalized it. In addition, Washington and Colorado have made marijuana legal for recreational use. Other states have pending legislations to legalize marijuana.

3. Psychic symptoms: alterations in mood (happy, sad, or irritable at varying times), tension, distorted time sense, difficulty in expressing thoughts, depersonalization, dreamlike feelings, and visual hallucinations

Although these are possible experiences from hallucinogens, in reality they are quite unpredictable and based on both the expectations of the user and the situation in which the drug is taken. This also makes research with the drugs more difficult to perform.

In order to conduct human research with hallucinogens, a self-administered rating scale, the "Altered States of Consciousness" (APZ) scale was developed (Dittrich, 1998). Dittrich suggested that the subjective effects of taking hallucinogens can be divided into three major components. The first is "Oceanic Boundlessness." This is similar to what have been described as mystical experiences such as depersonalization and derealization. The second component is "Anxious Ego Dissolution." This would include such experiences as anxiety, delusions, fear of losing control, and loss of a sense of self. The third component is "Visionary Restructuralization." This component includes visual hallucinations and illusions, synesthesia, and changes in the meaning of perceptions.

Although illegal in the United States, hallucinogens do not produce dependence and are relatively safe (Nichols, 2004). They also do not show withdrawal symptoms. However, as with any process, abuse and dependence are possible, although the pattern is not the same. Drugs that are addictive typically affect the dopamine system and the experience of reward. It is also possible to train animals to self-administer addictive drugs, but this is not the case with hallucinogens. Hallucinogens do not directly affect dopamine neurotransmission as do alcohol, cannabis, tobacco, and cocaine. They also appear to lack the toxic effects on human organs seen in alcohol or tobacco, for example. However, not all experiences with hallucinogens are positive. A so-called "bad trip" can include extreme anxiety and fearful psychotic-like experiences.

Structurally, the chemical makeup of hallucinogens is similar to the neurotransmitter *serotonin*. In fact, early theories suggested that hallucinogens produced their effects by increasing serotonin in specific brain areas. It is now known that hallucinogens bind to the 5-HT serotonin receptor.

LSD was first experienced on April 16, 1943. Albert Hoffmann, who worked for Sandoz Pharmaceuticals in Basel, Switzerland, was studying naturally occurring products and their modification in the laboratory. He was working on the ergot fungus, which is found on grains. On his way home from work, he experienced strange perceptual experiences including hallucinations. To determine if his experiences were due to LSD, Hoffmann purposely ingested LSD some 3 days later. Indeed, it was LSD that had given Hoffman the psychotic-like experiences. This was also confirmed by other scientists in the lab taking LSD. LSD has been shown to be the most potent of all hallucinogens with effects that can last up to 12 hours.

Whereas LSD is the most potent hallucinogen, mescaline is the least potent. Mescaline comes from the peyote cactus and has a history of being used by Native Americans in religious ceremonies. Even before that pre-Columbian Mexico used it and considered it magical and divine (Carson-DeWitt, 2001). From there, it spread to North America and Native American groups. In 1990, the U.S. Supreme Court ruled that mescaline could not be used legally for religious ceremonies. Mescaline produces vivid mental images and an altered sense of space and time with a loss of a sense of reality.

Psilocybin comes from a type of fungus often referred to as "magic mushrooms." These mushrooms are found throughout the world and have been used for centuries. Psilocybin affects the central nervous system through the functioning of serotonin, which it is chemically similar. The active ingredient was identified by Sandoz Pharmaceuticals and found to be similar to LSD with alteration in perception, mood, and thought (see Studerus, Kometer, Hasler, & Vollenweider, 2011, for an overview). It produces heightened sensory experiences and perceptual distortions but the lack of concrete cognitive functioning. It induces milder negative experiences such as anxiety and panic reaction. It is considered to be relatively safe in terms of dependence.

Erich Studerus and his colleagues (2011) examined a number of psilocybin sessions conducted in their lab using the APZ experiences scale. These are shown in *Figure 14-19*. This figure shows that the larger the dose, the greater the effect across the three domains of oceanic boundlessness, anxious ego dissolution, and visionary restructuralization. Note also that the placebo had no effect.

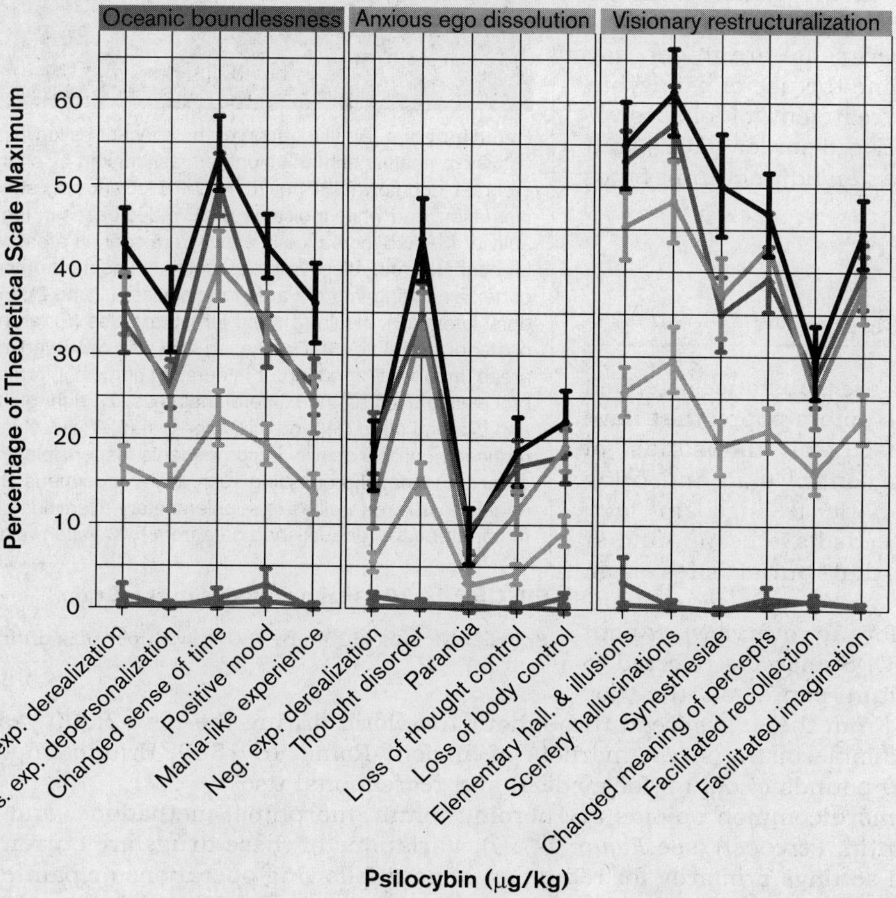

FIGURE 14-19 Altered States of Consciousness Rating Scale

Source: Studerus et al. (2011, p. 1440), with permission from Elsevier.

Brain blood flow research from this lab showed increases in the frontal areas of the brain, the insula, and the anterior and posterior cingulate (see *Figure 14-20*). These are areas involved in cognitive and affective processes including a sense of self. Decreased blood flow was found in areas related to integration of information such as the thalamus.

Current research is being directed at using hallucinogens in clinical treatment. For example, experiments are under way to examine the use of psilocybin in the treatment of obsessive-compulsive disorder (OCD) and MDMA as an adjunct to psychotherapy.

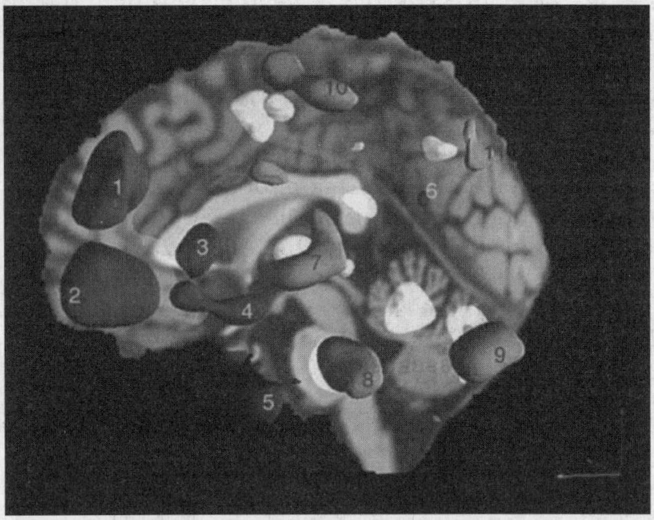

Hallucinogens. An illustration of the effect of psilocybin on brain activity in healthy human volunteers as indexed by changes in crebral blood flow (CBF) using H_2O-PET. Dark gray shows relative increases, and white indicates relative decreases in regional brain activity. Marked increases in activity are seen in areas important for cognitive and affective processes such as the frontomedial cortex extending into the anterior cingulate (1 and 2); the dorsolateral (3), insula (4), and temporal poles (5), and the left posterior cingulate (6). Decreased flow was observed in brain areas important for gating or integrating cortical information processing such as the bilateral thalamus (7), right globus pallidus and bilateral pons (8), and in cerebellum (9). Psilocybin also reduced neuronal activity in components responsible for higher order visuospatial processing such as the precuneus (11) and angular gyrus, as well as in supplementary eye fields of the pre-motor area (10) (unpublished data from F. X. Vollenweider).

FIGURE 14-20 Hallucinogens in the Brain

Source: Nichols (2004, p. 1806), with permission from Elsevier.

OPIOIDS

Opioids are substances derived from the opium poppy that have been used for thousands of years to control pain and bring on euphoric feelings. In fact, poppy seeds have been found at Neanderthal burial sites from 30,000 years ago (see Stuart, 2004, for an overview). About 3400 BC, Sumerians referred to the opium poppy as the "joy plant". From there, it spread throughout the world during the next 2,000 years. Opium was available in the street markets of ancient Rome. In 1860, Britain imported some 220,000 pounds of opium for medical and recreational use.

The more common opioids are heroin, opium, morphine, methadone, and oxycodone (OxyContin, Percocet) (see *Figure 14-21*). Variations of these drugs are currently used in medical settings primarily for reduction of pain following operations or pain experienced with some types of cancer. Opioids became popular in the United States after the Civil War for their ability to control pain. However, some individuals given these drugs became addicted to them. Abuse took the form of the opium den of the last century in which the drug was smoked. With the availability of the hypodermic needle, it was injected directly into the bloodstream. As noted earlier, before the early 1900s, opioids were available legally in the United States.

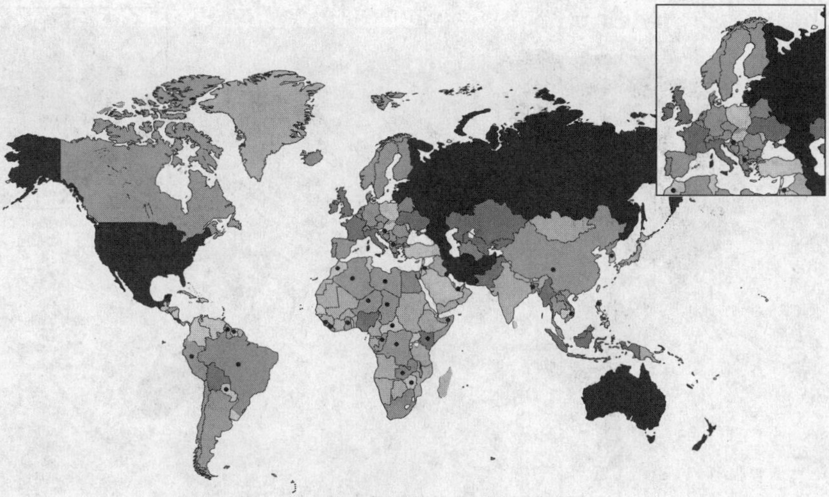

FIGURE 14-21 Prevalence of the Use of Opioids (Heroin, Opium, and Nonmedical Use of Synthetic Opioids) in 2010

Source: United Nations Office on Drugs and Crime (2012).
Disclaimer: This figure is not to scale. It does not represent any authentic national or international boundaries and is used for illustrative purposes only.

Do You Have Opium Receptors in Your Brain?

Surprisingly, you do have receptors in your brain that are sensitive to opioid drugs. The reason for this is that our bodies make a naturally occurring substance that also reduces the experience of pain and makes us feel good. *Endorphins* are produced at times of stress and allow individuals to continue in combat or a sports activity even when hurt. They also play a role in the placebo effect in relation to pain.

Cocaine

Cocaine comes from the naturally occurring coca plant. For thousands of years, individuals have chewed the leaves of the coca plant for its psychoactive experiences. It is largely grown in South America. As noted previously, it was even used to make Coca-Cola around 1900. About this time, Freud tried the drug and found it to be very pleasant. Its effects include a mental alertness including feelings of euphoria, energy, and a desire to talk. It also heightens the experience of sensory processes such as sound, touch, and sight.

Cocaine produces physiological effects such as increased heart rate and blood pressure. It has been administered by smoking, snorting through the nose, or injecting directly into the bloodstream. The form of cocaine that is smoked is referred to as crack. Crack refers to the sounds made when the white cocaine crystals are heated to turn it

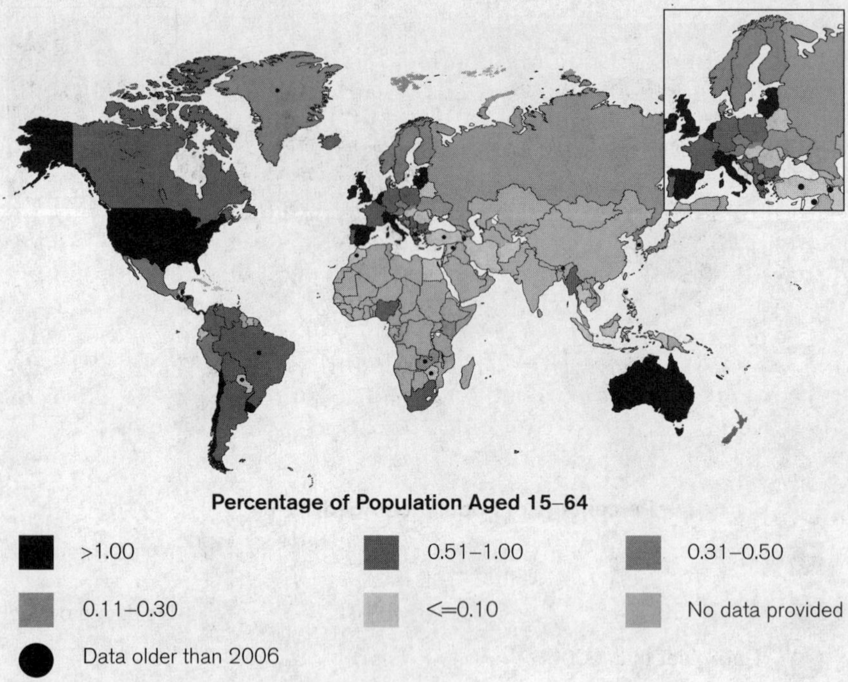

FIGURE 14-22 Prevalence of Cocaine Use in 2010

Source: United Nations Office on Drugs and Crime (2012).
Disclaimer: This figure is not to scale. It does not represent any authentic national or international boundaries and is used for illustrative purposes only.

into a form that can be smoked. Taking it through the nose results in a slower high than intravenously, which shows effects in 4 to 6 minutes. Cocaine has a shorter effect life in comparison with other drugs. That is, most of its effect is completed in 15 to 40 minutes. Like alcohol, individuals may use cocaine in binges.

In 2011, there were 1.4 million current cocaine users (SAMHSA, 2011) in the United States. That is about one half of 1% of the population. This is a drop from previous years. The UN estimates of cocaine use are a little higher, as shown in the map in *Figure 14-22*. You can note that rates of cocaine use in North America and Australia are some of the highest in the world.

Cocaine, Dopamine, and Your Brain

Normally, when there is an action potential, dopamine is released at the terminals. Dopamine is then removed from the receptors by a process called reuptake. However, the introduction of cocaine interferes with this natural process resulting in an increase of dopamine (see *Figure 14-23*). This increased dopamine signaling is involved in the effects experienced with cocaine.

The parts of your brain affected by dopamine depend on whether you are a new user or have taken it for a long time. In short-term users, the brain regions involved are primarily the nucleus accumbens and parts of the PFC. However, with long-term use more of the brain becomes involved, including the striatum, amygdala, hippocampus, and

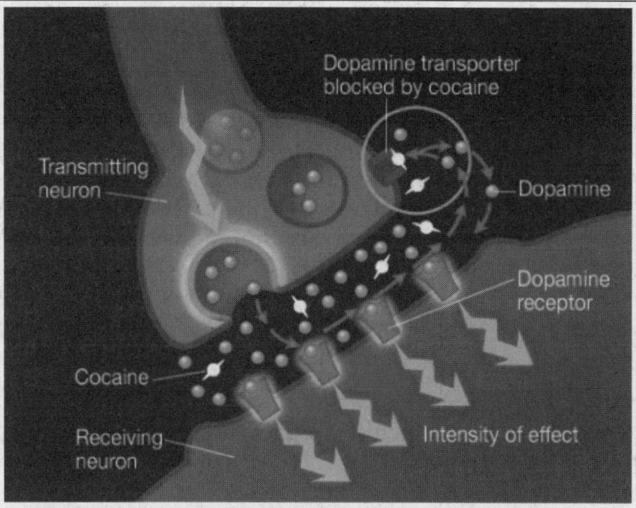

Cocaine in the brain: In the normal communication process, dopamine is released by a neuron into the synapse, where it can bind to dopamine receptors on neighboring neurons. Normally, dopamine is then recycled back into the transmitting neuron by a specialized protein called the dopamine transporter. If cocaine is present, it attaches to the dopamine transporter and blocks the normal recycling process, resulting in a buildup of dopamine in the synapse, which contributes to the pleasurable effects of cocaine.

FIGURE 14-23 Cocaine in the Brain

Source: National Institute on Drug Abuse (2010).

additional areas. What is different from some other drugs such as hallucinogens is that these brain changes are long lasting, even when the person ceases to use cocaine. This is shown in terms of positron emission testing (PET) in *Figure 14-24*. The top row depicts a non–cocaine user, which shows normal brain functioning in the area of the basal ganglia in four different brain slices. The middle row depicts a person who has not used cocaine

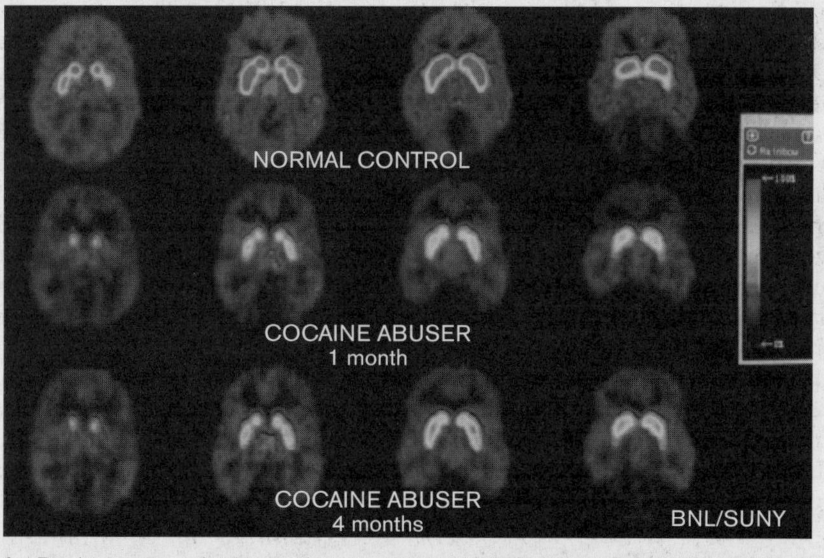

FIGURE 14-24 Brain Image of a Non–Cocaine User (Top Row) and a Cocaine User for 1 Month (Middle Row) and a Cocaine User for 4 Months (Bottom Row) After Ceasing to Use Cocaine

Source: Volkow et al. (1993, p. 172).

for a month. The bottom row depicts the same person after 4 months of not using cocaine. Note that there is still lower activity, which the researchers attribute to a continued blockage of dopamine receptors (Volkow et al., 1993).

Concept Check

- What is the primary psychoactive ingredient in cannabis? What are its impacts on an individual's body and brain?
- What is the relationship between cannabis and psychosis?
- Hallucinogens are not addictive, but in what other ways can they cause impairments to the individual using them?
- What are some common opioids? What is it about opioids that makes them sought after as medicines as well as substances to abuse?
- What factors impact the brain changes that occur from the use of cocaine?

AMPHETAMINES

Like cocaine, amphetamines are stimulants that result in positive feelings, a burst of energy, and alertness. However, unlike cocaine, it is a substance produced in the laboratory rather than found in nature. Amphetamine was first developed in the 1880s. It was not until the 1930s that it was introduced as a medicine in the form of an inhaler for the treatment of a stopped-up nose. Also during this time it was introduced in the form of pills with the name Benzedrine, which were called "bennies" (see Iversen, 2006; Koob, Kandel, & Volkow, 2008, for overviews).

Amphetamines as a Medicine

During the 1930s and 1940s, amphetamines were prescribed by health professionals for the treatment of more than 30 disorders, including epilepsy, Parkinson's disease, schizophrenia, migraine, and even behavioral problems in children. They were also prescribed to reduce addictions to other substances such as alcohol, morphine, and tobacco. During World War II, amphetamines were given to solders as "pep pills" to give them an edge in combat. The common ones were Benzedrine, Dexedrine, and Methedrine, the last one being methamphetamine. Although there are chemical differences in amphetamine and methamphetamine, they both function as stimulants.

As people experienced the stimulant effects, they began to abuse the use of amphetamines. In the 1950s, long-distance truck drivers would use them to drive farther. After they were publicized for use as a recreational drug from Hollywood to New York, the U.S. government began to pay attention. Amphetamines were also making their way into teenage parties. In 1959, the U.S. Food and Drug Administration (FDA) required that amphetamines would only be available by prescription.

The main reason people take amphetamines is that they believe they enhance performance and help them feel good. The common experience is euphoria, increased vigilance, and hyperactivity. The reactions from amphetamines are also similar to other stimulant drugs. They are easy to take in the form of a pill, which can be conveniently purchased one pill at a time on the illegal market. Amphetamines are not considered to be harmful by many individuals. Taking these drugs through intravenous injection or smoking increases the feeling of a rush.

In their 2011 global assessment, the United Nations suggests that amphetamine-type drugs are the second most widely used drugs throughout the world (United Nations Office on Drugs and Crime, 2011). The first is cannabis. This makes amphetamine use greater than heroin or cocaine worldwide. Amphetamine-like drugs do not require the cultivation of plants. Instead, they can be manufactured almost anywhere without an advanced knowledge of chemistry.

As with other stimulant drugs, amphetamines affect the dopamine system to produce the initial euphoric experience. In addition to the short-term experience, there are also less positive long-term effects (see Marshall & O'Dell, 2012, for an overview). These long-term effects, especially from methamphetamine, create brain changes in three areas. The first is the development of compulsive patterns of use. The second produces negative brain changes consistent with brain injury. And third, methamphetamine produces changes in the individual's cognitive functioning.

Cognitive deficits in people who use methamphetamine show problems with motor activities such as skill movements or perceptual speed. They also experience problems in the ability to shift attention. Finally, research also suggests memory, attention, and decision-making problems. These types of problems make it difficult for individuals to objectively see their addiction as well as be able to engage in therapy requiring cognitive responses. Methamphetamine also has a devastating effect on physical appearance, which can be seen in the before and after mug shots of the Oregon Multnomah County Detention Center (www.facesofmeth.us/main.htm).

One of the first studies to examine the effects of methamphetamine and methcathinone on the brain was performed by Una McCann and her colleagues (McCann, Szabo, Scheffel, Dannals, & Ricaurte, 1998). Methamphetamine is also known as "speed," "crystal meth," or "crank." Methcathinone is also known as "cat." Both of these drugs have been shown to be toxic to dopamine and serotonin neurons in animals. Parkinson's disease also shows a reduction in dopamine in the brain. *Figure 14-25* shows PET images from four individuals. The first is from a healthy control person. This person shows dopamine activity in the striatum as seen with the brighter colors. The next two PET images show a

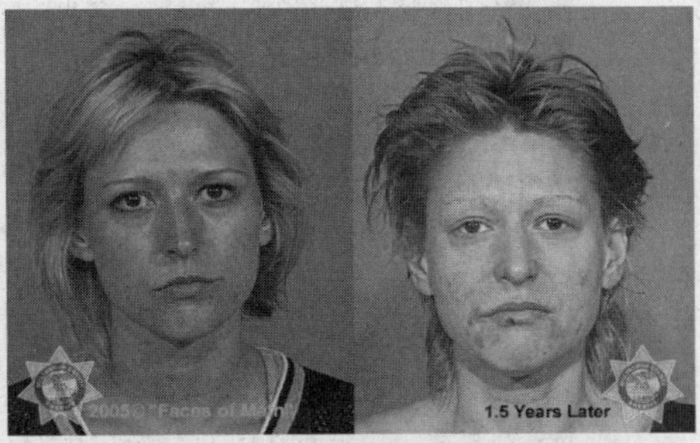

Jennifer

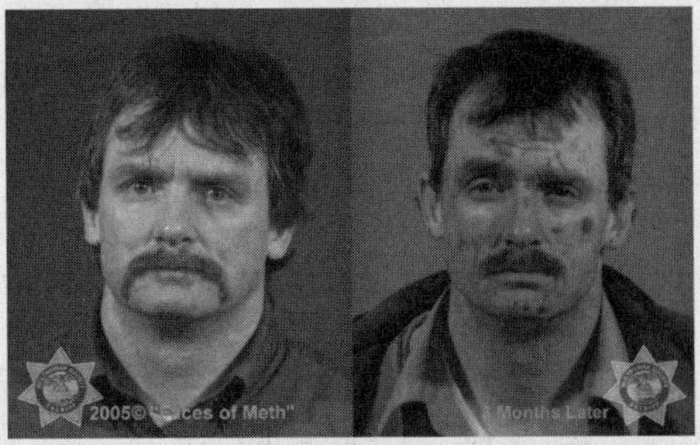

Joseph

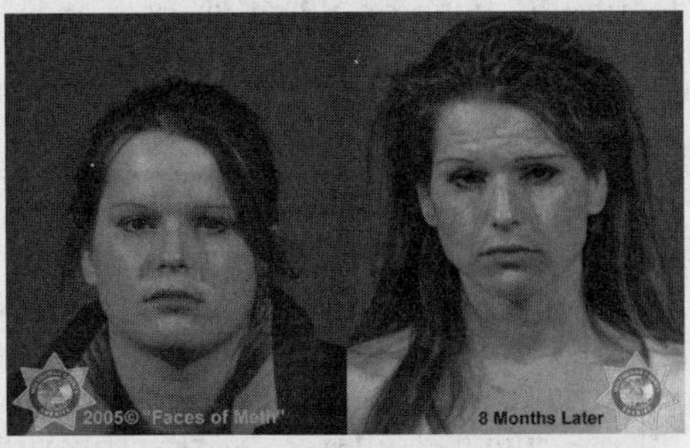

Esther

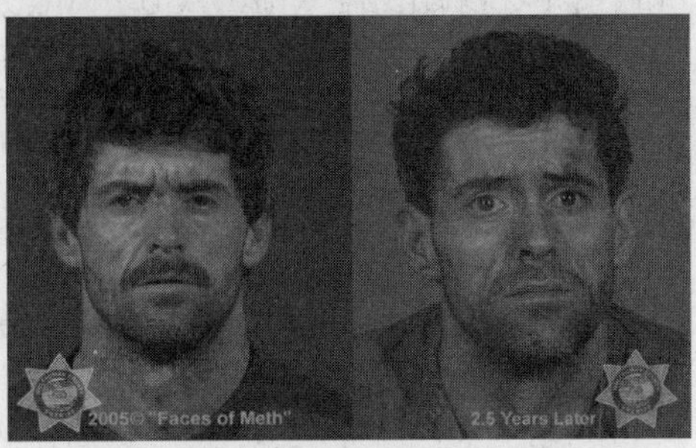

Patrick

Mug shots of individuals who were chronic users of methamphetamine

Source: Courtesy of Multnomah County Sheriff's *Faces of Meth*™ Program. Multnomah County Oregon.

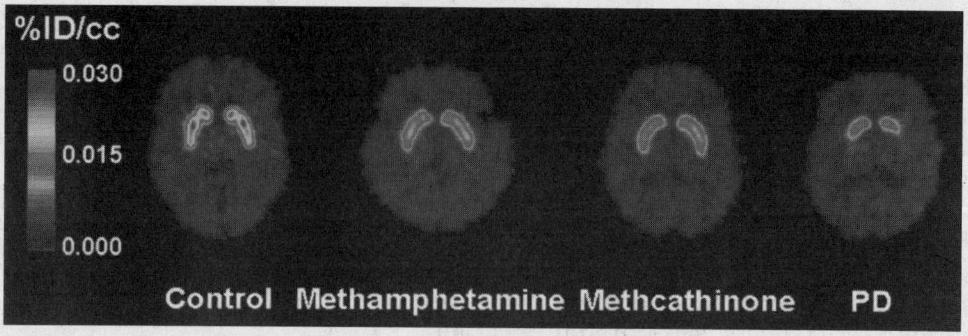

FIGURE 14-25 Positron Emission Testing Image From a Control Person, a Person Who Had Not Taken Methamphetamine, a Person Who Had Not Taken Methcathinone for 3 Years, and a Person Who Had Just Been Diagnosed With Parkinson's Disorder

Source: McCann et al. (1998, p. 8419).

person who had not taken methamphetamine for 3 years and a person who had not taken methcathinone for 3 years. Notice that there is less dopamine activity. The last image is from a person who had just been diagnosed with Parkinson's disorder and shows even less dopamine activity. This suggests damage to dopamine mechanisms is long lasting with methamphetamine users although improvement over time has been shown. Thus far, the focus has been on illegal substances, except for alcohol. In the next section, I move to legal substances: caffeine and tobacco.

CAFFEINE AND TOBACCO

There are two additional legal substances, caffeine and tobacco, that *DSM–5* includes in its substance-related and addictive disorders category. Caffeine is usually described as a stimulant although there are beneficial effects beyond stimulation (see Glade, 2010, for an overview). Caffeine works through the central nervous system and increases resting energy expenditure within 30 minutes of ingestion. Its effects will last for about 4 hours. Caffeine also increases serotonin concentration in the region of the brain stem. This, in turn, postpones fatigue and increases endurance. Overall, caffeine consumption increases alertness, ability to concentrate, problem solving, wakefulness, the feeling of energy, and elevated mood. These effects have also been shown in studies in which caffeine was compared with a placebo in a double-blind situation.

Caffeine comes from a number of sources. It is found naturally in different amounts in the leaves and seeds of various plants including coffee beans, tea leaves, and cocoa beans, which are used to make chocolate. Caffeine amounts even vary in different types of coffee beans. The average 8 oz. cup of coffee has about 100 milligrams of caffeine with tea having about half this amount and chocolate even less. It is also added to energy drinks, weight loss drugs, some sodas, and drugs for colds. It is estimated that over 85% of children and adults in the United States consume caffeine daily with adults consuming around 280 mg each day (APA, 2013). This equates to about 2 to 3 cups of coffee each day. Headaches are reported in about 10% of the people who have not used caffeine for the past 24 hours.

An Indian Study on Cognitive Dysfunction in Chronic Smokers

Chronic smoking has been associated with abnormalities in brain morphology, neurochemistry, cerebral blood flow as well as neurocognition.

Tobacco abuse is responsible for fifty percent of all the malignancies in males and one-fourth of all malignancies in females in India. Further, other forms of tobacco use in India include, typically tobacco chewing, *paan* chewing (piper betel leaf filled with sliced areca nut, lime, catechu, and other spices chewed with or without tobacco) *paan masala* or *gutkha* (a chewable tobacco containing areca nut), and *gulmanjan* (finely powdered tobacco rubbed on the gums as tooth paste). Tobacco may also be smoked in bidis (which do not filter the smoke) cigarettes and hookah.

In large-scale studies involving more than 100,000 individuals who were followed for up to 24 years, the consumption of coffee was related to the individuals having less risk for heart disease (see Glade, 2010, for a review). Even drinking six cups of coffee a day had no effect for developing heart disease. However, some individuals are more sensitive to caffeine than others. These individuals may experience stomach problems, trouble sleeping, anxiety, irritability, and nervousness from increased caffeine intake.

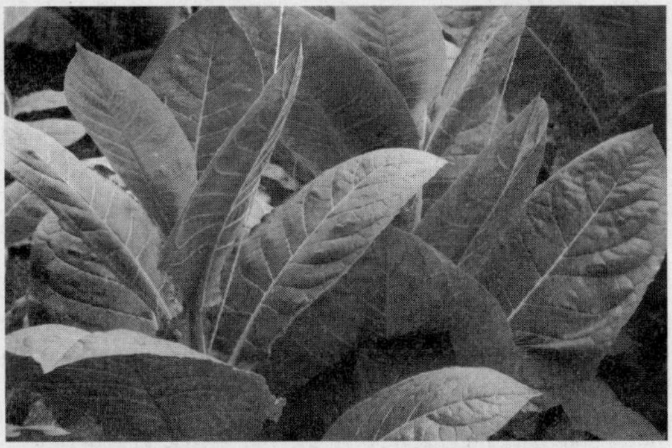

Tobacco leaf

© iStockphoto.com/vanbeets

In *DSM–5,* individuals who experience such symptoms along with clinically significant distress or impairment in important areas of functioning after ingesting a large dose of caffeine can be diagnosed with caffeine intoxication. There is also a caffeine withdrawal disorder in which the individual experiences clinically significant distress or impairment in important areas of functioning after an abrupt reduction in caffeine. In addition, the individual should also experience at least three of the following: headache, fatigue, depressed mood, difficulty concentrating, and flu-like symptoms. Although individuals can experience symptoms related to increased caffeine intake or abrupt reduction, there is little evidence that a person can become addicted to caffeine as with other drugs. However, individuals can become addicted to tobacco, which I will discuss next.

Tobacco originated in the Americas with native populations smoking or chewing the leaves of the plant (see Dani & Balfour, 2011, for an overview). After Columbus's trip to the new world in 1492, tobacco began to spread to Europe carried back by the sailors who came to the Americas. In 1623, the English scientist Francis Bacon described the addictive nature of tobacco. Also in the 1600s, tobacco was grown in the Jamestown colony. During the next few hundred years, it became a cash crop. After 1880, when the cigarette rolling machine was invented, billons of cigarettes and cigars were consumed worldwide.

In the 1950s, tobacco use was associated with cancer. Today, tobacco use is seen by the CDC as the leading cause of preventable disease, disability, and death in the United States (www.cdc.gov/nchs/data/hus/hus11.pdf). In 2010, 19% of adults 25 years of age and older in the United States were cigarette smokers. Cigarette smoking is related

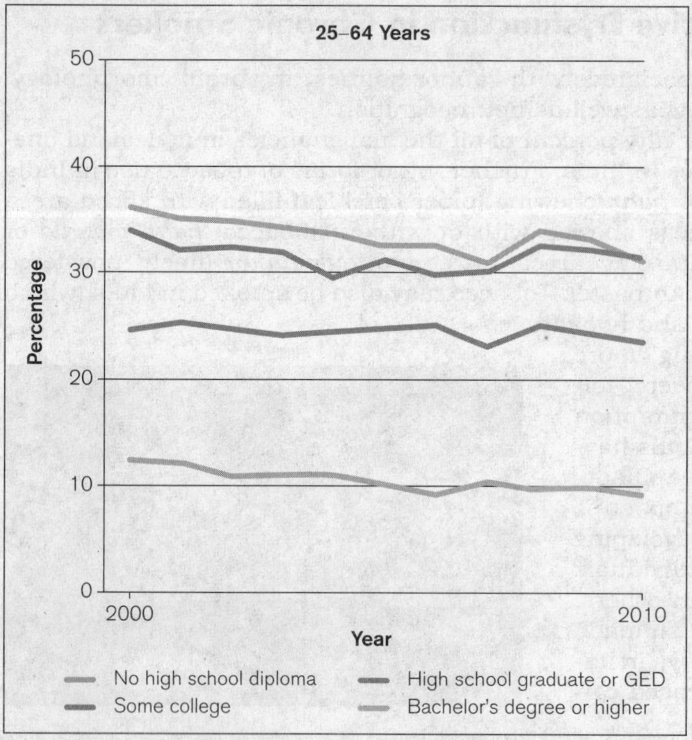

FIGURE 14-26 Cigarette Smoking Among Adults by Education Level

Source: National Center for Health Statistics. *Health, United States, 2011: With Special Feature on Socioeconomic Status and Health*. Hyattsville, MD. 2012.

to level of education (see *Figure 14-26*). The majority of tobacco use worldwide is in less developed countries.

The addictive substance in tobacco is nicotine (see Dani & Balfour, 2011, for an overview). Nicotine is a stimulant substance found in plants of the nightshade family. Like caffeine, nicotine may be produced by the plant to inhibit insects. In humans, research has shown that nicotine influences dopamine neurons in the midbrain. It increases dopamine and thus functions similarly to other drugs of addiction. Also similar to other drugs, the environmental cues associated with tobacco use play a critical role. For some, it is the smell of the smoke from another smoker. For others, it can be a cue such as finishing a meal or having sexual relations. Nicotine is able to alter the inhibitory effects of GABA and thus enhance the learning of external cues with tobacco use and experience. In terms of learning, nicotine acts throughout the brain and influences attention, memory, emotion, and motivation.

Nicotine can have varied effects on the body, which makes it function as both a stimulant and a depressant (www.nlm.nih.gov/medlineplus/ency/article/000953.htm). Some of these include the following:

- Decreases the appetite (for this reason, the fear of weight gain affects some people's willingness to stop smoking)
- Boosts mood and may even relieve minor depression; many people will feel a sense of well-being
- Raises the level of blood sugar (glucose) and increases insulin production
- Increases bowel activity, saliva, and phlegm
- Increases heart rate by around 10 to 20 beats per minute
- Increases blood pressure by 5 to 10 mmHg (because it tightens the blood vessels)
- May cause sweating, nausea, and diarrhea
- Stimulates memory and alertness; people who use tobacco often depend on it to help them accomplish certain tasks and perform well

As with other drugs of addiction, nicotine will affect changes in the brain that result in the experience of withdrawal if it is not available. These include the following:

- An intense craving for nicotine
- Anxiety, tension, restlessness, frustration, or impatience
- Difficulty concentrating
- Drowsiness or trouble sleeping, as well as bad dreams and nightmares
- Headaches
- Increased appetite and weight gain
- Irritability or depression

As with other addictive disorders, *DSM–5* includes tobacco use disorder and tobacco withdrawal disorder, which involve clinically significant distress or impairment in important areas of functioning.

GAMBLING

Gambling has been part of human existence worldwide—at least since the beginning of written history. Currently, lottery tickets are available throughout the world. Many countries have some form of legal gambling, such as seen in the United States in Las Vegas and many additional places. Poker tournaments are seen on TV, and online poker is available from many places on the Internet.

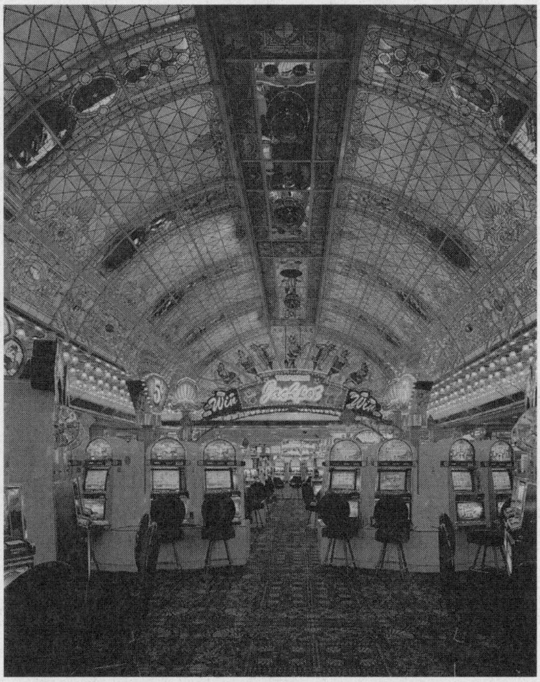

Slot machines

In one national community survey, four out of five respondents, or 78.4% of the more than 9,000 people in the sample, reported gambling at least once in their lifetime (Kessler et al., 2008). Some 54% gambled more than 10 times, 27% gambled more than 100 times, and 10.1% gambled more than 1,000 times. *Table 14-7* shows these data by type of gambling. In some individuals, gambling becomes a problem that appears similar to drug addiction.

Whereas *DSM–IV* categorized pathological gambling as an *impulse control disorder* (see Shaffer & Martin, 2011, for an overview), *DSM–5* considers pathological gambling an addictive disorder. Like drug addiction, pathological gambling continues even despite negative consequences such as consistent losses and an inability to control one's gambling behavior. The *DSM–5* criteria for gambling disorder have similarities to other addictive disorders. This includes at least

TABLE 14-7 Lifetime Prevalence by Gambling Type

	Prevalence	
	%	(Se)
I. Sports betting		
Office sports pool	44.3	(1.7)
Sports with bookie or parlay cards	5.8	(0.5)
Betting on horse/dog races or cock/dog fights	25.0	(1.3)
Gambling at a casino	44.7	(2.1)
II. Other types of gambling that involve some aspect of mental or physical skill		
Games involving mental skill (e.g., cards)	35.8	(1.2)
Games involving physical skill (e.g., pool)	22.7	(1.1)
Speculating on high-risk investments	8.4	(0.7)
Internet gambling	1.0	(0.2)
III. Types of gambling that largely involve chance rather than skill		
Playing numbers/lotto	62.2	(1.5)
Gambling machines (e.g., video poker)	26.1	(1.3)
Slot machines, bingo, or pull tabs	48.9	(1.8)

Source: Kessler et al. (2008, p. 1356).

four of the following: has a need to gamble with increasing amounts of money; is restless or irritable when attempting to cut down on gambling; has tried in the past to cut down on gambling; thinks about gambling; gambles when feeling distressed; tries to recoup loses; lies to conceal involvement in gambling; jeopardizes significant opportunities; and relies on others to supply money lost in gambling. The pattern of its development can be unpredictable and is not related to any age-group. It is seen to develop in adolescence, young adulthood, middle age, and even old age. Males tend to develop gambling disorder when younger whereas females develop it late in life. It has only recently been studied from a scientific standpoint.

In a study by Kessler and his colleagues (Kessler et al., 2008), those with pathological gambling symptoms showed a lifetime prevalence of 2.3% and a 12-month prevalence of less than 1% (0.3%). Those with pathological gambling symptoms also show comorbidity on a number of mental disorders. *Table 14-8* presents these data. Notice that individuals with pathological gambling show the highest comorbidity for other substance use disorders.

Psychological studies suggest that pathological gambling is more than just an impulse control disorder but is another

Concept Check

- What are some of the factors that promote the use and abuse of amphetamines?
- How do amphetamines affect the body?
- What are the primary effects of caffeine on the body? An individual can experience intoxication and withdrawal in regard to caffeine, but what about addiction?
- What is the addictive ingredient in tobacco and what are its impacts on an individual's body and brain?
- What are the characteristics of pathological gambling that make it an addictive disorder?

TABLE 14-8 Lifetime Comorbidity of Pathological Gambling With Other Mental Disorders

	Prevalence		
	%	(Se)	OR
I. Mood disorders			
Major depressive disorder or dysthymia	38.6	(9.1)	2.5
Bipolar disorder	17.0	(7.1)	4.6
Any mood disorder	55.6	(9.7)	3.7
II. Anxiety disorders			
Panic disorder	21.9	(6.7)	4.9
Generalized anxiety disorder	16.6	(7.0)	2.8
Phobia	52.2	(8.8)	3.2
PTSD	14.8	(7.8)	2.3
Any anxiety disorder	60.3	(9.1)	3.1
III. Impulse-control disorders			
ADHD	13.4	(8.1)	1.8
Oppositional-defiant disorder	15.4	(6.8)	1.9
Conduct disorder	24.9	(8.2)	3.1
Intermittent explosive disorder	27.0	(9.0)	3.1
Any impulse control disorder	42.3	(10.5)	2.2
IV. Substance use disorders			
Alcohol or drug abuse	46.2	(10.7)	4.5
Alcohol or drug dependence	31.8	(9.4)	5.8
Nicotine dependence	63.0	(9.0)	3.9
Any substance use disorder	76.3	(7.9)	5.5
V. Number of disorders			
Any disorder	96.3	(2.6)	17.4
Exactly one disorder	22.0	(10.2)	10.1
Exactly two disorders	9.9	(6.5)	9.1
Three or more disorders	64.4	(10.4)	30.0

Source: Kessler et al. (2008, p. 1357).
Note: SE = standard error; OR = odds ratio.

example of an addiction disorder (Wareham & Potenza, 2010). Individuals with both gambling and substance use disorder show **substance tolerance.** With drugs, individuals develop tolerance and must consume more of the drug to have the same effect. With gambling, the individual needs to bet more to keep the same level of excitement. Withdrawal is also a common factor in both gambling and substance use disorder. As the person cuts down or quits on either, he becomes anxious or irritable. Both gambling and substance use can lead to illegal activity to keep them available.

Researchers suggest that four cognitive–emotional processes play a role in pathological gambling (see van Holst, van den Brink, Veltman, & Goudriaan, 2010, for an overview).

The first is behavioral conditioning. People are sensitive to reward in their life. Early wins when playing games of chance will keep an individual gambling longer. Also, those who win are more likely to attribute the win to their behavior than those who lose. Finally, as seen in various studies of conditioning, a variable intermittent pattern of reinforcement, which is impossible to predict, is one of the most difficult to extinguish.

The second cognitive–emotional process to play a role in pathological gambling is the experience of cues, which bring forth urges to gamble. As with other addictive disorders such as alcohol use disorder, just seeing an item such as a glass of beer will produce arousal and increase the desire to drink. The same is true of gambling, and the person will show attentional processes in which he or she is quick to notice gambling-related items.

The third process is impulsivity. Studies of pathological gambling show more impulsiveness on behavioral inhibition tasks as well as questionnaires for pathological gamblers.

The fourth process is impaired executive functioning in pathological gamblers. Impaired executive function leads to decision making that results in an inaccurate evaluation of the situation; that is, they continue to gamble even when external factors show negative consequences. Pathological gamblers often ignore the long-term consequences over short-term experiences. One common research paradigm is to use the Iowa Gambling Task. In this task, individuals must choose between four decks of cards. Unknown to the person, two decks give low payouts but with fewer penalties. The other two give higher payout but also greater penalties. Since the task is to accumulate money, the best strategy is to consistently choose the low payout/low penalty decks. The Iowa Gambling Task is able to differentiate healthy individuals and individuals with frontal lobe disorders. People with a pathological gambling disorder also show a tendency to choose short-term gain over the more successful long-term strategy.

TREATMENT OF SUBSTANCE-RELATED DISORDERS

Addictive drugs create brain changes that affect one's ability to accurately see the way in which one is addicted. The person with an addiction will often deny that an addiction is present. Thus, those with addiction are slow to seek help until they experience the negative consequences of their situation. The changes that take place in the brain from taking psychoactive drugs on a prolonged basis also create an increased need for additional amounts of the drug to obtain the same effect. Further, physiological states of need such as feeling hungry are able to interfere with cognitive and emotional processes such that we tend to pay more attention to these need states. Likewise, drugs with their rewarding effects and withdrawal experiences make it difficult for an individual to reverse a drug addiction without help.

Treating addiction is a difficult process. Many individuals who engage in some type of substance abuse do not want to seek treatment. As noted, many have other comorbid mental disorders. This raises the question of what type of treatment is needed. Overall, there are two broad categories of treatment. The first is psychosocial approaches including cognitive behavioral therapy (CBT), motivational interviewing, and family or couple approaches. There are also community support and relapse prevention groups such as Alcoholics Anonymous (AA) that play a role. The second treatment approach involves using psychopharmacological agents. These agents can be directed at problems of withdrawal, relapse prevention, or comorbid mental disorders. Given the large number of approaches used in the clinical setting, systematic evaluation of these treatments has been limited.

The first step in treating addiction is to help the individual remove the drug from his or her system. For some, this requires a stay in a hospital or rehabilitation center during the initial phases of withdrawal and the craving that often follows. This is usually followed by some type of psychosocial treatment to help the person understand other factors related to the addiction and develop a plan for future action. One important goal is to help individuals gain the feeling of control over their substance use. For some, this may mean no further use of the substance. For others, this may result in using alcohol, for example, in a limited manner. In this section, some of the more effective means of treatment will be presented including both psychosocial and psychopharmacological approaches and the way in which they should be used.

Principles of Effective Treatment

In 2012, the National Institute on Drug Abuse, U.S. Department of Health and Human Services, examined the complex question of how to treat drug addiction (www.drugabuse.gov/PODAT/). In their summary publication, *Principles of Drug Addiction Treatment: A Research-Based Guide (Third Edition),* 13 principles are suggested. These principles are as follows:

1. *Addiction is a complex but treatable disease that affects brain function and behavior.* Drugs of abuse alter the brain's structure and function, resulting in changes that persist long after drug use has ceased. This may explain why drug abusers are at risk for relapse even after long periods of abstinence and despite the potentially devastating consequences.
2. *No single treatment is appropriate for everyone.* Treatment varies depending on the type of drug and the characteristics of the patients. Matching treatment settings, interventions, and services to an individual's particular problems and needs is critical to his or her ultimate success in returning to productive functioning in the family, workplace, and society.
3. *Treatment needs to be readily available.* Because drug-addicted individuals may be uncertain about entering treatment, taking advantage of available services the moment people are ready for treatment is critical. Potential patients can be lost if treatment is not immediately available or readily accessible. As with other chronic diseases, the earlier treatment is offered in the disease process, the greater the likelihood of positive outcomes.
4. *Effective treatment attends to multiple needs of the individual, not just his or her drug abuse.* To be effective, treatment must address the individual's drug abuse and any associated medical, psychological, social, vocational, and legal problems. It is also important that treatment be appropriate to the individual's age, gender, ethnicity, and culture.
5. *Remaining in treatment for an adequate period of time is critical.* The appropriate duration for an individual depends on the type and degree of the patient's problems and needs. Research indicates that most addicted individuals need at least 3 months in treatment and that the best outcomes occur with longer

durations of treatment. Recovery from drug addiction is a long-term process and frequently requires multiple episodes of treatment. As with other chronic illnesses, relapses to drug abuse can occur and should signal a need for treatment to be reinstated or adjusted. Because individuals often leave treatment prematurely, programs should include strategies to engage and keep patients in treatment.

6. *Behavioral therapies—including individual, family, or group counseling—are the most commonly used forms of drug abuse treatment.* Behavioral therapies vary in their focus and may involve addressing a patient's motivation to change, providing incentives for abstinence, building skills to resist drug use, replacing drug-using activities with constructive and rewarding activities, improving problem-solving skills, and facilitating better interpersonal relationships. Also, participation in group therapy and other peer support programs during and following treatment can help maintain abstinence.
7. *Medications are an important element of treatment for many patients, especially when combined with counseling and other behavioral therapies.* For example, methadone, buprenorphine, and naltrexone (including a new long-acting formulation) are effective in helping individuals addicted to heroin or other opioids stabilize their lives and reduce their illicit drug use. Acamprosate, disulfiram, and naltrexone are medications approved for treating alcohol dependence. For persons addicted to nicotine, a nicotine replacement product (available as patches, gum, lozenges, or nasal spray) or an oral medication (such as bupropion or varenicline) can be an effective component of treatment when part of a comprehensive behavioral treatment program.
8. *An individual's treatment and services plan must be assessed continually and modified as necessary to ensure that it meets his or her changing needs.* A patient may require varying combinations of services and treatment components during the course of treatment and recovery. In addition to counseling or psychotherapy, a patient may require medication, medical services, family therapy, parenting instruction, vocational rehabilitation, and/or social and legal services. For many patients, a continuing care approach provides the best results, with the treatment intensity varying according to a person's changing needs.
9. *Many drug-addicted individuals also have other mental disorders.* Because drug abuse and addiction—both of which are mental disorders—often co-occur with other mental illnesses, patients presenting with one condition should be assessed for the other(s). And when these problems co-occur, treatment should address both (or all), including the use of medications as appropriate.
10. *Medically assisted detoxification is only the first stage of addiction treatment and by itself does little to change long-term drug abuse.* Although medically assisted detoxification can safely manage the acute physical symptoms of withdrawal and can, for some, pave the way for effective long-term addiction treatment, detoxification alone is rarely sufficient to help addicted individuals achieve long-term abstinence. Thus, patients should be encouraged to continue drug treatment following detoxification. Motivational enhancement and incentive strategies, begun at initial patient intake, can improve treatment engagement.
11. *Treatment does not need to be voluntary to be effective.* Sanctions or enticements from family, employment settings, and/or the criminal justice system can

significantly increase treatment entry, retention rates, and the ultimate success of drug treatment interventions.

12. *Drug use during treatment must be monitored continuously, as lapses during treatment do occur.* Knowing their drug use is being monitored can be a powerful incentive for patients and can help them withstand urges to use drugs. Monitoring also provides an early indication of a return to drug use, signaling a possible need to adjust an individual's treatment plan to better meet his or her needs.
13. *Treatment programs should test patients for the presence of HIV/AIDS, hepatitis B and C, tuberculosis, and other infectious diseases, as well as provide targeted risk-reduction counseling, linking patients to treatment if necessary.* Typically, drug abuse treatment addresses some of the drug-related behaviors that put people at risk of infectious diseases. Targeted counseling focused on reducing infectious disease risk can help patients further reduce or avoid substance-related and other high-risk behaviors. Counseling can also help those who are already infected to manage their illness. Moreover, engaging in substance abuse treatment can facilitate adherence to other medical treatments. Substance abuse treatment facilities should provide on-site, rapid HIV testing rather than referrals to off-site testing—research shows that doing so increases the likelihood that patients will be tested and receive their test results. Treatment providers should also inform patients that highly active antiretroviral therapy (HAART) has proven effective in combating HIV, including among drug-abusing populations, and help link them to HIV treatment if they test positive.

These 13 principles seek to describe the reality of drug addiction. These principles suggest that addiction is a treatable disorder but one that requires an individualized approach. These principles also acknowledge that the person may have other disorders or problems and that these should be considered in the treatment. The principles also consider the complex nature of addiction. One of these realities is that those who use drugs may also engage in risky behavior including having unprotected sex, using dirty needles, and committing crime, which can result in getting HIV, hepatitis C, and other diseases. Pregnant females may also impact the health of their fetus through drug use. From a treatment standpoint, both behavioral approaches and medications should be considered for treating the problems.

Psychosocial Therapies and Addiction

Given the difficulty for most individuals to reduce drug use, a number of procedures have been developed. Some of these, such as an educational approach, have been shown not to be effective (see Miller, Sorensen, Selzer, & Brigham, 2006, for an overview). That is, just telling a person about the problems related to addiction does not change behavior. Other psychosocial approaches, such as those discussed previously in terms of other disorders, have also been utilized with substance abuse. However, the evaluation of these psychosocial approaches is complex as most of these psychosocial approaches are used in the context of other treatment types. Thus, it is difficult to determine which aspects of the treatment constitute the effective component.

One approach that has been found to have empirical support is CBT for individuals and for couples. CBT has mainly been used as a means to prevent relapse. As with CBT for other mental disorders, it is designed to help the person understand his or her thoughts toward substance abuse and create means to cope. One part of this is an exploration of positive and negative aspects of continued use. Another part of this is to anticipate problems associated with no longer using a substance and to consider alternative ways to act and reason in the situation. This would include teaching the person techniques of self-monitoring related to his or her emotions and internal sensations such that he or she is able to anticipate when craving will develop. Likewise, the person can consider which future situations would put him or her at risk for abuse.

The 12-Step Program

The **12-step program** forms the basis for AA. Variations of the approach have also been used with other addictions (e.g., Narcotics Anonymous, Gamblers Anonymous). The 12-step program and AA were established in the 1930s by William Wilson and Robert Holbrook Smith. These individuals are better known as "Bill W." and "Dr. Bob". They created a community in which individuals with alcohol problems would meet and follow the principles described in the 12 steps. AA is not considered a treatment in the usual sense since there is not a health care professional involved nor is there a desire to change their procedures based on empirical research.

AA groups are found throughout the world. According to AA (www.aa.org/pdf/products/p-48_membershipsurvey.pdf), in a 2011 survey, there are more than 114,000 groups worldwide. In the United States and Canada, 65% of the members are men and 35% women with an average age of 49 years. The average length of time since their last drink is around 10 years (see *Figure 14-27*). In this sense, AA is a support group designed to help an individual not drink or relapse.

The first step suggests that the individual is powerless over alcohol. Therefore, individuals must look to a higher power to help them. The Twelve Steps are presented here (www.aa.org/pdf/products/p-55_twelvestepsillustrated.pdf):

1. We admitted we were powerless over alcohol—that our lives had become unmanageable.
2. Came to believe that a Power greater than ourselves could restore us to sanity.

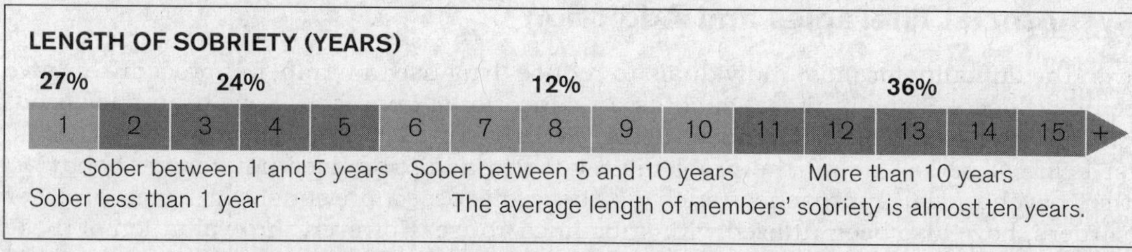

FIGURE 14-27 Length of Self-Reported Sobriety of Alcoholics Anonymous Members in the United States and Canada

Source: From ALCOHOLICS ANONYMOUS 2011 MEMBERSHIP SURVEY, http://www.aa.org/pdf/products/p-48_membershipsurvey.pdf.

3. Made a decision to turn our will and our lives over to the care of God *as we understood Him.*
4. Made a searching and fearless moral inventory of ourselves.
5. Admitted to God, to ourselves, and to another human being the exact nature of our wrongs.
6. Were entirely ready to have God remove all these defects of character.
7. Humbly asked Him to remove our shortcomings.
8. Made a list of all persons we had harmed, and became willing to make amends to them all.
9. Made direct amends to such people wherever possible, except when to do so would injure them or others.
10. Continued to take personal inventory, and when we were wrong, promptly admitted it.
11. Sought through prayer and meditation to improve our conscious contact with God *as we understood Him*, praying only for knowledge of His will for us and the power to carry that out.
12. Having had a spiritual awakening as the result of these steps, we tried to carry this message to alcoholics, and to practice these principles in all our affairs.

As the individual moves through these steps, he comes to see his own emotional reactions to the world as well as the manner in which his behavior has affected other individuals. The majority of individuals in AA have a sponsor who helps them consider their life. The typical person goes to two or three meetings a week. Although no formal evaluation of the program has been conducted, it appears to be useful for those committed to changing their relationship to drugs of addiction.

Controlled Drinking Approaches

Controlled drinking is based on the idea that a person can learn to use alcohol in moderation (see Saladin & Santa Ana, 2004, for an overview). This is in contrast to the AA approach, which suggests that total abstinence is required. It was commonly assumed in both the United States and Europe that a person with alcoholism could not learn to drink alcohol in moderation. This view was challenged in the United Kingdom when D. L. Davies published a paper in 1962 reporting that 7 of 97 individuals with serious alcoholism were able to control their consumption of alcohol over a 7- to 11-year period (Davies, 1962). There was also a Rand Report based on data from 45 treatment centers in the United States that suggested that around 20% of those who had been treated were able to drink moderately after 4 years (Polich, Armor, & Braiker, 1981). The controlled drinking approach gained additional scientific credibility when Mark and Linda Sobell conducted a study of men with an alcohol problem at a state hospital. Half of the men received a treatment group in which they were taught to drink in moderation whereas the other group focused on abstinence (see Sobell & Sobell, 1978, for an overview). These individuals were followed and at the end of 2 years, it was reported that the controlled drinking group was doing well 85% of the time whereas in the abstinence group, it was only 42% of the time. Clearly, in men picked because of their potential for a good prognosis, controlled drinking offered an alternative.

However, this conclusion was challenged in 1982 with a publication in the journal *Science* (Pendery, Maltzman, & West, 1982). These researchers reported that when they followed up on the individuals in the controlled drinking group some 10 years later, the results were not impressive. Only 1 out of 20 men had maintained a pattern of controlled drinking. However, they did not follow up with the abstinence-focused group. This stirred great debate in the research and treatment community as to whether controlled drinking works. In 1995, the Sobels wrote an editorial for the journal *Addiction* with the title "Controlled Drinking After 25 Years: How Important Was the Great Debate?" which was followed by eight commentaries on the editorial (Sobell & Sobell, 1995).

Although there was great debate during the end of the 1900s concerning whether an individual with alcohol problems could achieve controlled use of alcohol, more recent research suggests it is possible (see Saladin & Santa Ana, 2004, for an overview). Treatment alternatives to abstinence are known by a number of names besides controlled drinking, including moderated drinking, reduced-risk drinking, asymptomatic drinking, and behavioral self-control training. Various studies suggest these approaches are as effective as other approaches in treating those who experience problems with alcohol.

Overall, this points to the difficulty of treating individuals with alcohol abuse disorder long term.

Medications Used to Treat Addiction

Medications use at least three different approaches to treating addiction that utilize the manner in which the drug of addiction works in the brain. The first approach is to use agonists. An **agonist drug** is a substance that binds to the receptor and produces cellular activity. Methadone is an opioid agonist. When given, it functions like heroin at the receptor site. However, it does not give the same rush as heroin. If taken orally, it will also lessen the effects of using heroin or other opioids. Thus, if a person wants to lessen the withdrawal effect of heroin, methadone would offer that opportunity. By giving the body the molecular experience of taking a drug without the experience of a high, it aids in the reduction of opioids. Most states in the United States offer methadone treatment programs. Methadone maintenance works better if it is combined with a psychosocial treatment program.

The second approach is to use an **antagonist drug.** Where an agonist drug acts similar to the illicit drug, an antagonist drug blocks the receptor site so that the illicit drug does not produce an effect. By blocking or counteracting the effects of the illicit drug, it no longer has its rewarding and addictive effects. One such antagonist is naltrexone, which is used to treat opioid addiction. It is also used in emergency rooms to counteract opioid overdose. In terms of tobacco use, varenicline (Chantix) blocks the ability of nicotine to activate dopamine. By reducing the rewarding effects of tobacco use, it reduces craving. Naltrexone preforms a similar effect for alcohol.

The third approach is to use an **aversive drug** that becomes aversive when the drug of abuse is taken. One example is disulfiram (Antabuse). Antabuse interferes with the metabolism of alcohol and produces unpleasant reactions. If a person on Antabuse drinks alcohol, he or she will experience nausea and other physiological reactions such as increased heart rate. Other substances, such as those that leave a bad taste in one's mouth, have been used in reducing tobacco use.

Concept Check

- What are the primary steps in a treatment for drug addiction? Why is treating addiction such a difficult process?
- What are the principles for effective treatment as proposed by the National Institute of Drug Abuse?
- What psychosocial therapy approaches have been used with addiction?
- What are the primary characteristics that describe the 12-step program? Is it a treatment for addiction. Why or why not?
- What is the main principle behind the controlled drinking approach? Is it an effective treatment for alcohol addiction? Why or why not?
- It seems paradoxical to treat drug addiction with drugs. What three different approaches do pharmacological treatments use?

SUMMARY

The use of psychoactive substances has been part of our evolutionary history. From an evolutionary perspective, we can ask if taking psychoactive substances helps us protect ourselves, or mate, or engage in social activities. That is to say, how do these substances relate to fitness? Psychoactive substances use the same networks in the brain that are associated with a feeling of social well-being. In particular, the opioid system in the brain that is involved in the addiction to morphine and heroin is also involved in the satisfaction derived from social relationships, sexual stimulation, and eating tasty food. Many researchers make a distinction between drug use, drug abuse such as binge drinking, and addiction. In this chapter, the focus is on the addictive properties of the drug and the manner in which they are processed by our bodies, experienced in emotional and cognitive terms, and treated. Addiction is also described in terms of substance dependence. There are three major components to dependence: (1) the desire to seek and take a certain substance; (2) the inability to avoid or limit the intake of the substance; and (3) the experience of negative emotional states when the substance is not available. Substance abuse and addiction are burdens not only to the individual person but also to the family and society at large. There is no one answer as to what causes addiction, but related factors include (1) timing of first use; (2) genetic factors and their relationship with the environment; and (3) environmental factors such as stress and/or low socioeconomic level and their role in terms of epigenetics. There is a pattern seen in addiction: (1) intoxication—the initial positive experience of taking the drug leads to a compulsion to seek and take it; (2) bingeing—the individual loses control in the ability to limit intake of the drug; (3) withdrawal—emergence of a negative emotional state when the substance is unavailable or access to it is limited; and (4) what once gave a positive feeling now does little and the individual needs the drug to feel normal. There is a paradox in that by this last stage, people who are addicted want their psychoactive substance more than they enjoy it.

Drugs change the brain. This works in a manner similar to how all learning changes your brain, although drug addiction seems to last longer than simple learning. This sets up the possibility of relapse since the body has a difficult time forgetting the effects of the drug. Neuroscience studies show the rewarding effect of drugs is their ability to increase dopamine. More recent research has clarified dopamine's function is not so much associated with pleasure as with the expectation of pleasure. Thus, dopamine plays an important role in motivation, which includes activation, effort, and persistence. Drug addiction can be seen as one form of enhanced motivation. Not only can drugs change your brain; they can also take over the cognitive, emotional, and physiological mechanisms that we use for everyday life. They take over the brain mechanisms that are involved in reward. In addiction, compulsive drug use limits our level of human functioning. It is largely reduced to seeking means for obtaining the drug. This results in a decrease in social functioning as well as personal creativity and productivity. Additionally, brain changes in certain areas such as the frontal lobe lead us to deny we even have a problem and reduce our desire to make changes.

DSM–5 describes three substance-related disorders for each of the substances covered in this chapter: (1) substance use disorder, which is a pattern of use that leads to significant impairment or distress; (2) substance intoxication disorder, which develops during or shortly after substance ingestion; and (3) substance withdrawal disorder, which occurs following the cessation of, or reduction in, prolonged substance use.

In most humans, the experience of alcohol intake includes pleasant subjective experiences that may lead to increased social interactions. This is partly related to the effects of alcohol on such neurotransmitters as serotonin, endorphins, and dopamine. Alcohol will also decrease inhibition by reducing the effects of the GABA system, which is associated with anxiety. However, if the amount of alcohol intake is increased, it will increase the effects of GABA, which can lead to sedation, which is why alcohol is generally listed as a depressant. As an addictive substance, it can also lead to social, legal, and medical problems. An individual's alcohol intake is assessed at three levels: (1) moderate drinking of alcohol, especially wine, has been associated with better health outcomes; (2) heavy drinking, drinking more than the limits for moderate drinking, places individuals "at risk" for a number of health and other problems; and (3) binge drinking, which is defined as consuming enough alcohol in a 2-hour period to have a BAC of 0.08g/dL. Binge drinking is highest in college-age populations. Research suggests that heavy drinkers experience both a motivational system to want more alcohol and a hedonic reward system to experience it as pleasurable.

Individuals who use cannabis report a wide variety of experiences: (1) small doses produce enjoyable positive feelings; (2) larger doses can produce negative feelings such as anxiety and paranoia; and (3) long-term use is associated with cognitive impairment such as attention or memory. The main psychoactive ingredient in cannabis is THC. A persistent question about cannabis relates to its relationship to psychosis.

Hallucinogens are also called psychedelics and are able to alter perception, mood, and cognitive processes in often unpredictable ways. The subjective effects of taking hallucinogens can be divided into three major components: (1) "Oceanic Boundlessness," (2) "Anxious Ego Dissolution," and (3) "Visionary Restructuralization." Although illegal in the United States, hallucinogens do not produce dependence and are relatively safe. Drugs that are addictive typically affect the dopamine system and the experience of reward, whereas the chemical makeup of hallucinogens is similar to the neurotransmitter serotonin. They also do not show withdrawal symptoms. However, abuse is possible, and not all experiences with hallucinogens are positive. Current research is being directed at using hallucinogens in clinical treatment—experiments are under way to examine the use of (1) psilocybin in the treatment of OCD and (2) MDMA as an adjunct to psychotherapy.

Opioids are substances derived from the opium poppy that have been used for thousands of years to control pain and bring on euphoric feelings. Opioids are currently used in medical settings primarily for reduction of pain following operations or pain experienced with some types of cancer. There are receptors in the brain that are sensitive to opioid drugs; our bodies make a naturally occurring substance—endorphins—which also reduce the experience of pain and makes us feel good.

Cocaine comes from the naturally occurring coca plant. Its effects include (1) a mental alertness including feelings of euphoria, energy, and desire to talk; (2) a heightened experience of sensory processes such as sound, touch, and sight; (3) physiological effects such as increased heart rate and blood pressure; and (4) increased dopamine signaling in the brain. Brain changes are long lasting, even when the person ceases to use cocaine.

Amphetamines are stimulants produced in the laboratory that result in positive feelings, a burst of energy, and alertness. They have been used as a medicine and even prescribed to reduce addictions to other substances. Amphetamines affect the dopamine system to produce the initial euphoric experience but also less positive long-term brain changes: (1) development of compulsive patterns of use; (2) negative brain changes consistent with brain injury; and (3) changes in the individual's cognitive functioning.

Caffeine is usually described as a stimulant although there are beneficial effects beyond stimulation. Overall, caffeine consumption increases alertness, ability to concentrate, problem solving, wakefulness, the feeling of energy, and elevated mood. However, some individuals are more sensitive to caffeine than others and may experience stomach problems, trouble sleeping, anxiety, irritability, and nervousness from increased caffeine intake. In *DSM–5,* individuals who experience such symptoms along with clinically significant distress or impairment in important areas of functioning after ingesting a large dose of caffeine can be diagnosed with caffeine intoxication. There is also a caffeine withdrawal disorder. However, there is little evidence that a person can become addicted to caffeine. The addictive substance in tobacco is nicotine, which increases dopamine and thus functions similarly to other drugs of addiction. Similar to those for other drugs, the environmental cues associated with tobacco use play a critical role. Nicotine acts throughout the brain and influences attention, memory, emotion, and motivation. Nicotine can have varied effects on the body, which makes it function as both a stimulant and a depressant.

DSM–5 categorizes pathological gambling as an impulse control disorder. Like drug addiction, it continues despite negative consequences and because of an inability to control one's gambling behavior. The pattern of its development can be unpredictable. Individuals with pathological gambling show the highest comorbidity for other substance use disorders. Psychological studies suggest that pathological gambling is more than just an impulse control disorder but is another example of an addiction disorder. Researchers suggest that four cognitive–emotional processes play a role in pathological gambling: (1) behavioral conditioning, (2) the experience of cues that bring forth urges to gamble, (3) impulsivity, and (4) impaired executive functioning.

Treating addiction is a difficult process: (1) many do not want to seek treatment and (2) many have other comorbid mental disorders. There are several broad categories of treatment: (1) psychosocial approaches including CBT, motivational interviewing, and family or couple approaches; (2) community support and relapse prevention groups such as AA with its 12-step program; (3) controlled drinking approaches for alcohol; and (4) using psychopharmacological agents. Given the large number of approaches used, systematic evaluation of treatments has been limited. Steps in treating addiction include

(1) helping the individual remove the drug from his or her system and (2) some type of psychosocial treatment to help the person understand other factors related to the addiction and develop a plan for future action. In 2012, the National Institute on Drug Abuse suggested principles of effective treatment, including the following: (1) addiction is treatable but requires an individualized approach; (2) the treatment should consider other disorders or problems the person may have; (3) addiction is complex—those who use drugs may also engage in risky behavior; (4) pregnant females may impact the health of their fetus through drug use; and (5) both behavioral approaches and medications should be considered for treating the problems of addiction. Medications use at least three different approaches to treating addiction, which utilize the manner in which the drug of addiction works in the brain: (1) agonists, which bind to the receptor and produce cellular activity that lessens the effects of the illicit drug; (2) antagonists, which block the receptor site so that the illicit drug does not produce an effect; and (3) use of a drug that becomes aversive when the drug of abuse is taken.

STUDY RESOURCES

Review Questions

1. A number of the substances that have been covered in this chapter provide benefits as medicines—for example, opioids, cannabis, and amphetamines. On the other hand, it is clear that individuals can abuse or become addicted to these substances, which can lead to negative consequences. What principles would you use in developing a policy surrounding their use, including who could use them, what types of illnesses they could be used for, and who would regulate that use?
2. What are the similarities across substance-related and addictive disorders in terms of onset, diagnostic criteria, brain processes, and treatment?
3. Pathological gambling is the only addictive disorder considered in this chapter that is not substance-related. Are there other disorders that you think should be included as an addictive disorder?
4. What is it about substance-related and addictive disorders that make them so difficult to treat? If you were asked to put together an awareness program about these disorders targeting a college-age audience, what information would you include, and what approach would you take?

For Further Reading

Denizet-Lewis, B. (2009). *America anonymous: Eight addicts in search of a life.* New York: Simon & Schuster.

Levy, M. (2007). *Take control of your drinking . . . and you may not need to quit.* Baltimore: Johns Hopkins University Press.

Key Terms and Concepts

addiction
agonist drug
alcohol
amphetamines
antagonist drug
aversive drug
binge drinking
caffeine
cannabis
cocaine
craving
dependence
disordered use
hallucinogens
intoxication
nicotine
opioids
pathological gambling
substance tolerance
tobacco
12-step program
withdrawal

CHAPTER

15

Personality Disorders

CHAPTER OUTLINE

- INTRODUCING PERSONALITY DISORDERS 536
- PERSONALITY AND PERSONALITY DISORDERS 543
- SOCIOCULTURAL DIMENSIONS OF DELIBERATE SELF-HARM: A STUDY FROM MUMBAI 547
- ODD-ECCENTRIC PERSONALITY DISORDERS 547
- DRAMATIC EMOTIONAL PERSONALITY DISORDERS 551
- ANXIOUS FEARFUL PERSONALITY DISORDERS 568
- TREATMENT OF PERSONALITY DISORDERS 570
- *DSM* FUTURE CONSIDERATIONS OF PERSONALITY DISORDERS 574
- SUMMARY 574
- STUDY RESOURCES 576

You learn some psychological principles and concepts without even knowing you have learned them. We meet people early in life, we get some insight into their personality in our growing years and then, sometime much later, we get a chance to "fit" these observations and learnings into the neat framework of psychology and behavioral science.

Ever since I can remember, I have believed that people are basically good. They are doing what is correct and good, by their own lights. Their behavior is consistent. If you try to see things from their perspective, to put oneself into their shoes, you can completely understand why they do what they do.

If someone is mentally ill, they temporarily lose touch with reality. Their bonds with the world around them are loose and shaky. But once their receive medication and psychotherapy, they can think once again for themselves, pretty much as well as they could before they fell ill, and relationships are restored.

But as long as there is no mental illness, the psychological "graph" of each individual unfolds smoothly before us, and we "understand" or "decode" the person. I too learned quickly to decode the people I met in life.

Later, when I began to study psychology, I read that there was this great psychologist called Carl Rogers who too believed that people are by and large good.

If you observe them carefully, you can comprehend why they behave the way they do. If you try to see their behavior through their own eyes, from their own perspective, their reasoning may even appeal to you.

I feel the same way even today, even about "Difficult" People. But even back then, when I was young and had not yet studied psychology, I did realize that for certain people, this process of "decoding" and "understanding" is harder. It is far more difficult to get into their mindset to understand why they behave the way they do. It takes far more effort and you keep thinking you are falling short. There are points when you are almost "there" and then you lose them!

These are the people that "make you angry," "make you anxious" and "upset you." But actually, they are really "doing" nothing! They are just behaving the way they always do, much in the same consistent fashion as other people behave.

Just like other people, they too have firm opinions; they too have their own set of thoughts, beliefs, emotions, likes and dislikes. But then, why is it that they seem to draw this kind of negative reaction from us?

If we stick to our original premise and if people are really basically good, then why is it that we grow much angrier at these specific few? Why do they seem to "draw out" this reaction from us?

Then I realized that it is really very hard to think "like them." Well, it also hard to "think like" people who are extraordinarily brilliant, but that is because we are far less bright, and our mind cannot grasp concepts with as much speed and depth as their minds can. But with these "difficult people" the reason why we cannot easily comprehend their thinking is because of a strange twist in their personality. A kind of tangled web of logic that stumps us. They are rigid, inflexible. Their pattern of thinking is maladaptive, pervasive and enduring, which means that it tends to affect every aspect of their behavior and stays that way regardless of the circumstances.

These are people with Personality Disorders.

Are they mentally ill? Not at all. They are perfectly sane, like you and me. Not a trace of psychosis or any symptoms of mental illness. But is their behavior like other people? Not at all! It is strange, eccentric. In one word, "difficult."

It is difficult to get them to change their mind, difficult to convince them of anything new. Also difficult to understand their point of view about anything regarding which they are a hundred percent convinced; in short, they are difficult to live with.

But we cannot avoid them. They are everywhere. In the family, at our workplace, in our friends' group. By their own lights, their behavior is perfect, absolutely beyond reproach. They are "doing the right thing" in their interactions with others. But all this by their own standards, not ours!

How can we identify these people? They don't sprout horns! They look like you and me, ordinary, everyday people. They talk like us, work like us, travel-eat-sleep and converse just like us, but in the same rigid, set manner. Never is there a trace of flexibility, never any willingness to adapt.

Unfortunately, we figure out these aspects of their nature too late. Then there is no escape, one has to grin and bear it!

Picture this: you have gone for a factory inspection. The whole premises are sterile. You are given a disposable overall to cover your clothes, a cap, socks, shoes, gloves, to cover your hair, hands and feet. But only after you begin walking, you discover you have metal shoes on! Tight, binding, heavy shoes that weigh you down and make every step a punishment. And you have to wear them all day now; there is no escape. All day through, you will have to drag your feet in these terrible shoes that weigh a ton. Your feet ache, but you are not allowed to remove your shoes. How helpless you will feel, how frustrated and hopeless!

Or else, imagine we are all sitting around chatting, and eating some nuts. We laugh and relax, and pop a nut into our mouth now and then. This one nut looks just like the others ... one picks it up and pops it in, and whoa! This one is as hard as stone! The ache in your tooth seems to shoot up to your brain, brings tears to your eyes! Spitting out the nut brings no relief.

That is how it is for us when we are stuck with a difficult person, someone with a Personality Disorder. We make futile attempts to understand them, to be understood. But to no avail. We get caught into the web of their personality; get more and more enmeshed as we struggle to cut loose.

But it is not their fault! They are not being deliberately difficult! They don't even know they are behaving strangely, or that others are having such a hard time adjusting to the circumstances.

As I kept meeting more and more such Difficult People, I grew more curious about them. I met them not only in the course of my work, but in my day-to-day life as well! I encountered many such "puzzles," solved some quickly; others took time. I felt like sharing this journey through the landscape of Personality Disorders with others, my readers. I hoped this would help them solve their own "puzzles," deal with people with Personality Disorders around them, and this book took shape. It may perhaps prove to be a useful book for young psychologists in the making, as well! A well-informed guide through the maze of PDs!

Although the people are "difficult," the book is easy! See if you like it.

Source: Dr. Anuradha Sovani Preface of the book *Difficult People* (translated Avghad Maanse from Marathi). Unmesh Prakashan.

INTRODUCING PERSONALITY DISORDERS

As you read the Preface above, you probably had a number of reactions. You might have thought of others you know who react in similar ways. You might have thought about how you would react and what upsets you. You might have wondered why some people seem to be so dramatic in everything they do. Some people will tell you that they cut themselves or burn themselves when they experience psychological pain. Steven Westwood tells you that all he thinks about is suicide. However, he also tells you that he can have a relationship with a girlfriend. People who have these types of relationships with themselves and others are described in terms of personality disorders.

What Is a Personality Disorder?

The basic definition of a **personality disorder** is that it represents an enduring pattern of inner experience and behavior that deviates markedly from the expectations of the individual's culture (American Psychiatric Association [APA], 2013, p. 645). Further, the pattern is inflexible, stable, and generally begins in adolescence, and leads to distress or impairment. The characteristics of these disorders are especially apparent when these individuals find themselves in situations that are beyond their ability to cope. The fifth edition of the *Diagnostic and Statistical Manual of Mental Disorders (DSM–5)* (APA, 2013) identifies 10 personality disorders that form separate categories. These 10 disorders can be organized into three clusters.

The first cluster is referred to as *Cluster A* and includes *odd or eccentric disorders.* These include **schizoid personality disorder, paranoid personality disorder,** and **schizotypal personality disorder.** Individuals with these disorders typically feel uncomfortable or suspicious of others or restrict their relationships. Schizoid personality disorder is characterized by a pervasive pattern of detachment from social relationships and a restricted range of emotional expression. Paranoid personality disorder is characterized by a pervasive distrust and suspiciousness of others. Schizotypal personality disorder is characterized by odd beliefs and behaviors.

The second cluster is referred to as *Cluster B* and includes *dramatic, emotional, or erratic disorders.* These include **antisocial personality disorder, borderline personality disorder (BPD), histrionic personality disorder,** and **narcissistic personality disorder.** Individuals with these disorders show a wide diversity of patterns of social and emotional interactions with others. Antisocial personality disorder is characterized by a disregard for the other person. BPD is characterized by instability in relationships. Histrionic personality disorder is characterized by excessive emotional responding and the seeking of attention. Narcissistic personality disorder is characterized by grandiosity in terms of one's abilities and a lack of **empathy.**

The third cluster is referred to as *Cluster C* and includes *anxious or fearful disorders.* These include **avoidant personality disorder, dependent personality disorder,** and **obsessive-compulsive personality disorder.** Avoidant personality disorder is characterized by a pattern of social inhibition, feelings of inadequacy, and hypersensitivity to negative evaluation. Dependent personality disorder is characterized by an excessive need to be taken care of including clinging behavior. Obsessive-compulsive personality disorder is characterized by a preoccupation with orderliness, perfectionism, and interpersonal control.

In a number of community samples, personality disorders are found in 9% to 13% of the population (see Lawton, Shields, & Oltmanns, 2011; Lenzenweger, 2008, for overviews). This suggests that 1 in 10 people suffers from a personality disorder. Overall, similar numbers of males and females are seen in each personality disorder. The only exception is antisocial personality disorder, which is seen more frequently in men. In terms of the three clusters, Cluster A shows a prevalence of 5.7%, Cluster B shows a prevalence of 1.5%, and Cluster C shows a prevalence of 6% in a community sample (Lenzenweger, Lane, Loranger, & Kessler, 2007) although prevalence rates vary by a few percent in different studies. Estimates from World Health Organization (WHO) surveys of 13 countries suggest a worldwide prevalence of around 6.1% for any personality disorder and 3.6% for Cluster A, 1.5% for Cluster B, and 2.7% for Cluster C (Huang et al., 2009).

Comorbidity of Personality Disorders

A number of studies have shown that those with a personality disorder also meet criteria for other disorders—especially anxiety, mood, and substance use disorders (see Lenzenweger et al., 2007, for an overview). Lenzenweger and his colleagues used data from the National Comorbidity Survey Replication, which is a nationally representative, face-to-face household survey of 9,282 adults (ages 18 and older) in the continental United States. What these researchers did was to compute the percentage of individuals with a personality disorder who also met criteria for an anxiety disorder, mood disorder, impulse-control disorder, or substance use disorder. In *Table 15-1,* this is referred to as "column." These researchers also looked at the opposite relationship. That is, they looked at individuals who met criteria for an anxiety disorder, mood disorder, impulse control disorder, and substance use disorder to see if they also met criteria for a personality disorder. In *Table 15-1,* this is referred to as "row." What this shows for example is that a greater percentage of individuals with a personality disorder also have an anxiety disorder than individuals with an anxiety disorder are likely to have a personality disorder.

TABLE 15-1 Individuals With a Personality Disorder Who Also Meet Criteria for an Anxiety, Mood, Impulse Control, or Substance Disorder

			Cluster B									
	Cluster A		Antisocial		Borderline		Any cluster B		Cluster C		Any PD	
	Row[a]	Column[a]	Row[a]	Column[a]	Row[a]	Column[a]	Row[a]	Column[a]	Row[a]	Column[a]	Row[a]	Column[a]
	%(SE)	%(SE)	%(SE)	%(SE)	%(SE)	%(SE)	%(SE)	%(SE)	%(SE)	%(SE)	%(SE)	%(SE)
Anxiety												
GAD	11.6 (4.3)	8.1 (1.6)	2.7 (1.0)	20.2 (8.5)	6.9 (2.5)	20.3 (5.5)	7.9 (1.9)	22.0 (4.6)	17.3 (4.0)	11.9 (2.3)	34.0 (3.8)	15.2 (1.8)
Specific phobia	11.0 (3.6)	14.1 (2.8)	1.0 (.5)	12.5 (6.7)	5.7 (1.7)	30.3 (6.7)	5.3 (1.3)	26.7 (6.2)	16.9 (3.6)	21.1 (3.6)	28.8 (3.7)	23.4 (2.7)
Social phobia	12.1 (3.9)	11.4 (2.6)	2.0 (1.0)	19.5 (8.2)	7.3 (2.2)	28.4 (6.4)	7.2 (2.2)	26.4 (6.8)	25.2 (5.6)	22.8 (3.9)	44.5 (5.3)	26.3 (2.4)
Panic disorder	15.7 (6.4)	5.5 (1.5)	4.4 (1.8)	15.9 (6.8)	11.6 (4.1)	16.8 (4.7)	10.4 (3.1)	14.4 (4.3)	21.3 (5.2)	7.3 (1.7)	44.9 (5.7)	10.0 (1.4)
Adult separation anxiety disorder	12.8 (5.1)	4.3 (1.3)	3.9 (2.2)	13.0 (6.8)	8.9 (3.4)	12.4 (4.0)	12.4 (4.4)	15.9 (4.2)	16.7 (4.7)	5.4 (1.4)	42.5 (9.5)	8.9 (2.0)
PTSD	12.8 (5.0)	7.9 (1.8)	2.9 (1.2)	19.1 (8.3)	6.6 (2.2)	17.0 (4.5)	8.0 (2.3)	19.6 (5.5)	16.5 (3.9)	10.0 (2.1)	35.7 (4.6)	14.1 (2.1)
Any anxiety	10.7 (3.0)	31.0 (3.8)	1.6 (.5)	47.5 (10.4)	5.0 (1.2)	60.5 (7.8)	5.5 (1.2)	61.4 (6.5)	14.9 (3.2)	41.4 (5.0)	28.8 (3.0)	52.4 (3.8)
Mood												
Major depressive disorder	12.5 (4.1)	7.2 (1.7)	1.5 (.8)	9.1 (5.7)	6.7 (2.2)	16.1 (4.1)	5.8 (1.8)	13.1 (3.6)	16.4 (4.1)	9.1 (1.9)	36.9 (5.4)	13.4 (1.9)
Dysthymia	13.2 (5.1)	5.3 (1.5)	4.4 (1.8)	18.4 (8.3)	11.3 (3.3)	19.0 (4.9)	13.1 (3.3)	20.8 (5.1)	20.8 (4.8)	8.1 (1.8)	42.7 (5.4)	10.8 (1.6)
Bipolar I or II	13.4 (5.0)	3.4 (1.0)	5.8 (2.7)	15.1 (6.6)	14.8 (5.1)	15.5 (4.5)	14.8 (4.4)	14.5 (3.6)	22.0 (6.9)	5.3 (1.4)	50.7 (7.5)	8.1 (1.3)
Any mood	12.4 (3.7)	12.4 (2.2)	2.7 (.9)	27.7 (10.5)	8.2 (2.1)	34.3 (6.2)	8.4 (1.9)	33.0 (5.7)	17.4 (3.9)	16.8 (2.7)	38.1 (4.7)	24.1 (2.8)
Impulse-control												
Intermittent explosive disorder	13.4 (4.5)	10.1 (2.7)	4.5 (1.7)	34.2 (9.4)	12.3 (4.3)	38.0 (10.3)	12.0 (3.1)	35.0 (6.2)	13.0 (3.6)	9.4 (2.3)	33.8 (5.8)	15.9 (2.4)
Attention deficit disorder	11.2 (5.4)	5.2 (1.8)	5.6 (2.3)	22.4 (8.3)	12.5 (4.2)	21.5 (5.4)	13.6 (4.0)	21.5 (4.7)	15.7 (4.9)	7.0 (2.1)	41.5 (6.3)	11.0 (1.7)
Any impulse	12.7 (4.2)	13.5 (3.1)	3.8 (1.3)	41.4 (10.5)	11.2 (3.6)	49.0 (11.1)	11.0 (2.7)	45.1 (6.3)	13.4 (3.3)	13.7 (2.8)	34.8 (5.0)	23.2 (2.8)
Substance												
Alcohol abuse or dependence	10.4 (3.7)	5.8 (2.2)	4.5 (2.6)	23.9 (11.6)	12.0 (3.7)	27.0 (6.8)	12.8 (3.8)	26.7 (5.6)	10.4 (3.5)	5.4 (1.8)	32.1 (5.7)	10.9 (2.1)
Drug abuse or dependence	9.0 (5.3)	2.3 (1.3)	5.5 (3.0)	13.6 (6.8)	10.8 (3.4)	11.1 (3.9)	13.7 (5.2)	12.9 (3.9)	11.5 (5.3)	2.7 (1.4)	36.7 (9.9)	5.6 (1.4)
Tobacco dependence	8.9 (4.1)	6.2 (2.1)	2.9 (1.2)	21.0 (8.5)	4.6 (1.4)	13.7 (4.4)	5.6 (1.6)	15.5 (3.9)	9.9 (2.6)	6.8 (1.6)	26.4 (5.1)	11.8 (2.2)
Any substance	9.4 (3.1)	11.9 (2.8)	3.2 (1.3)	40.5 (11.5)	7.2 (1.9)	38.2 (6.9)	8.2 (2.1)	39.9 (5.4)	10.2 (2.6)	12.4 (2.8)	28.5 (4.8)	22.6 (3.4)

Source: Lenzenweger et al. (2007, p. 559).

TABLE 15-2 Correlations Between the Nine Personality Disorders

	NCS-RIPDE Clinical Data: Tetrachoric Correlation Estimates										
	Cluster A				*Cluster B*			*Cluster C*			
	PAR	*S'OID*	*STYP*	*ANY A*	*ANT*	*BOR*	*ANY B*	*AVO*	*DEP*	*OCD*	*ANY C*
Cluster A											
PAR											
S'OID	.77[a]										
S'TYP	.48	.96[a]									
ANY A	—	—	—								
Cluster B											
ANT	.73[a]	−.84[a]	.13	.56[a]	—						
BOR	.76[a]	.56[a]	.34	.58[a]	.64[a]						
ANY B	.83[a]	.46	.27	.65[a]	—	—	—				
Cluster C											
AVO	.70[a]	.55[a]	.53[a]	.60[a]	.05	.54[a]	.44				
DEP	.20[a]	−.84[a]	−.86[a]	.03	−.83[a]	.82[a]	.77[a]	.70[a]			
OCD	.59[a]	.40	49	.49[a]	.45	.67[a]	.59[a]	.63[a]	.80[a]		
ANY C	.67[a]	.49[a]	.46[a]	.55[a]	.24	.55[a]	.45	—	—	—	
Total											
PD NOS	.55	−.89[a]	−.10	.37	.90[a]	.55	.82[a]	−.27	−.79[a]	.64[a]	.43

NCS—R, National Comorbidity Survey Replication; PAR, paranoid; S'OID, schizoid; S'TYP, schizotypal; ANY A, any cluster A PD; ANT, antisocial; BOR, borderline; Any B, any cluster B PD; AVO, avoidant; DEP, dependent; OCD, obsessive-compulsive disorder; ANY C, any cluster C PD.
[a]Significant at the .05 level, two-sided test.

Source: Lenzenweger et al. (2007, p. 557).
Note: PD NOS refers to personality disorder not otherwise specified.

Not only do individuals with a personality disorder meet criteria for another non-personality disorder; they also met criteria for other personality disorders (Lenzenweger et al., 2007). Overall, the highest co-occurrence of personality disorders is seen within each of the clusters. That is, if a person has one Cluster A disorder he or she is more likely to have another Cluster A disorder than a Cluster C disorder. The relationships between different personality disorders are shown in *Table 15-2*. In the next section and throughout the chapter, I will discuss some of the implications of this comorbidity.

Personality Disorders and Normal Personality Traits

As you have just seen, the 10 separate personality disorders show considerable overlap with other mental disorders. These 10 separate personality disorders also show considerable overlap with traits found in normal personality patterns (see Costa & Widiger, 2002; Samuel & Widiger, 2008; South, Oltmanns, & Krueger, 2011, for overviews). In one study, measures of normal personality functioning and pathological personality functioning showed a shared dimensional structure (Samuel, Simms, Clark, Livesley, & Widiger, 2010). That is to say, personality characteristics reflected in personality disorders can be seen as an extreme version of normal personality characteristics.

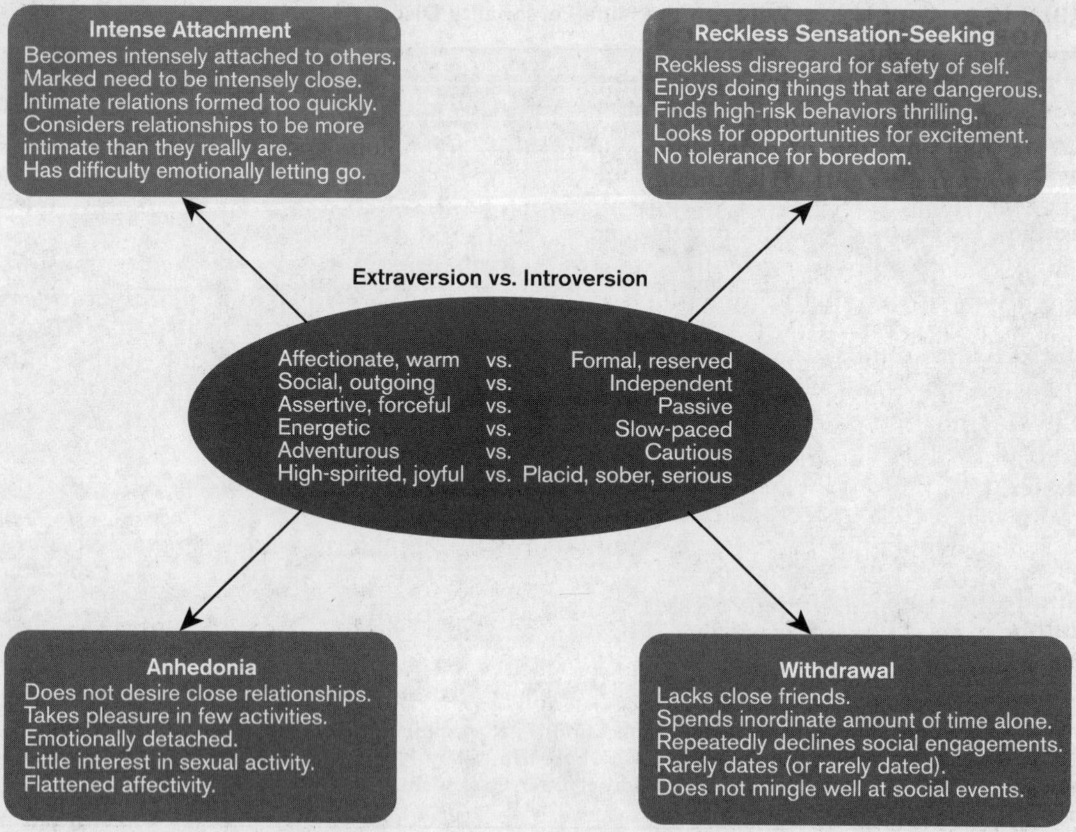

FIGURE 15-1 The Five-Factor Model Diagnosis of Maladaptive Extraversion Versus Introversion

Source: Widiger and Mullins-Sweatt (2009, p. 211).

Thus, there can be both healthy and maladaptive personality styles. An individual can be extraverted in a healthy manner by seeking relationships with others and developing warm and meaningful relationships. He can also enjoy large parties and feel fulfilled by meeting new people. This could also occur in a maladaptive manner in which the individual has a need to always be with others and to value himself only when in a relationship. An individual can also be introverted in a healthy way by valuing his inner experiences such as writing poetry or enjoying walks alone or with another friend. One could also be introverted in a maladaptive manner by avoiding or distrusting others and living a life without meaningful contact with others and one's self. *Figure 15-1* shows some of the maladaptive factors of introversion and **extraversion.**

The Characteristics of a Healthy Self

In order to understand personality disorders, one needs to consider what a healthy personality would look life. That is, what is a **healthy self?** One conceptualization suggested in *DSM–5* (APA, 2013) is to consider the healthy self in terms of a "Self and

Interpersonal Functioning Continuum." The first aspect of this continuum is **identity.** In terms of identity, the healthy person would see herself as a unique person with stable boundaries between herself and others. The self would have a history that the person understands. The person would also have an accurate sense of who she is and what she can accomplish. She also appreciates her abilities.

Another aspect of the self is **self-direction.** Healthy self-direction reflects the ability to have both meaningful short-term and long-term goals consistent with one's identity. Self-direction also includes a sense of what would be productive for society and how to interact with others. Internally, healthy self-direction also includes the ability to reflect on one's life in a productive manner.

The healthy personality also suggests the ability to have **positive interpersonal relationships.** One aspect of this is empathy. This includes understanding how another person experiences his life and what that person might want to accomplish. It also includes the ability to experience and accept different perspectives toward life and goals and how one's own behavior may influence others. In healthy relationships, **intimacy** is also critical. Intimacy includes having a relationship with another person that includes mutual connectedness and a valuing of that other person. The healthy personality values closeness and seeks it when appropriate.

Thus, a person can develop a stable self that has an identity and has the ability for self-direction and the fulfillment of goals. This person can also have positive interpersonal relationships in which the person relates to others in an intimate and empathetic manner. This person we would describe as healthy.

Not having a stable self and the ability to have intimate and empathetic relationships with others is a significant part of a personality disorder (Kernberg, 1984). One consideration for a future version of *DSM* is to place personality disorders on a continuum in terms of the person's disturbance of self and others as just described (Bender, Morey, & Skodol, 2011). That is, you could rate on 5-point scales the person's level of identity, self-direction, empathy, and intimacy. This would more clearly reflect those areas in which there are fundamental personality disturbances.

Another way to consider these relationships is from an evolutionary perspective by viewing personality disorders as a failure to solve adaptive life tasks relating to identity or self, intimacy and attachment, and prosocial behavior (see Livesley, 2007, for an overview). From this perspective, it has been the evolutionary task of a human to perform on three levels. The first level is the individual level and the development of a self. The second level is the interpersonal level, which reflects attachment processes. And the third is the group level and involves prosocial behavior, altruism, and the cooperation needed for the functioning of society.

Normal Personality Traits

In the early part of the 20th century, most psychologists who discussed personality used a theoretical perspective that emphasized the descriptive nature of specific traits. Outgoing individuals were described in terms of extraversion, for example. Those who frequently took risks in activities such as skydiving were referred to as sensation seekers. The problem was that there were far too many personality terms to describe a person's behavior and experiences. This made it difficult to create a coherent theory of personality. Using mathematical techniques that compared the similarity of responses between the different measure offered an alternative approach to that of a descriptive approach.

Such a psychometric approach was directed by Robert McCrae and Paul Costa (1987; see also McCrae, Gaines, & Wellington, 2013, for an overview). They used a factor analytic approach to personality, which suggested five major personality dimensions. This is referred to as the **five-factor model (FFM).** These five dimensions include extraversion, **neuroticism, openness, agreeableness,** and **conscientiousness.** Extraversion is associated with sociability, cheerfulness, energy, and a sense of fun. This dimension ranges from being passive, quiet, and inner-directed to being active, talkative, and outer-directed. Neuroticism is associated with a tendency to express distressing emotions and difficulty experiencing stressful situations. This dimension ranges from being calm, even-tempered, and comfortable to being worried, temperamental, and self-conscious. Openness as a personality trait is associated with curiosity, flexibility, and an artistic sensitivity, including imaginativeness and the ability to create a fantasy world. This dimension ranges from inventive and curious to cautious and conservative. Agreeableness is associated with being sympathetic, trusting, cooperative, modest, and straightforward. This dimension ranges from being friendly and compassionate to being competitive and outspoken. Conscientiousness as a personality trait is associated with being diligent, disciplined, well-organized, punctual, and dependable. This dimension ranges from being efficient and organized to easygoing and careless. These five dimensions are shown in *Table 15-3.*

Solid research on the FFM has also demonstrated that there is a consistency of results across a variety of cultures (McCrae, 2009). However, there are changes across the life span. In one study, McCrae and colleagues (1999) gave personality measures to individuals in five countries. They found that there were some changes in the levels of the five factors over the life span. These differences were found in all of the cultures studied (McCrae et al., 1999). Overall, life span data suggest that from age 18 to 30, individuals show declines in neuroticism, extraversion, and openness to experiences and increases in agreeableness and conscientiousness. McCrae and Costa (1996, 1999) suggested that the five factors of

TABLE 15-3 Five-Factor Model

Factor	*Low Scocers*	*High Scorers*
Extraversion (positive emotionality)	Passive Quiet Inward directed	Active Talkative Outwardly directed
Neuroticism (negative emotionality)	Calm Even-tempered Comfortable	Worried Temperamental Self-conscious
Openness	Not curious Less flexibility Down-to-earth	Curiosity Flexibility Imaginativeness
Agreeableness	Suspicious Aggressive Antagonistic	Trusting Sympathetic Cooperative
Conscientiousness	Less dependable Undisciplined Disorganized	Dependable Disciplined Well-organized

Source: From Thomas A. Widiger and Stephanie N. Mullins-Sweatt. "Five-Factor Model of Personality Disorder: A Proposal for DSM-V." *Annual Review of Clinical Psychology* Vol. 5: 197–220, 2009.

TABLE 15-4 Summary of Hypothesized Fitness Benefits and Costs of Increasing Levels of Each of the Five-Factor Personality Dimensions

Domain	*Benefits*	*Costs*
Extraversion	Mating success; social allies; exploration of environment	Physical risks; family stability
Neuroticism	Vigilance to dangers; striving and competitiveness	Stress and depression, with interpersonal and health consequences
Openness	Creativity, with effect on attractiveness	Unusual beliefs; psychosis
Conscientiousness	Attention to long-term fitness benefits; life expectancy and desirable social qualities	Missing of immediate fitness gains; obsessionality; rigidity
Agreeableness	Attention to mental states of others; harmonious interpersonal relationships; valued coalitional partner	Subject to social cheating; failure to maximize selfish advantage

Source: Nettle (2006, p. 628).

personality be considered as biologically based tendencies, as opposed to culturally conditioned characteristic adaptations. Genetic research has supported this perspective.

Evolution and Different Personality Characteristics

Nettle (2006) examined the FFM in relation to an evolutionary perspective. He suggested that each of the dimensions has a particular advantage given certain environmental conditions. Extraversion, for example, is associated with success in mating, having social allies, and exploration of the environment. Neuroticism, on the other hand, is associated with greater vigilance and labeling situations as dangerous. In times of little stress, extraversion would be a successful strategy. However, in dangerous times, it may not afford the necessary caution that would be found with neuroticism. Nettle's summary of the costs and benefits of each of the five-factor dimensions is presented in *Table 15-4.*

PERSONALITY AND PERSONALITY DISORDERS

As *DSM–5* was being developed, a large number of studies were addressing the question of how the personality dimensions of the FFM could be related to the personality disorder categories of *DSM* (see Widiger & Mullins-Sweatt, 2009, for an overview). The simple answer is that the three clusters representing 10 types of personality disorders can be understood as maladaptive variants of the FFM. Using data from clinicians and researchers, *Table 15-5* shows the relationship between different facets of each of the five factors and the 10 personality disorders described in the *DSM.* An *H* in the table means that this personality trait would be high for that particular personality disorder. An *L* would mean low occurrence. For example, individuals with antisocial personality disorder show high scores in the facets of extraversion and low scores in the facets of agreeableness and conscientiousness.

TABLE 15-5 ***DSM*** **Personality Disorder From the Perspective of the Five-Factor Model**

	PRN	*SZD*	*SZT*	*ATS*	*BDL*	*HST*	*NCS*	*AVD*	*DPD*	*OCP*
Neuroticism (vs. emotional stability)										
Anxiousness (vs. unconcerned)			H	L	H			H	H	H
Angry hostility (vs. dispassionate)	H			H	H		H			
Depressiveness (vs. optimistic)					H					
Self-consciousness (vs. shameless)			H	L	H	L	L	H	H	
Impulsivity (vs. restrained)				H	H	H				L
Vulnerability (vs. fearless)				L	H			H	H	
Extraversion (vs. introversion)										
Warmth (vs. coldness)	L	L	L				L		H	
Gregariousness (vs. withdrawal)	L	L	L	H		H		L		
Assertiveness (vs. submissiveness)				H			H	L	L	
Activity (vs. passivity)		L		H		H				
Excitement seeking (vs. dullness)		L		H		H	H	L		L
Positive emotionality (vs. anhedonia)		L	L			H				
Openness (vs. closedness)										
Fantasy (vs. concrete)						H				
Aesthetics (vs. disinterest)										
Feelings (vs. alexithymia)		L			H	H	L			L
Actions (vs. routine)	L	L		H	H	H	H	L		L
Ideas (vs. closed-minded)			H							L
Values (vs. dogmatic)	L									L
Agreeableness (vs. antagonism)										
Trust (vs. mistrust)	L		L	L	L	H	L		H	
Straightforwardness (vs. deception)	L			L			L			
Altruism (vs. exploitation)				L			L			
Compliance (vs. opposition, aggression)	L			L	L		L		H	
Modesty (vs. arrogance)				L			L	H	H	
Tender-mindedness (vs. tough-minded)	L			L			L			
Conscientiousness (vs. disinhibition)										
Competence (vs. ineptitude)									L	H
Order (vs. disordered)			L							H
Dutifulness (vs. irresponsibility)				L						H
Achievement striving (vs. lackadaisical)										H
Self-discipline (vs. negligence)				L		L				H
Deliberation (vs. rashness)				L	L	L				H

PRN, paranoid; SZD, schizoid; SZT, schizotypal; ATS, antisocial; BDL, borderline; HST, histrionic; NCS, narcissistic; AVD, avoidant; DPD, dependent; OCP, obsessive-compulsive; H, high; L, low.

Source: Costa and Widiger (2002).

One characteristic of personality disorders is the stable occurrence of the personality structure. This would lead one to expect only minor changes in the expression of these disorders over the life span. A number of studies have followed individuals with personality disorders over the life span. Overall, these studies have shown aspects of the disorders to remain stable until one's 20s or 30s and then to decrease over the life span. One exception to this is the schizoid personality disorder. *Figure 15-2* displays changes in diagnostic criteria for different age-groups (Gutiérrez et al., 2012).

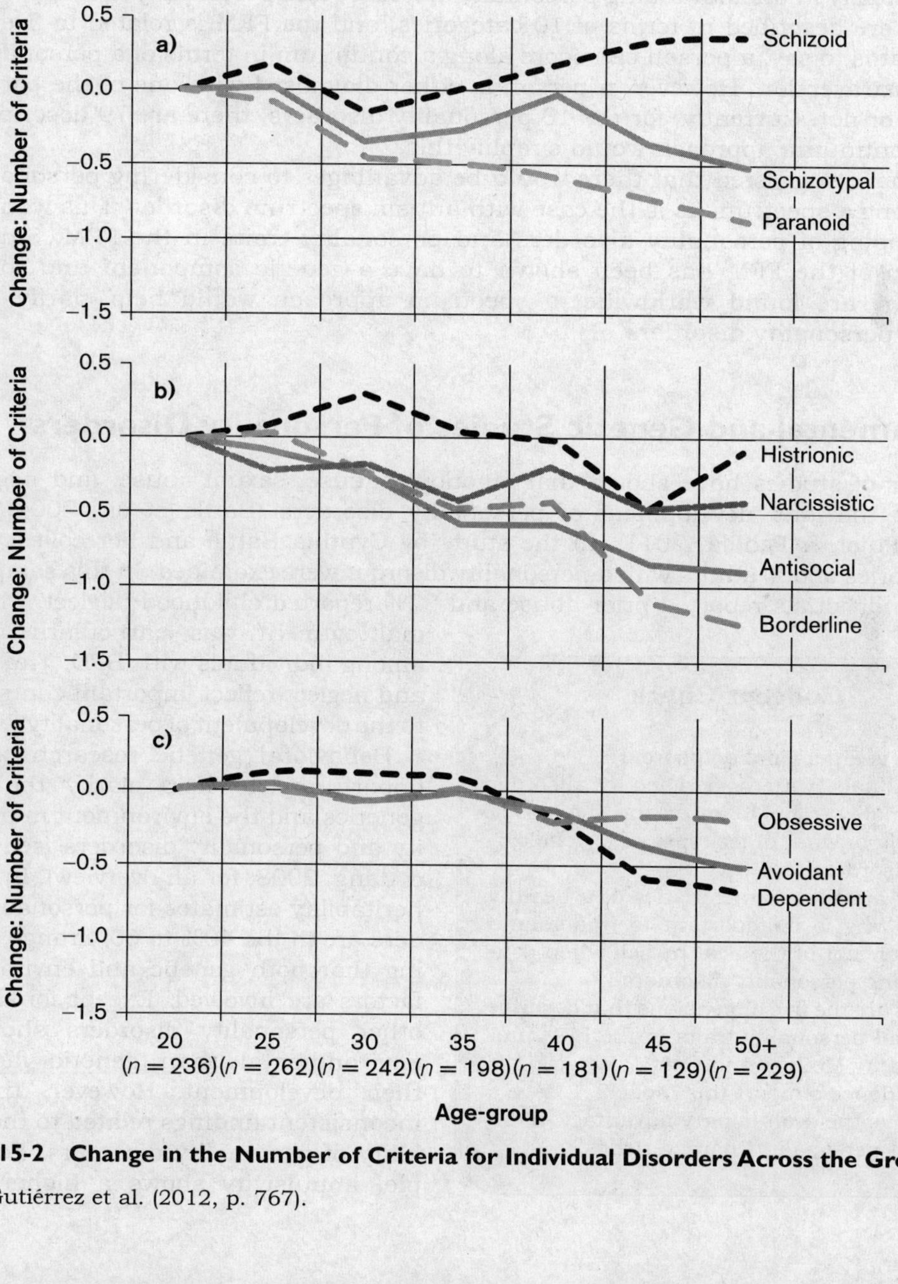

FIGURE 15-2 Change in the Number of Criteria for Individual Disorders Across the Groups

Source: Gutiérrez et al. (2012, p. 767).

"The field of personality disorders is at a nascent stage of development in India."

"An interesting observation in clinical epidemiology of personality disorders in India is the relatively narrow gap in prevalence between the genders, with respect to emotionally unstable personality disorders" Sharan (2010).

Categories and Dimensions

One complexity in understanding personality disorders and personality is that personality disorders are described in terms of 10 categories, and the FFM is related to five dimensions. That is to say, a person can score along a continuum in terms of a personality trait such as extraversion. However, a person is either diagnosed with one of the personality disorders or not. Currently, for the 10 personality disorders, there are 79 descriptive criteria. A continuum approach would simplify this.

Some have suggested that there would be advantages to considering personality disorders along a spectrum as is the case with autism spectrum disorder. This would allow for a mapping of personality disorders and personality traits in the FFM. Since each dimension of the FFM has been shown to have a genetic component and these five dimensions are found worldwide, a spectrum approach would help clarify another aspect of personality disorders.

Environmental and Genetic Studies of Personality Disorders

A number of studies have shown that emotional abuse, sexual abuse, and neglect are related to the later development of personality disorders (Battle et al., 2004; Pereda, Gallardo-Pujol, & Padilla, 2011). In the study by Cynthia Battle and her colleagues, the prior histories of 600 adults with a personality disorder were examined. In this sample, 73% of these individuals reported prior abuse and 82% reported childhood neglect. Childhood maltreatment was particularly common among individuals with BPD. Thus, abuse and neglect reflect important contributions to the development of personality disorders.

Behavioral genetic research offers an opportunity to help clarify the role of genetics and the environment in personality and personality disorders (see Livesley & Jang, 2008, for an overview). In general, heritability estimates for personality disorders are in the 40% to 60% range suggesting that both genetic and environmental factors are involved. Except for BPD, the other personality disorders show more environmental than genetic factors in their development. However, there are inconsistent findings related to the heritability of personality disorders. For example, impulsivity shows a higher genetic

Concept Check

- What is a personality disorder?
- Individuals with a personality disorder are more prone to meet the diagnostic criteria of what other types of psychological disorders?
- What are the characteristics of a healthy self? Why is it important to understand the concept of the healthy self when considering personality disorders?
- What are the five dimensions that describe normal personality traits in the FFM proposed by McCrae and Costa? What kinds of evidence support this model?
- What is the evolutionary advantage of different personality characteristics?

component than does BPD itself. At this point, future research is needed to clarify the role of genetic contributions to the development of a personality disorder.

SOCIOCULTURAL DIMENSIONS OF DELIBERATE SELF-HARM: A STUDY FROM MUMBAI

Dr. Shubhangi Parkar et al. from KEM Hospital, Mumbai, have reported an interesting study which "demonstrated the value of complementary psychiatric and cultural epidemiological assessments of suicidal behavior." SCID diagnostic interviews and a locally adapted EMIC interview were used to evaluate 196 patients admitted after DSH into a large tertiary care teaching hospital psychiatry department in Mumbai, India. The commonest diagnosis (38.8%) was major depression, followed by substance use disorders (16.8%). However, 44.4% of the patients did not meet criteria for an Axis I disorder and were labelled "no diagnosis," "V codes," or "adjustment disorders." They could perhaps have shown PD traits but this is not listed in the paper. The interesting term "psychache" is used, arising from patient identified sociocultural contexts (Parkar, Davani, & Weiss, 2006).

ODD-ECCENTRIC PERSONALITY DISORDERS

The three personality disorders included in the **odd-eccentric personality disorders (Cluster A)** grouping are paranoid personality disorder, schizoid personality disorder, and schizotypal personality disorder. The behavior of individuals with these disorders may seem similar to individuals with schizophrenia except that they show a greater grasp of reality. These disorders are sometimes seen in first-degree relatives of those with schizophrenia. Each of the three odd-eccentric personality disorders shows a prevalence rate of about 1%. However, these rates may be 10 times higher in relatives of those with schizophrenia.

Paranoid Personality Disorder

Paranoid personality disorder is characterized by a pervasive distrust and suspiciousness of others (see Bernstein & Useda, 2007, for an overview). If you were to meet an individual with this disorder, he would tell you how others are trying to exploit or deceive him. This may make him unwilling to confide in others. He may also focus much of his internal thought on the possible breaks in loyalty of his friends or spouses. Even if he were able to tell you about his concerns of loyalty or harm, you might find it difficult to understand how he reached the conclusions he did. He could be correct in all the details that he recounts concerning an interaction and in fact may be a better observer of the encounter than many people would be. However, you would have difficulty understanding how one could go from seeing a real event such as a smile or frown to the conclusion that a boss was about to fire him.

The interpersonal style of these individuals is often quarrelsome, stubborn, and rigid in their own beliefs. This can create a self-fulfilling prophecy in that if an individual acts cold to another, the other person will misinterpret his intentions. This leads to the other person breaking off the interaction. Although the individual with paranoid personality may interpret noise from a neighbor as an attempt to get back at him, he would not suggest that the neighbor was working for the CIA and gather information on him as might a person with schizophrenia. Prevalence rates vary from 4.4% in the National Epidemiologic Survey on Alcohol and Related Conditions (Grant et al., 2004) to 2.3% in the National Comorbidity Survey Replication (Lenzenweger et al., 2007).

The diagnostic criteria in *DSM–5* for paranoid personality disorder describe a person who is distrustful and suspicious of others such that the motives of others are seen as malevolent. This personality style should begin in early adulthood. Four specific characteristics should also be present. These characteristics include (1) believing that others are exploiting or deceiving the person, (2) having a preoccupation with unjustified doubts about the trustworthiness of a friend or colleague, (3) being reluctant to confide in others, (4) seeing simple statements as having hidden meanings, (5) bearing grudges, (6) seeing others as attacking the person's reputation, and (7) not trusting one's sexual partner as being faithful.

Schizoid Personality Disorder

Schizoid personality disorder is characterized by a pervasive pattern of detachment from social relationships and a restricted range of emotional expression (see Mittal, Kalus, Bernstein, & Siever, 2007; Triebwasser, Chemerinski, Roussos, & Siever, 2012, for overviews). These individuals are traditional loners. Others see them as unavailable, aloof, or detached. *DSM* has traditionally described these individuals as not desiring close relationships, lacking friends, and seeking solitary activities. Schizoid personality is one of the least studied disorders with very little empirical research. Prevalence rates vary from 3.1% in the National Epidemiologic Survey on Alcohol and Related Conditions (Grant et al., 2004) to 4.9% in the National Comorbidity Survey Replication (Lenzenweger et al., 2007).

The diagnostic criteria in *DSM–5* for schizoid personality disorder describe a person who shows a pattern of detachment in social relationships and a limited expression of emotions in social relationships. This personality style should begin in early adulthood. Four specific characteristics should also be present. These characteristics include (1) not desiring or enjoying social relationships, (2) mainly engaging in solitary activities, (3) showing little interest in sexual activities with others, (4) finding little pleasure in any activity, (5) having no close friends, (6) showing indifference to both praise and criticism, and (7) showing emotional coldness or detachment.

Schizotypal Personality Disorder

Schizotypal personality disorder is characterized by odd beliefs and behaviors (see Bollini & Walker, 2007, for an overview). An individual with schizotypal personality disorder may show excessive social anxiety as well as unusual ideas. This can include *magical thinking* such as the person believing that thinking about an event can actually make it happen. Historically, it was noted that first-degree relatives of those with schizophrenia had odd behavioral propensities. Early behavioral genetic studies also noted that oddities in social behavior, perception, and ideation were found in relatives of those with schizophrenia (see Gottesman, 1991, for a review).

Schizotypal personality disorder was first included in *DSM–III* in 1980. Currently, it is defined by odd behavior, cognitive distortions, and inappropriate affect. Although these behaviors, thoughts, and affects are similar to those seen in individuals with schizophrenia, the person with this disorder is not out of touch with reality. Unlike those with schizophrenia, although their speech may be odd or vague, you would still be able to understand it. Prevalence rates were found to be 3.3% in the National Comorbidity Survey Replication (Lenzenweger et al., 2007).

CASE OF DEPENDENT PERSONALITY DISORDER

Schizotypal Personality Disorder

Mr. Inamdar is a very capable, intelligent, and honest officer, on an excellent senior position in an international bank. He married, and was very pleased with his pretty, polite and very obedient wife. Mrs. Inamdar never, ever took any decision without consulting her husband. Whether it was purchasing any large item for the house, or giving her housemaid a day off, Mr. Inamdar had to be asked for his advice.

At first, Mr. Inamdar loved it. Other men's wives are so overconfident and brash. They are always giving their husband an earful. He loved it that all decisions taken in his home were taken by him. Later, their children were born. Mrs. Inamdar chose to be a homemaker. She always said in her sweet, soft manner that if she stayed at home and looked after the house, the children and the in-laws, her husband would be free to rise high in his profession, and to take up more and more responsibility at work. Citing this reason, she never worked, although she was a graduate.

Mr. Inamdar was often transferred to other offices in India. That used to present a problem, because he always had to do everything, right from looking for a new home, moving furniture and household stuff, appointing new servants, finding new schools for the children—everything.

"You do it all so well," Mrs. Inamdar would say. "I can't do this. I have never done it." Sometimes her husband was annoyed. "At least do some of these chores," he would say, but to no avail. He always had to do everything.

Once, on a Saturday afternoon, he called his colleagues home to lunch on an impulse. He called her up before coming. "Set up something quickly okay, dear?" he requested. "Four of my colleagues will drive home with me for lunch." Unfortunately, he never told her what to make, and hung up. He came with his friends and found to his horror, that not a morsel of food had been prepared. "What can I do?" his wife said. All the vegetable vendors go away by afternoon. And our maid had also left by then. So who will make rotis?" Mr. Inamdar was livid with rage by then, but he kept tight rein on his patience and said in a cajoling tone, "You should have made something else, pulav, pao-bhaji, whatever..."

"Oh, would that do? I did not know that! And anyway I could not think." She even refused to place a food delivery order at a restaurant, saying she did not know what to order, and finally Mr. Inamdar had to do that himself, and save the day. He was angry with his wife, but what was the use? He had no hopes of changing her.

The hardest hit of all came just last month. Mr. Inamdar was posted to Singapore. His children were delighted, and told everyone in school about it ... bragged about how they would now get chocolates and clothes from abroad! They were a little sad that their dad would be far away from the family, but Mr. Inamdar reassured them that he would come to India often, for work or even otherwise, just to see them. That was when Mrs. Inamdar dropped the bombshell on their dreams, "I can't do it."

(Continued)

(Continued)

What? Everybody was shocked, amazed. "It is a matter of a few years," Mr. Inamdar pleaded. "No, I cannot bear the thought of living away from you. Out of the question, dear. I can't look after this house alone." Everyone tried to coax her. Her parents, her in-laws, all offered to come and stay whenever she needed them. "We will even come and stay there till your husband comes back," they offered. Even the children said, "Mother, our grandparents are already offering to come stay with us. But even we will manage on our own, the three of us. It is not so very difficult."

But it was impossible to change Mrs. Inamdar's mind. She flatly refused. She also refused to go to Singapore with her husband and leave the children here with their grandparents. If Mr. Inamdar pressed her to agree, she would sit and cry helplessly, and that made everyone feel sorry for her. Finally, Mr. Inamdar gave up trying to convince her. He also gave up this wonderful job opportunity and things went back to normal in the Inamdar family. Mrs. Inamdar was unruffled. She had no remorse about her husband's missed opportunity. After all, she was helpless. What could she do? "Some ladies can handle all this. I can't," was her simple straightforward stance! And life went on.

Who does one blame for these circumstances? Did Mrs. Inamdar scotch her husband's career prospects on purpose? Of course not..." I would have loved for him to get this opportunity" she would say. "But what could I do? I was helpless. I can't cope." That was her only defense. She really regretted this lost opportunity, even cried about it. But did not change her mind!

That is why we say, some personalities are cast in stone!

Source: Translated from *Difficult People* by Dr. Sovani.

The diagnostic criteria in *DSM–5* for schizotypal personality disorder describe a person who shows a pattern of discomfort in social relationships and a limited expression of emotions in social relationships. This personality style should begin in early adulthood. Five specific characteristics should also be present. These characteristics include that the person (1) makes connections between ideas that are not related to one another, (2) holds odd beliefs or engages in magical thinking such as a belief in telepathy, (3) experiences unusual perceptual experience, (4) engages in odd thinking and speech, (5) is suspicious, (6) shows inappropriate affect, (7) appears odd to others, (8) does not have close friends, and (9) shows excessive social anxiety that does not become less as the situation becomes more familiar.

Brain imaging studies show a similarity between those with schizotypal personality disorder and schizophrenia (see Asami et al., 2013, for an overview). Both show a reduction of gray matter in the brain.

Concept Check

- What are the primary defining characteristics of paranoid personality disorder? How do they create a self-fulfilling prophecy in maintaining the disorder?
- Schizoid personality is one of the least studied disorders with very little empirical research. What is it about the characteristics of this disorder that contributes to this?
- How are the behaviors, thoughts, and affects in an individual with schizotypal personality disorder similar to an individual with schizophrenia? How are they different?

However, those with schizotypal personality disorder do not show more loss of grey matter volume with age as do those with schizophrenia. It can be noted that gray matter loss is seen in those areas that involve the default network, which is associated with internal tasks.

DRAMATIC EMOTIONAL PERSONALITY DISORDERS

There are four personality disorders included in the **dramatic emotional personality disorders (Cluster B)** grouping. These personality disorders include antisocial, borderline, histrionic, and narcissistic. The behavior of individuals with these disorders can be dramatic and impulsive. However, as you will see, there are also real differences between these four disorders.

Antisocial Personality Disorder and Psychopathy

Although the media interchange the words *antisocial personality disorder* and ***psychopathy,*** there are differences in the formal definitions of the terms. The *DSM–5* criteria for antisocial personality disorder emphasize the breaking of society's rules including laws. A majority of individuals in prisons would qualify for this disorder. The *DSM–5* criteria tend to focus on observable behaviors. As you will see, historically, psychopathy has been seen as an internal personality problem. It was initially referred to as "moral insanity." It has been estimated that only about 10% to 25% of individuals with an antisocial personality disorder would be classified as having psychopathy. Further, not all individuals who would be described as having psychopathy would show conduct disorders early in their life or have found themselves in trouble with the law. Psychopathy is not a formal definition of *DSM–5* but has been studied in both clinical and research settings for a number of years.

Antisocial Personality Disorder

The *DSM–5* criteria for antisocial personality disorder begin with the individual being at least 18 years of age. The person would also meet the requirements for a child conduct disorder before the age of 15. As described in the chapter on developmental disorders, child conduct disorder includes aggression toward animals or people, destruction of property, deception or stealing, and serious rule violations. The criteria for antisocial personality disorder include acts since the age of 15 such as repeated participation in illegal acts, deceitfulness, impulsiveness, hostility and aggression, engagement in dangerous acts, irresponsible behavior, and absence of remorse.

Using *DSM* criteria, the prevalence rate for antisocial personality disorder is around 3% with more males than females having the disorder. There is a high comorbidity of around 80% with substance use disorders (see Patrick, 2007, for an overview). However, the opposite is not the case. The prevalence of antisocial personality disorder also tends to be higher in correctional and forensic settings where base rates have been recorded between 50% and 80% (Hare, 2003). Often those who are mandated by the courts for treatment of sexual offences would qualify for an antisocial personality disorder.

CASE OF ANTISOCIAL PERSONALITY DISORDER

Mr. Chandrakant Vyavaharkar. He has been a charmer since childhood. Mischievous, active, with winning ways that drew people to him. A little sly too, to be very honest. His confidence in his abilities grew as one success followed another—as he succeeded in pulling wool over more and more people's eyes. As a schoolboy, he used to take other children's homework books without asking them, grab their snack boxes from their lockers, steal their pocket money. Once he went to college, he began his activity on a larger scale; he stole examination papers before the exam date on a bet, and sold them to other students. He would steal music systems from the parked vehicles of his teachers and sell those ... his mischief knew no limits. People know him by many different names, Chandu, Chandya, Chand, Chandrakant, Chandar, CV, ... many aliases!

Today, he belongs to a gang of like-minded youngsters. They all agree that "everyone behaves this way. There is nothing wrong with such behavior." They all have faith in Chandu. They are sure he will "handle it" if they are ever in trouble. What will he really do? Well, save his own skin, for sure!

Is there any aspect of life where his attitude does not permeate? None at all. His financial dealings, his friends' circle, his sexual relations, family bonds, one can see the traces of his callous indifference everywhere. He cannot get along with "boring" people who are "too straight." He feels contempt for them. He says they have "no guts."

There is really no point taking him to a psychologist. In his opinion, he has no problem. He firmly believes that problems will not occur and if they do, they can be easily handled.

He knows what he is like, but he does not think there is anything wrong with that. In fact, he often wonders why others do not behave the way he does! So, as we were saying, these are personalities "cast in stone," not willing to change themselves but ever ready to change others or pressurize them to change. They find it hard to comprehend another person's point of view. But they feel very strongly that others should understand them, in fact, they expect it! If that does not happen, they feel very angry and cheated. Whatever the situation, these "difficult people" remain immutable. Their basic personality traits permeate into their every action. For instance, Chandrakant, who we just described, can lie ever so easily. But if perchance he is nabbed by the police, and even if they threaten him and warn him to speak the truth, even then, he may just lie out of habit. He finds it hard to distinguish between truth and lies....that is how his mind works. There is always this schism between "the truth" and the "truth according to him."

These people behave much the same way even with people they love. No one can figure them out completely. It is almost as if, by default, they trot out a new story, a new "avatar," for every new person they meet. They enjoy it, and in the process, are perhaps even themselves unsure of what they "truly" are and how they truly feel. Hiding their real self becomes a challenge to them, and they delight in it.

Chandrakant, for one, never has any remorse. He never regrets what he has done, an according to him he has not erred! He is not particularly concerned about other people's emotions, nor does he dwell too long on his own feelings. His emotional life appears to be a little superficial. But when there is any advantage to be gleaned from putting these emotions on display, Chandrakant is a past master. He will go to any extreme to ensure that the other person feels sympathetic towards him. He will not even hesitate in making the other person feel guilty, so that Chandrakant can get his own way. Because he has always been such a "user," he has no close friends although his circle of acquaintances is large. Everyone is a "friend" because he or she may prove useful.

Source: Translated from *Difficult People* by Dr. Sovani.

The diagnostic criteria in *DSM–5* for antisocial personality disorder describe a person who shows a pattern of disregard for the rights of others. A person with this disorder must be 18 years old, and the personality style should have been present since 15 years of age. Before age 15, the person should meet criteria for a conduct disorder. Three specific characteristics should also currently be present. These characteristics include (1) a failure to observe social norms which can result in legal arrest, (2) a deceitfulness including lying to and using others, (3) a failure to plan ahead, (4) an irritability and aggressiveness that leads to physical fights, (5) a reckless disregard for the safety of others, (6) an irresponsibility such as a failure to pay debts or perform duties at work, and (7) a lack of remorse when another person is hurt.

Psychopathy

Individuals who display signs of psychopathy show emotional detachment with a lack of empathy for the experiences of others (see Patrick, 2010, for an overview). They also show impulsive behavior and a callousness concerning their actions. These patterns are stable and difficult to change. Although individuals with this disorder take a real toll on society, there is also a fascination by many with these individuals. They are portrayed in such movies as the *The Shining* and *The Silence of the Lambs,* although you don't need to be violent to be diagnosed as a psychopath. These are the classic "con men" who are able to manipulate others and get what they want. Often the victims find the con man charming and may not even know they are being taken.

Historically, in the early 1800s both Philippe Pinel in France and Benjamin Rush in America described individuals who experienced no shame or guilt in relation to their actions. In 1835, the British physician J. C. Pritchard used the term *moral insanity.* The basic idea was that these individuals had a deficit in moral reasoning, which led them to disregard the normal sense of decency, fairness, and responsibility. In 1891, the German psychiatrist J. L. Koch introduced the term *psychopathic,* which was followed by Emil Kraepelin in 1904 using the term *psychopathic personality* in his textbook of psychiatry. In 1909, the German psychiatrist Karl Birnbaum offered the term *sociopathic* to suggest that the condition resulted from environmental factors. However, the terms *psychopathic* and *sociopathic* have been used interchangeably over the years.

In the 1940s, the American psychiatrist Hervey Cleckley (1941/1988) published a major work on psychopaths, *The Mask of Sanity.* This was based on his work with a large number of patients at the VA hospital in Augusta, Georgia. One of his insights as implied by the title of his book was that beneath the appearance of being well adjusted and socially appealing, there exists severe pathology. Cleckley described these individuals in terms of 16 diagnostic criteria, which can be categorized in terms of three conceptual categories. The categories are positive adjustment, chronic behavioral deviance, and emotional-interpersonal deficits and are presented in *Table 15-6* on the next page.

Based on the descriptive characteristics of Cleckley, Robert Hare and his colleagues developed a checklist that serves as an assessment tool (Hare, 2003; Hare & Neumann, 2008). The checklist includes such items as glibness and superficial charm, grandiose sense of self-worth, pathological lying, lack of remorse, shallow affect, lack of empathy, need for stimulation, lack of long-term goals, poor behavioral control, and impulsivity. These can be divided into four facets, as shown in *Table 15-7.*

Psychopathy has often been described in terms of a deficit in emotional processing. Christopher Patrick and Edward Bernat (2009) have suggested two factors better explain

TABLE 15-6 Cleckley's 16 Diagnostic Criteria for Psychopathy

Item Category	No.	Description
Positive adjustment	1.	Superficial charm and good "intelligence"
	2.	Absence of delusions and other signs of irrational thinking
	3.	Absence of "nervousness" or psychoneurotic manifestations
	14.	Suicide rarely carried out
Behavioral deviance	7.	Inadequately motivated antisocial behavior
	8.	Poor judgment and failure to learn by experience
	4.	Unreliability
	13.	Fantastic and uninviting behavior with drink and sometimes without
	15.	Sex life impersonal, trivial, and poorly integrated
	16.	Failure to follow any life plan
Emotional-interpersonal deficits	5.	Untruthfulness and insincerity
	6.	Lack of remorse or shame
	10.	General poverty in major affective reactions
	9.	Pathologic egocentricity and incapacity for love
	11.	Specific loss of insight
	12.	Unresponsiveness in general interpersonal relations

Source: Patrick (2006); Skeem, Polaschek, Patrick, and Lilienfeld (2011).

TABLE 15-7 Psychopathy Checklist–Revised

Factor 1: Interpersonal-Affective Scale		*Factor 2: Antisocial Scale*	
Facet 1 Interpersonal	*Facet 2 Affective*	*Facet 3 Lifestyle*	*Facet 4 Antisocial*
Glibness/superficial charm Grandiose sense of self-worth Pathological lying Conning/manipulative	Lack of remorse or guilt Shallow affect Callousness/lack of empathy Failure to accept responsibility for own actions	Need for stimulation/proneness to boredom Parasitic lifestyle Lack of realistic long-term goals Impulsivity Irresponsibility	Poor behavioral controls Early behavioral problems Juvenile delinquency Revocation of conditional release Criminal versatility

Source: Hare (2003); Skeem et al. (2011).
Note: Two PCL-R items are not included in this factor structure: namely Promiscuous sexual behavior, Many short-term marital relationships.

psychopathy. These factors were determined from factor analytic studies. The first factor is fearlessness. This reflects an under-reactivity of the brain's defensive motivational system. The second factor is externalizing vulnerability. The second factor reflects impairments in the frontocortical system of the brain. This is the system involved in anticipation, planfulness, and affective/behavioral control. This model suggests there are two separate processes in the same individual. The first involves the lack of fear, and the second involves a weakness in impulse control. Further it should be noted that the *DSM* descriptions of antisocial personality disorder do not include such characteristics as superficial charm, which were included in a previous description of psychopathy. Thus, research may show inconsistencies depending on the measures used.

Evolutionary perspectives suggest that there is an advantage in certain environmental conditions for an individual who is cunning, manipulative, and not considerate of the well-being of others. Such an individual would create resources for himself and in certain situations do well in business and politics. He or she would also be able function well under conditions that would be extremely stressful for others. Such characteristics may be protective in terms of stress and anxiety disorders.

The Brain Involvement in Psychopathy

Unlike many other psychological disorders in which the brain volume of specific brain structures is shown to be smaller, the research with psychopathy shows the amygdala to be larger in psychopaths (Boccardi et al., 2011). Research also found larger white matter volumes in the parietal, occipital, and left cerebellar lobes. However, it has been found that gray matter reductions have been observed in the frontopolar, orbitofrontal, and anterior temporal cortices, superior temporal sulcus region, and insula (Oliveira-Souza et al., 2008). Other studies have also found reduced gray matter volume in relation to psychopathy, which may contribute to problems in decision making, emotional regulation, and moral judgments.

Reviews of current studies suggest two major brain areas are involved in both structural and functional approaches to the study of psychopathy (see Anderson & Kiehl, 2011, for an overview). The first area involves the frontal lobes, and the second involves temporal regions including the hippocampus and the amygdala. It may not be that the structures are not functioning but rather that they are being used for processing tasks for different purposes. One study showed pictures of people in pain (e.g., slamming a door on your finger) to those with psychopathy and control individuals (Decety, Skelly, & Kiehl, 2013). Participants in the psychopathy group exhibited significantly less activation in the ventromedial prefrontal cortex (vmPFC), lateral orbitofrontal cortex (OFC), and periaqueductal gray relative to controls.

There is some suggestion that psychopathy can be considered as a result of neurodevelopmental abnormalities (see Gao, Glenn, Schug, Yang, & Raine, 2009, for an overview). Specifically, psychopathic behaviors can be associated with the lack of frontal lobe development at a critical time. This might allow for the development of intellectual abilities but limit the development of social and moral development.

One intriguing study examined two adults who had prefrontal lesions before the age of a year and a half (Anderson, Bechara, Damasio, Tranel, & Damasio, 1999). The first person was run over by a vehicle at 15 months of age. She

Concept Check

- What are the differences between antisocial personality and psychopathy? How are they related?
- What is the organizing model Cleckley introduced to help us understand the diagnostic criteria for psychopathy? How did Hare and colleagues change the model in developing an assessment tool?
- Psychopathy has often been described in terms of a deficit in emotional processing. What are the factors in the competing model that Patrick and colleagues developed?
- What evidence exists to support the idea that psychopathy is the result of neurodevelopmental abnormalities?

recovered fully within days with no apparent abnormalities. However, at the age of 3, she was unresponsive to verbal or physical punishment. She became more disruptive and by the age of 14 was placed in a treatment facility. She was seen by her teachers to be intelligent, but she showed little moral development. She stole from others, lied to others, and was abusive. The second individual had a frontal lobe tumor at age 3 months. His recovery appeared to be normal, and he met normal developmental landmarks. By age 9, however, he showed a general lack of motivation. Although he graduated from high school, he would threaten others, lie often, and steal. He showed no guilt or remorse for his behavior. These case studies suggest that early dysfunction in the prefrontal cortex (PFC) is related to abnormal development of social and moral behavior.

Borderline Personality Disorder

BPD is characterized by an instability in mood, interpersonal relationships, and a sense of self (see Bradley, Conklin, & Westen, 2007, for an overview). These three factors interact with each other in such a manner that the person with BPD experiences a changing world without a solid sense of self. At one point, the person may feel rejected and abandoned due to a misinterpretation of an event and lash out in anger. At other times, she may see another person as perfect and form an intense relationship only to have that go to its opposite without warning. The movie *Fatal Attraction* shows this type of intense relationship seen in people with BPD. Arlene Roberson, at the beginning of this chapter, described her experiences as the following: "I go from feeling panicked and angry to feeling depressed and hurt to feeling anxious."

She also reported, "I have to react to this pain by lashing out at everything and everyone around me." This lashing out includes not only angry outbursts at others but also self-mutilating behaviors and suicide attempts. It is estimated that 75% of those with BPD engage in self-injurious behavior. Two common behaviors are to cut or burn themselves. Some say that the external pain from burning or cutting gives them an experience that they are alive compared with feeling that they do not exist. For those with BPD, feelings of emptiness and boredom are common as well as feelings of being special or having exceptional talents. *Table 15-8* shows some of the common functions of self-injurious behavior as reported by female inpatients.

Self-harm is closely related to attempts to regulate one's emotions. One review of the literature suggests three aspects of this relationship (Klonsky, 2007). The first aspect is that acute negative affect precedes self-injury. The second aspect is that after self-injury, individuals report relief. The third aspect is that individuals engage in self-injury as a means to reduce their experience of negative affect. Although many studies involve self-report, similar findings were seen in research studies performed in the lab.

TABLE 15-8 Functions of Self-Injurious Behavior

Feel pain	60%
Punish self	50%
Control feelings	40%
Exert control	22%
Express anger	22%
Feel	20%

Source: Shearer, Peters, Quaytman, and Wadman (1988).

Although self-harm is different from suicide, successful suicide is estimated to be about 9% in clinical samples. Also suicide threats or gestures are estimated to occur in 90% of clinical samples with BPD (Gunderson & Ridolfi, 2001).

Their view of self and others is sometimes described in terms of "splitting" or having things be all good or all bad without the nuance most individuals experience in their relationships. Thus, people with BPD have a sense of self that is fluid and can change quickly.

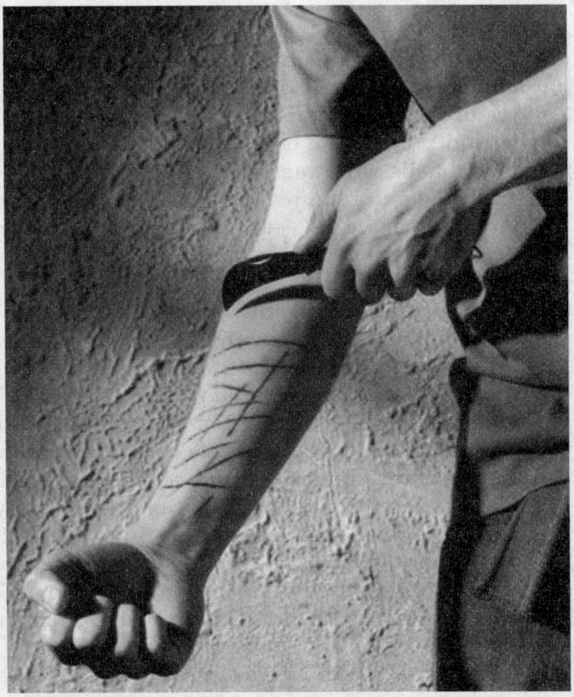

People With Borderline Personality Disorder May Cut Themselves or Do Other Acts of Self-Harm

Source: Raskin (2010, p. 46).

The conceptualization of BPD has been greatly influenced by the work of Kernberg (1984, 1995), who viewed these individuals as using immature ways of dealing with impulses and emotions. Historically, the term *borderline,* as the name implies, denoted individuals who were neither neurotic nor psychotic. Although not out of touch with reality, when under stress, these individuals can become disorganized in their view of self and others. On the other hand, their experiences go beyond those seen in anxiety or depression where the tendency is to withdraw when experiencing psychological distress.

One term that has been used to describe individuals with BPD is "fearful preoccupation" (Levy, 2005). This reflects an intense need for attention and closeness on the one hand and a deep fear of rejection and abandonment on the other. Thus, these individuals want to be close but become fearful and then angry when they experience closeness. Anger is also seen whenever individuals perceive they are being rejected. These characteristics can be seen in the case of Amy James (not her real name), which follows:

CASE OF AMY JAMES
Borderline Personality Disorder

Amy James is in her mid-20s. Amy has a history of multiple violent suicide attempts dating back to early adolescence. She reported that over time her suicide attempts have become more serious and aggressive. She describes her suicide attempts as more of a tantrum than a desire to die. She first entered therapy as a child for what she describes as an "unhappy childhood" and for being a "weird kid." However, it was not until she was 22 years old that she was first diagnosed with BPD.

She is the only child in a family that was chaotic and enmeshed, partly because of a major traumatic accident that occurred before her birth. She had a brother who was killed due to injuries sustained when a car hit him. Amy's mother developed a chronic illness and depended on her for emotional and physical caretaking. Her father, a research scientist, was an alcoholic who was alternatively cruel, seductive, and pathetic. The parents frequently separated and reunited during Amy's childhood, and both eroticized their relationship with her by engaging in a number of overt and covert sexualized interactions. In addition, she recollects various bizarre and traumatic incidents from her childhood, including witnessing her father drowning her pets.

Amy James is currently married and has no children. Amy describes being very unsatisfied in her relationship with her husband, whom she perceives as inept, unhelpful, or overly intrusive and irrelevant but whom she had frequent fantasies of being saved by. She has numerous affairs and would frequently torture her husband by telling him the details of the relationships. She states that she "did my best to ruin my marriage." One night, she even made a pass at her husband's brother, whom she dated before her husband.

Amy is very intelligent and college-educated but not working in her chosen field. At the time she entered therapy, she was underemployed working as a clerk. She did not enjoy her work, feeling that it is uninteresting. She calls in sick frequently and sometimes fails to show up for work due to overdoses. She describes the overdoses as a way of getting out of working while attempting to garner sympathy from her coworkers. However, because of these difficulties she is frequently fired from these jobs, despite the fact that they are relatively low-stress and low-level jobs.

Her prior psychotherapies all have a similar pattern. First, she would find the therapist helpful and begin to depend more on him or her. Then her dependency would put pressure on the therapist to be increasingly available. Nevertheless, there would always come a moment when she felt let down by the therapist and engaged in a nonsuicidal self-injurious behavior, some of which was very serious. During the current therapy, she also showed suicidal attempts—some resulting in hospitalization. After a year of treatment, she became more committed to her marriage and obtained a job consistent with her college degree. At the 3-year follow-up, she reported career success and giving birth to a child.

Clinical vignette provided by Kenneth Levy, PhD
Source: Adapted from Levy, Yeomans, and Diamond (2007).

Although genetic factors may play a role in terms of the trait of impulsivity, environmental factors play an important role. Around 70% of these individuals report some type of physical, emotional, or sexual abuse. Overall, there is evidence to suggest that the development of BPD is related to heightened risk from chaotic family life, increased stress experienced by the parents, and disruptive communications between the caregiver and the child.

The disorder is also related to attachment (see Levy, 2005, for an overview). In general, individuals with BPD show an insecure pattern of attachment. Only some 6% to 8% show secure attachment patterns. Studies that used dimensional measures of BPD show an inverse relationship between secure attachment and BPD. Further, studies that have looked at early loss or separation in children found that it occurred in 37% to 64% of individuals with BPD.

The diagnostic criteria in *DSM–5* for BPD describe a person who shows a pattern of instability and impulsivity in social relationships and his or her self-image. This personality style should begin in early adulthood. Five specific characteristics should also be present. These characteristics include (1) a frantic effort to avoid abandonment, whether real or imagined; (2) a pattern of unstable and intense interpersonal relationships characterized by alternating idealization and devaluation; (3) an unstable self-image and sense of self; (4) impulsivity in areas that can be damaging such as sexual relations, substance abuse, reckless driving, and binge eating; (5) recurrent suicidal behaviors or self-mutilating behaviors; (6) emotional instability lasting only a few hours; (7) chronic feelings of emptiness; (8) inappropriate anger and ability to control anger; and (9) short-term stress-related dissociative experiences or paranoid ideation. The current *DSM–5* criteria for BPD can be met in a variety of ways. Given the nine criteria, there are at least 150 different ways that a person can receive the diagnosis based on various combinations of the criteria. This suggests that the instability of the self and its functioning can be manifested in a number of ways.

One way the instability manifests for society is that individuals with BPD are high consumers of emergency room services, crisis lines, and referrals from health professionals to mental health services (see Bradley et al., 2007). It is estimated that individuals with BPD represent 20% of inpatients and 10% of outpatients in mental health clinics. Prevalence rates in community samples are around 1.6% as found in the National Comorbidity Survey Replication (Lenzenweger et al., 2007).

Comparing individuals with major depressive disorder (MDD) and BPD over a 10-year period, it was found that 85% of the individuals with BPD showed a reduction in their symptoms (Gunderson et al., 2011). However, they also found persistent impairment in social relationships. This study and Grilo et al. (2004) found that those with MDD showed a reduction in symptoms faster than those with personality disorders.

Brain Studies of Those With Borderline Personality Disorder

Studies looking at both structural and functional aspects of the brain have shown differences in those with BPD. Structurally, individuals with BPD have less volume in a number of brain areas (see Soloff et al., 2012). The regions with reductions include the insula, the middle and superior temporal cortex (Mid-Sup T), the fusiform gyrus (FG), the anterior cingulate cortex (ACC), the hippocampus and the parahippocampus, and the amygdala (Amyg) (see *Figure 15-3*).

In terms of functional processes, Uasbek Dziobek and his colleagues (2011) examined empathy using brain imaging tasks. These researchers divided empathy into two categories: cognitive empathy and emotional empathy. Cognitive empathy required participants to assess the mental states of individuals shown in pictures. Emotional empathy required participants to rate their concern for the person shown in the picture. Thus, a picture of a little girl standing in front of a destroyed house could be rated in terms of both how the little girl would feel as well as how much you would be concerned about her.

In terms of emotional empathy, individuals with BPD showed different responding from controls in the right insula (see *Figure 15-4*). The functional magnetic resonance imaging (fMRI) bold signal was larger in those with BPD suggesting greater arousal when performing empathy tasks (see *Figure 15-5*).

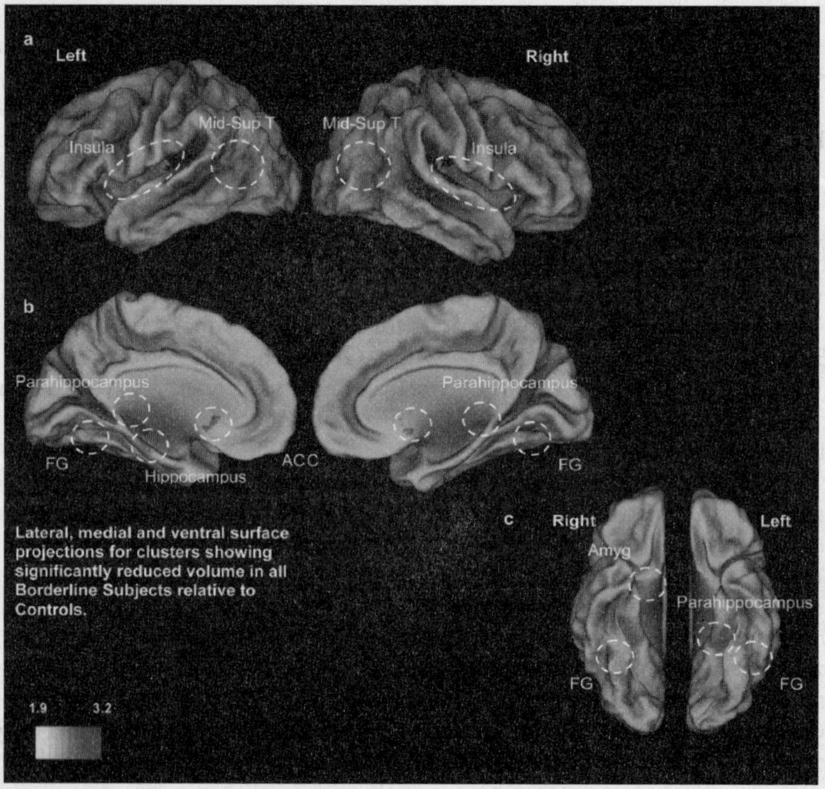

FIGURE 15-3 Areas That Show Less Volume in Those With Borderline Personality Disorder Compared With Controls

Source: Soloff et al. (2012, p. 520), with permission from Elsevier.

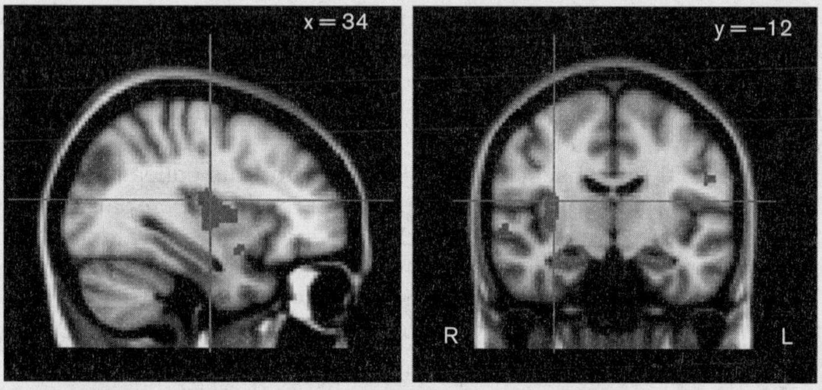

FIGURE 15-4 Areas Relating Differences Between Control Participants and Those With Borderline Personality Disorder Include the Right Insula

Source: Dziobek et al. (2011, p. 546), with permission from Elsevier.
Note: Figure uses radiological format in terms of right and left side.

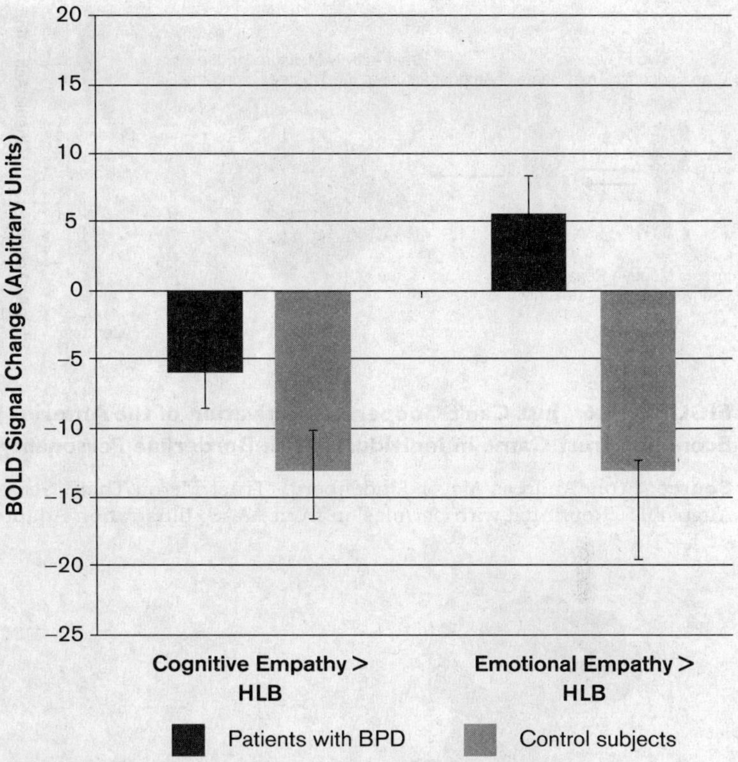

FIGURE 15-5 Bold Differences Between Control Participants and Those With Borderline Personality Disorder

Source: Dziobek et al. (2011, p. 546), with permission from Elsevier.

Trust and Borderline Personality Disorder

An important area of research is to have individuals with borderline personality play computer games. One of these games is the *trust game* (King-Casas et al., 2008). In this game, money is exchanged between an investor, who decides how much money to commit, and a trustee, who decides how much of the investment to repay the investor. During the game the investment is tripled. If both cooperate, then both the investor and the trustee benefit. However, this involves a degree of trust between the two. This trust builds up from playing the game a number of times. Individuals with BPD do not trust the situation and invest less money than do normal controls.

During the game, activity in the anterior insula was measured. This area is traditionally related to a sense of self and the physiological state of the body. It has also been shown to react to unfairness and the emotional states of others. With the healthy control, large activation of the anterior insula was related to the size of the investment. Small investments related to large activation and large investments corresponded to small activations. Thus, it is activated when the person does not cooperate. On the other hand, the insula of the person with BPD did not differentiate between the size of the offer. According to these researchers, those with BPD did not have the gut feeling that cooperation and thus the relationship was in jeopardy (see *Figure 15-6*).

Another game that is used to examine physiological responses of those with borderline personality is a simple ball toss game called cyberball. Imagine that you are sitting at a computer terminal and see *Figure 15-7* on the screen. You are told that there are two other people playing with you represented by the two cartoon characters on the screen.

At the beginning of the game, you see the other two people throwing to each other and then to you, and you, in turn, throw to them (see *Figure 15-8*). However, near the end of the game, the other two people throw only to each other. Individuals without personality disorders will experience distress and feel rejected. In one study, these individuals showed

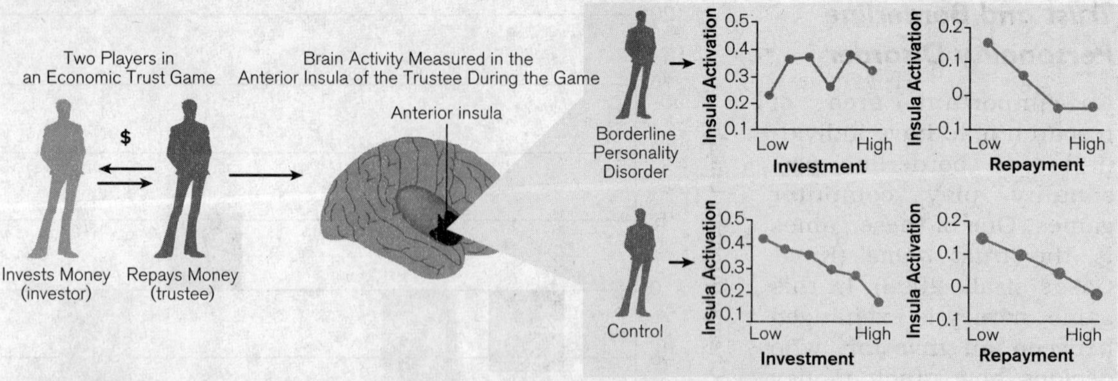

FIGURE 15-6 Just Can't Cooperate. Activation of the Anterior Insula Is Observed During an Economic Trust Game in Individuals With Borderline Personality Disorder and Healthy Controls

Source: From Andreas Meyer-Lindenberg, "Trust Me on This." *Science* Volume: 321, Issue: 5890. 2008, August 15. Reprinted with permission from AAAS. Illustration Adapted by N. Kevitiyagala/Science.

FIGURE 15-7 Image of Computer Screen Representing Two Other People Throwing a Ball. Your Hand Is Represented at the Bottom of the Screen

Source: Williams, Cheung, and Choi (2000).

greater activation of the ACC and right ventral prefrontal cortex (RVPFC) during exclusion (Eisenberger, Lieberman, & Kipling, 2003). Further, greater activity in the ACC was associated with more self-reported social distress, and the opposite was true for the RVPFC (see *Figure 15-9* and *Figure 15-10*). Interestingly, the experience of social distress paralleled those of physical pain. That is, activity in the ACC, which has been previously linked with pain, was also associated with social rejection. Likewise, increased activity in the RVPFC, previously linked with the regulation of pain, was associated with diminished distress after rejection.

When individuals with BPD played the cyberball game, they felt more excluded than controls whether it was the inclusion or exclusion condition (Renneberg et al., 2012). They also believed that fewer balls were thrown to them than did controls. In the inclusion condition, individuals with BPD reported more anger and sadness both before and after the

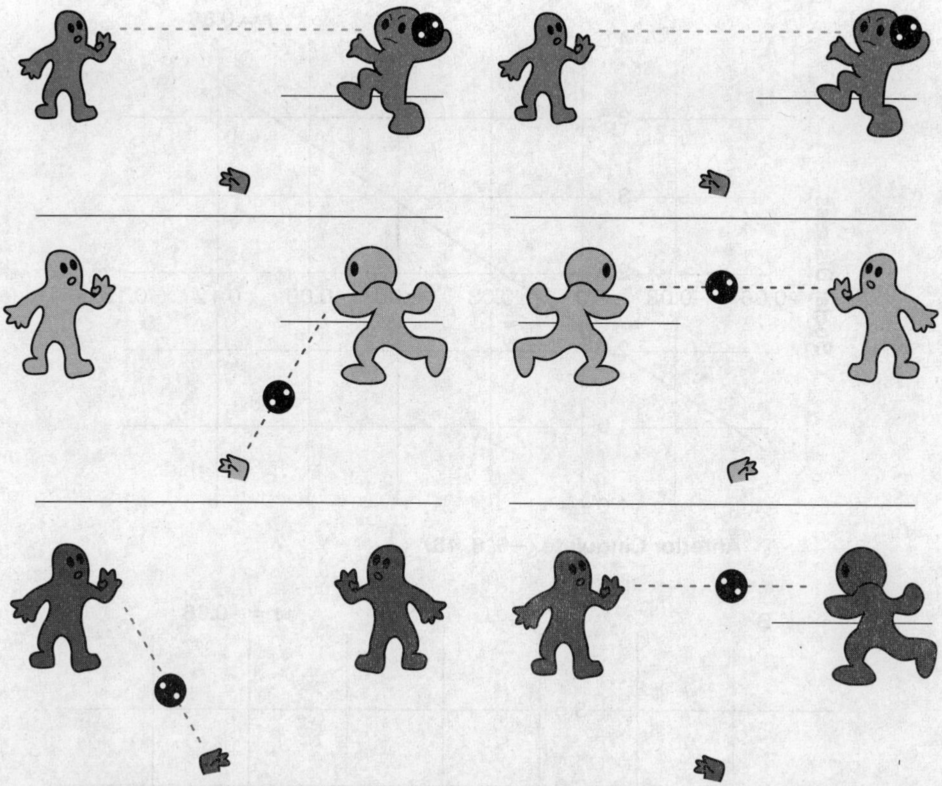

FIGURE 15-8 Cyberball Game in Which All Three Individuals Throw the Ball to Each Other

Source: Williams et al. (2000).

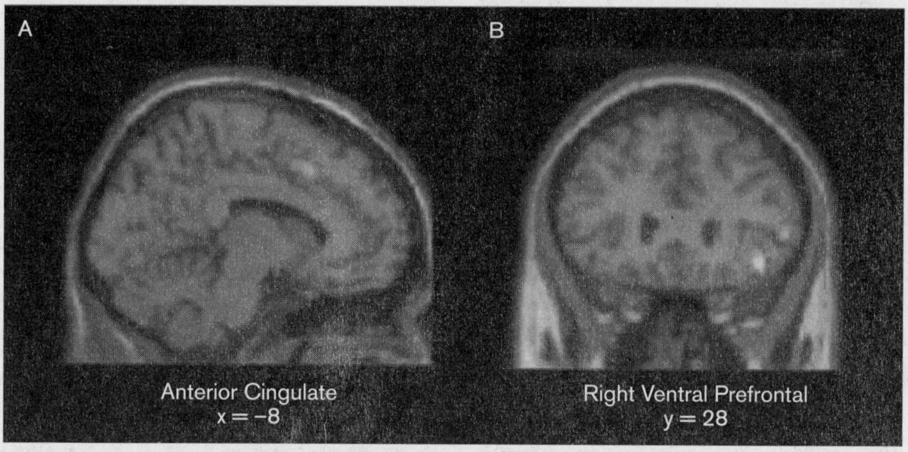

FIGURE 15-9 In A, Increased Activity in Anterior Cingulate Cortex During Exclusion. In B, Increased Activity in Right Ventral Prefrontal Cortex During Exclusion Relative to Inclusion

Source: Eisenberger et al. (2003, p. 291). Reprinted with permission from AAAS.

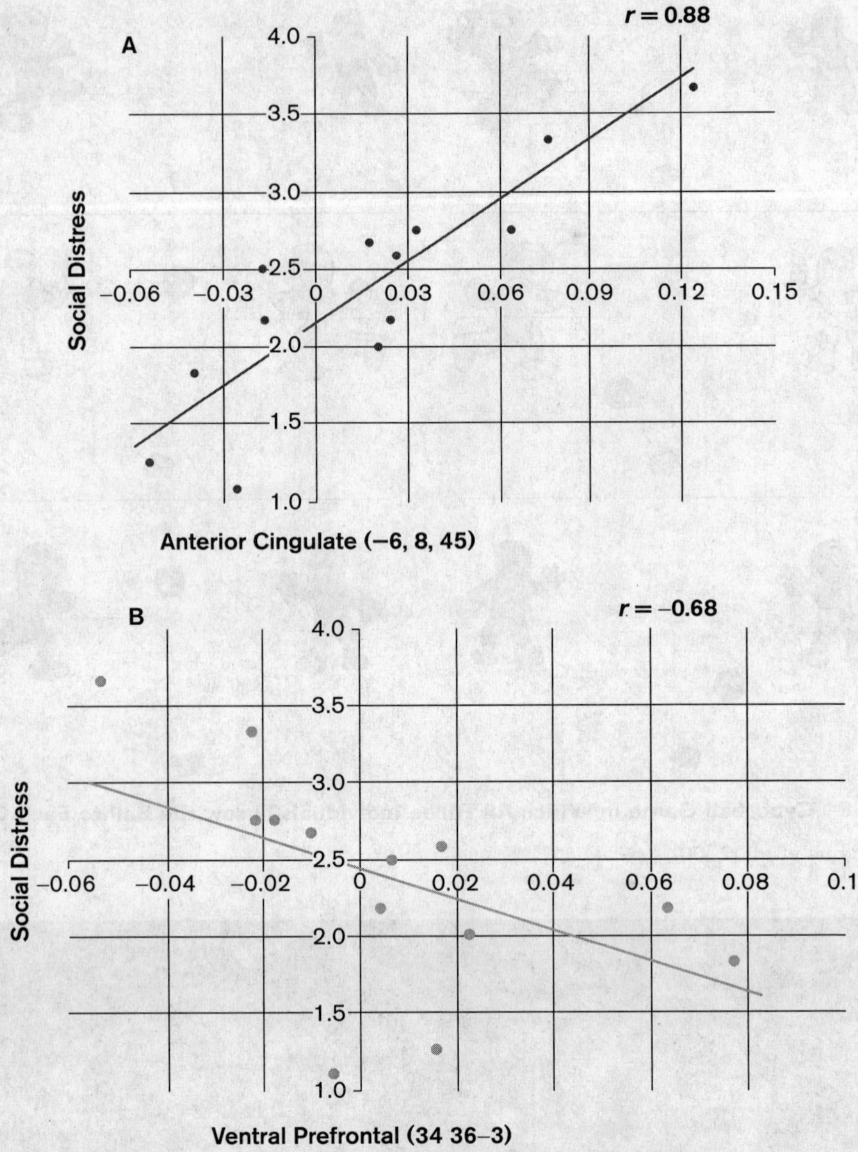

FIGURE 15-10 Scatterplots Showing the Relation During Exclusion, Relative to Inclusion, Between (A) Anterior Cingulate Cortex Activity and Self-Reported Distress and (B) Right Ventral Prefrontal Cortex and Self-Reported Distress

Source: Eisenberger et al. (2003, p. 292). Reprinted with permission from AAAS.

inclusion condition (see *Figure 15-11*). This was also true for the exclusion condition (see *Figure 15-12*). These figures show that whereas healthy controls show emotional reactions only to the situation in which they are actually excluded, individuals with BPD experience negative emotions in both situations.

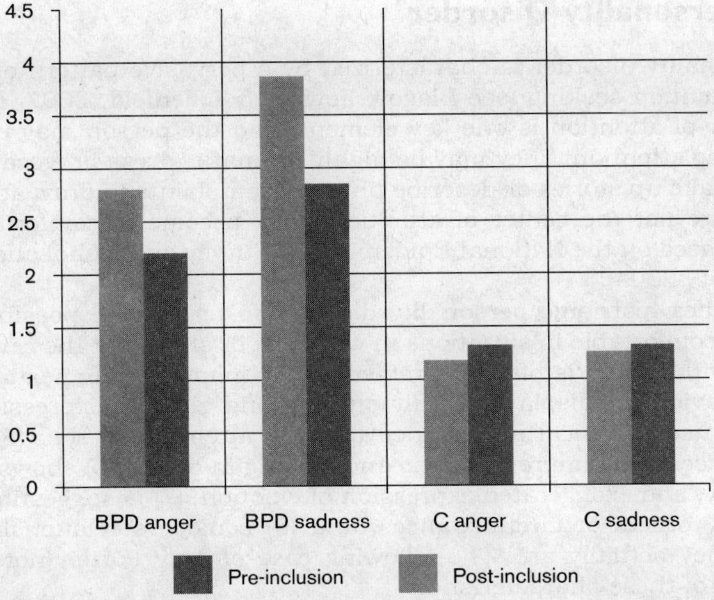

FIGURE 15-11 Anger and Sadness Before and After the Inclusion Condition for Those With Borderline Personality Disorder and Controls (C)

Source: Renneberg et al. (2012).

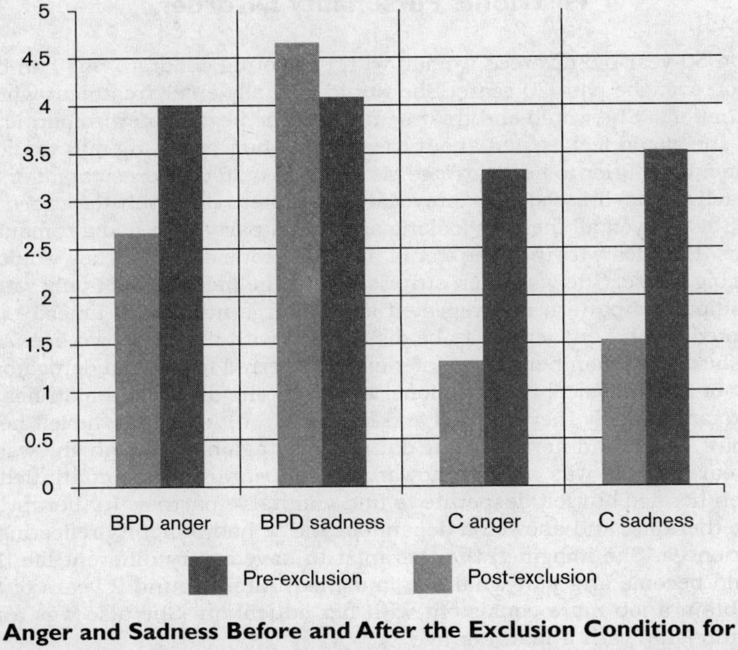

FIGURE 15-12 Anger and Sadness Before and After the Exclusion Condition for Those With Borderline Personality Disorder and Controls (C)

Source: Renneberg et al. (2012).

Histrionic Personality Disorder

Histrionic personality disorder is characterized by a pervasive pattern of excessive emotionality and attention seeking (see Blagov, Fowler, & Lilienfeld, 2007, for an overview). Being the center of attention is one key element, and the person may use a number of means for gaining attention. They may be highly dramatic, dress provocatively, be seductive, and even make up stories or describe physical complaints to draw attention to themselves. If they are not the center of attention, they become uncomfortable. Prevalence rates are 1.8% based on the National Epidemiologic Survey on Alcohol and Related Conditions (Grant et al., 2004).

DSM–5 describes histrionic personality disorder in terms of 8 possible facets. These include (1) is uncomfortable in situations in which he or she is not the center of attention; (2) interaction with others is often characterized by inappropriate sexually seductive or provocative behavior; (3) displays rapidly shifting and shallow expression of emotions; (4) consistently uses physical appearance to draw attention to self; (5) has a style of speech that is excessively impressionistic and lacking in detail; (6) shows self-dramatization, theatricality, and exaggerated expression of emotion; (7) is suggestible—that is, easily influenced by others or circumstances; and (8) considers relationships to be more intimate than they actually are. The following case of Amy Porter (not her real name) illustrates many of these characteristics.

CASE OF AMY PORTER
Histrionic Personality Disorder

Amy Porter is a 50-year-old divorced woman with two young children. She had been in treatment off and on over the past 20 years. She would typically enter treatment when distressed by difficult situations. She would end treatment when she began a new romantic relationship. At that point, she would feel excited about the person she was dating and would idealize the person and the future. Prior to her marriage Ms. Porter would date one man after another. She was very attractive and dressed in a provocative manner. She even described herself as a "Barbie doll." She enjoyed all the men looking at her at a party. She had a romance novel view of relationships. Her idea was that she would meet someone and that they would live happily ever after in a big house. She was often surprised that the men she met only wanted a short-term relationship. This pattern had repeated itself a large number of times. As she became older, she wanted a child but tended to be dissatisfied with men her own age. As she moved into her 40s, she viewed men her age as inferior and referred to them in derogatory terms and was intolerant of their physical imperfections. However, she did meet a man her age that she felt attracted to and quickly they married and had children. After that, he left her.

At some point, she found herself in the dating world again. Although she was still attractive as a 50-year-old, she was negative toward her appearance. She continued to be uninterested in men her age but felt desperate to find a suitable partner. In therapy, she wanted more from the therapist and showed a dependency. She had difficulty reflecting on her own internal experiences. She imagined the therapist to have a very different life than was the case and would become angry at what she imagined. After around 2 years of therapy, she was able to obtain a job more consistent with her education. She also was able to have a long-term relationship with a man her age.

Clinical vignette provided by Kenneth Levy, PhD

Narcissistic Personality Disorder

Narcissistic personality disorder is characterized by a pervasive pattern of grandiosity, a need for admiration, a sense of privilege or entitlement, and a lack of empathy for others (see Levy, Reynoso, Wasserman, & Clarkin, 2007, for an overview). Individuals with narcissistic personality disorder often think about how special they are and the ways in which they will succeed in all types of ways, including business, love, competiveness, and so forth. They may also make unreasonable demands on others in relation to their view of themselves. In doing so, they ignore the experiences or needs of others. Prevalence rates have been estimated as high as 6% in community samples (APA, 2013).

The diagnostic criteria in *DSM–5* for narcissistic personality disorder describe a person who shows a pattern of grandiosity, a need for admiration, and a lack of empathy for others. This personality style should begin by early adulthood. Five specific characteristics should also be present. These characteristics include (1) having a grandiose sense of self-importance; (2) being preoccupied with ideas of unlimited success or attractiveness; (3) seeing one's self as special and being understood by only other exceptional individuals; (4) needing excessive admiration; (5) having a sense of entitlement, which can include unreasonable expectations; (6) taking advantage of others for his or her own needs; (7) lacking empathy; (8) being envious of others or believing that others envy him or her; and (9) being arrogant.

The word *narcissism* comes from the Greek myth of Narcissus. Narcissus saw his image in a pool of water and fell in love with the image. Unable to remove himself from his own image, he died at the pool. In a similar manner, people with narcissistic personality disorder think only of their own image and lose close contact with others and the world. They may believe that they are so unique that they can be understood only by others who are similarly special. They need others only as someone to validate their own views. In fact, all the resources of the individual including regulating his or her emotions and interpersonal processes are directed at maintaining a positive self-image. This may be accomplished by seeking validation and self-enhancement experiences from others. When others cease to admire the person, an individual with narcissistic personality disorder will move on and seek someone who will. Although everyone likes to receive positive responses from others, those with narcissistic personality disorder take this to the extreme. The following case study of Dawn Nichols (not her real name) shows the characteristics of a person with narcissistic personality disorder.

CASE OF DAWN NICHOLS
Narcissistic Personality Disorder

Dawn Nichols was a tall, attractive married woman in her mid-30s with three children. A friend of hers helped her to find a therapist. Her chief complaints were feelings of long-term depression and a general feeling of anxiety. Others in her life reported that she could become angry quickly and that these outbursts could occur in businesses and when traveling with others. She grew up in a home in which her father was an extremely successful businessman. Her father was "all business" and too busy for his children. He was also hostile and derogatory toward her. Although her mother gave Dawn her basic needs as a child, her mother was emotionally distant and physically absent. Even after Dawn grew up, her mother sought to coerce her into doing what she wanted.

(Continued)

(Continued)

Dawn Nichols believed that she had superior intelligence and abilities. However, she also reported difficulty doing well in school and sticking with any of her activities such as horseback riding, acting, and singing. Overall, she blamed her parents for not helping her develop her abilities. Although she was in her 30s, she had little sense of what she wanted to do with her life. She would change her mind and become angry with others. She once sold a horse since she had not engaged in horseback riding for years only to buy another horse a few days later because she admired it.

In addition to feeling depressed and anxious, Dawn reported angry outbursts, significant alcohol and marijuana use, concerns about rapidly shifting interests, and unhappiness with the lack of success in her life. She also reported that her husband was concerned that she was disconnected from her three children and that she would often become angry with them for normal behaviors of children. She experienced this anger in spite of the fact that she had a housekeeper, a gardener, an au pair, and a number of babysitters to help her. She also blamed her husband for not helping her succeed. She was part of local acting workshops and sang with some local bands. She often fantasized about leaving her family and touring Europe with a younger man who would produce her music and help her achieve fame and fortune.

Clinical vignette provided by Kenneth Levy, PhD
Source: Adapted from Levy (2012).

ANXIOUS FEARFUL PERSONALITY DISORDERS

There are three personality disorders included in the **anxious fearful personality disorders (Cluster C)** grouping. These personality disorders include avoidant, dependent, and obsessive compulsive. The behavior of individuals with these disorders is one of fearfulness and avoidance.

Concept Check

- What three factors characterize BPD?
- What role do self-mutilating behaviors and suicide attempts play in individuals with BPD? What do we know about the prevalence of these behaviors?
- What evidence do we have that the brains of individuals with BPD differ from others?
- Two computer games—the trust game and a ball toss game—are used in research with individuals with BPD. What is the purpose of each of these games, and what have they revealed about personality disorder?
- What environmental factors play a role in the development of BPD?
- What is the defining characteristic of histrionic personality disorder? What eight facets do *DSM–5* use to describe the disorder?
- How would you explain the paradox that individuals with narcissistic personality disorder need other people at the same time that they have no empathy for others themselves?

Avoidant Personality Disorder

Avoidant personality disorder is characterized by a pervasive pattern of social inhibition, feelings of inadequacy, and hypersensitivity to negative evaluation (see Herbert, 2007, for an overview). Individuals with avoidant personality disorder avoid many social interactions, especially those involving close relationships with other people. One key feature is the fear of being criticized or evaluated by others. This, in turn, results in the person interacting only with her family or a few trusted others. Prevalence rates range between 2.3% based on the National Epidemiologic Survey on Alcohol and Related Conditions (Grant et al., 2004) and 5.1% in the National Comorbidity Survey Replication (Lenzenweger et al., 2007).

The diagnostic criteria in *DSM–5* for avoidant personality disorder describe a person who shows a pattern of social inhibition, feelings of inadequacy, and an increased sensitivity to negative evaluation. This personality style should begin by early adulthood. Four specific characteristics should also be present. These characteristics include (1) an avoidance of occupational activities that involve interpersonal contact that could lead to criticism; (2) an unwillingness to be involved with others unless it is certain that the person will be liked; (3) restraint within an intimate relationship for fear of being ridiculed; (4) a preoccupation with being criticized or rejected in social situations; (5) an inhibition in new interpersonal situations because of feelings of inadequacy; (6) a view of one's self as socially inept, unappealing, or inferior; and (7) a reluctance to take personal risks or engage in new activities for fear of being embarrassed.

Dependent Personality Disorder

Dependent personality disorder is characterized by a pervasive pattern of clinging and being submissive (see Bornstein, 2007, for an overview). The person with dependent personality disorder has difficulties making everyday decisions without reassurance from others. This results in a desire for others to assume responsibility for most areas of one's life. Their lack of experiencing a self who can plan and direct their behavior leaves them in a position that requires that they always be with another. Otherwise, they tend to feel anxious and helpless when alone. They tend not to be thoughtful in choosing a partner, which may result in choosing partners who are not reliable or empathic. Prevalence rates range from 0.4% based on the National Epidemiologic Survey on Alcohol and Related Conditions (Grant et al., 2004) to 0.6% in the National Comorbidity Survey Replication (Lenzenweger et al., 2007).

The diagnostic criteria in *DSM–5* for dependent personality disorder describe a person who shows a pattern of excessive need to be taken care of that leads to submissive and clinging behavior and fears of separation. This personality style should begin by early adulthood. Five specific characteristics should also be present. These characteristics include (1) an inability to make everyday decisions without an excessive amount of advice and reassurance from others; (2) a need for others to assume responsibility for one's life; (3) a difficulty to disagree with another person; (4) a difficulty to begin projects; (5) a need to work hard to receive support from others; (6) an uncomfortable feeling when alone, resulting from the idea that the person cannot take care of him- or herself; (7) beginning a new relationship when an old one is over as a source of care; and (8) feeling fearful that one cannot take care of one's self.

Obsessive-Compulsive Personality Disorder

Obsessive-compulsive personality disorder is characterized by a pervasive pattern of preoccupation with orderliness, perfectionism, and control of one's environment (see Bartz, Kaplan, & Hollander, 2007, for an overview). Individuals with obsessive-compulsive

Concept Check

- What are the similar characteristics that run through the personality disorders in Cluster C? What are the distinct characteristics of each disorder?
- How is obsessive-compulsive personality disorder similar to OCD? How is it different?

personality would be described as workaholics. They themselves would see little need for taking time off or just spending time with other people. In dealing with others, they may appear rigid and to be using standards not called for in the current situation.

One question is the manner in which obsessive-compulsive personality disorder is related to the obsessive-compulsive disorder (OCD) described in Chapter 10 since they appear to have similar characteristics. The traditional distinction between the two is the relation of the object of control to the person's self. In OCD, individuals typically attempt to control something that takes place outside of themselves. For example, some individuals with OCD fear germs and constantly wash their hands or clean their houses. However, in obsessive-compulsive personality disorder, the need for control is part of the individual's self in every domain that the person experiences. Thus, it is a way of life rather than a reaction to external processes. Prevalence rates range from 2.4% in the National Comorbidity Survey Replication (Lenzenweger et al., 2007) to 7.8% based on the National Epidemiologic Survey on Alcohol and Related Conditions (Grant et al., 2004). This disorder has one of the highest prevalence rates of any of the personality disorders.

The diagnostic criteria in *DSM–5* for obsessive-compulsive personality disorder describe a person who shows a pattern of being concerned with orderliness, perfectionism, and control. This control reduces flexibility and openness. This personality style should begin by early adulthood. Four specific characteristics should also be present. These characteristics include (1) a preoccupation with details, rules, lists, order, or schedules; (2) a perfectionism that interferes with task completion; (3) an excessive preoccupation with work rather than fun and friendships; (4) an inflexibility concerning morals and values; (5) an inability to discard worthless objects even when there is no emotional connection to the object; (6) a reluctance to delegate tasks to others unless they are performed in a particular way; (7) a hoarding of money; and (8) rigidity and stubbornness.

TREATMENT OF PERSONALITY DISORDERS

Personality disorders are difficult to treat. This is in part related to the fact that one individual with a personality disorder may show different signs and symptoms than another. Additionally, individuals with personality disorders find it difficult to maintain a close intimate relationship with their therapist. Because of this, psychotherapy for personality disorders is more individual focused than that for other disorders. At this point, research studies have shown that treatments based on both cognitive behavioral and dynamic perspectives have been effective. Although from different traditions, the effective approaches show many common factors.

BPD has been the focus of the most empirical treatment studies. One of the first researched treatment approaches for BPD is **dialectical behavior therapy (DBT).** DBT was developed by Marsha Linehan based on her work with suicidal clients and then expanded to those with BPD (Linehan, 1993; Linehan & Dexter-Mazza, 2008). The therapy begins with the acceptance of the fact that individuals with BPD experience extreme emotional reactions and are particularly sensitive to changes in the environment. Anger toward the therapist is not uncommon. Individuals with BPD take longer to return to baseline conditions after their emotional reactivity. They may be impulsive. Suicidal considerations are common. This makes these clients difficult to work with and therapy sessions are often very challenging.

DBT is described by Marsha Linehan and her colleagues as a blend of behavioral science, dialectical philosophy, and Zen practice. The cornerstone of DBT is based on problem solving and acceptance of the experience of the moment. That is, the therapist acknowledges and accepts that a person felt rejected at the moment but not that the response to the rejection would be to hurt herself. The therapy itself is conceptualized in terms of a number of stages.

The pretreatment stage is a time when the client and the therapist arrive at a mutually informed decision to work together. This includes an understanding of the person's history and decisions concerning which are the processes that should receive high priority. This pretreatment stage also includes a discussion concerning what can reasonably be expected from therapy and the roles of the therapist and the client. One emphasis is on the therapist and the client as a team, whose goal it is to help the client create a life worth living. In the service of creating a productive life, the individual will develop problem-solving skills for her own life.

The first stage of therapy is directed at helping the client develop a stable life. This includes reducing suicide-related behaviors and other behaviors that interfere with therapy and life. This stage typically lasts for 1 year. During this stage, dialectical thinking encourages clients to see reality as complex and not something that can be reduced to a single idea. This includes developing the ability to experience thoughts and feelings, which are experienced as contradictory. This is a difficult task for those with BPD. Four specific goals of Stage 1 include reducing suicidal ideation, reducing behavior that interferes with therapy, achieving a stable lifestyle, and developing skills in emotional regulation such as mindfulness. Stage 1 has been most researched in terms of empirically supported procedures.

The second stage of therapy moves to processing previously experienced traumatic events. One approach is to have the person reexperience prior trauma inside the therapy session. This stage can only occur once the person's life is stable and her emotional responding is under her control. The four specific goals of this stage include remembering and accepting the facts of earlier trauma, reducing any self-blame involving the earlier trauma, reducing the intrusive material associated with the earlier trauma as well as any denial associated with it, and resolving dialectical tensions associated with blame for the trauma.

The third stage is directed at helping the person develop a sense of self that allows her to live independently. The goal is to help the person experience both happiness and unhappiness with the ability to trust in her experiences. The fourth and final stage of treatment focuses on the ability to sustain joy and be part of an ever-changing world. The following LENS describes Marsha Linehan's own experiences, which led to the creation of DBT.

15-1 LENS
Marsha Linehan, Creating Dialectical Behavior Therapy From Her Own Experiences

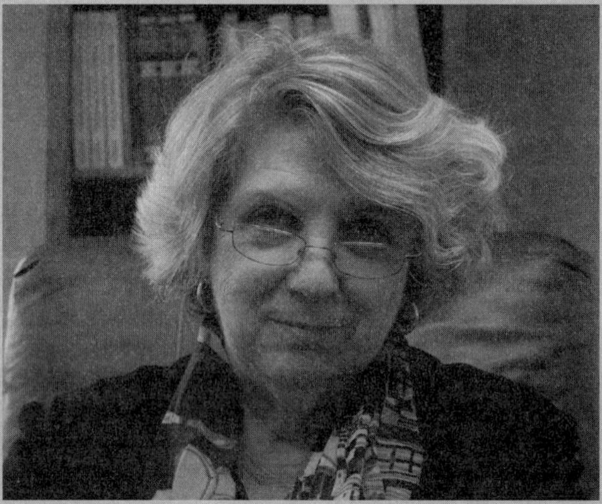

Source: Courtesy of University of Washington.

As she grew up in Tulsa, Oklahoma, Marsha Linehan was an excellent student and played the piano well. However, she felt deeply inadequate compared with others. She also found herself at odds with her parents and by her senior year in high school was taken to local mental health professionals. They recommended that she be institutionalized. Thus, at age 17, Marsha Linehan found herself on a locked ward at the Institute of Living in Hartford, Connecticut. Previously, she displayed the characteristics often seen in those with BPD. She burned herself and slashed her arms, legs, and other parts of her body. In the hospital without sharp objects, she hit her head on the wall or floor.

This is how she currently describes that time: "My whole experience of these episodes was that someone else was doing it; it was like 'I know this is coming, I'm out of control, somebody help me; where are you, God?'" She further stated, "I felt totally empty, like the Tin Man; I had no way to communicate what was going on, no way to understand it." After more than 2 years, she was released from the ward and returned home. While at home, she attempted suicide.

She later moved to Chicago in an attempt to start over. She lived at the YMCA and took a job as a clerk in an insurance company. She reports that her Catholic faith was critical to her and that she prayed often. A religious experience took her to a place where she accepted herself as she was. In Chicago, Marsha Linehan also took classes and was able to complete a PhD in psychology. As she continued her career, she became a therapist who worked with suicidal people who often were those with a personality disorder. She helped them to focus on life as it is rather than how the person thinks it should be. She also emphasized acceptance. She built on these principles to develop DBT and to test its empirical efficacy.

Marsha Linehan, along with Elyn Saks and Kay Jamison, has become a productive scholar and advocate of reforming our current mental health system with its frequently inadequate care. This also includes sharing an understanding of the experiences of those with mental disorders, including the way in which society stigmatizes these individuals. A growing number of voices, some of which are profiled in the *New York Times* series "Lives Restored," have demonstrated the reality of those with mental illness moving from distress to productivity (www.nytimes.com/interactive/science/lives-restored-series.html).

This LENS is based on a talk given by Dr. Linehan at the Institute of Living as reported in the *New York Times* (www.nytimes.com/2011/06/23/health/23lives.html?pagewanted=all&_r=0) (see Carey, 2011).

In addition to DBT, there are also a number of dynamic orientated therapies that are empirically supported. One of these is **dynamic deconstructive psychotherapy (DDP).** DDP was developed for clients who find therapy difficult as well as for those who may also have substance abuse problems (Gregory & Remen, 2008). This approach is partly based on neuroscience research, which shows that individuals with BPD show difficulties with memory, emotional regulation, and decision making. This is seen as preventing these individuals from building a coherent self-system independent of other people. DDP is designed to help individuals with BPD develop a coherent sense of self.

DDP is divided into four distinct stages. The first stage is for the client and the therapist together to identify the client's difficulties and establish a series of goals and tasks for working on these difficulties. They also create an agreement as to how the client will keep himself safe. By the end of this stage, the relationship between the therapist and client should be stable and give the client comfort. This stage is similar in both dynamic and cognitive behavioral approaches.

The second stage involves the development of the client's ability to maintain complex ideas related to his relationships with others. For example, when a relationship with another ended, he would be able to say, "I felt both horrified and relieved." As this stage ends, the client begins to give up an idealized image of himself. As his idealized image of himself and his abilities is given up, there can be a better understanding of self-limitations, which is the focus of the third stage. During this third stage, the client can learn to verbalize his or her disappointments and experience the loss associated with this. This can also lead to fears of personal incompetence. The final stage moves to the relationship between the client and therapist and how the person will experience the termination of therapy.

Another empirically supported therapy is **transference-focused psychotherapy (TFP).** This is a twice-weekly therapy based on Otto Kernberg's object relations model (Clarkin, Yeomans, & Kernberg, 2006; see also Levy & Scala, 2012). As with other approaches, TFP seeks to reduce symptoms of BPD, especially self-destructive behaviors. The technique involves an exploration of how the person views herself and may combine her identity with that of another. That is, she does not have a stable view of self. During the first year of treatment, behaviors involved with self-harm are limited and a therapy contract is developed. In the sessions, the therapist follows the affect that the client brings to the session. The emphasis is on the relationship between the client and therapist. Questions of whether this relationship can also be seen in the client's other relationships can be addressed. Many of these techniques are similar to those of Strupp and Bender described in Chapter 2.

Treatments for the Other Personality Disorders

Most of our knowledge of the treatment of personality disorders other than BPD is based on the experience of health care professionals, case studies, or simple descriptions of treatments. Thus, empirically validated treatments are not available at this time. As you can imagine, individuals with certain personality disorders such as schizoid or avoidant personality disorder rarely seek treatment, which makes systematic treatment studies more difficult. In addition to psychotherapy, medications have been used for specific aspects such as depression or impulsivity of different personality disorders. However, unlike psychotherapy, there are no medications that target all aspects of a personality disorder.

Concept Check

- What is it about personality disorders that makes them difficult to treat? What factors do effective treatments have in common to address those difficulties?
- BPD has been the focus of most empirical treatment studies. What is the state of knowledge about treatments for other personality disorders? What do you think should be the top priority in future treatment research?
- Personality disorders are said to involve problems with the person's sense of self. What are these problems? What conceptual models have been proposed for helping us understand how the sense of self is disrupted in personality disorders?

DSM FUTURE CONSIDERATIONS OF PERSONALITY DISORDERS

As described throughout this chapter, personality disorders involve problems with the person's sense of self. In many of the disorders, there is not a coherent sense of self as an independent identity. Further, the experience of being directed by one's goals and plans is missing. Instead, the experience of the moment may dictate the emotional reactions of the individual. In addition to a lack of a sense of self, there are also problems with interpersonal relationships. Specifically, there are problems with understanding others as well as being intimate with another person. This has led researchers to ask whether personality disorders could be conceptualized along a continuum based on ratings of each of these four dimensions: self-identity, self-direction, interpersonal empathy, and interpersonal intimacy. Thus, the health care professional would rate the person's level of personal functioning in these four areas. Current research is being directed at this goal.

SUMMARY

The basic definition of a personality disorder is that (1) it represents an enduring pattern of inner experience and behavior that deviates markedly from the expectations of the individual's culture; (2) the pattern is inflexible, stable, and generally begins in adolescence; and (3) the characteristics of these disorders are especially apparent when these individuals find themselves in situations that are beyond their ability to cope. Research has shown that those with a personality disorder also meet criteria for other disorders—especially anxiety, mood, and substance use disorders. Not only do individuals with a personality disorder meet criteria for another non-personality disorder; they also met criteria for other personality disorders where the highest co-occurrence of personality disorders is seen within each of the clusters. Some researchers have suggested that personality characteristics reflected in personality disorders can be seen as an extreme version of normal personality characteristics. Thus, there can be both healthy and maladaptive personality styles. A healthy self is considered to have the following characteristics: (1) identity, (2) self-direction, and (3) positive interpersonal relationships characterized by empathy and intimacy. Some researchers, from an evolutionary perspective, view personality disorders as a failure to solve adaptive life tasks relating to identity or self, intimacy and attachment, and prosocial behavior.

Normal personality traits can be described by the dimensions of the FFM, developed by McCrae and Costa encompassing earlier work by Eysenck. The five personality dimensions are (1) extraversion, which ranges from active and outer-directed on one end to passive and inner-directed on the other; (2) neuroticism, which ranges from being worried and temperamental on one side of the continuum to being even-tempered and confident on the other; (3) openness, which is associated with curiosity, flexibility, and an artistic sensitivity, including imaginativeness and the ability to create a fantasy world; (4) agreeableness, which is associated with being sympathetic, trusting, cooperative, modest, and straightforward; and (5) conscientiousness, which is associated with being diligent, disciplined, well-organized, punctual, and dependable. Nettle suggested, from an evolutionary perspective, that each of the personality dimensions has particular advantages—as well as disadvantages—in specific environmental conditions. Research has shown that personality disorders can be understood as maladaptive variants of the FFM. Some have suggested that there would be advantages to considering personality disorders along a spectrum, which would allow for a mapping of personality disorders and personality traits in the FFM. Since each dimension of the FFM has been shown to have a genetic component and these five dimensions are found worldwide, a spectrum approach would help clarify another aspect of personality disorders.

DSM–5 identifies 10 personality disorders that can be organized into three clusters. The first cluster of personality disorders is referred to as Cluster A and includes odd or eccentric disorders. Individuals with these disorders typically feel uncomfortable or suspicious of others or restrict their relationships: (1) schizoid personality disorder, which is characterized by a pervasive pattern of detachment from social relationships and a restricted range of emotional expression; (2) paranoid personality disorder, which is characterized by a pervasive distrust and suspiciousness of others; and (3) schizotypal personality disorder, which is characterized by odd beliefs and behaviors. The behavior of individuals with odd-eccentric personality disorders may seem similar to individuals with schizophrenia except that they show a greater grasp of reality. These disorders are sometimes seen in first-degree relatives of those with schizophrenia.

The second cluster of personality disorders is referred to as Cluster B and includes dramatic, emotional, or erratic disorders. Individuals with these disorders show a wide diversity of patterns of social and emotional interactions with others: (1) antisocial personality disorder, which is characterized by a disregard for the other person; (2) BPD, which is characterized by the three factors of an instability in mood, interpersonal relationships, and a sense of self, which interact with each other in such a manner that the person experiences a changing world without a solid sense of self; (3) histrionic personality disorder, which is characterized by a pervasive pattern of excessive emotionality and attention seeking; and (4) narcissistic personality disorder, which is characterized by a pervasive pattern of grandiosity, a need for admiration, a sense of privilege or entitlement, and a lack of empathy for others. Although the media interchange the words *antisocial personality disorder* and *psychopathy,* there are differences in the formal definitions of the terms. Psychopathy is not a formal definition of *DSM–5* but has been studied in both clinical and research settings. Individuals who display signs of psychopathy (1) show emotional detachment with a lack of empathy for the experiences of others and (2) show impulsive behavior and a callousness concerning their actions. These patterns are stable and difficult to change. Recent research suggests there are two separate processes in the same individual with psychopathy: (1) the lack of fear and (2) a weakness in impulse control that has the effect of externalizing vulnerability. Only about 10% to 25% of individuals with an antisocial personality disorder would be classified as having psychopathy, and not all individuals who would be described as having psychopathy would show conduct or antisocial personality disorder.

The third cluster of personality disorders is referred to as Cluster C and includes anxious or fearful disorders: (1) avoidant personality disorder, which is characterized by a pattern of social inhibition, feelings of inadequacy, and hypersensitivity to negative evaluation; (2) dependent personality disorder, which is characterized by an excessive need to be taken care of including clinging behavior; and (3) obsessive-compulsive personality disorder, which is characterized by a preoccupation with orderliness, perfectionism, and interpersonal control. In OCD, the individual typically attempts to control something that takes place outside of herself, whereas in obsessive-compulsive personality disorder, the need for control is part of the individual's self in every domain that the person experiences.

Personality disorders are difficult to treat: (1) one individual with a personality disorder may show different signs and symptoms than another, and (2) individuals with personality disorders find it difficult to maintain a close intimate relationship with their therapist. Most of our knowledge of the treatment of personality disorders other than BPD is based on the experience of health care professionals, case studies, or simple descriptions of treatments. Medications have been used for specific aspects of different personality disorders; however, there are no medications that target all aspects of a personality disorder. BPD has been the focus of the most empirical treatment studies. Research has shown that treatments based on both cognitive–behavioral and dynamic perspectives have been effective, including (1) DBT, whose cornerstone is based on problem solving and acceptance of the experience of the moment; (2) DDP, which was developed for clients who find therapy difficult as well as for those who may also have substance abuse problems; and (3) TFP, which seeks to reduce symptoms of BPD, especially self-destructive behaviors.

STUDY RESOURCES

Review Questions

1. A number of models have been presented in this chapter relating personality disorders to normal personality. What are those models? What evidence is presented to support them?
2. What are the advantages—and disadvantages—of describing personality disorders in terms of categories versus dimensions?
3. *DSM* places personality disorders in multiple groups. For each of the three groups, or clusters, of personality disorders, describe the cluster in terms of the following:
   a. The name and defining characteristics of the cluster
   b. The specific personality disorders included in the cluster, as well as the defining characteristics of each disorder
4. Historically, the term *borderline,* as the name implies, denoted individuals who were neither neurotic nor psychotic. From what you have read in this chapter, what additional meanings do you think the term *borderline* implies about that personality disorder?

5. What are three examples of effective treatment approaches for BPD? What is the overall approach of each therapy, the goals for each of the and what are/ therapies' stages? How are the therapies similar, and how are they different?

For Further Reading

Beck, A., Freeman, A., & Davis, D. (2004). *Cognitive therapy of personality disorders* (2nd ed.). New York: Guilford Press.

Gunderson, J., & Hoffman, P. (Eds.). (2005). *Understanding and treating borderline personality disorder.* Washington, DC: American Psychiatric Publishing.

Oldham, J., Skodol, A., & Bender, D. (Eds.). (2009). *Essentials of personality disorders.* Washington, DC: American Psychiatric Publishing.

Paris, J. (2007). *Half in love with death.* New York: Routledge.

Key Terms and Concepts

agreeableness
antisocial personality disorder
anxious fearful personality disorders (Cluster C)
avoidant personality disorder
borderline personality disorder (BPD)
conscientiousness
dependent personality disorder
dialectical behavior therapy (DBT)
dramatic emotional personality disorders (Cluster B)
dynamic deconstructive psychotherapy (DDP)
empathy
extraversion
five-factor model (FFM)
healthy self
histrionic personality disorder
identity
intimacy
narcissistic personality disorder
neuroticism
obsessive-compulsive personality disorder
odd-eccentric personality disorders (Cluster A)
openness
paranoid personality disorder
personality disorder
positive interpersonal relationships
psychopathy
schizoid personality disorder
schizotypal personality disorder
self-direction
transference-focused psychotherapy (TFP)

CHAPTER

16

Neurocognitive Disorders

CHAPTER OUTLINE

- ANNOUNCEMENT OF ALZHEIMER'S DISEASE BY PRESIDENT RONALD REAGAN 578
- CHANGES RELATED TO AGING ACROSS THE WORLD 580
- STUDIES FROM INDIA ON AGING CHANGES IN THE BRAIN 589
- DELIRIUM 590
- MILD AND MAJOR NEUROCOGNITIVE DISORDERS 592
- INDIAN WORK ON MILD COGNITIVE IMPAIRMENT 594
- SUMMARY 609
- STUDY RESOURCES 610

ANNOUNCEMENT OF ALZHEIMER'S DISEASE BY PRESIDENT RONALD REAGAN

November 5, 1994

My fellow Americans, I have recently been told that I am one of the millions of Americans who will be afflicted with Alzheimer's disease.

Upon learning this news, Nancy and I had to decide whether as private citizens we would keep this a private matter or whether we would make this news known in a public way. In the past, Nancy suffered from breast cancer and I had my cancer surgeries. We found through our open disclosures we were able to raise public awareness. We were happy that as a result, many more people underwent testing. They were treated in early stages and able to return to normal, healthy lives.

So now we feel it is important to share it with you. In opening our hearts, we hope this might promote greater awareness of this condition. Perhaps it will encourage a clearer understanding of the individuals and families who are affected by it.

At the moment I feel just fine. I intend to live the remainder of the years God gives me on this Earth doing the things I have always done. I will continue to share life's journey with my beloved Nancy and my family. I plan to enjoy the great outdoors and stay in touch with my friends and supporters.

Unfortunately, as Alzheimer's disease progresses, the family often bears a heavy burden. I only wish there was some way I could spare Nancy from this painful experience. When the time comes, I am confident that with your help she will face it with faith and courage.

In closing, let me thank you, the American people, for giving me the great honor of allowing me to serve as your president. When the Lord calls me home, whenever that day may be, I will leave with the greatest love for this country of ours and eternal optimism for its future.

I now begin the journey that will lead me into the sunset of my life. I know that for America there will always be a bright dawn ahead.

Thank you, my friends. May God always bless you.

Sincerely, Ronald Reagan

From Ronald Reagan's Letter to the American People Concerning His Alzheimer's Disease. Retrieved from http://www.reagan.utexas.edu/archives/reference/alzheimerletter.html

The loss of past memory was not as extreme as it is in amnesia. When I came out of the coma I had been in for 6 weeks, I knew who I was, and I knew that I was a husband, a father, and a psychologist. I knew my family, but I had difficulty recognizing some of my friends. In the beginning I thought I had two children, but I have but one. I thought my daughter was 13, but she was 15 at that point. I also thought I was 33, but I was 44.

During the drive home from the hospital (after 11 weeks), I saw that I did not recognize the route home, even though it was a route quite familiar to me. At that point, I realized that some of the geography of the city was lost to me. But I did recognize my home and the neighborhood when we arrived there. My house was familiar to me, but I didn't remember where some things were kept and how some things were used. I had to relearn how to play the stereo, set the alarm clock, use the calculator, change a razor blade, etc. All of these things were relearned, but because of the short-term memory problem, it often took several trials to relearn and keep these things in mind.

So, many things I had learned and that had made me feel like a competent person seemed to have been lost, and I wondered if I could be an adequate husband, father, or worker again. Combined with this, I felt to some extent that I had lost my identity. This was not total or extreme, but there were some questions in my mind about beliefs, values, and purposes in life. In addition, I felt that I had lost some of my cultural background when I had difficulty remembering some of the customs, traditions, and beliefs of the groups to which I belonged. This produces a feeling of being somewhat alone.

Reprinted from Malcolm Meltzer. (1983). Poor Memory: A Case Report. Journal of Clinical Psychology, 39, 3–10.

We all age. As we age, our mental and physical abilities change. Some of these changes happen gradually and appear to be related to genetic differences. **Huntington's disease** or Alzheimer's disease are examples of such disorders. The letter of Ronald Reagan shows that he understood that he was experiencing gradual memory changes. Other changes happen more quickly. Events such as a stroke or heart attack may lead to not only physical changes but also changes in mental processing. The description of Malcolm Meltzer, who was both the author and the subject of the case report, resulted from a heart attack that influenced brain function and was a sudden event.

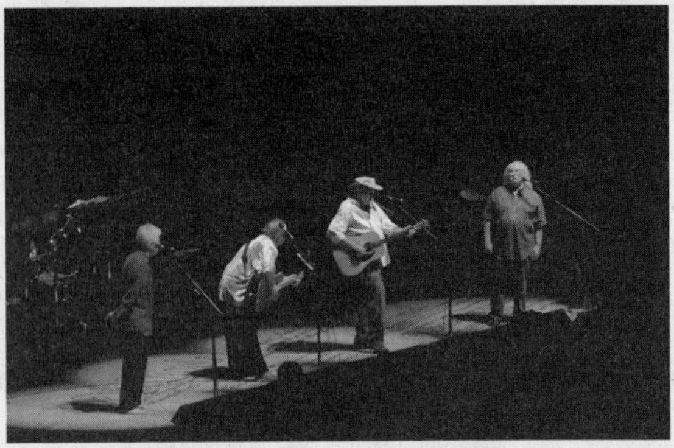

Crosby, Stills, and Nash are still performing

This chapter emphasizes **neurocognitive disorders** typically seen in older individuals. These disorders represent a loss of cognitive abilities not related to normal aging. Previously, these disorders were referred to as **dementias.**

We all know individuals or relatives who as they age show problems with memory or physical activities. Most of us also know individuals who continue to be productive well into their 80s and 90s. This has come to be called **successful aging** (Rowe & Kahn, 1987). The characteristics of successful aging include the following:

1. Freedom from disability and disease
2. High cognitive and physical functioning
3. Social activity including both having friends and being productive

The idea of successful aging emphasizes that life is more than just living a long time. It also includes a sense of connectedness and a close interaction with one's environment and self. Many of the performers associated with 1960s music, such as Bob Dylan and the group Crosby, Stills, and Nash, still perform.

The aging of each of us is related to a number of factors. These include the genes we received from our parents. These also include the experiences that happen to us, including the stresses of everyday life as well as the positive events in our lives. Aging also involves choices we make in terms of what we eat, how we exercise, and the type of work we do. To place neurocognitive changes in perspective, it is important to have an understanding of normal aging. I begin this chapter by noting the worldwide changes in aging. This is followed by research considerations of factors that may prevent or delay neurocognitive disorders. After a section on **delirium,** the **major neurocognitive disorders** are described with special attention given to Alzheimer's disease.

CHANGES RELATED TO AGING ACROSS THE WORLD

Throughout the world, better public health procedures, such as clean water and sanitation as well as medical and prevention procedures, have led to an increasing life expectancy. In the United States, individuals age 65 and older went from less than 2% of the population in 1900 to over 12% of the population in 2010 (see *Figure 16-1*). It is estimated that by 2020, there will be more people over 65 than children under 5 worldwide (see *Figure 16-2*). Data show that in North American, Europe, Russia, and Japan over 11% of the population is 65 and older (see *Figure 16-3*). Japan, Italy, and Germany have over 20% of their population 65 years of age and older.

With better public health conditions, it is noncommunicable diseases such as cardiovascular problems and cancer that are the major causes of death among older individuals in both developed and developing countries. With individuals living longer, there is also a greater chance of developing neurocognitive disorders such as Alzheimer's

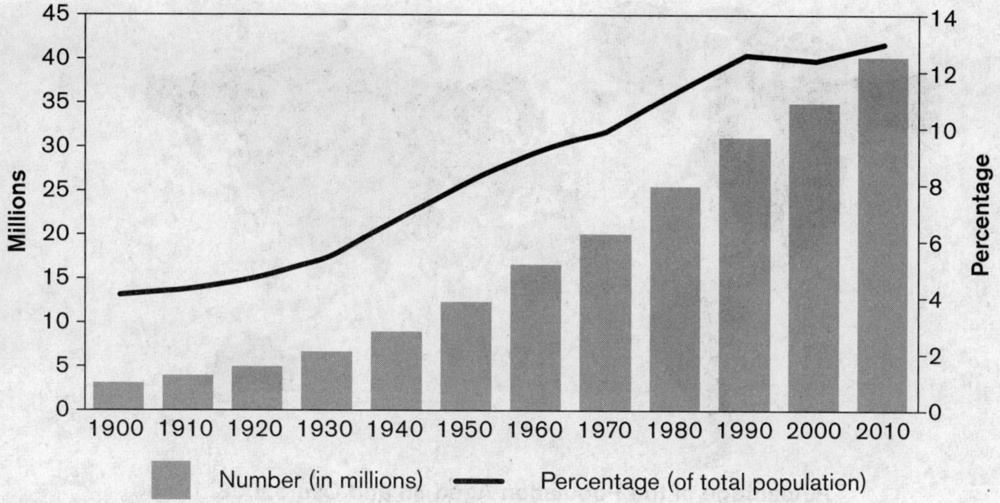

FIGURE 16-1 Population 65 Years and Up, 1900–2010

Source: Werner (2011, Figure 2).

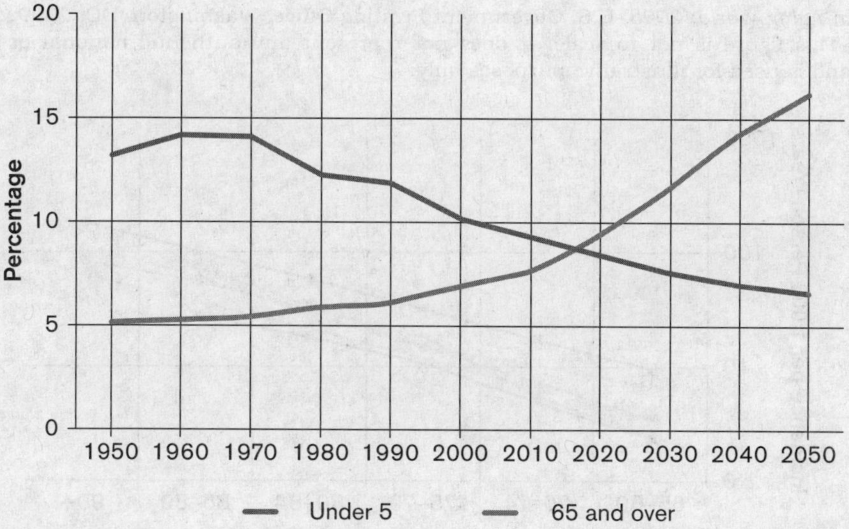

FIGURE 16-2 Young Children and Older People as a Percentage of the Global Population

Source: From Kinsella, Kevin and Wan He U.S. Census Bureau, International Population Reports, P95/09-1, *An Aging World: 2008*, U.S. Government Printing Office, Washington, DC, 2009.

and Parkinson's. Within the same age-group, mortality is higher for people with neurocognitive disorders than for those without. *Figure 16-4* shows the incidence of mild and moderate neurocognitive disorders from Europe, East Asia, and the United States. From this figure, one can note that the increase in neurocognitive disorders over the life span is similar throughout the world.

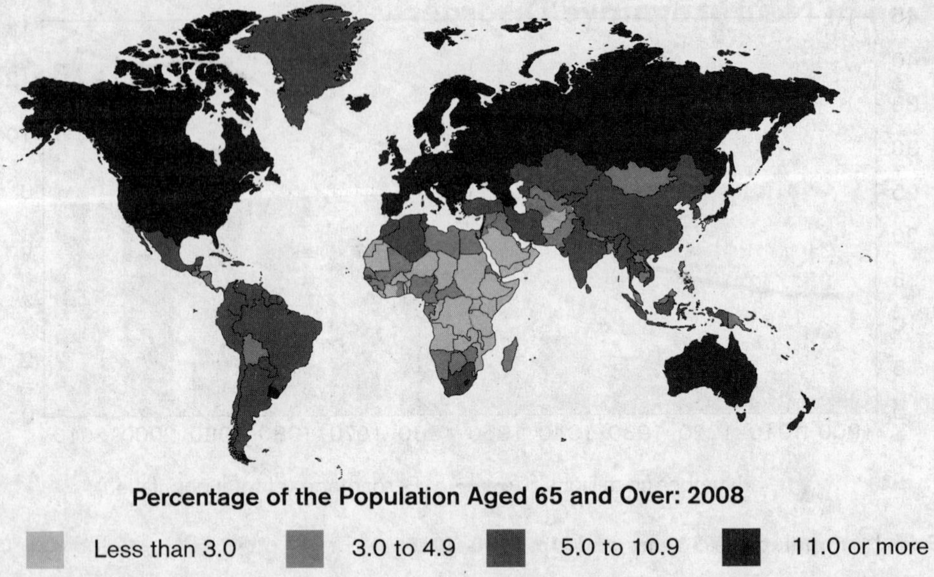

FIGURE 16-3 Percentage of Population Ages 65 and Over: 2008

Source: From Kinsella, Kevin and Wan He U.S. Census Bureau, International Population Reports, P95/09-1, *An Aging World: 2008*, U.S. Government Printing Office, Washington, DC, 2009.
Disclaimer: This figure is not to scale. It does not represent any authentic national or international boundaries and is used for illustrative purposes only.

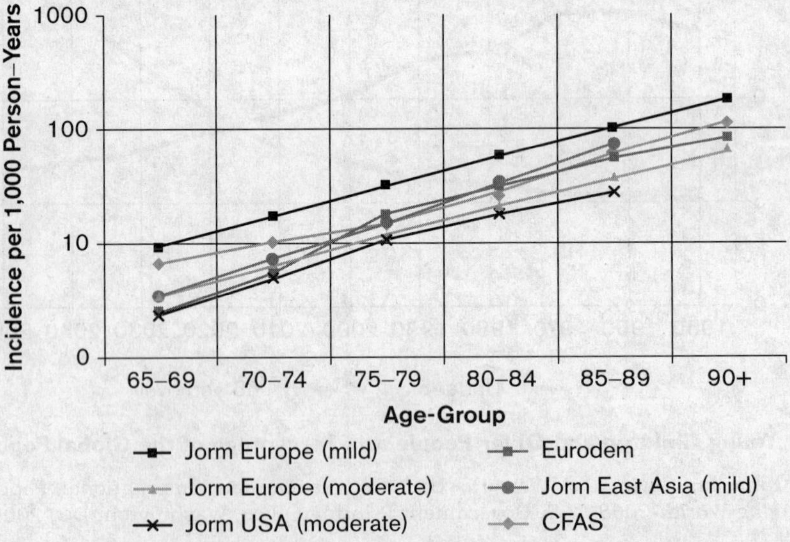

FIGURE 16-4 The Incidence of Mild and Moderate Neurocognitive Disorders From Europe, East Asia, and the United States

Source: Brayne (2007, p. 235).
Note: CFAS is a study from England and Wales. Eurodem is results from Europe. Jorm is based on research in Europe and Asia.

Prevention of Neurocognitive Disorders

Although many people assume that these disorders are a normal part of old age, it is suggested that perhaps 50% of neurocognitive disorders could be prevented (see Brayne, 2007, for an overview). Some of the prevention factors are related to lifestyle. Such life changes as exercising, eating better, and not using tobacco have been shown to be related to a reduction in both physical and mental health problems. Other prevention factors can be found through medical checkups. For example, studies that have examined blood pressure readings in childhood, midlife, and later life have shown that those with a higher blood pressure when young will have higher pressure throughout their life. High blood pressure at an earlier age, in turn, puts one at greater risk for neurocognitive disorders.

Do Cognitive Abilities Change with Age?

Cognitive abilities do change as one ages. In order to understand the changes seen in neurocognitive disorders, it is important to examine the normal changes in these cognitive abilities across the life span. Timothy Salthouse (2004, 2011) combined data from 33 separate studies with 6,832 individuals to follow cognitive changes in terms of five major categories. Although memory is often seen as a problem of aging, other abilities are also affected. As can be seen in the graphs (*Figure 16-5* through *Figure 16-9*), there is a consistent picture of change over the life span for each category with the sole exception of vocabulary ability, which does not decrease over the life span.

The first is vocabulary based on measures in which the individual provided definitions of words, or named an object in a picture, or selected antonyms or synonyms. As seen in *Figure 16-5*, vocabulary ability remains fairly constant across the life span with even a slight increase as individuals approach their 60s.

The second ability is perceptual speed. This reflects the ability to quickly compare patterns of letters or match symbols. As can be seen in *Figure 16-6*, this ability declines steadily from age 30 on.

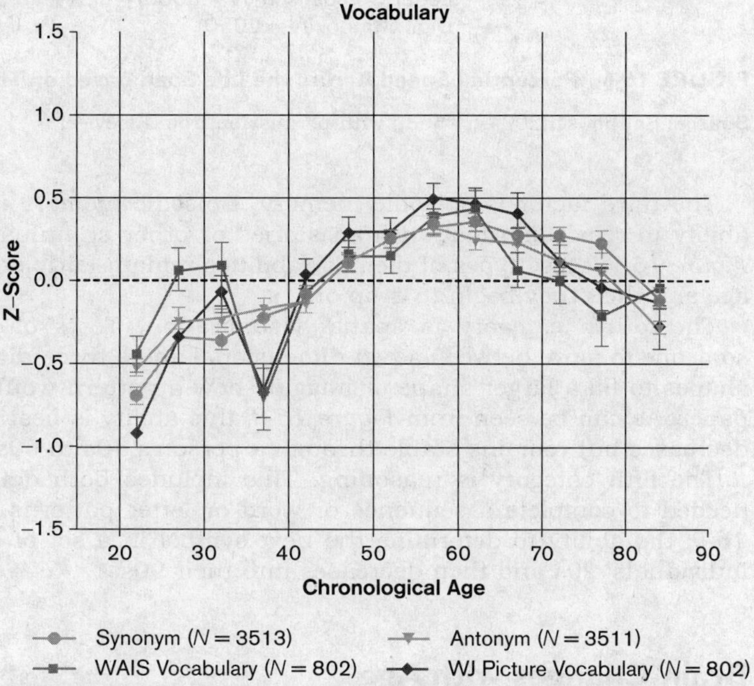

FIGURE 16-5 Vocabulary Abilities Across the Life Span Based on Four Different Measures

Source: Salthouse (2004, p. 553), with permission from Elsevier.

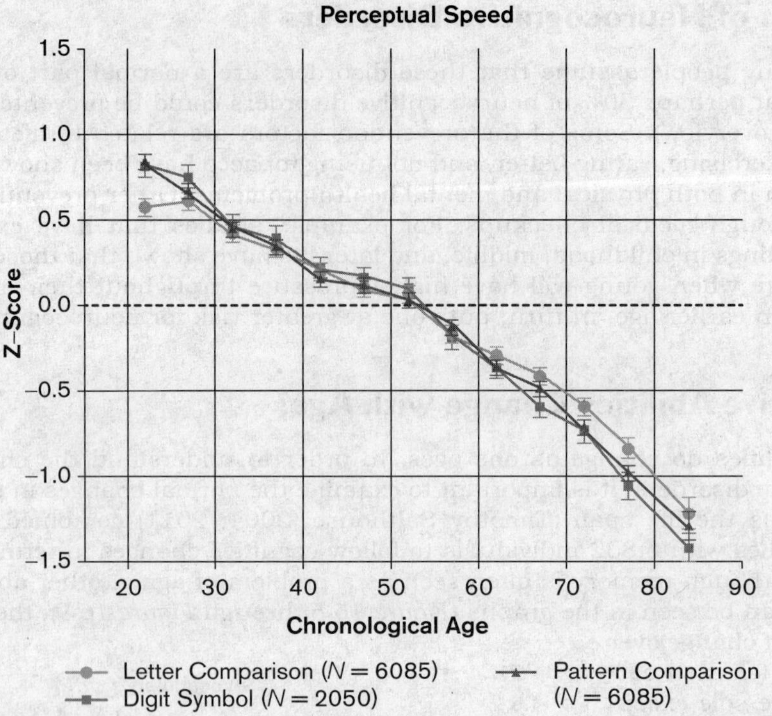

FIGURE 16-6 Perceptual Speed Across the Life Span Based on Three Different Measures

Source: Salthouse (2004, p. 553), with permission from Elsevier.

The third factor is episodic memory. Episodic memory in these studies refers to the ability to recall information from stories or other stimulus items. As can be seen from *Figure 16-7*, these types of memory abilities remain fairly stable until around 60 years of age and then they begin to drop off.

The fourth category is spatial visualization. Tests of spatial visualization require someone to move between a two-dimensional and a three-dimensional figure or determine shapes to fill a larger shape or imagine how a pattern would appear in a folded piece of paper. As can be seen from *Figure 16-8*, this ability is best in a person's 20s and 30s. It decreases but remains stable through a person's 40s to 60s. It then decreases rapidly.

The fifth category is reasoning. This includes both determining geometric patterns needed to complete a sequence or word or letter patterns. As can be seen from *Figure 16-9*, the ability to determine the next symbol in a set of geometric patterns is best in individuals' 20s and then decreases into their 90s.

Brain Changes with Age

Two consistent findings are that older adults show changes in brain structure and that they use their brains in different ways from younger adults (see Park & Reuter-Lorenz, 2009; Reuter-Lorenz & Park, 2010, for overviews). In terms of brain volume, volume reduction is seen in the hippocampus, cerebellum, prefrontal cortex (PFC), and caudate

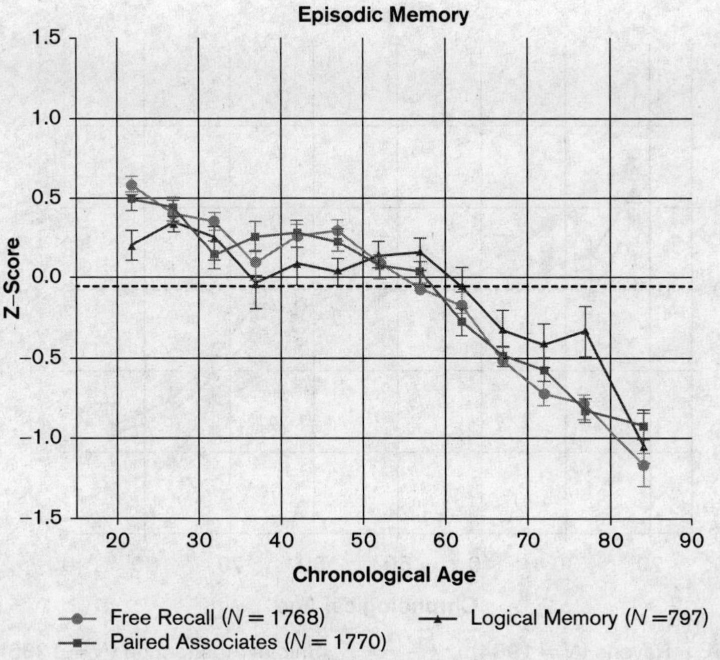

FIGURE 16-7 Episodic Memory Across the Life Span Based on Three Different Measures

Source: Salthouse (2004, p. 553), with permission from Elsevier.

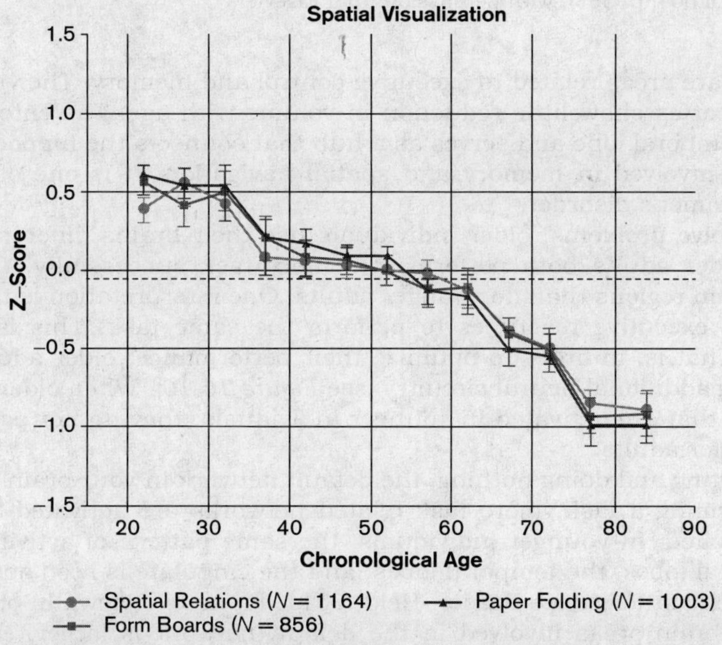

FIGURE 16-8 Spatial Visualization Across the Life Span Based on Three Different Measures

Source: Salthouse (2004, p. 553), with permission from Elsevier.

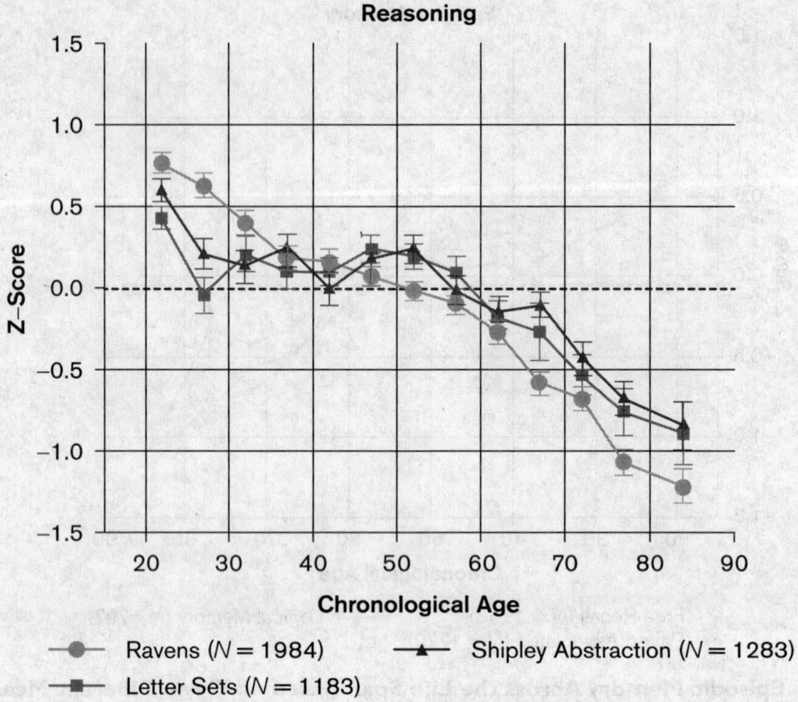

FIGURE 16-9 Reasoning Across the Life Span Based on Three Different Measures

Source: Salthouse (2004, p. 553), with permission from Elsevier.

nucleus, which are areas related to executive control and memory. The visual cortex and the entorhinal cortex show little reduction in volume with age. The entorhinal cortex is located in the temporal lobe and serves as a hub that connects the hippocampus and the neocortex. It is involved in memory and spatial navigation. It is one of the first areas affected in Alzheimer's disorder.

In order to solve problems, older individuals use their brains differently. Even when younger and older adults both perform a memory task successfully, the older adults recruit more brain regions than do younger adults. One interpretation is that older adults need additional executive resources to perform the same task. This is referred to as *compensation*. That is, in order to optimize their performance, older adults perform the same task using additional neural circuitry (see *Figure 16-10*). When older adults use just the brain areas that are activated in younger individuals, they do not perform the tasks as well as younger adults.

As you are sitting and doing nothing, the default network in your brain turns on. When you start performing a task, more task-related networks are activated and the default network is inhibited. In younger individuals, the same pattern of activity in the frontal lobes, the parietal lobes, the temporal lobes, and the cingulate is seen across a variety of tasks in numerous studies (see Beason-Held, 2011, for an overview). In older individuals, the number of brain areas involved in the default network is larger, especially in the frontal lobes. Older adults also have a more difficult time turning off the default network.

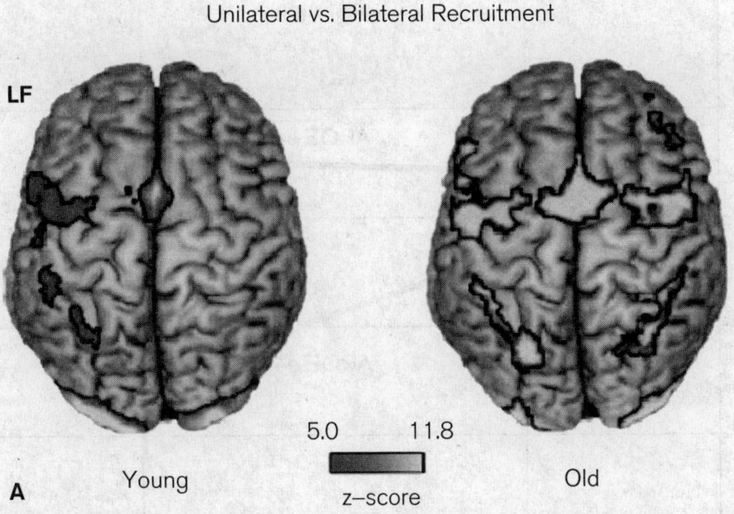

FIGURE 16-10 Older Adults Recruit More of Their Brain to Solve the Same Task as Younger Adults

Source: Schneider-Garces et al. (2010, Figure 4, p. 661). Reprinted by permission of MIT Press Journals © 2010, The MIT Press.

It is assumed that this is related to the problems some older adults have in shifting cortical resources to new tasks.

One interesting study followed a group of individuals in Scotland who were given an IQ test at age 11 and then again at age 79 (see www.lothianbirthcohort.ed.ac.uk/ for an overview). Beginning at age 79, they were also followed until they were 87, using a logical memory task. What the researchers discovered was that those individuals with a variant of the APOE gene referred to as the APOE4 allele showed more cognitive decline even in the absence of a neurocognitive disorder. *Figure 16-11* shows that at age 11, there was little difference in the IQ scores of those with and without the APOE4 allele. However, by age 79 those with the APOE4 allele showed a lower IQ score whereas those without this allele showed a similar IQ score to that seen when they were age 11. On the logical memory task, those with the APOE4 allele showed a decline over the next 8 years.

Can an Individual's Activities Be Protective in Brain Changes?

The answer to this question is yes. It was first noticed that not all individuals showed the same changes to similar neurocognitive disorders or brain injury. From this observation, the concept of **reserve** was developed. That is, high functioning individuals tend to show less loss of cognitive abilities in relation to neurocognitive disorders. The concept of reserve suggests that the brain can compensate for problems in neural functioning. This is illustrated by the case in which the brains of older individuals expand their networks to solve problems as shown in *Figure 16-10* earlier. High functioning or intelligence is often associated with greater reserve.

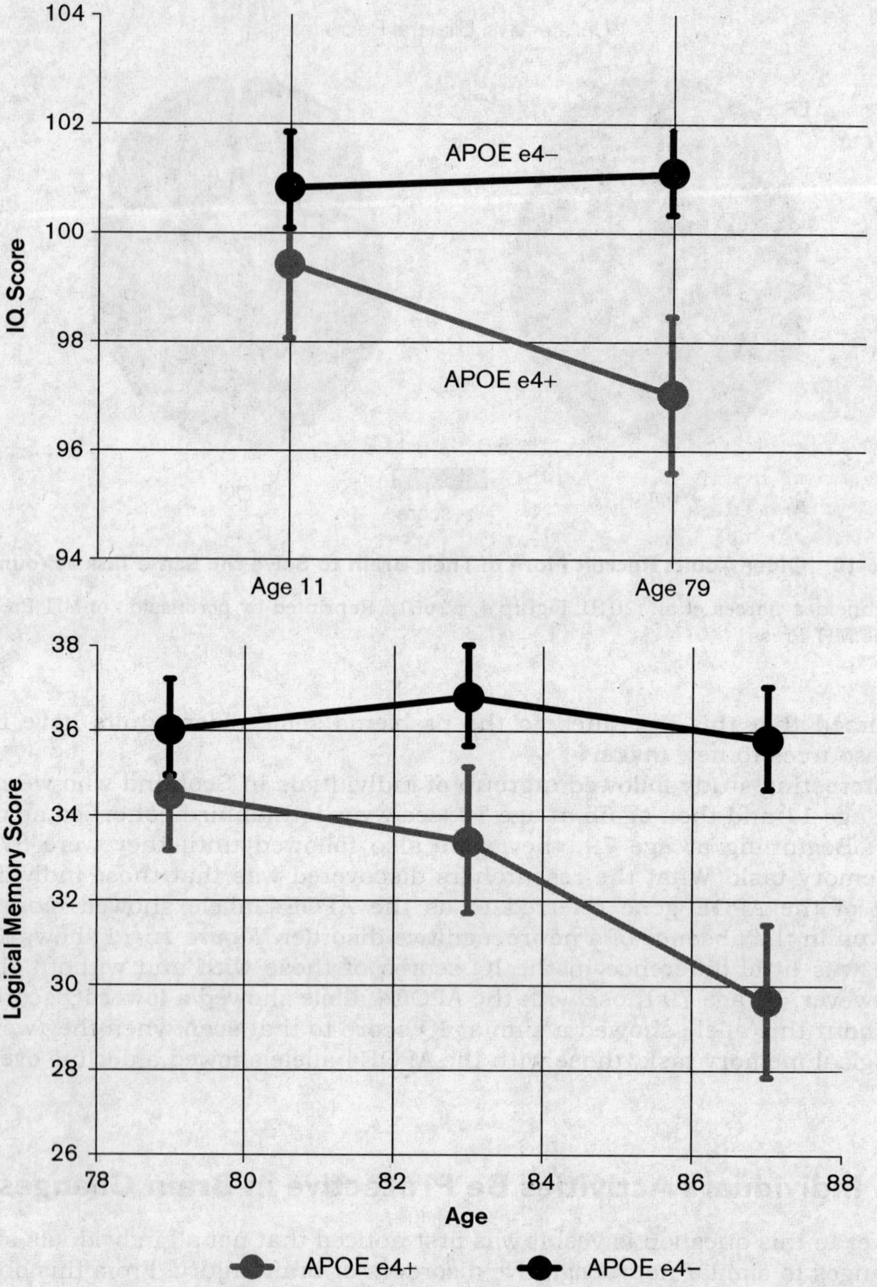

FIGURE 16-11 Presence of the APOE4 Allele Is Associated With Cognitive Decline in Individuals Without a Neurocognitive Disorder

Source: Harris and Deary (2011, p. 392), with permission from Elsevier.

Additional research has shown a role for exercise and social support. Exercise is thought to play an important role in aging by promoting healthy cardiovascular function. That is, exercise increases blood flow to the entire brain. Exercise has also been shown to slow the expression of Alzheimer's-like disorders in a mouse model. In a review of literature from different areas, Kramer & Erickson (2007) suggested that exercise provides multiple routes to enhancing cognitive vitality across the life span. These include the reduction of disease risk as well as improvement in molecular and cellular structures of the brain. This, in turn, increases brain function. Further, it is suggested that aerobic exercise affects executive function more than other cognitive processes.

Following more than 700 older individuals without neurocognitive disorders for several years, Aron Buchman and his colleagues (2012) found that daily physical activity slowed cognitive decline. Exercise was also associated with a lower risk for developing Alzheimer's disease. Although performing various types of cognitive tasks such as crossword puzzles or speaking a second language are also associated with successful aging, these brain effects appear to be more localized in those areas of the brain related to the specific task.

In order to better help articulate the causal role of exercise, Lindsay Nagamatsu and her colleagues (2013) randomly assigned older individuals who were beginning to show mild cognitive impairment to one of three groups. The first group received resistance training and lifted weights. The second group received aerobic training and walked outdoors at levels that increased their heart rate. The third group received balance and stretching exercises. The third group served as the control group. After 6 months of twice-weekly exercise, the first two groups showed improvement in memory functions. This was seen more strongly on a difficult spatial memory test. The aerobic group also improved performance on the verbal memory test. The important point of this study is that 6 months of exercise can improve memory in 70-year-olds.

Social support has also been associated with a reduced risk for neurocognitive disorders. Two of these factors are the size of one's network of friends and whether one is married or not. As suggested in studies of the social brain, understanding and maintaining networks of friends require a variety of cognitive resources, which in turn offer a reserve for dealing with brain pathologies. One study followed 16,638 individuals over the age of 50 for 6 years. Those individuals who were more socially integrated and active showed less memory loss during the 6-year period (Ertel, Glymour, & Berkman, 2008).

STUDIES FROM INDIA ON AGING CHANGES IN THE BRAIN

In a recent study, Apoorva, Kumar, and Marimuthu (2016) reported that a community sample of 90 healthy normal men and women participants between the age of 65 years and above, both literate and illiterate, were screened for dementia and psychiatric illness using Hindi mental Status Examination, Mini-international neuropsychiatric interview (MINI Screen) and Everyday Abilities Scale for India. Participants selected after screening were administered NIMHANS Neuropsychological Battery for elderly. Age-related cognitive decline were reported across the age groups on story memory, digit span, spatial span, wordlist learning, and recognition, stick construction and Go/No-Go tests.

In another interesting work reported from India (Jain and Kar, September 2014), focusing on the effect of cognitive aging on working memory consolidation, the researchers found using an attentional blink paradigm that decline in memory consolidation in aging may be determined by the reduction of inhibitory control processes. The decline in memory consolidation in an aging group may be due to difficulties in the early stages of perceptual processing, inhibitory control, and unsuccessful suppression of irrelevant stimuli. The authors report that these effects were also observed among middle-aged individuals.

Studying the molecular biology underlying dementia, Rao, Ramesh, Vasudevaraju, Rao (2010) opine that *DSM-IV* dementia criteria might underestimate dementia prevalence, especially in regions with low awareness. In this meta-analysis, they report a study from West Bengal where almost one-fourth (94/379, i.e., 24.5%) of all the patients with dementia were of young onset. Women constitute about one-third of these cases. The most common etiologies were Alzheimer disease (33%), fronto-temporal dementia (27%), and vascular dementia (20%). A positive family history was found in close to one-fifth of the patients. The authors also opine that dietary deficiencies of antioxidants and nutrients during aging precipitate dementias, perhaps due to failure of protective mechanisms.

Mild cognitive impairment is also often detected among aging patients, and reports from India also echo this finding. A research group from Mumbai (Nair, Urvashi Shah, et al., 2012) report the effectiveness of memory clinics for early detection. The authors of this study report that prevalence rates of dementia in India over the past two decades has ranged from approximately 1.4% among those 65 years and older to 3.5% among those 60 years and older in rural settings. In urban settings, prevalence rates have been reported at 2.44% among those 65 years and older. However, crude prevalence rates of dementia in India have been reported as high as 10.6% in persons 65 and older living in rural areas and 7.5% for those in urban areas. These findings underline the need for awareness-building and early detection. The paper is based on a cohort recruited between the years 2006 and 2010. A total of 212 participants were evaluated for cognitive complaints at a memory clinic at a large tertiary teaching hospital in Mumbai. Of these, as many as 58 patients, that is, 45.7%, had Alzheimer's disease (probable or possible); 28 (or 22%) had ischemic vascular dementia; and 15% and 11% respectively had mixed and fronto-temporal dementia. From among the non-dementia diagnoses, 43 (64.2%) had MCI.

DELIRIUM

Delirium is a short-term state of confusion. This short-term condition is characterized by a change in cognitive processing such as an inability to focus attention or problems with language, memory, or orientation. The idea of delirium dates back to at least the time of Hippocrates (see Caraceni & Grassi, 2011; Lindesay, Rockwood, & Macdonald, 2002, for overviews). In the 19th century, the term *confusion* was often used in relation to delirium. The role of physical illness, toxins including alcohol, and infections were historically seen as causes of delirium. The modern concept of delirium is based largely on the work of Lipowski (1980), who brought together a spectrum of acute cognitive problems that influence consciousness and are associated with medical illness. The fact that signs and symptoms associated with delirium fluctuate and are seen to be reversible has been used to differentiate it from more stable neurocognitive disorders.

The fifth edition of the *Diagnostic and Statistical Manual of Mental Disorders (DSM–5)* (APA, 2013) describes delirium as a disturbance in attention and awareness. That is, the person is less aware of his or her environment and has a reduced ability to direct and change the focus of attention. Additional cognitive disturbances such as memory, language, or perceptual disorders are seen. Further, delirium develops over a short period of time and shows fluctuations in severity during the day. In general, delirium develops in relation to another medical condition, including medication side effects or toxins.

Delirium occurs in up to 56% of older adults in general hospital populations (see Jones, Kiely, & Marcantonio, 2010, for an overview). It is seen in 15% to 53% of old individuals after a medical operation and in 70% to 87% of those in intensive care (American Psychiatric Association [APA], 2013). In a community sample, the prevalence of delirium is low (1%–2%) and increases with age to where the prevalence is 14% among those over 85 years of age. Overall, delirium is seen as a disturbance of consciousness that cannot be accounted for by neurocognitive disorders. Its onset is typically abrupt and lasts for only a few hours or days. It can be caused by a number of underlying physiological disturbances. As seen in the prevalence data, it is a frequent complication of hospitalization for older populations.

Delirium can manifest in a number of ways and be related to a number of causes. Problems with memory of recent events is one common manifestation of delirium. However, memory of older experiences is usually normal. Language problems are such that the person sounds incoherent, disorganized, and rambling. Writing problems may also be present. The person may also appear disoriented. Although delirium more often occurs in older individuals, it can also occur in young children. The following is the case study of Bobby Baldwin (not his real name).

CASE OF BOBBY BALDWIN
Delirium

Bobby Baldwin is a 7-year-old Caucasian male. He was taken to the hospital because he appeared to have ingested insecticide. While at the hospital, he was interviewed by a health care professional. When asked his address, he answered correctly but then spelled the name of the city and the word house. When asked about his birthday, he gave the wrong year for when he was born. He then said, "Jerry, get up and stand on this. Who said you could wear a blue jacket?" When asked about his hospital experience, he said, "Whose funeral—all the cars around mean a funeral—I was in the hospital 2 or 3 days." When asked about what he last ate, he said, "Today is Thursday—it's April—A B C. That is the alphabet. Jerry doesn't know the alphabet." He misperceived the 6'4", 200-pound health care worker as his mother. When identifying common objects, he answered all incorrectly—that is, a pen clip was a cross, a pen point was a cross and then a tent, and to the remaining objects he said, "How many hamburgers did you get?" He was unable to draw the geometric objects. Bobby also lost track in the middle of some of the tasks, such as counting backward.

When reexamined some three days later, Bobby was alert. He gave his correct birthday and address and knew what day it was. He could remember what he had last eaten. He could also draw geometric objects. He did complain of fatigue during the examination. The health care professional who examined Bobby concluded that there were no longer signs of delirium. Bobby did, however, show signs of mild central nervous system problems related to having ingested the insecticide.

Based on Dane G. Prugh, Samuel Wagonfeld, David Metcalf, and Kent Jordan. (1980). A Clinical Study of Delirium in Children and Adolescents [Supp.]. *Psychosomatic Medicine, 42*, 177–195.

MILD AND MAJOR NEUROCOGNITIVE DISORDERS

Neurocognitive disorders represent a condition in which a person shows cognitive deficits that are greater than those experienced with normal aging. These declines are typically shown in memory-related processes. Some older individuals call mild memory problems "senior moments" in which they cannot remember someone's name or a particular word. Some individuals show a progression in which it becomes more difficult to encode recent information or retrieve it from long-term memory. It is not uncommon for people with memory problems in old age to be able to remember events in great detail from their distant past while showing real problems remembering recent events.

In addition to memory problems, there can also be problems in a number of other cognitive processes. Complex attentional tasks in which the individual must divide her attention or pay attention to more than one process at a time may be difficult. Problems in executive functions that require planning, mental flexibility, and learning from mistakes can also be compromised. Declines in other tasks involving language and spatial abilities also decrease in neurocognitive disorders. In addition to cognitive tasks, the person may also show declines in social processes such as recognizing the intentions or emotions of others and being able to regulate one's own behavior.

As noted previously, a number of cognitive abilities are shown to decline with age. However, in many older individuals, these do not interfere with living a normal life. They may rely more on lists or friends to help them live independently. When cognitive or social deficits are greater than those seen with normal aging, this decline can be described in terms of **mild neurocognitive disorders** (see *Table 16-1*). If the declines are severe and interfere with one's ability to function independently, then these can be described in terms of major neurocognitive disorders (see *Table 16-2*). In *DSM–5*, the diagnosis of major neurocognitive disorder replaced the term *dementia*.

The diagnosis of a neurocognitive disorder is a two-step process. The first step is to determine if the person is showing normal changes related to aging, a mild neurocognitive disorder or a major neurocognitive disorder. With mild neurocognitive disorder, the person is

TABLE 16-1 Mild Neurocognitive Disorder

A.	Evidence of modest cognitive decline from a previous level of performance in one or more cognitive domains (complex attention, executive function, learning and memory, language, perceptual motor, or social cognition) based on: 1. Concern of the individual, a knowledgeable informant, or the clinician that there has been a mild decline in cognitive function; and 2. A modest impairment in cognitive performance, preferably documented by standardized neuropsychological testing or, in its absence, another quantified clinical assessment.
B.	The cognitive deficits do not interfere with independence in everyday activities (i.e., at a minimum, requiring assistance with complex instrumental activities of daily living such as paying bills or managing medications are preserved, but greater effort, compensatory strategies, or accommodation may be required).
C.	The cognitive deficits do not occur exclusively in the context of a delirium.
D.	The cognitive deficits are not better explained by another mental disorder (e.g., major depressive disorder, schizophrenia).

Source: Reprinted with permission from the *Diagnostic and Statistical Manual of Mental Disorders, Fifth Edition*, (Copyright 2013). American Psychiatric Association.

TABLE 16-2 Major Neurocognitive Disorder

A.	Evidence of significant cognitive decline from a previous level of performance in one or more of the domains (complex attention, executive function, learning and memory, language, perceptual-motor, or social cognition) based on: 1. Concerns of the individual, a knowledgeable informant, or the clinician that there has been a substantial decline in cognitive function; and 2. A substantial impairment in cognitive performance, preferably documented by standardized neuropsychological testing or, in its absence, another quantified clinical assessment.
B.	The cognitive deficits interfere with independence in everyday activities (i.e., at a minimum, requiring assistance with complex instrumental activities of daily living such as paying bills or managing medications).
C.	The cognitive deficits do not occur exclusively in the context of a delirium.
D.	The cognitive deficits are not better explained by another mental disorder (e.g., major depressive disorder, schizophrenia).

Source: Reprinted with permission from the *Diagnostic and Statistical Manual of Mental Disorders, Fifth Edition*, (Copyright 2013). American Psychiatric Association.

still able to function independently and do activities such as paying bills and taking medications on his or her own (see *Table 16-1*). When the person is no longer able to function independently, the diagnosis is major neurocognitive disorder. The second step is to determine what the neurocognitive disorder is due to. This includes Alzheimer's disease, frontotemporal lobar degeneration, Lewy body disease, vascular disease, substance/medication use, **human immunodeficiency virus (HIV)** infection, prion disease, **Parkinson's disease,** Huntington's disease, or another medical condition. I will describe the major causes of neurocognitive disorders in the next section. I begin with an extended discussion of Alzheimer's disease.

Concept Check

- What are the primary characteristics of successful aging? What can individuals and communities do to promote successful aging and why is that important?
- What is the relationship between cognitive changes in older adults and mental illness?
- What are the characteristics of each of the following in terms of triggering event, symptoms, treatment, and prevalence?
  - Delirium?
  - Mild neurocognitive disorder?
  - Major neurocognitive disorder?

It has been estimated that some type of neurocognitive disorder will impact around 15% of all individuals over age 65 and up to 45% of those over age 80. Since more extreme cases will require extensive care in a facility such as a nursing home, neurocognitive disorders require a large expenditure of resources on the part of the individual, his or her family, and society as a whole. Family members and caregivers in turn are at risk for a number of psychological problems including depression, anxiety, and stress. It has been estimated that about 10% of all health care costs are used for neurocognitive disorders. This is expected to increase in the future.

There is a complex relationship between cognitive changes in older adults and mental illness (see O'Hara, 2012, for an overview). One clear example is depression in older adults. With depression in this age range, memory and executive function are generally impaired. Similar findings are seen in anxiety in older populations. They show problems in cognitive performance, the ability to divide their attention, and memory recall. In one study looking at women 85 years of age and older, the researchers found that depressive symptoms were associated with cognitive impairment some 5 years later (Spira, Rebok, Stone, Kramer, & Yaffe, 2012). In fact, these individuals had 3 times the risk of developing mild neurocognitive impairment. Other studies have shown an increased prevalence of symptoms of mental illness in those with a mild neurocognitive disorder compared with similar age adults with normal cognitive processes (Teng, Tassniyom, & Lu, 2012). These symptoms of mental illness actually decreased the person's quality of life more than did decreases in their cognitive abilities.

INDIAN WORK ON MILD COGNITIVE IMPAIRMENT

There is a need to develop better measures to distinguish normal aging from MCI and both from Alzheimer's disease patients. In a study reported from NIMHANS (Balachandar, Tripathi, Bharath, & Kumar, 2015), the performance measures of cognitively normal group steeply worsened with increasing complexity. With receiver operating characteristic curve analysis, patients with mild Alzheimer's disease were poorly differentiated from cognitively normal group according to their Tower of Hanoi performance.

Another study from Hyderabad reported that a total of 12% of the cohort studied by them was classified by imaging biomarkers as having MCI with intermediate likelihood of AD, according to the NIA-AA criteria (Alladi, 2014).

Impact of MCI on caregiving is also studied (Trivedi, Subramanyam, Pinto, & Gambhire, 2013) and reports that the presence of behavioral problems in dementia results in higher caregiver distress for that group than the other two groups, and the presence of neuropsychiatric problems in MCI leads to greater caregiver distress than in caregivers of the normal aging.

An unpublished work, based on the doctoral thesis of Gauri Choudhary, shows that there often tend to be differences in the way an informant and the individual patient perceives the individual's capacity to perform a particular task or the improvement noticed.

In the study, it was seen that when asked specific questions about the subjects' cognitive functioning, the individuals have a different perception from their informant. One of the significant findings of this study is the importance of eliciting information from both, the individual and the informant. When a generic question is asked, checking if the person has become more forgetful, the patient is likely to respond in the affirmative but the caregiver will more likely be more specific.

Another finding was that cognitive retraining of persons with MCI can yield a marked advantage in the area of memory, helping to arrest the decline as compared to persons who have not availed of retraining (cited with permission from unpublished doctoral thesis of Dr. Gauri Chaudhary under the guidance of Dr. Anuradha Sovani).

Neurocognitive Disorder Due to Alzheimer's Disease

Neurocognitive disorder due to Alzheimer's disease is a progressive disorder characterized by problems with memory (see Selkoe, Mandelkow, & Holtzman, 2012, for an overview). It is associated with a loss of neurons and disruption of cortical networks, which result in cognitive problems. Initial memory problems may include forgetting names, misplacing household items, and forgetting the task one was about to undertake. As the disorder progresses, the person has more problems with finding words and may not be able to follow a familiar path from one location to another. The individual may also not undertake new tasks and withdraws socially. The health care professional may also see the person looking to his family for answers to personal questions that should be part of his own personal knowledge. In the later stages of the disorder, motor problems become apparent. This includes urinary incontinence. The person may also spend time in bed without acknowledging other people, including family, or speaking to those around her. Delusions and hallucinations are seen in a subset of individuals. On average, the full course of the disorder encompasses 10 to 20 years. The artist William Utermohlen drew self-portraits as his Alzheimer's disease developed.

As noted in President Reagan's letter to the American public, it is the family who experiences the greatest toll of the disorder as the person loses his memories and sense of self. At one point, his wife Nancy said, "Ronnie's long journey has finally taken him to a distant place where I can no longer reach him." It is hard for the children who had a relationship with their parent to lose this connection as well as watch it slowly disappear.

Alzheimer's disease is the most common neurodegenerative disorder in the world, and its prevalence is fairly similar worldwide (Prince, Bryce, Albanese, Wimo, Ribeiro, & Ferri, 2013). The prevalence for individuals in their 60s is between 1% and 2%, which increases to around 12% for people in their early 80s and then increases to over 40% for those in their 90s. It affects women about 3 times as often as men. In 2011, it was estimated that more than 5.4 million people in the United States had Alzheimer's disease. In the United States, Alzheimer's disease ranks sixth overall as the cause of death. At present, it is the only disorder in the top 10 causes of death that cannot be prevented, cured, or even slowed in its progression.

The disorder was first described by Alois Alzheimer in his report of a 51-year-old woman who displayed progressive memory loss and disorientation (Alzheimer, 1907; see Alzheimer, Stelzmann, Schnitzlein, & Murtagh, 1995, for English translation). Alzheimer had followed this woman for a number of years. After she died, Alzheimer examined her brain and identified two major factors that became hallmarks of Alzheimer's disorder. These are *neurofibrillary tangles* and *neuritic plaques* (see *Figure 16-12*). The tangles are found within the neuron whereas the plaques are extracellular deposits. Today, we know that β-amyloid (beta amyloid) is the core protein involved in extracellular amyloid plaques and that tau is the core protein of intracellular neurofibrillary tangles.

Alzheimer's disease is also associated with widespread synaptic and neuronal loss (see Nath et al., 2012, for an overview). During the progression of the disorder, the development of tangles follows a fixed pattern. The development of tangles begins in an area that is located in the temporal lobe and serves as a hub that connects the hippocampus and the neocortex, the entorhinal cortex. This then progresses to the hippocampus, which is associated with memory and then to other cortical areas along anatomical connections. The development of plaques does not follow a fixed pattern. The development of tangles is better correlated with cognitive decline than is

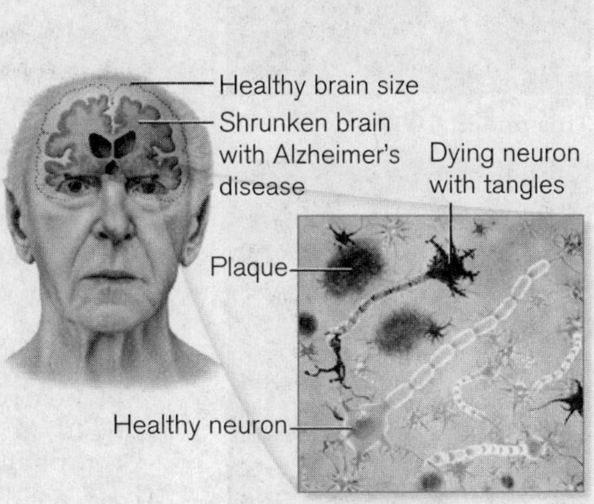

FIGURE 16-12 Brain Changes With Alzheimer's Disease—Neurofibrillary Tangles and Neuritic Plaques

Source: A.D.A.M., Inc.

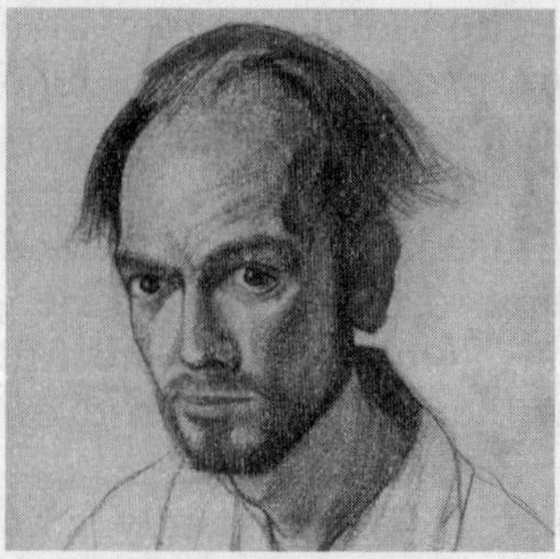

The Artist William Utermohlen Drew a self-portrait in 1967

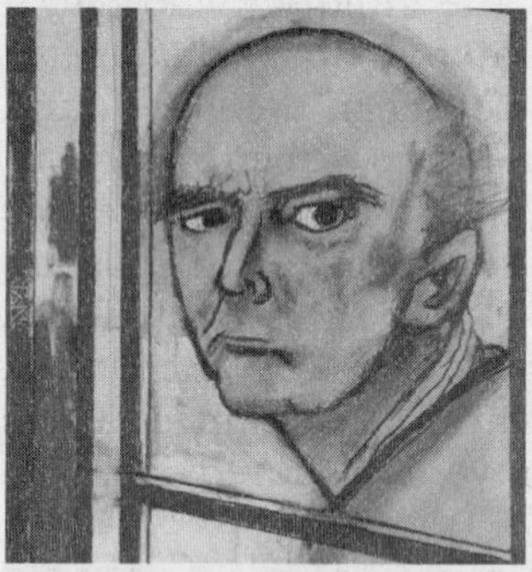

This one in 1996

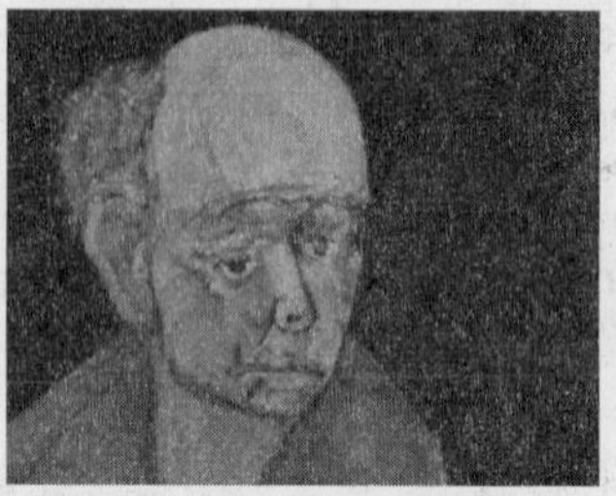

This one in 1997

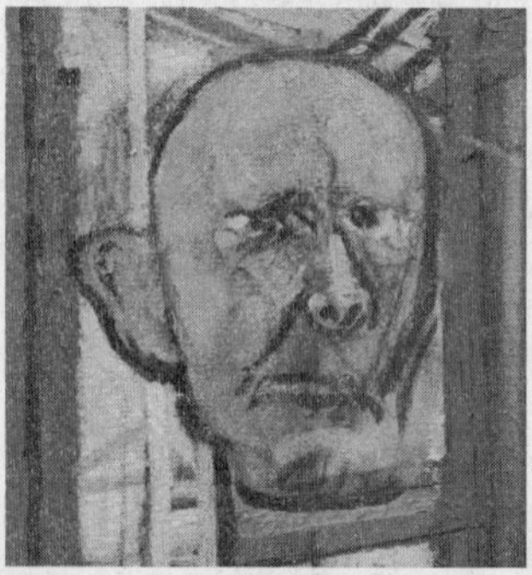

This one in 1998

Source: The above four images courtesy of galerie Beckel Odille Boico, Paris.

the development of plaques. Presently, Alzheimer's disease can only be diagnosed with certainty from brain studies after death although a number of imaging studies are suggesting alternatives to diagnosis for those still alive. See *Table 16-3* for the *DSM–5* diagnostic criteria for Alzheimer's disease.

TABLE 16-3 Neurocognitive Disorder Due to Alzheimer's Disease

A. The individual meets criteria for major or mild neurocognitive disorder.

B. There is insidious onset and gradual progression of impairment in one or more cognitive domains (for major neurocognitive disorder, at least two domains must be impaired).

C. Criteria are met for either probable or possible Alzheimer's disease as follows:

For major neurocognitive disorder:

Probable Alzheimer's disease is diagnosed if either of the following is present; otherwise, **possible Alzheimer's disease** should be diagnosed.

1. Evidence of a causative Alzheimer's disease genetic mutation from family history or genetic testing.
2. All three of the following are present:

A. Clear evidence of decline in memory and learning and at least one other cognitive domain (based on detailed history or serial neuropsychological testing).

B. Steadily progressive, gradual decline in cognition, without extended plateaus.

C. No evidence of mixed etiology (i.e., absence of other neurodegenerative or cerebrovascular disease, or another neurological, mental, or systemic disease or condition likely contributing to cognitive decline).

For mild neurocognitive disorder:

Probable Alzheimer's disease is diagnosed if there is evidence of a causative Alzheimer's disease genetic testing or family history.

Possible Alzheimer's disease is diagnosed if there is no evidence of a causative Alzheimer's disease genetic mutation from either genetic testing or family history, and all three of the following are present:

1. Clear evidence of decline in memory and learning.
2. Steadily progressive, gradual decline in cognition, without extended plateaus.
3. No evidence of mixed etiology (i.e., absence of other neurodegenerative or cerebrovascular disease, or another neurological, mental, or systemic disease or condition likely contributing to cognitive decline).

D. The disturbance is not better explained by cerebrovascular disease, another neurodegenerative disease, the effects of a substance, or another mental, neurological, or systemic disorder.

Source: Reprinted with permission from the *Diagnostic and Statistical Manual of Mental Disorders, Fifth Edition*, (Copyright 2013). American Psychiatric Association.

Genes and Alzheimer's Disease

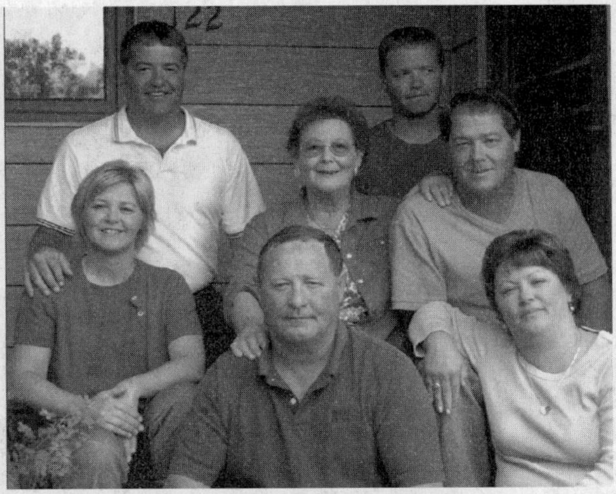

The DeMoe family from north Dakota; all of the family (except Karla at left) have a genetic makeup associated with early onset alzheimer's

Source: Shurkin (2009).

Family studies of those with Alzheimer's disease suggest that first-degree relatives (parents, siblings, and children) are at a greater risk for developing Alzheimer's. In fact, they have about 3 times the risk of developing the disorder. The photo to the left shows a portrait of the DeMoe family from North Dakota. All but one of the individuals pictured have a genetic makeup associated with early onset Alzheimer's.

Genetic studies also distinguish between those who show signs of the disorder before age 65 (early onset) and those who show signs of the disorder after age 65 (see Rademakers & Rovelet-Lecrux, 2009, for an overview). Individuals with early onset Alzheimer's show a stronger familial risk than the others. Early onset is associated with mutations in genes involved in encoding amyloid called APP and β-amyloid (beta amyloid) processing, especially the genes PSEN1 and PSEN2. That is, the presence of the β-amyloid protein is the primary component in the development of plaques (van Norden et al., 2012).

Late onset Alzheimer's has been consistently associated with an allele of the APOE gene. Individuals with one APOE4 allele have an increased risk that is about 2 to 3 times more than individuals without it. If an individual has two APOE4 alleles, the risk increases to between 7 and 15 times. By contrast, the APOE2 gene is associated with a longer life and not having Alzheimer's disease. The gene APOE is involved with removing β-amyloid. One current theory of Alzheimer's disease is that the substances involved in the development and removal of plaques are not functioning correctly allowing for their buildup. Current drug treatments for Alzheimer's disease seek to lower the production of β-amyloid. It has also been shown that those who engage in cognitively stimulating activities in their early and middle life show fewer problems associated with β-amyloid (Landau et al., 2012).

One surprising finding is that healthy older adults who do not show cognitive problems may also have abundant plaques. Additionally, plaques and tangles are found in individuals who do not show the loss of neurons seen in Alzheimer's disease. Cognitive reserve and the brain's ability to reorganize networks to compensate may play a role in these individuals. At this point, the role of plaques and tangles in Alzheimer's disease is still being worked out, although all individuals with Alzheimer's disease show tangles and plaques and a loss of neurons (see van Norden et al., 2012).

Neuroimaging of Alzheimer's Disease

There would be an advantage to know who would develop Alzheimer's disease in the future (see Koch et al., 2012; Mevel et al., 2011, for overviews). One promising approach is to study brain metabolism. In one study, it was found that those areas that correspond

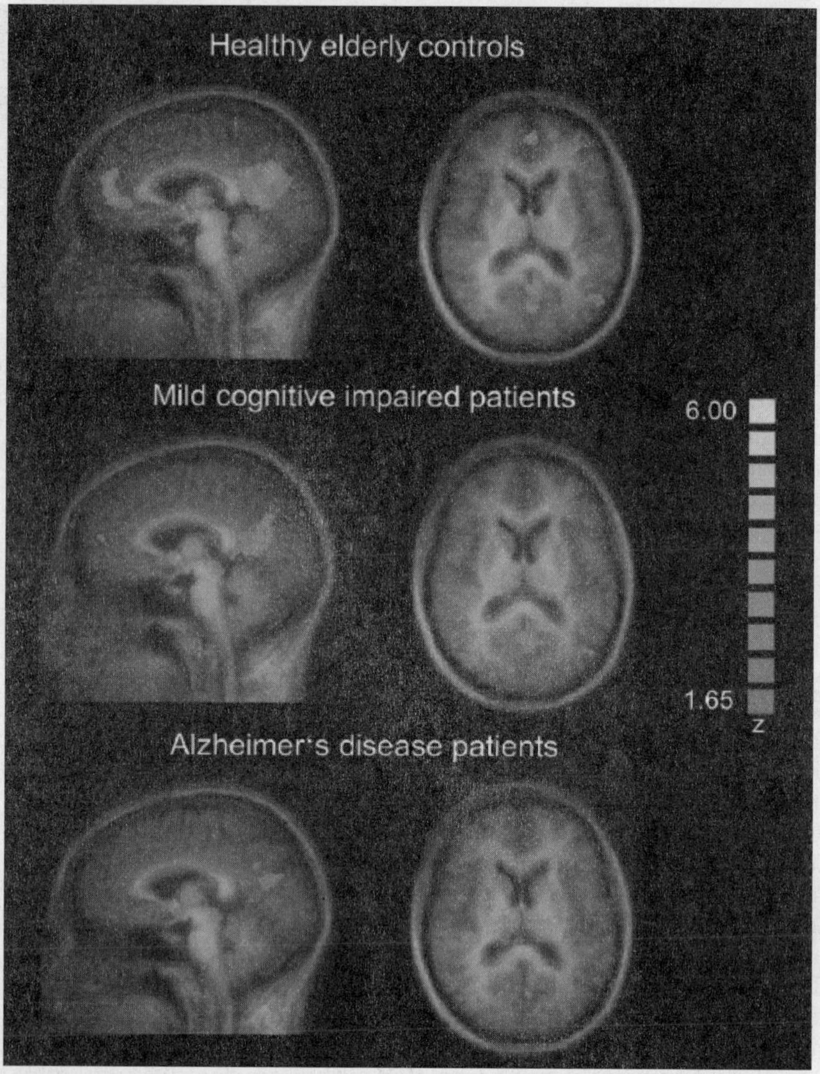

FIGURE 16-13 Magnitude of Impairment in the Brain for Patients with Alzheimer's Disease

Source: Koch et al. (2012, p. 471), with permission from Elsevier.

to the default network in young adults corresponded to those areas with amyloid deposits in elderly individuals with Alzheimer's (see *Figure 16-13*). In addition, the connection between the posterior cingulate and the hippocampus appears to be impaired in Alzheimer's disease. Individuals with Alzheimer's show less activation of the default network than healthy elderly controls. It is assumed that the deposit of amyloid plaques in these areas is related to lower glucose metabolism as well as atrophy. Thus, changes in the default network could be an important biomarker of those at risk for Alzheimer's disorder.

"Cultural considerations were key to engaging the community. Since this is a culture that holds high respect for elders, discussing what may be viewed as shortcomings (i.e., cognitive symptoms) can be viewed as a sign of disrespect. Thus, separate, private interviews with individual informants and family members were an important provision in order to collect unhindered information about true deficits. Additionally, same-gendered interviewers also facilitated more forthcoming discussion of behavioral symptoms that may be viewed as socially inappropriate (e.g., hypersexuality, abusive behaviors). In addition, some of the items of the basic and instrumental activities of daily living were not culturally relevant measures of functioning. For example, the item that measures the participant's ability to eat rates eating with one's hands as impaired, but among this population eating with one's hands is quite common and culturally normal.... The spoken version of many Indian languages lacks a term for dementia, and 'memory impairment' is frequently used to describe a wide range of deficits; thus, exhaustive interviews with informants were often required to obtain a clear understanding of the presentation."

The study from which quotes are reported is also partially supported by NIH grant to Mount Sinai Alzheimer's Disease Research Center (P50 AG05138; PI: M. Sano).

A study by Ravikesh Tripathi et al. (2015) concluded that word list learning with delayed recall component is a possible candidate for detecting MCI from normal aging. Persons with MCI performed significantly poorer than NC on word list (immediate and delayed recall), story recall test, stick construction delayed recall, fluency and Go/No-Go test. Measures of episodic memory especially word list delayed recall had the highest discriminating power compared with measures of semantic memory and executive functioning.

Vascular Neurocognitive Disorder

Concept Check

- What are the primary changes in the brain related to Alzheimer's disease?
- What is the characteristic progression of symptoms in Alzheimer's disease?
- What is the genetic risk for Alzheimer's disease?

Vascular problems such as strokes can lead to a neurocognitive disorder. It can be one large stroke or a series of smaller ones. Approximately 8% of individuals who have a stroke go on to develop a neurocognitive disorder. **Vascular neurocognitive disorder** is the second most frequent cause of neurocognitive disorder after Alzheimer's disease. Problems in cognitive performance are usually seen as abrupt changes following the stroke. These abrupt changes are one characteristic that differentiates vascular neurocognitive disorder from Alzheimer's disease although the symptoms may appear similar.

In the late 1800s, the disorder was referred to as "arteriosclerotic dementia" (see Erkinjuntti, 2005, for an overview). With increased research related to blood flow in the brain, it became apparent that a number of factors influence how blood is delivered to the brain and converted for cognitive and motor processes. Without blood flow, there is a lack of oxygen, which can lead to brain damage. The term *vascular neurocognitive disorder* reflects the role of blood flow in cognitive performance.

Frontotemporal Neurocognitive Disorder

Frontotemporal neurocognitive disorder was originally known as *Pick's disease* since Pick first described brain changes in those with this disorder in 1892. The disorder is characterized by a reduction of the anterior lobes of the frontal and temporal areas. The parietal and occipital lobes do not show this reduction. Prevalence rates are about 2 to 3 per 100,000 people (see Neary, 2005, for an overview). This disorder may be seen as early as the third decade of life.

Frontotemporal neurocognitive disorder is seen in different variants depending on the brain areas involved. Anne Adams, to whom I will introduce you in the next section, had a variant that shows a loss of language abilities. Another variant gives a pattern of impairment not unlike that seen in Phineas Gage, the railroad worker who received a rod through his brain (see Chapter 4). It is not so much cognitive impairment that is seen. Rather, there are behavioral and personality changes that come to the forefront. These include a lack of social awareness, a lack of insight, indifference, inappropriate behaviors, stereotyped behaviors, aggression, and a loss of inhibition. Some of these characteristics may be manifested in terms of eating. That is, the person will eat discriminately and may even take food from others' plates. The person may also show repetitive motor behaviors such as hand rubbing or foot tapping. He or she may also repeat the same phrase or do the same activity at the same time each day. Visuospatial skills tend not to be impaired, as you will see in the extended case study of Anne Adams (this is her real name).

The Development of Frontotemporal Neurocognitive Disorder in a Scientist and Artist

This section describes an extended case study in which an individual with frontotemporal neurocognitive disorder shows deficits in cognitive abilities, especially language. However, as she experienced these deficits, other areas of the brain became more active and increased her creativity. Dr. Anne Adams graduated from college with honors degrees in physics and chemistry. She taught college chemistry before taking time off to raise her children. After returning to work, she received a PhD in cell biology and taught for the next 4 years. At that point, her son was involved in a life-threatening motor vehicle accident. While taking care of her son, she went back to an old interest in art and began to paint. Surprisingly, her son recovered in 7 weeks but she continued to paint. She had a desire to paint and would spend all day in her studio.

Unknown to her, she was developing a neurocognitive disorder, which changed the relationship of networks in her brain. William Seeley and his colleagues followed these changes in her brain processes and in her art in the journal *Brain* (Seeley et al., 2008). Using structural and functional imaging, these researchers were able to show that as Anne Adams lost brain processing in the frontal and temporal areas, she was able to create enhanced connections in the right posterior areas including the right parietal, which is involved in spatial relationships as would be necessary for creativity in art. One intriguing scientific question relates to the manner in which loss in one area may increase abilities in another. In this case, the loss of language was associated with an increase in creativity and

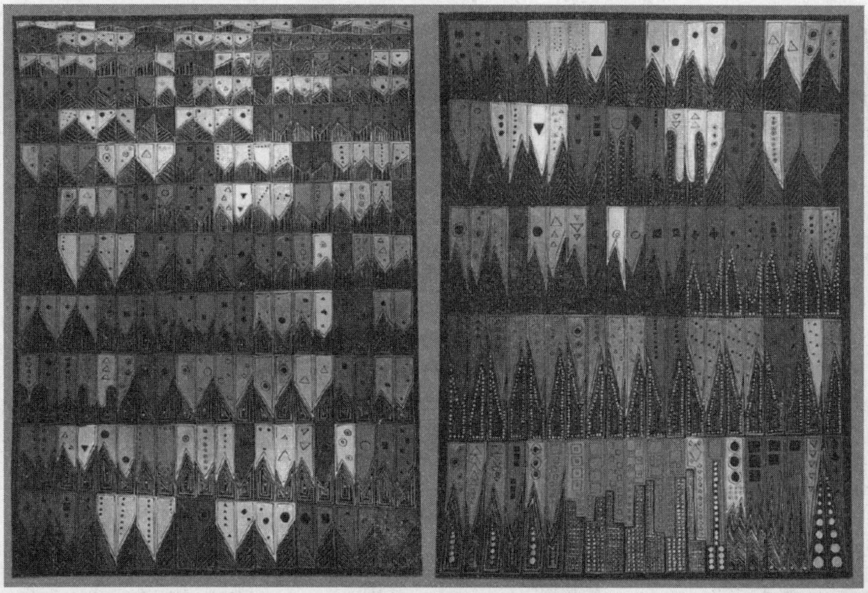

FIGURE 16-14 ***Unraveling Boléro*. Painting by Anne Adams**

Source: Courtesy of Robert A. Adams.

artistic abilities. Fortunately, Anne Adams kept extensive notes on the nature of her paintings, which detailed the manner in which she related her paintings to music and mathematics.

In a strange coincidence, Anne Adams became interested in the French composer Maurice Ravel (1875–1937), best known for his work *Boléro*. *Boléro* is a piece of music that is highly structured. The strange coincidence is that Ravel at the time in his life that he was writing *Boléro* may have begun to develop the same neurocognitive disorder that was to be manifested in Anne Adams a century later. At this point, at age 53, she turned the music of *Boléro* into art in the form of a visual analysis of the piece (see *Figure 16-14*). Each of the vertical panels represents a specific bar in the music. This was some seven years before any of her symptoms appeared.

At age 58, she moved from painting music to more abstract patterns such as those found in mathematics. One of Anne

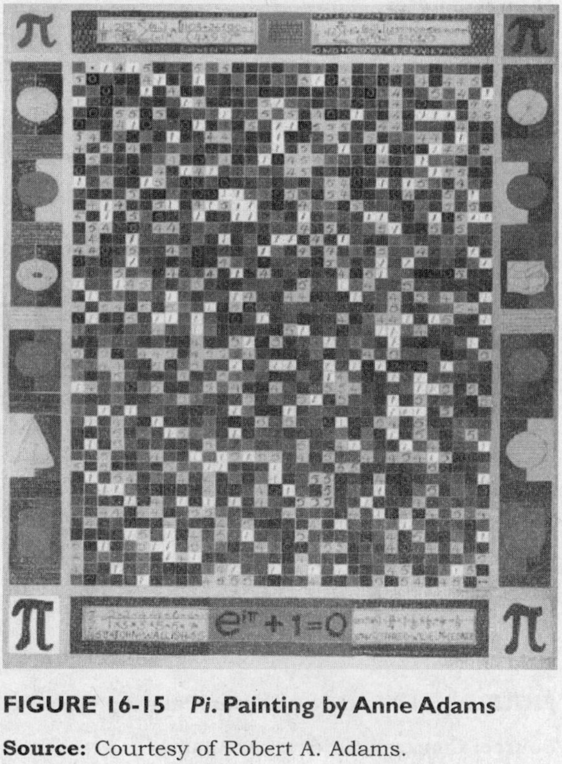

FIGURE 16-15 ***Pi*. Painting by Anne Adams**

Source: Courtesy of Robert A. Adams.

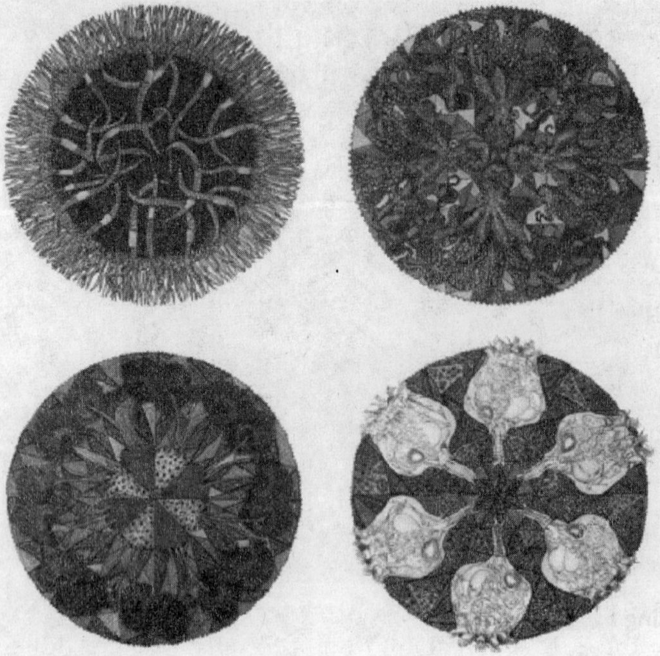

FIGURE 16-16 Examples from Anne Adams's *ABC Book of Invertebrates*

Source: Courtesy of Robert A. Adams.

Adams's paintings with this theme was called *Pi* (see *Figure 16-15*). This was 2 years before her symptoms appeared.

Anne Adams's symptoms began to appear around age 60 with difficulties in speech. However, comprehension remained intact. By age 64, she was nearly mute with only 3- or 4-word phrases at best. With the development of her symptoms, she also shifted her painting style to one of realism with high surface fidelity. Her paintings at this time were very symmetrical.

During the next 4 years, her paintings emphasized a certain type of realism (see *Figure 16-17*), including surfaces of buildings (see *Figure 16-18*).

Figure 16-19 shows the loss of brain areas in Anne Adams relative to the painting she was producing at the time.

The case of Dr. Anne Adams portrays a person with frontotemporal neurocognitive disorder who shows deterioration in language abilities over time. However, as she was losing language abilities she began to display greater creativity

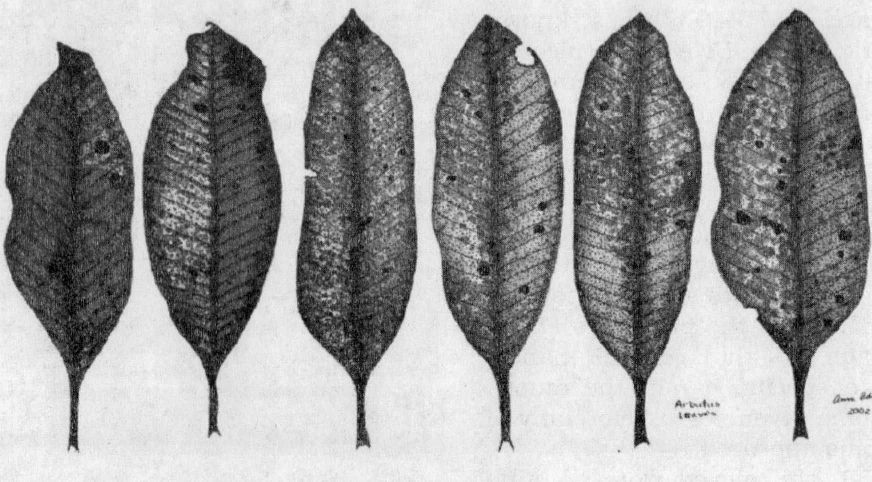

FIGURE 16-17 *Arbutus Leaves.* Painting by Anne Adams

Source: Courtesy of Robert A. Adams.

according to those who worked with her. Thus, she showed compensation and increased reliance on other areas of the brain related to creativity. Unlike the artist William Utermohlen, for whom you could see the deterioration of his artistic abilities in his painting due to Alzheimer's disorder, Anne Adams showed shifts in the types of images that she focused on and the levels of detail that she emphasized (Seeley et al., 2008). As she was losing her speech, she emphasized a spatial language in her paintings.

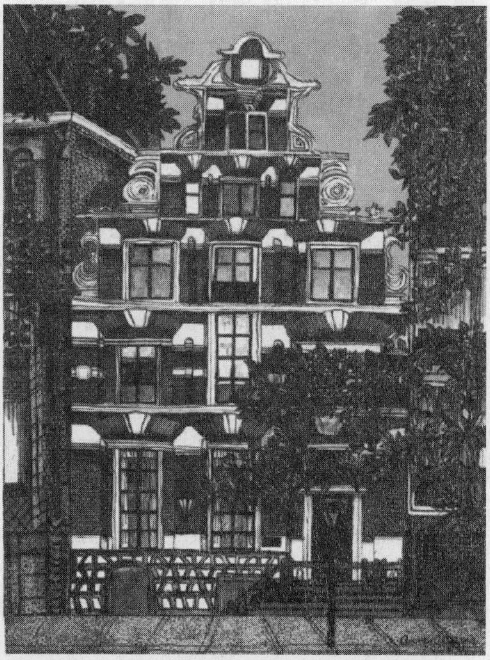

FIGURE 16-18 ***Amsterdam*. Painting by Anne Adams**

Source: Courtesy of Robert A. Adams.

Neurocognitive Disorder Due to Traumatic Brain Injury

Traumatic brain injuries (TBIs) are seen across the life span (see Silver, McAllister, & Yudofsky, 2011, for an overview). Acceleration and deceleration forces on the brain as it impacts with the skull commonly lead to injuries, which often produce diffuse microstructural injury. The severity of these injuries can range from mild to severe. Mild TBIs are often referred to as *concussions*. Common sources of

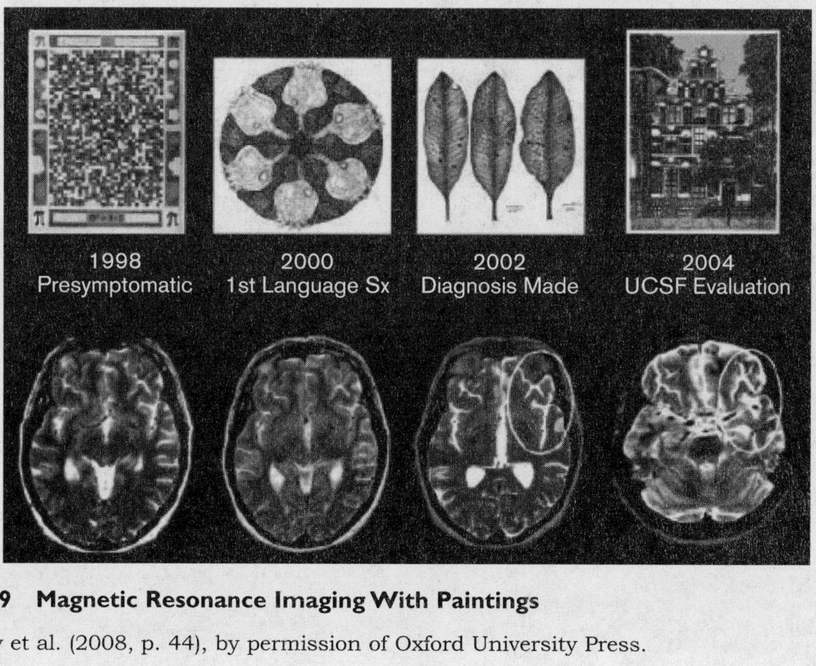

FIGURE 16-19 Magnetic Resonance Imaging With Paintings

Source: Seeley et al. (2008, p. 44), by permission of Oxford University Press.

TBIs are sports, transportation accidents, and falls in the elderly. Some are one-time-only events and others are repeated, such as concussions in contact sports. Boxers show a syndrome referred to as "punch-drunk." This is seen in aging boxers and characterized by slowed thought as well as changes in emotional processing. The National Football League (NFL) and college football associations in the United States have recently begun a number of studies to determine the long-term effects of concussions on the players. The U.S. military has also noted an increase in TBIs, at times along with post-traumatic stress disorder (PTSD), in soldiers involved in the conflicts in the Middle East. Worldwide, TBIs are a critical public health problem that can lead to a variety of neurocognitive and psychological problems.

These problems can include loss of consciousness, cognitive deficits, depression, and, at a later period, the onset of neurocognitive disorder. The types of deficits seen in individuals with TBI vary in terms of the areas of the brain affected by the injury. It is estimated by the Centers for Disease Control and Prevention (CDC) that in the United States, some 1.7 million occurrences of TBIs happen each year with about 2% of the population having TBI-related disabilities (Faul, Xu, Wald, & Coronado, 2010—www.cdc.gov/traumaticbraininjury/pdf/blue_book.pdf). The following LENS describes what has been called a silent epidemic: the presence of concussion in sports.

16-1 LENS
The Silent Epidemic of Concussion in Sports

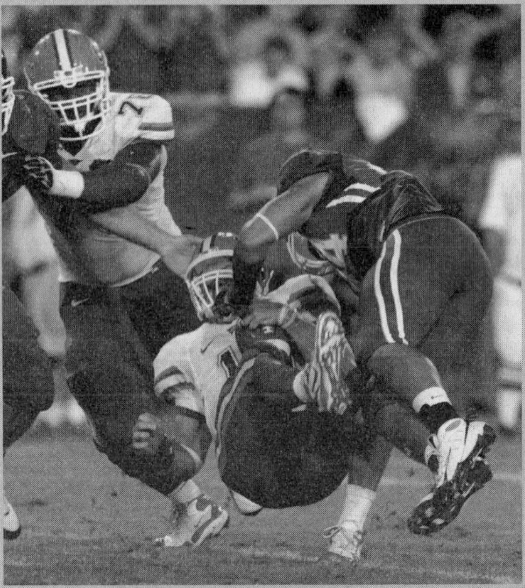

Florida quarterback Tim Tebow, center, is sacked and suffered a concussion that put him in the hospital.

© AP Photo/James Crisp

For years, few people paid attention to the encounters observed in contact sports. One of the most common injuries—concussion—has been referred to as a "silent epidemic." It was assumed that there were no long-term consequences of concussion. However, this has recently changed as more individuals have come forward to discuss the effects of playing such sports as football years ago. Ted Johnson, a former New England Patriots linebacker, had multiple concussions that resulted in significant memory and emotional problems throughout his 30s. Previously, athletes just "played through the pain." The former Denver Broncos and Washington Redskins running back Clinton Portis described his experiences as follows:

The truth is I had a lot of concussions. . . . It was just the way things were at the time. I'd get hit hard and be woozy. I'd be dizzy. I'd take a play off and then go back in. Sometimes when I went back into the game, I still couldn't see straight. This happened all the time. Sometimes once or twice a game. (Davenport, 2013)

It is now known that a person is most susceptible to another concussion for about 10 days after the first. Research has suggested that older retired professional football players experience neurocognitive disorders at 5 times the national rate. It is becoming more apparent that repetitive blows to the head affect the brain in negative ways, which can lead to neurocognitive disorders. Often, it is not contact with another person but a person's head hitting the ground that produces the concussion. Also, it is not limited to men; women who play such sports as field hockey are also at risk. The symptoms of concussion in men and women are very similar. Even a fall from a bicycle can result in a concussion.

In response to a new recognition of the effects of concussion, a number of groups have changed their approach. The NFL now supports studies of the long-term effects of concussion in professional athletes. Many universities have established centers for the study of concussion, and all but three states have established laws related to concussion assessment and management in high school athletics as well as return-to-play guidelines. High school athletes are particularly at risk since surveys suggest that this group believes that there is not a problem playing sports with a concussion. Returning to play before the concussion has been fully resolved can increase long-term injuries. Since adolescence is a time in which an individual's brain goes through a series of cortical reorganizations, brain insults at this time put the adolescent at greater risk for serious injury. Further, as risk takers, adolescent athletes may even deny there is a problem so they can continue to play. For college and professional athletes, different pressures may cause players to ignore information concerning the effects of concussion. Overall, this can lead to a lack of candor when athletes at all levels describe their symptoms.

The CDC now offers a number of programs directed at athletics at all levels for the care and prevention of concussion and also works with the National Collegiate Athletic Association (NCAA) (www.cdc.gov/concussion/sports/index.html). Professional football now has individuals in the press box who look for potential concussions on the field and immediately report this to team physicians. Many college programs engage in intensive baseline neuropsychological and neuroscience testing, which can be compared with a person's performance after a concussion to help determine when the person should return to play. It is no longer the case that a concussion should be seen as unimportant.

Based on Semyon Slobounov and Wayne Sebastianelli. (2014). *Concussions in Athletics: From Brain to Behavior.* New York: Springer Publishing.

Neurocognitive Disorder Due to Lewy Body Dementia

Lewy bodies are substances found in the neuron (see *Figure 16-20*). When these Lewy bodies build up, symptoms of a neurocognitive disorder, called **Lewy body dementia,** become apparent. The symptoms include changes in alertness and attention, which can result in drowsiness or staring into space. Other symptoms include visual hallucinations and Parkinson's-like symptoms, which begin a year after the cognitive impairment begins. The prevalence of this disorder is estimated to be less than 5% of the elderly population (APA, 2013). When autopsies have been conducted, Lewy bodies are seen in 20% to 35% of those with a neurocognitive disorder.

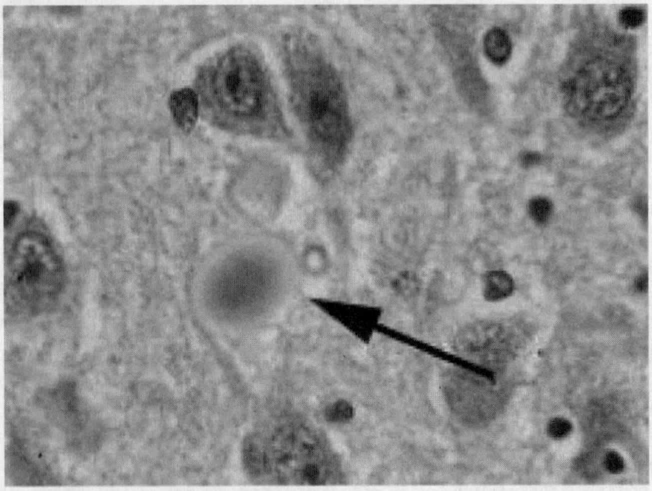

FIGURE 16-20 Lewy Body

Source: U.S. National Library of Medicine National Institutes of Health.

Neurocognitive Disorder Due to Parkinson's Disease

Parkinson's disease is a condition that affects the motor system. The symptoms generally include tremors, which may involve the hands, arms, legs, jaw, and face. In addition, the person shows a slowness of movement and stiffness in his limbs. Other motor problems such as poor balance and coordination may be present. In addition, there may be problems with sleep patterns. As the disorder progresses, the ability to walk may be lost and a wheelchair is required. Parkinson's disease typically begins after the age of 60 and affects about 1% of the people over age 60 and 3% over age 85. It affects men more often than women.

In Parkinson's disease, damaged nerve cells are found in the part of the brain stem referred to as the substantia nigra. There are two types of problems seen in this area. The first is a loss of neurons that create dopamine. Parkinson's disease does not become apparent until 60% of the dopamine neurons in the substantia nigra are lost or dopamine levels in the basal ganglia fall by 80%. Treatment of Parkinson's disease typically involves drugs that replace the lost dopamine. The second type of problem is the presence of Lewy bodies in the substantia nigra and locus coeruleus in the brain stem.

About a third of the individuals with Parkinson's disease continue to develop a neurocognitive disorder. Neurocognitive symptoms are generally not seen in the early stage of Parkinson's, but are found in about 40% of 70-year-olds. The cognitive characteristics are similar to those found in neurocognitive disorder due to Lewy body dementia. These include inflexibility and problems with executive functions. It is suggested that the progression of the neurocognitive disorder is related to the migration of the Lewy bodies from the motor areas to the cortex. Hallucinations may also be seen but this may be related to the increase of dopamine in the brain. These hallucinations tend to be of a visual rather than auditory nature.

Indian Work on Parkinson's Disease

Much work is also being done in India on Parkinson's disease. A study from NIMHANS reports poor prospective memory performance in PD (Ramanan & Kumar, 2013) "more likely due to failure in self-initiated retrieval of intention to be executed, rather than forgetting the content of the intention itself."

A research group from Mumbai working with Parkinson's Disease and Motor Disorder Society (PDMDS) has attempted to set up community-based Parkinson's rehabilitation centers across various urban, rural, and tribal settings—41 urban, 3 peri-urban, 1 tribal and 3 rural centers working on community-based rehabilitation for Parkinson's disease patients have emerged from this project. The group has presented their work summarizing the comparisons across such settings and the challenges posed by them.

Interestingly, they have attempted the use of dance movements in the rehabilitation of person with Parkinson's disease, and specifically have used Indian dance techniques. Data of 16 participants from the Indian dance group and 11 from traditional exercise group has been analyzed. The findings show that participants in the dance intervention group improved significantly on mood as measured by PANAS ($p = 0.02$) and HADS ($p = 0.02$) as compared to participants in traditional exercise group, leading to the conclusion that dance intervention using Indian dance techniques can be used as an alternative or supportive therapy along with traditional exercises, with the added benefits that it helps improve mood and alleviate depression of persons with Parkinsonism. (reported with permission of authors, Sovani, Kumawat, & Joshi, 2012).

Another important contribution of the group has been to create standardized multidisciplinary models for the care of persons with Parkinsonism. Studies have showed this model to be clear and novel in content. It was seen to be easily deliverable by lay facilitators, who had never worked with this population earlier. It was reported by users to be comprehensible and relevant to persons with Parkinson's disease as well as their caregivers. It was time efficient and generated interest and could be adapted to the needs of different groups. It was rated as practical, beneficial, and logical in its flow and sequencing of sessions. Effective if delivered in a group format, such a model has high utility in underserved areas of a vast and low resource setting such as India.

The research group has also been working on segments if the population that was irregular in their attendance of support groups and are attempting to develop an approach that focuses on patient engagement and ownership right from the induction. They opine that this can promote better adherence to community neuro-rehabilitative services.

In a paper, Wandrekar, D'souza and Barretto (2014) researched, 50 individuals with Parkinson's disease were administered the Movement Disorder Society's Unified Parkinson's Disease Rating Scale, Hoehn and Yahr's Scale, Mini Mental Status examination, and their caregivers were asked to complete the Zarit Burden Interview. The researchers report that caregivers suffering from ill health and the patients' MDS-UPDRS scores significantly affected caregiver burden ($p < 0.03$). Simultaneous multiple regression analysis showed that MDS-UPDRS Parts I, II, and III were significant predictors of burden ($R2 = 0.72$, $p < 0.0001$) of which the motor examination emerged as the most significant predictor of burden.

Neurocognitive Disorder Due to HIV Infection

HIV is a virus that can be passed on by coming in contact with the bodily fluids of an infected person. Common means of contact include unprotected sex or sharing a needle for drug use or tainted blood. It can also be seen in infants born to infected women. The virus affects the person's immune system in a negative manner. In the later stages, this is referred to as **acquired immune deficiency syndrome (AIDS).** About a third of the individuals with AIDS will also show neurocognitive problems such as slowing in both cognitive and motor functions. These include memory problems, confusion, depression, and difficulty with fine motor tasks. Prior to the development of AIDS drugs, many individuals died of disorders related to a compromised immune system. Today, drug treatments have successfully increased life span and reduced neurocognitive problems of those with HIV/AIDS.

Substance-Induced Neurocognitive Disorder

The abuse of drugs over a period of time can lead to neurocognitive deficits, referred to as **substance-induced neurocognitive disorder.** These drugs can include illegal substances as well as medications. Toxins such as lead, mercury, and carbon monoxide are also included as potential causes of neurocognitive problems. One common substance that can lead to cognitive changes is alcohol. This is especially the case when combined with poor nutrition. There is also some suggestion that the toxic effects of alcohol make the person more susceptible to the negative effects of a head injury. Alcohol is seen as the third leading cause of neurocognitive disorder and affects more women than men.

Neurocognitive Disorder Due to Huntington's Disease

Huntington's disease is a genetic disorder that causes a degeneration of neurons in the brain (see Gusella & MacDonald, 2006). It is one of the few disorders that has a single cause—a gene—in all people. A child of an individual with Huntington's disease has a 50-50 chance of inheriting the gene that produces the disorder. Typically, this disorder does not become apparent until around 40, which is after the childbearing years. This loss of brain cells results in cognitive, emotional, and motor disturbances. The cognitive deficits include problems with executive function, memory, arithmetic, and spatial ability. There are fewer problems with language functions. Emotional disturbances include mood swings and depression. Motor problems include both voluntary movements in which the person may appear clumsy and involuntary movements such as jerking of the body.

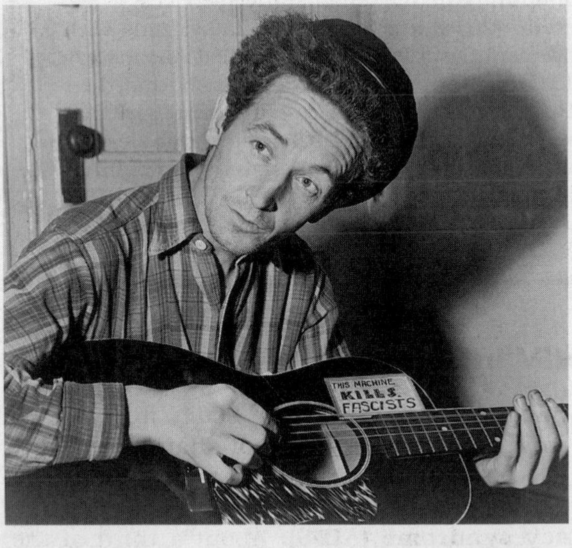

The Folk Singer Woody Guthrie, who wrote such songs as "this land is your land," suffered from Huntington's disease

Neurocognitive Disorder Due to Prion Disease

Prions are infectious pathogens that are different in structure and the diseases they cause from other pathogens such as bacteria, fungi, parasites, and viruses. They produce tiny holes in the brain, which give it a spongy appearance and result in **neurocognitive disorder due to prion disease.** Prion proteins occur in natural form in all brains and are harmless. The general public became aware of prions with the advent of "mad cow disease," also called *bovine spongiform encephalopathy*, which spread through the food chain to humans in the United Kingdom in the 1990s. It is not infectious in the usual sense of the word but is spread through eating the brain tissue of a diseased organism. A similar disorder was found in an isolated tribe in Papua New Guinea whose members ate brains as a part of funeral rites.

A related disease that also causes brain degeneration is Creutzfeldt–Jakob Disease, a disorder described by Creutzfeldt and Jakob in the 1920s. This disorder can also have a genetic component that is estimated to be related to 10% of the occurrences of the disorder. Overall, these disorders affect about 1 in a million people. Creutzfeldt–Jakob Disease typically occurs in individuals over 60 with about 90% dying within a year. During this time, there are cognitive impairments including memory loss, motor problems, personality changes, and impaired judgment. Although the cognitive problems may be similar to other neurocognitive disorders, it has a more rapid course of development and can be distinguished on autopsy by the spongelike changes in the brain.

Concept Check

- What are the defining characteristics of each of these neurocognitive disorders, including triggering event, time of onset, symptoms, and treatment?
  - Vascular neurocognitive disorder?
  - Frontotemporal neurocognitive disorder?
  - Neurocognitive disorder due to TBI?
  - Neurocognitive disorder due to Lewy body dementia?
  - Neurocognitive disorder due to Parkinson's disease?
  - Neurocognitive disorder due to HIV infection?
  - Substance-induced neurocognitive disorder?
  - Neurocognitive disorder due to Huntington's disease?
  - Neurocognitive disorder due to prion disease?

SUMMARY

As we age, our mental and physical abilities change. Some of these changes happen gradually and appear to be related to genetic differences. Other changes happen more quickly. They may lead to not only physical changes but also changes in mental processing, including neurocognitive disorders. This contrasts with what has come to be called normal successful aging. Perhaps 50% of neurocognitive disorders could be prevented through lifestyle changes and preventive medical care. In order to understand the changes seen in neurocognitive disorders, it is important to examine the normal changes in cognitive abilities across the life span, including (1) vocabulary, (2) perceptual speed, (3) episodic memory, (4) spatial visualization, and (5) reasoning. Two consistent findings are that older adults show changes in brain structure and that they use their brains in different ways from younger adults, using compensation to improve their performance. High functioning or intelligence, exercise, and social support are all associated with a greater reserve and overall brain health to provide for compensation.

There is a complex relationship between cognitive changes in older adults and mental illness. Studies have shown that symptoms of mental illness actually decreased the person's quality of life more than did decreases in their cognitive abilities. Delirium is a short-term condition characterized by a change in cognitive processing and can be caused by a number of underlying physiological disturbances. When cognitive or social deficits are greater than those seen with normal aging, this decline can be described in terms of a mild neurocognitive disorder. If the declines are severe and interfere with one's ability to function independently, then these can be described in terms of major neurocognitive disorders. *DSM–5* defines a variety of neurocognitive disorders.

Neurocognitive disorder due to Alzheimer's disease is a progressive disorder characterized by problems with memory. It is associated with a loss of neurons and disruption of cortical networks, which result in cognitive problems. Alzheimer's disease is the most common neurodegenerative disorder in the world, and its prevalence is fairly similar worldwide. Neurofibrillary tangles and neuritic plaques as well as widespread synaptic and neuronal loss in the brain are the hallmarks of Alzheimer's disorder. There is a genetic risk for developing Alzheimer's disease. Changes in the default network, as shown in neuroimaging studies, could prove to be an important biomarker or predictor of those at risk for Alzheimer's disorder.

Vascular neurocognitive disorder can result from vascular problems such as strokes—either one large stroke or a series of smaller ones. Frontotemporal neurocognitive disorder has different variants depending on the brain areas involved. It can present as cognitive impairment or behavioral and personality changes. Neurocognitive disorder due to TBI occurs across the life span as a result of a one-time-only traumatic event or a series of smaller injuries. It results in slowed thought as well as changes in emotional processing. Neurocognitive disorder due to Lewy body dementia results in a buildup of Lewy bodies in the neuron. Symptoms include changes in alertness and attention. Parkinson's disease is a condition that affects the motor system. About a third of the individuals with Parkinson's disease continue to develop a neurocognitive disorder. The cognitive characteristics are similar to those found in neurocognitive disorder due to Lewy body dementia. About a third of individuals with AIDS will also show neurocognitive problems, referred to as neurocognitive disorder due to HIV infection, such as slowing in both cognitive and motor functions. The abuse of drugs or alcohol over a period of time can lead to neurocognitive deficits, referred to as substance-induced neurocognitive disorder. Huntington's disease is a genetic disorder that causes a degeneration of neurons in the brain, referred to as neurocognitive disorder due to Huntington's disease, resulting in cognitive, emotional, and motor disturbances. It is one of the few disorders that has a single cause—a gene—in all people. Prions are infectious pathogens that produce tiny holes in the brain, which give it a spongy appearance and result in neurocognitive disorder due to prion disease. A related disease that also causes brain degeneration is Creutzfeldt–Jakob Disease, which can have a genetic component. These two diseases have a rapid course of development, and cognitive impairments include memory loss, motor problems, personality changes, and impaired judgment.

STUDY RESOURCES

Review Questions

1. This chapter on neurocognitive disorders talks a lot about the process of aging and the diseases experienced by older adults. Does that mean it has no personal meaning for you or your friends—at least for a few more years? Present an argument that this information is vitally important for young people to know.

What evidence would you cite to support your position and convince them that they should care?

2. Alzheimer's disease is the most common neurodegenerative disorder in the world, and currently, it is the only disorder in the top 10 causes of death that cannot be prevented, cured, or even slowed in its progression. What would be your focus of research in each of these three important areas: prevention, cure, and slow progression? Which one would you start with?
3. "One intriguing question relates to the manner in which loss in one area may increase abilities in another." This question arises in relation to the case of Anne Adams, whose creativity and artistic abilities increased at the same time she was developing frontotemporal neurocognitive disorder. Using this example, as well as the concepts of brain reserve and compensation presented at the beginning of the chapter, what can we say about the plasticity of the brain, that is, the brain's ability to reorganize and repurpose itself to be able to function?

For Further Reading

Arnett, P. (Ed.). (2013). *Secondary influences on neuropsychological test performance.* New York: Oxford University Press.

Bayley, J. (1999). *Elegy for Iris.* New York: Picador.

Favdin, L., & Katzen, H. (Eds.). (2013). *Handbook on the neuropsychology of aging and dementia.* New York: Springer.

Lipton, A., & Marshall, C. (2013). *The common sense guide to dementia for clinicians and caregivers.* New York: Springer.

Key Terms and Concepts

acquired immune deficiency syndrome (AIDS)
delirium
dementias
frontotemporal neurocognitive disorder
human immunodeficiency virus (HIV)
Huntington's disease
Lewy body dementia
major neurocognitive disorders
mild neurocognitive disorders
neurocognitive disorder due to Alzheimer's disease
neurocognitive disorder due to prion disease
neurocognitive disorders
Parkinson's disease
reserve
substance-induced neurocognitive disorder
successful aging
traumatic brain injuries (TBIs)
vascular neurocognitive disorder

CHAPTER

17

The Law and Mental Health

CHAPTER OUTLINE

- THE LEGAL SYSTEM AND THE INSANITY DEFENSE 615
- ETHICAL AND LEGAL ISSUES IN TREATMENT 618
- NEW DEVELOPMENTS ON THE INDIAN LEGAL SCENARIO 622
- NEUROSCIENCE AND EVOLUTIONARY PERSPECTIVES ON THE LEGAL ASPECTS OF PSYCHOPATHOLOGY 628
- SUMMARY 630
- STUDY RESOURCES 631

3/30/81
12:45 P.M.
Dear Jodie,

There is a definite possibility that I will be killed in my attempt to get Reagan. It is for this very reason that I am writing you this letter now.

As you well know by now I love you very much. Over the past seven months I've left you dozens of poems, letters and love messages in the faint hope that you could develop an interest in me. Although we talked on the phone a couple of times I never had the nerve to simply approach you and introduce myself. Besides my shyness, I honestly did not wish to bother you with my constant presence. I know the many messages left at your door and in your mailbox were a nuisance, but I felt that it was the most painless way for me to express my love for you.

I feel very good about the fact that you at least know my name and know how I feel about you. And by hanging around your dormitory, I've come to realize that I'm the topic of more than a little conversation, however full of ridicule it may be. At least you know that I'll always love you.

Jodie, I would abandon this idea of getting Reagan in a second if I could only win your heart and live out the rest of my life with you, whether it be in total obscurity or whatever.

I will admit to you that the reason I'm going ahead with this attempt now is because I just cannot wait any longer to impress you. I've got to do something now to make you understand, in no uncertain terms, that I am doing all of this for your sake! By sacrificing my freedom and possibly my life, I hope to change your mind about me. This letter is being written only an hour before I leave for the Hilton Hotel. Jodie, I'm asking you to please look into your heart and at least give me the chance, with this historical deed, to gain your respect and love.

I love you forever,
John Hinckley

Source: law2.umkc.edu/faculty/projects/ftrials/hinckley/hinckleytrial.html

The story goes that John Hinckley became obsessed with the film Taxi Driver *in which a character played by Robert De Niro plans to kill a presidential candidate. After watching the film a number of times, John Hinckley became infatuated with the actress Jodie Foster, who was in the film. He followed her when she went to college at Yale. He left her notes, but she did not respond. After a period of time, he decided that he would need to do something serious to get her attention. He considered a number of extreme situations to get her attention. As his letter to Jodie Foster states,* "Jodie, I would abandon this idea of getting Reagan in a second if I could only win your heart and live out the rest of my life with you, whether it be in total obscurity or whatever. I will admit to you that the reason I'm going ahead with this attempt now is because I just cannot wait any longer to impress you."

The next day, John Hinckley tried to kill President Reagan. At his trial, John Hinckley was found not guilty by reason of insanity.

As we watch and listen to the media, we are at times told about horrific events. Just in 2011 and 2012, three such events happened in the United States. A U.S. House of Representatives member, Gabby Giffords, was shot outside a grocery store in Tucson, Arizona, along with six other people being killed. Someone appeared inside a movie theater during a midnight showing in Aurora, Colorado, in tactical clothes. The audience initially thought it was part of the movie event. But then James Holmes began to shoot people randomly. A young adult went into a school in Newtown, Connecticut, and shot children and teachers. Before going to the school, Adam Lanza shot and killed his mother at their home. Each of these individuals clearly was involved in a crime. As with any other crime, the person would have the opportunity for a trial and be found guilty or innocent. However, the media labels these individuals as "mentally ill." If they do have a

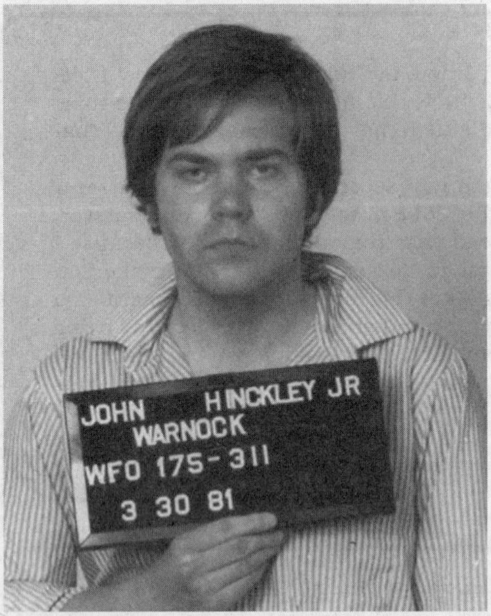

John Hinckley

mental illness, how does this influence the manner in which the justice system views the actions of these three individuals who shot someone else? This attempted assassination indeed became world news and all of us globally need to think about what definitions we wish to have in place vis-a-vis mental illness and the term "insanity" as it is used in law.

An interesting book, Amita Dhanda (2000) begins the Introduction with the words, "Mental illness is a medical problem—what has law got to do with it?"

In reality, although there may be a gap in the terminology used in legal and mental health contexts, the concept of unsoundness of mind may indeed impinge upon a number of crucial activities we undertake, including our personal liberty, family life, economic affairs, and political status.

What is in legal contexts labelled insanity may impinge upon capacity to litigate, to enter contractual agreements, capacity to marry, adopt a child, vote, or hold public office.

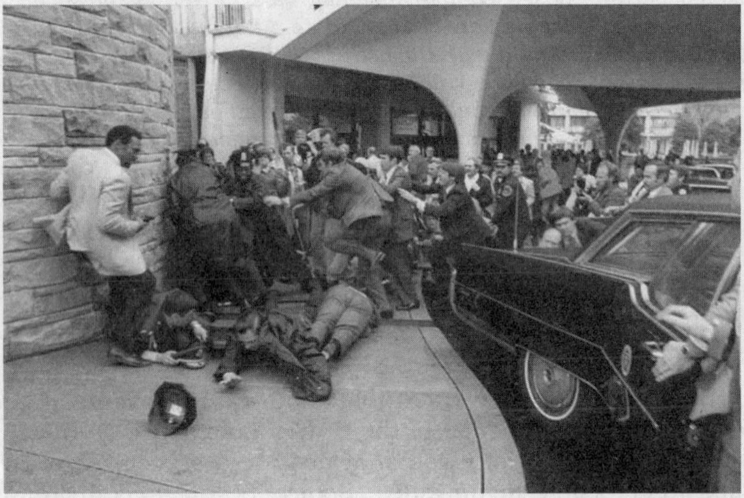
Scene outside a Washington, D.C., hotel as John Hinckley was trying to kill the president of the United States

Another equally important issue is the care and treatment of the mentally ill. Indian laws have witnessed many changes around this issue over the years. The year 1858 witnessed the Indian Lunatic Asylums Act and in the current context, it is easy to see that even the nomenclature of this act was pejorative and stigmatizing. The Indian Lunacy Act came in existence in the year 1912.

As we know, the Indian Constitution contains a chapter on Fundamental Rights, including the right to personal liberty and equality. The Mental Health Act, 1987, which had been passed on 22 May 1987, thus came into being and of late has seen a lot of rethinking and revision.

India also has the Code of Criminal Procedure (CrPC), 1973, which requires the accused to be informed of the accusation against him or her, which is where again unsoundness of mind may come into play.

One of the most recent developments on the Indian legal as well as mental health scene is the Indian Mental Healthcare Act, 2017, seen as a highly progressive piece of legislation (Duffy & Kelly, 2017). So also, India already had the PWD or Persons with Disabilities (Equal Opportunities, Protection of Rights, Full Participation) Act, 1995, in place, which was replaced by another significant Indian Legislative reform, the Rights of Persons with Disabilities Act, 2016, which is explicitly in lieu with the United Nations Convention on the Rights of Persons with Disabilities (UNCRPD), 2006.

The Mental Healthcare Act, which was passed on April 7, 2017, is still under a lot of discussion, and there have been voices of praise as well as dissent. However, it does have several positive features that are being highlighted in several publications. The key features seem to be the right to access to mental health services, the right to confidentiality, to live with dignity, right to personal contacts and communication, the right to protection from cruel, inhuman, or degrading treatment, and the right to treatment equal to persons with physical illness, among others. There is also provision made for advanced directives, and mental health promotion and mental illness prevention programs, all of which mark a positive change.

Insanity is a legal term, not a psychological one. Law courts are designed to determine who is responsible for an event. The level of analysis is the individual. Is the individual responsible for the event or not? Legal determinations focus on the individual level whereas considerations in this book have emphasized a number of levels ranging from the genetic level to the cultural one. Neuroscience perspectives view mental illness as a complex process that is influenced by a number of factors. Legal considerations focus on determining if an individual is responsible or not. The underlying assumption is that a person has free will and should be held accountable for his or her actions. If she breaks the law, then she is found guilty. The law is one way in which societies regulate themselves. What if the person does not have free will? Is he still responsible for his actions? This has been a question that societies have debated.

THE LEGAL SYSTEM AND THE INSANITY DEFENSE

All cultures throughout time have sought to determine the role of an individual's responsibility in committing criminal acts. The American system of justice in relation to insanity was initially influenced by an event that happened in England more than 170 years ago. An individual named Daniel M'Naghten (pronounced *McNaughton*) believed that he was being persecuted by the Tory party, one of the political parties of England. In response to this belief, M'Naghten planned to kill the British prime minister Sir Robert Peel. However, he ended up attacking and killing the prime minister's secretary rather than the prime minister himself. When M'Naghten was tried for the crime, medical experts said he was psychotic. Today, he would be described as someone with paranoid schizophrenia. He was acting under the delusion of believing that the pope and the prime minister were conspiring against him. The court found M'Naghten not guilty by reason of insanity. There was some concern about the verdict on the part of the public, which resulted in a more formal definition of mental insanity. However, in 1843 it was determined that mental insanity could be used as a defense only if the following was found:

> At the time of the committing of the act, the party accused was labouring under such a defect of reason, from a disease of the mind, as not to know the nature and quality of the act he was doing;

> or, if he did know it, that he did not know he was doing what was wrong. (*Queen v. M'Naghten*, 8 Eng. Rep. 718 [1843])

This came to be known as the **M'Naghten rule.** The two basic conditions for the M'Naghten rule to apply are that there is the presence of a mental disorder and that there is a lack of comprehension of the nature or wrongfulness of the act. As you can imagine, it is difficult to determine someone's state of mind at a previous time, such as when the crime was committed. Further, it is difficult to determine if a disease of the mind is present and what is a disease of the mind. Generally, psychosis is thought of in these cases. However, many of the disorders you have considered in this book, such as post-traumatic stress disorder (PTSD), substance abuse, and bipolar disorder, could all impair judgment and action.

In the United States, a number of variations based on capacity and knowledge have been applied in determining sanity. In the 1880s, the state of Alabama found an individual not guilty by reason of insanity because mental illness made the person unable to control himself even though he knew the difference between right and wrong. This came to be known as the **volitional test.** This was often described as the elbow test. That is, if a policeman was standing next to the person, would she still commit the crime? Again, it is difficult to determine an individual's state of mind after the fact. In fact, this has been a rarely used legal principle in modern times.

In the 1950s, a decision based on an 1871 New Hampshire ruling became known as the **Durham rule,** or "product test." The basic idea is that an individual is not "criminally responsible if his unlawful act is the product of a mental disease or defect." One problem with this approach is that a person could understand that he was committing a crime and still be found not guilty by reason of insanity. As with other approaches, it was hard to define and limit the definition of a mental disease. Most states in the United States dropped this approach by the 1970s, and federal judges rejected the approach in 1972.

With all of the problems experienced with the insanity plea, the American Law Institute (ALI) in 1962 developed a broader approach to not guilty by reason of insanity. Their formulation, known as the **ALI rule,** is defined as follows:

> A person is not responsible for criminal conduct if at the time of such conduct as the result of mental disease or defect he lacks substantial capacity either to appreciate the criminality (wrongfulness) of his conduct or to conform his conduct to the requirements of the law.

This approach broadens the M'Naghten rule. Instead of requiring a defendant to have no understanding whatsoever of the nature of his acts or the difference between right and wrong, the ALI rule requires merely that he or she lack a "substantial capacity" to understand right from wrong and expands the M'Naghten rule to include an "irresistible impulse" component. Other parts of the ALI rule also eliminated criminal antisocial acts as being covered.

The insanity defense was changed drastically by an event on March 30, 1981. On that day in Washington, D.C., John Hinckley tried to kill the president of the United States, Ronald Reagan. Rushed to the hospital with a serious chest wound, President Reagan survived the shooting. John Hinckley was a person who after 2 years of college where he played his guitar, listened to music, and watched television dropped out and moved to Hollywood. He planned to make it as a songwriter although he had no musical training. While in Hollywood, John Hinckley saw the movie *Taxi Driver*, the story of a psychotic taxi driver who contemplates political assassination and rescues a young prostitute who was played by the actress Jodie Foster. This movie influenced John Hinckley, who saw the

After her death, the parents of Tatiana sued the campus police, health service employees, and regents of the University of California for failing to warn them that their daughter was in danger. The trial court initially dismissed the suit. At the time, most courts had ruled that a doctor had a duty to a patient but not to a third party. The appeals court supported the dismissal. An appeal was then taken to the California Supreme Court.

In 1974, the California Supreme Court reversed the appeals court ruling. The court held that a therapist bears a duty to use reasonable care to give threatened persons such warnings as are essential to avert foreseeable danger arising from a patient's condition. This is known as the Tarasoff I decision. The Tarasoff I decision meant that the trial court was instructed to hear the lawsuit against the police and various employees of the University of California. Due to great uproar among psychiatrists and policemen, the California Supreme Court took the very unusual step of rehearing the same case in 1976. This case came to be known as Tarasoff II.

The legal statement that the court issued was as follows:

> When a therapist determines, or pursuant to the standards of his profession should determine, that his patient presents a serious danger of violence to another, he incurs an obligation to use reasonable care to protect the intended victim against such danger. The discharge of this duty may require the therapist to take one or more of various steps. Thus, it may call for him to warn the intended victim, to notify the police, or to take whatever steps are reasonably necessary under the circumstances.

Following the California decision, a number of states in the United States have adopted the **duty to protect** provision of the Tarasoff decision.

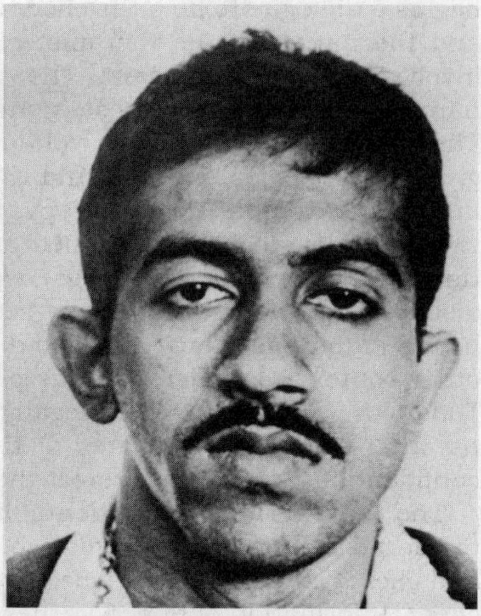

Prosenjit Poddar

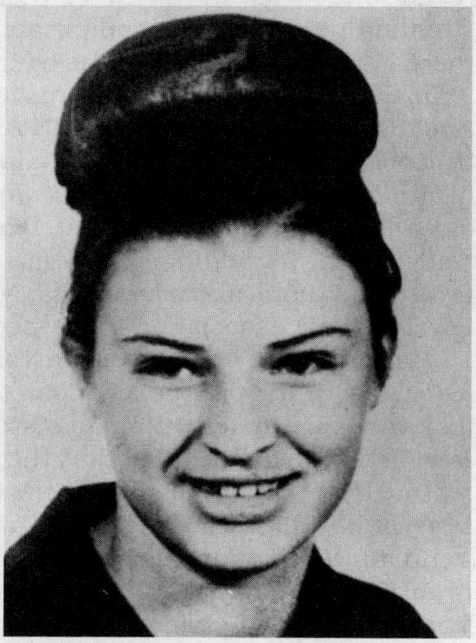

Tatiana Tarasoff

The Ethical and Legal Aspects of the Initial Contract for Treatment

Ethical and legal considerations are part of every professional interaction. This is particularly true in relation to the mental health system. Let's use psychotherapy as an example. After the client describes the initial reason for seeking treatment, the therapist begins a dialogue to help the client understand what will take place in the therapy session and the nature of the therapist–client relationship. One major aspect of this dialogue involves **informed consent.** That is to say, the client has the right to know what will happen during the therapy sessions, what is expected of her, and the potential outcomes. The client also has the right to know the experience and expertise of the therapist with a given psychological problem and if there are alternative choices for treatment. After being informed of the nature of therapy, the client can consent or not.

In addition to being informed about the nature of therapy, the client also needs to understand the ethical and legal aspects of therapy. The first point is that the information discussed in the psychotherapy session is confidential. **Confidentiality** means that the health care professional is not to discuss information learned in a therapy session in any other context. Confidentiality as part of treatment has a long history in many cultures. Today, this confidentiality is legally required for those who are legally licensed to practice psychotherapy. All 50 states of the United States and the District of Columbia have confidentiality laws that protect the information revealed in therapy.

The legal term for confidentiality is **privileged communication.** In most states, a privileged communication takes place in a number of situations including an attorney and client, a husband and wife, a priest and penitent, and a health care professional and client. Information obtained in these situations cannot be released in court. Thus, a court could not compel a therapist to reveal information learned in the therapy session. However, the privilege is controlled by the client. Thus, if a client wants the therapist to reveal what was discussed in therapy in court, then the therapist must comply. The situation becomes more complicated if a couple was seen together in family therapy or if there is a child involved in the court or custody proceedings.

In addition, health care records are protected by the **Health Insurance Portability and Accountability Act of 1996 (HIPAA).** HIPAA regulates the manner in which medical and psychological records are maintained and shared with insurance companies and other health care professionals. If you wanted your current therapist to have access to work you did with a previous therapist, you would need to consent to having these records transferred. In addition to legal laws, which determine what information must be protected, there are also ethical guidelines from such organizations as the American Psychological Association (APA) (see *Table 17-2*).

Based on the findings of the Tarasoff and other court rulings, the therapist needs to discuss with the client exceptions to confidentiality. One of these is duty to protect. This may vary slightly from state to state, but the general statement is that the therapist must take action if she believes that the client will harm another person or himself. This may require that the therapist warn the other person, talk with the authorities or the police, or suggest hospitalization. This was a direct consequence of the Tarasoff court ruling.

Another exception to confidentiality is related to the legal requirement for **mandated reporting.** Mandated reporting is the requirement that when health care professionals learn firsthand of child abuse or neglect, they report this information to the appropriate state agency. More specific information by state is available from the U.S. Department of Health and Human Services (www.childwelfare.gov/systemwide/sgm/index.cfm).

Emergency Commitment

Most mental health professionals rarely are required to make emergency commitments. In therapy, they work closely with their clients who are at risk to themselves to prevent suicide attempts. When there is concern for imminent danger, the first approach is to

TABLE 17-2 Ethical Principles From the American Psychological Association—Some Highlights

Privacy and Confidentiality

Maintaining Confidentiality

Psychologists have a primary obligation and take reasonable precautions to protect confidential information obtained through or stored in any medium, recognizing that the extent and limits of confidentiality may be regulated by law or established by institutional rules or professional or scientific relationship. (See also Standard 2.05, Delegation of Work to Others.)

Discussing the Limits of Confidentiality

(a) Psychologists discuss with persons (including, to the extent feasible, persons who are legally incapable of giving informed consent and their legal representatives) and organizations with whom they establish a scientific or professional relationship (1) the relevant limits of confidentiality and (2) the foreseeable uses of the information generated through their psychological activities. (See also Standard 3.10, Informed Consent.)

(b) Unless it is not feasible or is contraindicated, the discussion of confidentiality occurs at the outset of the relationship and thereafter as new circumstances may warrant.

(c) Psychologists who offer services, products, or information via electronic transmission inform clients/patients of the risks to privacy and limits of confidentiality.

Therapy

Informed Consent to Therapy

(a) When obtaining informed consent to therapy as required in Standard 3.10, Informed Consent, psychologists inform clients/patients as early as is feasible in the therapeutic relationship about the nature and anticipated course of therapy, fees, involvement of third parties and limits of confidentiality and provide sufficient opportunity for the client/patient to ask questions and receive answers. (See also Standards 4.02, Discussing the Limits of Confidentiality, and 6.04, Fees and Financial Arrangements.)

Source: *Ethical Principles of Psychologists and Code of Conduct* (2010).

help the client to place herself in a mental health facility on a voluntary basis. When this is not possible, an emergency commitment may be required. If the person refuses the treatment, mental health professionals will involve the courts. The courts may require a civil commitment to an inpatient facility. Many states allow for an initial 72-hour involuntary commitment in an inpatient facility if the person is dangerous to herself or others. If after 72 hours, health care professionals believe the person is still in need of inpatient treatment, then they request that the person be committed for a longer period of time through the court system.

A civil commitment is the legal process by which a court orders the involuntary commitment of an individual (see Zander, 2005, for an overview). In general, the court needs to determine that the person has a mental illness, is dangerous to himself or others, or is unable to care for himself. The ability not to take care of one's self is legally referred to as "*grave disability.*" The goal of a civil commitment is to protect the public or to protect, or treat the person.

The legal precedence for civil commitment is based on two legal principles. The first legal principle is based on the government's need to invoke police powers to ensure public health, safety, welfare, and morals. Thus, it is the task of the government to protect the public. The second legal principle is referred to as *parens patriae* authority. This means parent of the nation and is derived from English common law. Since the 1500s, the king or queen held the authority to take care of those who could not take care of themselves. In the United States, courts have held this authority to take care of children in certain situations or those with certain types of mental disorders.

Concept Check

- How do confidentiality and informed consent work together to provide legal and ethical protections for individuals seeking psychological treatment?
- When should an individual be committed to a mental health facility? What are the rights and responsibilities of both the client and the mental health professionals in that situation?

Until the 1970s, involuntary commitment of individuals with mental illness required only that there was a need for treatment. This was changed in a landmark federal court decision in 1972 referred to as *Lessard v. Schmidt.* This was the first of many court decisions based on the due process requirements of the Fourteenth Amendment to the U.S. Constitution, which concluded that civil commitment could not be solely justified based on the *parens patriae* authority. That is, a court needed to meet additional requirements other than just the person's need for treatment.

The additional requirement was to show individuals about to be involuntarily committed were dangerous to themselves or others. By showing that there was danger, the court could draw upon another responsibility of the government. Legally, this is referred to as the police power authority. It is the job of government to ensure safety of the people, which is traditionally performed by the police. For involuntary commitment, the person must also be shown to be dangerous to him- or herself or others. Thus, needing treatment is not enough for a civil commitment. This was formally decided by the U.S. Supreme Court in 1975 in the *O'Connor v. Donaldson* decision. Basically, the court ruled that there is no constitutional basis for confining people involuntarily if they are dangerous to no one and can live safely in freedom. In the 1980s, the Supreme Court ruled that being dangerous to self and others also applied to sexual offenders.

From the 1970s until today, those with mental illness have gained more rights within the law. Even if involuntarily committed to an inpatient facility, the person still retains the right to be considered competent and be involved in her own treatment. This includes the right in many states to refuse medication. If the health care professionals deem that medication is critical, they, in turn, can involve the courts or their representatives.

In health care, the **Patient Self-Determination Act (PSDA) of 1991** was introduced. This is a set of federal requirements intended to implement advance directive policies at all health care facilities that receive federal funding through Medicaid and Medicare programs. Today, many individuals have "living wills" that direct how they will be treated if they become seriously ill or near death. What became apparent was that this approach could also be applied to mental health.

This approach is referred to as **psychiatric advance directives (PADs).** PADs have been written into law in a number of states. These directives allow a person to submit directives or designate individuals to consent on his behalf. This allows a person who has a history of periods in which he would not be competent to make a rational decision to direct the types of treatments he would accept or refuse. Thus, an individual with schizophrenia, mania, or suicide attempts could, when experiencing periods of incapacity, direct how he would be treated when he is not able to make rational decisions on his own. This would reduce the need to use courts to mandate treatment.

NEW DEVELOPMENTS ON THE INDIAN LEGAL SCENARIO

Several interesting new legislations mark a progressive trend in Indian society vis-a-vis delivery of safety and justice to many groups within the community.

The Protection of Children from Sexual Offences Act, 2012 (POCSO)

This act has been one of the first very clearly formulated child-friendly legislations in India with well-defined modes of implementation and rapid redressal.

The said act attempts to protect children from offences of sexual assault, sexual harassment, and pornography and provides for establishment of special courts for trial of such offences and for matters connected with such incidents as soon as they are reported (http://indiacode.nic.in/amendmentacts2012/The%20Protection%20of%20Children%20From%20Sexual%20Offences%20Act.pdf).

There is a clearly spelt-out procedure for the reporting of cases and for recording the statement of the child in a sensitive manner.

The Sexual Harassment of Women at Workplace (Prevention, Prohibition And Redressal) Act, 2013 (POSH)

This act clearly spells out duties of the employer and constitution of the local or internal complaints committee (http://lawmin.nic.in/ld/P-ACT/2013/The%20Sexual%20Harassment%20of%20Women%20at%20Workplace%20(Prevention,%20Prohibition%20and%20Redressal)%20Act,%202013.pdf).

The Juvenile Justice (Care and Protection of Children) Act, 2015 (JJ Act)

This act outlines general principles of care and protection of children and outlines the formation of Juvenile Justice Boards or JJBs. Rehabilitation and social reintegration is the prime focus, rather than stigmatization and exclusion of children whose behavior has required corrective action (http://wcd.nic.in/acts/juvenile-justice-care-and-protection-children-act-2015).

Narcotic Drugs and Psychotropic Substances (NDPS) Act, 1985

This is a relatively old legislation and currently seems to require some attention since there is an epidemic of drug usage and dependence among young populations, also coupled with non-substance addictions due to the overuse of social media and the Internet in an unhealthy manner (http://dor.gov.in/sites/default/files/Narcotic-Drugs-and-Psychotropic-Substances-Act-1985.pdf).

17-2 LENS
Global Mental Health—Prisoners and Mental Health

The sole survivor of the terror attacks was subsequently psychometrically assessed by the author and her colleagues and the paper, which was published in the Archives of Indian Psychiatry of 2012, is reproduced here with their permission (Sovani, Kumawat, & Joshi, 2013).

Case Report Terrorism and the 'utility' of people with ASPD trait patterns Forensic significance of MCMI III and Rorschach Inkblot assessment

Anuradha Sovani
Sanjay Kumawat
Geeta Joshi

Abstract

Terrorist attacks have become the bane of the state of Maharashtra in particular, and India in general, in the recent past. Many cases have remained sub judice and hence it has often not been possible to share psychometric test findings of the same with the academic community of psychiatrists and psychologists.

This paper presents a case study of one such profile, which clearly reveals a profile of an ASPD personality style (301.7) with the use of the Millon Clinical Multiaxial Inventory – 3rd edition (MCMI III) and the Rorschach Inkblot Test. The assessment for the prison inmate was completed in April 2011 and is published now since the case is no longer sub judice. The report reveals the equal importance that must be laid on both, empirical and projective testing, as well as on a carefully obtained history and mental status examination findings. (**Key words:** terrorism, antisocial personality disorder, Millon Clinical Multiaxial Inventory, Rorschach Inkblot Test)

Introduction

Terrorism is a phenomenon that is spreading its tentacles worldwide. The role that extremist subcultures play in the induction of young people into the ranks of terrorist groups is well documented. Fanaticism and fundamentalism, aggression and frustration, inequality and extreme poverty, all have their role to play in drawing people into this net. India in general, and the state of Maharashtra, with Mumbai as its capital has perhaps become an easy target for terrorist groups.[1]

A strong socialization process by the mentors of these young terrorists helps to dehumanize and stigmatize potential victims, and fan the flames of ambition and the desire in young recruits into terrorism to seek a niche for themselves. Use of technology is certainly a marker of 21st century terrorism and there is no doubt now that recruiters are now adept at recognizing certain characteristics in those to be enlisted.

Various observations about recruitment into terrorist activity have been made by experts. "A principal reason for the lack of psychometric studies of terrorism is that researchers have little, if any, direct access to terrorists, even imprisoned ones. Individuals who become terrorists often are unemployed, socially alienated individuals who have dropped out of society. Increasingly, terrorist organizations in the developing world are recruiting younger members. The only role models for these young people to identify with are often terrorists and guerrillas."[2]

Forensic psychological profiling of those terrorists who have been apprehended can give us some insight into these profiles. This paper presents a single case study of one such young terrorist whose psychometric assessment was completed using MCMI – III and Rorschach Inkblot Test.

The MCMI – III consists of 175 statements which require a Yes-No format of response, and takes about 35–45 minutes to complete. In the current case, the questions were asked of the respondent in Hindi and his Yes/No responses were recorded and later scored.

Ideally, the MCMI III should be administered to individuals of 18 years or above, if there is evidence of some psychological disturbance. In this instance, psychological assessment was recommended by a government appointed psychiatrist and hence the investigation was undertaken. The MCMI III consists of 14Personality Disorder scales of which 3 are considered severe personality disorders, 10 Clinical Syndrome scales, of which 3 are severe clinical syndromes, as well as one validity scale and three modifying indices, X, Y and Z.[3]

The Rorschach Inkblot Method is perhaps the best known of the various projective techniques of personality assessment.[4] This consists of ten plates of which five are black and white and five are colored. Once again, three of the latter are multihued, and two have black, white and red designs. There are various approved methods of scoring the Rorschach, of which the Klopfer approach was used in this case. The Rorschach inkblot method has been critiqued for the apparent subjectivity of its interpretations, and at the same time lauded for the flexibility of its use and application, and the sheer volume of its usage over the years.[4, 5]

The Klopfer approach allows for a judgment about the speed with which the client responded, indicative of depressive pointers if any, as well as an insight into reality testing of the respondent, in addition to many other aspects of interpretation based on the location, determinants and content of the responses.[6]

Case Study and Findings

Observations and interview

The respondent was small built, compact and agile, although he walked slowly to the testing room. He gave his age correctly, indicating good orientation. He was coherent and relevant and answered to the point. His time orientation was also reflected in his awareness of meal and prayer times, even if there was no clock in the testing room. He showed discipline and declined a second cup of tea, and also kneeled and prayed without seeking permission, showing motor agility. He looked down often, avoided eye contact and needed to be coaxed to respond.

His memory was unimpaired, since he could report his age, name of school, names and marital statuses of siblings, lack of relationship with parents, site of incidents for which he was apprehended, as well as date of departure from his country and arrival here, number and names of people accompanying him, equipment and cards, currency they carried, etc. although several years had elapsed since these incidents occurred.

The respondent admitted to occasional use of alcohol, charas, ganja, bhang and cocaine in the past and claimed to be a vegetarian. He had contradicted this claim on past occasions, and could be using such contradictions purposefully. He also claimed knowledge about brewing local liquor, crafts such as bag making, as well as expertise at weaponry and knowledge of English without attempt to feign, possibly reflecting some overconfidence.

He responded appropriately to all questions although he tried to stall on some by feigning lack of comprehension or smiling to delay answering. He spoke in a thin, soft voice, again probably purposefully produced since he sang later in a full-throated voice. He shows a sense of humor, and occasionally tried to joke at the expense of the doctor who regularly visits him. He spoke as if he had a higher status than her, conceding that "she works very hard."

The respondent showed absolutely no remorse for any deaths, either of his colleagues or victims, attributing it to divine will. In fact, at a point he spoke of people in his group in glorifying terms. Further, he showed alertness and intelligence in admitting to the reason he was trained and sent to this country, but totally and consistently denying any involvement in the deaths attributed to him. Psychologist Jerrold Post opines that the most

(Continued)

(Continued)

dangerous terrorist is likely to be the religious terrorist, "who can justify the most heinous acts" in the name of faith, and can still maintain a cool and unruffled demeanor.[7]

Test Findings

Millon Clinical Multiaxial Inventory, 3rd ed (MCMI III) and the Rorschach Inkblot Method (RIM) were used, and the respondent co-operated with testing. Attempts were made to put him at ease during the assessment, and also to achieve results in the minimum possible time for security purposes. The police personnel in charge at the institution extended full support and were present throughout, as was the referring psychiatrist deputed by the government authorities. Their presence in no way restricted responsivity of the testee who was much at ease and relaxed throughout. The assessment lasted for approximately three hours, with breaks given for the respondent to rest, take tea or water, visit the toilet, etc. Due consent was taken before testing was done, and no pressure was put on him to respond. Notes were maintained, the latter process being visible to the respondent. The interview and testing was done mainly in Hindi, since the inmate expressed comfort with this language, although he seemed comfortable with English and Marathi as well, and often used these languages interchangeably.

MCMI III profile:

V = 1	X = (152) 87	Y = (14)65	Z = (19)76
1 = 71		A = 85	
2A = 67		H = 65	
2B = 67		N = 61	
3 = 70		D = 74	
4 = 36		B = 80	
5 = 49		T = 77	
R = 65			
6A = 79		SS = 66	
6B = 66		CC = 67	
7 = 32		PP = 69	
8A = 48			
8B = 62			
S = 65			
C = 70			
P = 58			

MCMI III Note: Elevated scales: 6A : ASPD personality style; A = Anxiety; B and T = respectively alcohol and drug dependence, usually also indicative of impulsivity.

Impressions: V = 1 usually invalidates a profile. However, it must be kept in mind that the respondent is facing a high public profile case in court, which has sensitized him and at the same time, has been kept incarcerated continuously living in very unreal conditions.

His high X is probably the reflection of his need to speak and communicate after remaining in solitary confinement and being in the glare of the media. It would also be a reflection of his need to impress. Scores under 85 are not indicative of any personality disorder.

The only significant elevations seen were on ASPD personality style (8A = 79) and high impulsivity reflected on B = 80. A = 85 seems to be a natural outcome of his current legal status and impending punishment (possibly death penalty).

(RORSCHACH findings on next page ... they are getting misaligned if moved.)

RORSCHACH Profile

∑Time	**12 min 35 sec**	**∑R 25**	**Populars 6**
	Mean RT 7.8 sec	Chr RT 5 sec	Achr RT 10.5 sec

FLR: F+=16 F– = nil F+/- =9; F+%=64%; Ext F+=100%

Loc	**Determinants**	**Content**
W = 10	F = 10	H = 1
D = 13	M = nil	A = 8
Dd = nil	FM = 1	Hd = nil
S = 4 (one was pure S)	FC = 2	Ad = 1
Cut off W = 1	CF = 2	Obj = 13
	FC' = 4	
	Fc = 3, Fk = 1, KF = 1	(H) = 1; (A) = 1
	FK = 1	

Notes: Adequate card turning. Some perseveration of "bat" and "bag" responses since the latter, i.e. bag making, was his trade prior to his current assignment.

Interpretation: Excellent FLR reflects totally intact reality testing, and no diagnosis is made on axis I. No psychotic pointers seen. This is supported by 6 Populars, which reflect touch with reality and strong adherence to norms (in this case subcultural norms) and even 3 original responses which reflects creativity and out of box thinking in the presence of intelligence. Determinants and content present a wide variety reflecting rich associational life and emotional health. The total number of responses (25) is also adequate, especially given his low scholastic exposure and low test sophistication.

Very "clean" protocol, no double scoring, each response usually yielded single determinant or content. Balance of W, D and S reflects normal pattern. 4 S responses reflect rebellious tendency, following one's own set of rules. Nil M and only 1 FM reflects almost an absence of relationships or human affectional bonds. The normal FC' responses (4) rule out depression, as does the quick mean RT (7.8 seconds) and quicker chromatic than achromatic RT (5 and 10.5 seconds respectively.) The 25 responses were given in 12.5 minutes, showing alert yet unhurried responding. "A" responses seem to reflect impulsivity, and immediate need gratification, (A) and (H) reflect fantasy responses.

Summary

The profile on both tests clearly reflected absence of any psychopathology, yet presence of Antisocial personality pattern traits which would render the respondent easily trainable into a terrorist regime. Hudson writes that "In addition to having a normal personality and not being diagnosably mentally disturbed, a terrorist's other characteristics make him or her practically indistinguishable from normal people at least in terms of outward appearance..... terrorists tend to be in their twenties, healthy and strong, with no particular demands about social background or educational level." Maxwell Taylor also opines that mental illness has little utility in terrorism. Even psychopathy, if at all, should be present only to a limited extent, so that the person does not become unreliable and uncontrolled. There should be

(Continued)

(Continued)

no personal purposefulness to his or her acts, and they should follow the group will, remain discreet, careful, and be capable of detailed planning and well timed execution.[8]

Conclusion

The purpose of this paper was to outline an interesting case study to provoke academic interest in the forensic applications of psychometric assessment and psychiatric interviewing with a view to better understanding the phenomenon of terrorism and recruitment of young people into groups that create havoc in the lives of citizens the world over.

References

1. Karan, Vijay. (1997). *War by Stealth: Terrorism in India.* New Delhi: Viking (Penguin Books India).
2. Hudson, R.A. (1999). The sociology and psychology of terrorism: who becomes a terrorist and why? Federal research Division, Library of Congress, Washington, D.C.
3. Strack, Stephen. (2008). Essentials of Millon Inventories assessment, 3rd edition. New Jersey: John Wiley and Sons Inc.
4. Rorschach, Hermann. (1927). Rorschach Test. Psychodiagnostic plates. Hogrefe.
5. Goldstein, G. and Hersen, M. (ed.). (2000). *Handbook of Psychological Assessment.* Amsterdam: Pergammon press.
6. Klopfer, B., Ainsworth, M.D., Klopfer, W.G., & Holt, R.R. (1954). *Developments in the Rorschach Technique: Vol. 1, Technique and Theory.* World Book Co: Yonkers-on-Hudson.
7. Post, Jerrold. (1990). Current understanding of terrorist motivation and psychology implications for a Differentiated Antiterrorist policy. *Terrorism, 13*(1), 65–71.
8. Taylor, Maxwell. (1988). *The Terrorist.* UK: Brassey's.

NEUROSCIENCE AND EVOLUTIONARY PERSPECTIVES ON THE LEGAL ASPECTS OF PSYCHOPATHOLOGY

The legal profession and the courts have been greatly influenced by neuroscience discoveries and methods (Roskies, Schweitzer, & Saks, 2013). Today, deoxyribonucleic acid (DNA) is commonly used to help to convict or demonstrate innocence in court trials. Hundreds of individuals who were previously serving prison sentences have been exonerated through DNA and other types of biological testing. The legal system is also seeking information from neuroscience researchers. In 2012, the Connecticut Medical Examiner asked geneticists at the University of Connecticut to examine the DNA of Adam Lanza, the 20-year-old who killed 27 at Sandy Hook Elementary School in Newtown, Connecticut. Although Adam Lanza committed suicide, the medical examiner is seeking to determine if there are clues in the DNA to help explain the killings. Using neuroscience to arrive at answers to legal questions is a field referred to as *forensic neuroscience.*

Neuroscience information also requires that the legal system ask questions it is not used to asking. For example, how should we understand the fact that Charles Whitman, who was an Eagle Scout and marine, killed at least 14 people from the University of Texas tower with a rifle? Had he lived and gone to court, juries would have likely said he was responsible for the killings. Yet, should we consider the fact that he had a brain tumor that pressed on his amygdala? The relationship between neuroscience research and the law is not easy, especially when the task is to determine responsibility.

Concept Check

- What is the purpose of SVP laws?
- What have communities put in place to try to prevent pedophilia and other sexual offences?

Neuroscience research is currently being included in legal decisions. It has been used to help establish responsibility. The U.S. Supreme Court has used neuroscience data to help determine if an individual is responsible for his or her actions (see Steinberg, 2013, for an overview). In this case, it was the question of whether an adolescent who killed another person should be treated as an adult. Sixteen- and 17-year-olds could receive the death penalty in some states before 2005, and those even younger could be sentenced to life in prison without parole for killing another person. In 2005, the U.S. Supreme Court in the *Roper v. Simmons* case abolished the death penalty for crimes committed while under the age of 18. In 2012, in the *Miller v. Alabama* and the *Jackson v. Hobbs* cases, the Supreme Court banned the use of the life without parole sentence for adolescents on constitutional grounds. In these cases, it was noted that neuroscience research shows the adolescent brain to be different from an adult's, as you read in Chapter 6. Thus, an adolescent should be held responsible for his or her actions to a different degree than should an adult. This, in turn, should be reflected in the sentencing of the convicted individual.

Another situation in which neuroscience research has changed legal procedures is in terms of memory and the ability to influence another individual's recollection of an event (Loftus, 2003; Schacter & Loftus, 2013). Schacter and Loftus described a crime that happened in Camden, New Jersey, on New Year's Day 2003. Larry Henderson was accused of holding a gun on James Womble while another man shot Rodney Harper to death. Almost 2 weeks after the murder, Womble identified Henderson from a photograph. Womble again identified Henderson at trial, and Henderson was easily convicted of reckless manslaughter and aggravated assault, among other charges. The case was appealed to the New Jersey Supreme Court, which resulted in the court issuing a new set of guidelines that reflected the reconstructive nature of memory and the various factors that can influence it. Specifically, jurors are now to be told that memory is not like a video recording, and it is not foolproof but can be influenced. This also included a statement that those of a different race may be harder to identify than a person of your own race. These are common findings from neuroscience research. By the way, in the original trial, the jury was never told that the victim who identified Larry Henderson had used crack cocaine and drank wine and champagne on that New Year's Day when the crime happened.

Although neuroscience approaches have potential for clarifying legal questions in relation to mental illness, as noted previously, the ability to diagnose a given individual from neuroscience techniques is not available at this time. Even in areas in which neuroscience research has been directed at criminal behavior, such as convicted criminals with antisocial personality disorder, it is still impossible to predict which individual will commit another crime from brain imaging studies (see Eastman & Campbell, 2006, for an overview). At this time, neither neuroscience nor brain imaging research can determine if a specific individual person is telling a lie or not (Langleben & Moriarty, 2013). Research can of course suggest which groups of individuals, such as those with antisocial personality disorder, are more likely to seek to deceive others.

As you have seen in this book, neuroscience research is largely characterized by research studies that reflect the differences between one group of individuals with specific psychopathologies and another group of individuals without the disorder. These data represent the average of measures from all individuals in a given group and the probability of these results being found if the study was performed again. These results are described in terms of statistical probabilities. On the other hand, courts do not say a person has a 95% probability of being guilty. The legal system seeks a different type of answer than does neuroscience research. Of course, as with the U.S. Supreme Court, neuroscience has extremely important information to help the legal system make informed judgments.

Evolutionary perspectives in relation to the legal system have been less well studied. However, we know that our long history of social relationships has resulted in a rich calculus of how we make moral judgments and exact punishments on others. For example, if you are asked who you would save from a burning building—a 2-year-old or a 70-year-old—all people quickly answer a 2-year-old. It is a gut reaction with little thinking required. What if you see someone hurt a helpless animal? How do you respond? It is also a quick response, unless you have an antisocial personality or a conduct disorder. Our evolutionary history leads us to approach social and moral situations in a particular manner. It does not matter if we are out in the world or part of a jury.

Someone who thinks that rape or killing is wrong does not think that this only applies to his or her hometown but to the entire world. In this sense, moral judgments are experienced differently from cultural ones. It is also the case that humans believe that committing immoral acts should be followed by punishment. People often say it is wrong to let someone "get away with it." Thus, humans not only make moral judgments but also believe that what they consider to be immoral behavior should be punished. These are two critical elements that juries consider, although often out of awareness, as they determine guilt and innocence. Thus, neuroscience and evolutionary perspectives have the potential to help inform the legal system in relation to the types of questions it considers.

SUMMARY

Individuals seeking treatment for a psychological disorder have both legal and ethical protections, including (1) informed consent; (2) confidentiality, or in legal terms, privileged communication; and (3) protection of health care records through HIPAA. Exceptions to confidentiality include (1) duty to protect and (2) mandated reporting. Commitment to a mental health facility may be necessary if it is determined that the person has a mental illness, is dangerous to himself or others, or is unable to care for himself. Even if involuntarily committed to an inpatient facility, the person still retains the right to be considered competent and be involved in her own treatment. A new approach, referred to as PADs, allows a person with a psychological disorder to submit directives or designate individuals to consent on his behalf and direct how he would be treated when he is not able to make rational decisions on his own.

Insanity is a legal term, not a psychological one. All cultures throughout time have sought to determine the role of responsibility in committing criminal acts. In the United States, a number of variations based on capacity and knowledge have been applied in determining sanity, including (1) the M'Naghten rule, (2) the volitional test, (3) the Durham rule, (4) the ALI rule, and (5) the Comprehensive Crime Control Act of 1984. In reality, the insanity defense is used less than 1% of the time. The first step before a trial is to determine if a person is competent to stand trial. Four factors have been used for determining decision-making competence: (1) ability to communicate a choice, (2) ability to understand relevant information, (3) ability to appreciate the nature of the situation and its consequences, and (4) ability to rationally manipulate information.

SVP or SDP statutes generally allow for a person who committed a sexual crime to be held after his or her sentence has been completed. The idea is that these individuals represent a threat to public safety if they are released. A number of groups, including the American Psychiatric Association, have opposed these laws. Pedophilia and other sexual offenses greatly concern a community that seeks various ways to prevent such behaviors. Although research suggests that these laws may reduce sexual incidents in those who know the sexual predator personally, they do not increase overall public safety. It is currently a critical question to determine the role of mental illness in committing sexual crimes.

STUDY RESOURCES

Review Questions

1. Think about the terror attacks on India and the psychometric report in Lens and discuss whether psychopathology or cultural/religious and social conditioning had a larger role to play in the shaping of the terrorists?
2. The impact of mental illness on an individual's ability to think rationally and make rational decisions is an important consideration in his or her interactions within both the legal system and the mental health system. What are some situations where this is most problematic, and what are some ideas for improving those situations?
3. Why is it critical to both individuals and communities to determine the role of mental illness in committing sexual crimes?

For Further Reading

Eagleman, D. (2011). *Incognito: The secret lives of the brain.* New York: Pantheon Books.
Morse, S., & Roskies, A. (Eds.). (2013). *A primer on criminal law and neuroscience.* New York: Oxford University Press.
Tottey, E. (2008). *The insanity offense.* New York: Norton.

Key Terms and Concepts

ALI rule
confidentiality
Durham rule
duty to protect
Health Insurance Portability and Accountability Act of 1996 (HIPAA)
informed consent
insanity
mandated reporting
M'Naghten rule
Patient Self-Determination Act (PSDA) of 1991
privileged communication
psychiatric advance directives (PADs)
sexually violent predator (SVP) or sexually dangerous person (SDP) statutes
volitional test

to understand relevant information, (b) ability to appreciate the nature of the situation and its consequences, and (c) ability to rationally manipulate information.

SVP or SDP statutes generally allow for a person who committed a sexual crime to be held after his/her sentence has been completed. The idea is that these individuals represent a threat to public safety if they are released. A number of groups, including the American Psychiatric Association, have opposed these laws. Pedophilia and other sexual [illegible] [illegible] a continuum that [illegible] to prevent such behaviors. Although research suggests that these laws may reduce sexual incidents in those who [illegible] [illegible] personality, they do not [illegible] overall public safety. It is currently a [illegible] question to determine the role of mental illness in committing sexual crimes.

STUDY RESOURCES

Review Questions

1. Think about the terror attacks on India and the psychometric reports in news and discuss whether psychopathology of cultural, religious and social conditioning has [illegible] to play in the shaping of the terrorists.

2. The impact of mental illness on an individual's ability to think rationally and make rational decisions is an important consideration in his or her interactions with both the legal system and the mental health system. What are some situations where this is most problematic, and what are some ways to improve those situations?

3. Why is it critical for both individuals and communities to determine the role of mental illness in committing sexual crimes?

For Further Reading

[illegible], [illegible] (20[illegible]). [illegible]. New York: [illegible] Books.

[illegible], S., [illegible], [illegible] (20[illegible]). [illegible]. New York: Oxford University Press.

[illegible], E. (200[illegible]). *The [illegible]*. New York: Norton.

Key Terms and Concepts

ALI rule	informed consent	psychiatric advance
confidentiality	insanity	directives (PADs)
Durham rule	mandated reporting	sexually violent predator
duty to protect	M'Naghten rule	[illegible]
Health Insurance Portability	Patient Self-Determination	dangerous person (SDP)
and Accountability Act of	Act (PSDA) of 1991	statutes
1996 (HIPAA)	privileged communication	[illegible]

GLOSSARY

12-step program: a community in which individuals with addiction problems meet and follow the principles described in the 12 steps; forms the basis for Alcoholics Anonymous (AA), and variations of the approach have been used with other addictions; not considered a treatment in the usual sense since there is not a health care professional involved

abnormal psychology: the study of mental disorders; this includes psychological dysfunctions that the person experiences in terms of distress; a complete definition of abnormal behavior compares the behaviors and experiences in terms of those accepted in the person's culture.

acquired immune deficiency syndrome (AIDS): a disorder caused by the human immunodeficiency virus (HIV), which affects the person's immune system in a negative manner; characterized by neurocognitive problems such as slowing in both cognitive and motor functions including memory problems, confusion, depression, and difficulty with fine motor tasks

acute stress disorder: a short-term reaction to traumatic events that last from 3 days to 1 month

addiction: the situation of using psychoactive substances in which individuals experience a stronger motivation that results in a active wanting and seeking of the substance as opposed to a simple choice of when and where to have the experience

adjustment disorders: disorders in which reactions to events are out of proportion to the severity of the event

adoption study: the situation where dizygotic (DZ) and monozygotic (MZ) twins have been raised apart; by studying those children who were twins and were raised in different environments, it was possible to better determine the environmental and genetic influences in terms of development

agonist drug: as a treatment for addiction, it is a substance that binds to the receptor in the brain and produces cellular activity that mimics the function of the illicit drug without producing the high; methadone is an opioid agonist

agoraphobia: the condition in which a person experiences fear or anxiety when in public

agreeableness: associated with being sympathetic, trusting, cooperative, modest, and straightforward; as a dimension in the five-factor model (FFM), this dimension ranges from being friendly and compassionate to being competitive and outspoken

alcohol: a liquid created through a process of fermentation; in most humans, the experience of alcohol intake includes pleasant subjective experiences, which is partly related to the effects of alcohol on such neurotransmitters as serotonin, endorphins, and dopamine; alcohol will also decrease inhibition by reducing the effects of the GABA system, which is associated with anxiety

ALI rule: a broader approach to not guilty by reason of insanity developed by the American Law Institute (ALI) in 1962 that states the following: A person is not responsible for criminal conduct if at the time of such conduct as the result of mental disease or defect he lacks substantial capacity either to appreciate the criminality (wrongfulness) of his conduct or to conform his conduct to the requirements of the law

allele: the alternative molecular form of the same gene

allostasis: the body's ability to achieve stability through change

allostatic load: cumulative wear and tear on the body by responding to stressful conditions

alogia: lack of interest in talking with others or answering questions with more than a one or two word answer

amphetamines: stimulants produced in the laboratory which result in positive feelings, a burst of energy, and alertness

anhedonia: the inability to experience pleasure

anonymity: a principle that requires that the personal identity of a given participant be kept separate from his or her data

anorexia nervosa: the fifth edition of the Diagnostic and Statistical Manual of Mental Disorders (*DSM–5*) criteria for a diagnosis of anorexia nervosa include a restriction of food, which results in a weight that is below normal, a fear of gaining weight, and a lack of seriousness of current body weight and a distortion of how body weight is experienced

antagonist drug: as a treatment for addiction, it is a substance that blocks the receptor site in the brain so that the illicit drug does not produce an effect; by blocking or counteracting the effects of the illicit drug, it no longer has its rewarding and addictive effects; naltrexone is an antagonist used to treat opioid addiction

antisocial personality disorder: classified in dramatic emotional personality disorders (Cluster B).; the criteria include acts since the age of 15 such as repeated participation in illegal acts, deceitfulness, impulsiveness, hostility and aggression, engagement in dangerous acts, irresponsible behavior, and absence of remorse

anxious fearful personality disorders (Cluster C): A grouping of personality disorders within the fifth edition of the Diagnostic and Statistical Manual of Mental Disorders (*DSM–5*); these include avoidant personality disorder, dependent personality disorder, and obsessive-compulsive personality disorder; the behavior of individuals with these disorders is one of fearfulness and avoidance

anxious/ambivalent attachment pattern: an attachment style in which the infant appears preoccupied with having access to the mother and shows protest on her separation; when she returns, the infant may show anger or ambivalence to her

Asperger's syndrome: individuals with this syndrome tend to be more intelligent and display higher functioning in terms of social processes than those diagnosed with autism, which can include social impairment in the form of egocentricity; a narrowing of interests;

compulsive need for introducing routines; speech and language peculiarities; nonverbal communication in the form of limited facial and gesture expression; and motor clumsiness; this category is used in the International Classification of Diseases (ICD-10) but not the Diagnostic and Statistical Manual of Mental Disorders (*DSM–5*)

assessment: the process of gathering information about a person so that you can make a clinical decision about a person's symptoms

attachment: the infant–mother relationship

attention deficit/hyperactivity disorder (ADHD): a disorder of childhood that includes two major dimensions: inattention, and hyperactivity and impulsivity

autism spectrum disorders: a group of neurodevelopmental disorders; individuals with autism spectrum disorders have difficulty in connecting and communication with others and with behavioral processes, often displaying stereotypical behaviors and the desire to engage in the same behavior in a repetitive manner

autonomic nervous system (ANS): a brain pathway that innervates a variety of organs including the adrenal medulla that results in the release of catecholamines (norepinephrine and epinephrine) from the terminal of sympathetic nerves

aversive drug: as a treatment for addiction, it becomes aversive when the drug of abuse is taken; Antabuse is an aversive drug that interferes with the metabolism of alcohol and produces unpleasant reactions

avoidant attachment pattern: an attachment style in which the infant shows more interest in the toys than the mother and shows less distress when the mother leaves and less positive emotion when she returns

avoidant personality disorder: classified in anxious fearful personality disorders (Cluster C); characterized by a pervasive pattern of social inhibition, feelings of inadequacy, and hypersensitivity to negative evaluation. Individuals avoid many social interactions, especially those involving close relationships with other people; one key feature is the fear of being criticized or evaluated by others

Avoidant/restrictive food intake disorder: the condition in which an individual does not eat certain foods, which leads to such conditions as weight loss or nutritional deficiency

avolition: lack of will or volition

Beck Depression Inventory (BDI): a questionnaire useful for determining the level of depressive symptoms that a person is reporting

behavioral and experiential perspective: examines the behavior and experience observed in psychopathology, especially the manner in which the signs and symptoms of a particular disorder are seen in a similar manner throughout the world

behavioral genetics: the study of genetic and environmental contributions to organisms' behavior

behavioral perspective: an approach focused on the level of actions and behaviors

binge drinking: defined by the National Institute on Alcohol Abuse and Alcoholism (NIAAA) as consuming enough alcohol in a 2-hour period to have a blood alcohol concentration (BAC) of 0.08 g/dL

binge eating disorder: characterized by the consumption of large amounts of food and the sense that one cannot control his or her eating behavior

bipolar disorder: previously known as manic depression; a mood disorder characterized by the experience of both depression and mania

blind controls: research participants who do not know whether they are in the experimental group or the control (placebo) group

borderline personality disorder (BPD): classified in dramatic emotional personality disorders (Cluster B); characterized by an instability in mood, interpersonal relationships, and a sense of self; these three factors interact with each other in such a manner that the person with borderline personality disorder experiences a changing world without a solid sense of self

bulimia nervosa: the main characteristics are periods of overeating in which the person feels out of control followed by purging

caffeine: a substance that acts as a stimulant although there are beneficial effects beyond stimulation; caffeine is found naturally in different amounts in the leaves and seeds of various plants including coffee beans, tea leaves, and cocoa beans

cannabis: a plant species also referred to as marijuana; the resin is referred to as hashish; the main psychoactive ingredient in cannabis is THC

case study: a method for studying individual participants

catatonic subtype: a type of schizophrenia characterized by non-normal activity of the motor system

categorical: the situation in which objects or concepts are defined as part of a category; categorical definitions of mental disorder results in the person either having a disorder or not; can be contrasted with dimensional definitions

central executive network: the neural network involved in performing such tasks as planning, goal setting, directing attention, performing, and inhibiting the management of actions, and the coding of representations in working memory

chromosomes: a deoxyribonucleic acid (DNA) molecule along with the proteins attached to it

classical conditioning: given that an unconditioned stimulus, such as food, results in an unconditioned response, such as salivation, classical conditioning is the pairing of the unconditioned stimulus, a neutral stimulus such as a bell a number of times; then the neutral stimulus will produce the response such as salivation

classification: a way to organize the diversity seen in mental disorders

client-centered therapy: also called person-centered therapy; an approach characterized by the therapist's empathic understanding, unconditional positive regard, genuineness and congruence

clinically significant: this refers to the question of whether the results of a study even if statistically significant would influence clinical outcomes

cocaine: comes from the naturally occurring coca plant largely grown in South America; for thousands of years, individuals have chewed the leaves of the coca plant for its psychoactive experiences.; its effects include a mental alertness, heightening the experience of sensory processes, and physiological effects such as increased heart rate and blood pressure

cognitive avoidance model: a theoretical model that proposes that worry is the manner in which an individual with GAD attempts to reduce the negative emotional experiences associated with GAD

cognitive behavioral perspective: a perspective that suggests that dysfunctional thinking is common to all psychological disturbances; by learning in therapy how to understand one's thinking, it is possible to change the way one thinks as well as one's emotional state and behaviors

cognitive behavioral therapy (CBT): a therapy based on the cognitive behavioral perspective, directed at changing the individual's faulty logic and maladaptive behaviors

cognitive bias: having more sensitivity than others to the possibility of potential threat

cognitive model of depression: a model that suggests that individuals with depression display a bias in the way they search for information and process this information

comorbid: this refers to an individual having more than one disorder at the same time

compulsions: behaviors that one uses to respond to obsessive thoughts

conduct disorder (CD): a disorder in which individuals display more extreme behaviors that reflect little regard for those around them; they actively violate the rights of others

confidentiality: a principle that requires that the scientist not release data of a personal nature to other scientists or groups without the participant's consent

confound: something that systematically biases the results of our research

confound hypothesis: a conceptual question that asks if our results could be the result of a factor other than the independent variable (IV)

confounding variables: unintended variables not chosen by the experimenter that influence the independent variable (IV)

connectivity: a concept that asks how different areas of the brain work together in specific conditions

conscientiousness: as a personality trait it is associated with being diligent, disciplined, well-organized, punctual, and dependable; as a dimension in the five-factor model (FFM), this dimension ranges from being efficient and organized to easy going and careless

Continuous Performance Test (CPT): a test that measures attentional characteristics.

control group: a group that is treated exactly like the experimental group except for the independent variable (IV) factor being studied

conversion disorders: the situation in which a person shows the signs of a disorder but the disorder does not follow what we know to be the underlying physiology; previously referred to as hysteria

conversion reaction: refers to Freud's idea that psychic energy was converted into physical symptoms; the basic concept is that painful memories or trauma are not consciously experienced in an emotional manner but rather converted into physical processes

correlation coefficient: a statistical technique to determine if an association exists in a relationship

correlational approach: an approach designed to help us understand how specific factors are associated with one another

cortisol: a hormone which is released in response to stress

covary: the degree to which variables are related to one another

craving: a step in the addiction pattern in which the individual loses control in the ability to limit intake of the drug

Cultural Formulation Interview (CFI): a set of questions developed to help mental health professionals obtain information concerning the person's culture and its influence on behavior and experience

cultural perspective: examines the social world in which a person lives and from which a person learns skills, values, beliefs, attitudes, and other information

default or intrinsic network: neural network that is active during internal processing

delayed ejaculation: the situation (over a 6-month period) in which a male shows a delay in ejaculation or shows a lack of ejaculation and that this causes significant distress

delirium: a short-term state of confusion characterized by a change in cognitive processing such as an inability to focus attention, problems with language, memory, or orientation

delusional thinking: an unrealistic pattern of thoughts forming a theme

delusions: beliefs without support for their occurrence and which are at odds with the individual's current environment

demand characteristics: bias that occurs when a participant's response is influenced more by the research setting than by the independent variable (IV)

dementias: term previously used to refer to a loss of cognitive abilities not related to normal aging; currently called neurocognitive disorders

deoxyribonucleic acid (DNA): provides information necessary to produce proteins

dependence: a way to describe addiction to a substance; three major components are (1) the desire to seek and take a certain substance, (2) the inability to avoid or limit the intake of the substance, and (3) the experience of negative emotional states when the substance is not available

dependent personality disorder: classified in anxious fearful personality disorders (Cluster C); characterized by a pervasive pattern of clinging and being submissive; the person with has difficulties making everyday decisions without reassurance from others resulting in a desire for others to assume responsibility for most areas of one's life; their lack of experiencing a self who can plan and direct their behavior leaves them in a position that requires that they always be with another; otherwise, they tend to feel anxious and helpless when alone

dependent variable (DV): depends on or is influenced by the independent variable (IV)

depersonalization: the experience of not experiencing the reality of one's self; this experience can include feeling detached or observing one's self as if you were an outside observer

depression in terms of attachment: suggestion that depression is a protective mechanism that prevents further critical losses, as depressed mood reduces the desire of the individual to immediately enter a social relationship in which there could be an adverse outcome, and secondly, as the outward signs of depressed mood, including changes in voice tone, reaction time, eye contact and facial expression, signal to others signs of submission and helplessness

depression in terms of resource conservation: suggestion that depressive mood protects the organism by conserving energy; by reducing energy expenditure, the organism can both protect itself in the present situation and conserve energy that can be used in future productive situations

depression in terms of social competition: suggestion that depression is seen in the context of hierarchies as an involuntary deescalating strategy, which signals to the other individual that he has won

derealization: the experience that the external world is not solid; one's world is experienced with a sense of detachment or as if in a fog, dream, or in other ways distorted or unreal

Diagnostic and Statistical Manual of Mental Disorders (*DSM*): publication of criteria for diagnosis by the American Psychiatric Association (APA), used in North America

dialectical behavior therapy (DBT): one of the first researched treatment approaches for borderline personality disorders; it was developed by Marsha Linehan, who describes it as a blend of behavioral science, dialectical philosophy, and Zen practice; cornerstone of DBT therapy is based on problem solving and acceptance of the experience of the moment.

diffusion tensor imaging (DTI): use of the magnetic resonance imaging (MRI) magnet to measure cortical connections in the brain, a procedure for showing fiber tracts (white matter) in the brain

dimensional: the situation in which objects or concepts are defined along a continuous scale; dimension definitions of mental disorder reflect that a person can experience the disorder in terms of differing degrees; temperature is an example of a dimensional definition whereas ice and stream represent categorical definitions.

disinhibited social engagement disorder: a disorder in which the child is willing to accept strangers who are not attachment figures

disordered use: the condition in the use of the psychoactive substance in which the person experiences significant impairment or distress

disorganized subtype: a type of schizophrenia characterized by disorganized speech patterns and behavior

disorganized/controlling attachment pattern: an attachment style in which the infant show disruptions in processing during a strange situation

disruptive, impulse control, and conduct disorders: a category of childhood disorders referred to as externalizing disorders

dissociation: the common experience of "spacing out" shared by most people; overall, this is the situation in which there is a disruption in our normal ability to integrate information from our sensory and psychological processes such as memory and awareness

dissociative amnesia: the main diagnostic element is an inability to recall important autobiographical information

dissociative fugue: a sudden, unexpected travel away from one's home or place of work with an inability to recall one's past

dissociative identity disorder (DID): a developmental disorder where one consistent sense of self does not occur—that is, the person does not experience her thoughts, feelings, or actions in terms of a well-developed "I" or sense of self or rather, the person experiences different "personalities" at different times; previously referred to as multiple personality disorder

dizygotic (DZ) twins: twins who arise from the situation in which two different eggs are fertilized by two different spermatozoa; these are called fraternal twins since their shared genes are approximately 50%—the same as that between any two siblings

dopamine: a neurotransmitter in the brain

double-blind experiment: research participants who do not know whether they are in the experimental group or the control (placebo) group is one aspect of a double blind experienter; the other aspect is that the researcher involved in the study do not know whether the participants are in the experimental group or the control (placebo) group thus both the participants and the researchers are blind to the experimental conditions

doubt: to question our ideas and our research and ask whether factors other than the ones that we originally considered might have influenced our results

Down syndrome: a disorder resulting in both physical and intellectual problems found in individuals with an extra copy of chromosome 21

dramatic emotional personality disorders (Cluster B): a grouping of personality disorders within the fifth edition of the Diagnostic and Statistical Manual of Mental Disorders (*DSM–5*); include antisocial personality disorder, borderline personality disorder, histrionic personality disorder, and narcissistic personality disorder; individuals with these disorders show a wide diversity of patterns of social and emotional interactions with others

Durham rule: also called the "product test"; a decision based on an 1871 New Hampshire ruling that an individual is not "criminally responsible if his unlawful act is the product of a mental disease or defect"

duty to protect: an exception to the principle of confidentiality; the general statement is that the therapist must take action if she believes that the client will harm another person or himself—a direct consequence of the Tarasoff court ruling

dynamic deconstructive psychotherapy (DDP): developed for clients who find therapy difficult as well as for those who may also have substance abuse problems; designed to help individuals with borderline personality disorder develop a coherent sense of self

early ejaculation: diagnosed when a man experiences an ejaculation within approximately the first minute of sexual activity and that this causes significant distress over a 6-month period

eating disorders: the three major eating disorders in the fifth edition of the Diagnostic and Statistical Manual of Mental Disorders (*DSM–5*) are anorexia nervosa, bulimia, and binge eating disorder.

effect size: the measured magnitude that a treatment has on the dependent variable (DV)

electroconvulsive therapy (ECT): a treatment for depression in which electrical current is passed through the brain for a brief period

electroencephalography (EEG): a technique for recording electrical activity from the scalp related to cortical activity, which reflects the electrical activity of the brain at the level of the synapse

emotion-focused therapy: also known as process-experiential therapy; in this therapy, emotion is viewed as centrally important in the experience of self, as either adaptive or maladaptive, and as the crucial element that brings about change and management of emotional experiences

empathizing-systemizing theory of autism: coupled with the inability to empathize is the superior ability to systemize in autism

empathy: one aspect of a healthy self and positive personal relationships; it includes understanding how another person experiences his life and what that person might want to accomplish as well as the ability to experience and accept different perspectives toward life and goals and how one's own behavior may influence others

empiricism: the acceptance of sensory information as valid

encephalization: the principle by which more recently evolved higher level systems in the brain control the older lower level centers

encode: to lay out the process by which a particular protein is made; this is the job of a gene

endophenotypes: patterns of processes that lie between the gene (the genotype) and the manifestations of the gene in the external environment (the phenotype)

epidemiology: the study of the distribution and determinants of the frequency of a disorder in humans

epigenetic inheritance: another form of inheritance by which factors largely influenced by the environment of the organism that turn the genes on and off can be passed on to the next generation without influencing DNA itself

epigenetic marks or tags: that which influences whether a segment is relaxed and able to be activated or condensed resulting in no action

epigenetics: study of the factors that turn the genes on and off and are passed on to the next generation; these are largely influenced by the environment of the organism

erectile disorder: requires that a male has a problem in one of three areas: (1) he cannot obtain an erection during sexual activity; (2) he cannot maintain an erection until the completion of sexual activity; and (3) he has a decrease in the rigidity of the penis in a way that interferes with sexual activity; further, the experience of erectile problem produces significant distress

ethics: the study of proper action

event-related potentials (ERPs): also known as evoked potentials (EP), show electroencephalography (EEG) activity in relation to a particular event

evoked potentials (EP): also known as event related potentials (ERPs), show electroencephalography (EEG) activity in relation to a particular event

evolutionary perspective: examines psychological disorders in terms of how certain ways of seeing or being in the world might be adaptive, asking if there is any advantage to behaving and feeling in certain ways that others consider abnormal or if the disordered behavior is secondary to another process that is beneficial

executive functions: cognitive functions involved in planning, understanding new situations and cognitive flexibility

exhibitionistic disorder: the case in which a person becomes sexually aroused by exposing his genitals to an unsuspecting stranger

existential-humanistic perspective: the existential-humanistic approach focuses on the experience of the person in the moment and the manner in which he or she interprets the experiences; it emphasizes processing and understanding both internal and external experiences of human life

experimental group: a group that receives the independent variable (IV) in a study

experimental method: an approach in which the influence of the independent variable (IV) on the dependent variable (DV) is determined with random selection and random assignment of participants

experimenter effects: bias that occurs due to the experimenter's expectations

exposure therapy for PTSD: a therapy designed to have the individual with post-traumatic stress disorder (PTSD) reexperience the original trauma; the person confronts her fears and expectations such that they are reduced

external validity: also known as generalizability, the possibility of applying the results from an internally valid experiment to other situations and other research participants

externalizing disorders: disorders that are manifested in the external world and include conduct disorder (CD), oppositional defiant disorder (ODD), antisocial personality disorder, substance use disorder, and in some studies attention deficit/hyperactivity disorder (ADHD)—contrast with internalizing disorders

extinction: the process by which, after a period of time, the conditioned stimulus, when presented alone, will no longer produce the response

extraversion: as a personality trait, it is associated with sociability, cheerfulness, energy, and a sense of fun; as a dimension in the five-factor model (FFM), this dimension ranges from being passive, quite, and inner-directed to being active, talkative, and outer-directed

factitious disorder imposed on another: a type of factitious disorder in which typically a caregiver such as a parent would produce symptoms in his or her child; historically referred to as Munchausen syndrome by proxy.

factitious disorder: the situation in which a person creates the symptoms seen by the health care professional

factitious disorder imposed on self: a type of factitious disorder in which the person produces symptoms in himself or herself; historically referred to as Munchausen syndrome.

facts: General conclusions drawn from observations

falsification: the approach by which a claim is shown to be wrong; in philosophy of science, it is the position that goal of science is to falsify hypotheses

feeding and eating disorders: the fifth edition of the Diagnostic and Statistical Manual of Mental Disorders (*DSM–5*), unlike *DSM–IV*, combines feeding and eating disorders into one category

feeding disorders: the three major feeding disorders in the fifth edition of the Diagnostic and Statistical Manual of Mental Disorders (*DSM–5*) are pica, rumination disorder, and avoidant/restrictive food intake disorder; previously considered part of a category of disorders usually first diagnosed in infancy, childhood, and adolescence

female orgasmic disorder: the condition in which a woman either does not experience an orgasm or has a reduced intensity of the sensation of the orgasm; this causes significant distress

female sexual interest/arousal disorder: requires significant distress or impairment along with at least three specific symptoms including a reduction or absence of interest in: sexual activity, sexual fantasies, sexual activity, excitement or pleasure during sex, internal or external sexual cues or sexual sensations

fetishistic disorder: involves an erotic fixation on an object or body part that is not sexual in nature and that lasts for over six months and results in clinically significant distress or impairment in important areas of functioning

fight-or-flight response: the overall stress reaction in which the body prepares you either to fight or to leave the scene

five-factor model (FFM): a model of personality based on a factor analytic approach to personality developed by Robert McCrae and Paul Costa, which suggested five major personality dimensions: extraversion, neuroticism, openness, agreeableness, and conscientiousness

flight of ideas: responses that are not related to the question asked or to tell a narrative in which each sentence is not related to the one that came before it

fMRI (functional magnetic resonance imaging): based on the fact that blood flow increases in active areas of the cortex; because hemoglobin, which carries oxygen in the bloodstream, has different magnetic properties before and after oxygen is absorbed, by measuring the ratio of hemoglobin with and without oxygen, the fMRI is able to map changes in cortical blood and infer neuronal activity

fragile X syndrome: a chromosome disorder that results in intellectual developmental disorder due to the FMR1 gene producing too little of a protein needed for brain development

frontotemporal neurocognitive disorder: a disorder characterized by a reduction of the anterior lobes of the frontal and temporal areas; it is seen in different variants depending on the brain areas involved

frotteuristic disorder: the condition in which an individual gains sexual arousal from touching or rubbing against another nonconsenting person

functional neurological symptom disorder: common term in neurology adopted by the fifth edition of the Diagnostic and Statistical Manual of Mental Disorders (*DSM–5*) to refer to conversion disorder

gamma-aminobutyric acid (GABA): the major inhibitory neurotransmitter in the brain and one of the major neurotransmitters involved in anxiety

gender dysphoria: the situation where individuals feel that they are in the wrong body; they may have been born as a male in terms of their body, but their internal experience is that they feel like a female; a smaller number of those born in a female body feel that they are really a male

gender identity: the internal experience of knowing that you are male or female

gender roles: typically defined by one's culture in terms of the kinds of activities boys and girls are expected to engage in

gene by environment correlations: how certain genotypes and certain environments occur together

gene by environment interaction: the possibility that individuals with different genotypes may respond to the same environment in different ways

general adaptation syndrome (GAS): the body reacts similarly to a variety of different stressors in three stages: the alarm stage, the resistance stage, and the exhaustion stage

generalizability: also known as external validity, the possibility of applying the results from an internally valid experiment to other situations and other research participants

generalized anxiety disorder (GAD): characterized by excessive anxiety and worry that has been present for more than three months

genes: form the blueprint that determines what an organism is to become

genito-pelvic pain/penetration disorder: refers to conditions associated with dyspareunia or vaginismus or the fear or anxiety associated with these conditions

genotype: genetic material

glove anesthesia: a specific example of the general phenomenon in which the person reports sensory or motor symptoms such as not being able to hear or see or feel pain or move a part of the body, however, the symptoms do not follow known physiological or neurological patterns

glutamate: an excitatory neurotransmitter in the brain

hallucinations: sensory experiences which can involve any of the senses which are at odds with the individual's current environment

hallucinogens: drugs that are able to alter perception, mood, and cognitive processes in often unpredictable ways; also called psychedelics; some of these drugs occur in nature and have been used by various cultures for thousands of years—e.g., mescaline, which comes from the peyote cactus; although the ergot fungus is naturally occurring, LSD was first made in the laboratory; other laboratory-made drugs include MDMA, commonly known as ecstasy

Health Insurance Portability and Accountability Act of 1996 (HIPAA): U.S. law that protects health care records; regulates the manner in which medical and psychological records are maintained and shared with insurance companies and other health care professionals

healthy self: one conceptualization suggested in the fifth edition of the Diagnostic and Statistical Manual of Mental Disorders (*DSM–5*) is to consider it in terms of a "Self and

Interpersonal Functioning Continuum," which includes the aspects of identity, self-direction, empathy, and intimacy

heterozygotes or heterozygous: when a person has two different alleles for a particular gene

hierarchical integration: through inhibitory control, the various levels of the brain, such as the brain stem, the limbic system and the neocortex, are able to interact with each other, and the type of interaction from the higher levels is restricting or inhibiting the lower levels

hierarchy of needs: Abraham Maslow's theoretical concept for understanding the nature of human needs, which states that one meet lower-level needs (hunger, thirst, and safety) before attaining higher-level needs (belongingness and love, esteem, and self-actualization)

histrionic personality disorder: classified in dramatic emotional personality disorders (Cluster B); characterized by a pervasive pattern of excessive emotionality and attention seeking; being the center of attention is one key element and the person may use a number of means for gaining attention; if they are not the center of attention, they become uncomfortable

hoarding: an excessive acquisition of objects and an inability to discard these objects

homozygotes or homozygous: when a person has two copies of the same allele

human immunodeficiency virus (HIV): a virus that can be passed on by coming in contact with the bodily fluids of an infected person; the virus affects the person's immune system in a negative manner; in the later stages, this is referred to as acquired immune deficiency syndrome (AIDS).

Huntington's disease: a genetic disorder that causes a degeneration of neurons in the brain; one of the few disorders that has a single cause—a gene—in all people; characterized by the loss of brain cells resulting in cognitive, emotional, and motor disturbances

hypothalamic-pituitary-adrenal (HPA) axis: the hypothalamus, pituitary, and adrenal pathway, which is activated in times of stress

hypothalamus, pituitary, and adrenal pathway: a stress pathway referred to as the hypothalamic-pituitary-adrenal (HPA) axis

hypothesis: a formally stated expectation

identity: one aspect of a healthy self; this includes (1) seeing oneself as a unique person with stable boundaries between herself and others; (2) having a history that the person understands; (3) having an accurate sense of who she is and what she can accomplish; and (4) appreciating her abilities

Illness anxiety disorder: occurs when a person is preoccupied with the possibility of having a serious illness; however, the person experiences few if any symptoms; previously referred to as hypochondriasis.

imitation learning: on a brain level, each time an individual sees an action done by another, the neurons that would be involved in that action are activated, creating a motor representation of the observed action, essentially turning a visual image into a motor plan

immune system: the body's system to recognize foreign agents in the body and then destroy them

incidence: the number of new cases of a disorder that develop during a certain period of time

independent variable (IV): the manipulated variable in an experimental study

Individuals with Disabilities Education Act (IDEA): the act by which the Department of Education in the United States defined the services required to be provided to students with learning disabilities

inference: the process by which we look at the evidence available to us and then use our powers of reasoning to reach a conclusion

inferential statistics: a study that concerns the relationship between the statistical characteristics of the population and those of the sample

informed consent: the principle that the client has the right to know what will take place in the therapy session and the nature of the therapist–client relationship. After being informed of the nature of therapy, the client can consent or not.

insanity: a term used in the legal system instead of "mental illness"

institutional review board (IRB): a committee to determine whether the participants are adequately protected in terms of both welfare and rights, and to determine when a risk is unreasonable

intellectual developmental disorder (IDD): a disorder characterized by intellectual disabilities in which the person does not meet normal developmental milestones

intergenerational transmission of depression: the idea that depression in an individual is influenced by having one or more parents who are depressed

internal validity: the ability to make valid inferences between the independent variables (IVs) and dependent variables (DVs)

internalizing disorders: disorders that are experienced internally such as anxiety and depression

International Classification of Diseases (ICD): a publication of criteria for diagnosis by the World Health Organization (WHO), used in Europe

intimacy: one aspect of a healthy self and positive personal relationships; it includes having a relationship with another person that include mutual connectedness and a valuing of that other person; it values closeness and seeks it when appropriate

intoxication: refers to the effects of the psychoactive substance on the individual; effects are substance-related but typically involve psychological changes and behavioral abilities

learning disabilities: the situation in which a child's achievement is lower than that expected from his or her scores on achievement or intelligence tests

levels of analysis: examination of psychopathology ranging from culture and society at a higher level to the individual at a middle level and physiology and genetics at the lower levels

Lewy body dementia: a neurocognitive disorder caused by the buildup of a substance called Lewy bodies in the neurons; the symptoms include changes in alertness and attention, which can result in drowsiness or staring into space as well as visual hallucinations and Parkinson's-like symptoms

lifetime prevalence: the percentage of a specific population that had the disorder at some point in their life even if they no longer show symptoms of the disorder currently

linkage analysis: an examination of generations of families that looks for the association between particular deoxyribonucleic acid (DNA) marker alleles and particular traits

logic: a tool to help us answer questions of inference

longitudinal design: a research design that allows the researcher to follow a specific group of individuals across a period of time to document any changes that take place during that time

M'Naghten rule: a rule adopted in the British legal system in 1843 stating that mental illness could be used as a defense only if (1) there is the presence of a mental disorder and (2) there is a lack of comprehension of the nature or wrongfulness of the act

macrophage theory of depression: the suggestion that cytokines malfunction may be involved in depression

magnetoencephalography (MEG): measures the small magnetic field gradients exiting and entering the surface of the head that are produced when neurons are active

major depressive disorder (MDD): a mood disorder characterized by depressed mood in which one feels sad or empty without any sense of pleasure in one's activities

major neurocognitive disorders: term used to describe cognitive or social deficits that are severe and interfere with one's ability to function independently

male hypoactive sexual desire disorder: refers to the situation in which a male has little desire for sexual activity or even erotic thoughts for 6 months, and this condition causes significant distress

mandated reporting: an exception to the principle of confidentiality; requirement that when health care professionals learn firsthand of child abuse or neglect, they report this information to the appropriate state agency

manic depression: now known as bipolar disorder; a mood disorder characterized by the experience of both depression and mania

match subjects design: a design type in psychopathology research in which the closer a scientist can match individuals in the individual and control groups, the stronger the logic of the design

melancholia: now known as depression; described by ancient Greek writers as in terms of despondency, dissatisfaction with life, problems sleeping, restlessness, irritability, difficulties in decision making, and a desire to die

memory: a process including specific brain areas such as the hippocampus and the biochemical and structural changes among neurons as new information is retained

Mendel's first law or the law of segregation: for the trait to appear, both nondominant elements must be present

Mendel's second law or the law of independent assortment: the inheritance of the gene of one trait is not affected by the inheritance of the gene for another trait

mental retardation: a disorder in which the person shows intellectual disabilities; term no longer used in the Diagnostic and Statistical Manual of Mental Disorders (*DSM–5*)

mental status exam: clinical interview organized into major categories designed to determine a person's cognitive processes

meta-analysis: statistical examination of the results of studies taken together and treated as one study

mild neurocognitive disorders: term used to describe cognitive or social deficits in an individual greater than those declines seen with normal aging

mindfulness: a meditation technique involving an increased, focused, nonjudgmental, purposeful awareness of the present moment to observe thoughts without reacting to them in the present

Minnesota Multiphasic Personality Inventory (MMPI): a test with 567 items of a true–false nature to help determine if a person endorses more or less of a category of experiences than the general population; used to assess broad mental disorders

mirror neurons: neurons in your brain that fire as if you had performed the same actions as you observe

mitochondrial DNA (mtDNA): Deoxyribonucleic acid (DNA) of mitochondria structures within a cell; because mtDNA does not recombine sections of DNA from the mother and father, it is very stable and mutates very slowly

mitochondrial inheritance: generally mitochondrial DNA (mtDNA) is inherited only from the mother

modeling: also known as observational learning; when organisms imitate the behaviors of others even without reinforcement

modularity: describes how specific areas of the brain are dedicated to certain types of process

monozygotic (MZ) twins: identical twins resulting from the zygote (fertilized egg) dividing during the first two weeks of gestation

narcissistic personality disorder: classified in dramatic emotional personality disorders (Cluster B); characterized by a pervasive pattern of grandiosity, a need for admiration, a sense of privilege or entitlement, and a lack of empathy for others; individuals often think about how special they are and the ways in which they will succeed in all types of ways including business, love, competiveness, and so forth; they may also make unreasonable demands on others in relation to their view of themselves. In doing so, they ignore the experiences or needs of others

National Institute of Mental Health (NIMH): one large organization of the U.S. government that advances the understanding and treatment of mental disorders; NIMH emphasizes the utilization of neuroscience information to understand mental illness

natural selection: Darwin's idea that if an individual has even a slight variation that helps it to compete successfully for survival, then over time the species will be made up more and more of members with these characteristics and less and less of individuals lacking these features

naturalistic observation: observing and describing the phenomenon occurring naturally without manipulating any variables

negative cognitive triad: the self, the personal world, and the future as they contribute to a negative schema

negative correlation: the correlation statistic is a technique to determine if to variables are related to each other; a negative correlation is when the two measures show an inverse relationship

negative symptoms: lack of affect in situations which call for it, poor motivation, and social withdrawal

neurocognitive disorder due to Alzheimer's disease: a progressive disorder characterized by problems with memory; associated with a loss of neurons and disruption of cortical networks that result in cognitive problems

neurocognitive disorder due to prion disease: neurocognitive disorder caused by prions that are infectious pathogens that produce tiny holes in the brain, which give it a spongy appearance; it has a rapid course of development and is characterized by cognitive impairments including memory loss, motor problems, personality changes and impaired judgment

neurocognitive disorders: decline in brain function typically seen in older individuals but that represent a loss of cognitive abilities not related to normal aging

neurodevelopmental disorders: a category of childhood disorders including autism spectrum disorder; attention deficit/hyperactivity disorder (ADHD); disorders of learning, intelligence, and communication; and motor disorders such as tics and Tourette's disorder

neuroethics: a field of ethical inquiry that is asking how brain processes are involved in making moral decisions as well as who should have access to your internal processes

neuroscience perspective: examines what we know about particular psychopathological experience from the standpoint of a neuroscience, including the structure and function of the brain, the autonomic nervous system, and a genetic and epigenetic consideration as it relates to psychopathology

neuroticism: as a personality trait, it is associated with a tendency to express distressing emotions and difficulty experiencing stressful situations; as a dimension in the five-factor model (FFM), this dimension ranges from being calm, even-tempered, and comfortable to being worried, temperamental and self-conscious

neurotransmitters: chemicals which are involved in increasing or decreasing the potential for action potentials to be produced; they also maintain the communication across the synapse

nicotine: the addictive substance in tobacco; it is a stimulant substance found in plants of the nightshade family; it can have varied effects on the body which makes it function both as a stimulant and a depressant

null hypothesis: a statistical hypothesis that is tested to determine if there are differences between the experimental and control groups; the null hypothesis states that there is no difference

obesity: seen to result from a mismatch between the amount of calories that we eat and the amount of energy that we expend; it is influenced by factors such as are the environment in which we live, psychological factors and biological factors

observational learning: also known as modeling; when humans imitate the behaviors of others even without reinforcement

obsessional thinking: a pattern of repeated thoughts beyond the control of the person

obsessions: generally unwelcomed thoughts that come into one's head

obsessive-compulsive disorder (OCD): characterized by repetitive thoughts and feelings usually followed by behaviors in response to them

obsessive-compulsive personality disorder: classified in anxious fearful personality disorders (Cluster C); characterized by a pervasive pattern of preoccupation with orderliness, perfectionism, and control of one's environment; individuals would be described as workaholics; they themselves would see little need for taking time off or just spending time with other people; in dealing with others, they may appear rigid and using standards not called for in the current situation

odd-eccentric personality disorders (Cluster A): a grouping of personality disorders within the fifth edition of the Diagnostic and Statistical Manual of Mental Disorders (*DSM–5*); these include schizoid personality disorder, paranoid personality disorder, and schizotypal personality disorder; individuals with these disorders typically feel uncomfortable or suspicious of others or restrict their relationships

openness: as a personality trait, it is associated with curiosity, flexibility, and an artistic sensitivity, including imaginativeness and the ability to create a fantasy world; as a dimension in the five-factor model (FFM), this dimension ranges from inventive and curious to cautious and conservative

operant conditioning: the idea that behavior can be elicited or shaped if reinforcement followed its occurrence

operational definition: the definition of events in terms of the operations required to measure them and thus gives an idea a concrete meaning

opioids: substances derived from the opium poppy that have been used for thousands of years to control pain and bring on euphoric feelings; more common opioids are heroin, opium, morphine, methadone, and oxycodone (oxyContin, Percocet).

oppositional defiant disorder (ODD): a disorder in which individuals mainly show anger and defiance, but do not act aggressively toward other people or animals or destroy property

panic attack: comes quickly and carries with it an intense feeling of apprehension, anxiety, or fear; happens without an actual situation that would suggest danger

paranoid personality disorder: classified in odd-eccentric personality disorders (Cluster A); characterized by a pervasive distrust and suspiciousness of others; the interpersonal style of these individuals is often quarrelsome, stubborn, and rigid in their own beliefs, which can create a self-fulfilling prophecy

paranoid subtype: a type of schizophrenia characterized by delusions whose themes generally center on ideas of grandiosity or persecution

paraphilia: refers to nontraditional sexual practices that exist alongside of the traditional expressions of love

paraphilic disorders: for a sexual desire or sexual behavior to qualify as a disorder, it must cause distress to the person involved, and may cause distress or harm to others; in general, they are also long term in nature

parasympathetic division: the element of the autonomic nervous system involved in the restoration of bodily reserves and the elimination of bodily waste; it connects through the upper and lower parts of the spinal cord

Parkinson's disease: a condition that affects the motor system; symptoms generally include tremors that may involve the hands, arms, legs, jaw, and face; in addition, the person shows a slowness of movement and stiffness in his limbs

pathological gambling: a disorder in which gambling continues even despite negative consequences such as consistent losses and an inability to control one's gambling behavior

Patient Self-Determination Act (PSDA) of 1991: a set of federal requirements intended to implement advance directive policies at all health care facilities that receive federal funding through Medicaid and Medicare programs

pedophilic disorder: involves a persistent sexual interest in prepubescent or early pubescent children; the clinical definition of pedophilic disorder does not require an actual sexual act although this can be the case

personality disorder: represents an enduring pattern of inner experience and behavior that deviates markedly from the expectations of the individual's culture; the pattern is inflexible, stable, and generally begins in adolescence and leads to distress or impairment; characteristics of these disorders are especially apparent when these individuals find themselves in situations that are beyond their ability to cope; the fifth edition of the Diagnostic and Statistical Manual of Mental Disorders (*DSM–5*) identifies 10 personality disorders that form separate categories, which can be organized into three clusters

person-centered therapy: also called client-centered therapy; an approach characterized by the therapist's empathic understanding, unconditional positive regard, genuineness, and congruence

phenotype: organism's observable characteristics

pica: a feeding disorder in which the person eats something that would not be considered food

placebo effect: the phenomenon that some people show psychological and physiological changes just from the suggestion that a change will take place

population: in a research study, this is the larger group of individuals to which the results can be generalized

positive correlation: the correlation statistic is a technique to determine if to variables are related to each other; a positive correlation is when two measures vary together

positive interpersonal relationships: one aspect of a healthy self; characterized by interpersonal relationships in which the person relates to others in an intimate and empathetic manner

positive symptoms: hallucinations, delusions, disorganized thinking, and disorganized behavior

positron emission tomography (PET): a measure related to blood flow in the brain that reflects cognitive processing; PET systems measure variations in cerebral blood flow that are correlated with brain activity

prevalence: the proportion of individuals who have a particular disorder at a particular time period

private personality: the private thoughts of a person

privileged communication: the legal term for confidentiality; the privilege is controlled by the client

probability: whether a set of results differed from what would be expected by chance

process experiential therapy: also known as emotion-focused therapy; in this therapy, emotion is viewed as centrally important in the experience of self, as either adaptive or maladaptive, and as the crucial element that brings about change and management of emotional experiences

projective instruments: ambiguous stimuli are used to elicit the internal cognitive and emotional organization of a person's psychological processes

proteins: do the work of the body and are involved in a variety of processes; functionally, proteins in the form of enzymes are able to make metabolic events speed up, whereas structural proteins are involved in building body parts

psychiatric advance directives (PADs): These directives allow a person to submit directives or individuals to consent on his behalf; allows a person who has a history of periods in which he would not be competent to make a rational decision to direct the types of treatments he would accept or refuse; written into law in a number of states

psychoanalysis: treatment developed by Freud based on the search for ideas and emotions that are in conflict on an unconscious level; this also includes the manner in which the person repeats negative relationships with other people based on past history rather than current interactions; one early procedure was free association in which an individual lay on a couch with the therapist behind him and said whatever came to mind; it was the therapist's job to help the client connect ideas and feelings that were out of awareness. Freud was searching for was connections within the person's psyche when external stimulation was reduced; dreams were also analyzed in this way since they are produced outside of the external stimulation of daily life; although a person may not be able to change their initial reactions, they can learn to process these in a cognitive manner

psychodynamic perspective: this perspective suggests that current behavior and experience result from internal conflicts based on previous experiences including instinctual processes and cultural directives; psychodynamic therapy is designed to help the individual understand their reactions based on prior experiences and relationships

psychogenic disorders or functional disorders: terms used in the medical literature in reference to conversion reactions

psychological stress: an experience when something we do not expect and cannot control happens to us

psychoneuroimmunology: the study of how psychological factors can influence the immune system

psychopathology: the study of mental illness; this is in contrast with pathophysiology, or pathology of our physiology

psychopathy: a disorder characterized by showing emotional detachment with a lack of empathy for the experiences of others; also showing impulsive behavior and a callousness concerning their actions

psychotic disorders: disorders that involve a loss of being in touch with reality and are characterized by abnormal thinking and sensory processes

purging: an aspect of bulimia where a person eliminates food from the body by such means as vomiting, taking laxatives, diuretics, or enemas

randomization: a process that controls for both known and unknown potentially confounding variables; randomization leaves solely to chance the assignment of our participants to a group

reactive attachment disorder (RAD): a disorder that is the result of inadequate caregiving, which may include institutional settings

real self: self includes who one is and what one appreciates

reinforcement: rewards that follow behaviors and increase their occurrence

reliability: consistency of the instrument

replicated: when a study is performed in different laboratories with different participants and obtains the same results

Research Domain Criteria (RDoC): five domains established by the National Institute of Mental Health (NIMH) to better clarify our understanding of psychopathology, which are negative affect, positive affect, cognition, social processes, and regulatory systems

research hypothesis: the formal statement of the manner in which the dependent variable (DV) is related to the independent variable (IV)

reserve: concept that suggests that the brain can compensate for problems in neural functioning since not all individuals showed the same changes to similar neurocognitive disorders or brain injury; high functioning or intelligence is often associated with greater reserve; additional research has shown a role for exercise and social support

reward system: particular brain structures, especially the nucleus accumbens part of the ventral striatum, influenced by an increase in dopamine during reward

ribonucleic acid (RNA): information that determines the sequence of amino acids which are the building blocks of proteins; it is made up single strands rather the dual strands in deoxyribonucleic acid (DNA)

right to privacy: the right to spend time by oneself or with others of one's choosing, without being disturbed, and the right to have private thoughts

risk: a way of thinking about incidence, which asks how likely someone in a specific population is to develop a particular disorder in a given time period

Rorschach Inkblot: inkblots developed by Herman Rorschach; they were made by dripping ink on a piece of paper and then folding it in half to create a symmetrical design; it functions as a projective technique

rumination disorder: the condition in which a person regurgitates his food; this swallowed food is then re-chewed, re-swallowed, or spit out

salience network: the neural network involved in monitoring and noting important changes in biological and cognitive systems

sample: participants in a study

schizoid personality disorder: classified in odd-eccentric personality disorders (Cluster A); characterized by a pervasive pattern of detachment from social relationships and a restricted range of emotional expression; these individuals are traditional loners; others see them as unavailable, aloof, or detached

schizophrenia: a debilitating psychotic disorder in which individuals may hear voices, see images not seen by others, believe that others wish to harm or control them, and have bizarre thoughts

schizotypal personality disorder: classified in odd-eccentric personality disorders (Cluster A); characterized by odd beliefs and behaviors; an individual may show excessive social anxiety as well as show unusual ideas

schizotypal traits: schizophrenic-like traits

SCID-D: a screening device for dissociative disorders developed by Marlene Steinberg

science: a process of understanding the world through observation and research, which includes developing theories

scientific knowledge: the known facts about a particular subject derived from the scientific method

secure attachment pattern: an attachment style characterized by the following pattern in the strange situation in which the infant (1) engages in active exploration, (2) is upset when the mother leaves, and (3) shows positive emotions when the mother returns

self-actualization: the situation in which one lives one's life to the fullest

self-direction: one aspect of a healthy self; it reflects the ability to have both meaningful short-term and long-term goals consistent with one's identity as well as a sense of what would be productive for society and how to interact with others; internally, healthy self-direction also includes the ability to reflect on one's life in a productive manner

self-realization: recognition of who one is and what one appreciates in terms of their connections with themselves and others

separation anxiety disorder: a situation where children as they develop do not show a normal sense of independence and continue to feel distress when not with their caregivers

sexual dysfunction disorders: a category of the fifth edition of the Diagnostic and Statistical Manual of Mental Disorders (*DSM–5*) in which there are problems in sexual functioning, the condition exists for at least six months, and it causes significant distress or impairment

sexual masochism disorder: present when the person experiences sexual arousal from the act of being humiliated, beaten, bound, or otherwise made to suffer, as manifested by fantasies, urges, or behaviors for over six months, and these urges or behaviors cause distress or impairment in their life

sexual sadism disorder: involves deriving sexual pleasure from inflicting pain or humiliation on others. It is required that the person has acted out these impulses with a non-consenting individual or experienced distress or impairment from these impulses, and it must have been present for at least six months.

sexual selection: the manner in which males and females choose a mate

sexually violent predator (SVP) or sexually dangerous person (SDP) statutes: laws that allow for a person who committed a sexual crime to be held after his or her sentence has been completed. The idea is that these individuals represent a threat to public safety if they are released. Since the 1990s, 19 states and the federal government have passed laws that allow for such civil commitment of individuals.

signs: features observed by the clinician

single subject designs: also referred to as small-N designs, use the data from each participant without averaging it as part of a group of participants

small world framework: this is a model of brain connections based on idea that the ability to socially contact any two random individuals in the world can be accomplished in a limited number of connections; neurons have numerous short-distance local connections, which taken together can be considered as a hub or module; from these hubs are more long-distance connections to other hubs; the small world perspective suggests that the connections between any two nodes in the brain can be represented by only a limited number of connections

social anxiety disorder (SAD): characterized by marked fear or anxiety about one or more social situations in which the individual is exposed to possible scrutiny by others

somatic symptom and related disorders: situation in which individuals are certain something is wrong with them; they may continue to search for organic problems or may feel anxiety that the simple symptoms they have are really something serious

specific learning disorder: a disorder in which a child shows problems in one of the major school tasks

specific phobia: the condition in which an individual experiences fear or anxiety to a particular condition or object

statistically significant: the probability that the independent variable (IV) influences the dependent variable (DV) by chance; by using statistics, we ask if we performed the same experiment 100 times, what is the probability we would obtain the results seen in the present study?

stigma: negative attitudes and beliefs that cause the general public to avoid others including those with a mental illness

Stroop test: a psychological test used to study cognitive bias; the traditional Stroop test has color names in ink of a different color

Structured Clinical Interview for *DSM* Disorders (SCID): an interview that directly probes for the existence of the criteria for disorders within the current classification manual, the Diagnostic and Statistical Manual of Mental Disorders (*DSM–5*)

structured interview: an interview that is highly structured in terms of the questions asked, allowing for better consistency across interviewers and clients

substance tolerance: the situation in which the individual must consume more of the drug to have the same effect, or with gambling, the individual needs to bet more to keep the same level of excitement

substance-induced neurocognitive disorder: neurocognitive deficits caused by the abuse of drugs over a period of time

successful aging: individuals who continue to be productive well into their 80s and 90s; characterized by (1) freedom from disability and disease, (2) high cognitive and physical functioning, and (3) social activity including both having friends and being productive

suicidal ideation: thinking often about suicide

suicide: to kill oneself

sympathetic division: the element of the autonomic nervous system that connects with its target organs through the middle part of the spinal cord, responsible for the fight-or-flight response

symptoms: features observed by the patient

syndrome: determination of which signs and symptoms go together

tend-and-befriend response: a response to stress associated with the tendency of females to take care of others and form social connections in times of stress

Thematic Apperception Test (TAT): a testing instrument composed of 30 black-and-white drawings of various scenes and people; by noting the content and emotionality of the individual's responses, it is possible to gain insight into his or her thoughts, emotions, and motivations including areas of conflict

theory of mind: the study of one's ability to understand one's own or another person's mental state

tobacco: a plant that originated in the Americas with native populations smoking or chewing its leaves

transcranial magnetic stimulation (TMS): a treatment for depression in which an electromagnetic coil is placed on the scalp; from the coil, a magnetic field induces a small electrical current in the first few centimeters of the brain which depolarizes the neurons

transference-focused psychotherapy (TFP): a twice-weekly therapy based on Otto Kernberg's object relations model; as with other approaches, TFP seeks to reduce symptoms of borderline personality disorder, especially self-destructive behaviors

transgender: individuals who have the anatomy of one sex and the gender identity of the other

transsexual: the situation in which a transgendered individual has sought medical intervention such as hormone treatment and sexual reassignment surgery to change his or her body into that of the opposite sex

transvestic disorder: characterized by recurrent and intense sexual arousal from cross-dressing, as manifested by fantasies, urges, or behaviors which lasts for a period of at least six months and causes distress or impairment

trauma- and stressor-related disorders: a category of childhood disorders, including disorders of attachment

traumatic brain injuries (TBI): acceleration and deceleration forces on the brain as it impacts with the skull commonly lead to injuries, which often produce diffuse microstructural injury; the severity of these injuries can range from mild to severe; seen across the life span

twin studies: a major paradigm of behavioral genetics involving examination and understanding of critical factors related to genetic influences by studying twins

unipolar depression: the mood disorder characterized by the experience of depression without mania

vagal nerve stimulation (VNS): a treatment for depression in which an electrical stimulator is surgically implanted next to the vagus, then connected to a pulse generator in the person's chest; like a pacemaker in the heart, the pulse generator can be programmed to deliver electrical pulses at desirable frequencies and currents

validity: truth and capability of being supported

variation: the assumption that heritable variations can and do occur in nature

vascular neurocognitive disorder: neurocognitive disorder caused by vascular problems such as strokes; problems in cognitive performance are usually seen as abrupt changes

volitional test: a test adopted in Alabama in the 1880s for not guilty by reason of insanity in which mental illness made the person unable to control himself even though he knew the difference between right and wrong

voluntary participation: a principle stating that a person should participate in an experiment only by free choice, and should be free to leave an experiment at any time, whether or not the experiment has been completed

voyeuristic disorder: involves obtaining sexual arousal from watching unsuspecting people when they are undressing, performing sexual acts, or going to the bathroom; it lasts for a period of at least six months and causes distress or impairment

Wechsler Adult Intelligence Scale (WAIS): a common intelligence test with a number of subscales designed to measure verbal and performance tasks

Wisconsin Card Sorting Test (WCST): a test that requires that an individual sort cards into four piles; each card has a specific shape on it such as a circle or square, and each card has a specific number of these shapes and each card is printed in a specific color; thus, you could sort the cards by shape, by number, or by color

withdrawal: the symptoms experienced when a psychoactive substance is reduced or no longer used

REFERENCES

Abel, J. L., & Borkovec, T. D. (1995). Generalizability of DSM-III-R generalized anxiety disorders to proposed DSM-IV criteria and cross-validation of proposed changes. *Journal of Anxiety Disorders, 9,* 303–315.

Abi-Dargham, A., & Grace, A. (2011). Dopamine and schizophrenia. In D. Weinberger & P. Harrison (Eds.), *Schizophrenia.* New York: Wiley.

Abramowitz, J., Deacon, B., & Whiteside, S. (2011). *Exposure therapy for anxiety.* New York: Guilford Press.

Ader, R. (Ed.). (2007). *Psychoneuroimmunology* (4th ed., 2 vols.). New York: Elsevier.

Adolphs, R. (2003). Cognitive neuroscience of human social behaviour. *Nature Reviews Neuroscience, 4,* 165–178.

Adolphs, R. (2009). The social brain: Neural basis of social knowledge. *Annual Review of Psychology, 60,* 693–716.

Adrian, E. (1928). *The basis of sensation.* New York: W. W. Norton & Co.

Agan, A. (2011). Sex offender registries: Fear without function? *Journal of Law and Economics, 54,* 207–239.

Agarwal, S.M., Jose, D., Baruah, U. Shivkumar, V., et al. (2013). Neurohemodynamic Correlates of Washing Symptoms in Obsessive-compulsive Disorder: A Pilot fMRI Study Using Symptom Provocation Paradigm. *Indian Journal of Psychological Medicine,* 35 (1), 67–74.

Agras, W., Walsh, T., Fairburn, C., Wilson, G., & Kraemer, H. (2000). A multicenter comparison of cognitive-behavioral therapy and interpersonal psychotherapy for bulimia nervosa. *Archives of General Psychiatry, 57,* 459–466.

Aguiar, A., Eubig, P., & Schantz, S. (2010). Attention deficit/hyperactivity disorder: A focused overview for children's environmental health researchers. *Environmental Health Perspective, 118,* 1646–1653.

Ainsworth, M., Blehar, M., Waters, E., & Wall, S. (1978). *Patterns of attachment: A psychological study of the Strange Situation.* Hillsdale, NJ: Lawrence Erlbaum.

Albert, P. (2010). Epigenetics in mental illness: Hope or hype? *Journal of Psychiatry and Neuroscience, 35,* 366–368.

Allen, A. J., Griss, M. E., Folley, B. S., Hawkins, K. A., & Pearlson, G. D. (2009). Endophenotypes in schizophrenia: A selective review. *Schizophrenia Research, 109,* 24–37.

Allen, N. & Badcock, P. (2003). The social risk hypothesis of depressed mood: Evolutionary, psychosocial, and neurobiological perspectives. *Psychological Bulletin, 129,* 887–913.

Allen, P., Larøi, F., McGuire, P., & Aleman, A. (2008). The hallucinating brain: A review of structural and functional neuroimaging studies of hallucinations. *Neuroscience and Biobehavioral Reviews, 32,* 175–191.

Alzheimer, A. (1907). Uber eine eigenartige Erkrankung der Hirnrinde. *Allgemeine Zeitschrift fur Psychiatrie und phychish-Gerichtliche Medizin, 64,* 146–148.

Alzheimer, A., Stelzmann, R. A., Schnitzlein, H. N., & Murtagh, F. R. (1995). An English translation of Alzheimer's 1907 paper, "Uber eine eigenartige Erkankungder Hirnrinde." *Clinical Anatomy, 8,* 429–431.

Amaral, D., Schumann, C., & Nordahl, C. (2008). Neuroanatomy of autism. *Trends in Neurosciences, 31,* 137–145.

Ambady, N., & Bharucha, J. (2009). Culture and the brain. *Current directions in psychological science, 18,* 342–345.

American Psychiatric Association. (2013). *Diagnostic and statistical manual of mental disorders* (5th ed.). Washington, DC: Author.

Amudhan, S., Gururaj, G., & Satishchandra, P. (2015). Epilepsy in India I: Epidemiology and public health. *Annals of Indian Academy of Neurology, 18*(3), 263.

Anastopoulos, A., & Farley, S. (2003). A cognitive-behavioral training program for parents of children with attention-deficit/hyperactivity disorder. In A. Kazdin & J. Weisz (Eds). *Evidence-based psychotherapies for children and adolescents.* New York: Guilford Press.

Anderson, D., & Maloney, K. (2001). The efficacy of cognitive-behavioral therapy on the core symptoms of bulimia nervosa. *Clinical Psychology Review, 21,* 971–988.

Anderson, N., & Kiehl, K. (2011). The psychopath magnetized: Insights from brain imaging. *Trends in Cognitive Sciences, 16,* 52–60.

Anderson, S., Bechara, A., Damasio, H., Tranel, D., & Damasio, A. (1999). Impairment of social and moral behavior related to early damage in human prefrontal cortex. *Nature Neuroscience, 2,* 1032–1037.

Andreasen, N. (2001). *Brave new brain.* New York: Oxford University Press.

Andreasen, N. (2005). *The creating brain: The neuroscience of genius.* New York: Dana Press.

Andrews, P. (2007). Reconstructing the evolution of the mind is depressingly difficult. In S. Gangestad & J. Simpson (Eds.), *The evolution of mind* (pp. 45–52). New York: Guilford Press.

Antony, M. M., & Barlow, D. H. (2002). Specific phobia. In D. H. Barlow, *Anxiety and its disorders: The nature and treatment of anxiety and panic* (2nd ed., pp. 380–417). New York: Guilford Press.

Appelbaum, P. S., & Grisso, T. (1995). The MacArthur Treatment Competence Study: I. Mental illness and competence to consent to treatment. *Law and Human Behavior, 19,* 105–126.

Asami, T., Whitford, T., Bouix, S., Dickey, C., Niznikiewicz, M., Shenton, M., . . . McCarley, R. (2013). Globally and locally reduced MRI gray matter volumes in neuroleptic-naive men with schizotypal personality disorder. *JAMA Psychiatry, 70,* 361–372.

Ballmaier, M., Toga, A., Blanton, R., Sowell, E., Havretsky, H., Peterson, J., . . . Kumar, A. (2004). Anterior cingulate, gyrus rectus, and orbitofrontal abnormalities in elderly depressed patients. *American Journal of Psychiatry, 161,* 99–108.

Bang, R. (1989). Why do women hide them? Rural women's viewpoints on reproductive tract infections. *Manushi, New Delhi, 69*(1), 27–63.

Bang, R., & Bang, A. (1994). Perception of rural women on white discharge: Ethnographic data from rural Maharashtra. In J. Gittelsohn (ed.), *Listening to women talk about their health issues: Evidence from India.* New Delhi: Har-Anand Publication/Ford Foundation.

Baranek, G., Watson, L., Boyd, B., Poem M., David, F., & McGuire, L. (2013). Hyporesponsiveness to social and nonsocial sensory stimuli in children with autism, children with developmental delays, and typically developing children. *Development and Psychopathology, 25,* 307–320.

Barber, J., Muran, J., McCarthy, K., & Keefe, J. (2013). Research on dynamic therapies. In M. Lambert (Ed.), *Handbook of psychotherapy and behavior change* (6th ed.). Hoboken, NJ: Wiley.

Barch, D., & Ceaser, A. (2012). Cognition in schizophrenia: Core psychological and neural mechanisms. *Trends in Cognitive Science, 16,* 27–34.

Bardin, J. (2012). Unlocking the brain. *Nature, 487,* 24–26.

Barlow, D. (1988). *Anxiety and its disorders: The nature and treatment of anxiety and panic.* New York: Guilford Press.

Barlow, D. (2002). *Anxiety and its disorders: The nature and treatment of anxiety and panic* (2nd ed.). New York: Guilford Press.

Baron-Cohen, S. (2005). The empathizing system. In B. Ellis & D. Bjorklund (Eds.), *Origins of the social mind: Evolutionary psychology and child development.* New York: Guilford Press.

Baron-Cohen, S. (2009). Autism: The empathizing-systemizing (E-S) theory. *Annals of the New York Academy of Science, 1156,* 68–80.

Baron-Cohen, S., Ashwin, E., Ashwin, C., Tavassoli, T., & Chakrabarti, B. (2008). Talent in autism: Hyper-systemizing, hyper-attention to detail and sensory hypersensitivity. *Philosophical Transactions of the Royal Society B, 364,* 1377–1383.

Baron-Cohen, S., & Belmonte, M. (2005). Autism: A window onto the development of the social and the analytic brain. *Annual Review of Neuroscience, 28*, 109–126.

Barrowclough, C., & Lobban, F. (2008). Family intervention. In K. Meser & D. Jeste (Eds.), *Clinical handbook of schizophrenia* (pp. 214–225). New York: Guilford Press.

Bartz, J., Kaplan, A., & Hollander, E. (2007). Obsessive-compulsive personality disorder. In W. O'Donohue, K. A. Fowler, & S. O. Lilienfeld (Eds.), *Personality disorders: Toward the DSM-V* (pp. 325–352). Thousand Oaks, CA: SAGE.

Basco, N., & Rush, A. (2005). *Cognitive-behavioral therapy for bipolar disorder* (2nd ed.). New York: Guilford Press.

Bassett, D. S., Nelson, B. G., Mueller, B. A., Camchong, J., & Lim, K. O. (2012). Altered resting state complexity in schizophrenia. *NeuroImage, 59,* 196–207.

Battle, C. L., Shea, M. T., Johnson, D. M., Yen, S., Zlotnick, C., Zanarini, M. C., . . . Morey, L. C. (2004). Childhood maltreatment associated with adult personality disorders: Findings from the Collaborative Longitudinal Personality Disorders Study. *Journal of Personality Disorders, 18*(2), 193–211.

Beason-Held, L. (2011). Dementia and the default mode. *Current Alzheimer Research, 8,* 361–365.

Beck, A. (1967). *Depression: Clinical, experimental, and theoretical aspects.* New York: Harper & Row.

Beck, A. T., & Alford, B. A. (2009). *Depression: Causes and treatments* (2nd ed.). Philadelphia: University of Pennsylvania Press.

Beck, A. T., & Beck, R. W. (1972). Screening depressed patients in family practice: A rapid technic. *Postgraduate Medicine, 52,* 81–85.

Beck, A. T., & Rector, N. A. (2005). Cognitive approaches to schizophrenia: Theory and therapy *Annual Review of Clinical Psychology, 1,* 577–606.

Beck, J. (2011). *Cognitive behavioral therapy* (2nd ed.). New York: Guilford Press.

Becker, A. (2011). Cutlure and eating disorders classification. In R Struegek-Moore, S. Wonderlich, B. Walsh, & J. Mitchell (Eds.), *Developing an evidence-based classification of eating disorders.* Arlington, VA: American Psychiatric Association.

Bell, J., & Spector, T. (2011). A twin approach to unraveling epigenetics. *Trends in Genetics, 27,* 116–125.

Bellivier, F., Golmard, J., Rietschel, M., Schulze, T., Malafosse, A., Preisig, M., . . . Leboyer, M. (2003). Age at onset in bipolar I affective disorder: Further evidence for three subgroups. *American Journal of Psychiatry, 160,* 999–1001.

Belsky, J. (2005). Differential susceptibility to rearing influence: An evolutionary hypothesis and some evidence. In B. Ellis & D. Bjorklund (Eds.), *Origins of the social mind: Evolutionary psychology and child development.* New York: Guilford Press.

Bender, D., Morey, L., & Skodol, A. (2011). Toward a model for assessing level of personality functioning in DSM–5, Part I: A review of theory and methods. *Journal of Personality Assessment, 93,* 332–346.

Berger, H. (1969). Über das Elektrekephalogramm des Menschen. *Electroencephalography and Clinical Neurophysiology* (Supp. 28). (Reprinted from *Archive für Psychiatrie und Nervenkrankheiten, 87,* 527–570, 1929)

Bernstein, D., & Useda, J. (2007). Paranoid personality disorder. In W. O'Donohue, K. Fowler, & S. Lilienfeld (Eds.), *Personality disorders: Toward the DSM-V.* Thousand Oaks, CA: SAGE.

Berntson, G. G., Cacioppo, J. T., & Quigley, K. S. (1991). Autonomic determinism: The modes of autonomic control, the doctrine of autonomic space, and the laws of autonomic constraint. *Psychological Review, 98,* 459–487.

Berntson, G. G., Cacioppo, J. T., & Quigley, K. S. (1993). Cardiac psychophysiology and autonomic space in humans: Empirical perspectives and conceptual implications. *Psychological Bulletin, 114,* 296–322.

Beutel, M., Weidner, W. & Brähler, E. (2006). Epidemiology of sexual dysfunction in the male population. *Andrologia, 38,* 115–121.

Bhugra, D. (1992). Psychiatry in ancient Indian texts: A review. *History of Psychiatry, 3*(10), 167–186. Retrieved from http://journals.sagepub.com/doi/abs/10.1177/0957154X9200301002

Bidwell, L., McClernon, F., & Kolins, S. (2011). Cognitive enhancers for the treatment of ADHD. *Pharmacology, Biochemistry and Behavior, 99,* 262–274.

Bienvenu, O., Samuels, J., Wuyek, L., Liang, K., Wang, Y., Grados, M., . . . Nestadt, G. (2012). Is obsessive-compulsive disorder an anxiety disorder, and what, if any, are spectrum conditions? A family study perspective. *Psychological Medicine, 42,* 1–13.

Bishop, S. (2007). Neurocognitive mechanisms of anxiety: An integrative account. *Trends in Cognitive Sciences, 11,* 307–316.

Bissada, H., Tasca, G., Barber, A., & Bradwejn, J. (2008). Olanzapine in the treatment of low body weight and obsessive thinking in women with anorexia nervosa: A randomized, double-blind, placebo-controlled trial. *American Journal of Psychiatry, 165,* 1281–1288.

Bisson, J., & Andrew, M. (2007). Psychological treatment of post-traumatic stress disorder (PTSD). *Cochrane Database,* Jul 18(3):CD003388.

Blagov, P. S., Fowler, K., & Lilienfeld, S. (2007). Histrionic personality disorder. In W. O'Dononue, S. O. Lilienfeld, and K. A. Fowler (Eds.), *Personality disorders: Toward DSM-V* (pp. 203–232). Thousand Oaks, CA: SAGE.

Blackmore, S. (2013). Teenage kicks: Cannabis and the adolescent brain. *Lancet, 381,* 888–889.

Blashfield, R., & Dragus, J. (1976). Toward a taxonomy of psychopathology: The purpose of psychiatric classification. *British Journal of Psychiatry, 129,* 574–583.

Blashfield, R. K., Flanagan, E. H., & Raley, K. (2010). Themes in the evolution of the 20th century DSMs. In T. Millon, R. Krueger, & E. Simonsen (Eds.), *Contemporary directions in psychopathology* (2nd ed.). New York: Guilford Press.

Bloch, M. H., Landeros-Weisenberger, A., Rosario, M. C., Pittenger, C., & Leckman, J. F. (2008). Systematic review of the factor structure of obsessive-compulsive disorder. *American Journal of Psychiatry, 165,* 1532–1542.

Blumberger, D., Mulsant, B., & Daskalakis, Z. (2013). What is the role of brain stimulation therapies in the treatment of depression? *Current Psychiatry Reports, 15,* 368.

Boccardi, M., Frisoni, G., Hare, R., Cavedo, E., Najt, P., Pievani, M., . . .Tiihonen, J. (2011). Cortex and amygdala morphology in psychopathy. *Psychiatry Research, 193,* 85–92.

Bodas, J, Ollendick, T.H., and Sovani A.V. (2008). Test anxiety in Indian children: A cross-cultural perspective. *Anxiety, Stress and Coping, 21*(4), 387–404.

Bodnar, R., Commons, K., & Pfaff, D. (2002). *Central neural states relating sex and pain.* Baltimore: Johns Hopkins Press.

Boland R. J., & Keller, M. B. (2009). Course and outcome of depression. In I. H. Gotlib & C. L. Hammen (Eds.), *Handbook of depression* (2nd ed.). New York: Guilford Press.

Bollini, A., & Walker, E. (2007). Schizotypal personality disorder. In W. O'Donohue, K. Fowler, & S. Lilienfeld (Eds.), *Personality disorders: Toward the DSM-5.* Thousand Oaks, CA: SAGE.

Bono, C. (2011). *Transition, The story of how I became a man.* New York: Dutton.

Boring, E. (1950). *A history of experimental psychology* (2nd ed.). New York: Appleton-Century-Crofts.

Borkovec, T. D. (1994). The nature, functions, and origins of worry. In G. C. L. Davey & F. Tallis (Eds.), *Worrying: Perspectives on theory, assessment and treatment* (pp. 5–33). Oxford, UK: Wiley.

Borkovec, T. D. (2006). Treatment of generalized anxiety disorder and its central worry process. In S. Sassaroli & G. Ruggerio (Eds.), *Worry, need of control, and other core cognitive constructs in anxiety and eating disorders.* New York: Wiley.

Borkovec, T. D., Alcaine, O., & Behar, E. S. (2004). Avoidance theory of worry and generalized anxiety disorder. In R. Heimberg, D. Mennin, & C. Turk (Eds.), *Generalized anxiety disorder: Advances in research and practice* (pp. 77–108). New York: Guilford Press.

Borkovec, T. D., & Ruscio, A. (2001). Psychotherapy for generalized anxiety disorder. *Journal of Clinical Psychiatry, 62,* 37–42.

Bornstein, R. (2007). Dependent personality disorder. In W. O'Donohue, K. A. Fowler, & S. O. Lilienfeld (Eds.), *Personality disorders: Toward the DSM–V* (pp. 307–324). Thousand Oaks, CA: SAGE.

Bouchard, C. (2010). Genetics and genomics of obesity: Current status. *Progress in Molecular Biology and Translational Science, 94,* 1–8.

Bouchard, T., Lykken, D., McGue, M., Segal, N. & Tellegen, A. (1992). Sources of human psychological differences: The Minnesota study of twins reared apart. *Science, 250,* 223–228.

Bowlby, J. (1951). *Maternal care and mental health.* World Health Organization, Monograph Series No. 2.

Bowlby, J. (1982). Attachment and loss: retrospect and prospect. *American Journal of Orthopsychiatry, 52,* 664–678.

Bowlby, J. (1988). *A Secure Base: Clinical Applications of Attachment Theory.* London: Routledge.

Bowlby, J. (1961). Childhood mourning and its implications for psychiatry. The Adolf Meyer Lecture. *American Journal of Psychiatry, 118,* 481–497.

Bowlby, J. (1969). *Attachment and loss: Vol 1. Attachment.* London: Hogarth.

Boxer, P., & Flick, P. (2008). Treating conduct problems, aggression, and antisocial behavior in children and adolescents: An integrated view. In R. Steele, T. Elkin, & M. Roberts (Eds.), *Handbook of evidence-based therapies for children and adolescents.* New York: Springer.

Bradley, R., Conklin, C. Z., & Westen, D. (2007). Borderline personality disorder. In W. O'Donohue, K. Fowler, & S. Lilienfeld (Eds.), *Sage handbook of personality disorders.* Thousand Oaks, CA: SAGE.

Bradley, R., Greene, M., Russ, E., Dutra, L., & Westen, D. (2005). A multidimensional meta-analysis of psychotherapy for PTSD. *American Journal of Psychiatry, 162,* 214–227.

Brayne, C. (2007). The elephant in the room—Healthy brains in later life, epidemiology and public health. *Nature Reviews Neuroscience, 8,* 233–239.

Brendgen, M., Vitaro, F., Bukowski, W., Dionne, G., Tremblay, R., & Boivin, M. (2013). Can friends protect genetically vulnerable children from depression? *Development and Psychopathology, 25,* 277–289.

Bressler, S., & Menon, V. (2010). Large scale brain networks in cognition emerging methods and principles. *Trends in Cognitive Sciences, 14,* 277–290.

Brinkmeyer, M., & Eyberg, S.M. (2003). Parent-child interaction therapy for oppositional children. In A. E. Kazdin & J. R. Weisz (Eds.), *Evidence-based psychotherapies for children and adolescents.* New York: Guilford Press.

Brody, J. (2007, February 20). Out of control: A true story of binge eating. *The New York Times.*

Bromley, D. (1986). *The case-study design in psychology and related disciplines.* New York: Wiley.

Brothers, L. (1990). The social brain: A project for integrating primate behaviour and neurophysiology in a new domain. *Concepts in Neuroscience, 1,* 27–51.

Brown, A., & Patterson, P. (2011). Maternal infection and schizophrenia: Implications for prevention. *Schizophrenia Bulletin, 37,* 284–290.

Brown, T. A., Campbell, L. A., Lehman, C. L., Grisham, J. R., & Mancill, R. B. (2001). Current and lifetime comorbidity of the DSM-IV anxiety and mood disorders in a large clinical sample. *Journal of Abnormal Psychology, 110,* 585–599.

Bruce, S., Buchholz, K., Brown, W., Yan, L., Durbin, A., & Sheline, Y. (2013). Altered emotional interference processing in the amygdala and insula in women with post- traumatic stress disorder. *NeuroImage: Clinical, 2,* 43–49.

Bryant, R., Friedman, M., Spiegel, D., Ursano, R., & Strain, J. (2011). A review of acute stress disorder in DSM-5. *Depression and Anxiety, 28,* 802–817.

Bryant-Waugh, R., Markham, L., Kreipe, R., & Walsh, B. (2010). Feeding and eating disorders in childhood. *International Journal of Eating Disorders, 43,* 98–111.

Bryk, M., & Siegel, P. T. (1997). My mother caused my illness: The story of a survivor of Munchausen by proxy syndrome. *Pediatrics, 100,* 1–7.

Buchen, L. (2010). In their nurture. *Nature, 467,* 146–148.

Buchman, A., Boyle, P., Yu, L., Shah, R., Wilson, R., & Bennett, D. (2012). Total daily physical activity and the risk of AD and cognitive decline in older adults. *Neurology, 24,* 1323–1329.

Buchsbaum, M., & Haier, R. (1987). Functional and anatomical brain imaging: Impact on schizophrenia research. *Schizophrenia Bulletin, 13,* 115–132.

Buckner, R. L., Andrews-Hanna, J. R., & Schacter, D. L. (2008). The brain's default network: Anatomy, function, and relevance to disease. *Annals of the New York Academy of Science, 1124,* 1–38.

Buhrich, N. & Beaumont, T. (1981). Comparison of transvestism in Australia and America. *Archives of Sexual Behavior, 26,* 589–605.

Burgmer, M., Konrad, C., Jansen, A., Kugel, H., Sommer, J., Heindel, W., . . . Knecht, S. (2006). Abnormal brain activation during movement observation in patients with conversion paralysis. *NeuroImage, 29,* 1336–1343.

Burnett, S., Sebastian, C., Kadosh, K., & Blakemore, S. (2011). The social brain in adolescence: Evidence from functional magnetic resonance imaging and behavioural studies. *Neuroscience and Biobehavioral Reviews, 35,* 1654–1664.

Burnette, M., & Cicchetti, D. (2012). Multilevel approaches toward understanding antisocial behavior: Current research and future directions. *Development and Psychopathology, 24,* 703–704.

Burns, J. (2004). An evolutionary theory of schizophrenia: Cortical connectivity, metarepresentation, and the social brain. *Behavioral and Brain Sciences, 27,* 831–885.

Buss, D. (Ed.). (2005). *The handbook of evolutionary psychology.* Hoboken, NJ: Wiley.

Butler, A., Chapman, J., Forman, E., & Beck, A. (2005). The empirical status of cognitive-behavioral therapy: a review of meta-analyses. *Clinical Psychology Review, 26,* 17–31.

Byne, W., Bradley, S., Coleman, E., Eyler, A., Green, R., Menvielle, E., . . . Tompkins, D. (2012). Report of the American Psychiatric Association Task Force on Treatment of Gender Identity Disorder. *Archives of Sexual Behavior, 41,* 759–796.

Callahan, L., Steadman, H., Tillman, S., & Vesselinov, R. (2012). A multi-site study of the use of sanctions and incentives in mental health courts. *Law and Human Behavior, 37,* 1–9.

Calhoun, L.G., & Tedeschi, R.G. (2001). Posttraumatic growth: The positive lessons of loss. In R. A. Neimeyer (Ed.), *Meaning reconstruction and the experience of loss* (pp. 157–172). Washington, D.C: American Psychological Association.

Campbell, D. T., & Stanley, J. C. (1963). *Experimental and quasi-experimental designs for research.* Chicago: Rand McNally.

Cannon, W. (1932). *The wisdom of the body.* New York: W. W. Norton & Co.

Caraceni, A., & Grassi, L. (2011). *Delirium: Acute confusional states in palliative medicine* (2nd ed.). New York: Oxford University Press.

Carey, B. (2011, June 23). Expert on mental illness reveals her won fight. *The New York Times.*

Carey, G. (2003). *Human genetics for the social sciences.* Thousand Oaks, CA: SAGE.

Carhart-Harris, R., & Friston, K. (2010). The default-mode, ego-functions and free-energy: A neurobiological account of Freudian ideas. *Brain, 133,* 1265–1283.

Carone, B., Fauquier, L., Habib, N., Shea, J., Hart, C., Li, R., . . . Rando, O. (2010). Paternally induced transgenerational environmental reprogramming of metabolic gene expression in mammals. *Cell, 143,* 1084–1096.

Carpenter, L. Janicak, P., Aaronson, S., Boyadjis, T., Brock, D., Cook, I., . . . Demitrack, M. (2012). Transcranial magnetic stimulation (TMS) for major depression: A multisite, naturalistic, observational study of acute treatment outcomes in clinical practice. *Depression and Anxiety, 29,* 587–596.

Carson-DeWitt, R. (2001). Mescaline. In *Encyclopedia of drugs, alcohol, & addictive behavior* (2nd ed., pp. 714–715). Durham, NC: Macmillan Reference.

Caspi, A., McClay, J., Moffitt, T., Mill, J., Martin, J., Craig, I., . . . Poulton, R. (2002). Role of genotype in the cycle of violence in maltreated children. *Science, 297,* 851–854.

Caspi, A., Hairi, A., Holmes, A., Uher, R., & Mofitt, T. (2010). Genetic sensitivity to the environment: The case of the serotonin transporter gene and its implications for studying complex diseases and traits. *American Journal of Psychiatry, 167,* 509–527.

Castellanos, F., & Proal, E. (2012). Large-scale brain systems in ADHD: Beyond the prefrontal–striatal model. *Trends in Cognitive Science, 16,* 17–26.

Castonguay, L., Nelson, D., Boswell, J., Nordberg, S., McAleavey, A., Newman, M., & Borkovec, T. (2012). Corrective experiences in cognitive behavior and interpersonal–emotional processing therapies: A qualitative analysis of a single case. In L. Castonguay & C. Hill (Eds.), *Transformation in* *psychotherapy: Corrective experiences across cognitive behavioral, humanistic, and psychodynamic approaches* (pp. 245–279). Washington, DC: American Psychological Association.

Castrén, E., & Hen, R. (2013). Neuronal plasticity and antidepressant actions. *Trend in Neuroscience, 36,* 259–267.

CBS News. (2009, February 11). *Donny Osmond confronts panic.* Retrieved from www.cbsnews.com/8301-18559_162-164444.html

Centers for Disease Control and Prevention. (2012). *Attitudes toward mental illness: Results from the Behavioral Risk Factor Surveillance System.* Atlanta, GA: Author.

Centers for Disease Control and Prevention. (2013). *Percent of obese (BMI > 30) in U.S. adults* [Animated map]. Retrieved from http://www.cdc.gov/obesity/data/adult.html#Prevalence– slide%20show

Cerny, J., & Janssen, E. (2011). Patterns of sexual arousal in homosexual, bisexual, and heterosexual men. *Archives of Sexual Behavior, 40,* 687–697.

Chamberlain, S., Menzies, L., Hampshire, A., Suckling, J., Fineberg, N., del Campo, N., . . . Sahakian, B. (2008). Orbitofrontal dysfunction in patients with obsessive- compulsive disorder and their unaffected relatives. *Science, 321,* 421–422.

Chartrand, T. L., & Bargh, J. A. (1999). The chameleon effect: The perception-behavior link and social interaction. *Journal of Personality and Social Psychology, 76,* 893–910.

Chaudhury, S., Augustine, M., Saldanha, D., Srivastava, K., Kundeyawala, S. M., Pawar, A. A., & Ryali, V. S. S. R. (2006). Norms of the Rorschach test for Indian subjects. *Medical Journal Armed Forces India, 62*(2), 153–160.

Chaturvedi, S. K. (1988). Psychasthenic syndrome related to leucorrhoea in Indian women. *Journal Psychosomatic Obstetrics & Gynecology, 8,* 67–72.

Chauhan, P., & Widom, C. (2012). Childhood maltreatment and illicit drug use in middle adulthood: The role of neighborhood characteristics. *Development and Psychopathology, 24,* 723–738.

Chein, J., Albert, D., O'Brien, L., Uckert, K., & Steinberg, L. (2011). Peers increase adolescent risk taking by enhancing activity in the brain's reward circuitry. *Developmental Science, 14,* F1–F10.

Cheney, T. (2008). *Manic.* New York: William Morrow.

Chiao, J. (2009). Cultural neuroscience: A once and future discipline. *Progress in Brain Research, 178,* 287–304.

Chiao, J. (2011). Cultural neuroscience: Visualizing culture-gene influences on brain function. In J. Decety & J. Cacioppo (Eds.), *The Oxford handbook of social neuroscience* (pp. 742–761). New York: Oxford University Press.

Chivers, M., Pittini, R., Grigoriadis, S., Villegas, L., & Ross, L. (2011). The relationship between sexual functioning and depressive symptomatology in postpartum women: a pilot study. *Journal of Sexual Medicine, 8,* 792–799.

Choudhary, G. (2016). *Relevance of Informant and subjective complaints and effects of cognitive intervention in individuals with mild cognitive impairment.* Thesis submitted to University of Mumbai for a PhD degree in Psychology.

Chowdhury, U. (1960). An Indian modification of the thematic apperception test. *The Journal of Social Psychology, 51*(2), 245–263.

Christopoulou-Aletra, H., & Niki Papavramidou, N. (2004). Methods used by the Hippocratic physicians for weight reduction. *World Journal of Surgery, 28,* 513–517.

Clarkin, J. F., Yeomans, F. E., & Kernberg, O. F. (2006). *Psychotherapy for borderline personality: Focusing on object relations.* Washington, DC: American Psychiatric Publishing, Inc.

Cleckley, H. (1988). *The mask of sanity: An attempt to clarify some issues about the so called psychopathic personality* (5th ed.). St. Louis, MO: Mosby. (Original work published 1941).

Cohen, S., & Herbert, T. (1996). Health psychology: Psychological factors and physical disease from the perspective of human psychoneuroimmunology. *Annual Review of Psychology, 47,* 113–142.

Cojan, Y., Waber, L., Carruzzo, A., & Vuilleumier, P. (2009). Motor inhibition in hysterical conversion paralysis. *NeuroImage, 62,* 862–875.

Colas, E. (1998). *Just checking: Scenes from the life of an obsessive-compulsive.* New York: Washington Square Press.

Coleman, M., & Glillberg, C. (2012). *The autisms* (4th ed.). New York: Oxford University Press.

Copeland W., Shanahan L., Worthman C., Angold A., & Costello E. J. (2012). Cumulative depression episodes predict later C-reactive protein levels: A prospective analysis. *Biological Psychiatry, 71,* 15–21.

Coryell, W., Endicott, J., Winokur, G., Akiskal, H., Solomon, D., Leon, A., . . . Shea, T. (1995). Characteristics and significance of untreated major depressive disorder. *American Journal of Psychiatry, 152,* 1124–1129.

Costa, P. T, & Widiger, T. (Eds.). (2002). *Personality disorders and the five factor model of personality* (2nd ed.). Washington, DC: American. Psychological Association.

Courtet, P., Gottesman, I. I., Jollant, F., & Gould, T. D. (2011). The neuroscience of suicidal behaviors: What can we expect from endophenotype strategies? *Translational Psychiatry, 1,* e7. doi:10.1038/tp.2011.6

Craddock, N., & Sklar, P. (2009). Genetics of bipolar disorder: Successful start to a long journey. *Trends in Genetics, 25,* 95–105.

Craske, M. G., Kircanski, K., Epstein, A., Wittchen, H. U., Pine, D. S., Lewis-Fernández, R., Hinton, D., . . . Posttraumatic and Dissociative Disorder Work Group. (2010). Panic disorder: A review of DSM-IV panic disorder and proposals for DSM-V. *Depression and Anxiety, 27,* 93–112.

Crean, R., Crane, N., & Mason, B. (2011). An evidence based review of acute and long-term effects of cannabis use on executive cognitive functions. *Journal of Addiction Medicine, 5,* 1–8.

Crichton-Browne, J. (1879). On the weight of the brain and its component parts in the insane. *Brain, 2,* 42–67.

Cristea, I., Montgomery, G., Szamoskozi, S., & David, D. (2013). Key constructs in "classical" and "new wave" cognitive behavioral psychotherapies: Relationships among each other and with emotional distress. *Journal of Clinical Psychology, 69,* 584–599.

Cronbach, L. J., & Meehl, P. (1955). Construct validity in psychological tests. *Psychological Bulletin, 52,* 281–302.

Cropley, J., Suter, C., Beckman, K., & Martin, D. (2006). Germ-line epigenetic modification of the murine Avy allele by nutritional supplementation. *Proceedings of the National Academy of Science, 103,* 17308–17312.

Cross-Disorder Group of the Psychiatric Genomics Consortium, Smoller, J. W., Craddock, N., Kendler, K., Lee, P. H., Neale, B. M., . . . Sullivan, P. F. (2013). Identification of risk loci with shared effects on five major psychiatric disorders: A genome-wide analysis. *Lancet, 381,* 1371–1379.

Crow, S., Peterson, C., Swanson, S., Raymond, N., Specker, S., Eckert, E., & Mitchell, J. (2009). Increased mortality in bulimia nervosa and other eating disorders. *The American Journal of Psychiatry, 166,* 1342–1346.

Crow, T. (2000). Schizophrenia as the price that Homo sapiens pays for language: A resolution of the central paradox in the origin of the species. *Brain Research Reviews, 31,* 118–129.

Cubells J., & Zabetian C. (2004). Human genetics of plasma dopamine beta-hydroxylase activity: Applications to research in psychiatry and neurology. *Psychopharmacology 174,* 463–476.

Cuijpers, P., Clignet, F., van Meijel, B., van Straten, A., Li, J., & Andersson, G. (2011). Psychological treatment of depression in inpatients: A systematic review and meta-analysis. *Clinical Psychology Review, 31,* 353–360.

Curley, J., Davidson, S., Bateson, P., & Champagne, F. (2009). Social enrichment during postnatal development induces transgenerational effects on emotional and reproductive behavior in mice. *Frontiers in Behavioral Neuroscience, 3.* doi: 10.3389/neuro.08.025.2009

Cuthbert, B., & Insel, T. (2010). Classification issues in women's mental health: clinical utility and etiological mechanisms. *Archives of Women's Mental Health, 12,* 57–59.

Damasio, H., Grabowski, T., Frank, R., Galaburda, A. M., & Damasio, A. (1994). The return of Phineas Gage: Clues about the brain from the skull of a famous patient. *Science, 264,* 51–62.

Dani, J., & Balfour, D. (2011). Historical and current perspective on tobacco use and nicotine addiction. *Trends in Neuroscience, 34,* 383–392.

Dantzer, R. (2012). Depression and inflammation: An intricate relationship. *Biological Psychiatry, 71,* 4–5.

Dantzer, R., O'Connor, J., Freund, G., Johnson, R., & Kelley, K. (2008). From inflammation to sickness and depression: When the immune system subjugates the brain. *Nature Reviews Neuroscience, 9,* 46–57.

Dapretto, M., Davies, M., Pfeifer, J., Scott, A., Sigman, M., Bookheimer, S., & Iacoboni, M. (2006). Understanding emotions in other: Mirror neuron dysfunction in children with autism spectrum disorder. *Nature Neuroscience, 8,* 781–789.

Darcangelo, S. (2008). Fetishism: Psychopathology and theory. In D. R. Laws & W. O'Donohue (Eds.), *Sexual deviance: Theory, assessment and treatment* (2nd ed.). New York: Guilford Press.

Darwin, C. (1859). *On the origin of species by means of natural selection.* London: J Murray.

Davenport, G. (2013, July 1). Why the NFL's concussion problem is bigger than you think. *Bleacher Report.* Retrieved from http://bleacherreport.com/articles/1690768-why-the-nfls-concussion-problem-is-bigger-than-you-think

Davidson, J., Baldwin, D., Stein, D., Kuper, E., Benattia, I., Ahmed, S., . . . Musgnung, J. (2006). Treatment of posttraumatic stress disorder with venlafaxine extended release: A 6-month randomized controlled trial. *Archives of General Psychiatry, 63,* 1158–1165.

Davidson, N. (1999). *Goodbye, Jonnie Walker.* In N. Shange (Ed.), *Beacon best of 1999: Creative writing by women and men of all colors.* Boston: Beacon Press.

Davies, D. (1962). Normal drinking in recovered alcoholics. *Quarterly Journal of Studies on Alcohol, 23,* 94–104.

Dawson, G., Sterling, L., & Faja, S. (2009). Autism. In M. De Haan & M. Gunnar (Eds.), *Handbook of developmental social neuroscience* (pp. 435–458). New York: Guilford Press.

Dawson, M., Soulières, I., Gernsbacher, M., & Mottron, L. (2007). The level and nature of autistic intelligence. *Psychological Science, 18,* 657–662.

Decety, J., Skelly, L., & Kiehl, K. (2013). Brain response to empathy-eliciting scenarios involving pain in incarcerated individuals with psychopathy. *JAMA Psychiatry, 70,* 638–645.

DeKlyen, M., & Greenberg, M. (2008). Attachment and psychopathology in childhood. In J. Cassidy, & P. Shaver (Eds.), *Handbook of attachment: Theory, research, and clinical applications* (2nd ed.). New York: Guilford Press.

Denizet-Lewis, B. (2009). *America anonymous: Eight addicts in search of a life.* New York: Simon & Schuster.

DeRubeis, R., Siegle, G., & Hollon, S. (2008). Cognitive therapy versus medication for depression: Treatment outcomes and neural mechanisms. *Nature Reviews Neuroscience, 9,* 788–796.

Deshpande, S. N., Rao, G. P., & Nimgaonkar, V. L. (2016). Advances in schizophrenia genetics bring new challenges for clinicians and researchers. Indian Journal of Psychiatry, *58,* 4–5. doi: 10.4103/0019-5545.174353

Dietrich, M., & Horvath, T. (2013). Hypothalamic control of energy balance: insights into the role of synaptic plasticity. *Trends in Neuroscience, 36,* 65–73.

Difede, J., & Eskra, D. (2002). Cognitive processing therapy for PTSD in a survivor of the World Trade Center bombing: A case study. *Journal of Trauma Practice, 1,* 155–165.

DiLalla, L. (ed.) (2004). *Behavior genetics principles: Perspectives in development, personality, and psychopathology.* Washington, DC: American Psychological Association.

Dima, D., Roiser, J. P., Dietrich, D. E., Bonnemann, C., Lanfermann, H., Emrich, H. M., & Dillo, W. (2009). Understanding why patients with schizophrenia do not perceive the hollow-mask illusion using dynamic causal modelling. *NeuroImage, 15,* 1180–1186.

Disner, S., Beevers, C. G., Haigh, E. P., & Beck, A. T. (2011). Neural mechanisms of the cognitive model of depression. *Nature Reviews Neuroscience, 12,* 467–477.

Dittrich, A. (1998). The standardized psychometric assessment of altered states of consciousness (ASCs) in humans. *Pharmacopsychiatry, 31,* 80–84.

Diwadkar, V. A., Wadehra, S., Pruitt, P., Keshavan, M. S., Rajan, U., Zajac-Benitez, C., & Eickhoff, S. B. (2012). Disordered corticolimbic interactions during affective processing in children and adolescents at risk for schizophrenia revealed by functional magnetic resonance imaging and dynamic causal modeling. *Archives of General Psychiatry, 69,* 231–242.

Dozier, M., Stovall-McClough, K., & Albus, K. (2008). Attachment and psychopathology in adulthood. In J. Cassidy, & P. Shaver (Eds.), *Handbook of attachment: Theory, research, and clinical applications* (2nd ed.). New York: Guilford Press.

Draguns, J. (1973). Comparisons for psychopathology across cultures: Issues, findings, directions. *Journal of Cross-Cultural Psychology, 4,* 9–47.

Draguns, J., & Tanaka-Matsumi, J. (2003). Assessment of psychopathology across and within cultures: issues and findings. *Behavior Research and Therapy, 41,* 755–776.

Drewnowski, A. (1997). Taste preferences and food intake. *Annual Review of Nutrition, 17,* 237–253.

Duman, R., & Aghajanian, G. (2012). Synaptic dysfunction in depression: Potential therapeutic targets. *Science, 338,* 68–72.

Durex global sex surveys. (1996). London: London International Group.

Durex global sex surveys. (1998). London: London International Group.

Dyer, K., Dunlap, G., & Winterling, V. (1990). Effects of choice making on the serious problem behaviors of students with severe handicaps. *Journal of Applied Behavior Analysis, 23,* 515–524.

Dykens, E., & Hodapp, R. (2001). Research in mental retardation: toward an etiologic approach. *Journal of Child Psychology and Psychiatry, 42,* 49–71.

Dziobek, I., Preissler, S., Grozdanovic, Z., Heuser, I., Heekeren, H. R., & Roepke, S. (2011). Neuronal correlates of altered empathy and social cognition in borderline personality disorder. *NeuroImage, 57,* 539–548.

Eastman, N., & Campbell, C. (2006). Neuroscience and legal determination of criminal responsibility. *Nature Reviews Neuroscience, 7,* 311–318.

Ecker, C., Rocha-Rego, V., Johnston, P., Mourao-Miranda, J., Marquand, A., Daly, E., . . . the MRC AIMS Consortium (2010). Investigating the predictive value of whole-brain structural MR scans in autism: A pattern classification approach. *NeuroImage, 49,* 44–56.

Eckmanns, T., Bessert, J., Behnke, M., Gastmeier, P., & Rüden, H. (2006). Compliance with antiseptic hand rub use in intensive care units: The Hawthorne Effect. *Infection Control and Hospital Epidemiology, 27,* 931–934.

Ehlers, A., & Clark, D. (2003). Early psychological interventions for adult survivors of trauma: A review. *Biological Psychiatry, 53,* 817–826.

Eisenberg, D., & Berman, K. (2010). Executive function, neural circuitry, and genetic mechanisms in schizophrenia. *Neuropsychopharmacology, 35,* 258–277.

Eisenberger N., & Lieberman M. (2004). Why rejection hurts: A common neural alarm system for physical and social pain. *Trends in Cognitive Sciences, 8,* 294–300.

Eisenberger, N., Lieberman, M., & Kipling, K. (2003). Does rejection hurt? An FMRI study of social exclusion. *Science, 302,* 290–292.

Ekman, P., & Oster, H. (1979). Facial expression of emotion. *Annual Review of Psychology, 30,* 527–554.

Elbert, T., Pantev, C., Wienbruch, C., Rockstroh, B., & Taub, E. (1995). Increased cortical representation of the fingers of the left hand in string players. *Science, 270,* 305–307.

Elder, J. P., & Arredondo, E. M. (2013). Strategies to reduce obesity in the U.S. and Latin America: Lessons that cross international borders. *American Journal of Preventive Medicine, 44*(5), 526–528.

Ellenberger, H. F. (1970). *The discovery of the unconscious: The history and evolution of dynamic psychiatry.* New York: Basic Books.

Ellicott, A., Hammen, C., Gitlin, M., Brown, G., & Jamison, K. (1990). Life events and the course of bipolar disorder. *American Journal of Psychiatry, 147,* 1194–1198.

Elliott, R., Greenberg, L., Watson, J., Timulak, L., & Freire, E. (2013). Humanistic-experiential psychotherapies. In M. Lambert (Ed.), *Handbook of psychotherapy and behavior change* (6th ed.). Hoboken, NJ: Wiley.

Ellis, A. (2010). *All out.* New York: Prometheus Books.

Elsabbagh, M., Mercure, E., Hudry, K., Chandler, S., Pasco, G., Charman, T., . . . BASIS Team. (2012). Infant neural sensitivity to dynamic eye gaze is associated with later emerging autism. *Current Biology, 22,* 338–342.

Engel, G. (1977). The need for a new medical model: A challenge for biomedicine. *Science, 196,* 129–136.

English, H. (1929). Three cases of the "conditioned fear response." *Journal of Abnormal Psychology, 24,* 221–225.

Erdelyi, M. (1985). *Psychoanalysis: Freud's cognitive psychology.* New York: Freeman.

Erkinjuntti, T. (2005). Vascular cognitive impairment. In A. Burns, J. O'Brien, & D. Ames (Eds.), *Dementia* (3rd ed.). London: Hodder Arnold.

Ertel, K., Glymour, M. & Berkman, L. (2008). Effects of social integration on preserving memory function in a nationally representative US elderly population. *American Journal of Public Health, 98,* 1215–1220.

Etkin, A., & Wager, T. D. (2007). Functional neuroimaging of anxiety: A meta-analysis of emotional processing in PTSD, social anxiety disorder, and specific phobia. *American Journal of Psychiatry, 164,* 1476–1488.

Ewing, C., & McCann, J. (2006). *Minds on trial: Great cases in law and psychology.* New York: Oxford University Press.

Exner, J. E. (1986). *The Rorschach: A comprehensive system: Vol. I. Basic foundations* (2nd ed.). New York: Wiley.

Exner, J. E. (2003). *The Rorschach: A comprehensive system* (4th ed.). New York: Wiley.

Fairburn, C. G. (2008). *Cognitive behavior therapy and eating disorders.* New York: Guilford Press.

Fairburn, C. G., Agras, W., Walsh, B., Wilson, G., & Stice, E. (2004). Prediction of outcome in bulimia nervosa by early change in treatment. *American Journal of Psychiatry, 161,* 2322–2324.

Fairburn, C. G., Cooper, Z., & Shafran, R. (2003). Cognitive behaviour therapy for eating disorders: A "transdiagnostic" theory and treatment. *Behaviour Research and Therapy, 41,* 509–528.

Fairburn, C. G., Cooper Z., & Shafran, R. (2008). Enhanced cognitive behavior therapy for eating disorders ("CBT-E"): An overview. In C. Fairburn (Ed.), *Cognitive behavior therapy and eating disorders.* New York: Guilford Press.

Fairburn C. G., Cooper Z., & Doll H. A. (2009). Transdiagnostic cognitive behavioral therapy for patients with eating disorders: A two-site trial with 60-week follow-up. *American Journal of Psychiatry, 166,* 311–319.

Fairchild, G., Passamonti, L., Hurford, G., Hagan, C., von dem Hagen, E., van Goozen, S., . . . Calder, A. (2011). Brain structure abnormalities in early-onset and adolescent-onset conduct disorder. *American Journal of Psychiatry, 168,* 624–633.

Faith, M., & Ray, W. (1994). Hypnotizability and dissociation in a college age population: Orthogonal individual differences. *Personality and Individual Differences, 17,* 211–216.

Fallon, A., & Rozin, P. (1985). Sex differences in perceptions of desirable body shape. *Journal of Abnormal Psychology, 94,* 102–105.

Faludi, G., & Mirnics, K. (2011). Synaptic changes in the brain of subjects with schizophrenia. *International Journal of Developmental Neuroscience, 29,* 305–309.

Faul, M., Xu, L., Wald, M. M., & Coronado, V. G. (2010). Traumatic brain injury in the United States: Emergency department visits, hospitalizations and deaths 2002–2006. Centers for Disease Control and Prevention, National Center for Injury Prevention and Control. Retrieved from http://www.cdc.gov/traumaticbraininjury/tbi_ed.html

Fava, G. (2003). Can long-term treatment with antidepressant drugs worsen the course of depression? *Journal of Clinical Psychiatry, 64,* 123–133.

Fava, L., & Morton, J. (2009). Causal modeling of panic disorder theories. *Clinical Psychology Review, 29,* 623–637.

Fazel, S., & Danesh, J. (2002). Serious mental disorder in 23,000 prisoners: A systematic review of 62 surveys. *Lancet, 359,* 545–550.

Ferretti, A., Caulo, M., Del Gratta, C., Di Matteo, R., Merla, A., Montorsi, F., . . . Romani, G. (2005). Dynamics of male sexual arousal: distinct components of brain activation revealed by fMRI. *NeuroImage, 26,* 1086–1096.

Feygin, D., Swain, J., & Leckman, J. (2006). The normalcy of neurosis: Evolutionary origins of obsessive-compulsive disorder and related behaviors. *Progress in Neuropsychopharmacology & Biological Psychiatry, 30,* 854–864.

Field, M., & Behrman, R. (Eds.) (2004). *Ethical conduct of clinical research involving children.* Washington, DC: National Academies Press.

Finer, L. (2007). Trends in premarital sex in the United States, 1954–2003, *Public Health Reports, 122,* 73–78.

Finger, S. (2000). *Minds behind the brain: A history of the pioneers and their discoveries.* New York: Oxford University Press.

Fink, M., Shorter, E., & Taylor, M. (2010). Catatonia is not schizophrenia: Kraepelin's error and the need to recognize catatonia as an independent syndrome in medical nomenclature. *Schizophrenia Bulletin, 36,* 314–320.

Firestone, P., Kingston, D., Wexler, A., & Bradford, J. (2006). Long-term follow-up of exhibitionists: Psychological, phallometric, and offense characteristics. *Journal of the American Academy of Psychiatry and Law, 34,* 349–359.

Fisher, M., Loewy, R., Hardy, K., Schlosser, D., & Vinogradov, S. (2013). Cognitive interventions targeting brain plasticity in the prodromal and early phases of schizophrenia. *Annual Review of Clinical Psychology, 9,* 435–463.

Fisher, R. (1935). *The design of experiments.* Edinburgh: Oliver & Boyd.

Fisher, T., Moore, Z., & Pittenger, M. (2012). Sex on the brain?: An examination of frequency of sexual cognitions as a function of gender, erotophilia, and social desirability. *Journal of Sex Research, 49,* 69–77.

Fisher, W., Geller, J., & Pandiani, J. (2009). The changing role of state psychiatric hospital. *Health Affairs, 28,* 676–684.

Fletcher, P., & Frith, C. (2009). Perceiving is believing: A Bayesian approach to explaining the positive symptoms of schizophrenia. *Nature Reviews Neuroscience, 10,* 48–58.

Flinn, M. V. (2008). Why words can hurt us: Social relationships, stress, and health. In W. Trevathan, E. Smith, & J. McKenna (Eds.), *Evolutionary medicine and health.* New York: Oxford University Press.

Foa, E., Gillihan, S., & Bryant, R. (2013). Challenges and successes in dissemination of evidence-based treatments for posttraumatic stress: Lessons learned from prolonged exposure therapy to PTSD. *Psychological Science in the Public Interest, 14,* 65–111.

Foa, E., & Kozak, M. (1986). Emotional processing of fear: Exposure to corrective information. *Psychological Bulletin, 99,* 20–35.

Folks, D., Ford, C., & Regan, W. (1984). Conversion symptoms in a general hospital. *Psychosomatics, 25,* 285–289.

Fong, G. C. Y., Shah, P. U., Gee, M. N., Serratosa, J. M., Castroviejo, I. P., Khan, S., ... & Medina, M. T. (1998). Childhood absence epilepsy with tonic-clonic seizures and electroencephalogram 3–4-Hz spike and multispike–slow wave complexes: Linkage to chromosome 8q24. The American Journal of Human Genetics, *63*(4), 1117–1129.

Ford, J., & Hoffman, R. (2013). Functional brain imaging of auditory hallucinations: From self-monitoring deficits to co-opted neural resources. In R. Jardri, A. Cachia, P. Thomas, & D. Pins (Eds.), *The neuroscience of hallucinations.* New York: Springer.

Ford, J. M., Mathalon, D. H., Whitfield, S., Faustman, W. O., & Roth, W. T. (2002). Reduced communication between frontal and temporal lobes during talking in schizophrenia. *Biological Psychiatry, 21,* 485–492.

Ford, J. M., Roach, B. J., Faustman, W. O., & Mathalon, D. H. (2007). Synch before you speak: Auditory hallucinations in schizophrenia. *American Journal of Psychiatry, 164,* 456–466.

Foussias, G., & Remington, G. (2010). Negative symptoms in schizophrenia: Avolition and Occam's razor. *Schizophrenia Bulletin, 36,* 359–369.

Franklin, J., Schiele, B., Brozek, J., & Keys, A. (1948). Observations on human behavior in experimental semistarvation and rehabilitation. *Journal of Clinical Psychology, 4,* 28–45.

Franklin, M., & Foa, E. (2008). Obsessive-compulsive disorder. In D. Barlow (Ed.), *Clinical handbook of psychological disorders: A step-by-step treatment manual* (4th ed., pp. 164–215). New York: Guilford Press.

Franklin, M., & Foa, E. (2011). Treatment of obsessive-compulsive disorder. *Annual Review of Clinical Psychology, 7,* 229–243.

Fredriksen, M., Halmøy, A., Faraone, S., & Haavik, J. (2013). Long-term efficacy and safety of treatment with stimulants and atomoxetine in adult ADHD: A review of controlled and naturalistic studies. *European Neuropsychopharmacology, 23,* 508–527.

Friese, B., & Grube, J. (n.d.). *Youth drinking rates and problems: A comparison of European countries and the United States.* Washington, DC: U.S. Department of Justice.

Frese, F., Knight, E., & Saks, E. (2009). Recovery from schizophrenia: with views of psychiatrists, psychologists, and others diagnosed with this disorder. *Schizophrenia Bulletin, 35,* 370–380.

Frick, P., Barry, C., & Kamphaus, R. (2010). *Clinical assessment of child and adolescent personality and behavior.* New York: Springer.

Frick, P., & Nigg, J. (2012). Current issues in the diagnosis of attention deficit hyperactivity disorder, oppositional defiant disorder, and conduct disorder. *Annual Review of Clinical Psychology, 8,* 77–107.

Fries, E., Moragues, N., Caldji, C., Hellhammer, D. H., & Meaney, M. J. (2004). Preliminary evidence of altered sensitivity to benzodiazepines as a function of maternal care in the rat. *Annals of the New York Academy of Science, 1032,* 320–324.

Frith, U., & Frith, C. (2010). The social brain: Allowing humans to boldly go where no other species has been. *Philosophical Transactions of the Royal Society B, 365,* 165–175.

Frith, U., Happé, F., Amarakm, D., & Warren, S. (2013). Autism and other neurodevelopmental disorders affecting cognition. In E. Kandel, J. Schwartz, T. Jessell, S. Siegelbaum, & A. Hudspeth (Eds.), *Principles of neural science* (5th ed.). New York: McGraw-Hill.

Galván, A. (2013). The teenage brain: Sensitivity to rewards. *Current Directions in Psychological Science, 22,* 88–93.

Garb, H. N., Wood, J. M., Lilienfeld, S. O., & Nezworski, M. T. (2005). Roots of the Rorschach controversy. *Clinical Psychology Review, 25,* 97–118.

Garner, D. M., & Garfinkel, P. E. (1997). *Handbook of treatment for eating disorders* (2nd ed.). New York: Guilford Press.

Garrett, B. (2010). *Brain & behavior: An introduction to biological psychology.* Thousand Oaks, CA: Sage.

Gao, Y., Glenn, A., Schug, R., Yang, Y., & Raine, A. (2009). The neurobiology of psychopathy: A neurodevelopmental perspective. *Canadian Journal of Psychiatry, 54,* 813–823.

Gaudio, S., & Quattrocchi, C. (2012). Neural basis of a multidimensional model of body image distortion in anorexia nervosa. *Neuroscience and biobehavioral reviews, 36,* 1839–1847.

Gerard, D. (1997). Chiarugi and Pinel considered: Soul's brain/person's mind. *Journal of the History of the Behavioral Sciences, 33,* 381–403.

Geddes, J., Burgess, S., Hawton, K., Jamison, K., & Goodwin, G. (2004). Long-term lithium therapy for bipolar disorder: Systematic review and meta-analysis of randomized controlled trials. *American Journal of Psychiatry, 161,* 217–222.

Geschwind, D. (2009). Advances in autism. *Annual Review of Medicine, 60,* 367–380.

Ghaffar, O., Staines, W., & Feinstein, A. (2006). Unexplained neurologic symptoms: An fMRI study of sensory conversion disorder. *Neurology, 67,* 2036–2038.

Gilbert, A., Gilbert, A., de Almeida, J., & Szeszko, P. (2011). In M. Shenton & B. Turetsky (Eds.), *Understanding neuropsychiatric disorders: Insights from neuroimaging.* New York: Cambridge University Press.

Gilbert, P. (2005). Evolution and depression: Issues and implications. *Psychological Medicine, 36,* 287–297.

Gilbertson, M. (2011). Structural imaging of post-traumatic stress disorder. In M. Shenton & B. Turetsky (Eds.), *Understanding neuropsychiatric disorders: Insights from neuroimaging.* New York: Cambridge University Press.

Gillberg, C. (1991). Clinical and neurobiological aspects of Asperger's syndrome in six families studied. In U. Frith (Ed.), *Autism and Asperger's syndrome.* Cambridge, UK: Cambridge University Press.

Gilmore, J. H., Kang, C., Evans, D. D., Wolfe, H. M., Smith, J. K., Lieberman, J. A., . . . Gerig, G. (2010). Prenatal and neonatal brain structure and white matter maturation in children at high risk for schizophrenia. *American Journal of Psychiatry, 167,* 1083–1091.

Giromini, L., Porcelli, P., Viglione, D., Parolin, L., & Pineda, J. (2010). The feeling of movement: EEG evidence for mirroring activity during the observations of static, ambiguous stimuli in the Rorschach cards. *Biological Psychology, 85,* 233–241.

Gitlin, M. (2009). Pharmacotherapy and other somatic treatments for depression. In I. Gotlib & C. Hammen (Eds.), *Handbook of depression* (2nd ed.). New York: Guilford Press.

Glade, M. (2010). Caffeine—Not just a stimulant. *Nutrition, 26,* 932–938.

Glasser, R. J. (1976). *The body is the hero.* New York: Random House.

Gleaves, D., May, M., & Cardena, E. (2001). An examination of the diagnostic validity of dissociative identity disorder. *Clinical Psychology Review, 21,* 577–608.

Goghari, V., Sponheim, S., & MacDonald, A. (2010). The functional neuroanatomy of symptom dimensions in schizophrenia: A qualitative and quantitative review of a persistent question. *Neuroscience and Biobehavioral Review, 34,* 468–486.

Gogtay, N., Vyas, N., Testa, R., Wood, S., & Pantelis, C. (2011). Age of onset of schizophrenia perspectives from structural neuroimaging studies. *Schizophrenia Bulletin, 37,* 504–513.

Goldfried, M., Castonguay, L., Hayes, A., Drozd, J., & Shapiro, D. (1997). A comparative analysis of the therapeutic focus in cognitive-behavioral and psychodynamic-interpersonal sessions. *Journal of consulting and clinical psychology, 65,* 740–748.

Goldsmith, S. (2001). *Rick factors for suicide.* Washington, DC: National Academy Press.

Goldstein, R., & Volkow, N. (2002). Drug addiction and its underlying neurobiological basis: Neuroimaging evidence for the involvement of the frontal cortex. *American Journal of Psychiatry, 159,* 1642–1652.

Gonzalez-Liencres, C., Shamay-Tsoory, S., & Brüne, M. (2013). Towards a neuroscience of empathy: Ontogeny, phylogeny, brain mechanisms, context and psychopathology. *Neuroscience and Biobehavioral Research, 37,* 1537–1548.

Goodman, A. (2007). Neurobiology of addiction. An integrative review. *Biochemical Pharmacology, 75,* 266–322.

Goodwin, F., & Jamison, K. (2007). *Manic depressive illness* (2nd ed.). New York: Oxford University Press.

Goodyer, I. (2001). *Depressed child and adolescent* (2nd ed.). New York: Cambridge University Press.

Gordon, R. (1990). *Anorexia and bulimia: Anatomy of a social epidemic.* Cambridge, MA: Basil Blackwell.

Gottesman, I. (1991). *Schizophrenia genesis: The origin of madness.* New York: Freeman.

Gottesman, I., & Hanson, D. (2005). Human development: Biological and genetic processes. *Annual Review of Psychology, 56,* 263–286.

Gottesman, I., & Shields J. (1972). *Schizophrenia and genetics: A twin study vantage point.* New York: Academic Press.

Grace, A. (2010). Ventral hippocampus, interneurons, and schizophrenia: A new understanding of the pathophysiology of schizophrenia and its implications for treatment and prevention. *Current Directions in Psychological Science, 19,* 232–237.

Graeff, F., & Del-Ben, C. (2008). Neurobiology of panic disorder: From animal models to brain neuroimaging. *Neuroscience and Biobehavioral Review, 32,* 1326–1235.

Graham, C. (2009). The DSM diagnostic criteria for female orgasmic disorder. *Archives of Sexual Behavior, 39,* 256–270.

Grandin, T. (2002, May 6). Myself. *Time, 159*(18), 56.

Grandin, T. (2009). How does visual thinking work in the mind of a person with autism? A personal account. *Philosophical Transactions of the Royal Society B, 364,* 1437–1442.

Grandin, T. (2010). *Thinking in pictures, expanded edition: My life with autism.* New York: Vintage.

Grant, B., Stinson, F., Dawson, D., Chou, S., Dufour, M., Compton, W., . . . Kaplan, K. (2004). Prevalence and co-occurrence of substance use disorders and independent mood and anxiety disorders: Results from the National Epidemiologic Survey on Alcohol and Related Conditions. *Archives of General Psychiatry, 61,* 807–816.

Gray, J. A., & McNaughton, N. (2000). *The neuropsychology of anxiety* (2nd ed.). Oxford, UK: Oxford University Press.

Grazia, D. (2010). *On the outside looking in: My life with social anxiety disorder.* Bradenton, FL: BookLocker.com, Inc.

Greenberg, L. (2002). *Emotion-focused therapy: Coaching clients to work through their feelings.* Washington DC: American Psychological Association.

Greenberg, L. S., & Watson, J. C. (2006). *Emotion-focused therapy for depression.* Washington, DC: American Psychological Association.

Gregory, R. J., & Remen, A. L. (2008). A manual-based psychodynamic therapy for treatment-resistant borderline personality disorder. *Psychotherapy Theory, Research, Practice, Training, 45,* 15–27.

Grilo, C., Sanislow, C., Gunderson, J., Pagano, M., Yen, S., Zanarini, M., . . . McGlashan, T. (2004). Two-year stability and change of schizotypal, borderline, avoidant, and obsessive-compulsive personality disorders. *Journal of Consulting and Clinical Psychology, 72,* 767–775.

Grob, G. (1991). Origins of *DSM-I*: A study in appearance and reality. *American Journal of Psychiatry, 148,* 421–431.

Groover, S. (2005, October 19). The storm: A first-hand account of Katrina [Letter to the editor]. *By George!* Retrieved from www.gwu.edu/~bygeorge/oct1905/letter.html

Gross, C., & Hen, R. (2004). The developmental origins of anxiety. *Nature Reviews Neuroscience, 5,* 545–552.

Grossman, P., Niemann, L., Schmidt, S., & Walach, H. (2004). Mindfulness-based stress reduction and health benefits: A meta-analysis. *Journal of Psychosomatic Research, 57,* 35–43.

Gruber, H. (1974). *Darwin on Man: A psychological study of scientific creativity.* New York: Dutton.

Gu, B., Kang, D., & Kwon, J. (2011). Functional imaging of obsessive-compulsive disorder. In M. Shenton & B. Turetsky (Eds.), *Understanding neuropsychiatric disorders: Insights from neuroimaging.* New York: Cambridge University Press.

Gull, W. (1874). Anorexia nervosa. *Transactions of the Clinical Society of London, 7,* 22–28.

Gunderson, J., & Ridolfi, M. (2001). Borderline personality disorder: Suicidality and self-mutilation. *Annals of the New York Academy of Science, 932,* 61–77.

Gunderson, J., Stout, R., McGlashan, T., Shea, M., Morey, L., Grilo, C., . . . Skodol, A. (2011). Ten-year course of borderline personality disorder: psychopathology and function from the Collaborative Longitudinal Personality Disorders study. *Archives of General Psychiatry, 68,* 827–837.

Gusella, J., & MacDonald, M. (2006). Huntington's disease: Seeing the pathogenic process through a genetic lens. *Trends in Biochemical Sciences, 31,* 533–540.

Gutiérrez, F., Vall, G., Peri, J., Baillés, E., Ferraz, L., Gárriz, M., & Caseras, X. (2012). Personality disorder features through the life course. *Journal of Personality Disorders, 26,* 763–774.

Häggström, M. (2009). Possible long-term effects of ethanol. *Wikipedia.org.* Retrieved from http://en.wikipedia.org/wiki/File:Possible_long-term_effects_of_ethanol.svg

Hahn, A., Stein, P., Windischberger, C., Weissenbacher, A., Spindelegger, C., Moser, E., . . . Lanzenberger, R. (2011). Reduced resting-state functional connectivity between amygdala and orbitofrontal cortex in social anxiety disorder. *NeuroImage, 56,* 881–889.

Hallett, M., Lang, A., Jankovic, J., Fahn, S., Halligan, P., Voon, V., & Cloninger, C. (Eds.) (2011). *Psychogenic movement disorders and other conversion disorders.* New York: Cambridge University Press.

Hallgrímsson, B., & Hall, B. (Eds.). (2011). *Epigenetics: Linking genotype and phenotype in development and evolution.* Berkeley: University of California Press.

Halligan, P., & David, A. (2001). Cognitive neuropsychiatry: towards a scientific psychopathology. *Nature Reviews Neuroscience, 2,* 209–215.

Halmi, K. (2005). Psychopathology of anorexia nervosa. *International Journal of Eating Disorders, 37,* S20–S21.

Halmi, K., Agras, W., Crow, S., Mitchell, J., Wilson, G., Bryson, S., & Kraemer, H. (2005). Predictors of treatment acceptance and completion in anorexia nervosa: implications for future study designs. *Archives of General Psychiatry, 62,* 776–781.

Hammen, C. (2009). Children of depressed parents. In I. Gotlib & C. Hammen (Eds.), *Handbook of depression* (2nd ed.). New York: Guilford Press.

Hare, R. (2003). *The Hare Psychopathy Checklist-Revised.* Toronto, ON: Multi-Health System.

Hare, R., & Neumann, C. (2008). Psychopathy as a clinical and empirical construct. *Annual Review of Clinical Psychology, 4,* 17–46.

Harlow, H. (1958). The nature of love. *American Psychologist, 13,* 673–685.

Harlow, H., McGaugh, J., & Thompson, R. (1971). *Psychology.* San Francisco: Albion Publishing.

Harpending, H., & Sobus, J. (1987). Sociopathy as an adaptation. *Ethology and Sociobiology, 8,* 63–72.

Harris, S., & Deary, I. (2011). The genetics of cognitive ability and cognitive ageing in healthy older people. *Trends in Cognitive Sciences, 15,* 388–394.

Harrow, M., & Jobe, T. (2010). How frequent is chronic multiyear delusional activity and recovery in schizophrenia: A 20-year multi-follow-up. *Schizophrenia Bulletin, 36,* 192–204.

Hart, H., Radua, J., Nakao, T., Mataix-Cols, D., & Rubia, K. (2013). Meta-analysis of functional magnetic resonance imaging studies of inhibition and attention in attention-deficit/ hyperactivity disorder. *JAMA Psychiatry, 70,* 185–198.

Hartocollis, A. (2011, October 6). Nearly 8 years later, guilty plea in subway killing. *The New York Times.* Retrieved from http://www.nytimes.com/2006/10/11/nyregion/11kendra.html?_r=0

Hasin, D. S., Stinson, F. S., Ogburn, E., & Grant, B. F. (2007). Prevalence, correlates, disability, and comorbidity of DSM-IV alcohol abuse and dependence in the United States: Results from the National Epidemiologic Survey on Alcohol and Related Problems. *Archives of General Psychiatry, 64,* 830–842.

Hayden, B., Canuel, N., & Shanse, J. (2013). What was brewing in the Natufian? An archaeological assessment of brewing technology in the Epipaleolithic. *Journal of Archaeological Method and Theory, 20,* 102–150.

Hayes, S. C. (2004). Acceptance and commitment therapy, relational frame theory, and the third wave of behavioral and cognitive therapies. *Behavior Therapy, 35,* 639–665.

Heiman, J., & Pfaff, D. (2011). Sexual arousal and related concepts: an introduction. *Hormones and Behavior, 59,* 613–615.

Herbenick, D., Reece, M., Schick, V., Sanders, S. A., Dodge, B., & Fortenberry, J. D. (2010). Sexual behavior in the United States: Results from a national probability sample of men and women ages 14–94 [Issue supplement S5]. *The Journal of Sexual Medicine, 7,* 255–265. Retrieved from www.nationalsexstudy.indiana.edu/graph.html

Herbert, J. (2007). Avoidant personality disorder. In W. O'Donohue, K. A. Fowler, & S. O. Lilienfeld (Eds.), *Personality disorders: Toward the DSM-V.* Thousand Oaks, CA: Sage.

Hersen, M., & Bellack, A. S. (1976). A multiple-baseline analysis of social-skills training in chronic schizophrenia. *Journal of Applied Behavior Analysis, 9*(3), 239–245.

Hettema, J., Neale, M., & Kendler, K. (2001). A review and meta-analysis of the genetic epidemiology of anxiety disorders. *American Journal of Psychiatry, 158,* 1568–1578.

Hiday, V., Wales, H., & Ray, B. (2013). Effectiveness of a short-term mental health court: Criminal recidivism one year postexit. *Law and Human Behavior.*

Higgins, E. (2008). The new genetics of mental illness. *Scientific American,* pp. 42–42.

Hiller, W., Leibbrand, R., Rief, W., & Fichter, M. (2005). Differentiating hypochondriasis from panic disorder. *Journal of Anxiety Disorders, 19,* 29–49.

Hippocrates; Translated by Francis Adams (400 B.C.E). *On the Sacred Disease.* http://classics.mit.edu/Hippocrates/sacred .html

Hofman, M. (2001). Brain evolution in hominids: Are we at the end of the road? In D. Falk & K Gibson (Eds.), *Evolutionary anatomy of the primate cerebral cortex.* New York: Cambridge University Press.

Hofmann, S. G., & Barlow, D. H. (2002). Social phobia (social anxiety disorder). In D. H. Barlow (Ed.), *Anxiety and its disorders: The nature and treatment of anxiety and panic* (2nd ed.). New York: Guilford Press.

Hofmann, S., Grossman, P., & Hinton, D. (2011). Loving-kindness and compassion meditation: Potential for psychological interventions. *Clinical Psychology Review, 31,* 1126–1132.

Hofmann, S., Sawyer, A., Witt, A., & Oh, D. (2010). The effect of mindfulness-based therapy on anxiety and depression: A meta-analytic review. *Journal of Consulting and Clinical Psychology, 78,* 169–183.

Hogarty, G., & Goldberg, S. (1973). Drugs and sociotherapy in the after care of schizophrenic patients: one year relapse rates. *Achieves of General Psychiatry, 28,* 54–64.

Hoge, E. A., Bui, E., Marques, L., Metcalf, C. A., Morris, L. K., Robinaugh, D. J., . . .Simon, N. M. (2013). Randomized controlled trial of mindfulness meditation for generalized anxiety disorder: Effects on anxiety and stress reactivity. *Journal of Clinical Psychiatry, 74.*

Hollister, L. E. (1984). Effects of hallucinogens in humans. In B. L. Jacobs (Ed.), *Hallucinogens: Neurochemical, behavioral, and clinical perspectives* (pp. 19–33). New York: Raven Press.

Hollon, S., & Beck, A. (2013). Cognitive and cognitive-behavioral therapies. In M. Lambert (Ed.), *Handbook of psychotherapy and behavior change* (6th ed.). Hoboken, NJ: Wiley.

Holton, G. (1952). *Introduction to concepts and theories in physical science.* Boston: Addison Wesley Press.

Holtzheimer, P., Kosel, M., & Schlaepfer, T. (2012). Brain stimulation therapies for neuropsychiatric disease. In M. Aminoff, F. Boller, & D. Swaab (Eds.), *Handbook of clinical neurology* (pp. 681–695). New York: Elsevier.

Holub, C., Elder, J., Arredondo, E., Barquera, S., Eisenberg, C., Sánchez Romero, L., . . . Simoes, E. (2013). Obesity control in Latin American and U.S. Latinos: A systematic review. *American Journal of Preventive Medicine, 44,* 529–537.

Hölzel, E., Hoge, D., Greve, D., Gard, T., Creswell, J., Brown, L., . . . Lazar, S. (2013). Neural mechanisms of symptom improvements in generalized anxiety disorder following mindfulness training. *NeuroImage: Clinical, 2,* 448–458.

Hornbacher, M. (1998). *Wasted: A memoir of anorexia and bulimia.* New York: HarperFlamingo.

Horney, K. (1950). *Neurosis and human growth.* New York: W. W. Norton & Co.

Hoza, B., Kaiser, N., & Hurt, E. (2008). Evidence-based treatments for attention-deficit/hyperactivity disorder (ADHD). In R. Steele, T. Elkin, & M. Roberts (Eds.), *Handbook of evidence-based therapies for children and adolescents: Bridging science and practice.* New York: Springer.

Huang, Y., Kotov, R., de Girolamo, G., Preti, A., Angermeyer, M., Benjet, C., . . . Kessler, R. (2009). DSM-IV personality disorders in the WHO World Mental Health Surveys. *British Journal of Psychiatry, 195,* 46–53.

Hudson, J., Hiripi, E., Pope, H. Jr., & Kessler, R. (2007). The prevalence and correlates of eating disorders in the National Comorbidity Survey Replication. *Biological Psychiatry, 61,* 348–358.

Huizink, A., Mulder, E., & Buitelaar, J. (2004). Prenatal stress and risk for psychopathology: Specific effects or induction of general susceptibility? *Psychological Bulletin, 130,* 115–142.

Hunsley, J., & Mash, E. (2007). Evidence-based assessment. *Annual Review of Clinical Psychology, 3,* 29–51.

Huxley, J., Mayr, E., Osmond, H., & Hoffer, A. (1964). Schizophrenia as a genetic morphism. *Nature, 204,* 220–221.

Hyman, S. (2007). Can neuroscience be integrated into the *DSM–V*? *Nature Reviews Neuroscience, 8,* 725–732.

Hyman, S. (2010). The diagnosis of mental disorders: The problem of reification. *Annual Review of Clinical Psychology, 6,* 155–179.

Hyman, S., & Cohen, J. (2013). Disorders of thought and volition: Schizophrenia. In E. Kandel, J. Schwartz, T. Jessell, S. Siegelbaum, & A. Hudspeth (Eds.), *Principles of neural science* (5th ed.). New York: McGraw-Hill.

Hyman, S., Malenka, R., & Nestler, E. (2006). Neural mechanisms of addiction: The role of reward-related learning and memory. *Annual Review of Neuroscience, 29,* 565–598.

Iacoboni, M. (2009). Imitation, empathy, and mirror neurons. *Annual Review of Psychology, 60,* 653–670.

Illes, J., & Bird, S. (2006). Neuroethics: a modern context for ethics in neuroscience. *TRENDS in Neurosciences, 29,* 511–517.

Insel, T. (2009). Translating scientific opportunity into public health impact: A strategic plan for research on mental illness. *Archives of General Psychiatry, 66,* 128–133.

Insel, T. (2010). Rethinking schizophrenia. *Nature, 468,* 187–193.

Insel, T., & Cuthbert, B. (2009). Endophenotypes: Bridging genomic complexity and disorder heterogeneity. *Biological Psychiatry, 66,* 988–989.

Iversen, L. (2006). Neurotransmitter transporters and their impact on the development of psychopharmacology. *British Journal of Pharmacology, 147,* S82–S88.

Iwamoto, K., & Kato, T. (2009). Epigenetic profiling in schizophrenia and major mental disorders. *Neuropsychobiology, 60,* 5–11.

Jackson, J. (1894). The factors of insanities. *The medical press and circular, 108,* 615–619.

Jackson, J. (1932). Evolution and dissolution of the nervous system. In J. Taylor (Ed.), *Selected writing of John Hughlings Jackson* (Vol. 2). London: Hodder & Stroughton.

Jadhav, S. (2004). Dhat syndrome: A re-evaluation. *Psychiatry, 3*(8), 14–16.

Jadhav, S., Littlewood, R., Ryder, A. G., Chakraborty, A., Jain, S., & Barua, M. (2007). Stigmatization of severe mental illness in India: Against the simple industrialization hypothesis. Indian Journal of Psychiatry, *49*(3), 189. Retrieved from https://www.ncbi.nlm.nih.gov/pmc/articles/PMC2902092/

Jain, S. and Kar, B.R. (2014). Effect of cognitive aging on working memory consolidation. *Psychological Studies*, 59 (4) 383–393.

Jamison, K. (1995). *An unquiet mind.* New York: Random House.

Janssen, E. (2011). Sexual arousal in men: A review and conceptual analysis. *Hormones and Behavior, 59,* 708–716.

Jardri, R., & Summer, I. (2013). Functional brain imaging of hallucinations: Symptom capture studies. In R. Jardri, A. Cachia, P. Thomas, & D. Pins (Eds.), *The neuroscience of hallucinations.* New York: Springer.

Jeremy P. (2010, February 21). Fighting the war at home. *New America Media.* Retrieved from newamericamedia.org/2010/02/fighting-the-war-at-home.php

Jobe, T., & Harrow, M. (2010). Schizophrenia course, long-term outcome, recovery, and prognosis. *Current Directions in Psychological Science, 19,* 220–225.

Johnson, J., Cohen, P., Kasen, S., & Brook, J. (2006). Dissociative disorders among adults in the community, impaired functioning, and Axis I and Axis II comorbidity. *Journal of Psychiatric Research, 40,* 131–140.

Johnson, S. (2005). Mania and dysregulation in goal pursuit: A review. *Clinical Psychology Review, 25,* 241–262.

Johnson, S., Cuellar, A., & Miller, C. (2009). Bipolar and unipolar depression: A comparison of clinical phenomenology, biological vulnerability and psychosocial predictors. In I. Gotlib & C. Hammen (Eds.), *Handbook of depression* (2nd ed., pp. 142–160). New York: Guilford Press.

Johnson, S., Murray, G., Fredrickson, B., Youngstrom, E., Hinshaw, S., Bass, J., . . . & Salloum, I. (2012). Creativity and bipolar disorder: Touched by fire or burning with questions? *Clinical Psychology Review, 32,* 1–12.

Jolles, D. D., van Buchem, M. A., Crone, E. A., & Rombouts, S. A., (2010). A comprehensive study of whole-brain functional connectivity in children and young adults. *Cerebral Cortex, 21,* 385–391.

Jones, R., Kiely, D., & Marcantonio, E. (2010). Prevalence of delirium on admission to postacute care is associated with a higher number of nursing home deficiencies. *Journals of the American Medical Directors Association, 11,* 253–256.

Jones, R., Yates, W., & Zhou, M. (2002). Readmission rates for adjustment disorders: comparison with other mood disorders. *Journal of Affective Disorders, 71,* 199–203.

Joshipura, M.K., Shah, H.S., Patel, P.R., & Divatia, P.A. (2014). Trauma care systems in India—An overview. *Indian Journal of Critical care Medicine,* 8, 93–97.

Junginger, J. (1990). Predicting compliance with command hallucinations. *American Journal of Psychiatry, 147,* 245–247.

Kabat-Zinn, J. (1990). *Full catastrophe living.* New York: Delta Publishing.

Kalivas, P. (2009). The glutamate homeostasis hypothesis of addiction. *Nature Reviews Neuroscience, 10,* 561–572.

Kamio, Y., Tobimatsu S., & Fukui, H. (2011). Developmental disorders. In J. Decety & J. Cacioppo (Eds.), *The handbook of social neuroscience.* New York: Oxford University Press.

Kandel, E. (2005). *Psychiatry, psychoanalysis, and the new biology of mind.* Washington, DC: American Psychiatric Publications.

Kanner L. (1943). Autistic disturbances of affective contact._*Nervous Child, 2,* 217–250.

Kar, B. R., Rao, S. L., Chandramouli, B. A., & Thennarasu, K. (2004). NIMHANS neuropsychological battery for children. Bangalore: NIMHANS Publication Division.

Karlsgodt, K. H., Sun, D., & Cannon, T. D. (2010). Structural and functional brain abnormalities in schizophrenia. *Current Directions in Psychological Science, 19,* 226–231.

Katsnelson, A. (2010). Epigenome effort makes its mark. *Nature, 467,* 646.

Kaufman, J., Yang, B., Douglas-Palumberi, H., Grasso, D., Lipschitz, D., Houshyar, S., . . . Gelernter, J. (2006). Brain-derived neurotrophic factor-5-HTTLPR gene interactions and environmental modifiers of depression in children. *Biological Psychiatry, 59,* 673–680.

Kaye, W., Fudge, J., & Paulus, M. (2009). New insights into symptoms and neurocircuit function of anorexia nervosa. *Nature Reviews Neuroscience, 10,* 573–584.

Kaye, W., Wierenga, C., Bailer, U., Simmons, A., & Bischoff-Grethe, A. (2013). Nothing tastes as good as skinny feels: The neurobiology of anorexia nervosa. *Trends in Neurosciences, 36,* 110–120.

Kazdin, A. E. (2005). *Parent management training: Treatment for oppositional, aggressive, and antisocial behavior in children and adolescents.* New York: Oxford University Press.

Keane, T., Marshall, A., & Taft, C. (2006). Posttraumatic stress disorder: Etiology, epidemiology, and treatment outcome. *Annual Review of Clinical Psychology, 2,* 161–197.

Keel, P., Brown, T., Holland, L., & Bodell, L. (2012). Empirical classification of eating disorders. *Annual Review of Clinical Psychology, 8,* 381–404.

Kellner, R. (1985). Functional somatic symptoms and hypochondriasis. A survey of empirical studies. *Archives of General Psychiatry, 42,* 821–833.

Kelly, A., Uddin, L., Biswal, B., Castellanos, F., & Milham, M. (2008). Competition between functional brain networks mediates behavioral variability. *Neuroimage, 39,* 527–537.

Kelly, C., Biswal, B., Craddock, R., Castellanos, F., & Milham, M. (2012). Characterizing variation in the functional connectome: Promise and pitfalls. *Trends in Cognitive Sciences, 16,* 181–188.

Kemeny, M., & Schedlowski, M. (2007). Understanding the interaction between psychosocial stress and immune- related diseases: A stepwise progression. *Brain, Behavior, and Immunity, 21,* 1009–1018.

Kendler, K., & Baker, J. (2007). Genetic influences on measures of the environment: A systematic review. *Psychological Medicine, 37,* 615–626.

Kendler, L., Jaffee. S., & Romer, D. (Eds). (2011). *The dynamic genome and mental health: The role of genes and environments in youth development.* New York: Oxford University Press.

Kendler, K. S., Neale, M. C., Kessler, R. C., Heath, A. C., & Eaves, L. J. (1992). Major depression and generalized anxiety disorder: same genes, (partly) different environments? *Archives of General Psychiatry, 49,* 716–722.

Kendler, K., Thornton, L., & Gardner, C. (2000). Stressful life events and previous episodes in the etiology of major depression in women: An evaluation of the "kindling" hypothesis. *American Journal of Psychiatry, 157,* 1243–1251.

Kernberg, O. (1984). *Severe personality disorders: Psychotherapeutic strategies.* New Haven, CT: Yale University Press.

Kernberg, O. (1995). *Love relations: Normality and pathology.* New Haven, CT: Yale University Press.

Kessler, R. C., Aguilar-Gaxiola, S., Alonso, J., Chatterji, S., Lee, S., Ormel, J., . . . Wang, P. S. (2009). The global burden of mental disorders: An update from the WHO World Mental Health (WMH) surveys. *Epidemiologia e Psichiatria Sociale, 18*(1), 23–33.

Kessler, R., Avenevoli, S., Costello, E., Georgiades, K., Green, J., Gruber, M., . . . Merikangas, K. (2012). Prevalence, persistence, and sociodemographic correlates of DSM-IV disorders in the National Comorbidity Survey Replication Adolescent Supplement. *Archives of General Psychiatry, 69,* 372–380.

Kessler, R. C., Berglund, P., Demler, O., Jin, R., Merikangas, K. R., & Walters, E. E. (2005). Lifetime prevalence and age-of-onset distributions of DSM-IV disorders in the National Comorbidity Survey Replication. *Archives of General Psychiatry, 62,* 593–602.

Kessler, R., Chiu, W., Jin, R., Ruscio, A., Shear, K., & Walters, E. (2006). The epidemiology of panic attacks, panic disorder, and agoraphobia in the National Comorbidity Survey Replication. *Archives of General Psychiatry, 63,* 415–424.

Kessler, R. C., Green, J. G., Gruber, M. J., Sampson, N. A., Bromet, E., Cuitan, M., . . . Zaslavsky, A. M. (2010). Screening for serious mental illness in the general population with the K6 screening scale: Results from the WHO World Mental Health (WMH) survey initiative. *International Journal of Methods in Psychiatric Research, 19(S1),* 4–22.

Kessler, R. C., Hwang, I., LaBrie, R., Petukhova, M., Sampson, N., Winters, K., & Shaffer, H. (2008). The prevalence and correlates of DSM-IV Pathological Gambling in the National Comorbidity Survey Replication. *Psychological Medicine, 38,* 1351–1360.

Kessler, R. C., McGonagle K., Zhao S., Nelso, C. B., Hughes, M., Eshleman, S., . . . Kendler, K. S. (1994). Lifetime and 12-month prevalence of *DSM-III-R* psychiatric disorders in the United States. Results from the National Comorbidity Survey. *Archives of General Psychiatry 51,* 8–19.

Kessler, R. C., Merikangas, K., & Wang, P. (2007). Prevalence, comorbidity, and service utilization for mood disorders in the United States at the beginning of the twenty-first century. *Annual Review of Clinical Psychology, 137,* 137–158.

Kessler, R. C., Petukhova, M., Sampson, N., Zaslavsky, A., & Wittchen, H. (2012). Twelve-month and lifetime prevalence and lifetime morbid risk of anxiety and mood disorders in the United States. *International Journal of Methods in Psychiatric Research, 21,* 169–184.

Kessler R. C., & Wang P. S. (2009). Epidemiology of depression. In I. H. Gotlib & C. L. Hammen (Eds.), *Handbook of depression* (2nd ed.). New York: Guilford Press.

Keyes, K., Schulenberg, J., O'Malley, P., Johnston, L., Bachman, J., Li, G., & Hasin, D. (2012). Birth cohort effects on adolescent alcohol use: The influence of social norms from 1976 to 2007. *Archives of General Psychiatry, 69,* 1304–1313.

Khambaty, M., and Parikh, R.M. (2017). Cultural aspects of anxiety disorders in India. *Dialogues in Clinical Neuroscience, 19*(2), 117–126.

Kiecolt-Glaser, J., Garner, W., Speicher, C., Penn, G., Holliday, J., & Glaser, R. (1984). Psychosocial modifiers of immunocompetence in medical students. *Psychosomatic Medicine, 46,* 7–14.

Kiecolt-Glaser, J., Gouin, J., & Hantsoo, L. (2010). Close relationships, inflammation, and health. *Neuroscience and Biobehavioral Review, 35,* 33–38.

Kiecolt-Glaser, J., McGuire, L., Robles, T., & Glaser, R. (2002). Psychoneuroimmunology: Psychological influences on immune function and health. *Journal of Consulting and Clinical Psychology, 70,* 537–547.

King, A., de Wit, H., McNamara, P., & Cao, D. (2011). Rewarding, stimulant, and sedative alcohol responses and relationship to future binge drinking. *Archives of General Psychiatry, 68,* 389–399.

King, S., St-Hilaire, A., & Heidkamp, D. (2010). Prenatal factors in schizophrenia. *Current Directions Psychological Science, 19,* 209–213.

King-Casas, B., Sharp, C., Lomax-Bream, L., Lohrenz, T., Fonagy, P., & Montague, P. (2008). The rupture and repair of cooperation in borderline personality disorder. *Science, 321,* 806–810.

Kingdon, D., & Turkington, D. (1994). Cognitive behaviour therapy of schizophrenia. The amenability of delusions and hallucinations to reasoning. *British Journal of Psychiatry, 164,* 581–587.

Kinselia, K., & He, W. (2009, June). An aging world: 2008. *International Population Reports.* Washington, DC: U.S. Government Printing Office. Retrieved from http://www.census.gov/prod/2009pubs/p95-09-1.pdf

Kinsey, A. (1948). *Sexual behavior in the human male.* Bloomington: Indiana University Press.

Kinsey, A. (1953). *Sexual behavior in the human female.* Bloomington: Indiana University Press.

Kitayama, S., & Cohen, D. (2007). *The handbook of cultural psychology.* New York: Guilford Press.

Klonsky, E. (2007). The functions of deliberate self-injury: A review of the evidence. *Clinical Psychology Review, 27,* 226–239.

Knyazev, G. (2007). Motivation, emotion, and their inhibitory control mirrored in brain oscillations. *Neuroscience and Biobehavioral Reviews, 31,* 377–395.

Koch, W., Teipel, S., Mueller, S., Benninghoff, J., Wagner, M., Bokde, A., . . . Meindl, T. (2012). Diagnostic power of default mode network resting state fMRI in the detection of Alzheimer's disease. *Neurobiology of Aging, 33,* 466–478.

Koob, G., Kandel, D., & Volkow, N. (2008). Pathophysiology of addiction. In A. Tasman, J. Kay, J. Lieberman, M. First, & M. Maj (Eds.), *Psychiatry* (3rd ed.). New York: Wiley.

Kramer, A., & Erickson, K. (2007). Capitalizing on cortical plasticity: influence of physical activity on cognition and brain function. *Trends in Cognitive Sciences, 11,* 342–348.

Kring, A., & Elis, O. (2012). Emotion deficits in people with schizophrenia. *Annual Review of Clinical Psychology, 9,* 409–433.

Krishnamurthy, K., Venugopal, D., & Alimchandani, A. K. (2000). Mental hospitals in India. Indian journal of psychiatry, *42*(2), 125–132. Retrieved from https://www.ncbi.nlm.nih.gov/pmc/articles/PMC2957702/pdf/IJPsy-42-125.pdf

Krystal, J., & Moghaddam, B. (2011). Contributions of glutamate and GABA systems to the neurobiology and treatment of schizophrenia. In D. Weinberger & P. Harrison (Eds.), *Schizophrenia.* New York: Wiley.

Krystal, J., Perry, E. B., Gueorguieva, R., Belger, A., Madonick, S. H., Abi-Dargham, A., . . . D'Souza, D. C. (2005). Comparative and interactive human psychopharmacologic effects of ketamine and amphetamine: Implications for glutamatergic and dopaminergic model psychoses and cognitive function. *Archives of General Psychiatry, 62,* 985–995.

Kuepper, R., van Os, J., Lieb, R., Wittchen, H., Höfler, M., & Henquet, C. (2011). Continued cannabis use and risk of incidence and persistence of psychotic symptoms: 10 year follow-up cohort study. *BMJ, 342.* doi: 10.1136/bmj.d738

Kulka, R. A., Schlenger, W. E., Fairbank, J. A., Hough, R. L., Jordan, B. K., Marmar, C. R., & Weiss, D. S. (1990). *Trauma and the Vietnam generation: Report of findings from the National Vietnam Veterans Readjustment Study.* New York: Brunner/Mazel.

Kupka, R. W., Luckenbaugh, D. A., Post, R. M., Suppes, T., Altshuler, L. L., Keck, P. E., Jr., . . . Nolen, W. A. (2005). Comparison of rapid-cycling and non-rapid-cycling bipolar disorder based on prospective mood ratings in 539 outpatients. *American Journal of Psychiatry, 162,* 1273–1280.

Kutscher, E. (2008). Antipsychotics. In K. Meser & D. Jeste (Eds.), *Clinical handbook of schizophrenia* (pp. 159–167). New York: Guilford Press.

Lacey, E. (1990). Broadening the perspective of pica: literature review. *Public Health Reports, 105,* 29–35.

Lahey, B., Rathouz, P., Applegate, B., Hulle, C., Garriock, H., Urbano, R., & Waldman, I. (2008). Testing structural models of DSM-IV symptoms of common forms of child and adolescent psychopathology. *Journal of Abnormal Child Psychology, 36,* 187–206.

Lahey, B., Van Hulle, C., Singh, A., Waldman, I., & Rathouz, P. (2011). Higher-order genetic and environmental structure of prevalent forms of child and adolescent psychopathology. *Archives of General Psychiatry, 68,* 181–189.

Lahey, B., & Waldman, I. (2012). Phenotypic and causal structure of conduct disorder in the broader context of prevalent forms of psychopathology. *Journal of Child Psychology and Psychiatry, 53,* 536–557.

Lahey, B., & Willcutt, E. (2010). Predictive validity of a continuous alternative to nominal subtypes of attention-deficit hyperactivity disorder for *DSM-V. Journal of Clinical Child Adolescence Psychology, 39,* 761–775.

Lai, C. (2011). Gray matter deficits in panic disorder. *Journal of Clinical Psychopharmacology, 31,* 287–293.

Lamers, F., Vogelzanga, N., Merikangas, K., de Jonge, P., Beekman, A., & Penninz, B. (2013). Evidence for a differential role of HPA-axis function, inflammation and metabolic syndrome in melancholic versus atypical depression. *Molecular Psychiatry, 18,* 692–699.

Landau, S., Marks, S., Mormino, E., Rabinovici, G., Oh, H., O'Neil, J., . . . Jagust, W. (2012). Association of lifetime cognitive engagement and low β-amyloid deposition. *Archives of Neurology, 69,* 623–629.

Langleben, D., & Moriarty, J. (2013). Using brain imaging for lie detection: Where science, law and research policy collide. *Psychology and Public Policy Law, 19,* 222–234.

Långström, N., & Zucker, K. (2005). Transvestic fetishism in the general population: prevalence and correlates. *Journal of Sex and Marital Therapy, 31,* 87–95.

Large, M., Sharma, S., Compton, M., Slade, T., & Nielssen, O. (2011). Cannabis use and earlier onset of psychosis: A systematic meta-analysis. *Archives of General Psychiatry, 68,* 555–561.

Laughlin, S., & Sejnowski, T. (2003). Communication in neuronal networks. *Science, 301,* 1870–1974.

Laumann, E., Paik, A., Glasser, D., Kang, J., Wang, T., Levinson, B., . . . Gingell, C. (2006). A cross-national study of subjective sexual well-being among older women and men: findings from the Global Study of Sexual Attitudes and Behaviors. *Archives of Sexual Behavior, 35,* 145–161.

Laumann, E., Paik, A., & Rosen, R. (1999). Sexual dysfunction in the United States: Prevalence and predictors. *Journal of the American Medical Association, 281,* 537–544.

Lauzon, N., Bechard, M., Ahmad, T., & Laviolette, S. (2013). Supra-normal stimulation of dopamine D1 receptors in the prelimbic cortex blocks behavioral expression of both aversive and rewarding associative memories through a cyclic-AMP-dependent signaling pathway. *Neuropharmacology, 67,* 104–114.

Lawton, E., Shields, A., & Oltmanns, T. (2011). Five-factor model personality disorder prototypes in a community sample: Self- and informant-reports predicting interview-based DSM diagnoses. *Personality Disorders, 2,* 279–292.

Lazary, J., Viczena, V., Dome, P., Chase, D., Juhasz, G., & Bagdy, G. (2012). Hopelessness, a potential endophenotpye for suicidal behavior, is influenced by TPH2 gene variants. *Progress in Neuropsycholpharmacology and Biological Psychiatry, 36,* 155–160.

LeBeau, R., Glenn, D., Liao, B., Wittchen, H., Beesdo-Baum, K., Ollendick, T., & Craske, M. (2010). Specific phobia: A review of DSM-IV specific phobia and preliminary recommendations for DSM-V. *Depression and Anxiety, 27,* 148–167.

Leckman, J., Denys, D., Simpson, H., Mataix-Cols, D., Hollander, E., Saxena, S., . . . Stein, D. (2010). Obsessive-compulsive disorder: A review of the diagnostic criteria and possible subtypes and dimensional specifiers for DSM-V. *Depression and Anxiety, 27,* 507–527.

LeDoux, J. (1994, June). Emotion, memory, and the brain. *Scientific American,* pp. 62–71.

LeDoux, J. (2000). Emotion circuits in the brain. *Annual Review of Neuroscience, 23,* 155–184.

LeDoux, J. (2003). The self: Clues from the brain. *Annals of the New York Academy of Science, 1001,* 295–304.

Lee, J., Pilli, S., Gebremariam, A., Keirns, C., Davis, M., Vijan, S., . . . Gurney, J. (2010). Getting heavier, younger: trajectories of obesity over the life course. *International Journal of Obesity, 34,* 614–623.

Leff, J., Wig, N. N., Ghosh, A., Bedi, H., Menon, D. K., Kuipers, L., ... & Sartorius, N. (1987). Expressed emotion and schizophrenia in north India. III. Influence of relatives' expressed emotion on the course of schizophrenia in Chandigarh. The British Journal of Psychiatry, *151*(2), 166–173.

Le Grange, D., & Eisler, I. (2009) Family interventions in adolescent anorexia nervosa. *Child and Adolescent Psychiatric Clinics of North America, 18,* 159–173.

Lemos, J. C., Wanat, M. J., Smith, J. S., Reyes, B. A. S., Hollon, N. G., Van Bockstaele, E. J., . . . Phillips, P. (2012). Severe stress switches CRF action in the nucleus accumbens from appetitive to aversive. *Nature, 490,* 402–406.

Lenoir, M., Serre, F., Cantin, L., & Ahmed, S. H. (2007). Intense sweetness surpasses cocaine reward. *PLOS ONE, 2,* e698.

Lenzenweger, M. (2008). Epidemiology of personality disorders. *Psychiatric clinics of North America, 31,* 395–403.

Lenzenweger, M., Lane, M., Loranger, A., & Kessler, R. (2007). DSM-IV personality disorders in the National Comorbidity Survey Replication. *Biological Psychiatry, 62,* 553–564.

Levay, S., & Baldwin, J. (2012). *Human sexuality* (4th ed.). Sunderland, LA: Sinauer Associates.

Levy, B., & Sidel, V. (2009). Health effects of combat: A life-course perspective. *Annual Review of Public Health, 30,* 123–136.

Levy, K. N. (2005). The implications of attachment theory and research for understanding borderline personality disorder. *Development and Psychopathology, 17,* 959–986.

Levy, K. N. (2012). Subtypes, dimensions, levels, and mental states in narcissism and narcissistic personality disorder. *Journal of Clinical Psychology: In Session, 8,* 886–897.

Levy, K. N., Reynoso, J., Wasserman, R. H., & Clarkin, J. F. (2007). Narcissistic personality disorder. In W. O'Donohue, K. A. Fowler, & S. O. Lilienfeld (Eds.), *Personality disorders: Toward the DSM–V* (pp. 233–277). Thousand Oaks, CA: Sage.

Levy, K. N., & Scala, J. W. (2012). Transference, transference interpretations, and transference-focused psychotherapies. *Psychotherapy, 49,* 391–403.

Levy, K. N., Yeomans, F. E., & Diamond D. (2007). Psychodynamic treatments of self-injury. *Journal of Clinical Psychology, 63*(11), 1105–1120.

Lichtenstein, P., Carlstrom, E., Råstam, M., Gillberg, C., & Anckarsäter, H. (2010). The genetics of autism spectrum disorders and related neuropsychiatric disorders in childhood. *Archives of General Psychiatry, 167,* 1357–1363.

Lieberman, J. & Stroup, T. (2011). The NIM H-CAT IE Schizophrenia Study: What Did We Learn? *American Journal of Psychiatry, 168,* 770–775.

Liebe, S., Hoerzer, G., Logothetis, N. K., & Rainer, G. (2012). Theta coupling between V4 and pre-frontal cortex predicts visual short-term memory performance. *Nature Neuroscience, 15,* 456–464.

Lindesay, J., Rockwood, K., & Macdonald, A. (2002). *Delirium in old age.* New York: Oxford University Press.

Linehan, M. M. (1993). *Cognitive-behavioral treatment of borderline personality disorder.* New York: Guilford Press.

Linehan, M. M., & Dexter-Mazza, E. T. (2008). Dialectical behavior therapy for borderline personality disorder. In D. H. Barlow (Ed.), *Clinical handbook of psychological disorders: a step-by-step treatment manual* (pp. 365–420). New York: The Guilford Press.

Linscott, R., Allardyce, J., & van Os, J. (2010). Seeking verisimilitude in a class: a systematic review of evidence that the criterial clinical symptoms of schizophrenia are taxonic. *Schizophrenia Bulletin, 36,* 811–829.

Lipowski, Z. (1980). *Delirium.* Springfield, IL: Charles C. Thomas.

Liu, Z., Zhu, F., Wang, G., Xiao, Z., Wang, H., Tang, J., . . . Li, W. (2006). Association of corticotropin-releasing hormone receptor1 gene SNP and haplotype with major depression. *Neuroscience Letters, 404,* 358–362.

Livesley, J. (2007). A framework for integrating dimensional and categorical classifications of personality disorders. *Journal of Personality Disorders, 21,* 199–224.

Livesley, W., & Jang, K. (2008). The behavioral genetics of personality disorder. *Annual Review of Clinical Psychology, 4,* 247–274.

Lock, J., Le Grange, D., Agras, W., & Dare, C. (2001). *Treatment manual for anorexia nervosa: A family-based approach.* New York: Guilford Press.

Loftus, E. (2003). Our changeable memories: Legal and practical implications. *Nature Reviews Neuroscience, 4,* 231–234.

Lombardo, N., Chakrabarti, B., Bullmore, E., Sadk, S., Pasco, G., Wheelwright, S., . . . Baron-Cohen, S. (2010). Atypical neural self-representation I autism. *Brain, 133,* 611–624.

Loo, C., & Mitchell, P. (2005). A review of the efficacy of transcranial magnetic stimulation (TMS) treatment for depression, and current and future strategies to optimize efficacy. *Journal of Affective Disorders, 88,* 255–267.

López, S., & Guarnaccia, P. (2000). Cultural psychopathology: Uncovering the social world of mental illness. *Annual Review of Psychology, 51,* 571–598.

Lovaas, O., & Smith, T. (2003). Early and intensive behavioral intervention in autism. In A. Kazdin & J. Weisz (Eds.), *Evidence-based psychotherapies for children and adolescents.* New York: Guilford Press.

Lucassen, P., Fitzsimons, C., Korosi, A., Hoels, M., Belzung, C., & Abrous, D. (2013). Stressing new neurons into depression? *Molecular Psychiatry, 18,* 396–397.

Luck, S. J., Woodman, G. F., & Vogel, E. K. (2000). Event-related potential studies of attention. *Trends in Cognitive Sciences, 11,* 432–440.

Luders, E., Sánchez, F., Tosun, D., Shattuck, D., Gaser, C., Vilain, E., & Toga, W. (2012). Increased cortical thickness in male-to-female transsexualism. *Journal of Behavioral and Brain Science, 2,* 357–362.

Lukens, S., & Ray, W. (1995) Dissociative experiences and their relation to psychopathology. Paper presented at the *Society for Psychopathology Research* annual meeting, Iowa City, IA.

Luria, A. R. (1972). *The man with a shattered world.* New York: Basic Books.

Lussier, P., & Piché, L. (2008). Frotteurism: Psychopathology and theory. In D. R. Laws & W. O'Donohue (Eds.), *Sexual deviance: Theory, assessment and treatment* (2nd ed.). New York: Guilford Press.

Lykins, A., Meana, M., & Kambe, G. (2006). Detection of differential viewing patters to erotic and non-erotic stimuli using eye-tracking methodology. *Archives of Sexual Behavior, 35,* 569–575.

Lynch, W. C., Crosby, R. D., Wonderlich, S. A., & Striegel-Moore, R. H. (2011). Eating disorder symptoms of Native American and white adolescents. In R. H. Striegel-Moore, S. A. Wonderlich, B. T. Walsh, & J. E. Mitchell (Eds.), *Developing an evidence-based classification of eating disorders: Scientific findings for DSM-5.* Arlington, VA: American Psychiatric Association.

Mack, K., & Mack, P. (1992). Induction of transcription factors in somatosensory cortex after tactile stimulation. *Brain Research: Molecular Brain Research, 12,* 141–147.

MacLeod, C., & Mathews, A. (2012). Cognitive bias modification approaches to anxiety. *Annual Review of Clinical Psychology, 8,* 189–217.

Magistretti, P. J. (2009). Low-cost travel in neurons. *Neuroscience Science, 325*(5946), 1349–1351. doi:10.1126/science.118102 Retrieved from http://www.sciencemag.org/content/325/5946/1349.short

Mahan, A., & Ressler, K. (2012). Fear conditioning, synaptic plasticity and the amygdala: Implications for posttraumatic stress disorder. *Trends in Neuroscience, 35,* 24–35.

Main, M., & Solomon, J. (1990). Procedures for identifying infants as disorganized/disoriented during the Ainsworth Strange Situation. In M. Greenberg, D. Cicchetti, & E. M. Cummings (Eds.), *Attachment in the preschool years: Theory, research and intervention* (pp. 121–160). Chicago: University of Chicago Press.

Maiti, S., Kumar, K., Castellani, C., O'Reilly, R., & Singh, S. (2011). Ontogenetic de novo copy number variations (CNVs) as a source of genetic individuality: Studies on two families with MZD twins for schizophrenia. *PLOS ONE, 6.*

Maldonado, J. R., & Spiegel, D. (2008). Dissociative disorders. In R. E. Hales, S. C. Yudofsky, & G. O. Gabbard (Eds.), *The American psychiatric publishing textbook of psychiatry* (5th ed.). Arlington, VA: American Psychiatric Publishing.

Malhi, G. (2009). The impact of lithium on bipolar disorder. *Bipolar Disorders, Supplement, 2,* 1–3.

Malhotra, H. K., & Wig, N. N. (1975). Dhat syndrome: A culture-bound sex neurosis of the orient. *Archives Sexual Behavior, 4*(5), 519–528.

Manzano, O., Cervenka, S., Karabanov, A., Farde, L., & Ullén, F. (2010). Thinking outside a less intact box: Thalamic dopamine D2 receptor densities are negatively related to psychometric creativity in healthy individuals. *PLOS ONE, 5*(5), e10670. doi:10.1371/journal.pone.0010670

Marchand, W. & Yurgelun-Todd, D. (2011). Functional imaging of bipolar illness In M. Shenton & B. Turetsky (Eds.), *Understanding neuropsychiatric disorders: Insights from neuroimaging.* New York: Cambridge University Press.

Markon, K. E., & Krueger, R. F. (2005). Categorical and continuous models of liability to externalizing disorders: A direct comparison in NESARC. *Archives of General Psychiatry, 62,* 1352–1359.

Marsella, A. J., & Yamada, A. (2000). Culture and mental health: An introduction and overview of foundations, concepts, and issues. In I. Cuellar & F. Paniagua (Eds.), *Handbook of multicultural mental health* (pp. 3–24). New York: Academic Press.

Marshall, J., & O'Dell, S. (2012). Methamphetamine influences on brain and behavior: Unsafe at any speed? *Trends in Neurosciences, 35,* 536–545.

Masters, W., & Johnson, V. (1966). *Human sexual response.* New York: Little, Brown.

Masters, W., & Johnson, V. (1970). *Human sexual inadequacy.* New York: Little, Brown.

Masters, W., & Johnson, V. (1979). *Homosexuality in perspective.* New York: Little Brown.

Masters, W., Johnson, V., & Kolodny, R. (1986). *Masters and Johnson on sex and human loving.* New York: Little, Brown.

McAnulty, R. (2012). *Sex in college.* New York: Praeger.

McCabe, R. E., Antony, M. M., Summerfeldt, L. J., Liss, A., & Swinson, R. P. (2003). Preliminary examination of the relationship between anxiety disorders in adults and self-reported history of teasing or bullying experiences. *Cognitive Behaviour Therapy, 32,* 187–193.

McCann, U., Szabo, Z., Scheffel, U., Dannals, R., & Ricaurte, G. (1998). Positron emission tomographic evidence of toxic effect of MDMA ("Ecstasy") on brain serotonin neurons in human beings. *Lancet, 352,* 1433–1437.

McCrae, R. (2009). Personality profiles of cultures: Patterns of ethos. *European Journal of Personality, 23,* 205–227.

McCrae, R., & Costa, P. (1987). Validation of the five-factor model of personality across instruments and observers. *Journal of Personality and Social Psychology, 52,* 81–90.

McCrae, R & Costa, P. (1996). Toward a new generation of personality theories: Theoretical contexts for the five- factor model. In J. S. Wiggins (Ed.), *The five-factor model of personality.* New York: Guilford Press.

McCrae, R. R., & Costa, P. T., Jr. (1999). A five-factor theory of personality. In L. A. Pervin & O. P. John (Eds.), *Handbook of personality: Theory and research* (2nd ed., pp. 139–153). New York: Guilford Press.

McCrae, R. R., Costa, P. T., Jr., Lima, M. P., Simões, A., Ostendorf, F., Angleitner, A., . . . Piedmont, R. L. (1999). Age differences in personality across the adult life span: Parallels in five cultures. *Developmental Psychology, 35,* 466–477.

McCrae, R., Gaines, J., & Wellington, M. (2013). The five- factor model in fact and fiction. In I. Weiner (Ed.), *Handbook of psychology* (2nd ed.). New York: Wiley.

McEwen, B. S. (1998). Protective and damaging effects of stress mediators. *New England Journal of Medicine, 338,* 171–179.

McEwen, B. (2010). Stress, sex, and neural adaptation to a changing environment: mechanisms of neuronal remodeling. *Annals of the New York Academy of Science, 1204,* E38–E59.

McGovern, P. (2009). *Uncorking the past: The quest for wine, beer, and other alcoholic beverages.* Berkeley: University of California Press.

McGowan, P., Sasaki, A., D'Alessio, A., Dymov, S., Labonté, B., Szyf, M., . . . Meaney, M. (2009). Epigenetic regulation of the glucocorticoid receptor in human brain associates with childhood abuse. *Nature Neuroscience, 12,* 342–348.

McGrath, J., Burne, T., Féron, F., Mackay-Sim, A., & Eyles, D. (2010). Developmental vitamin D deficiency and risk of schizophrenia: A 10 year update. *Schizophrenia Bulletin, 36,* 1073–1078.

McLaughlin, K., Greif-Green, J., Gruber, M., Sampson, N., Zaslavsky, A., & Kessler, R. (2012). Childhood adversities and first onset of psychiatric disorders in a national sample of US adolescents. *Archives of General Psychiatry, 69,* 1151–1160.

McLean, R. (2003). *Recovered, not cured: A journey through schizophrenia.* Australia: Allen Unwin.

McMahon, R. J., & Kotler, J. S. (2008). Evidence-based therapies for oppositional behavior in young children. In R. G. Steele, T. D. Elkin, & M. C. Roberts (Eds.), *Handbook of evidence-based therapies for children and adolescents.* New York: Springer.

McNaughton, N., & Corr, P. J. (2004). A two-dimensional neuropsychology of defense: Fear/anxiety and defensive distance. *Neuroscience and Biobehavioral Reviews, 28,* 285–305.

Mefford, H., Batshaw, M., & Hoffman, E. (2012). Genomics, intellectual disability, and autism. *New England Journal of Medicine, 366,* 733–743.

Mehrotra, S., & Sukumar, P. (2007). Sources of strength perceived by women caring for relatives diagnosed with Cancer. An Exploratory study from India. *Support Care Cancer, 15,* 1357–1366.

Mello, C., Vicario, D., & Clayton, D. (1992). Song presentation induces gene expression in the songbird forebrain. *Proceedings of the National Academy of Sciences, 89,* 6818–6822.

Meltzer, M. (1983). Poor memory: A case report. *Journal of Clinical Psychology, 39,* 3–10.

Menon, V. (2011). Large scale brain networks and psychopathology: A unifying triple network model. *Trends in Cognitive Sciences, 15,* 483–506.

Menzies, L., Chamberlain, S., Laird, A., Thelen, S., Sahakian, B., & Bullmore, E. (2008). Integrating evidence from neuroimaging and neuropsychological studies of obsessive-compulsive disorder: The orbitofronto-striatal model revisited. *Neuroscience and Biobehavioral Review, 32,* 525–549.

Metcalf, P., Scragg, R., Willoughby, P., Finau, S., & Tipene-Leach, D. (2000). Ethnic differences in perceptions of body size in middle-aged European, Maori and Pacific People living in New Zealand. *International Journal of Obesity, 24,* 593–599.

Mevel, K., Chételat, G., Eustache, F., & Desgranges, B. (2011). The default mode network in healthy aging and Alzheimer's disease. *International Journal of Alzheimer's Disease.* doi: 10.4061/2011/535816

Meyer, G. (2001). Introduction to the final Special Section in the Special Series on the utility of the Rorschach for clinical assessment. *Psychological Assessment, 13,* 419–422.

Meyer, G., & Archer, R. (2001). The hard science of Rorschach research: What do we know and where do we go? *Psychological Assessment, 13,* 486–502.

Meyer, G., Erdberg, P., & Shaffer, T. (2007). Toward international normative reference data for the comprehensive system. *Journal of Personality Assessment, 89,* S201–S216.

Meyer-Lindenberg, A. (2008). Psychology. Trust me on this. *Science, 321,* 778–780.

Meyer-Lindenberg, A. (2010). From maps to mechanisms through neuroimaging of schizophrenia. *Nature, 468,* 194–202.

Mihura, J. L., Meyer, G. J., Dumitrascu, N., & Bombel, G. (2013). The validity of individual Rorschach variables: Systematic reviews and meta-analyses of the Comprehensive System. *Psychological Bulletin.* Advance online publication. doi: 10.1037/a0029406

Miklowitz, D. J., Goldstein, M. J., Nuechterlein, K. H., Snyder, K. S., & Mintz, J. (1988). Family factors and the course of bipolar affective disorder. *Archives of General Psychiatry, 45,* 225–231.

Miklowitz, D., & Johnson, S. (2006). The psychopathology and treatment of bipolar disorder. *Annual Review of Clinical Psychology, 2,* 199–235.

Millan, M. (2003). The neurobiology and control of anxious states. *Progress in Neurobiology, 70,* 83–244.

Miller, G. (2010). The seductive allure of behavioral epigenetics. *Science, 329,* 24–27.

Miller, G., & Rockstroh, B. (2013). Endophenotypes in psychopathology research: Where do we stand? *Annual Review of Clinical Psychology, 9,* 1–15.

Miller, M., Azrael, D., & Barber, C. (2012). Suicide mortality in the United States: The importance of attending to method in understanding population-level disparities in the burden of suicide. *Annual Review of Public Health, 33,* 393–408.

Miller, S., & Byers, E. (2004). Actual and desired duration of foreplay and intercourse: Discordance and misperceptions within heterosexual couples. *Journal of Sex Behavior, 41,* 301–309.

Miller, W., Sorensen, J., Selzer, J., & Brigham, G. (2006). Disseminating evidence-based practices in substance abuse treatment: A review with suggestions. *Journal of Substance Abuse and Treatment, 31,* 25–39.

Minshew, N., & Williams, D. (2007). The new neurobiology of autism. *Archives of Neurology, 64,* 945–950.

Minzenberg, M., Laird, A., Thelen, S., Carter, C., & Glahn, D. (2009). Meta-analysis of 41 functional neuroimaging studies of executive function in schizophrenia. *Archives of General Psychiatry, 66,* 811–822.

Minzenberg, M., Yoon, J., & Carter, C. (2010). Schizophrenia and other psychotic disorders. In R. Hales & S. Yudofsky (Eds.), *Essentials of psychiatry*. Arlington, VA: American Psychiatric Press.

Miklowitz, D., Goldstein, M. J., Nuechterlein, K. H., Snyder, K. S., & Mintz, J. (1988). Family factors and the course of bipolar affective disorder. *Achieves of General Psychiatry, 45,* 225–231.

Miklowitz, D., & Johnson, S. (2006). The psychopathology and treatment of bipolar disorder. *Annual Review of Clinical Psychology, 2,* 199–235.

Mirsky, A., Bieliauskas, L., French, L., Van Kammen, D., Jönsson, E., & Sedvall, G. (2000). A 39-year followup of the Genain quadruplets. *Schizophrenia Bulletin, 26,* 699–708.

Miskovic, V., & Schmidt, L. (2012). Social fearfulness in the human brain. *Neuroscience and Biobehavioral Reviews, 36,* 459–478.

Mittal, V., Kalus, O., Bernstein, D., & Siever, L. (2007). Schizoid personality disorder. In W. O'Donohue, K. Fowler, & S. Lillenfeld (Eds.), *Personality disorder: Toward the DSM-V.* Thousand Oaks, CA: Sage.

Mitte, K. (2005). A meta-analysis of the efficacy of psycho- and pharmacotherapy in panic disorder with and without agoraphobia. *Journal of Affective Disorders, 88,* 27–45.

Moffitt, T. (1993). Adolescence-limited and life-course-persistent antisocial behavior: A developmental taxonomy. *Psychological Review, 100,* 674–701.

Moffitt, T., & Scott, S. (2008). Conduct disorders of childhood and adolescence. In M. Rutter, D. V. M. Bishop, D. S. Pine, S. Scott, J. Stevenson, E. Taylor, & A. Thapar (Eds.), *Rutter's child and adolescent psychiatry* (5th ed.). London: Blackwell Publishing.

Mora, G. (1959). Vincenzo Chiarugi (1759–1820) and his psychiatric reform in Florence in the late 18th century. *Journal of the history of medicine and allied sciences, 14,* 424–433.

Morin, J., & Levenson, J. (2008). Exhibitionism: Assessment and treatment. In D. R. Laws & W. O'Donohue (Eds.), *Sexual deviance: Theory, assessment and treatment* (2nd ed.). New York: Guilford Press.

Morley, T., & Moran, G. (2011). The origins of cognitive vulnerability in early childhood: Mechanisms linking early attachment to later depression. *Clinical Psychology Review, 31,* 1071–1082.

Morrison, A. (2008). Cognitive-behavioral therapy. In K. Meser & D. Jeste (Eds.), *Clinical handbook of schizophrenia* (pp. 226–239). New York: Guilford Press.

Morrison, B. (2008). Depression: Disease, loneliness social isolation, suicide, negative thoughts. *Social Alternative, 27,* 312–328.

Mosher, W. D., Chandra, A., & Jones, J. (2005, September 15). Sexual behavior and selected health measures. Men and women 15–44 years of age, United States, 2002. *CDC advance data from vital and health statistics,* 362. Retrieved from www.cdc.gov/nchs/data/ad/ad362pdf

Moustafa, J., & Froguel, P. (2013). From obesity genetics to the future of personalized obesity therapy. *Nature Reviews Endocrinology, 9,* 402–413.

Mukundan, C. R. (2016). Emotion–Arousal and control. International Journal of Indian Psychology, *3*(2).

———. (2017). Emotion — The driving force. Lunawada, Gujarat: RED'SHINE Publication.

Muñoz, R. F., Le, H. N., Clarke, G. N., Barrera, A. Z., & Torres, L. D. (2008). Preventing first onset and recurrence of major depressive episodes. In I. H. Gotlib & C. L. Hammen (Eds.), *Handbook of depression* (2nd ed., pp. 533–553). New York: Guilford Press.

Murad, M., Elamin, M., Garcia, M., Mullan, R., Murad, A., Erwin, P., & Montori, V. (2010). Hormonal therapy and sex reassignment: A systematic review and meta- analysis of quality of life and psychosocial outcomes. *Clinical Endocrinology, 72,* 214–231.

Murphy, J. (1976). Psychiatric labeling in cross-cultural perspective. *Science, 191,* 1019–1028.

Murphy, W., & Page, I. (2008). Exhibitionism: Psychopathology and theory. In D. R. Laws & W. O'Donohue (Eds.), *Sexual deviance: Theory, assessment and treatment* (2nd ed.). New York: Guilford Press.

Murray, R., Morrison, P., Henquet, C., & Di Forti, M. (2007). Cannabis, the mind and society: The hash realities. *Nature Reviews Neuroscience, 8,* 885–895.

Murthy, R. Srinivasa. (2014). Mental health of survivors of 1984 Bhopal disaster: A continuing challenge. *Industrial Psychiatry Journal, 23*(2), 86–93.

Murthy, R. Srinivasa. (2015). *From institutions, to clinics, to community: Development of community mental health in the last 50 years and looking to the future. In* Developments in psychiatry in India: clinical research and policy perspectives. Chapter 21. (eds.) Malhotra, S. and Chakrabarti, S. New Delhi: Springer (pp. 419–438).

Murthy, S. (2012). Farmer suicide: Need for mental health interventions. *Indian Journal of Social Psychiatry, 28*(1–2), 26–35.

Musto, D. (1991). Opium, cocaine and marijuana in American history. *Scientific American, 265,* 40–47.

Nagamatsu, L., Chan, A., Davis, J., Beattie, B., Graf, P., Voss, M., . . . Liu-Ambrose, T. (2013). Physical activity improves verbal and spatial memory in older adults with probable mild cognitive impairment: A 6-month randomized controlled trial. *Journal of Aging Research.*

Naglieri, J. A., Salter, C., & Rojahn, J. (2008). Specific learning and intellectual disabilities. In J. E. Maddux & B. A. Winstead (Eds.), *Psychopathology: Contemporary theory, research, and issues* (2nd ed.). Mahwah, NJ: Lawrence Erlbaum.

Nadkarni, A., Velleman, R., Dabholkar, H., Shinde, S., Bhat, B. McCambridge, J., Murthy, P., Wilson, T. Weobong, B., and Patel, V. (2015). The systematic development and pilot randomized evaluation of counselling for alcohol problems, a lay counselor-delivered psychological treatment for harmful drinking in primary care in India: The premium study. *Alcoholism: Clinical and Experimental Research, 39*(3), 522–531.

Nasar, S. (1998). *A beautiful mind.* New York: Simon & Schuster.

Nashold Jr., B.S., Wilson, N. P., & Slaughter, G. S. (1974). The midbrain and pain. In J. J. Bonica (Ed.), *Advances in neurology, international symposium on pain* (Vol. 4, pp. 191–196). New York: Raven Press.

Nasser, M., Katzman, M. A., & Gordon, R. A. (Eds.). (2001). *Eating disorders and cultures in transition.* New York: Taylor & Francis.

Nath, S., Agholme, L., Kurudenkandy, F. R., Granseth, B., Marcusson, J., & Hallbeck, M. (2012). Spreading of neurodegenerative pathology via neuron-to-neuron transmission of β-amyloid. *Journal of Neuroscience, 32,* 8767–8777.

National Center for Health Statistics. (2012). *Health, United States, 2011: With special feature on socioeconomic status and health.* Retrieved from www.cdc.gov/nchs/data/hus/hus11.pdf

National Institute on Drug Abuse. (2010, September). *Cocaine: Abuse and addiction. How does cocaine produces its effects?* Retrieved from www.drugabuse.gov/publications/research-reports/cocaine-abuse-addiction/how-does-cocaine-produce-its-effects

Neary, D. (2005). Frontotemporal dementia. In A. Burns, J. O'Brien, & D. Ames (Eds.), *Dementia* (3rd ed.). London, UK: Hodder Arnold.

Neel, J. V. (1962). Diabetes mellitus: A thrifty genotype rendered determined by progress? *American Journal of Human Genetics, 14,* 353–363.

Nelson, E., Leibenluft, E., McClure, E., & Pine, D. (2005). The social re-orientation of adolescence: a neuroscience perspective on the process and its relation to psychopathology. *Psychological Medicine, 35,* 163–174.

Nesse, R. M. (1990). Evolutionary explanations of emotions. *Human Nature, 1,* 261–289

Nesse, R., & Williams, G. (1994). *Why we get sick: The new science of Darwinian Medicine.* New York: Vintage.

Nestler, E. (2011). Hidden switches in the mind. *Scientific American, 305,* 76–83.

Nestler, E., & Malenka, R. (2004). The addictive brain. *Scientific American, 290,* 78–85.

Nettle, D. (2006). The evolution of personality variation in humans and other animals. *American Psychologist, 61,* 622–631.

Newring, K., Wheeler, J., & Draper C. (2008). Transvestic fetishism: Assessment and treatment. In D. R. Laws & W. O'Donohue (Eds.), *Sexual deviance: Theory, assessment and treatment* (2nd ed.). New York: Guilford Press.

Newschaffer, C., Croen, L., Daniels, J., Giarelli, E., Grether, J., Levy, S., . . . Windham, G. (2007). The epidemiology of autism spectrum disorders. *Annual Review of Public Health, 28,* 235–258.

Nieuwenstein, M. R., Aleman, A., & de Haan, E. H. (2001). Relationship between symptom dimensions and neurocognitive functioning in schizophrenia: A meta-analysis of WCST and CPT studies.

Wisconsin Card Sorting Test. Continuous Performance Test. *Journal of Psychiatric Research, 35,* 119–125.

Newton, I. (1969). *Mathematical principles* (F. Cajori, Trans.). New York: Greenwood. (Translation first published 1729).

Ng, S., Lin, R., Laybutt, D., Barres, R., Owens, J., & Morris, M. (2010). Chronic high-fat diet in fathers programs β-cell dysfunction in female rat offspring. *Nature, 467,* 963–966.

Nichols, D. (2004) Hallucinogens. *Pharmacology & Therapeutics, 101,* 131–181.

Nielsen, J., & Pernice, K. (2008). *Eyetracking web usability.* Berkeley, CA: New Riders Press.

Nikulina, V., Widom, C. S., & Brzustowicz, L. M. (2012). Child abuse and neglect, MAOA, and mental health outcomes: A prospective examination. *Biological Psychiatry, 71,* 350–357.

Nizamie, S. H., & Goyal, N. (2010). History of psychiatry in India. Indian Journal of Psychiatry, *52*(Suppl1), S7. Retrieved from https://www.ncbi.nlm.nih.gov/pmc/articles/PMC3146221/

Northcutt, R. G., & Kaas, J. H. (1995). The emergence and evolution of mammalian neocortex. *Trends in Neuroscience, 18,* 373–379.

Nowak, D., & Fink, G. (2009). Psychogenic movement disorders: aetiology, phenomenology, neuroanatomical correlates and therapeutic approaches. *NeuroImage, 47,* 1015–1025.

Nunez, P., & Srinivasan, R. (2006). *Electrical fields of the brain: The neurophysics of EEG.* New York: Oxford University Press.

Oathes, D. J., & Ray, W. J. (2006). Depressed mood, index finger force, and motor cortex stimulation: A transcranial magnetic stimulation (TMS) study. *Biological Psychology, 72,* 278–290.

Oathes, D. J., Ray, W. J., Yamasaki, A. S., Borkovec, T. D., Newman, M. G., & Castonguay, L. G. (2008). Worry, generalized anxiety disorder, and emotion: Evidence from the EEG gamma band. *Biological Psychology, 79,* 165–170.

O'Connor, E., Bureau, J., McCartney, K., & Lyons-Ruth, K. (2011). Risks and outcomes associated with disorganized/controlling patterns of attachment at age three in the NICHD Study of Early Child Care and Youth Development. *Infant Mental Health Journal, 32,* 450–472.

Office of the U.S. Surgeon General & National Action Alliance for Suicide Prevention. (2012). *2012 national strategy for suicide prevention: Goals and objectives for action.* A report of the U.S. Surgeon General and of the National Action Alliance for Suicide Prevention. Washington, DC: U.S. Department of Health and Human Services.

Office on Women's Health. (2009a, June 15). *Jen's story.* Washington, DC: U.S. Department of Health and Human Services. Retrieved from http://www.womenshealth.gov/publications/our-publications/fact-sheet/anorexia-nervosa .html

Office on Women's Health. (2009b, June 15). *Jen's story.* Washington, DC: U.S. Department of Health and Human Services. Retrieved from www.womenshealth.gov/publications/our-publications/fact-sheet/bulimia-nervosa .cfm

O'Hara, R. (2012). The reciprocal relationship of neurocognitive and neuropsychiatric function in late life. *American Journal of Geriatric Psychiatry, 20,* 1001–1005.

Öhman, A. (1986). Face the beast and fear the face: Animal and social fears as prototypes for evolutionary analyses of emotion. *Psychophysiology, 23,* 123–145.

Öhman, A., (2009). Of snakes and faces: An evolutionary perspective on the psychology of fear. *Scandinavian Journal of Psychology, 50,* 543–552.

Öhman, A., & Mineka, S. (2001). Fears, phobias, and preparedness: toward an evolved module of fear and fear learning. *Psychological Review, 108,* 483–522.

Oliveira-Souza, R., Hare, R., Bramati, I., Garrido, G., Azevedo, F, Tovar-Moll, F., & Moll, J. (2008). Psychopathy as a disorder of the moral brain: Fronto-temporo-limbic grey matter reductions demonstrated by voxel-based morphometry. *Neuroimage, 40,* 1202–1213.

Ollendick T., Yang, B., King, N., Dong, Q., & Akande, A. (1996). Fears in American, Australian, Chinese, and Nigerian children and adolescents: A cross-cultural study. *Journal of Child Psychology and Psychiatry, 37,* 213–220.

Öst, L., (1989). One-session treatment for specific phobias. *Behavior Research and Therapy, 27,* 1–7.

Öst, L., (1996). One-session treatment for specific phobias. *Behavior Research and Therapy, 34,* 707–715.

Palacios, S., Castaño, R., & Grazziotin, A. (2009). Epidemiology of female sexual dysfunction. *Maturitas, 63,* 119–123.

Palmer, R., Young, S., Corley, R., Hopfer, C., Stallings, M., & Hewitt, J. (2013). Stability and change of genetic and environmental effects on the common liability to alcohol, tobacco, and cannabis DSM–IV dependence symptoms. *Behavioral Genetics, 43*(5), 374–385.

Panksepp, J. (1998). *Affective neuroscience: The foundations of human and animal emotions.* New York: Oxford University Press.

Panksepp, J. (Ed.) (2004). *Testbook of biological psychiatry.* New York: Wiley.

Panksepp, J., Knutson, B., & Burgdorf, J. (2002). The role of brain emotional systems in addictions: A neuro- evolutionary perspective and new "self-report" animal model. *Addiction, 97,* 459–469.

Pardo, C., Vargas, D., & Zimmerman, A. (2005). Immunity, neuroglia and neuroinflammation in autism. *International Review of Psychiatry, 17,* 485–495.

Park, D., & Reuter-Lorenz, P. A. (2009). The adaptive brain: Aging and neurocognitive scaffolding. *Annual Review of Psychology, 60,* 173–196.

Passamonti, L., Fairchild, G., Goodyer, I. M., Hurford, G., Hagan, C. C., Rowe, J. B., & Calder, A. J. (2010). Neural abnormalities in early-onset and adolescence-onset conduct disorder. *Archives of General Psychiatry, 67,* 729–738.

Patel, V., Araya, R., Chatterjee, S., Chisholm, D., Cohen, A., De Silva, M., . . . van Ommeren, M. (2007). Treatment and prevention of mental disorders in low-income and middle-income countries. *The Lancet, 370*(9591), 991–1005.

Patel, V., Chatterji, S., Chisholm, D., Ebrahim, S., Gopalakrishna, G., Mathers, C., ... & Reddy, K. S. (2011). Chronic diseases and injuries in India. The Lancet, *377*(9763), 413–428.

Patel, V., DeSouza, N., & Rodrigues, M. (2003). Postnatal depression and infant growth and development in low income countries: a cohort study from Goa, India. *Archieves of Diseases in Childhood,* 88, 34–37.

Patel, V., Farooq, S., & Thara, R. (2007). What is the best approach to treating schizophrenia in developing countries? *PLOS Medicine, 4*(6), 963–966.

Patel, V., Ramasundarahettige, C., Vijayakumar, L., Thakur, J. S., Gajalakshmi, V., Gururaj, G., ... Jha, P. (2012). Suicide mortality in India: A nationally representative survey. The Lancet, *379*(9834), 2343–2351. Retrieved from http://www.thelancet.com/journals/lancet/article/PIIS0140-6736(12)60606-0/fulltext

Pato, M., Fanous, A., Eisen, J., & Phillips, K. (2008). Obsessive-compulsive disorder. In A. Tasman, J. Kay, J. Lieberman, M. First, & M. Maj (Eds.), *Psychiatry* (3rd ed.). New York: Wiley.

Patrick, C. J. (2006). Back to the future: Cleckley as a guide to the next generation of psychopathy research. In C. J. Patrick (Ed.), *Handbook of psychopathy* (pp. 605–617). New York: Guilford Press.

Patrick, C. J. (2007). Antisocial personality disorder and psychopathy. In W. O'Donohue, K. A. Fowler, & S. O. Lilienfeld (Eds.), *Personality disorders: Toward the DSM-V* (pp. 325–352). Thousand Oaks, CA: Sage.

Patrick, C. J. (2010). Conceptualizing psychopathic personality: Disinhibited, bold, or just plain mean? In R. J. Salekin & D. R. Lynam (Eds.), *Handbook of child and adolescent psychopathy* (pp. 15–48). New York: Guilford Press.

Patrick, C. J., & Bernat, E. M. (2009). Neurobiology of psychopathy: A two-process theory. In G. G. Berntson & J. T. Cacioppo (Eds.), *Handbook of neuroscience for the behavioral sciences* (pp. 1110–1131). New York: Wiley.

Paus, T., Keshavan, M., & Giedd, J. (2008). Why do many psychiatric disorders emerge during adolescence? *Nature Reviews Neuroscience, 9,* 947–957.

Pavlov, I. P. (1941). *Conditioned reflexes and psychiatry (Lectures on conditioned reflexes* (Vol. 2). (W. H. Gantt, Trans.). New York: International Publishers.

Pearlson, G. (2011). Functional imaging of schizophrenia. In M. Shenton & B. Turetsky (Eds.), *Understanding neuropsychiatric disorders: Insights from neuroimaging.* New York: Cambridge University Press.

Pechtel, P., & Pizzagalli, D. (2011). Effects of early life stress on cognitive and affective function: An integrated review of human literature. *Psychopharmacology, 214,* 55–70.

Pelham, V. (2013, July 7). Michael Boatwright awakes in Palm Springs with apparent amnesia. *The Desert Sun.* Retrieved from www.mydesert.com/article/20130706/LIFESTYLES03/307060025/Michael-Boatwright-awakes-Palm-Springs-apparent-amnesia?nclick_check=1

Pelphrey, K., & Carter, E. (2008). Brain mechanisms for social perception. *Annals of the New York Academy of Sciences, 1145,* 283–299.

Pelphrey, K. & McPartland, J. (2012). Brain development: Neural signature predicts autism's emergence. *Current Biology, 22*(4), R127–R128.

Peluso, M., Lewis, S., Barnes, T., & Jones, P. (2012). Extrapyramidal motor side-effects of first- and second- generation antipsychotic drugs. *British Journal of Psychiatry, 200,* 387–392.

Pembrey, M., Bygren, L., Kaati, G., Edvinsson, S, Northstone, K, Sjostrom, M., . . . ALSPAC Study Team. (2006). Sex-specific, male-line transgenerational responses in humans. *European Journal of Human Genetics, 14,* 159–166.

Pendery, M., Maltzman, & West, L. (1982). Controlled drinking by alcoholics? New findings and a reevaluation of a major affirmative study. *Science, 217,* 169–175.

Penfield, W., & Rasmussen, T. (1978). *The cerebral cortex of man.* New York: Macmillan.

Pereda, N., Gallardo-Pujol, D., & Padilla, R. (2011). Personality disorders in child sexual abuse victims. *Actas Españolas de Psiquiatría, 39,* 131–139.

Pershad, D., & Verma, S. K. (1990). Hand-book of PGI Battery of Brain Dysfunction (PGI-BBD). National Psychological Corporation.

Perrin, J., Merz, S., Bennetta, D., Curriea, J., Steele, D., Reida, I., . . . Schwarzbauer, C. (2012). Electroconvulsive therapy reduces frontal cortical connectivity in severe depressive disorder. *Proceedings of the National Academy of Science, 109,* 5464–5468.

Peterson, B., & Weissman, M. (2011). A brain-based endophenotype for major depressive disorder. *Annual Review of Medicine, 62,* 461–474.

Petronis A. (2004). The origin of schizophrenia: Genetic thesis, epigenetic antithesis, and resolving synthesis. *Biological Psychiatry, 55,* 965–970.

Pfäfflin, F., & Junge, A. (1998). *Sex reassignment. Thirty years of international follow-up studies after sex reassignment surgery: A comprehensive review, 1961–1991.* Retrieved from http://classic-web.archive.org/web/20070503090247/http:/www.symposion.com/ijt/pfaefflin/1000.htm.

Phan, K. L., Fitzgerald, D. A., Nathan, P. J., & Tancer, M. E. (2006). Association between amygdala hyperactivity to harsh faces and severity of social anxiety in generalized social phobia. *Biological Psychiatry, 59,* 424–429.

Phillips, O., Nuechterlein, K., Asarnow, R., Clark, K., Cabeen, R., Yang, Y., . . . Narr, K. (2011). Mapping corticocortical structural integrity in schizophrenia and effects of genetic liability. *Biological Psychaitry, 70,* 680–689.

Pine, D. (2009). A social neuroscience approach to adolescent depression. In M. De Haan & M. Gunnar (Eds.), *Handbook of developmental social neuroscience.* New York: Guilford Press.

Pittenger, C., & Etkin, A. (2008). Are there biological commonalities among different psychiatric disorders? In A. Tasman, J. Kay, J. A. Lieberman, M. B. First, & M. Maj (Eds). *Psychiatry* (3rd ed.). New York: Wiley.

Plomin, R., DeFries, J., & Loehlin, J. (1977). Genotype-environment interaction and correlation in the analysis of human behavior. *Psychological Bulletin, 84,* 309–322.

Plomin, R., DeFries, J., McClearn, G., & McGuffin, P. (2008). *Behavioral genetics* (5th ed.). New York: Worth

Poeppl, T., Nitschke, J., Santtila, P., Schecklmann, M., Langguth, B., Greenlee, M., . . . Mokros, A. (2013). Association between brain structure and phenotypic characteristics in pedophilia. *Journal of Psychiatric Research, 47,* 678–685.

Polich, J., Armor, D., & Braiker, H. (1981). *The course of alcoholism: Four years after treatment.* New York: Wiley.

Portner, M. (2008, April/May). The orgasmic mind. *Scientific American Mind,* 67–71.

Pos, A., & Greenberg, L. (2007). Emotion-focused therapy: The transforming power of affect. *Journal of Contemporary Psychotherapy, 37,* 25–31.

Prescott, J., & Rockoff, J. (2011). Do sex offender registration and notification laws affect criminal behavior? *Journal of Law and Economics, 54,* 161–206.

Preuss, T., & Kaas, J. (1999). Human brain evolution. In F. Bloom, S. Landis, J. Roberts, L. Squire, & M. Zigmond (Eds.). *Fundamental neuroscience.* New York: Academic Press.

Price, D. D. (2000) Psychological and neural mechanisms of the affective dimension of pain. *Science, 288,* 1769–1772.

Price, P. (1996). *Biological evolution.* Pacific Grove, CA: Brooks/Cole.

Prince, M. (1913). *The dissociation of a personality: A biographical study in abnormal psychology.* New York: Longmans, Green, and Co.

Prince, M., Bryce, R., Albanese, E., Wimo, A., Ribeiro, W., & Ferri, C. (2013). The global prevalence of dementia: A systematic review and metaanalysis. *Alheizmer's & Dementia, 9,* 63–75.

Prugh, D. G., Wagonfeld, S., Metcalf, D., & Jordan, K. (1980). A clinical study of delirium in children and adolescents [Supp.]. *Psychosomatic Medicine, 42,* 177–195.

Purves, D., Cabeza, R., Huettel, S., LaBar, K., Platt, M., & Woldorff, M. (2013). *Principles of cognitive neuroscience* (2nd ed.). Sunderland, MA: Sinauer Associates.

Queen v. *M'Naghten,* 8 Eng. Rep. 718 (1843).

Rademakers, R, & Rovelet-Lecrux, A. (2009). Recent insights into the molecular genetics of dementia. *Trends in Neurosciences, 32,* 451–461.

Radtke, K., Ruf, M., Gunter, H., Dohrmann, K., Schauer, M., Meyer, A., & Elbert T. (2011). Transgenerational impact of intimate partner violence on methylation in the promoter of the glucocorticoid receptor. *Translational Psychiatry, 1.* doi:10.1038/tp.2011.21

Raebhausen, O. M., & Brim, O. G. (1967). Privacy and behavioral research. *American Psychologist, 22,* 423–437.

Raguram, R., & Jadhav, S. (1994). Historical perspectives on Dhat syndrome. *NIMHANS J, 12,* 117–124.

Raha, S., Shah, U., & Udani, V. (2012). Neurocognitive and neurobehavioral disabilities in Epilepsy with Electrical Status Epilepticus in slow sleep (ESES) and related syndromes. Epilepsy & Behavior, *25*(3), 381–385.

Raichle, M. (2011). The restless brain. *Brain Connectivity, 1,* 3–12.

Raichle, M., MacLeod, A., Snyder, A., Powers, W., Gusnard, D., & Shulman, G. (2001). A default mode of brain function. *Proceedings of the National Academy of Sciences of the United States of America, 98,* 676–682.

Raichle, M., & Snyder, A. (2007). A default mode of brain function: A brief history of an evolving idea. *NeuroImage, 37,* 1083–1090.

Rais, M., Cahn, W., Schnack, H. G., Hulshoff Pol, H. E., Kahn, R. S., & van Haren, N. E. (2012). Brain volume reductions in medication-naïve patients with schizophrenia in relation to intelligence quotient. *Psychosomatic Medicine, 42,* 1847–1856.

Raj, A., Kuceyeski, A., & Weiner, M. (2010). A network diffusion model of disease progression in dementia. *Neuron, 73,* 1204–1215.

Ramachandran, V. S. (1998). Consciousness and body image: Lessons from phantom limbs, Capgras syndrome and pain asymbolia. *Transitions of the Royal Society of London, B, 353,* 1851–1859.

Ramachandran, V. S., & Blakeslee, S. (1998). *Phantoms in the brain.* New York: William Morrow and Company.

Rametti, G., Carrillo, B., Gómez-Gil, E., Junque, C., Segovia, S., Gomez, A., & Guillamon, A. (2011). White matter microstructure in female to male transsexuals before cross-sex hormonal treatment. A diffusion tensor imaging study. *Journal of Psychiatric Research, 45,* 199–204.

Rampon, C., Jiang, C., Dong, H., Tang, Y., Lockhart, D., Schultz, P., . . . Hu, Y. (2000). Effects of environmental enrichment on gene expression in the brain. *Proceedings of the National Academy of Sciences, 97,* 12880–12884.

Rankinen, T., & Bouchard, C. (2006). Genetics of food intake and eating behavior phenotypes in humans. *Annual Review of Nutrition, 26,* 413–434.

Rapee, R., Schniering, C., & Hudson, J. (2009). Anxiety disorders during childhood and adolescence: Origins and treatment. *Annual Review of Clinical Psychology, 5,* 311–341.

Raskin, M. (2010). Passion is the enemy. *Scientific American Mind.*

Ratiu, P., Talos, O., Haker, S., Lieberman, D., & Evert, P. (2004). The tale of Phineas Gage, Digitally remastered. *Journal of Neurotrauma, 21,* 637–643.

Rauch, S., Shin, L., & Phelps, E. (2006). Neurocircuitry models of posttraumatic stress disorder and extinction: Human neuroimaging research—Past, present, and future. *Biological Psychiatry, 60,* 376–382.

Ravi, A., Rao, V., & Klein, J. (2013). Dystextia: Acute stroke in the modern age. *JAMA, Neurology, 70,* 404.

Ray, W. J. (2012). *Methods toward a science of behavior and experience* (10th ed.). Belmont, CA: Wadsworth Publishing.

Ray, W. J. (2013). *Evolutionary psychology: Neuroscience determinants of human behavior and experience,* Thousand Oaks, CA: Sage.

Ray, W. J., & Cole, H. W. (1985). EEG alpha reflects attentional demands, Beta reflects emotional and cognitive processes. *Science, 228,* 750–752.

Ray, W., Odenwald, M., Neuner, F., Schauer, M., Ruf, M., Wienbruch, C., . . . Elbert, T. (2006). Decoupling neural networks from reality: Dissociative experiences in torture victims are reflected in abnormal brain waves in left frontal cortex. *Psychological Science, 17,* 825–829.

Redlich, A., & Han, W. (2013). Examining the links between therapeutic jurisprudence and mental health court completion. *Law and Human Behavior.* Advance online publication. doi: 10.1037/lhb0000041

Regenold, W., Phatak, P, Marano, C., Sassan, A, Conley, R., & Kling, M. (2009). Elevated cerebrospinal fluid lactate concentrations in patients with bipolar disorder and schizophrenia: Implications for the mitochondrial dysfunction hypothesis. *Biological Psychiatry, 65,* 489–494.

Renneberg, B., Herm, K., Hahn, A., Staebler, K., Lammers, C., & Roepke, S. (2012). Perception of social participation in borderline personality disorder. *Clinical psychology and Psychotherapy, 19,*473–480.

Repetti, R. L. (1989). Effects of daily workload on subsequent behavior during marital interaction: The roles of social withdrawal and spouse spouse support. *Journal of Personality and Social Psychology, 57,* 651–659.

Reuter-Lorenz, P. A., & Park, D. C. (2010). Human neuroscience and the aging mind: a new look at old problems. *Journal of Gerontology: Psychological Sciences, 65B,* 405–415.

Reuters Staff. (2009, November 9). *Future of food: Daily calorie intake* [Web log post]. Retrieved from http://blogs.reuters.com/commodity-corner/page/3/

Ribeiro, S., & Mello, C. (2000). Gene expression and synaptic plasticity in the auditory forebrain of songbirds. *Learning and Memory, 7,* 235–243.

Rich, B. A., Carver, F. W., Holroyd, T., Rosen, H. R., Mendoza, J. K., Cornwell, B. R., . . . Leibenluft, E. (2011). Different neural pathways to negative affect in youth with pediatric bipolar disorder and severe mood dysregulation. *Journal of Psychiatry Research, 45,* 1283–1294.

Richards, R. (1983). *Second serve.* New York: Stein and Day.

Richerson, P., & Boyd, R. (2005). *Not by genes alone: How culture transformed human evolution.* Chicago: University of Chicago Press.

Rief, W., Hiller, W., & Margraf, J. (1998). Cognitive aspects of hypochondriasis and the somatization syndrome. *Journal of Abnormal Psychology, 107,* 587–595.

Rieke, F., Warland, D., van Steveninck, R., & Bialek, W. (1999). *Spikes: Exploring the neural code.* Cambridge, MA: MIT Press.

Rizzolatti, G., & Craighero, L. (2004). The mirror-neuron system. *Annual Review of Neuroscience, 27,* 169–192.

Roberson, A., (2010). *Borderline traits: Her life with borderline personality disorder.* Bloomington, IN: Xlibris Corporation.

Roberts, R., Deleger, S., Strawbridge, W., & Kaplan, G. (2003). Prospective association between obesity and depression: Evidence from the Alameda County Study. *International Journal of Obesity, 27,* 514–521.

Robison, A., & Nestler, E. (2011). Transcriptional and epigenetic mechanisms of addiction. *Nature Reviews Neuroscience, 12,* 623–637.

Robison, J. (2007). *Look me in the eye: My life with Asperger's.* New York: Crown Publishers.

Rocha-Rego, V., Jogia, J., Marquand, A., Mourao-Miranda, J., Simmons, A. & Frangou, S. (2013). Examination of the predictive value of structural magnetic resonance scans in bipolar disorder: A pattern classification approach. *Psychological Medicine, 5,* 1–14.

Rockstroh, B., & Elbert, T. (2010). Traces of fear in the neural web—Magnetoencephalographic responding to arousing pictorial stimuli. *International Journal of Psychophysiology, 78,* 14–19.

Rockstroh, B., Wienbruch, C., Ray, W.J. & Elbert, T. (2007). Abnormal oscillatory brain dynamics in schizophrenia: A sign of deviant communication in neural network? *BMC Psychiatry, 7,* 44.

Rodebaugh, T., Holaway, R., & Heimberg, R. (2004). The treatment of social anxiety disorder. *Clinical Psychology Review, 24,* 883–908.

Rodrigues, M., Patel, V., Jaswal, S., & de Souza, N. (2003). Listening to mothers: qualitative studies on motherhood and depression from Goa, India. Social Science and Medicine, 57, 1797–1806.

Roemer, L., Orsillo, S. M., & Barlow, D. H. B. (2002). Generalized anxiety disorder. In D. Barlow (Ed.), *Anxiety and its disorders: The nature and treatment of anxiety and panic* (2nd ed., pp. 477–515). New York: Guilford Press.

Rogers, J., Raveendran, M., Fawcett, G., Fox, A., Shelton, S., Oler, J., . . . Kalin, N. (2013). CRHR1 genotypes, neural circuits and the diathesis for anxiety and depression. *Molecular Psychiatry, 18,* 700–707.

Rogers, S., & Vismara, L. (2008). Evidence-based comprehensive treatments for early autism. *Journal of Clinical Child & Adolescent Psychology, 37,* 8–38.

Roggers, A., Morgan, C., Bronson, S., Revello, S., & Bale, T. (2013). Paternal stress exposure alters sperm microRNA content and reprograms offspring HPA stress axis regulation. *Journal of Neuroscience, 33,* 9003–9012.

Rorschach, H. (1942). *Psychodiagnostik [Psychodiagnostics].* Bern, Switzerland: Bircher. (Original work published 1921)

Roskies, A., Schweitzer, N., & Saks, M. (2013). Neuroimages in court: Less biasing than feared. *Trends in Cognitive Sciences, 17,* 99–101.

Ross, C. (1997). *Dissociative identity disorder: Diagnosis, clinical features, and treatment of multiple personality disorder.* New York: Wiley.

Ross, C., Joshi, S., & Currie, R. (1990). Dissociative experiences in the general population. *American Journal of Psychiatry, 147,* 1547–1552.

Rossignol, D., & Frye R. (2012). Mitochondrial dysfunction in autism spectrum disorders: A systematic review and meta-analysis. *Molecular Psychiatry, 17,* 290–314.

Roth, T., & Sweatt, J. (2011). Annual research review: Epigenetic mechanisms and environmental shaping of the brain during sensitive periods of development. *Journal of Child Psychology and Psychiatry, 52,* 398–408.

Rowe, J., & Kahn, R. (1987). Human aging: Usual and successful. *Science, 237,* 143–149.

Roy, A., Hodgkinson, C. A., Deluca, V., Goldman, D., & Enoch, M. A. (2012). Two HPA axis genes, CRHBP and FKBP5, interact with childhood trauma to increase the risk for suicidal behavior. *Journal of Psychiatric Research, 46,* 72–79.

Rudolf, K. (2009). Adolescent depression. In I. Gotlib & C. Hammen (Eds.), *Handbook of depression* (2nd ed.). New York: Guilford Press.

Rupp, H., & Wallen, M. (2007). Sex differences in viewing sexual stimuli: An eye-tracking study in men and women. *Hormones and Behavior, 51,* 524–533.

Russell, G. (1979). Bulimia nervosa: An ominous variant of anorexia nervosa. *Psychological Medicine, 9,* 429–448.

Russell, M. (2008). Scientific resistance to research, training and utilization of eye movement desensitization and reprocessing (EMDR) therapy in treating post-war disorders. *Social Science and Medicine, 67,* 1737–1746.

Russo, S., & Nestler, E. (2013). The brain reward circuitry in mood disorders. *Nature Reviews Neuroscience, 14,* 609–625.

Rutter, M. (2006). *Genes and behavior: Nature-nurture interplay explained.* Malden, MA: Blackwell Publishing.

Saah, T. (2005). The evolutionary origins and significance of drug addiction. *Harm Reduction Journal, 2,* 2–8.

Sachs, B. D. (2007). A contextual definition of male sexual arousal. *Hormones and Behavior, 51,* 569–578.

Sacher-Masoch, L. (2013). *Venus in furs.* New York: Dover Publications. (Original work published 1888)

Saks, E. (2007). *The center cannot hold: My journey through madness.* New York: Hyperion.

Saladin, M., & Santa Ana, E. (2004). Controlled drinking: More than just a controversy. *Current Opinion in Psychiatry, 17,* 175–187.

Salthouse, T. (2004). Localizing age-related individual differences in a hierarchical structure. *Intelligence, 32,* 541–561.

Salthouse, T. (2011). Neuroanatomical substrates of age-related cognitive decline. *Psychological Bulletin, 137,* 753–784.

Samuel, D. B., Simms, L. J., Clark, L. A., Livesley, W. J., & Widiger, T. A. (2010). An item response theory integration of normal and abnormal personality scales. *Personality Disorders: Theory, Research, and Treatment, 1,* 5–21.

Samuel, D., & Widiger, T. (2009). A meta-analytic review of the relationships between the five-factor model and the DSM-IV-TR personality disorders: A facet level analysis. *Clinical Psychology Review, 28,* 1326–1342.

Sanislow, C., Pine, D., Quinn, K, Kozak, M., Garvey, M., Heinssen, R., . . . Cuthbert, B. N. (2010). Developing constructs for psychopathology research: Research domain criteria. *Journal of Abnormal Psychology, 199,* 631–639.

Santhosh, N. S., Sinha, S., & Satishchandra, P. (2014). Epilepsy: Indian perspective. Annals of Indian Academy of Neurology, *17*(Suppl 1), S3–S11.

Sanyal, D. and Majumdar, A. (2016). Presentation of gender dysphoria: A perspective from Eastern India. *Indian Journal of Endocrinology and Metabolism, 20,* 129–133.

Sapolsky, R. (2003, September). Taming stress. *Scientific American,* pp. 87–95.

Sartorius, N., Jablensky, A., Korten, A., Ernberg, G., Anker, M., Cooper, J. E., & Day, R. (1986). Early manifestations and first-contact incidence of schizophrenia in different cultures. A preliminary report on the initial evaluation phase of the WHO Collaborative Study on determinants of outcome of severe mental disorders. *Psychological Medicine, 16,* 909–928.

Savitz, J., & Drevets, W. (2009). Bipolar and major depressive disorder: Neuroimaging the developmental-degenerative divide. *Neuroscience and Biobehavioral Reviews, 333,* 699–771.

Sovani, A., & Apte, S. (2012). Intervention for burnout experienced by caregivers of people with schizophrenia. Archives of Indian Psychiatry, *14*(1), 30–36.

Sovani, A., & Thatte, S. (1994). Interpersonal interaction in groups of schizophrenics: A psychosocial intervention. Indian Journal of Clinical Psychology, *21,* 33–37.

Sax, K., & Strakowski, S. (2001). Behavioral sensitization in humans. *Journal of Addiction Disorders, 20,* 55–65.

Saxena, S., Thornicroft, G., Knapp, M., & Whiteford, H. (2007). Global Mental Health 2 Resources for mental health: Scarcity, inequity, and inefficiency. *Lancet, 370,* 878–889.

Schacter, D., & Loftus, E. (2013). Memory and law: What can cognitive neuroscience contribute? *Nature Neuroscience, 16,* 119–123.

Schiller, L., & Bennett, A. (1994). *The quiet room.* New York: Warner Books.

Schneider-Garces, N., Gordon, B., Brumback-Peltz, C., Shin, E., Lee, Y., Sutton, B., . . . Fabiani, M. (2010). Span, CRUNCH, and beyond: Working memory capacity and the aging brain. *Journal of Cognitive Neuroscience, 22,* 655–669.

Schott, G. (2011). Freud's *Project* and its diagram: Anticipating the Hebbian synapse. *Journal of Neurology, Neurosurgery & Psychiatry, 82,* 122–125.

Seeley, W., Matthews, B., Crawford, R., Gorno-Tempini, M., Foti, D., Mackenzie, I., & Miller, B. (2008). Unravelling Boléro: Progressive aphasia, transmodal creativity and the right posterior neocortex. *Brain, 131,* 39–49.

Segraves, R. (2010). Considerations for an evidence-based definition of premature ejaculation in the DSM-V. *Journal of Sexual Medicine, 7,* 672–679.

Segerstrom, S., & Miller, G. (2004). Psychological stress and the human immune system: A meta-analytic study of 30 years of inquiry. *Psychological Bulletin, 130,* 601–630.

Sehlmeyer, C., Schöning, S., Zwitserlood, P., Pfleiderer, B., Kircher, T., Arolt, V., & Konrad, C. (2009). Human fear conditioning and extinction in neuroimaging: A systematic review. *PLOS ONE, 4,* e5865.

Seto, M. (2008). Pedophilia: Psychopathology and theory. In D. R. Laws & W. O'Donohue (Eds.), *Sexual deviance: Theory, assessment and treatment* (2nd ed.). New York: Guilford Press.

Sex education for adults: Researchers Masters and Johnson [Cover]. (1970, May 25). *Time, 95*(21). Retrieved from http://www.time.com/time/covers/0,16641,19700525,00.html

Schweckendiek, J., Klucken, T., Merz, C., Tabbert, K., Walter, B., Ambach, W., . . . Stark, R. (2011). Weaving the (neuronal) web: Fear learning in spider phobia. *NeuroImage, 54,* 681–688.

Selfe, L. (2011). *Nadia revisited.* New York: Psychology Press.

Selkoe, D., Mandelkow, E., & Holtzman, D. (**2012**). *The biology of Alzheimer Disease.* Cold Spring Harbor, NY: Cold Spring Harbor Laboratory Press.

Serretti, A., Calati, R., Mandelli, L., & De Ronchi, D. (2006). Serotonin transporter gene variants and behavior: A comprehensive review. *Current Drug Targets, 7,* 1659–1669.

Shaffer, H., & Martin, R. (2011). Disordered gambling: Etiology, trajectory, and clinical considerations. *Annual Review of Clinical Psychology, 7,* 483–510.

Shapiro, B. K., & Batshaw, M. L. (2011). Intellectual disability. In R. M. Kliegman, R. E. Behrman, H. B. Jenson, B. F. Stanton (Eds.), *Nelson textbook of pediatrics* (19th ed., chap. 33). Philadelphia, Pa: Saunders Elsevier.

Shapiro, F. (2001). *Eye movement desensitization and reprocessing: Basic principles, protocols, and procedures* (2nd ed.). New York: Guilford Press.

Shapiro, F. (2013). The case: Treating Jared through eye movement desensitization and reprocessing therapy. *Journal of Clinical Psychology, 69,* 494–496.

Shearer, S., Peters, C., Quaytman, S., & Wadman, B. (1988). Intent and lethality of suicide attempts among female borderline inpatients. *American Journal of Psychiatry, 145,* 1424–1427.

Shenton, M., Dickey, C., Frumin, M., & McCarley, R. (2001). A review of MRI finding in schizophrenia. *Schizophrenia Bulletin, 49,* 1–52.

Shenton, M., & Turetsky, B. (Eds). (2011). *Understanding neuropsychiatric disorders: Insights from neuroimaging.* New York: Cambridge University Press.

Sheridan, M. (2003). The deceit continues: An updated literature review of Munchausen Syndrome by Proxy. *Child abuse and Neglect, 27,* 431–451.

Shidhaye, R., Mendenhall, E., Sumathipala, K., Sumathipala, A., & Patel, V. (2013). Association of somatoform disorders with anxiety and depression in women in low and middle income countries: a systematic review. International Review of Psychiatry, *25*(1), 65–76.

Shidhaye, R., Murhar, V., Gangale, S., Aldridge, L., Shastri, R., Parikh, R., ... & Patel, V. (2017). The effect of VISHRAM, a grass-roots community-based mental health programme, on the treatment gap for depression in rural communities in India: a population-based study. The Lancet Psychiatry, *4*(2), 128–135.

Shidhaye, R., Mendenhall, E., Sumathipala, K., Sumathipala, A., & Patel, V. (2013). Association of somatoform disorders with anxiety and depression in women in low and middle income countries: a systematic review. International Review of Psychiatry, 25(1), 65–76.

Shidhaye, R., Murhar, V., Gangale, S., Aldridge, L., Shastri, R., Parikh, R., ... & Patel, V. (2017). The effect of VISHRAM, a grass-roots community-based mental health programme, on the treatment gap for depression in rural communities in India: a population-based study. The Lancet Psychiatry, 4(2), 128–135.

Shin, L., Brohawn, K., Pfaff, D., & Pitman, R. (2011). Functional imaging of post-traumatic stress disorder. In M. Shenton, & B. Turetsky (Eds), *Understanding neuropsychiatric disorders: Insights from neuroimaging.* New York: Cambridge University Press.

Shrivastava, A. (2010). Initiatives in biological research in Indian Psychiatry. *Indian Journal of Psychiatry,* 52, S110.

Shurkin, J. (2009). Alzheimer's update: New insight may speed therapies. *Scientific American,* p. 58.

Sierra, M. (2008). Depersonalization disorder: Pharmacological approaches. *Expert Review of Neurotherapeutics, 8,* 19–26.

Sierra, M., Senior, C., Dalton, J., McDonough, M., Bond, A., Phillips, M., . . . & David, A. (2002). Autonomic response in depersonalization disorder. *American Journal of General Psychiatry, 59,* 833–838.

Sigman, M., Spence, S., & Wang, A. (2006). Autism from developmental and neurpsychological perspectives. *Annual Review of Clinical Psychology, 2,* 327–355.

Silva, D. (1990). Pedophilia: An autobiography. In J. Feierman (Ed.), *Pedophilia: Biosocial dimensions.* New York: Springer.

Silver, J., McAllister, T., & Yudofsky, S. (2011). *Textbook of traumatic brain injury* (2nd ed.). Washington, DC: American Psychiatric Publishing.

Simeon, D., Gross, S., Guralnik, O., Stein, D. J., Schmeidler, J., & Hollander, E. (1997). Feeling unreal: 30 cases of DSM-III-R depersonalization disorder. *American Journal of Psychiatry, 154,* 1107–1113.

Simeon, D., Guralnik, O., Hazlett, E., Spiegel-Cohen, J., Hollander, E., & Buchsbaum, M. (2000). Feeling unreal: A PET study of depersonalization disorder. *American Journal of Psychiatry, 157,* 1782–1788.

Singer, W. (2009). Distributed processing and temporal does in neuronal networks. *Cognitive Neurodynamics, 3,* 189–196.

Singer, W., & Gray, C. (1995). Visual feature integration and the temporal correlation hypothesis. *Annual Review of Neuroscience, 18,* 555–586.

Sinigaglia, C., & Rizzolatti, G. (2011). Through the looking glass: Self and others. *Consciousness and Cognition, 20,* 64–74.

Skeem, J. L., Polaschek, D. L. L., Patrick, C. J., & Lilienfeld, S. O. (2011). Psychopathic personality: Bridging the gap between scientific evidence and public policy. *Psychological Science in the Public Interest, 12,* 95–162.

Skinner, B. (1938). *The behavior of organisms.* New York: Appleton-Century-Crofts.

Skinner, M. (2010). Fathers' nutritional legacy. *Nature, 467,* 922–923.

Slavich, G. M., O'Donovan, A., Epel, E. S., & Kemeny, M. E. (2010). Black sheep get the blues: A psychobiological model of social rejection and depression. *Neuroscience and Biobehavioral Reviews, 35,* 39–45.

Slobounov, S., & Sebastianelli. W. (2014). *Concussions in athletics: From brain to behavior.* New York: Springer Publishing

Smith, L., Nathan, P., Juniper, U., Kingsep, P., & Lim, L. (2003). *Cognitive behavioural therapy for psychotic symptoms: A therapist's manual.* Perth, Australia: Centre for Clinical Interventions.

Smith, M. (2005). Bilateral hippocampal volume reduction in adults with post-traumatic stress disorder: A meta-analysis of structural MRI studies. *Hippocampus, 15,* 798–807.

Smith, R. (1991). The macrophage theory of depression. *Medical Hypotheses, 35,* 298–306.

Snaith, R., & Collins, S. (1981). Five exhibitionists and a method of treatment. *British Journal of Psychiatry, 138,* 126–130.

Sobel, C., & Li, P. (2013). *The cognitive sciences* (2nd ed.). Thousand Oaks, CA: Sage.

Sobell, M., & Sobell, L. (1995). Controlled drinking after 25 years: How important was the great debate? [editorial]. *Addiction, 90,* 1149–1154.

Solanki, R. K., Kumar, A., Satija, Y., Gupta, S., & Singh, P. (2016). An Indian experience of neurocognitive endophenotypic markers in unaffected first-degree relatives of schizophrenia patients. Indian journal of psychiatry, *58*(1), 20–26.

Soloff, P., Pruitt, P., Sharma, M., Radwan, J., White, R., & Diwadkar, V. (2012). Structural brain abnormalities and suicidal behavior in borderline personality disorder. *Journal of Psychiatric Research, 46,* 16–25.

South, M., Ozonoff, S., & Schultz, R. (2008). Neurocognitive development in autism In C. Nelson & M. Luciana (Eds.), *Handbook of developmental cognitive neuroscience* (2nd ed., pp. 701–715). Cambridge, MA: MIT Press.

South, S., Oltmanns, T., & Krueger, R. (2011). The spectrum of personality disorders. In D. Barlow (Ed.), *The Oxford handbook of clinical psychology* (pp. 530–550). New York: Oxford University Press.

Sovani, A.V., Kumawat, S., and Joshi. G.S. (2012). Case Report :Terrorism and the 'utility' of people with ASPD trait patterns Forensic significance of MCMI III and Rorschach Inkblot assessment. *Archives of Indian Psychiatry, 14*(2), 1–6.

Sovani, Thatte, and Nadkarni. (2000). in Bodas, J. and Ollendick, T.H. (2005). *Test anxiety: A cross-cultural perspective.* https://www.ncbi.nlm.nih.gov/pubmed/15898305. *Clinical Child and Family Psychology, 8*(1), 65–88.

Spiegel, D., Lewis-Fernández, Lanius, R., Vermetten, E., Simeon, D., & Friedman, M. (2013). Dissociative disorders in DSM-5. *Annual Review of Clinical Psychology, 9,* 299–326.

Spira, A., Rebok, G., Stone, K., Kramer, J., & Yaffe, K. (2012). Depressive symptoms in oldest-old women: Risk of mild cognitive impairment and dementia. *American Journal of Geriatric Psychiatry, 20,* 1006–1015.

Sporns, O. (2011). *Networks of the brain.* Cambridge, MA: MIT Press.

Stice, E., Marti, C., & Rohde, P. (2012). Prevalence, Incidence, Impairment, and Course of the Proposed DSM-5 Eating Disorder Diagnoses in an 8-Year Prospective Community Study of Young Women. *Journal of Abnormal Psychology, 122,* 445–457.

Stice, E., Spoor, S., Bohon, C., Veldhuizen, M. G., & Small, D. M. (2008). Relation of reward from food intake and anticipated food intake to obesity: a functional magnetic resonance imaging study. *Journal of Abnormal Psychology, 117,* 924–935.

State, M., & Levitt, P. (2011). The conundrums of understanding genetic risks for autism spectrum disorders. *Nature Neuroscience, 14,* 1499–1506.

Sreenivasan, S., Frances, A., & Weinberger, L. (2010). Normative versus consequential ethics in sexually violent predator laws: An ethics conundrum for psychiatry. *The Journal of the American Academy of Psychiatry and the Law, 38,* 386–391.

Steadman, H., Davidson, S., & Brown, C. (2001). Mental health courts: Their promise and unanswered questions. *Psychiatric Services, 52,* 457–458.

Stebbins G., & Murphy C. (2009). Diffusion tensor imaging in Alzheimer's disease and mild cognitive impairment. *Behavioral Neurology, 21,* 39–49.

Steele, K., & Berman, C. (2001). *The day the voices stopped.* New York: Basic Books.

Stein, M., Keller, S. E., & Schleifer, S. J. (1985). Stress and immunomodulation: the role of depression and neuroendocrine function. *Journal of Immunology, 135(Suppl),* 827s–833s.

Steinberg, L. (2013). The influence of neuroscience on US Supreme Court decisions about adolescents' criminal culpability. *Nature Reviews Neuroscience, 14,* 513–518.

Steinberg, M. (1994). *Interviewer's guide to the structured clinical interview for DSM-IV dissociative disorders (SCID-D).* Washington, DC: American Psychiatric Publishing.

Steinberg, M., & Schnall, M. (2000). *The stranger in the mirror.* New York: Cliff Street Books.

Stokes, T. (2006). The earth-eaters. *Nature, 444,* 543–544.

Strakowski, S. (2011). Structural imaging of bipolar illness. In M. Shenton & B. Turetsky (Eds.), *Understanding neuropsychiatric disorders: Insights from neuroimaging.* New York: Cambridge University Press.

Strakowski, S. M., Adler, C. M., Holland, S. K., Mills, N., & DelBello, M. P. (2004). A preliminary FMRI study of sustained attention in euthymic, unmedicated bipolar disorder. *Neuropsychopharmacology, 29,* 1734–1740.

Striegel-Moore, R., & Franko, D. (2008). Should binge eating disorder be included in the DSM-V? A critical review of the state of the evidence. *Annual Review of Clinical Psychology, 4,* 305–324.

Straube, T., Glauer, M., Dilger, S., Mentzel, H., & Miltner, W. (2006). Effects of cognitive-behavioral therapy on brain activation in specific phobia. *NeuroImage, 29,* 125–135.

Strupp, H. (1971). *Psychotherapy and the modification of abnormal behavior.* New York: McGraw-Hill.

Strupp, H., & Binder, J. (1984). *Psychotherapy in a new key: A guide to time-limited dynamic psychotherapy.* New York: Basic Books.

Stuart, D., (2004). *Dangerous garden.* Cambridge, MA: Harvard University Press.

Studerus, E., Kometer, M., Hasler, F., & Vollenweider, F. (2011). Acute, subacute and long-term subjective effects of psilocybin in healthy humans: A pooled analysis of experimental studies. *Journal of Psychopharmacology, 25,* 1434–1452.

Stunkard, A. (1959). Eating patterns and obesity. *Psychiatry Quarterly, 33,* 284–295.

Sturman, D. A., & Moghaddam, B. (2011). The neurobiology of adolescents: Changes in brain architecture, functional dynamics, and behavioral tendencies. *Neuroscience and Behavioral Reviews, 35,* 1704–1712.

Substance Abuse and Mental Health Services Administration. (2011). Utilization of mental health services by adults with suicidal thoughts and behavior. National Survey on Drug Use and Health. The NSDUH Report. Rockville, MD: Author.

Substance Abuse and Mental Health Services Administration. (2012). *Results from the 2011 national survey on drug use and health: Summary of national findings,* NSDUH Series H-44, HHS Publication No. (SMA) 12-4713. Rockville, MD: Author.

Suicide warning signs. (n.d.). Retrieved from reportingonsuicide.org.

Suliman, S., Troeman, Z., Stein, D. J., & Seedat, S. (2013). Predictors of acute stress disorder severity. *Journal of Affective Disorders, 149,* 277–281.

Sulloway, F. (1979). *Freud, biologist of the mind.* New York: Basic Books.

Sumathipala, A. (2007). What is the evidence for the efficacy of treatments for somatoform disorders? A critical review of previous intervention studies. *Psychosomatic Medicine, 69,* 889–990.

Suomi, S. (1999). Attachment in rhesus monkeys. In J. Cassidy & P. Shaver (Eds.), *Handbook of attachment: Theory, research, and clinical applications.* New York: Guilford Press.

Swanson, J. W., Tepper, M. C., Backlar, P. B., & Swartz, M. S. (2000). Psychiatric advance directives: An alternative to coercive treatment? *Psychiatry, 63,* 160–172.

Swanson, J., Van Dorn, R., Swartz, M., Robbins, P., Steadman, H., McGuire, T., & Monahan, J. (2013). The cost of assisted outpatient treatment: Can it save states money? *American Journal of Psychiatry.*

Sylvester, C., Corbetta, M., Raichle, M., Rodebaugh, T., Schlaggar, B., Sheline, Y., . . . Lenze, E. (2012). Functional network dysfunction in anxiety and anxiety disorders. *Trends in Neuroscience, 35,* 527–535.

Tabarés-Seisdedos, R., & Rubenstein, J. (2013). Inverse cancer comorbidity: a serendipitous opportunity to gain insight into CNS disorders. *Nature Reviews Neuroscience, 14,* 293–304.

Takeda, T., Ambrosini, P., deBerardinis, R., & Elia, J. (2012). What can ADHD without comorbidity teach us about comorbidity? *Research in Developmental Disabilities, 33,* 419–425.

Tallon-Baudry, C., & Bertrand, O. (1999). Oscillatory gamma activity in humans and its role in object representation. *Trends in Cognitive Sciences, 3,* 151–162.

Tanielian, T., & Jaycox, L. (2008). *Invisible wounds of war.* Santa Monica, CA: RAND Corporation.

Tandon, S., Mehrotra, S., & Vallikad, E. (2010). Illness meanings in the context of cancer: An Indian perspective. Psychological Studies, *55*(3), 230–238.

Tandon, R., Nasrallah, H. A., & Keshavan, M. S. (2009). Schizophrenia,"Just the facts": Clinical features and conceptualization. *Schizophrenia Research, 110,* 1–23.

Tasman, A., Kay, J., Lieberman, J. A., First, M. B., & Maj, M. (Eds.). (2008). *Psychiatry* (3rd ed.). New York: Wiley.

Tau, G., & Peterson, B. (2010). Normal development of brain circuits. *Neuropsychopharmacology Reviews, 35,* 147–168.

Taylor, K. (Ed.). (2008). *Going hungry.* New York: Anchor Books.

Taylor, S. (2011). Pathways linking early life stress to adult health. In J. Decety & J. Cacioppo (Eds.), *The Oxford handbook of social neuroscience* (pp. 776–786). New York: Oxford University Press.

Taylor, S. E., Dickerson, S. S., & Klein, L.C. (2002). Toward a biology of social support. In C.R. Snyder & S.J. Lopez (Eds.), *Handbook of positive psychology.* New York: Oxford University Press.

Taylor, S. E., Klein, L. C., Lewis, B. P., Gruenewald, T. L., Gurung, R. A. R., & Updegraff, J. A. (2000). Biobehavioral responses to stress in females: Tend-and-befriend, not fight-or-flight. *Psychological Review, 107,* 411–429.

Teicher, M. H., Samson, J. A., Sheu, Y.-S., Polcari, A., McGreenery, C. E. (2010). Hurtful words: Association of exposure to peer verbal abuse with elevated psychiatric symptom scores and corpus callosum abnormalities. *American Journal of Psychiatry, 167,* 1464–1471.

Teng, E., Tassniyom, K., & Lu, P. (2012). Reduced quality of life ratings in mild cognitive impairment: Analyses of subject and informant responses. *American Journal of Geriatric Psychiatry, 20,* 1016–1025.

Thase, M., & Denko, T. (2008). Pharmacotherapy of mood disorders. *Annual Review of Clinical Psychology, 4,* 53–91.

Thomason, M., & Thompson, P. (2011). Diffusion imaging, white matter, and psychopathology. *Annual Review of Clinical Psychology, 7,* 63–85.

Thompson, P., Vidal, C., Giedd, J., Gochman, P., Blumenthal, J., Nicolson, R., . . . Rapoport, J. (2001). Mapping adolescent brain change reveals dynamic wave of accelerated gray matter loss in very early-onset schizophrenia. *Proceedings of the National Academy of Science, 98,* 11650–11655.

Tillfors, M., Furmark, T., Marteinsdottir, I., Fischer, H., Pissiota, A., Langstrom, B., & Fredrikson, M. (2001). Cerebral blood flow in subjects with social phobia during stressful speaking tasks: A PET study. *American Journal of Psychiatry, 158,* 1220–1226.

Tolin, D., Stevens, M., Villavicencio, A., Norberg, M., Calhoun, V., Frost, R., . . . Pearlson, G. (2012). Neural mechanisms of decision making in hoarding disorder. *Archives of General Psychiatry, 69,* 832–841.

Tolstoy, L. (1882). *My confession: My life had some to a sudden stop.* New York: Crowell.

Tomko, R., Brown, W., Tragesser, S., Wood, P., Mehl, M., & Trull, T. (2012). Social Context of Anger in Borderline Personality Disorder and Depressive Disorders: Findings from a Naturalistic Observation Study. *Journal of Personality Disorders, 26,*

Torrey, E. (1994). *Schizophrenia and manic depressive disorder.* New York: Basic Books.

Torrey, E. (1997). *Out of the shadows: Confronting America's mental illness crisis.* New York: Wiley.

Torrey, E., Kennard, A., Eslinger, D., Lamb, R., & Pavle, J. (2010). More mentally ill persons are in jails and prisons than hospitals: A survey of the states. *Report for National Sheriffs Association, & Treatment Advocacy Center.*

Travers, J., & Milgram, S. (1969). An experimental study of small world problem. *Sociometry, 32,* 425–443.

Treffert, D. (2009). The savant syndrome: an extraordinary condition. A synopsis: past, present, future. *Philosophical Transition of the Royal Society of London, B, 364,* 1351–1357.

Tripathi, R., Kumar, J. K., Bharath, S., Marimuthu, P., & Varghese, M. (2013). Clinical validity of NIMHANS neuropsychological battery for elderly: A preliminary report. Indian Journal of Psychiatry, 55(3), 279.

Tripathi, R., & Mehrotra, S. (2015). Pseudo-dementia: A neuropsychological review. Annals of Indian Academy of Neurology, *18*(1), 123–124.

Treutlein, J., Cichon, S., Ridinger, M., Wodarz, N., Soyka, M., Zill, P., . . . Rietschel, M. (2009). Genome-wide association study of alcohol dependence. *Archives of General Psychiatry, 47,* 2016–2022.

Triebwasser, J., Chemerinski, E., Roussos, P., & Siever, L. (2012). Schizoid personality disorder. *Journal of Personality Disorders, 26,* 919–926.

Tsuang, M., Cohen, M., & Zahner, G. (Eds.). (1996). *Textbook of psychiatric epidemiology.* New York: Wiley.

Turecki, G., Ernst, C., Jollant, F., Labonté, B., & Mechawar, N. (2012) The neurodevelopmental origins of suicidal behavior. *Trends in Neurosciences, 35,* 14–23.

Turkington, D., Kingdon, D., & Weiden, P. (2006) Cognitive behavior therapy for schizophrenia. *American Journal of Psychiatry, 163,* 365–373.

Turner, J., & Reid, S. (2002). Munchausen's syndrome. *Lancet, 359,* 346–349.

Uhlhaas, P. (2011). The adolescent brain: Implications for the understanding, pathophysiology, and treatment of schizophrenia. *Schizophrenia Bulletin, 37,* 480–483.

Uhlhaas, P., Roux, F., Singer, W., Haenschel, C., Sireteanu, R., & Rodriguez, E. (2009). The development of neural synchrony reflects late maturation and restructuring of functional networks in humans. *Proceedings of the National Academy of Sciences, 106,* 9866–9871.

Uhlhaas, P., & Singer, W. (2011). The development of neural synchrony and large-scale cortical networks during adolescence: Relevance for the pathophysiology of schizophrenia and neurodevelopmental hypothesis. *Schizophrenia Bulletin, 37,* 514–523.

Uhlhaas, P., & Singer, W. (2012). Neuronal dynamics and neuropsychiatric disorders: Toward a translational paradigm for dysfunctional large-scale networks. *Neuron, 75,* 963–980.

Ulrich-Lai, Y., & Herman, J. (2009). Neural regulation of endocrine and autonomic stress responses. *Nature Reviews Neuroscience, 10,* 397–409.

United Nations Office on Drugs and Crime. (2011). *Amphetamines and ecstasy.* New York: United Nations. Retrieved from www.unodc.org/documents/ATS/ATS_Global_Assessment_2011.pdf

United Nations Office on Drugs and Crime. (2012). *World drug report 2012.* Retrieved from www.unodc.org/documents/data-and-analysis/WDR2012/WDR_2012_web_small.pdf

Ursano, R., Li, H., Zhang, L., Hough, C., Fullerton, C., Benedek, D., . . . Holloway, H. (2008). Models of PTSD and traumatic stress: The importance of research "from bedside to bench to bedside." *Progress in Brain Research, 167,* 203–215.

Ursekar, M. (2008) Imaging in Epilepsy. *Journal of Pediatric Neurosciences,* 3, 48–54. Online full text atHYPERLINK "https://www.dropbox.com/referrer_cleansing_redirect?hmac=9UJtg3WEAxrc903cjuPXWFHmUB9l9VwtJEyaFosGmuI%3D&url=http%3A%2F%2Fwww.pediatricneurosciences.com"http://www.pediatricneurosciences.com

Uys, J., & Reissner, K. (2011). Glutamatergic neuroplasticity in cocaine addiction. *Progress in Molecular Biology and Translational Science, 98,* 367–400.

Vahia.V.N., Shetty.H.K., Motiwala, S., Thakkar, G., Fernandes, L., Sharma, C.J. (1993). Effect of Meditation. *Generalised Anxiety Disorder, 35*(2), 87–92.

Van der Horst, F., LeRoy, H., & van der Veer, R. (2008). "When stranger meet": John Bowlby and Harry Harlow on attachment behavior. *Integrative Psychology and Behaviorial Science, 42,* 370–388.

van Ewijk, H., Heslenfeld, D., Zwiers, M., Buitelaar, J., & Oosterlaan, J. (2011). Diffusion tensor imaging in attention deficit/hyperactivity disorder: A systematic review and meta-analysis. *Neuroscience and Biobehavioral Reviews, 36,* 1093–1106.

van Holst, R., van den Brink, W., Veltman, D., & Goudriaan, A. (2010). Brain imaging studies in pathological gambling. *Current Psychiatry Reports, 12,* 418–425.

Van Horn, J. D., Irimia, A., Torgerson, C. M., Chambers, M. C., Kikinis, R., & Toga, A. (2012). Mapping connectivity damage in the case of Phineas Gage. *PLOS ONE, 7*(5), e37454. doi:10.1371/journal.pone.0037454

van Norden, A., van Dijk, E., de Laat, K., Scheltens, P., Olderikkert, M., & de Leeuw, F. (2012). Dementia: Alzheimer pathology and vascular factors: From mutually exclusive to interaction. *Biochimica et Biophysica Acta, 1822,* 340–349.

van Os, J. (2010). Are psychiatric diagnoses of psychosis scientific and useful? The case of schizophrenia. *Journal of Mental Health, 19,* 305–317.

van Os, J., Kenis, G., & Rutten, B. P. (2010). The environment and schizophrenia. *Nature, 468,* 203–212.

van Winkel, R., van Beveren, N., Simons, C., & Genetic Risk and Outcome of Psychosis (GROUP) Investigators. (2011). AKT1 moderation of cannabis-induced cognitive alterations in psychotic disorder. *Neuropsychopharmacology, 36,* 2529–2537.

Ventriglio, A., Ayonrinde, O., & Bhugra, D. (2016). Relevance of culture-bound syndromes in the 21st century. Psychiatry and Clinical Neurosciences, *70*(1), 3–6. doi: 10.1111/pcn.12359

Varghese, K.M., Bansal, R. Kekre, K.N. and Jacob K. (2012). Sexual dysfunction among young married women in southern India. *International Urogynecology Journal, 23*(12), 1–6.

Vermetten, E., & Lanius, R. A. (2012). Biological and clinical framework for posttraumatic stress disorder. *Handbook of Clinical Neurology, 106,* 291–342.

Vermetten, E., Schmahl, C., Lindner, S., Loewenstein, R., & Bremner, J. (2006). Hippocampal and amygdalar volumes in dissociative identity disorder. *American journal of psychiatry, 163,* 630–636.

Vita A, de Peri L, Silenzi C, Dieci M (2006). Brain morphology in first-episode schizophrenia: A meta-analysis of quantitative magnetic resonance imaging studies. *Schizophrenia Research, 82,* 75–88.

Volkow, N., Fowler, J., Wang, G., Hitzemann, R., Logan, J., Schlyer, D., . . . Wolf, A. (1993). Decreased dopamine D2 receptor availability is associated with reduced frontal metabolism in cocaine abusers. *Synapse, 14,* 169–177.

Volkow, N., & Li, T. (2005). The neuroscience of addiction. *Nature, 8,* 1429–1430.

Volkow, N., Wang, G., Fowler, J., & Tomasi, D. (2012). Addiction circuitry in the human brain. *Annual Review of Pharmacology and Toxicology, 52,* 321–336.

Volkow, N., Wang, G., Tomasi, D., & Baler, R. (2013). Obesity and addiction: Neurobiological overlaps. *Obesity Reviews, 14,* 2–18.

Voon, V., & Fox, S. (2007). Medication-related impulse control and repetitive behaviors in Parkinson disease. *Archives of Neurology, 64,* 1089–1096.

Waite, L.J., Laumann, E.O., Das, A., & Schumm, L.P. (2009). Sexuality: Measures of partnerships, practices, attitudes, and problems in the national social life, health, and aging study. *Journal of Gerontology: Social Sciences, 64B*(S1), i56–i66. doi:10.1093/geronb/gbp038.

Waheed, K. (n.d.). *Honoring the person I am.* Retrieved from Anxiety and Depression Association of America website: www.adaa.org/living-with-anxiety/personal-stories/ honoring-person-i-am

Waldinger, M. (2008). Recent advances in the classification, neurobiology and treatment of premature ejaculation. In R. Balon (Ed.), *Sexual dysfunction: The brain-body connection* (pp. 50–69). Basel: Karger.

Walker, E., McMillan, A., & Mittal, V. (2005). Neurohormones, neurodevelopment and the prodrome of psychosis in adolescence. In D. Romer & E. Walker (Eds.), *Adolescent psychopathology and the developing brain: Integrating brain and prevention science.* New York: Oxford University Press.

Walker, E., Shapiro, D., Esterberg, M., & Trotman, H. (2010). Neurodevelopment and schizophrenia, broadening the focus. *Current Directions in Psychological Science, 19,* 204–208.

Walsh, B. (2008). Eating disorders. In A. Tasman, J. Kay, J. Lieberman, M. First, & M. Maj (Eds.), *Psychiatry* (3rd ed.). New York: Wiley.

Walsh, P., Elsabbagh, M., Bolton, P., & Singh, I. (2011). In search of biomarkers for autism: Scientific, social and ethical challenges. *Nature Reviews Neuroscience, 20,* 603–612.

Wang, L., Zhu, C., He, Y., Zang, Y., Cao, Q., Zhang, H., . . . Wang, Y. (2009). Altered small-world brain functional networks in children with attention-deficit/hyperactivity disorder. *Human Brain Mapping, 30,* 638–649.

Wang, O., Su, T., Zhou, Y., Chou, K., Chen, I., Jiang, T., & Lin, C. (2012). Anatomical insights into disrupted small-world networks in schizophrenia. *Neuroimage, 59,* 1085–1093.

Wardle, J., Haase, A., & Steptoe, A. (2006). Body image and weight control in young adults: International comparisons in university students from 22 countries. *International Journal of Obesity, 30,* 644–651.

Wareham, J., & Potenza, M. (2010). Pathological gambling and substance use disorders. *The American Journal of Drug and Alcohol Abuse, 36,* 242–247.

Watanabe, N., Churchill, R., & Furukawa, T. (2009, January). Combined psychotherapy plus benzodiazepines for panic disorder. *Cochrane Database Systematic Reviews.*

Waterhouse, L. (2012). *Rethinking autism.* New York: Academic Press.

Watkins, L., & Maier, S. (2002). Beyond neurons: Evidence that immune and glial cells contribute to pathological pain states. *Physiological Review, 82,* 981–1011.

Watson, J. (1913). Psychology as the behaviorist views it. *Psychological Review, 20,* 158–177.

Watson, J. (1924). *Behaviorism.* New York: People's Institute Publishing Company.

Watson, J., & Rayner, R. (1920). Conditioned emotional reactions. *Journal of Experimental Psychology, 3,* 1–14.

Weaver, I., Cervoni, N., Champagne, F., D'Alessio, A., Sharma, S., Seckl, J., . . . Meaney, M. (2004). Epigenetic programming by maternal behavior. *Nature Neuroscience, 7,* 847–854.

Weck, F., Neng, J., Richtberg, S., & Stangier, U. (2012). The restrictive concept of good health in patients with hypochondriasis. *Journal of Anxiety Disorders, 26,* 792–798.

Wedeen, V. J., Rosene, D. L., Wang, R., Dai, G., Mortazavi, F., Hagmann, P., . . .Tseng, W. Y. (2012). The geometric structure of the brain fiber pathways. *Science, 335,* 1628–1634.

Weinberger, D. (1987). Implications of normal brain development for the pathogenesis of schizophrenia. *Archives of General Psychiatry, 44,* 660–669.

Weiss, B., Hope, D., & Cohn, L. (2010). Treatment of social anxiety disorder: A treatments-by-dimensions review. In S. Hofmann & P. DiBartolo (Eds.), *Social anxiety* (2nd ed.). New York: Elsevier.

Weiss, M. (1986). History of psychiatry in India: Toward a culturally and historiographically informed study of indigenous traditions. Samiksa, *40*, 31–45. Retrieved from http://cscs.res.in/dataarchive/textfiles/volume-40-number-2-1986.pdf

Weiss, M. G. (1997). Explanatory Model Interview Catalogue (EMIC): framework for comparative study of illness. Transcultural Psychiatry, *34*(2), 235–263.

———. (2001). Cultural epidemiology: An introduction and overview. Anthropology & Medicine, *8*(1), 5–29.

———. (2011). Explanatory models in psychiatry. In D. Bhugra & K. Bhui (Eds.), Textbook of Cultural Psychiatry (2nd ed.). Cambridge University Press.

———. (2017). The Promise of Cultural Epidemiology. Taiwanese Journal of Psychiatry, *31*(1), 8–24.

Weiss, M. G., Doongaji, D. R., Siddhartha, S., Wypij, D., Pathare, S., Bhatawdekar, M., ... & Fernandes, R. (1992). The Explanatory Model Interview Catalogue (EMIC). Contribution to cross-cultural research methods from a study of leprosy and mental health. The British Journal of Psychiatry, *160*(6), 819–830.

Welham, J., Isohanni, M., Jones, P., & McGrath, J. (2009). The antecedents of schizophrenia: A review of birth cohort studies. *Schizophrenia Bulletin, 35,* 603–623.

Werner, C. (2011, November). *The older population: 2010. 2010 census briefs* (Figure 2). Washington, DC: U.S. Government Printing Office. Retrieved from http://www.census.gov/prod/cen2010/briefs/c2010br-09.pdf

Westen, D., Gabbard, G. O., & Ortigo, K. (2008). Psychoanalytic approaches to personality. In O. John, R. Robins, & L. Pervin (Eds.), *Handbook of personality: Theory and research* (4th ed., pp. 61–113). New York: Guilford Press.

Westwood, S. (2007). *Suicide junkie*. Brentwood, Essex, UK: Chipmunkapublishing.

Whelan, R., Conrod, P. J., Polines, J.-B., Lourdusamy, A., Banaschewski, T., Barker, G. J., . . . the IMAGEN Consortium. (2012). Adolescent impulsivity phenotypes characterized by distinct brain networks. *Nature Neuroscience, 15,* 920–927.

White, T., Magnotta, V., Bockholt, H., Williams, S., Wallace, S., Ehrlich, S., ... Lim, K. (2011). Global white matter abnormalities in schizophrenia: A multisite diffusion tensor imaging study. *Schizophrenia Bulletin, 37,* 222–232.

Whitfield-Gabrieli, S., Thermenos, H. W., Milanovic, S., Tsuang, M. T., Faraone, S. V., McCarley, R. W., . . .Seidman, L. J. (2009). Hyperactivity and hyperconnectivity of the default network in schizophrenia and in first-degree relatives of persons with schizophrenia. *Proceedings of the National Academy of Sciences of the United States of America, 106,* 1279–1284.

Whitford, T., & Kubicki, M., & Shenton, M. (2011). Structural imaging of schizophrenia. In M. Shenton, & B. Turetsky (Eds), *Understanding neuropsychiatric disorders: Insights from neuroimaging.* New York: Cambridge University Press.

Whittingstall, K., & Logothestis, N. (2009). Frequency band coupling I surface EEG reflects spiking activity in monkey visual cortex. *Neuron, 64,* 281–289.

Wicker, B., & Gomot, M. (2011). The Asperger syndrome. In J. Decety & J. Cacioppo (Eds.), *The Oxford handbook of social neuroscience.* New York: Oxford University Press.

Widiger, T., & Mullins-Sweatt, S. (2009). Five-factor model of personality disorder: A proposal for DSM-V. *Annual Review of Clinical Psychology, 5,* 197–220.

Wig, N. N. (1960). Problems of mental health in India. *Journal of Social and Clinical Psychology, 17,* 48–53.

Wilens, T., Biederman, J., & Spencer, T. (2002). Attention deficit/hyperactivity disorder across the lifespan. *Annual Review of Medicine, 53,* 113–131.

Wilkinson, P. K., Sedman, A. J., Sakmar, E., Kay, D. R., & Wagner, J. G. (1977). Pharmacokinetics of ethanol after oral administration in the fasting state. *Journal of Pharmacokinetics and Biopharmaceutics, 5*(3), 207–224.

Williams, J. H. G., Whiten, A., Suddendorf, T., & Perrett, D. I. (2001). Imitation, mirror neurons and autism. *Neuroscience and Biobehavioral Reviews, 25,* 287–295.

Williams, K. D., Cheung, C. K. T., & Choi, W. (2000). Cyberostracism: Effects of being ignored over the Internet. *Journal of Personality and Social Psychology, 79,* 748–762.

Williamson, P. C., & Allman, J. M. (2011). *The human illnesses: Neuropsychiatric disorders and the nature of the human brain.* New York: Oxford University Press.

Wincze, J., & Carey, M. (2001). *Sexual dysfunction: A guide for assessment and treatment* (2nd ed.). New York: Guilford Press.

Wise, R. A. (1998). Drug-activation of brain reward pathways. *Drug and Alcohol Dependence, 51,* 13–22.

Wittchen, H., Gloster, A., Beesdo-Baum, K., Fava, G., & Craske, M. (2010). Agoraphobia: A review of the diagnostic classificatory position and criteria. *Depression and Anxiety, 27,* 113–133.

Wolosin, S., Richardson, M., Hennessey, J., Denckla, M., & Mostofsky, S. (2009). Abnormal cerebral cortex structure in children with ADHD. *Human Brain Mapping, 30,* 175–184.

Woo, S., & Keatinge, C. (2008). *Diagnosis and treatment of mental disorders across the lifespan.* New York: Wiley.

Woolfolk, R., Allen, L., & Tiu, J. (2007). New directions in the treatment of somatization. *Psychiatric Clinics of North America, 30,* 621–644.

World Health Organization. (2002). Self-directed violence. In *World report on violence and health.* Geneva, Switzerland: Author.

World Health Organization. (2005). *Mental health atlas.* Geneva, Switzerland: Author.

World Health Organization. (2011). *Global status report on alcohol and health.* Geneva Switzerland: Author.

Wray, N., & Visscher, P. (2010). Narrowing the boundaries of the genetic architecture of schizophrenia. *Schizophrenia Bulletin, 36,* 14–23.

Young, S. (2010). Pica in pregnancy: New ideas about an old condition. *Annual Review of Nutrition, 30,* 403–422.

Young, S. (2011). *Craving earth: Understanding pica.* New York: Columbia University Press.

Zander, T. (2005). Civil commitment without psychosis: The law's reliance on the weakest links in psychodiagnosis. *Journal of Sexual Offender Civil Commitment: Science and the Law, 1,* 17–82.

Zeanah, C., & Gleason, N. (2010). *Reactive attachment disorder: A review for DSM–V.* Report presented to American Psychiatric Association, Washington, DC.

Zerwas, S., Lund, B., Von Holle, A., Thornton, L., Berrettini, W., Brandt, H., . . . Bulik, C. (2013). Factors associated with recovery from anorexia nervosa. *Journal of Psychiatric Research, 47,* 972–979.

Zhou, J., Hofman, M., Gooren, L., & Swaab, D. (1995). A sex difference in the human brain and its relation to transsexuality. *Nature, 378,* 68–70.

Zimmer, C. (2001). *Evolution: The triumph of an idea.* New York: HarperCollins.

INDEX

A Beautiful Mind (Nash), 1
Abraham, Aju, 71t, 73t
Acamprosate, 524
ACC. *See* Anterior cingulate cortex (ACC)
Acquired immune deficiency syndrome (AIDS), 607–608
Acute stress disorder, 331t–332t, 335
Adams, Robert A., 601–603
Ade, Robert, 322
ADHD. *See* Attention deficit/ hyperactivity disorder (ADHD)
Adjustment disorders, 334
Adolescence
  anorexia nervosa, 421
  depression, developmental aspects of, 273
  peer influence, 196
  risk taking, 197–198
  schizophrenia, 245
  social brain, 197
Adolphs, R., 200
Adoption study, 148
Adrenal pathway, 324
Adrenergic, 325
Adrenocorticotropic hormone (ACTH), 324
Affective-conceptual information, 201
Affective disorders, 22
Affect, schizophrenia, 239
Agarwal, A., 74t
Agarwal, A. K., 68t, 75t
Agarwal, S., 70t
Agarwal, S. S., 72t
Agashe, Mohan, 2
Agonist drug, 528
Agoraphobia, 366
Agrawal, A. K., 71t
Agreeableness, 542
AIIMS. *See* All India Institute of Medical Sciences (AIIMS)
Ainsworth, Mary, 192
Ajmani, Virender, 202
Albert, Little, 367–368
Alcohol, 480, 491–492
  DSM–5, 492–496, 493t, 494t, 495f
  effects on human body, 496–497, 497f, 498f
  moderate, heavy, and binge drinking, 498, 499f, 500f, 500t
  neuropsychological rehabilitation, 492
  rates of drinking, 498, 500, 501t, 502f
Alcoholics Anonymous (AA), 522, 526, 527
Alcohol intoxication, 482–483, 494t
Alcoholism: Clinical and Experimental Research, 503
Alcohol use disorders, 492–496, 493t, 494t, 495f, 496, 503
Alcohol withdrawal, 483, 494t
Ali Yavar Jung National Institute of Speech and Hearing Disabilities (Divyangjan) (AYJNISHD), 226
Allele, 100
Allen, N., 279, 280, 307
All India Institute of Medical Sciences (AIIMS), 68
All India Institute of Speech and Hearing (AIISH), 226
Allostasis, 327
Allostatic load, 327, 328
Allostatic systems, 327
Alogia, 236
Altered States of Consciousness (APZ), 508, 509
Alternative form reliability, 165
Alzheimer, Alois, 595
Alzheimer's disease, 84, 578–580, 586, 589, 590, 593, 594
  DSM–5 diagnostic criteria, 596t
  genes, 597
  neurofibrillary tangles and neuritic plaques, 595, 595f
  neuroimaging, 597–599, 598f
  prevalence for, 595
  synaptic and neuronal loss, 595
Ambivalence, schizophrenia, 239
Amresh, Shrivastava, 69t
American Association for the Advancement of Science (AAAS), 98
American Law Institute (ALI) rule, 616
American Psychiatric Association (APA), 23, 49, 76, 150, 620

Amphetamines, 480, 514–516, 516f
Amplitude, 87
Amygdala, 339
Amyotrophic lateral sclerosis (ALS), 42
Anand, L., 70t
Ananthanarayanan, C. V., 69t
Ananth, J. V., 75t
Anderson, Mc C. W., 69t
Andrade, Chitra, 70t
Andrade, Chittaranjan, 68t, 69t, 70t, 71t, 75t
Andreasen, N., 242–243
Andrews, P., 278
Anhedonia, 236
Animal spirits, 31
anorexia nervosa, 418
  adolescents, 421
  causes of, 423
  characteristics, 420
  cultural factors, 424
  daily calorie allowance table, 425t
  DSM–5 criteria, 420–421
  functional magnetic resonance imaging studies, 422, 423f
  genetics, 423
  outward signs of, 421
  risk factors, 423–424, 424f
  semi-starvation period, 425
  serotonin and dopamine systems, 423
  starvation, 424–425
  time course and phenomenology, 421, 422f
  treatment, 426–427
ANS. *See* Autonomic nervous system (ANS)
antagonist drug, 528
anterior cingulate cortex (ACC), 276, 317–318, 491, 562
antibodies, 322
antidepressant medication, 282, 283
antipsychotic medications, schizophrenia, 262–263
antisocial personality disorder, 67, 537, 551–553
anxiety complaints, 117
anxiety disorders, 80, 196, 348–351, 349f, 437, 451
  cognitive processes, 351–352
  developmental aspects, 353–355, 354tf–355t
  global mental health anxiety disorders, 357t
  Indian work on, 359
  neurobiology, 352–353, 353f
  twelve-month prevalence, 356t, 358t
  types of
    agoraphobia, 366
    GAD, 360–364
    panic disorder, 370–372, 371t
    SAD, 364–366
    separation anxiety disorder, 359–360
    specific phobia, 367–370
anxious ego dissolution, 508
anxious fearful personality disorders
  avoidant personality disorder, 568–569
  dependent personality disorder, 569
  obsessive-compulsive personality disorder, 569–570
anxious or fearful disorders, 537
APOE4 allele, 587, 588f, 597
APZ. *See* Altered States of Consciousness (APZ)
Aretaeus of Cappadocia, 291
Aristotle, 34
Asian diets, 16
Asperger, Hans, 204
Asperger's syndrome, 204, 209
assessing cultural dimensions, 162–164
assessment, 159
  empirical tests, India, 170
  neuropsychological tests, 174–175
  neuroscience techniques, 175–176
  personality tests, 167–170
  projective instruments, 170–173
  projective tests, India, 174
  symptom questionnaires, 167
associations, schizophrenia, 239
Astu, 2
attachment, 186
attachment disorders, 202–203
attention, 276
attention deficit/hyperactivity disorder (ADHD), 67, 142, 175, 187
  DSM–5 diagnostic criteria for, 214t–215t
  emotional–behavioral disorder, 215
  genetic component, 216
  hyperactivity and impulsivity, 214
  inattention, 213
  response inhibition, 216
  spatial working memory, 216
  treatment for, 217–218
  verbal working memory, 216
atypical antipsychotics, 262
autism, 80, 239
autism spectrum disorders (ASD), 79
  behavioral processes, 203
  communication patterns, 203
  DSM–5 diagnostic criteria for, 204, 207t
  intellectual disabilities, 210
  pattern thinking, 205
  Raven's Progressive Matrices, 205, 206f

social interactions, 203
special abilities, 210–211
specialized thinkers, 205
traditional IQ tests, 205
traditional symptoms, 206
treatment for, 211–213
visual thinking, 205
word and fact thinking, 205
autistic disorder, 204
autonomic nervous system (ANS), 66, 318, 323, 325–327, 326f
autopsies, 42
aversive drug, 529
avoidant personality disorder, 537, 568–569
avoidant/restrictive food intake disorder, 410
avolition, 236
azapirones, 364

Babinski reflex, 40
Bacon, Francis, 517
Badcock, P., 279, 280, 307
Bagadia, V. N., 68t, 72t
Baker, David, 206
Baldwin, J., 447
Banyan, 48
Baron-Cohen, Simon, 195, 196
Baron of Lying, 403
Barry, C., 173
Basco, Monica, 301
Battle, Cynthia, 546
Bayer aspirin, 477
BDI. *See* Beck depression inventory (BDI)
BDNF. *See* Serum Brain-derived neurotrophic factor (BDNF)
Beck, Aaron, 59f, 275, 286
Beck depression inventory (BDI), 127, 167
Beck's cognitive triad, 60f
befriending response, 329
behavioral therapies, 524
Bellack, A. S., 141, 143f
Belmont report, 150
Belsky, Jay, 317
Bennies, 514
Benzedrine, 514
Benzodiazepines, 352, 361–362, 364, 372, 479
Berger, Hans, 86
Bernat, Edward, 553
Bhadoria, Rano, 74t
Bharathi, P., 72t
Bhargava, Subhash C., 72t
Bhatia, M. S., 70t
Bhatia, Triptish, 72t
Bhatt, A. D., 70t
Bhave, Sumitra, 2, 266
Bhugra, D., 31
Bill, W., 526
binge drinking, 482, 498, 502f
binge eating disorder, 418, 430–431
binge-eating/purging type, 421
biopsychosocial approach, 15
bipolar disorders, 32, 35, 79, 270, 290–291
brain imaging, 297–298, 298f
and creativity, 297
diagnosis, 291, 292t–293t, 294
bipolar I, 294
bipolar II, 295
cyclothymic disorder, 295–296, 295f, 296f
environmental factors, 299–300
genetics of, 296–297
neurotransmitter dysregulation, 298–299
treatment, 300–302
Birnbaum, Karl, 553
Bisexual males, 441–442
Biswas, P. K., 73t
Blair, Clancy, 206
Bleuler, Eugene, 239, 390
blind controls, 132
blood alcohol concentration (bac) level, 496, 497, 499f, 500f
bodily symptoms, 360
body mass index (BMI), 414, 415, 415f
Bono, Chaz, 465, 466
Boral, G. C., 73t
borderline personality disorder (bpd), 122, 537, 546, 547, 557–558
brain studies of, 559–560, 560f, 561f
diagnostic criteria in *DSM-5,* 559
fearful preoccupation, 557
self-injurious behavior, 556t
trust and, 561–565, 562f–565f
Borkovec, T. D., 363
Bouillaud, Jean-Baptiste, 38
Bourne, Reverend Ansel, 387–388
Boveri, Theodore, 100
Bovine spongiform encephalopathy, 609
Bowlby, John, 19, 186, 190
BPD. *See* Borderline personality disorder (BPD)
brain
changes seen in schizophrenia, 252–253, 253f, 254f, 255
imaging, 13
networks
auditory network, 95
central executive network, 95
connectivity, 98
default/intrinsic network, 95–96
dorsal attentional network, 95
executive functions, 96
modularity, 97
neurotransmitters, 98–99
salience network, 95, 97
schizophrenia and, 255–256, 256f
sensorimotor network, 95

small world framework, 94
visual network, 95
white matter, 95
schizophrenia and, 249–251, 250f, 251t, 252f
structures, 198–199
brain Electrical Oscillation Signature profiling (BEOS), 618
Brayne, C., 582
Breuer, Josef, 397
Briquet, Paul, 397
Broca, Paul, 38, 243
Broca's area, 38f, 39, 93
Brody, Jane, 430–431
Browne, Thomas, 302
Brown, G., 299
Brown, Wilson J., 91
Bruce, Steven E., 91
Buchholz, Katherine R., 91
Buchman, Aron, 589
Bulimia nervosa, 418
DSM–5, 429
secondary medical problems, 429
treatment, 430
twelve-month prevalence, 428
typical onset, 428
Buprenorphine, 524
Burgmer, Markus, 399
Burns, Jonathan, 243, 244
Buspirone, 364
Buss, David, 280

caffeine, 483, 516–519, 518f
Campbell, Donald, 131
cannabis, 480
cannabinoids, 505
hallucinogens, 506–510, 509f, 510f
history of, 503, 504f
prevalence of, 503f
psychosis, 505–506, 506t
THC (Δ9-tetrahydrocannabinol), 505
Cannon, Walter, 324–325
Capgras syndrome, 66
Cardena, E., 390
Carhart-Harris, R., 51, 77
Case study, 120–122
Caspi, A., 79, 186, 316
Castellani, C., 246–247
Catatonic, 238
Catatonic subtype, 241
Catharsis, 342
CBT. *See* Cognitive behavioral therapy (CBT) approach
Center for Sexual Health Promotion study, 439
Central executive network, 80
Central Institute, Ranchi, 68
Cereal box, 195
CFI. *See* Cultural formulation interview (CFI)
Chandra, A., 438
Chandra, S., 71t
Chaplin, Charlie, 258
Characteristics of healthy self, 540–541
Charcot, Jean-Martin, 42
Charles Bonnet syndrome, 235
Chatterjee, A. K., 69t, 72t
Chatterjee, S. B., 73t
Chattopadyay, Subhagata, 74t
Chaturvedi, Santosh, 72t
Chaudhury, S., 70t, 74t
Chein, Jason, 198
Chemical synapse, 82
Cheney, Terri, 290
Cherian, Alice, 69t, 73t
Cheung, C. K. T., 562, 563
Chiarugi, Vincenzo, 44, 45
Childhood development
adolescence, 196–198
anxious/ambivalent attachment pattern, 192
attachment patterns, 193
avoidant attachment pattern, 192
brain development, 188–189
cloth and wire surrogate, 191f
disorganized/controlling attachment pattern, 192
DSM–5, 187t
early life stress, 189–190
general characteristics, attachment, 192
imitation learning, 193–194
infant–mother relationship, 186
insula and limbic system, 194
malnutrition, 188
mother–infant bonding, 190
peer verbal abuse, 187
secure attachment pattern, 192
social–emotional behavior, 190
theory of mind, 194–196
Childhood disorders
ADHD
DSM–5 diagnostic criteria for, 214t–215t
emotional–behavioral disorder, 215
genetic component, 216
hyperactivity and impulsivity, 214
inattention, 213
response inhibition, 216
spatial working memory, 216
treatment for, 217–218
verbal working memory, 216
ASD
behavioral processes, 203
communication patterns, 203
DSM–5, 204
DSM–5 diagnostic criteria for, 207t
intellectual disabilities, 210
pattern thinking, 205
Raven's Progressive Matrices, 205, 206f

social interactions, 203
special abilities, 210–211
specialized thinkers, 205
traditional IQ tests, 205
traditional symptoms, 206
treatment for, 211–213
visual thinking, 205
word and fact thinking, 205
attachment disorders, 202–203
CD, 203, 218–219, 221
IDD
chromosomes and, 223–224
gestation and, 224–225
metabolism and, 224
treatment of, 225–226
learning disabilities, 220–222
ODD, 67, 216, 219–220
Children's apperception test (CAT), 174
Chlorpromazine, 262
Choi, W., 562, 563
Cholinergic, 326
Choudhary, Gauri, 594
Chromosomes, 100, 101f
Chronic diseases and injuries, 6
Chronic stress, 272
Cialis, 456
Cingulo-opercular network, 353
Circumstantiality, 234
Classical conditioning, 57
Classification, 162
anxiety disorders, 179
bipolar disorder, 180
character disorders, 179
dimensional assessment, 180
DSM–I, DSM–II and *DSM–III,* 179
DSM–IV, 180
DSM–IV–TR, 180
DSM–5, 180
Huntington's chorea, 179
ICD and *DSM* criteria, 177
ICD-8 and *DSM–II,* 179
ICD-10, 177
neurocognitive disorders, 179
psychotic disorders, 179
Cleckley, Hervey, 553
Client-centered approach, 54
Clinical Antipsychotic Trials of Intervention Effectiveness (CATIE) study, 262
Clinical neurology, 42
Cluster A, 536
Cocaine, 476–478, 480, 489, 511–512, 512f, 513, 513f
Code of Criminal Procedure (CrPC), 614
Cognitive avoidance model, 361
Cognitive behavioral orientations, 465
Cognitive behavioral therapy (CBT) approach, 60–62, 263, 264, 281–282, 282f, 286–287, 342, 363, 366, 427, 456, 525
Cognitive bias, 351
Cognitive dysfunction in chronic smokers, 517–519, 518f
Cognitive empathy, 559
Cognitive model of depression, 275–276, 276f, 307
Cognitive processes, changed in schizophrenia, 258–259
Cognitive restructuring, 342, 344
Cognitive therapy-continuation, 287
Cojan, Yann, 400
Coleridge, Samuel Taylor, 477
Collins, S., 458
Combat fatigue, 336
Community-based intervention, 281
Community Mental Health Act, 1963, 46
Comorbid, 67
Compensation, 586
Comprehensive Crime Control Act of 1984, 617
Compulsions, 373
Computerized axial tomography (CAT), 121
Concomitant psychological stress, 320–321
Concurrent validity, 166
Concussions, 603
Conduct disorder (CD), 203, 218–219, 221
Confidentiality, 620
Confounding variables, 128
Connectivity, 98
Conscientiousness, 542
Construct validity, 166
Content validity, 166
Continuous performance test (CPT), 174
Control group, 127
Controlled drinking approaches, 527–528
Conversion disorder, 393, 396–401, 396f, 398f–400f, 401f
Conversion reaction, 397
Copy number variations, 246
Corpus striatum, 35
Correlation coefficient, 124
Cortical networks, 94
Cortical pathways, 349
Corticotropin-releasing factor (CRF), 272, 372
Corticotropin-releasing hormone (CRH), 324
Cortisol, 273, 324, 372
Costa, P.T., 542, 544
Covary, 128
CPT. *See* Continuous performance test (CPT)
Craving, 486, 491
C-reactive protein (CRP), 277
Creutzfeldt–Jakob disease, 609
Crichton-Browne, J., 243

Crick, Francis, 104
Crow, Tim, 243
Cultural formulation interview (CFI), 164
Cultural sensitivity, 162–163
Cultural variations, 160–161
Culture, obesity, 418
Cyber-suicide, 275
Cyclothymic disorder, 295–296, 295f, 296f
Cytokines, 322

Dadheech, Gora, 70t
Darwin, Charles, 41, 122, 437, 470
Das, A., 425
Das, Mrinmay, 73t
Davidson, Neil, 492
Davies, D. L., 527
Davis, R. B., 69t
Deary, I., 588
Deep brain stimulation (DBS), 285–286, 286f
Default network, 95, 353
Deinstitutionalization, 46f–47f
de la Salpêtrière, Hospice, 45
Delayed ejaculation, 453
Delirium, 580, 590–591
Delirium tremens (DT), 483
Delusional thinking, 161
Delusions, 32, 40, 233, 235
Demand characteristics, 131
Dementia, 44, 80
Dementia praecox, 238, 239
Dementias, 580
Deoxyribonucleic acid (DNA), 81, 297, 318–320
Department of Nuclear Medicine, 93
Department of Science and Technology (DST), 68
Dependent personality disorder, 537, 569
Dependent variable (DV), 128
Depersonalization, 383
Depersonalization–derealization disorder, 385–386, 387f
Depressive complaints, 117
Depressive disorders, 32, 80, 270–271, 331, 437, 449, 464, 593
  around world, 271–273
  cognitive model of depression, 275–276
  developmental aspects of, 273–275
  evolutionary perspective concerning depression, 278–279
    resource conservation theories, 279
    social competition theories, 280
    social risk hypothesis, 280
  in families, 277–278
  Indian statistics on, 272
  and inflammation, 277
  prevention and treatment, 280–281
    DBS, 285–286, 286f
    ECT, 283–284, 284f
    medications, 282
    TMS, 285, 285f
    VNS, 284–285
  psychological treatments, 286
    cognitive therapy, 286–287
    EFT, 288
    psychodynamic therapy, 288–289
Derealization, 383
DeRubeis, R., 77, 282
de Sade, Marquis, 462
Desai, N. G., 73t, 75t
Deshpande, Smita, 148
Descartes, René, 33
Deshmukh, D. K., 68t
Devasis Ghosh, 71t
Devi, Parvathi S., 73t
Devrai (film), 1–2, 265
Dhanda, Amita, 614
Dhar, M. K., 70t
Dhat syndrome, 116, 359, 437, 439
Diabetes, 15
Diagnostic and Statistical Manual of Mental Disorders (DSM), 76, 144
Diagnostic and Statistical Manual of Mental Disorders (DSM–III), 549
Diagnostic and Statistical Manual of Mental Disorders (DSM-4) dementia criteria, 590
Diagnostic and Statistical Manual of Mental Disorders (DSM-5), 23, 161, 187, 273, 449, 457, 482–483, 536, 590
  anxiety disorders, 348
  criteria, 519
  diagnostic criteria, 596t
Dialectical behavior therapy (DBT), 49, 570–572
Diffusion tensor imaging (DTI), 92, 255. 258
Di Forti, M., 504, 505
Disability Adjusted Life Years (DALYs), 4t–6t, 7f
Disinhibited social engagement disorder, 203
Disordered use, 482
Disorganized subtype, 241
Disruptive, 187
Dissociation, 125, 383, 385
Dissociative amnesia, 383, 387–388, 388f
Dissociative disorders, 383–385, 392t
  depersonalization–derealization disorder, 385–386, 387f
  DID, 389–391, 390f, 391t
  dissociative amnesia, 387–388, 388f
  factitious disorder, 402–403
  prevalence, 384t
  treatment, 392–393, 404
  work in India, 391–392
Dissociative fugue, 387

Dissociative identity disorder (DID), 383, 389–391, 390f, 391t
Disulfiram, 524, 529
Divine madness, 297
Dix, Dorothea, 46
Dizygotic (DZ) twins, 147, 207
DNA methylation, 320
Doongaji, Dinshaw R., 72t
Dopamine, 250, 257f, 487–489, 497, 512, 514–516
Dopamine imbalance hypothesis, 257
Dorsolateral prefrontal cortex (DLPFC), 250
Double-blind experiment, 132
Double insanity, 291
Doubt, 119
Down syndrome, 223
Dramatic emotional personality disorders
  antisocial personality disorder, 551–553
  BPD, 557–558
    brain studies of, 559–560, 560f, 561f
    diagnostic criteria in *DSM–5,* 559
    fearful preoccupation, 557
    self-injurious behavior, 556t
    trust and, 561–565, 562f–565f
  histrionic personality disorder, 566
  psychopathy, 551, 553–556, 554t
Drug De-addiction and Treatment Centre, 479
Drugs, 412
du Bois-Reymond, Emil, 37
Duhkha, 31
Durbin, Anthony, 91
Durham rule, 616
Duty to protect provision, 619
Dylan, Bob, 580
Dynamic deconstructive psychotherapy (DDP)., 573
Dyspareunia, 454
Dziobek, I., 560, 561
Dziobek, Uasbek, 559

Early ejaculation, 451, 453
Eating disorders, 196, 408
  feeding disorders, 408, 409
    avoidant/restrictive food intake disorder, 410
    DSM–5, 409t
    pica, 409–410
    rumination disorder, 410
  major eating disorders, 418
    anorexia nervosa, 418, 420–427
    binge eating disorder, 430–431
    bulimia nervosa, 418, 428–430
    DSM–IV, 418
    lifetime prevalence rates, 419t
    prevalence and standard error, 419t
  obesity, 408, 410
    BMI, 412–415, 415f, 416f
    environmental factors, 410, 412
    evolutionary history, 411
    interconnected systems, 412, 412f
    psychological factors, and biological factors, 411
    risk, 415
    thrifty gene hypothesis, 410
    in United States, 414, 415f
    weights, males and females, 417–418
    worldwide, 413–414
Echolalia, 241
Echopraxia, 241
Eckmanns, T., 118
Ecological validity, 166
EDA. *See* Electrodermal activity (EDA)
Edwin, Tony, 71t
EEG. *See* Electroencephalography (EEG)
Effect size, 148
Einstein, Albert, 205
Eisenberger, N., 563, 564
Elbert, Thomas, 128
Electroconvulsive therapy (ECT), 283–284, 284f
Electrodermal activity (EDA), 66
Electroencephalography (EEG), 78, 81, 86–87, 150, 176, 209, 243, 441
Electroencephalography frequency bands, 251t
Ellicott, A., 299
Ellis, Albert, 436
Ellis, Havelock, 437, 441, 470
Elsabbagh, Mayada, 209
Emotional empathy, 559
Emotional response, 66
Emotion—arousal and control, 318
Emotion focused therapy (EFT), 55, 286, 288
Emotions, schizophrenia and, 259
Empathizing-systemizing theory of autism, 208
Empathy, 537
Empiricism, 31, 120
Encephalization, 41
Endophenotypes, 78, 304
Endorphins, 511
Engel, George, 15
Environmental risk factors, 67
Environmental stress, 273
Epidemiology, 144–145
Epigenetic inheritance, 104
Epigenetic marks, 104
Epigenetics, 79, 318–320, 485

Epinephrine, 323, 325
Eraser tags, 319
Erectile disorder, 452–453
Erickson, K., 589
Eswaraiah, G., 72t
Ethical relationship, 154
European diets, 16
Event-related potentials (ERPs), 87–88, 209
Everyday Abilities Scale for India, 589
Evoked potentials (EP), 87–88
Evolutionary psychologists, 22
Executive functions, 96
Exhibitionism, 458
Exhibitionistic disorder, 458
Experimental group, 127
Experimenter effects, 132
Explanatory Model Interview Catalogue (EMIC), 166
Exposure therapy, 342, 365
Externalizing disorders, 67, 216
External validity, 131
Extinction, 57
Extraversion, 53, 540, 542
Eye movement desensitization and reprocessing (EMDR), 342

Factitious disorder, 394, 402–403
Factitious disorder imposed on another, 403
Factitious disorder imposed on self, 403
Facts, 119
False-belief task, 195
Falsification, 119
Feeding disorders, 408, 409
  avoidant/restrictive food intake disorder, 410
  DSM–5, 409t
  pica, 409–410
  rumination disorder, 410
Feierman, Jay, 460
Feinstein, A., 397
Female dyspareunia, 439
Female external sexual anatomy, 445, 446f
Female orgasmic disorder, 453
Female reproductive system, 445, 446f
Female sexual interest/arousal disorder, 454
Fernandez, Antony, 69t
Ferretti, Antonio, 443, 444
Fetal alcohol syndrome (FAS), 224–225
Fetishistic disorder, 459
Feygin, D., 375
FFM. *See* Five-factor model (FFM)
Fiber tracts, 37
Fight-or-flight response, 325, 329
Firestone, P., 458
First-generation antipsychotics, 262
Five-factor model (FFM), 542, 542t, 543, 544t, 546
Flasher, 458
Flight of ideas, 161
Flinn, M. V., 330
Fluoxetine, 430
fMRI. *See* Functional magnetic resonance imaging (fMRI)
Foa, E., 379
Folie circulaire, 239
Forensic neuroscience, 628
Fragile X syndrome, 224
Franklin, Benjamin, 37, 477
Freud, Sigmund, 43, 49, 50f, 170, 397, 437, 441, 470
Frick, P., 173
Friends' Asylum, 45f
Friese, B., 484
Friston, K., 51, 77
Frontal lobe, 36
Frontoparietal network, 353
Frotteuristic disorder, 459
Functional magnetic resonance imaging (fMRI), 90–91, 150, 176, 198, 255–256, 256f, 397, 401, 441, 443, 559
Functional neurological symptom disorder, 397
Fusiform face area (FFA), 66

Gada, M. T., 73t
Gage, Phineas, 121
Galen, 30, 31, 408
Galgali, R. B., 73t
Galileo, 34
Gall, Joseph, 37
Gall's head structure, 37, 38f
Galvani, Luigi, 37
Gambling, 480, 483
  behavioral conditioning, 522
  cognitive–emotional process, 522
  DSM–5 criteria, 519
  impaired executive functioning, 522
  impulse control disorder, 519
  impulsivity, 522
  lifetime comorbidity of pathological, 520, 521t
  lifetime prevalence, 520t
  substance tolerance, 521
Gamma-aminobutyric acid (GABA), 257f, 352
Gamson, David, 206
Ganesan, V., 74t
Gangadhar, B. N., 69t, 71t
Gaur, R. K., 69t
Gautam, Shiv, 75t
Gender dysphoria, 466
  in adolescents and adults, 466
  in children, 466
  gender identity, 465
  gender roles, 465
  Indian cultural context, 469
  non-dysphoria conditions, 467
  prevalence, 466
  transgender, 466
  treatment
    cortical thickness examination, 467, 468f

family therapy and child based therapy, 467
gender transition surgery, 467
sex change procedure, 468
Gender dysphoria. *See* Sexuality disorders
Gender identity, 436, 465, 466, 469
Gender roles, 465
General adaptation syndrome (GAS), 327
Generalizability, 131
Generalized anxiety disorder (GAD), 134, 196, 348
General pervasive developmental disorder, 204
Genetics, 101f
allele, 100
behavior and experience, 103–106
chromosomes, 100, 101f
DNA, 101f, 102
heterozygotes/heterozygous, 101
homozygotes/homozygous, 101
Mendel's first law, 100
Mendel's second law, 100
proteins, 101
Genito-pelvic pain/penetration disorder, 454
Genotype, 102
Ghaffar, O., 397
Ghulam, R., 73t, 74t
Giffords, Gabby, 613
Gilbert, P., 278
Gilmore, John, 252
Girish, K., 69t, 74t
Gitlin, M., 299
Gleaves, D., 390
Global Assessment of Functioning Scale score, 299
Glove anesthesia, 396
Glutamate, 99, 250, 257–258, 257f
Gogtay, N., 245
Goldstein, R., 486, 491
Gong, S. L., 74t
Goodman, A., 486
Goodwin, Frederick, 297
Gopinath, P. S., 72t
Goswami, 300
Gottesman, I., 147
Government of India, 6, 68
Goyal, N., 31
Gradual exposure, 370
Grandin, Temple, 185, 204, 205
Grave disability, 621
Gray matter, 35f, 36
reduction, 253
Greenberg, Leslie, 55, 55f
Gross, C., 352
Grossman, P., 56
Grube, J., 484
Gull, William, 420
Gupta, A. K., 70t
Gurnani, K. C., 74t
Guthrie, Woody, 608

Hallucinations, 32, 40, 234, 235
Hallucinogens, 480, 506–510, 509f, 510f
altered states of consciousness rating scale, 508, 509f
anxious ego dissolution, 506
LSD (*d*-lysergic acid diethylamide), 506, 508
mescaline, 506
oceanic boundlessness, 506
perceptual symptoms, 506
psilocybin, 508–509, 510f
psychedelics, 506
psychic symptoms, 508
serotonin, 508
somatic symptoms, 506
visionary restructuralization, 508
Haloperidol, 262
Hammen, C., 299
Haque, S., 73t
Hare, Robert, 553, 554
Hariharasubrmanian, N., 73t
Harlow, Harry, 190
Harpending, H., 109
Harris, S., 588
Harvey, William, 33
Hathaway, S. R., 167
Health Insurance Portability and Accountability Act of 1996 (HIPAA), 620
Hebb, Donald, 51
Hebephrenia, 238
Hebephrenic schizophrenia, 241
Hecker, Ewald, 238
Heiman, J., 439
Hemingway, Ernest, 297
Hemisphere, 35
Henquet, C., 504, 505
Hen, R., 352
Heroin, 480
Hersen, M., 141, 143f
Heterosexual males, 441, 462
Heterozygotes, 101
Heterozygous, 101
Hierarchical integration, 40
Hierarchy of needs, 54
Highly active antiretroviral therapy (HAART), 525
Hinckley, John, 235, 616, 617
Hindi mental Status Examination, 589
Hippocampus, 325, 338
Hippocrates, 29, 30, 291, 408
Histones, 318
Histrionic personality disorder, 537, 566
Hoarding, 375
Hoffman, Dustin, 210
Hoffmann, Albert, 508
Hofmann, S., 56
Hollon, S., 77
Holmes, James, 613
Holmes, Sherlock, 130
Holton, Gerald, 34
Homeostasis, 326
Homeostatic system, 411

Homosexuality in Perspective (Masters and Johnson), 445
Homozygotes, 101
Homozygous, 101
Hormonal changes, 196
Horney, Karen, 52, 53, 53f
Human brain, 85
Human culture, 16
Human immunodeficiency virus (HIV) infection, 593
Humanistic-experiential therapies, 53
Human Sexual Inadequacy (Masters and Johnson), 445, 455, 471
Human sexual response, 446
  excitement phase, 447
  orgasm phase, 448
  plateau phase, 447, 448
  resolution phase, 448
Human Sexual Response (Masters and Johnson), 445
Humors, 30
Huntington's disease, 579
Hygienic performance, 118
Hyman, S., 488
Hypnosis, 385
Hypoactive sexual desire disorder (HSDD), 439
Hypochondriasis, 395
Hypomanic episode, 292t–293t
Hypothalamic-pituitary-adrenal (HPA) axis, 318, 323–325, 323f, 324f, 372
Hypothalamus, 324
Hypothesis testing, 117
Hysteria, 393, 397
Hysterical neurosis, 394

ICMR Center of Research, 68
IConS. *See* International Conference on Schizophrenia (IConS)
Idiocy, 45
IHBAS, 48
Illicit drug, 480, 481f, 528
Illness anxiety disorder, 395
Immune system, 318, 321–322
Impastato, David J., 68t
Impressionists, 8
Impulse control, 187
Incidence, 144
Indecent exposure, 458, 471
Independent variable (IV), 128
Indian epidemiological data, 439
Indian Journal of Endocrinology and Metabolism, 2016, 469
Indian Journal of Medical Research (2014), 479
Indian Lunatic Asylums Act, 614
Indian medical system of Ayurveda, 116
Indian Mental Healthcare Act, 2017, 615
Indian Ocean tsunami, 315f
Indian Scale for Assessment of Autism (ISAA), 218
Individuals with Disabilities Education Act (IDEA), 221
Inference, 129
Inflammation, 277
Informed consent, 152, 620
Institute for Psychological Health (IPH), 3
Institutional Review Board (IRB), 153–154
Insula and limbic system, 194
Intellectual developmental disorder (IDD)
  chromosomes and, 223–224
  gestation and, 224–225
  metabolism and, 224
  treatment of, 225–226
Intergenerational transmission of depression, 273
Internalizing disorders, 67, 216
Internal reliability, 165
Internal validity, 130
International Classification of Diseases (ICD), 177
  ICD-10, 482–483
International Conference on Schizophrenia (IConS), 95
International Urogynecological Journal of 2012, 439
Internet, 262
Interpersonal transactions, 52
Inter-rater reliability, 165
Intimacy, 541
Intoxication, 482, 483, 484f
Intrinsic network, 80
Introversion, 53
Invisible Wounds of War (Tanielian & Jaycox), 340
Iowa Gambling Task, 522
IVF treatments, 470

Jackson, John Hughlings, 39, 40f, 50, 243
Jadhav, Sushrut, 10
Jagadisha, 73t
Jain, R. K., 68t
Jainer, Ashok Kumar, 74t
Jambur Ananth, 69t
James, William, 95
Jamison, Kay, 290, 297, 299
Jaslok Hospital and Research Center, 93
Jayaswal, S. K., 74t
Jhingan, H. P., 72t
Joffe-Ellis, Debbie, 436
John, John P., 69t, 73t
John, Sajiv, 71t
Johnson, Sheri, 297, 384
Johnson, Ted, 604
Johnson, Virginia, 445–447, 449f, 455, 459, 470
Jones, J., 438
Joshi, Geeta, 624
Journal of Ethnicity in Substance Abuse, 485
Jung, Carl, 52, 81, 171
The Juvenile Justice (Care and Protection of Children) Act, 2015 (JJ Act), 623

Kaasav (film), 2, 265
Kahlbaum, Karl Ludwig, 238
Kamphaus, R., 173
Kandel, Eric, 51
Kanner, Leo, 203
Kellogg, John, 437
Kennedy, John F., 46
Kernberg, Otto, 557, 573
Kessler, R. C., 355, 520
Khandelwal, S. K., 74t
Khanna, Sumant, 71t, 74t
Kiecolt-Glaser, Janice, 321
Kiloh, L. G., 68t
Kimball, John W., 445, 446
King Henry VIII, 43
Kinsey, Alfred, 437, 438
Kirpal Singh, 72t
Klopfer approach, 625
Koch, J. L., 553
Koch, W., 598
Kohli, Adarsh, 71t
Kolodny, R., 459
Kozak, M., 379
Kraepelin, Emil, 238, 239, 553
Kramer, A., 589
K. S. Wani Memorial Trust, 2
Kulkarni, M. R., 68t
Kumar, K., 246–247
Kumar, Pradeep, 69t
Kumar, Ratanendra, 72t, 74t
Kumar, S., 73t
Kumawat, Sanjay, 624
Kunigiri, Girish, 74t
Kuruvilla, K., 73t, 74t

la belle indifférence, 396
Lactose tolerance, 17
Lakshmi Reddy, P., 70t
The Lancet (Patel), 503
Långström, N., 462
Larger protein molecules, 99
Laumann, E. O., 425
Law and mental health
  ethical and legal issues in treatment, 618–619
    emergency commitments, 620–622
    initial contract for treatment, 619–620, 621t
  Indian legal scenario
    The Juvenile Justice (Care and Protection of Children) Act, 2015, 623
    Narcotic Drugs and Psychotropic Substances Act, 1985, 623
    The Protection of Children from Sexual Offences Act, 2012, 623
    The Sexual Harassment of Women at Workplace (Prevention, Prohibition And Redressal) Act, 2013, 623
  insanity, 614, 615
  legal aspects of psychopathology, 628–630
  legal system and insanity defense, 615–618
The law of independent assortment, 100
The law of segregation, 100
Learning disabilities, 220–222
LeDoux, Joseph, 349
Left-hand movement, 400
Left prefrontal cortex (LPFC), 198
Lemos, Julia, 272
Lenzenweger, M., 537, 539
Leonardo da Vinci's drawings, 32f
Lesbian, gay, bisexual, and transgender (LGBT) community, 469
Lessard v. Schmidt, 622
Levay, S., 447
Levitra, 456
Lifetime prevalence, 144
Lilienfeld, S. O., 554
Limbic system, 349
Lincoln, Abraham, 271
Linehan, Marsha, 571, 572
Linkage analysis, 148
Logic, 129–130
Longitudinal design, 142–144
Lord Adrian, 85
Lorenz, Konrad, 192
Lou Gehrig's disease, 42
Lovaas treatment program, 212
Luders, E., 468
Lukens, S., 384
Luria, A.R., 120, 121

MacArthur Foundation, 9
Macrophage theory of depression, 277
Mad cow disease, 608
Magic mushrooms, 508
Magistretti, P. J., 98
Magnetic resonance imaging (MRI), 176
Magnetoencephalography (MEG), 88, 176, 385
Malhotra, Savita, 74t
Mahendru, R. K., 68t
Maier, S., 330
Maiti, S., 246–247
Major depressive disorder (MDD), 271, 274, 274t, 277, 306, 559
Major depressive episode, 293t
Major eating disorders, 418
  anorexia nervosa, 418, 420–426
    adolescents, 421
    causes of, 423
    characteristics, 420
    cultural factors, 424
    daily calorie allowance table, 425t
    DSM–5 criteria, 420–421
    functional magnetic resonance imaging studies, 422, 423f
    genetics, 423
    outward signs of, 421

risk factors, 423–424, 424f
semi-starvation period, 425
serotonin and dopamine systems, 423
starvation, 424–425
time course and phenomenology, 421, 422f
treatment, 426–427
binge eating disorder, 430–431
bulimia nervosa, 418
DSM–5, 429
secondary medical problems, 429
treatment, 430
twelve-month prevalence, 428
typical onset, 428
DSM–IV, 418
lifetime prevalence rates, 419t
prevalence and standard error, 419t
Major neurocognitive disorders, 580, 592–594, 593t
Male hypoactive sexual desire disorder, 454
Malenka, R., 488
Male reproductive system, 445f
Malhotra, H. K., 116
Malin, Fr., 174
Malingering, 394
Malleus Maleficarum, 32
Mandated reporting, 620
Mania
with delirium, 44
without delirium, 44
and melancholia, 35
Manic depression, 35, 270
Manic episode, 292t
Margoob, Mushtaq A., 72t
Marijuana, 478, 480
intoxication, 483, 507
legalization of, 507
The Mask of Sanity (Cleckley, Hervey), 553
Maslow, Abraham, 53, 54
Masters, William, 445–447, 449f, 455, 459, 470
Maternal infection, 245
Mathew, Kuruvilla, 70t
Mathew, Roy J., 69t
Maudsley approach, 426
May, M., 390
McCann, Una, 515, 516
McCrae, R., 542
McEwen, Bruce, 327, 328
McKinley, J. C., 167
McLean, Richard, 235
MDMA, 510
Measles, mumps, and rubella (MMR) vaccine, 130, 207
Mechanical models, 33, 33f
Medical disorders, 325, 450
Mehrotra, S., 343
Mehta, C. H., 69t
Melancholia, 44, 270
Meltzer, Malcolm, 579
Mendel, Gregor, 99
Mendel's first law, 100
Mendel's second law, 100
Menon, V., 96, 97f
Mental disorders/illness, 2, 302, 449, 463
alcohol misuse, 6
behavioral perspective, 56–59
biopsychosocial approach, 15
categorical and a dimensional manner, 67
classification systems for, 177, 178f
clinical interventions, 7
cognitive behavioral perspective, 59–62
dementia, 44
devil/supernatural forces, 48
empirically based principles and treatments, 49
evidence-based medicine, 49
existential-humanistic perspective, 52–56
idiocy, 45
mania with delirium, 44
mania without delirium, 44
melancholia, 44
mental hospitals, 46–48
neuropsychological tests, 175
neuroscience techniques, 175–176
psychodynamic perspective, 49–52
psychology and physiology, 48
stigma of, 8–12
St. Mary of Bethlehem, 43
trauma producing, 316–317
Western industrial culture, 21
Mental Healthcare Act, 614, 615
Mental health professionals, 18f–19f
Mental health services, 18f–19f
Mental retardation, 222
Mental status exam, 160
Mescaline, 506, 508
Meta-analysis, 149
Methadone, 524, 528
Methamphetamines, 489, 514–516
Methcathinone, 515
Meyer-Lindenberg, Andreas, 562
Microscope, 34
Miklowitz, D. J., 299
Mild cognitive impairment (MCI), 590
Mild neurocognitive disorders, 592–594, 592t
Alzheimer's disease (*see* Alzheimer's disease)
frontotemporal neurocognitive disorder, 600–603, 601f, 602f, 603f
HIV infection, 607–608
Huntington's disease, 608

Lewy Body dementia, 605–606, 606f
Parkinson's disease, 606–607
prion disease, 608–609
substance-induced neurocognitive disorder., 608
traumatic brain injuries (TBIs), 603–605
vascular neurocognitive disorder, 599–600
Milgram, Stanley, 94
Millon Clinical Multiaxial Inventory, 3rd ed (MCMI III), 625, 626
Mind–body problem, 34
Mindfulness-based cognitive therapy, 287
Mindfulness techniques, 56
Mini-international neuropsychiatric interview (MINI screen), 589
Minimal brain dysfunction, 220
Ministry of Health and Family Welfare, 6, 68
Minnesota multiphasic personality inventory (MMPI), 167–168
MMPI-2 profile, 169f
Mirror neurons, 193, 194
Mirsky, Allan, 175
Mishra, B. P., 71t
Mishra, T. K., 70t
Mitochondria, 297
Mitochondrial DNA (mtDNA), 105–106
Mitochondrial dysfunction hypothesis, 106
Mitochondrial inheritance, 105–106
MMPI. *See* Minnesota multiphasic personality inventory (MMPI)
MMR vaccine. *See* Measles, mumps, and rubella (MMR) vaccine
M'Naghten, Daniel, 615
M'Naghten rule, 616
Modularity, 97
Mohandas, E., 72t
Monoamine oxidase (MAO) inhibitor, 282–283, 366
Monoamine oxidase A (MAO-A) gene, 79, 146, 316–317
Monozygotic (MZ) twins, 147, 207
Mood disorders, 196
bipolar disorders
bipolar I, 294
bipolar II, 295
brain imaging, 297–298, 298f
and creativity, 297
cyclothymic disorder, 295–296, 295f, 296f
diagnosis, 291, 292t–293t, 294
environmental factors, 299–300
genetics of, 296–297
neurotransmitter dysregulation, 298–299
treatment, 300–302
depressive disorders, 270–271, 278–281, 286
around world, 271–273
cognitive model of depression, 275–276
cognitive therapy, 286–287
DBS, 285–286, 286f
developmental aspects of, 273–275
ECT, 283–284, 284f
EFT, 288
in families, 277–278
Indian statistics on, 272
and inflammation, 277
medications, 282
psychodynamic therapy, 288–289
resource conservation theories, 279
social competition theories, 280
social risk hypothesis, 280
TMS, 285, 285f
VNS, 284–285
risk factors, 306f
suicide, 302
cultural differences, 303
endophenotypes and, 304
gender differences and type of attempts, 303–304, 304t
prevention, 305
short-term and long-term factors, 304–305
warning signs, 305t
Mood symptoms, 234
Moore, Brian P., 71t
Moral insanity, 551
Morgan, Christiana, 172
Morrison, P., 504, 505
Morton, Richard, 420
Mosher, W. D., 438
Motor symptoms, 234
mtDNA. *See* mitochondrial DNA (mtDNA)
Muktaangan, 48
Mukundan, C. R., 108, 318, 618
Mullins-Sweatt, Stephanie N., 540, 542
Multiple sclerosis, 42
Multisystemic therapy (MST), 220
Munchausen syndrome, 403
Munch, Edvard, 291
Murphy, Jane, 21, 22
Murray, Henry, 172
Murray, R., 504, 505
Murthy, Pratima, 72t
Murthy, S. K., 72t
Murthy, Srinivasa, 321, 343, 618
Musical instrument, 128
Musto, D., 477, 478
Myotonia, 447

Nadel, George, 463, 464
Nagamatsu, Lindsay, 589
Nainian, M. R., 71t
Naltrexone, 524, 528
Nand, Satya D., 69t
Narasimha Rao, I. V. L., 70t
Narayanan, H. S., 70t
Narayan Murthy, H., 68t

Narcissism, 566
Narcissistic personality disorder, 537
Narcotic Drugs and Psychotropic Substances (NDPS) Act, 1985, 623
Nash, John, 1–2, 235
Nathawat, S. S., 72t
National Commission on Farmers (NCF), 9
National Comorbidity Replication Adolescent Supplement, 354
National Comorbidity Survey, 67, 196
National Data Sharing and Accessibility Policy (NDSAP), 6t
National Institute of Mental Health (NIMH), 144, 180
National Institute of Mental Health and Neurosciences (NIMHANS), 68
National Institute on Alcohol Abuse and Alcoholism (NIAAA), 498
National Sample Survey Organization, 3
National Survey of Sexual Health and Behavior (NSSHB), 438
Natural disasters, 334
Naturalistic observation method, 122–123
Natural selection, 41
Natural spirits, 31
Negative cognitive triad, 275
Negative correlation, 124
Negative symptoms, 234, 236
Neocortex, 200
Nerve impulse, 37
Nervous system, 36, 37f
Nestler, E., 488
Nettle, D., 543
Neural model, 276
Neuritic plaques, 595, 595f
Neurocognitive disorders
  brain changes with age, 584, 586–587, 587f
  cognitive abilities change with age, 583–584, 583f, 584f–586f
  delirium, 580, 590–591
  dementias, 580
  Huntington's disease, 579
  incidence of mild and moderate, 581, 582f
  India on aging changes in brain, 589–590
  individual's activities, 587–589
  major, 592–594, 593t
  mild, 592–594, 592t
    Alzheimer's disease (*see* Alzheimer's disease)
    frontotemporal neurocognitive disorder, 600–603, 601f, 602f, 603f
    HIV infection, 607–608
    Huntington's disease, 608
    Lewy Body dementia, 605–606, 606f
    Parkinson's disease, 606–607
    prion disease, 608–609
    substance-induced neurocognitive disorder., 608
    traumatic brain injuries (TBIs), 603–605
    vascular neurocognitive disorder, 599–600
  percentage of global population, 580, 581f
  population ages 65 and over, 580, 582f
  population 65 years and up, 580, 581f
  prevention of, 583
Neurodevelopmental disorders, 187
Neurodevelopmental hypothesis, 245
Neuroethics, 110–111
Neurofibrillary tangles, 595, 595f
Neurons
  characteristics of, 81, 82f
  encoding information, 84–85
  levels of firing, 84f
  local hubs, 94
  low-cost travel, 98
  mirror, 193, 194
  passing information, 83–84
  white matter, 95
Neuropeptides, 99
Neuroscience approach
  behavior and experience, 76
  biochemical and electrophysiological processes, 76
  brain imaging, 76
  brain networks (*see* Brain, networks)
  DSM, 76
  DTI, 92
  electroencephalography, 86–87
  endophenotypes, 78
  ERPs, 87
  fMRI, 90–91
  genes, 78–79
  genetics, 76 (*see* Genetics)
  human brain, 85
  ICD, 76
  levels of analysis, 80–81
  MEG, 88
  neural networks, 79–80
  neuroethics, 110–111
  PET, 88–90
  reward system, 76, 76f
  spatial and temporal resolution, 92–93
  themes of evolution, 106–107
Neuroticism, 542, 543
Neurotransmitter dysregulation, 298–299
Neurotransmitters, 79, 98–99, 257–258, 257f, 323
Newton, Isaac, 205
"New wave"/"third wave" approaches, 286

Nichols, D., 510
Nicotine, 489, 518
Nimgaonkar, Vishwajit L., 72t, 148
NIMH. *See* National Institute of Mental Health (NIMH)
NIMHANS. *See* National Institute of Mental Health and Neurosciences (NIMHANS)
Nizamie, Alaka, 71t
Nizamie, S. H., 31
Noradrenaline, 99
Norepinephrine, 323, 325
Norepinephrine-SSRI venlafaxine, 366
Normalcy, 22
Norris, James, 43

Obesity, 408, 410
  BMI, 412–415, 415f, 416f
  environmental factors, 410, 412
  evolutionary history, 411
  interconnected systems, 412, 412f
  psychological factors, and biological factors, 411
  risk, 415
  thrifty gene hypothesis, 410
  in United States, 414, 415f
  weights, males and females, 417–418
  worldwide, 413–414
Observational learning, 59
Obsessional thinking, 161
Obsessions, 373
Obsessive-compulsive disorder (OCD), 348, 374t, 510
  brain processes associated with, 376–377
  hoarding, 375–376
  Indian studies on, 378
  manifestation, 375
  obsessions and compulsions, 373–375
  treatment, 378–379
  types of symptoms, 373
Obsessive-compulsive personality (OCP) disorder, 537, 569–570
Occipital lobe, 36
Oceanic Boundlessness, 506
O'Connor *vs.* Donaldson decision, 622
Odd-eccentric personality disorders
  paranoid personality disorder, 547–548
  schizoid personality disorder, 548
  schizotypal personality disorder, 548–551
Odd/eccentric disorders, 536
Öhman, Arne, 59
OPD treatment, 116
Openness, 542
Operant conditioning, 58
Operational definition, 127
Opiates, 477, 478
Opioids, 479, 480
  cocaine, 511–512, 512f, 513, 513f
  dopamine, 512, 514
  endorphins, 511
  peptides, 99
  prevalence of, 510, 511f
  system, 485
Oppositional defiant disorder (ODD), 67, 216, 219–220
Orbitofrontal cortex (OFC), 491
O'Reilly, R., 246–247
Orgasmic disorder, 453
Orwell, George, 205
Öst, Lars, 369, 370
Other specified paraphilic disorder, 463
Ouyang, Daniel, 72t
Overlapping genetic risk factors, 67
Oxytocin, 329

Palaniappun, V., 75t
Pandey, R. S., 70t
Panic attack, 348
Panic disorder, 348, 370–372, 371t
Panksepp, Jaak, 350
Pantelis, C., 245
Pappenheim, Bertha, 397
Paranoid, 238
  subtype, 240
Paranoid personality disorder, 536, 537, 547–548
Paraphilic disorders, 457
  exhibitionistic disorder, 458
  fetishistic disorder, 459
  frotteuristic disorder, 459
  pedophilic disorder, 459–461
  sexual masochism disorder, 461
  sexual sadism disorder, 462
  specified paraphilic disorder, 463
  transvestic disorder, 462–463
Parasympathetic division, 325–326
Parens patriae authority, 621
Parietal lobe, 36
Parkar, Shubhangi, 547
Parkinson's disease, 42, 516, 593, 606–607
Parvathi Devi, S., 73t, 74t
Patel, Vikram, 265, 280–281
Pathological gambling, 485
Patient Self-Determination Act (PSDA) of 1991, 622
Patrick, C. J., 553, 554
Pattern of addiction, 486–487, 486f
Pattern thinking, 205
Pavlov, Ivan, 56, 57, 397
Pawar, A. A., 71t
Pedophilic disorder, 459–461
Peduncle, 35
Peel, Sir Robert, 615
Pendulum-type timing device, 34
Penfield, Wilder, 401, 402

Perfectionism, 421
Performance anxiety, 455
Perrin, J., 284
Personality disorders, 196, 534–536
  anxious fearful personality disorders
    avoidant personality disorder, 568–569
    dependent personality disorder, 569
    obsessive-compulsive personality disorder, 569–570
  categories and dimensions, 546
  characteristics of healthy self, 540–541
  comorbidity of, 537–539, 538t, 539t
  definition of, 536–537
  different age-groups, diagnostic criteria for, 545f
  dramatic emotional personality disorders
    antisocial personality disorder, 551–553
    BPD (*see* Borderline personality disorder (BPD))
    histrionic personality disorder, 566
  psychopathy, 551, 553–556, 554t
  DSM-5, 543
  DSM future considerations, 574
  environmental and genetic studies, 544–547
  evolution and different personality characteristics, 543, 543t
FFM, 544t
  normal personality traits, 539–540, 540f, 541–543, 542t
  odd-eccentric personality disorders
    paranoid personality disorder, 547–548
    schizoid personality disorder, 548
    schizotypal personality disorder, 548–551
  sociocultural dimensions of deliberate self-harm, 547
  treatment of
    DBT, 570–572
    DDP, 573
    TFP, 573
Personality traits, 305
Person-centered therapy, 54
Persons with Disabilities (PWD) Act, 615
Peters, C., 556
Pfaff, D., 439
PFC. *See* Prefrontal cortex (PFC)
PGIMER Chandigarh, 48
Phenelzine sulfate, 366
Phenotype, 102
Physical illness, 320–321
Physical pain, 14
Physiological needs, 54
Pica, 409–410
Pierce, Franklin, 46
Pinel, Philippe, 44, 553
Pinto, Charles, 75t
Pituitary pathway, 324
Placebo effect, 132
Plath, Sylvia, 297
POCSO Act. *See* Protection of Children from Sexual Offenses (POCSO) Act, 2012
Polaschek, D. L. L., 554
Pollock, Jackson, 297
Ponnudurai, R., 72t
Positive correlation, 124
Positive interpersonal relationships, 541
Positive symptoms, 234–236
Positron emission tomography (PET), 88–90, 386, 442, 515, 516f
Post-traumatic stress disorder (PTSD), 91, 121, 196, 315, 332t–333t, 334–337, 385, 604
  physiological aspects, 337–339, 339f
  stressors, 336t
  and suicide, 340
  treatment, 339–343
Pradhan, N., 70t
Prakashdoot, 502
Prakashdoot (messenger of light), 9
Prasad Rao, G., 73t, 148
Predictive validity, 166
Prefrontal cortex (PFC), 200, 338, 491, 512, 556
Premorbid phase, 237
Prevalence, 144
Price, P., 280
Prince, Morton, 120
Pritchard, J. C., 553
Privileged communication, 620
Problem-solving skills training (PSST), 220
Process experiential therapy, 55
Prodromal phase, 237
Product test, 616
The Protection of Children from Sexual Offences Act, 2012 (POCSO), 623
Projective instruments, 170
Projective tests, 173t
Protection of Children from Sexual Offenses (POCSO) Act, 2012, 189, 469
Proteins, 79
Prozac, 283
Psilocybin, 508–509, 510f
Psychedelics. *See* Hallucinogens
Psychiatric advance directives (PADs), 622
Psychoanalysis, 51
Psychodynamic therapy, 288–289
Psychogenic disorders/functional disorders, 397
Psychological disorder, symptoms and signs, 13
Psychological stress, 315–316, 321–323, 323f

Psychoneuroimmunology, 322
Psychopathic personality, 553
Psychopathology, 315–316
abnormal processes, 21
affective disorders, 22
Ancient Greek and Roman influences, 29–31
from Ancient India, 31
behavior and, 13, 35–36
cultural perspective, 16
DALY, 4t–6t
definition, 2
diagnostic considerations of, 67–75
1800s and evolution, 41–42
environmental situation, 21
evolutionary and cultural perspectives, 17, 19
evolutionary perspective, 14, 107–110
experiential perspective, 13, 22–23
external and internal levels, 21
genetic processes, 20
historical experience, 21
human culture, 16
internal experiences, 20
intrapersonal relationship, 3
lactose tolerance, 17
levels of analysis, 14–15
mental health disorders, 6–8
mental health professionals, 18f–19f
mental illness, prevalence of, 3
in Middle ages, 31–32
neuroscience approach (*See* Neuroscience approach)
neuroscience perspective, 13
psychosis and learning disabilities, 3
reliability and validity, 164–166
renaissance to 1700s, 32–34
search for organization, 42–43
1700s to 1900s, 36–41
social learning, 16
social processes, 20
societal and cultural perspectives, 20
Psychopathy, 551, 553–556, 554t
Psychopharmacological approaches, 366
Psychosis, 196, 238, 505–506, 506t
Psychosomatic disorder, 393
Psychotic disorders, 233
Psychotic phase, 237
PTSD. *See* Post-traumatic stress disorder (PTSD)
Punch-drunk, 604
Purging, 420, 428–429
Puri, V. N., 70t
Pyramid, 35
Pythagoras, 29

Qualitative methodology, 8
Quaytman, S., 556

Rachmaninoff, Sergei, 297
Radtke, K., 319–320
Raj Mohan, V., 69t
Rakesh Kumar Jangid, 72t
Ramachandran, V.S., 65
Ramprasad, Gayatri, 3
Ram Sharan, 69t
RAND Corporation, 340
Randomization, 133
Randomized controlled trials (RCTs), 139t–141t
Rao, Murti D. L. N., 68t
Rao, Sankara A., 69t
Rao, Sheelaa, 2
Rapid cycling, 296
Rasmussen, Theodore, 402
Ravel, Maurice, 601
Raven's Progressive Matrices, 205, 206f
Ray, W., 384
RDoC. *See* Research Domain Criteria (RDoC)
Reactive attachment disorder (RAD), 202
Reagan, Ronald, 235, 578–579, 595, 616, 617
Real self, 53
Reinforcement, 58
Reliability, 165
Religio Medici (Browne), 302
Renneberg, B., 565
Repetitive TMS (rTMS), 285
Repetti, R. L., 329
Replication, 149
Repression, 50
Research Domain Criteria (RDoC), 77
Research methods
anonymity, 152
behavioral genetics, 146–148
blind controls, 132
case study, 120–122
clinically significant, 148–149
confidentiality, 152
confound hypothesis, 137–138
correlational approach, 123–126
demand characteristics, 131
designing study, 135–136
double-blind experiment, 132
empiricism, 120
epidemiological research, 144–145
ethical relationship, 154
ethics, 149–151
experimental method, 126–129
experimenter effects, 132
hypothesis, 119
informed consent, 152
IRB, 153–154
logic and inference, 129–130
longitudinal design, 142–144

match subjects design, 134
naturalistic observation method, 122–123
Nazi medical experiments, 151
null hypothesis, 136–137
participant assignment, 132, 133
participant selection, 132, 133
placebo effect, 132
private personality, 152
randomization, 133
RCTs, 139t–141t
replication and meta-analysis, 149
research hypothesis, 138–139
right to privacy, 152
single subject designs, 141–142
statistically significant, 148–149
traditional genetics studies, 145–146
validity, 130–131
voluntary participation, 151–152
Reserve, 587
Residual subtype, 241
Resilience, 343
Resource conservation theories, 279
Response inhibition ability, 318
Restraint stress, 273f
Reward system, 76, 76f
Ribonucleic acid (RNA), 102
Richards, Renée, 465, 466
Right-hand movement, 400
Rights of Persons with Disabilities Act, 2016, 615
Right ventral prefrontal cortex (RVPFC), 562
Risk, 145
Risk taking, 197
Roberson, Arlene, 556
Robison, John Elder, 185
Rogers, Carl, 54
Rogers, S., 212
Rooting reflex, 190
Rorschach, Herman, 171
Rorschach Inkblot method (RIM), 170, 625, 626
Rorschach performance assessment system (R-PAS), 171–172
Rothko, Mark, 297
Rumination disorder, 410
Ruscio, A., 363
Rush, Benjamin, 44, 553
Rush, John, 301

Sabhesan, S., 69t, 71t
Sachdev, K. S., 70t
Sahu, R. N., 71t
Saikumar Reddy, M., 73t
St. Mary of Bethlehem, 43
Saks, Elyn, 27–29, 158, 235
Salience network, 80
Salthouse, Timothy, 583, 584
SAM. *See* Severe acute malnutrition (SAM)
Same-sex competition, 42
Sanyal, R. K., 69t
Sargunaraj, D., 73t
Saxena, Jalaj, 74t
Schizoid personality disorder, 536, 545, 548
Schizophrenia, 14, 17, 79, 80, 107, 108, 233–234, 505, 548, 550, 615
antipsychotic medications, 262–263
brain changes, 252–253, 253f, 254f, 255
and brain function, 249–251, 250f, 251t, 252f
and brain networks, 255–256, 256f
cognitive processes changed in, 258–259
course of, 237, 237f
DSM–5 diagnostic criteria, 242t
and emotions, 259
endophenotypes associated with, 247–249, 248f, 249f
evolutionary perspective, 242–244
evolution of concept, 238f
factors in development, 244–245
facts of, 259–260, 260t
genetic factors in, 245–247, 246f
historical perspective, 238–239
natural history, 237, 237f
negative symptoms, 236
neurotransmitters involved in, 257–258, 257f
positive symptoms, 235–236
psychosocial interventions for, 263–266
subtypes of, 239–241
symptoms, 234
treating individuals with, 260–262
Schizotypal personality disorder, 536, 537, 548–551
Schizotypal traits, 242
Schneider-Garces, N., 587
School shootings, 201–202
Schultz, Thomas, 92
Schumm, L. P., 425
Schweckendiek, Jan, 369
Scientific knowledge, 119
Sea stars, 41
Sebastianelli, Wayne, 605
Second-generation antipsychotics, 262
Seeley, William, 600, 603
Seethalakshmi, R., 74t
Selective serotonin reuptake inhibitors (SSRIs), 283, 372, 458, 464
Self-actualization, 54, 55
Self-direction, 541
Self-injurious behavior, 556t
Self-realization, 53
Selye, Hans, 327
Separation anxiety disorder, 348, 360–361
Serotonin, 99, 423, 508, 515
SERT gene, 78

Serum Brain-derived neurotrophic factor (BDNF), 213
Sethi, B. B., 74t
Sethi, N., 72t, 74t
Seth, T. H., 69t
Severe acute malnutrition (SAM), 188
Sexual activities, 449, 451
Sexual behavior, 457
Sexual Behavior in the Human Female (Kinsey), 437
Sexual Behavior in the Human Male (Kinsey), 437
Sexual behaviors, 443, 457, 464
Sexual desire, 457
Sexual dysfunction disorders
- in *DSM–5,* 450
- early ejaculation, 451, 453
- epidemiological data, 451
- erectile disorder, 452–453
- female orgasmic disorder, 453
- female sexual interest/arousal disorder, 454
- genito-pelvic pain/penetration disorder, 454
- male hypoactive sexual desire disorder, 454
- medical and biological factors, 450
- performance anxiety, 451
- prevalence of sexual problems by age and gender, 451, 452t
- treatment approaches
  - directed masturbation, 455
  - paraphilic disorders, 457
  - pharmacological approaches, 456
  - psychological factors, 455
  - sensate focus, 455
  - sexual therapy, 455
  - squeeze technique, 456

Sexual excitement, 463
The Sexual Harassment of Women at Workplace (Prevention, Prohibition And Redressal) Act, 2013 (POSH), 623
Sexual instinct, 20
Sexual intercourse, 436
Sexuality disorders
- gender dysphoria
  - in adolescents and adults, 466
  - in children, 466
  - cortical thickness, 467, 468f
  - family therapy and child based therapy, 467
  - gender identity, 465
  - gender roles, 465
  - gender transition surgery, 467
  - Indian cultural context, 469
  - non-dysphoria conditions, 467
  - prevalence, 466
  - sex change procedure, 468
  - transgender, 466
- India, land of the Kamasutra, 436–438
- infertility treatment in India, 470
- normal sexual functioning
  - female external sexual anatomy, 445, 446f
  - female reproductive system, 445, 446f
  - human sexual response, phases of, 446–448, 449f
  - male reproductive system, 445f
  - men, genital changes in, 446, 447f
  - sexual activities, 449
  - women, genital changes in, 446, 448f
- paraphilic disorders
  - exhibitionistic disorder, 458
  - fetishistic disorder, 459
  - frotteuristic disorder, 459
  - other specified paraphilic disorder, 463
  - pedophilic disorder, 459–461
  - sexual masochism disorder, 461
  - sexual sadism disorder, 462
  - transvestic disorder, 462–463
  - treatment approaches, 464–465
  - unspecified paraphilic disorder, 463
  - voyeuristic disorder, 463
- psychosocial consequences, 470
- sexual activities of America
  - Indian epidemiological data, 439
  - sexual behaviors in past year, 440f
  - sexual contact, 438f
- sexual arousal and drive, 439
  - brain imaging techniques, 441, 442
  - cortical areas, 443, 444f
  - definition, 444
  - sexuality and clashing of cultures, 442–443
  - sexual motivation, 441
  - sexual orientation, 441–442
- sexual dysfunction disorders
  - in *DSM–5,* 450
  - early ejaculation, 451, 453
  - epidemiological data, 451
  - erectile disorder, 452–453
  - female orgasmic disorder, 453
  - female sexual interest/arousal disorder, 454

genito-pelvic pain/ penetration disorder, 454
male hypoactive sexual desire disorder, 454
medical and biological factors, 450
performance anxiety, 451
prevalence of sexual problems by age and gender, 451, 452t
treatment approaches, 454–457
sexual reassignment surgery, 469
Sexual masochism disorder, 461
Sexual motivation, 441
Sexual reassignment surgery, 469
Sexual sadism disorder, 462
Sexual selection, 41
Shadows in the Sun (Gayatri), 3
Shah, A. V., 68t
Shah, Nilesh, 70t
Shaji, K. S., 69t
Sharan, Ram, 546
Sharma, I., 70t, 71t
Sharma, Mukul, 75t
Shastri Grant, 8
Shearer, S., 556
Sheline, Yvette I., 91
Shell shock, 336
Sherrington, Charles, 35
Shoba Srinath, 75t
Short-term stress, 272, 325
Shrivastava, Amresh, 74t
Shukla, G. D., 68t, 69t
Shukla, R., 73t
Sickle-cell anemia, 14
Siddiqui, Shazia Veqar, 72t
Siegle, G., 77
Signs, 42
Silva, Donald, 460
Silva, Melvin Chagas, 72t
Singh, Baljinder, 74t
Singh, Gurmeet, 70t
Singh, Om Prakash, 70t
Singh, P. M., 73t
Singh, R., 73t
Singh, S., 246–247
Single subject designs, 141–142
Sissies, 465
Skeem, J. L., 554
Skin conductance response, 386, 387f
Skinner, B. F., 58
Skull, 37
Slobounov, Semyon, 605
Small molecule neurotransmitters, 99
Small-N designs. *See* Single subject designs
Snaith, R., 458
SNRIs, 283
Sobell, Linda, 527
Sobus, J., 109
Social anxiety disorder (SAD), 20, 348, 364–365
neuroscience aspects, 365
treatment, 365–366
Social brain regions, 197, 365
Social competition theories, 280
Social learning, 16
Social pain, 317–318
Social phobia, 352, 364
Social relationships, 13
Social risk hypothesis, 280
Social skills training, 366
Social stress, 330–331
Society of Clinical Psychology, 287
Sociopathic, 553
Soloff, P., 560
Somatic symptom and related disorders, 393–394
conversion disorder, 396–401, 396f, 398f–400f, 401f
illness anxiety disorder, 395
Indian studies on, 394–395
somatic symptom disorder, 394
Somatoform disorders, 393
Sovani, Anuradha, 536, 624
Specialized thinkers, 205
Specific learning disorder, 221
Specific phobia, 367
clinical features, 368t
neuroscience aspects of, 367–369
specific fears, lifetime prevalence and standard error of, 369t
treatment, 369–370, 370f
Spencer, W., 84f
Spirituality, 343
Squeeze technique, 456
Sridhara, B. S., 70t
Sridhara Rama Rao, B. S., 69t, 70t
Srinivasa Murthy, R., 9, 75t, 189
Srivastava, J. S., 75t
SSRIs. *See* Selective serotonin reuptake inhibitors (SSRIs)
Stable phase, 237
Staines, W., 397
Steele, Ken, 234, 235
Steinberg, Marlene, 390
Stice, Eric, 419
Stigma, 8–12
Stigmatization, 469
Stoplight driving game, 198
Straube, Thomas, 370
Stress
fight-or-flight response, males and females, 329–330
and hypothalamic-pituitary-adrenal axis, 323–325, 323f, 324f
physiological mechanisms related to, 318
study of, 327–328, 328f
Srinivasan, Latha, 71t
Stroop test, 351, 351f
Structured Clinical Interview for DSM Disorders (SCID), 161–162

Structured interview, 161–162
Strupp, Hans, 51f
Studerus, Erich, 509
Studies in the Psychology of Sex (Ellis, Havelock), 437
Subbakrishna, D. K., 68t
Subcortical pathways, 349
Subrahmanyan, P., 69t
Substance abuse, 196
Substance-related and addictive disorders
- alcohol, 491–492
  - *DSM–5,* 492–496, 493t, 494t, 495f
  - effects on human body, 496–497, 497f, 498f
  - moderate, heavy, and binge drinking, 498, 499f, 500f, 500t
  - neuropsychological rehabilitation, 492
  - rates of drinking, 498, 500, 501t, 502f
- alcoholic beverages, 477
- amphetamines, 514–516, 516f
- Bayer aspirin, 477
- binge drinking, 482
- brain reward circuitry, 487, 488f
- caffeine and tobacco, 516–519, 518f
- cannabis
  - cannabinoids, 505
  - hallucinogens, 506–510, 509f, 510f
  - history of, 503, 504f
  - prevalence of, 503f
  - psychosis, 505–506, 506t
  - THC (Δ9-tetrahydrocannabinol), 505
- cocaine, 476–478, 489
- crisis of addiction, 478
- dopamine, 487, 488, 488f, 489
- drug use
  - Indian statistics on, 478–479
  - in United States, 479–482, 480f, 481f
- *DSM–5* and *ICD-10,* 482–483
- environmental factors, 484–485
- epigenetics, 485
- explanatory models for alcohol use, 483
- gambling
  - behavioral conditioning, 522
  - cognitive–emotional process, 522
  - *DSM–5* criteria, 519
  - impaired executive functioning, 522
  - impulse control disorder, 519
  - impulsivity, 522
  - lifetime comorbidity of pathological, 520, 521t
  - lifetime prevalence, 520t
  - substance tolerance, 521
- genetics, 484
- internet addiction, 475–476
- intoxication, 483, 484f
- marijuana, 478
- methamphetamines, 489
- model of brain and behavior, 491f
- nicotine, 489
- opioids
  - cocaine, 511–512, 512f, 513, 513f
  - dopamine, 512, 514
  - endorphins, 511
  - prevalence of, 510, 511f
- pathological gambling, 485
- PFC disrupted in addiction, 489, 490f
- PREMIUM study, 502–503
- psychoactive substances use, 485
- qualitative study from India, 486–487, 486f
- substance abuse and addiction, 482
- substance dependence, 482
- treatment of, 522–523
  - agonist drug, 528
  - Alcoholics Anonymous, 522
  - antagonist drug, 528
  - aversive drug, 529
  - controlled drinking approaches, 527–528
  - principles of effective treatment, 523–525
  - psychosocial therapies and addiction, 525–526
  - 12-step program, 526–527, 526f
- U.S. opiate consumption, 477, 478f

Substance tolerance, 521
Substance use disorder, 67
Successful aging, 580
Suicidal ideation, 284
Suicide, 270, 302
- cultural differences, 303
- endophenotypes and, 304
- gender differences and type of attempts, 303–304, 304t
- prevention, 305
- short-term and long-term factors, 304–305
- warning signs, 305t

Suicide mortality, India, 9
Sukthankar, Sunil, 2, 266
Superconducting quantum interference device (SQUID), 88
Suresh Kumar, P. N., 72t
Sutton, Walter, 100
Sylvester, Chad, 353
Sympathetic division, 325
Sympathetic nervous system, 31
Symptoms, 42
Synapses, 82
Syndrome, 42

Taj, Mubeen, 71t
Tandon, Rajiv, 259
Tandon, Rajul, 71t
Tangentiality, 234
Tarafder, Sreemoyee, 71t
Tarasoff I decision, 619
Tardive dyskinesia, 262
Taylor, Maxwell, 627
Taylor, Shelley, 329
Tchaikovsky, Peter, 297
Temporal lobe, 36
Tend-and-befriend response, 327
Tending response, 329
Testa, R., 245
Test-retest reliability, 165
Thara, R., 127, 265
Tharyan, Prathap, 69t, 74t
Thematic apperception test (TAT), 170–171, 174
Therapeutic relationship, 52
Theravada Buddhism, 56
Thorne, Steven, 206
Thornicroft, Graham, 234, 265
Thrifty gene hypothesis, 410
Tiwari, S. C., 70t
Tobacco, 479, 480, 516–519, 518f
Tolin, David, 377
Tomboys, 465
Tomko, Rachel, 122
Torrey, E. Fuller, 134
Tourette's disorder, 42, 187
Traditional genetics studies, 145–146
Traditional IQ tests, 205
Transcranial magnetic stimulation (TMS), 285
Transference, 52
Transference-focused psychotherapy (TFP), 573
Transgender, 471
Transsexual, 462, 466
Transvestic disorder, 462–463
Trauma
  epigenetics, 318–320
  physiological mechanisms related to, 318
  producing mental illness, 316–317
Trauma-and stressor-related disorders, 187, 331, 334
  acute stress disorder, 331t–332t, 335
  adjustment disorders, 334
  post-traumatic growth, 334
  post-traumatic stress disorder, 332t–333t
Trauma Network, 341
Tricyclic antidepressants, 282, 364
Tripathi, Ravikesh, 343, 599
Tripathi, S. K., 74t
Trivedi, J. K., 70t, 71t, 75t
Tuke, William, 45
Twin studies, 147

Uma Choudhury, 174
Undifferentiated subtype, 241
Unipolar depression, 270, 291
Unmaada, 31
U.S. Department of Health and Human Services, 49
U.S. Food and Drug Administration (FDA), 514
U.S. opiate consumption, 477, 478f
U.S. Substance Abuse and Mental Health Services Administration (SAMHSA), 49, 479
Utermohlen, William, 595, 596f, 603

Vagal nerve stimulation (VNS), 284–285
Vaginismus, 454
Vahia, N. S., 72t, 73t
Vahia, Vihang N., 73t
Validity, 128, 166
Van Horn, J. D., 122
Varenicline (Chantix), 528
Variation, 41
Varma, S. L., 73t
Vascular neurocognitive disorder, 599–600
Vasocongestion, 447
Venkoba Rao, A., 71t, 73t, 74t, 75t
Ventral attentional network, 353
Ventral striatum (VS), 198
Ventral tegmental area (VTA), 442, 491
Ventrolateral prefrontal cortex (VLPFC), 250
Ventromedial prefrontal cortex (vmPFC), 201
Verghese, Abraham, 73t
Verma, Harish, 69t
Verma, Sandeep, 70t
Viagra, 456
Vikram Patel, 6, 9, 75t, 483
Virginia Twin Registry, 272
Visionary restructuralization, 508
Vismara, L., 212
Visual thinking, 205
Vital spirits, 31
Vitamin D deficiency, 245
Volitional test, 616
Volkow, N., 486, 491, 514
Voluntary actions, 34
Voluntary participation, 151–152
Volunteering, 343
von Helmholtz, Hermann, 37
von Krafft-Ebing, Richard Freiherr, 460
von Sacher-Masoch, Leopold, 461, 462
VTA. *See* Ventral tegmental area (VTA)
Vyas, N., 245

Wadman, B., 556
Waheed, K., 336
WAIS. *See* Wechsler Adult Intelligence Scale (WAIS)
Waite, L. J., 425
Walker, Johnnie, 492
War neurosis, 336
Warren Anatomical Museum, 122

Watkins, L., 330
Watson, John, 57f, 367–368
Wavelet analysis, 88f
Waxy flexibility, 241
WCST. *See* Wisconsin Card Sorting Test (WCST)
Wechsler Adult Intelligence Scale (WAIS), 174
Weinberger, Daniel, 245
Weiss, Mitchell, 31, 117, 166
Wellbeing, 343
Well-being therapy, 287
Wells, H. G., 205
Werner, C., 581
Wernicke, Carl, 39
Wernicke's area, 39, 39f
Westwood, Steven, 536
White matter, 35f, 36
WHO. *See* World Health Organization (WHO)
WHO-CHOICE analysis, 6
WHO collaborative center, 68
Widiger, Thomas A., 540, 542, 544
Wig, N. N., 116
Williams, K. D., 562, 563
Willis, Thomas, 35
Wisconsin Card Sorting Test (WCST), 174
Withdrawal, 482, 483
Wood, S., 245
Woolf, Virginia, 297
Word and fact thinking, 205
Word salad, 234
Working memory, 258
World Health Organization (WHO), 7, 76, 177, 192, 433, 436, 495, 537
Writer tags, 319

Yan, Laura, 91

Zucker, K., 462